"The child clinician is in for a treat when reading *The Handbook of Complex Trauma and Dissociation in Children*. With well-written contributions that span theory, diagnosis, treatment, and special issues, the handbook's thought-provoking chapters are filled with clinical anecdotes and case histories that make the pages come alive. Readers will find in-depth analysis of the ways in which different theories apply to a child population, including (but not limited to) polyvagal theory, the theory of interpersonal neurobiology, betrayal trauma theory, and the theory of structural dissociation. The editors have assembled an impressive collection of top experts who approach difficult issues with clarity, sensitivity, and depth. Whether you are a researcher, theorist, or practicing therapist, this book is bound to spark new, creative ideas that will help enrich this growing field. This comprehensive compendium belongs on the shelf of every clinician who deals with childhood complex trauma and dissociation. It will enrich professionals' thinking and expand awareness of multiple treatment options."

Joyanna Silberg, PhD, author of *The Child Survivor: Healing Developmental Trauma and Dissociation, 2nd edition*

"This comprehensive handbook provides a nuanced exploration of the theories, research, and therapeutic approaches pertaining to complex trauma and dissociation in children. The depth and breadth of this book make it an invaluable resource for all clinicians and researchers dedicated to addressing developmental trauma."

Ruth A. Lanius, MD, PhD, coauthor *of Healing the Traumatized Self: Consciousness, Neuroscience, Treatment*, and co-editor of *The Impact of Early Life Trauma on Health and Disease: The Hidden Epidemic*

"Trauma and dissociation are alarmingly common, affecting a vast number of children. Yet children experiencing complex trauma are often misdiagnosed, leading to years of ineffective treatment and continued suffering. Ana Gómez and Jillian Hosey have provided an exceptional review of theory, assessment, best treatment practices, and research, essential for all professionals working with children impacted by complex trauma. This handbook is an invaluable resource for clinicians and researchers worldwide."

Marlene Steinberg, MD, author of *The SCID-D Interview: Dissociation Assessment in Therapy, Forensics, and Research and The Stranger in the Mirror: Dissociation—The Hidden Epidemic*

THE HANDBOOK OF COMPLEX TRAUMA AND DISSOCIATION IN CHILDREN

The Handbook of Complex Trauma and Dissociation in Children: Theory, Research, and Clinical Applications is a comprehensive and truly vital text for both experienced professionals and novice clinicians alike. In these pages, dozens of experts and pioneers thoroughly cover the complex nuances of theory, assessment, research, and clinical practice. Specific sections cover etiology, neurobiology, and various theoretical and conceptual models for working with the complexities of cumulative and chronic traumatization in childhood.

Additional sections cover standardized and non-standardized assessment and diagnostic tools, as well as the formulation and organization of the clinical interview with children and caregivers. Other chapters provide systematic and comprehensive reviews of current treatment modalities and effective approaches for treating children with complex trauma and dissociation across different stages of early development. The book's co-editors bookend the volume with thorough explorations of the nuanced and multifaceted issues impacting children with complex trauma and dissociative symptoms and features.

Ana M. Gómez, MC, LPC, is the director of the AGATE Institute, a leading expert and global speaker on complex trauma and dissociation in youth, and the author of multiple books, therapeutic tools, and training programs.

Jillian Hosey, MSW, RSW, LICSW, is a clinical consultant, trainer, and social worker. She is faculty with the ISSTD's Center for Advanced Studies and the AGATE Institute and is also a fellow of the ISSTD.

THE HANDBOOK OF COMPLEX TRAUMA AND DISSOCIATION IN CHILDREN

Theory, Research, and Clinical Applications

Edited by Ana M. Gómez and Jillian Hosey

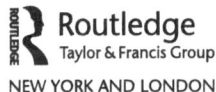

Designed cover image: Shutterstock

First published 2025
by Routledge
605 Third Avenue, New York, NY 10158

and by Routledge
4 Park Square, Milton Park, Abingdon, Oxon, OX14 4RN

Routledge is an imprint of the Taylor & Francis Group, an informa business

© 2025 selection and editorial matter, Ana M. Gómez and Jillian Hosey; individual chapters, the contributors

The right of Ana M. Gómez and Jillian Hosey to be identified as the authors of the editorial material, and of the authors for their individual chapters, has been asserted in accordance with sections 77 and 78 of the Copyright, Designs and Patents Act 1988.

All rights reserved. No part of this book may be reprinted or reproduced or utilised in any form or by any electronic, mechanical, or other means, now known or hereafter invented, including photocopying and recording, or in any information storage or retrieval system, without permission in writing from the publishers.

Trademark notice: Product or corporate names may be trademarks or registered trademarks, and are used only for identification and explanation without intent to infringe.

Library of Congress Cataloging-in-Publication Data
Names: Gomez, Ana M., editor. | Hosey, Jillian, editor.
Title: The handbook of complex trauma and dissociation in children : theory, research, and clinical applications / edited by Ana M. Gómez and Jillian Hosey.
Description: New York, NY : Routledge, 2025. | Includes bibliographical references and index. |
Identifiers: LCCN 2024045196 (print) | LCCN 2024045197 (ebook) | ISBN 9781032389011 (hbk) | ISBN 9781032388908 (pbk) | ISBN 9781003350156 (ebk)
Subjects: MESH: Stress Disorders, Traumatic | Dissociative Disorders | Child
Classification: LCC RJ506.P66 (print) | LCC RJ506.P66 (ebook) | NLM WM 172.5 | DDC 618.92/8521—dc23/eng/20250121
LC record available at https://lccn.loc.gov/2024045196
LC ebook record available at https://lccn.loc.gov/2024045197

ISBN: 978-1-032-38901-1(hbk)
ISBN: 978-1-032-38890-8 (pbk)
ISBN: 978-1-003-35015-6 (ebk)

DOI: 10.4324/9781003350156

Typeset in Times New Roman
by codeMantra

*To my husband Jim, for being my unwavering companion on this journey
of being, becoming and unbecoming
To my parents, my family, and my furry children, for your love that has
strengthened and sustained me
Ana M. Gómez*

*To my beloved husband, family, friends, and animals for your support
on this incredible journey
Jillian Hosey*

*To the children we have been privileged to walk beside on their paths of healing,
discovery and growth. We are inspired by your courage every day!*

CONTENTS

Foreword xv
Acknowledgments xxv
List of Contributors xxvii

1 Setting the Stage: An Introduction to Child Complex Trauma
  and Dissociation 1
  Ana M. Gómez and Jillian Hosey

PART 1
Theory, Conceptual Models, and Neurobiology **15**

2 Epidemiology of Dissociation in Children 17
  Colin A. Ross

3 The Discrete Behavioral States/States of Being Model 23
  John Lovern

4 Traumatic Attachment: Clinical Reasoning for Attachment Trauma 38
  Benedetto Farina and Adriano Schimmenti

5 Affect Regulation, Attachment, and the Developing Social Brain:
  Implications for Assessment and Treatment of Dissociative Disorders 56
  Richard M. Cross

6 Structural Dissociation: Developmental Pathways and Treatment
  Implications 73
  Kathy Steele

7	The Autohypnotic Model of Dissociation *D. Michael Coy*	89
8	Knowledge Isolation, Protective Adaptation, and Long-Term Impacts: Betrayal Trauma Theory's Contribution to Our Understanding of Complex Trauma and Dissociation in Childhood *Laura K. Noll*	107
9	Interpersonal Neurobiology *Robyn Gobbel*	124
10	Polyvagal Theory and the Autonomic Nervous System *George S. Thompson*	143
11	The Innate Connection System and Sensory-Affective Orienting: Relevance to Deep Brain Reorienting (DBR) *Jessica Christie-Sands and Frank Corrigan*	167

PART 2
Symptomatology, Assessment, and Diagnosis — 185

12	Symptomatology *Betsy de Thierry*	187
13	Considerations in Screening, Assessment, and Clinical Interviewing *Alexis Arbuthnott, Billie Jo Bennett, Jillian Hosey, and Patti van Eys*	206
14	Differential and Co-occurring Diagnoses, Neurodivergence, and the Complexity of Dissociative Features in Children *Patti van Eys and Alexis Arbuthnott*	237
15	Working Considerations in Building the Road Map to Treatment: Case Conceptualization, Treatment Guidelines, and Treatment Planning *Jillian Hosey*	264
16	Clinical Applications of the Star Theoretical Model *Frances S. Waters*	287

PART 3
Treatment Modalities for Children with Complex Trauma and Dissociation — 307

17	Trauma-Informed Child Psychoanalytic Psychotherapy *Valerie Sinason*	309

18	Dyadic Developmental Psychotherapy *Kim S. Golding*	328
19	The Attachment Video-Feedback Intervention (AVI): Reducing Dysregulated Parental Behavior, Attachment Disorganization and Dissociation *Valérie Langlois, Gabrielle Myre and Chantal Cyr*	345
20	A Multimodal-Integrative Approach to EMDR Therapy *Ana M. Gómez*	364
21	Psycho-Sensory Intervention®: An Occupational Therapy Approach *Kim Barthel*	389
22	A Sensorimotor Psychotherapy Perspective on Family Interventions *Bonnie Goldstein*	424
23	Somatic Experiencing® *Maggie Kline*	441
24	Clinical Neurofeedback *Anna K. Morrell*	460
25	Trauma-Focused Cognitive-Behavioral Therapy: Not Just for Acute Trauma Anymore! *Matthew D. Kliethermes*	483
26	Animal-Assisted Therapy *Michael Remole*	501
27	Child-Centered Play Therapy *Kristi L. Perryman*	520
28	TraumaPlay™: An Integrative Play Therapy Model *Paris Goodyear-Brown and Eleah Hyatt*	539
29	Theraplay and Parts Work *Karen Andor and Dafna Lender*	560
30	A Synergetic Play Therapy Approach *Lisa Dion*	575
31	An Integrative and Phase-Oriented Approach to Sandtray Therapy *Ana M. Gómez and Marshall Lyles*	590

32	Art Therapy *Elizabeth Davis*	612

PART 4
Important Treatment Considerations — **635**

33	The Therapeutic Relationship *Jillian Hosey and Eva Teirstein Young*	637
34	Boundaries and Ethics *David S. Prescott*	658
35	Sociocultural Determinants, Anti-Oppressive and Culturally Responsive Practices *LaKaavia Taylor and Krystal K. Turner*	673
36	Prenatal Reform: Complex Trauma, Dissociation, and Bonding with the Calming Womb Model *Rosita Cortizo*	690
37	Fractured Bonds: Healing Trauma in the Caregiving System *Maria Zaccagnino, Martina Cussino and Cristina Civilotti*	709
38	Intersecting Timelines: Generational Perspectives *Rebeca Chow*	725
39	Shame and Guilt *Paula Moreno and Sandra Baita*	735
40	The Trauma-Formed Defense and Self-Protective System *Ana M. Gómez*	752
41	Self-Harm and Suicidality *Alexis E. Arbuthnott*	774
42	Complex Trauma and Dissociation in the Face of Ongoing Stress and Trauma: Child Refugees and Asylum Seekers *Safa Kemal Kaptan, Betül Yılmaz, Tania Bosqui and Trudy Mooren*	791
43	Listening to the Body Speak: Conversion Issues and Functional Neurological Symptoms *Nicole Black*	808

44 Chronic Pain, Medical Issues, and Complicated Clinical Presentations 824
    Christine C. Forner

45 "Mind Control" in Ritualistic and Other Extreme and
    Dissociation-Savvy Abuse 839
    Ellen Lacter

46 Psychiatry and Pharmacology 861
    *Darren Bingham, Helen Milroy, Guilia Pace, Pradeep Rao
    and Alix Woolard*

47 Conclusion 880
    Jillian Hosey and Ana M. Gómez

Index *887*

FOREWORD

What Does a Profoundly Abused Child Do to Cope and Survive, and How Do We Help Them?

Christine A. Courtois

I am honored to have been invited to write the Foreword to this *Handbook of Complex Trauma and Dissociation in Children: Theory, Research, and Clinical Applications*, edited by Ana Gómez, MC, LPC and Jillian Hosey, MSW, RSW, LICSW. It has been more than a decade since Dr. Julian Ford and I co-edited *Treating Complex Traumatic Stress Disorders in Children and Adolescents* which, along with several other texts, can be regarded as antecedents to this handbook. It is gratifying to see in this text the continuation and extension of information about the population of complexly traumatized and dissociative children and adolescents and the most current information about their treatment. It is urgently needed information, as this population continues to expand in response to the wide array of experiences and events that are now understood to be traumagenic or potentially so. And, despite its introduction of the complex trauma conceptualization in 1992, mental health and other professionals continue to be ill-informed about it and its myriad potential consequences. Obviously and tragically, this impacts the likelihood of appropriately focused and effective treatment.

Let me begin by presenting some background, even though it is likely to be familiar to some readers. The contemporary study of child abuse—especially child sexual and physical abuse and its impact—has developed over the course of the past 50 years and counting. Along with the study of war trauma, it anchored the development of the now robust field of traumatic stress studies. Early research efforts documented the effects of abuse on child victims at the time and later, many over the course of their adult years. Treatment methods were developed before research substantiation was available. And, as the aforementioned texts on complex trauma emphasize, despite the many advances that took place, traumatized children and abused women too often were not recognized and many of their symptoms were misunderstood and stigmatized, often by those they turned to for help, creating a second injury. Unfortunately, that remains the case for many to this day, making informed treatment difficult to find.

PTSD

The new diagnosis of Posttraumatic Stress Disorder (PTSD; American Psychiatric Association, 1980) was included in the *DSM*-III. Its development was jumpstarted by the alarming psychological condition of many returning Vietnam veterans and was developed from the study of these and other veterans, mostly males in late adolescence and early adulthood. Their traumatic exposure took place in the line of duty and was not directed at them personally, and therefore could be understood as horrific but *impersonal* in origin. PTSD included three main criteria, reexperiencing, numbing, and hyperarousal, each associated with a listing of the most pronounced symptoms. When this diagnosis was first encoded in the *DSM-III*, it was met with both enthusiasm and relief by clinicians and researchers who were then studying many different types of traumas and their sequelae. There was finally a diagnosis that accounted for the effects of exposure to overwhelming events *experienced by* the individual and that *were not purely intrapsychic in origin* (i.e., did not follow the then prevalent Freudian perspective). That was an important new paradigm in mental health. Other social movements of the times added to this shift, namely the women's liberation, sexual revolution, racial equality, anti-war, and human potential movements, each of which challenged the social status quo and the inequities within. As part of their overall critique, they questioned Freudian psychoanalytic orthodoxy and its general disregard for the impact of real events and for its sexist and prejudicial positions toward women.

Before long, feminists and others studying childhood incest, sexual and physical abuse and other familial forms of trauma, and other violence against women such as rape and domestic and community violence and their aftereffects, found that these were most often perpetrated against female children and adults, often at the hands of intimates and other responsible parties and less often by total strangers. They increasingly noticed that the criteria for the new PTSD diagnosis were less than a good fit, especially regarding the consequences of pervasive interpersonal trauma during childhood. To account for additional symptoms found in child victims and adult survivors of childhood abuse based on a compilation of the then available research, Dr. Judith Herman introduced the concept of *complex trauma* and proposed a new diagnosis of Complex PTSD (CPTSD; Herman, 1992a, 1992b). She noted the contextual differences between impersonal versus interpersonal forms of trauma and their consequences, and between PTSD and her proposed CPTSD diagnosis. These differences included its perverse interpersonal and intentional perpetration by someone in close relationship or proximity to the child who had responsibility for their well-being and protection, its frequent initiation in early childhood, its likely repetition and escalation over time, the child's dependent status and their mind/body immaturity and vulnerability. These were not benign occurrences and had a wide-ranging impact on the child's physical and emotional maturation at the time and later. The occurrence of trauma in childhood meant that the child's healthy development was put at great risk. Their posttraumatic symptoms intertwined in complex ways with the child victim's and later the adolescent's and then the adult's neuropsychophysiological development, maturation, and functioning.

Herman organized these consequences into seven criteria categories, all of which differed from the core symptoms of PTSD. She proposed a separate and freestanding diagnosis to account for these differences and to direct treatment. The proposed diagnosis was meant to be an encompassing one that accounted for these criteria categories and some, if not many, of the co-occurring disorders found in the population of polyvictimized children and later adults. This diagnosis was to provide an umbrella under which the symptoms and co-occurring conditions all fit and was intended to put an end to the multiple and sometimes opposing diagnoses typically applied to these (especially female) clients in ways that were judgmental and discriminatory. To quote Herman (2014) and to illustrate her pragmatism, "Sometimes the whole is more than the sum of its parts" (p. xiii). This diagnostic conceptualization along with its approach to treatment was immediately embraced by clinicians treating adult survivors of complex trauma as it had face validity and provided a solution to the problem of multiple diagnoses spanning several axes of the *DSM*.

The diagnosis of CPTSD was proposed as a stand-alone diagnosis to the *DSM-IV* update, whose working group voted it in, and whose decision was reversed at a higher level, seemingly by those who believed there was only one type of PTSD. It was instead codified as an associated feature of PTSD, where it remains to this day. In the latest edition (*DSM-5 & 5-TR;* American Psychiatric Association, 2017, 2022), the criteria for PTSD expanded from three to four main categories—numbing responses were differentiated from avoidance to make a fourth criteria that included additional cognitive and emotional consequences—in ways that made it more like the complex PTSD criteria. It also included two new subtypes: (1) the dissociative and (2) the child before age 6. Although another alternative diagnosis, Developmental Trauma Disorder, was proposed, it too was not included. It is noteworthy that, *up until the present, the DSM has not included a separate diagnosis for children who have had extensive trauma exposure*, a significant gap given the high prevalence and the severity and extent of the mental health, medical, and psychosocial consequences that have been documented. Research has consistently shown that abused children respond in developmentally specific ways and according to their age and stage at the time of the abuse and other factors.

Fully 26 years after its introduction by Herman, in counterpoint to this position and based on newly available research data (Cloitre et al., 2013), the *International Classification of Diseases (ICD-11,* World Health Organization, 2018) included a new diagnosis of Complex Posttraumatic Stress Disorder (CPTSD) as a "sibling diagnosis" to PTSD. To be diagnosed with CPTSD, individuals must meet criteria for the ICD diagnosis of PTSD and additional criteria in three categories of CPTSD: (1) emotional dysregulation (including dissociation), (2) identity development, and (3) difficulties in relationships, designated as Disturbances in Self Organization (DSOs). The diagnostic system of the *ICD* has always been more streamlined than that of the *DSM*; however, the reduction to three criteria, each with several symptoms, has been called into question as overly condensed (Frewen et al., 2023). Additional research studies are underway to continue to determine the scope of complex trauma aftereffects, including dissociation (Fung et al., 2022). In a nod to the complexity of sequelae not reflected in the current CPTSD diagnosis, Courtois and Ford (2014) suggested the use of the more wide-ranging terms such as "complex traumatic stress disorders," "complex developmental traumatic stress disorders," "complex dissociative traumatic stress disorders" in addition to or exclusive of CPTSD.

Research findings from developmental psychology, particularly longitudinal and attachment studies, and ongoing studies of abused children, have added another cross-cutting element to the understanding of complex trauma and its short- and long-term effects. Early in life *attachment and relational forms of trauma*, without protection or effective intervention, were found to have profound impact in many major life domains. Attachment deficits and difficulties can result in insecure styles of attachment (*fearful/anxious* and its opposite, *detached/avoidant*) that can unfortunately make children more vulnerable to revictimization at the time or in later life. The most pathogenic attachment style has been labeled as *disoriented/dissociative* and is the result of caregiving styles that alternate between periods of abuse/neglect and more normal interactions. Children caught in what Spiegel (1986) identified as a "macabre double bind" of being dependent upon and needing the very individuals who are victimizing them—with intention and often at severe levels of physical intrusion and with the use of psychological coercion—typically are so entrapped and powerless to escape physically that they escape psychologically, via dissociation or shifts in self-state or state of being. In fact, Frank Putnam (1997), one of the pioneer researchers in dissociation and child abuse, was quoted as making the comment "dissociation is the means of escape when there is no escape." Clinical researcher Liotti (2004) discussed how three different strands, trauma, attachment disorganization, and dissociation, are braided together in the aftereffects of severe and repeated polyvictimization during childhood These strands need to be anticipated and considered together by therapists treating clients with a background of relational/attachment trauma and the resultant compromised attachment style. They must also be mindful of client safety and their vulnerability to the possibility of additional traumatic experiences (revictimization). Jennifer Freyd (1996) introduced *betrayal trauma theory (BTT)* in recognition of the powerful role that betrayal by intimates and caregivers plays in the development of more severe aftereffects that interfere with victim's ability to recognize interpersonal danger (Freyd & Birrell, 2013). She and her colleagues coined the term "betrayal blindness" as being due to the original perfidy and the conditioning involved in chronic abuse that resulted in victim confusion and naivete regarding other dangerous or coercive relationships.

Findings from neuroscience and affect theory have provided additional strands that intertwine with the others in Liotti's braid analogy, providing more nuanced understanding of multiply traumatized children and adults. Important findings about the function, structure, and network connectivity of the traumatized brain have been and continue to be investigated, especially focused on those whose abuse began early in life and those who have experienced layered and cumulative forms of trauma at different times in their lives. It stands to reason that those whose trauma experiences and exposures have been most severe, longstanding in duration, repeated, and high in betrayal trauma would be most associated with the use of dissociative defenses and processes, up to and including dissociative identity disorder (DID). This continues to be investigated.

Dissociation

Beginning in the late 1960s and early 1970s, the contemporary study of dissociation and dissociative disorders began and a crossover between the fields of child abuse and dissociation was once again re-discovered. Dissociation came to be identified as a posttraumatic condition, especially prominent in children who experienced the pervasive and prolonged abuse that characterizes complex trauma. A recently published scoping review (Fung et al., 2022) aimed to summarize the existing research on the relationship between dissociation and CPTSD. After a systematic review and exclusions of studies that did not meet criteria, 26 studies were included. Ten of them reported that subjects with CPTSD scored significantly higher on a dissociation measure than those without and 11 reported a positive correlation between symptoms and psychoform/somatoform dissociation scores. The researchers reported that a considerable subgroup of those with CPTSD have clinically significant levels of dissociative symptoms (e.g., 28.6–76.9%) and that dissociation may be involved with other comorbidities. They recommend the need for more studies in line with the recommendation made in Chapter 2 of this handbook by Dr. Colin Ross (another pioneer clinical researcher in dissociation and a coauthor of the scoping review). A recently published clinical commentary on the neuroscience of dissociative identity disorder reviewed the significance of neuroimaging in addressing the question of dissociation (Lebois et al., 2022). The authors commented on the research of neuroscientists Drs. Ruth Lanius and Simone Reinder whose neuroimaging work has provided scientific support for the dissociative subtype of PTSD, PTSD, CPTSD, and DID as being on a continuum of severity, depending on different dimensions of the traumatization endured, including its duration and overall degree of severity. In neuroimaging studies, conventional PTSD shows hyperarousal, while the dissociative subtype additionally shows derealization and depersonalization. Both patterns of arousal have been found to occur in CPTSD and DID. They concluded:

> After more than a century, science is finally catching up with the experience of front-line clinicians. [Pierre] Janet's original formulation was prescient. DID is, in fact, a complex biopsychosocial syndrome—an alternative neurodevelopmental pathway that can emerge with chronic child maltreatment. The core clinical feature is a disruption to the sense of self and mind. Under ordinary conditions, children gradually coalesce a cohesive sense of self; however, in the context of trauma, individuals with the capacity to dissociate (perhaps based on genetic factors) can be left with discrete self-states that patients describe as feeling they're "not me".

Why Have Complex Trauma and Dissociation Been Such a "Hard Sell" in Mental Health?

Despite all of the discoveries across these decades, complex trauma and dissociation did not receive much by way of legitimacy in academic research settings. In the absence of an evidence-base for treatment, clinicians developed consensus-based approaches to treatment that are only now being researched. Likely for many reasons (including conflicts of interest in some cases, misinformation or ignorance about childhood abuse and bias and discrimination against adult survivors and their confusing symptoms and manner of presentation, lack of adequate training about trauma and dissociation in the professional curriculum, overfascination with multiple personality disorder (MPD) later DID, and a reversal based on the "false memory" challenges of the 1990s that dramatically upended some of the clinical advances that were being made), complex (developmental) trauma, CPTSD, and the DDs have been a "hard sell" in mental health and with those whose allegiance was to the classic or conventional form of PTSD.

This only began to give way in more recent times when efforts at identifying the definitions and dimensions of complex trauma and dissociation continued (see Chapter 1 for a discussion) despite the ongoing critique of the "purists" that no data were available to support the concept of complex trauma. As the number and types of potentially traumatizing events and experiences increased and were documented (e.g., climate-related disasters and outcomes; the global ubiquity of colonialism and historical/ancestral trauma and its intergenerational transmission and impact; the COVID pandemic and resultant deaths and debilities; mass shootings; global conflicts and resultant displacement of populations), it became obvious that many fit some of the defining characteristics of complex trauma. Additional assessment methods and instruments were developed and revised (Cloitre et al., 2018). Herman (1992a, 1992b) rehabilitated Janet's original sequenced treatment model developed at the turn of the last century.

During this period, evidence-based treatment methods for PTSD were identified through efficacy studies; preliminary treatment guidelines followed. There are now approximately a dozen available US and international clinical practice guidelines for the treatment of PTSD in adults. All have coalesced around what are described as trauma-focused treatments since they have the most evidence of efficacy for the amelioration of the symptoms of PTSD. These are predominantly cognitive-behavioral interventions and include prolonged exposure, cognitive processing therapy, cognitive therapy, narrative exposure therapy, and eye movement desensitization and reprocessing. Most of the available guidelines did not include attention to children or to CPTSD, or only did so tangentially, and the question of their applicability arose, especially when clients with a complex trauma history were not among the samples that were studied, due to their instability and symptom severity. Several of the most recently published guidelines for adults were compared and contrasted by Hamblen et al. (2019), a helpful resource for clinicians.

Practice guidelines for complex trauma based on a survey of identified experts were first published by the International Society for Traumatic Stress Studies (Cloitre et al., 2011, 2012) to fill the gap and two sets of in-depth Australian consensus and research-based complex trauma practice guidelines were published (Kezelman & Stavropolous, 2012, 2019) in addition to shorter documents on dimensions of particular concern when treating complex trauma, one of which was on dissociation. The International Society for the Study of Trauma and Dissociation developed several sets of consensus and research-based guidelines for the treatment of dissociation and DID in children (ISSTD, 2003) as well as adults (ISSTD, 2011; under revision). A Professional Practice Guideline jointly developed by Division 56 of the American Psychological Association and the ISSTD has been recently published (American Psychological Association, 2024).

The ISSTD (formerly the International; Society for the Study Multiple Personality Disorder (ISSMPD) and later the International Society for the Study of Dissociation (ISSD) was founded in the 1980s to support the study of dissociation and to develop treatment approaches. In recent times, it again changed its name to the International Society for the Study of Trauma and Dissociation (ISSTD) this time in recognition of the connection between childhood adversity and trauma and dissociative processes and disorders. It is of note that many of the chapter authors in the current volume are or have been active members of this association, as theoreticians, researchers, and clinicians. In addition to the treatment guidelines published by the organization, two handbooks summarizing research and clinical findings on dissociation have been published and are recognized as essential and definitive documents in the field (Dell & O'Neil, 2009; Dorahy et al., 2022). The organization also sponsors a continuing education sequence of clinical training in the treatment of CPTSD and the DDs that fill in what typical clinical training programs continue to omit (Foltz et al., 2023).

One more endeavor deserves mention, that of the Trauma-Informed Care (TIC) movement that began as a grassroot effort organized by traumatized clients and their advocates who were misdiagnosed, mistreated, and misunderstood while seeking treatment. TIC is a philosophy of care that acknowledges the likelihood that a high percentage of mental health clients have a history of some sort of trauma in their backgrounds that clinicians, administrators, and policy makers need to recognize rather than ignore. TIC has had a considerable impact on service delivery in some organizations and agencies and as social policy in some states but remains to be fully implemented. Building on this initiative, we can also suggest that *complex trauma-informed care* is needed as both the application and the duration of treatment tend to differ from the treatment for conventional PTSD. Both can provide the context for treatment that is trauma-responsive as well as trauma-informed and within which evidence-based trauma-focused treatments (TFTs) and empirically supported treatments are applied in a sequence that is flexibly adapted to the needs of the client.

This Handbook

This overview brings us up to the present and provides background for the status of the field and thus to the significance of this handbook. The various linkages between childhood complex trauma, dissociation, and neuro-biopsychophysiological development are now well-established and are well-represented in this text. The impact of childhood trauma and its developmental trajectory are at the core of this text which is laid out in a very organized way. It begins with a chapter on definitions and theoretical formulations of complex trauma and dissociation followed by a chapter on the paucity of research on the epidemiology of dissociation in children and the ongoing lack of focus on dissociation and the dissociative disorders in children in the fields of child psychology, psychiatry, and social work. Although, as noted in almost every chapter, much remains to be investigated and new discoveries made, the remainder of the handbook offers a broad overview that brings the reader up to date on what has been learned most recently. Updated conceptual, theoretical, and neurobiopsychosocial information indicates the complexity of circumstances and reactions that are possible following experiences of ongoing childhood victimization and the scope of what the clinician who treats these children will face.

The second section provides an overview of symptomatology, assessment, diagnosis, and treatment planning for children with CT histories. It begins with a chapter that provides an overview of the symptomatology typically seen in children with complex trauma and dissociation. It emphasizes the need for this information to get incorporated into training on children's development and mental health to rehabilitate traumatized children in hopes of alleviating their present and future suffering. The chapter on advances in screening and clinical interviews in the assessment of dissociation in these children is followed by one on the complexity created by comorbidities and the need for careful attention to differential diagnosis. Another dimension, family systems theory and therapeutic applications, is discussed as part of the Five Star Theoretical Model in Chapter 16.

Treatments from a variety of theoretical orientations and modalities ranging from psychoanalytic to animal-assisted therapy are included in the third section, the centerpiece of the book. The various authors describe a broad scope of interventions that have been developed and applied to the treatment of traumatized children and adolescents. This, in turn, supports new theoretical developments in understanding and treating these children. The treatments described attend to issues of body and mind, the child's unique subjective experience, and the impact of complex trauma on a child's development. Authors recommend different forms of treatment whose application is individualized to the child and to dyadic treatment. The intersections of developmental trauma with identity, culture, ethnicity, and family dynamics are also emphasized, along with multi-modal and integrative applications. There is significant attention paid to different forms of play and expressive therapies. A thread running through these chapters is the focus on helping dissociated children express themselves and become more integrated through a variety of techniques designed for the purpose of exposure to and narration of the trauma in various modes of expression. All are aimed at the re-integration of self-experience and identity and a lessening of the use of dissociation to cope. However it is achieved, such personal integration interrupts the intergenerational transmission patterns in families and is preventive of additional traumatization of the child victim over their life course. Additionally, several chapters are devoted to strengthening of parent-child attachment bonds in recognition of the critical importance of relational security to the healing process. Although research remains to be conducted on many of these treatments, their reliance on various theoretical underpinnings and their integration are noteworthy advances.

Section 4 brings the focus to key professional and process considerations that also fortify this treatment for children and adolescents. The emphasis here is on the relational component between child and therapist as the foundation of the treatment. As clinical and ethical issues can abound in this treatment compared to treatment with non-traumatized children, a chapter is devoted to these issues. Sociocultural influences and determinants have been found to have major influence on the susceptibility of children from marginalized and minoritized populations, pointing to the requirement for cultural responsiveness on the part of the therapist. Many of the emotional and neurological consequences are discussed in several chapters with some novel approaches to their treatment. All begins with an appreciation for trauma-formed defenses and self-protective strategies as adaptive responses to past and ongoing adversity, danger, and traumatization. These include self-harm and suicidality that must be recognized as possibilities and even probabilities in some children, especially those in conditions of ongoing traumatization, including profound and highly damaging emotional abuse. Thus, safety monitoring needs to be ongoing. Dissociation is implicated in these responses and in conversive and functional neurologic systems as well as medical illnesses and pain that make up other complicated clinical presentations. The issue of coercive control in some forms of abuse is something therapists who treat these children must be aware of. A rich discussion of the mechanisms of mind control and gaslighting works and strategies for their reversal is included. Finally, pharmacology considerations are discussed, especially important given how abused children tend to receive diagnoses of ADHD, ODD, conduct disorders, and bi-polar disorders without consideration of a past or present trauma history and their influence on the child. Not infrequently, this leads to misdiagnosing and mismedicating the child, putting some at risk for medical consequences in later development.

Caregivers receive needed attention in this section as well, especially important as many of them often have their own unrecognized and unresolved trauma histories, as identified primarily in attachment studies and in other research studies as well. The intergenerational transmission of violence and victimization and the difficulty with providing children with secure attachment is an important point of prevention (as illustrated in the chapter on working with high-risk caregivers and the calming womb family therapy model) and intervention for the child therapist, either separately for the caregiver or in conjunction with the child. Such active, present-day interventions are proving to be important components of treating traumatized children and in preventing additional victimization. The impact of this work on the therapist or others in the treatment team is also addressed. Collaborative treatment in the context of agencies or other organizations that are trauma-informed can help with the monitoring of therapist risk, countertransference, and burnout. This, in turn, may provide the opportunity to be deeply satisfying to the treatment personnel.

Foreword

Altogether, the reader of this book will be introduced to an up-to-date overview of the world of the abused child and what they need to do to protect, defend against, and separate themselves from ongoing and complex forms of trauma. The range of treatment issues and treatment modalities makes for very interesting and informative reading that paves the way in learning how to treat this challenging population. Brava to the two co-editors for organizing such a rich compilation!

References

American Psychiatric Association. (1980). *Diagnostic and statistical manual of mental disorders* (3rd ed.). Author.
American Psychiatric Association. (2022). *Diagnostic and statistical manual of mental disorders-5 TR* (5th ed.). Author.
American Psychological Association (APA). (2017). *Clinical practice guidelines for the treatment of PTSD in adults*. Author.
American Psychological Association (2024). *Guidelines for Working with Adults with Complex Trauma Histories*. Retrieved from https://www.apa.org/practice/guidelines/adults-complex-trauma-histories.pdf
Cloitre, M., Shevlin, M., Brewin, C. R., Bisson, J. I., Roberts, N. P., Maercker, A., Karatzias, T., & Hyland, P. (2018). The international trauma questionnaire: Development of a self-report measure of ICD-11 PTSD and complex PTSD. *Acta Psychiatrica Scandinavica, 138*(6), 536–546. https://doi.org/10.1111/acps.12956
Cloitre, M. K., Courtois, C. A., Charuvastra, A., Carapezza, R., Stolbach, B. C., & Green, B. L. (2011). Treatment of complex PTSD: Results of the ISTSS expert clinician survey on best practices. *Journal of Traumatic Stress, 24*(6), 615–627.
Cloitre, M. K., Courtois, C. A., Ford, J. D., Green, B L., Alexander, P. L., Briere, J., & Van der Hart, O. (2012). *The ISTSS Expert Consensus Treatment Guidelines for complex PTSD in adults*. https://citeseerx.ist.psu.edu/document?repid=rep1&type=pdf&doi=c5eaffe436518684793cb359a7856797853b512c
Cloitre, M. K., Garvert, D. W., Brewin, C. R., Bryant, R. A., & Maercker, A. (2013). Evidence for proposed ICD-11 PTSD and complex PTSD: A latent profile analysis. *European Journal of Psychotraumatology, 4*, 1–12.
Courtois, C. A., & Ford, J. D. (Eds.). (2014). *Treating complex traumatic stress disorders: Scientific foundations and therapeutic models* (Paperback ed.). Guilford.
Dell, P. F., & O'Neil, J. A. (2009). *Dissociation and the dissociative disorders: DSM-V and beyond*. Routledge, Taylor & Francis Group.
Dorahy, M. J., Gold, S. N., & O'Neil, J. A. (Eds.). (2022). *Dissociation and the dissociative disorders: Past, present, future* (2nd ed.) Routledge.
Foltz, R., Kaeley, A., Kupchan, J., Mills, A., Murray, K., Pope, A., Rahman, H., & Rubright, C. (2023). Trauma-informed care? Identifying training deficits in accredited doctoral programs. *Psychological Trauma: Theory, Research, Practice, and Policy*. Advance online publication. https://doi.org/10.1037/tra0001461
Frewen, P., Wong, S., Bailey, T., Courtois, C., & Lanius, R. (2023). As simple as possible, but not simpler: Revisiting the International Trauma Questionnaire (ITQ) complex PTSD items omitted in the shortened version. *Child Abuse & Neglect, 141*, 106207. https://doi.org/10.1016/j.chiabu.2023.106207
Freyd, J. J. (1996). *Betrayal trauma: The logic of forgetting childhood abuse*. Harvard University Press.
Freyd, J. J., & Birrell, P. (2013). *Blind to betrayal: Why we fool ourselves we aren't being fooled*. Wiley.
Fung, H. W., Chien, W. T., Lam, S. K. K., & Ross, C. A. (2022). The relationship between dissociation and complex post-traumatic stress disorder: A scoping review. *Trauma, Violence, and Abuse*, 1–17. https://doi.org/10.1.11771524838022112835
Hamblen, J. L., Norman, S. B., Sonis, J. Phelps, A., Bisson, J, Delgado Nunes, V., Megnin-Viggars, O., Forbes, D., Riggs, D., & Schnurr, P. P. (2019). A guide to PTSD guidelines. *Psychotherapy, 56*(3), 359–373.
Herman, J. L. (1992a). Complex PTSD: A syndrome in survivors of prolonged and repeated trauma. *Journal of Traumatic Stress, 3*, 377–391.
Herman, J. L. (1992b). *Trauma and recovery: The aftermath of violence-from domestic to political terror*. Basic Books.
Herman, J. L. (2014). Forward. In C. A. Courtois & J. D. Ford (Eds.), *Treating complex traumatic stress disorders: Scientific foundations and therapeutic models* (p. xiii). Guilford.
International Classification of Diseases, Eleventh Revision (ICD-11), World Health Organization (WHO) 2019/2021. (2018). https://icd.who.int/browse11

Foreword

International Society for the Study of Dissociation Task Force on Children and Adolescents. (2003). *Guidelines for the evaluation and treatment of dissociative symptoms in children and adolescents*. Author.

International Society for the Study of Trauma and Dissociation [Chu, J. A., Dell, P. F., Van der Hart, O., Cardeña, E., Barach, P. M., Somer, E., Loewenstein, R. J., Brand, B. L., Golston, J. C., Courtois, C. A., Bowman, E. S., Classen, C. C., Dorahy, M., Şar, V., Gelinas, D. J., Fine, C. G., Paulsen, S., Kluft, R. P., Dalenberg, C. J., Jacobson-Levy, M., Nijenhuis, E. R. S., Boon, S., Chefetz, R. A., Middleton, W., Ross, C. A., Howell, E., Goodwin, G., Coons, P. M., Frankel, A. S., Steele, K., Gold, S. N., Gast, U., Young, L. M., & Twombly, J.]. (2011). *Guidelines for treating Dissociative Identity Disorder in adults*. Author.

Kezelman, C. & Stavropolous, P. (2012). *The last frontier: Practice guidelines for treatment of complex trauma and trauma informed care and service delivery*. Adults Surviving Child Abuse (ASCA). www.asca.org.au

Kezelman, C. & Stavropolous, P. (2019). *Practice guidelines for clinical treatment of complex trauma*. Blue Knot Foundation. www.blueknot.org.au

Lebois, L. A. M., Ross, D. A., & Kaufman, M. L. (2022). "I am not I": The neuroscience of dissociative identity disorder. *Biological Psychiatry, 91*, e11–e13. https://doi.org/10.1016/j.biopsych 2021.11.004

Liotti, G. (2004). Trauma, dissociation and disorganized attachment: Three strands of a single braid. *Psychotherapy: Theory, Research, Practice, Training, 41*, 472–486.

Putnam, F. W. (1997). *Dissociation in children and adolescents: A developmental perspective*. Guilford Press.

Spiegel, D. (1986). Dissociation, double binds, and posttraumatic stress in multiple personality disorder. In B. G. Braun (Ed.), *Treatment of multiple personality disorder* (pp. 61–77). American Psychiatric Press, Inc.

ACKNOWLEDGMENTS

Writing and editing a book is a journey that demands companionship, inspiration, encouragement, and support from many. We want to extend an earnest appreciation and gratitude to the contributors of this book for all the time, work, and energy that went into building your chapters. Your insight, wisdom, and expertise have been instrumental in shaping this book. To all pioneers in the field of complex trauma and dissociation, your contributions have cemented the way for our endeavors. We stand upon the shoulders of your legacy.

We want to especially thank Christine Courtois for reviewing this volume and for writing our foreword, as well as to Joyanna Silberg, Ruth Lanius, and Marlene Steinberg, for your endorsements and feedback. To our editor, Steph VanderMeulen, thank you for walking with us through every step of this book's development and providing invaluable guidance. To Anna Moore and the team from Routledge, thank you for believing in us and our vision of what could be possible.

To the thousands of children, consultees, and students who have crossed our paths, your willingness to share the depths and intricacies of your human experience has been the cornerstone of this book. To all of our mentors for your guidance!

Ana M. Gómez

Jill Hosey, I am immensely grateful for our journey together and our friendship. Your wise and honest presence was such an anchor for me during the highs and lows of the writing process.

To my husband Jim, your unwavering support, love, and your ability to bring humor even in the most challenging times created a safe space for me as I embarked on the long days and nights of reading, writing, and editing.

To my mother, Elizabeth, your love and guidance have been a constant presence in my life. Even now that you are not in the physical realm, your influence continues to shape every step of my journey. I am grateful for all my family, my father, and especially my sister Oderay. Dear Sister, your unconditional love has been a source of strength and inspiration throughout this process. To my beloved Lady and Candy, whose loyal companionship infused my days with love, laughter, and warmth.

To my students, consultees, and colleagues, each of you has enriched my personal and professional life in unique ways. I am especially grateful to Kathy Steele for your insightful feedback, valuable contributions, and friendship. To the children and their caregivers that have shaped my journey

Acknowledgments

as a therapist and entrusted me with their life stories. Walking by your side has been a privilege and a journey of mutual discovery and transformation.

Lastly, to the place of knowing within, a source that exists beyond time and space, and the guiding whispers whose subtle prompts have inspired me throughout my travels.

Jillian Hosey

I want to thank my partner in this journey, Ana Gómez. Thank you for being such a wonderful friend, mentor, colleague, chosen family member, and human being. There is no one else I could have undertaken such a book with, and I am grateful for this shared adventure and profound learning experience. I appreciate you and I treasure our friendship beyond what words can convey.

To my husband, Joe, thank you for your support, understanding, and flexibility as I undertook this long process. Thank you for the space you created for me to take on this project, and being by my side. Thank you to my family, as well as friends and colleagues for your friendship, support, and tolerance throughout this incredibly arduous process that brought moments of absence, but no shortage of love! To A.B., thank you for allowing me to show up perfectly imperfect to weather the storms; there isn't a day that goes by that I am not proud of you. Thank you to my consultants for your ongoing support and guidance, which I am extremely grateful for. To Maurice P., thank you for always believing in me and modeling how to think more critically. Finally, and of utmost importance, I want to thank my clients, who continue to inspire me and bring hope amidst turmoil. You have been my greatest teachers, helping me to better understand the complexity of what it means to be human and in relationship. Thank you for allowing me to support you through the process of healing the immense burdens of harm you have carried.

CONTRIBUTORS

Karen Andor, BA, BA (hons), BEd (hons), MEd, Educational Psychologist, Learning Support Specialist, and Psychotherapist in Private Practice Therapist in Dorset, England.

Alexis E. Arbuthnott, PhD, RD Psych, Assistant Professor with the Department of Psychiatry at the University of Saskatchewan, Psychologist in the Adolescent Psychiatry Unit, Saskatchewan Health Authority, Regina, Saskatchewan, Canada.

Sandra Baita, LCP, Licensed Clinical Psychologist, Author and Presenter, ISSTD Fellow and Faculty, Owner and Moderator "Trauma infantil" Listserv and Psychotherapist in Private Pratcie in Buenos Aires, Argentina.

Kim Barthel, BMR, OTR, Multi-Disciplinary Teacher and Trainer in Neuro-developmental Treatment and Occupational Therapy, Mentor, Author, Past Professor at the University of Manitoba, and Founder of Relationship Matters Consultancy Inc. in British Columbia, Canada.

Billie Jo Bennett, MSW, RSW, CPT-S, EMDR-AC, Clinical Director and owner of Purple Butterfly Healing Centre in Cambridge, Ontario, Canada.

Darren Bingham, MD, MRC Psych, Consultant Child and Adolescent Psychiatrist, Family Pathways, Western Australia.

Nicole Black, PhD, LPC-S, LCDC, RPT, Consultant, Supervisor, Expert Witness, and Author, Founder of Phoenix Arise and Phoenix Arise Consulting in Lubbock, Texas.

Tania Bosqui, PhD, Clinical Psychologist and Assistant Professor at the Trinity Centre for Global Health, Trinity College Dublin and at the American University of Beirut.

Rebeca Chow, PhD, LPC, LCPC, RPT-S, Chair-Elect of the Association for Play Therapy Board of Directors, Consultant for Sesame Street in Communities, and Clinician, Play Therapy Supervisor in Missouri and Kansas, USA.

Contributors

Jessica Christie-Sands, PhD, CPsych, CSci, AFBPsS, Senior Trainer in Deep Brain Reorienting and Clinical Director of DBR Training and Certification, Researcher and Clinical Director of an independent Multidisciplinary Psychology in the UK.

Cristina Civilotti, PhD, Lecturer for the Faculty of Psychology of the University of Turin, Psychologist and Psychotherapist, Milan, Italy.

Frank Corrigan, MD, FRC Psych, Author, Developer of Deep Brain Reorienting (DBR), and Independent Psychiatrist in Private Practice in Scotland.

Rosita Cortizo, PsyD, MFT, MA, Author, Presenter, ISSTD Fellow, and Creator of the Calming Womb Family Therapy Model, Psychotherapist in Private Practice and Public Health in California, USA.

D. Michael Coy, MA, LICSW, Author and Presenter, ISSTD Fellow, and therapist in Private Practice, Seattle, Washington State.

Richard M. Cross, UKCP, Fellow and Faculty Member of ISSTD and a Trustee of the Bowlby Centre, Director of MCTS and Registered Psychotherapist and Child Psychotherapist with the United Kingdom Council for Psychotherapy and the European Association for Psychotherapy and World Council for Psychotherapy.

Martina Cussino, PhD Past senior researcher at the Italian Swiss University of Lugano, Psychologist and Psychotherapist in Private practice in Milan, Italy (Centro di Terapia EMDR per l'Anoressia).

Chantal Cyr, PhD, Canada Research Chair in Child Attachment and Development, Université du Québec à Montréal, Canada.

Elizabeth Davis, MFA, MS, LCAT, ATR-BC, Author, EMDR Consultant and Trainer, Art Therapist, Director of the Buffalo NY Satellite Site, and Supervisor of Intake for Trauma Institute, in New York State, USA.

Betsy de Thierry, MA, MBACP Psychotherapist, Author, and Founder of The Childhood Trauma Recovery Network, United Kingdom.

Lisa Dion, LPC, RPT-S, Author, International Teacher, Creator of Synergetic Play Therapy and Founder and President of the Synergetic Play Therapy Institute, Co-founder of the Synergetic Education Institute, and host of the Lessons from the Playroom Podcast.

Benedetto Farina, MD, PhD in Neuroscience, psychiatrist and psychotherapist, full professor of Psychopathology and Psychotherapy at European University of Rome, Janet Clinical Centre, Scientific Advisory Board of the International Society for the Study of Trauma and Dissociation, Editorial Board of the *Journal of Trauma and Dissociation and of Clinical Neuropsychiatry*.

Christine C. Forner, BA, BSW, MSW, RSW, Author, Trainer and Presenter, Public Educator, ISSTD Fellow and Past President, and Private Practice Clinician in Calgary, Alberta, Canada.

Contributors

Robyn Gobbel, MSW, Past Faculty in the Foundations of Interpersonal Neurobiology Certificate Program at Portland Community College Author, Trainer, Consultant, and Therapist in Grand Rapids, MI.

Kim S. Golding, CBE, D Clin Psy AFBPsS, Author, Researcher and Associate Lecturer, Certified Consultant and Trainer in DDP and Board of Director Member for DDP Connects UK, Clinical Psychologist with the NHS in England.

Bonnie Goldstein, PhD, EdM, LCSW, Author, Sensorimotor Psychotherapy Institute Faculty, Professor of Social Work at USC, and founder and director of Lifespan Psychological Services in Los Angeles, California.

Paris Goodyear-Brown, LCSW, RPT-S, Author, Trainer, Ted Talk Speaker, creator of TraumaPlay™, Executive Director of the TraumaPlay Institute, Clinical Director of Nurture House, Adjunct Instructor of Psychiatric Mental Health at Vanderbilt University, and founder of Nurture House in Tennessee, USA.

Eleah Hyatt, LMFT, RPT-S is a Marital and Family therapist, AAMFT Approved Supervisor, Registered COSPTM Facilitator through the Circle of Security International and TraumaPlay TM Supervisor in Tennessee, USA.

Safa Kemal Kaptan, PhD Candidate in Clinical Psychology at the University of Manchester, UK, author, clinician, and researcher in traumatic reactions and parenting practices among war-affected individuals.

Matthew D. Kliethermes, PhD, Author, Trainer, and Supervisor, Training Director at Children's Advocacy Services of Greater St. Louis (CASGSL) and a Clinical Professor in the Department of Psychological Sciences at the University of Missouri-St. Louis (UMSL).

Maggie Kline, LMFT, Senior Somatic Experiencing Instructor for the Somatic Experiencing Institute, Author and Presenter, and Marriage, Family and Child Therapist in California, USA.

Ellen Lacter, PhD, Author, Presenter, Registered Play Therapy Supervisor, and past Academic Coordinator of the Play Therapy Certificate program at University of California San Diego, Division of Extended Studies for 25, in California, USA.

Valérie Langlois, PhD/PsyD, Researcher, Educator, Presenter, and Doctoral Student in Developmental Psychology at the Université du Québec à Montréal.

Dafna Lender, LCSW, Author, International Trainer and Clinical Supervisor in Theraplay and Dyadic Developmental Psychotherapy, Founder and Chief Consultant of Dafna Lender LLC Psychotherapy Training and Consulting in Evanston, Illinois.

John Lovern, PhD, Author, Researcher, Teacher, ISSTD Faculty, and Adjunct Faculty in the Psychology Department at Georgia Gwinnett College. Psychologist Veterans Healthcare System, Atlanta, Georgia, USA.

Contributors

Marshall Lyles, LPC-S, LMFT-S, RPT-S, Author, Presenter, Trainer and Teacher in the use of Sand Tray Therapies, and Psychotherapist in Private Practice in Texas, USA.

Helen Milroy, MBBS, RANZCP, CATCAP, descendant of the Palyku people of the Pilbara region of Western Australia, Stan Perron Professor of Child and Adolescent psychiatry with the Child and Adolescent Mental Health Service of Western Australia, Honorary Research Fellow with the Telethon Kids Institute, 2013–2017 Commissioner on the Royal Commission into Institutional Responses to Child Sexual Abuse.

Trudy Mooren, PhD, Clinical Psychologist and systemic therapist at ARQ Centrum'45, professor by special appointment at the Department of Clinical Psychology of the Faculty of Social Sciences at Utrecht University, Netherlands.

Paula Moreno, LCP, Licensed Clinical Psychologist, Author, Consultant and Trainer, and Psychotherapist in Child Abuse Assistance Program, General Directorate of Women, Government of the City of Buenos Aires, Argentina.

Anna K. Morrell, MA, LMHC, BCN, Mental Health Counselor and Neurofeedback Consultant and Trainer, Asheville, NC area.

Gabrielle Myre, PhD/Psy D Candidate in developmental psychology at the Université du Québec à Montréal, Author, Researcher, and Clinician.

Laura K. Noll, PhD, Author, Researcher and Prevention Scientist, Assistant Professor in the Department of Psychological Sciences and Director of the Interdisciplinary Health PhD program at Northern Arizona University.

Guilia Pace, MD, RANZCP, Clinical Psychologist, Touchstone, Child and Adolescent Mental Health Service in Western Australia.

Kristi L. Perryman, PhD, LPC, RPT-S, Author and Researcher, Associate Professor of Counseling at the University of Arkansas, and Founder of the Missouri State University Institute for Play Therapy and the University of Arkansas Office of Play Therapy Research and Training.

David S. Prescott, LICSW, Author and Editor, International Trainer, Director of the Safer Society Continuing Education Center, Vermont, USA.

Pradeep Rao, MBBS MD FRC Psych. FRANZCP CCT, Consultant Child and Adolescent Psychiatrist and Head of Service at the Complex Attention and Hyperactivity Disorders Service in the Child and Adolescent Mental Health Service in Western Australia, Clinical Lecturer at the University of Western Australia.

Michael Remole, MA, LCPC, NCC, Clinical Director, Children's Pastor, and Speaker, Former Natural Lifesmanship Trainer, Founder of Gateway Family Services of Illinois and present Executive Director of Hooves of Hope.

Colin A. Ross, MD, Author and Researcher, Founder of the Ross Institute Trauma Program and The Trauma Recovery Institute, Austin, Texas.

Contributors

Adriano Schimmenti, PhD, Professor at UKE – Kore University of Enna, President of the Italian Academic Scholars in Psychodynamic Psychology, Scientific Director of the Italian Institute of Psychoanalytic Psychotherapy (IIPP), Associate editor for *Clinical Neuropsychiatry* and *the European Journal of Trauma and Dissociation*.

Valerie Sinason, PhD, PGTC, MACP, Poet, Author, Researcher, Child Psychotherapist and Adult Psychoanalyst, and Past Consultant Child Psychotherapist at the Tavistock Clinic and Consultant Psychotherapist at both the Anna Freud and Portman Clinics, Founding Director of the Clinic for Dissociative Studies (CDS) in the UK.

Kathy Steele, MN, CS, Author, Presenter, ISSTD Fellow, Consultant and Supervisor, and Adjunct Faculty at Emory University, in Private Practice in Atlanta, Georgia, USA.

LaKaavia Taylor, PhD, LPC, NCC, RPT, Presenter, Clinician, Supervisor and Researcher, Associate Professor at Southern Methodist University, Texas.

George S. Thompson, MD, Author, Researcher, Associate Professor of Psychiatry at the University of Missouri-Kansas City School of Medicine, Medical Director at St. Francis Ministries Psychiatric Residential Treatment Facility, and Executive Director and Medical Director at the Treatment and Recovery Center, Inc., in Lawrence, KS.

Krystal K. Turner, M.A., LPC-Associate, NCC, Author and Presenter, Founding Board Member of Minorities in Counseling and Coalition of Black Counselors, Clinician and Assistant Director and School Outreach Coordinator for the Center for Play Therapy, and Doctoral Student in Counseling and Play Therapy at the University of North Texas.

Patti van Eys, PhD, past Assistant Professor of Psychology and Psychiatry at Vanderbilt University and past Clinical Director of the Vanderbilt University Center of Excellence for Children in State Custody, Expert Witness and Lead Psychologist at van Eys Mental Health in Nashville, Tennessee.

Frances S. Waters, DCSW, LMSW, LMFT, Author and International Trainer, Contributing Editor for the Journal of Child & Adolescent Trauma, and Consultant and Clinician in Private Practice in Michigan, USA.

Alix Woolard, PhD., Senior Research Fellow and Provisional Clinical Psychologist at the Telethon Kids Institute and the University of Western Australia.

Betül Yılmaz, MSc, PhD Candidate in Clinical Psychology at the University of Manchester, UK, Complex Trauma and Resilience Research Unit and the Global Mental Health and Cultural Psychiatry Research Group.

Eva Teirstein Young, MFA, MPS, ATR-BC, LCAT, Author and Presenter, Private Practice Therapist, Faculty with the William Alanson White Institute, and Assistant Professor at Pratt Institute in Brooklyn, New York.

Maria Zaccagnino, PhD, past senior researcher at the Italian Swiss University of Lugano, Psychologist and Psychotherapy, Director of Centers of EMDR Therapy for Eating Disorders and Children and Adolescents in Milan, Italy.

1
SETTING THE STAGE
An Introduction to Child Complex Trauma and Dissociation

Ana M. Gómez and Jillian Hosey

This book has been a labor of love, born out of a desire to expand the available literature and collate the various dimensions of dissociation as it manifests in children under the age of 12, which remain minimal and fragmented. Suitable for students, clinicians, researchers, and writers alike, this volume intends to offer an ample view of how generational wounds may be acknowledged in the genesis of dissociation and other mental health issues deriving from chronic traumatization. In the sensitive years of childhood, experiences of chronic trauma result in enduring bio-emotional, affective, and somatic trajectories that give rise to behaviors that challenge the child and those who seek to understand and support them. This volume represents a journey into the labyrinth of complex traumatization and its intricate relationship with dissociation in children. It also represents our unwavering dedication to the well-being and healing of our youngest and most vulnerable. Throughout our lives as clinicians, we have been witnesses and active participants in the often convoluted and intricate work that complex trauma demands. It is imperative to recognize the multifaceted nature of how the human mind interacts and is shaped by early experiences of adversity, trauma, and hardship. These life encounters are characterized by wounding acts of commission (what happened) and acts of omission (missing developmental experiences) that chronically flood the child's systems and subsequently shape neurodevelopment in profound and enduring ways.

The organization of this volume integrates the contributions of experts in the field, highlighting advances and theoretical frameworks as they pertain to the landscape of research, assessment, diagnosis, and clinical practice. With strides forward, divergent perspectives on what complex trauma and dissociation are and how they manifest still lack unification and clear pathways that link research to treatment. Post-secondary education continues to be inconsistent when it comes to dissociation as a consequence of child maltreatment. A recent quantitative content analysis of ten undergraduate textbooks found substantial differences in the adequacy, comprehensiveness, and balance of coverage on child maltreatment and dissociation, with minimal attention given to empirical research on dissociation (Nester et al., 2024). This book, however, serves as a testament to the remarkable advances that have been made while acknowledging the gaps that challenge our field. In presenting a comprehensive view of complex trauma and dissociation in children, we hope to inspire critical thinking around the magnitude and impact trauma has on the developing mind. We endeavor to cultivate awareness, change, and growth that can result in cohesive, effective, and efficient pathways for children to access culturally responsive assessment, diagnostic, and treatment practices.

Complex Trauma

Across this volume and the literature, complex trauma has received multiple definitions and labels that speak to its extensive and pervasive effects on children's neurodevelopment (Perry, 2008; Perry & Pollard, 1998; Gabowitz et al., 2008). Multiple terms and constructs exist that attempt to define complex trauma and its associated symptoms and phenomena as they manifest in children and adults (Herman, 1992; Cook et al., 2005; Kliethermes et al., 2014). Terr (1991) proposed typologies of trauma, including Type I (single incident trauma) and Type II (prolonged or repeated trauma experiences resulting in more nuanced and complex symptoms). Solomon and Heide (1999) later added Type III to address the impact of childhood-onset experiences of multiple and pervasive violent traumatic events that continue over long periods of time. Different terms utilized to define the phenomena of complex trauma in children include interpersonal trauma, relational trauma, cumulative trauma, developmental trauma, attachment trauma (Schore, 2003; Liotti, 2004; Spinazzola et al., 2021), and "polytraumatization" to refer to the exposure to multiple forms and types of trauma (Ford, 2021). Most of these terms speak about the child's early and repetitive exposure to disruptions in the parent-child relationship and an abdicated caregiving system unable to fulfill its protective and regulating functions. We now have a much greater awareness of the recurrent misdiagnosis and subsequent treatment that is askew and asynchronous to the actual needs of children affected by chronic traumatization. How we comprehend the impact of complex trauma continues to evolve alongside our understanding of its etiology; symptomatology; and cognitive, emotional, behavioral, and somatic manifestations.

Grounded in attachment theory, the concept of developmental trauma embodies an evolving understanding of how early and chronic exposure to adversity and trauma profoundly shapes long-term psychological, emotional, and physical well-being. Informed by studies on adverse childhood experiences (ACEs) (Felitti, 2012), developmental and complex trauma highlights the lasting impact of early, repeated trauma on neurodevelopment, emotional regulation, relationships, identity, and somatic symptoms. Despite its exclusion from the DSM-5, the concept has fueled trauma-informed care approaches and continues to shape the understanding and treatment of early-life adversity and trauma. It gained prominence through the work of van der Kolk and colleagues, leading to a proposal for a DSM diagnosis of developmental trauma disorder (DTD) (van der Kolk et al., 2009) containing four domains of diagnostic criteria, including exposure to interpersonal victimization or disrupted attachment, with emotion/somatic/attentional/behavioral/relational symptoms, or self-dysregulation (Cook et al., 2005; Spinazzola et al., 2021). While PTSD has been found to be associated with physical violence and traumatic loss (Norris & Slone, 2007), DTD is associated with attachment disruptions with primary caregiving figures occurring in emotionally abusive and physically violent environments (Spinazzola et al., 2021). Isolated traumatic events result in discrete behavioral and biological responses in comparison to children who experience complex trauma. These children often face profound effects on emotion processing and regulatory capacities, disrupting fundamental overarching biopsychosocial, neurodevelopmental processes (Novick et al., 2018; Morelli & Villodas, 2022). Growing literature and research attest to how exposure to multiple and chronic caregiver-related trauma has a more significant association with a higher severity of traumatic stress and mental health symptoms, high-risk behaviors, and day-to-day functioning challenges (Kisiel et al., 2020). According to Schore (2019), "Caregiver-induced relational trauma is qualitatively and quantitatively more potentially phytopathogenic than any other social or physical stressor" (p. 43). Internal working models and synaptic systems holding cognitive, emotional, behavioral, and sensorimotor schemas emerge from complex trauma, keeping the child in survival. They defend against the invisible assaults that live within that interfere with the formation of close bonds and the capacity for play, imagination, and learning (van der Kolk, 2014).

It is relevant to note that not all children exposed to chronic trauma develop severe symptomatology, instead displaying significant malleability and resilience (Racine et al., 2020). For instance, a third of at-risk foster and adopted children follow a typical developmental trajectory, a third develop mild mental health issues, and a third show an increased risk for more complex and pervasive symptomatology (Vliegen et al., 2023). This volume seeks to recognize each child's unique characteristics, resilience, and capacities and how trauma impacts their development differently. Trauma does not exist in isolation in the child's biology. Instead, it interacts with their environment, strengths, and vulnerabilities. As such, the expressions of genetic, epigenetic, environmental, and experiential factors cohabit and interact actively in how trauma manifests in each child's unique biological and environmental characteristics.

Dissociation

In the simplest sense, dissociation is the separation of typically integrated mental processes (Spiegel & Cardeña, 1991). Through our own growth and learning journeys, we have found ourselves coming back to similar questions. What do we actually mean when speaking of dissociation? How can this be understood in children, who are in a continual process of growth and development? Dissociation presents as a multi-layered, multidimensional phenomenon, encompassing a spectrum from mild disengagement or absorption to acute fragmentation of identity. Defying a single definition, the complexity of the term "dissociation" encompasses perspectives from multiple disciplines, cultures, and fields of study, including trauma, neurobiology, and hypnosis. Definitions of dissociation may describe it as a process, a condition, or a phenomenon (Howell, 2011). Each definition offers multiple avenues of understanding within the extensive tapestry of the mind exposed to chronic traumatization. Embracing the multitude of, at times, divergent voices compels us to realize the true complexity involved in defining, assessing, and treating dissociation.

Pierre Janet is often considered the originator of the term "dissociation," or désagrégation (Scalabrini et al., 2020), both through his development of a theory of Psychological Automatism and in establishing connections between the division of the personality and exposure to trauma and traumatic stress (van der Hart & Dorahy, 2009). With the earliest cases of "multiple personality states" in adults dating back to the 1500s (Brand et al., 2016), interest in dissociation and dissociative states has waxed and waned over time and across disciplines. In her text that focuses on the relational treatment of dissociative identity disorder, Howell (2011) offers a concise review of the history of the concept of dissociation, exploring the intersections of relationality, trauma, dissociation, and multiplicity, and highlights important differences between the concepts of repression, suppression, and dissociation.

The study of dissociation has not been without controversy, signaling the discomfort that arises when we turn toward the painful realities of what causes dissociation in the first place. Despite contemporary neurobiological research into the veracity of dissociation (see Dorahy et al., 2022; Lebois et al., 2021), issues related to trauma, memory, and dissociation have proliferated across time, invalidating and revictimizing those already most vulnerable (Crook, 2022; Sinason & Conway, 2021). Two enduring yet diametrically opposed theories of dissociation and dissociative disorders represented in the literature are the trauma model and the socio-cognitive model (Loewenstein, 2018). The trauma model postulates that dissociation is a psychobiological state and/or trait that serves to protect and defend against traumatic experiences that overwhelm the ability to cope. The socio-cognitive model sees dissociation as a condition created in fantasy-prone, highly suggestible clients by therapists or cultural and social influence (Loewenstein, 2018). Sar et al. (2013) share that the trauma model and the socio-cognitive model may not be as opposed as some believe due to the varying, dynamic factors and contexts within which dissociative disorders develop.

Holmes et al. (2005) identified in a literature review that dissociation may be described through its nosology or etiology, as pathological or non-pathological, as the subjectively different processes of detachment and compartmentalization, or as a wide-ranging term in the PTSD literature that seems to span a variety of dissociative symptoms and phenomena. Inextricable from complex trauma (van Dijke et al., 2015), dissociation in the adult literature is often described phenomenologically (Dell, 2009), through its etiology (Cardeña, 1997), or as a theoretical or conceptual process-based description of what is happening and how (Ludwig, 1983; Braun, 1988). Dell (2009) highlights that "there are at least three important levels or domains of explanation and description for dissociation: a neuroanatomical-neurophysiological explanation, a psychological explanation, and phenomenological description" (p. 225). Spiegel (1963) proposed a bidirectional model of dissociation (e.g., a dissociation/association continuum), which offered a way to conceptualize dissociation on a continuum from normative to pathological in nature. Braun (1984) stated that dissociation and the previously termed multiple personality disorder (re-termed dissociative identity disorder in the DSM-IV in 1994) represent an extreme on the continuum. Decades of research have helped us better understand that at this severe end of the continuum, "Dissociative identity disorder (DID) is a complex, posttraumatic, developmental disorder" (Brand et al., 2016, p. 257). In a deep dive into the various ways the term dissociation is used, Cardeña (1994) wisely observed that "the domain of dissociation can be thought of as a constellation, or a way of thinking about dissociation and its related phenomena, with boundaries that define what lies inside and outside the domain" (p. 15). Each definition brings different treatment implications (Holmes et al., 2005). The process of clarifying dissociation as a concept more generally, let alone specifically as experienced by children, has resulted in fragmentation and conflict.

Putnam's groundbreaking work in the contemporary literature on dissociation (see Chapter 3) helped us begin to better understand what this means for children, describing,

> The range of potential manifestations of dissociation in childhood, including problems with (a) memory and amnesia; (b) sense of self; (c) trance-like states; (d) rapidly shifting mood/behaviors; (e) inconsistencies or perplexing shifts in awareness, memory, and abilities; (f) auditory/visual hallucinations; and (g) vivid imaginary companions.
>
> *(Putnam, 1997, as cited in Kisiel et al., 2020, p. 191)*

Richard Kluft (1985) published an edited book titled *Childhood Antecedents of Multiple Personality Disorder*, within which he detailed four criteria for the development of DID, stating:

> The child who will develop multiple personality disorder has the capacity to dissociate (factor 1), which is enlisted in defending that child against any of a variety of overwhelming experiences usually (but not invariably) involving abuse (factor 2). Any of a number of naturally occurring substrates are enlisted to provide the structure of an alter or alters, leading to the remarkable diversity encountered among multiple personality disorder patients (factor 3). The failure of significant others to help the child process his experiences and prevent retraumatization (factor 4) results in a transient pathological adaptation's [sic] becoming relatively fixed and further elaborated.
>
> *(pp. 186–187)*

This way of understanding the pathway to the development of dissociative symptomatology in children highlights the complex interaction between early and later abuse-related experiences and characteristics, individual factors (hypnotizability or the capacity to dissociate), and interactions with others (relational, attachment-based contributors). Interest in childhood dissociation research and practice has been limited, a situation that seems not to have changed much in the past 30 years since Peterson

(1991) identified the then-problematic lack of attention to child dissociation in the psychiatric community. Texts published by Wieland (2011, 2015), Waters (2016), and Silberg (2012, 2021) have led the way, offering child clinicians various relevant theories and dissociation-specific approaches to treatment. Despite theoretical advances in the adult realm, research on the treatment of childhood dissociation continues to be limited in scope and availability, which leaves the field with ongoing challenges in assessment and diagnosis and without a clear therapeutic framework for treatment (Woolard et al., 2024).

The Organization and Structure of This Volume

Theory, Conceptual Models, and Neurobiology

In the first section of this volume, experts in the field address multiple theoretical models, neurodevelopmental trajectories, and alterations associated with exposure to complex trauma and resulting dissociation (see Chapters 2–11). These initial chapters present multiple perspectives and theoretical models elucidating the etiology and progression of complex trauma and dissociation in children. Following this introduction, Chapter 2 brings awareness to the scarcity of scientific data or large-scale studies on the epidemiology of dissociation in children.

Chapter 3 thoroughly explores the groundbreaking *Discrete Behavioral States Model*, which is central to our current understanding and conceptualization of dissociation. It explores how exposure to early trauma alters pathways between states that disrupt the accessibility of autobiographical memory and a coherent sense of self.

Chapter 4 is devoted to the study of the enduring consequences of continued and severe ruptures in the caregiver-child attachment bond resulting in attachment trauma. It delves into the dimensional impact of child maltreatment that goes beyond a single diagnosis or symptomatology.

Chapter 5 offers an overview of the intricate connection between regulation, attachment, and the evolving social brain and how early caregiving experiences shape the child's emotional development.

The theory of structural dissociation (Chapter 6) offers a comprehensive model to conceptualize fragmentation in the child's emerging personality in response to exposure to complex traumatization. The author differentiates alterations in attention and consciousness (spaciness, absorption, maladaptive daydreaming) from divisions in the child's emerging personality that will signal the presence of structural dissociative processes.

The autohypnotic model of dissociation follows in Chapter 7, bringing a thorough review of the literature on how hypnotizability and hypnotic abilities are associated with the development and maintenance of dissociative disorders. It is important to highlight that this model does not come without controversies.

The contributions of betrayal trauma theory to the current understanding of dissociation in children are addressed in Chapter 8. This chapter offers insight into the significant impact of violations of trust in the caregiver-child relationship across the lifespan and the ways in which the human mind is designed to "not know" when betrayal is perpetrated by those we also depend on. The author brings awareness to the impact of betrayal on children, its prevalence in childhood, and its impact on development.

Chapter 9 delves into complex trauma and dissociation through the lens of interpersonal neurobiology (IPNB). The author conceptualizes integration and dissociation through four of the nine domains of integration delineated in IPNB: interpersonal integration, vertical integration, state integration, and integration of consciousness.

Polyvagal Theory has revolutionized the field with research on heart rate variability and the multi-branched vagus nerve, representing an integrated autonomic nervous system. Chapter 10 thoroughly addresses how trauma resets the nervous system and turns off social engagement, disrupting integration. This chapter elucidates the complex interplay of chronic traumatization and the disruption of autonomic states of safety and homeostasis.

This section ends with Chapter 11, which is dedicated to a neurobiological exploration of a mid-brain-based model of traumatic dissociation, which explores the interrelationship of the innate connection system to initial sensory-affective orienting responses. Using a Deep Brain Reorienting approach, this chapter explores the connection between early life shock and pre-attachment wounding; shock-induced derealization and depersonalization; and experiences of neurochemical, structural, and supracortical dissociation.

Assessment, Symptomatology, and Diagnosis

The second section of this volume delves into important considerations in assessment, diagnosis, and treatment planning. We intend to honor current advances and challenge existing paradigms in the assessment, diagnosis, and conceptualization of child complex trauma and dissociation. New perspectives confront the pathologizing, evaluative, and diagnostic stance (Carel, 2023) borrowed from the medical model and its effectiveness and necessity in guiding the treatment of child complex trauma and dissociation. Prescriptive treatment delivery solely founded on diagnosis may miss each child's individual and unique characteristics while overfocusing on the label. However, without empirical research and needed advances in the assessment and diagnostics of dissociation in children, clinicians are without a clear clinical understanding of the nuances of complex trauma and dissociative symptomatology—such a lack risks children receiving inadequate treatment, perpetuating the legacy of trauma across generations.

This section begins with Chapter 12, which presents an overview of dissociative symptomatology in children under 12 across different developmental phases, offering readers a means of conceptualizing the myriad of ways dissociation manifests in children, which is qualitatively different from adults. Chapter 13 explores essential considerations in the processes of screening, assessment, and clinical interviewing with children, while Chapter 14 addresses considerations related to comorbidity, neurodiversity, and differential diagnosis. Readers are encouraged to think critically, examining what our measures may miss and whether they can truly capture the complexity of the human experience, connection, and the impact of complex trauma and dissociation in children. Inclusion of lived experience research, and advocating for its inclusion in what becomes the evidence base, is also asserted to be essential. This section finishes off with an exploration into case conceptualization and treatment planning (Chapter 15), which includes core treatment principles and guidelines, and a chapter that illustrates the use of the Five-Star Theoretical Model (Chapter 16) as a way of bringing together theory, assessment, conceptualization, and treatment planning.

Treatment Modalities and Clinical Applications

There is a scarcity of literature and research that compares treatment model components, the degree to which they focus on complex trauma, and the evidence and efficacy of these methodologies (Lawson & Quinn, 2013; Dorsey et al., 2017). Most studies with children under 12 years of age focus on symptoms related to PTSD rather than complex trauma and dissociation. However, there is emerging interest in studying treatment outcomes for this population (Arvidson et al., 2011; Chen et al., 2018; Hébert et al., 2020; Lichtenstein & Brager, 2017). We cannot deny the important contributions of clinical observation, practice-based evidence, and emerging quantitative studies highlighted in this book. The psychotherapeutic process is nuanced, with moment-to-moment explicit and implicit processes between two (or more) embodied minds that are not easily operationalizable or quantitatively segmented into parts to study them. Once the therapeutic phenomenon is segmented, it risks the loss of its fundamental essence and contributions to the treatment outcome. Connection, reciprocity, compassion, the clinician's capacities for holding the child's mind in mind, the creation of a safe therapeutic relational environment, and attention to the autonomic patterns of activation occurring throughout the therapeutic moments are not easily taken into the lab. As such, new qualitative and phenomenological approaches to research need development.

Several approaches in this volume adhere to a phase approach endorsed by the International Society for the Study of Trauma and Dissociation (ISSD, 2004). The controversy and tension in the field about whether a stabilization phase is needed and useful are worth recognition (Bongaerts et al., 2017). The issue at the center is if trauma-related material is tolerable and in equilibrium with the child's capacities. However, the lack of compelling evidence with children leaves this debate open. We invite the recognition of children's diverse responses to trauma and the unique adaptations each child has to support (survival). The intersectionality of identities and contextual and individual influences underscores the importance of tailoring assessment, diagnosis, and treatment approaches to the child's unique individual and environmental characteristics and capacities. For some children, the rapid entrance into traumatogenic experiences may prove to be the most effective portal. In contrast, others may benefit from a titrated and gradual approach with enough work allocated to building homeostatic capacities and safety. Polarizations that force binary views and methodologies may bypass and override individual and contextual variances.

This section extensively explores different treatment methodologies employed with dissociative children, offering a wide range of therapeutic possibilities (see treatment modalities section, Chapters 17–32). It brings a comprehensive view of what exists in the literature, research, and clinical practice while acknowledging the prevailing gaps, dilemmas, and challenges in treating children impacted by trauma. Considering the interpersonal nature of complex trauma and the presence of ruptures in the protective and regulating role of the caregiver, multiple therapeutic methodologies in this book involve the caregiver as an active therapeutic partner. Across the spectrum of therapeutic modalities, there is a fundamental consensus around restoring developmental rhythms and trajectories and the importance of repairing and cultivating co-regulation in the caregiver-child and clinician-child relationship. Clinicians are more actively assuming the role of the external psychobiological regulator for the child (Schore, 2019) and caregiver, diligently working to restore relational shared coherence, reciprocity, and connectedness in the caregiver-child relationship. Systemic and dyadic models that recognize and work with the transmission of generational wounds and the pivotal contributions of the parent-child attachment bond in the child's neurodevelopment are increasing exponentially.

The relational environment shapes the child's neural landscape (Siegel, 2023) and, as such, the relational milieu is prominent and is included across all therapeutic approaches in this book. Parent-based methodologies and family interventions are integrated throughout the treatment chapters, and some dive deep into the fundamental but often intricate therapeutic work with families and caregivers. Bottom-up and top-down practices are utilized and incorporated actively as the field is arriving at a much greater understanding of the biological imprint left by complex trauma and the need to work with methodologies that merge body-based interventions (for example, sensorimodulating strategies and approaches). Multiple chapters present ways in which treatment can support the restoration of the interconnected rhythms of the brain and the viscera through therapeutic embodiments, play, movement, and connectedness.

Treatment delivery is moving into a more integrated, biopsychosocial field (Gilbert, 2009), and all treatment models addressed in this book reflect this and incorporate developmentally sound approaches to treatment that recognize and work with the heterogeneity of symptoms emerging from exposure to complex traumatization. New understandings of the functioning of the autonomic nervous system and the often necessary restorative work to repattern previously ruptured autonomic states are moving our field to acknowledge the importance of restoring safety and homeostasis. Throughout the treatment section, most approaches incorporate and highlight the therapeutic value of play, focusing on therapeutic methodologies centered around play therapy, including Child-Centered Play Therapy (CCPT), Theraplay, Synergetic Play Therapy, and Trauma Play. Each underscores the transformative power of play in promoting healing to the traumatized child. Expressive arts therapies and sand tray therapies also offer abundant opportunities for play, expression, integration, and the developing relationship with self. Animal-Assisted Therapy harnesses the profound bond between humans and animals that awaken abundant corrective relational possibilities. They include opportunities for co-regulation, connectedness, empathy, mentalization, and the forging of new relationships with sentient beings that challenge trauma-formed relational working models.

Vliegen et al. (2023) propose that, besides the active work with children and parents, systemic work with the network caring for the child is paramount to have a lasting impact. Clinicians must often work on scaffolding the child's environment to promote developmental recovery. The caregiving environment that encompasses the parent (biological, adoptive, and foster), extended family, teachers, and all the professional and para-professional teams often involved (i.e., case managers, therapists, clinicians, parenting training specialists) calls for a shift into a more collaborative and synchronic approach that ensures safety across multiple domains, predictability, connectedness, and co-regulation to the child who had none. Due to the high emotional investment, the child's care system may, at times, become exhausted, hopeless, dysregulated, or disengaged and shut down. After working for many years with children in the foster care system, we have been witnesses to the burnout that may result from caring for children with complex clinical symptomatology. Often, the large number of stakeholders that maintain multiple views, perspectives, and goals and partake in the creation of the child's treatment plan may lead to complete disorganization that recreates the unpredictable and chaotic environment that wounded the child. The treating clinician is part of a collective network and, as such, work should be allocated to providing psychoeducation designed to upsurge accessibility to information on complex trauma and dissociation and increase the team's synchrony in their decision-making and approaches to supporting the child's developmental recovery. The lives of these children are often nuanced by frequent changes in their home placements, the potential of parental severance, crisis, and medical issues. Ineffective treatment may lead to a constant rotation of clinicians, leading to the severance of treatment and absolute hopelessness of all participating actors, especially the child.

This volume acknowledges the merit that exists in the capacity of the child's mind to dissociate and compartmentalize in the face of chronic exposure to severe traumatization. We also want to underscore the long history of marginalization and stigmatization of the child that has to coexist with insufficient, wounding, abusive, abdicated, and traumatizing relational, caregiving, and institutional systems. We have closely witnessed how children often have had to carry the burden of generational wounds by becoming the identified patient. The overuse and emphasis on pharmacological management (Correll et al., 2011; Olfson et al., 2014) with this population can further marginalize these children, masking their pain while releasing the relational and institutional systems from their responsibility to change.

Despite all the advances, we still have abundant work ahead of us to give childhood dissociation and symptomatology emerging from complex trauma a much greater recognition and effective early identification and interventions. The field still struggles to "integrate the intricacies of child's circumstances into a trauma-informed framework" (Zilberstein, 2022).

Setting the Stage

Important Considerations in the Treatment of Complex Trauma and Dissociation

The concluding section of this volume examines the intricate tapestry of special issues surrounding childhood complex trauma and dissociation. This portion begins with a journey into the role of the therapeutic relationship (Chapter 33), bringing together psychoanalytic, attachment, attunement, neurobiological, and relational perspectives. Additional concepts related to the (re)development of a felt sense of relational safety and trust and the role of play in the development of the self, relationship, and the healing milieu are explored. This chapter premises the healing relationship as the foundation from which all interventions flow, serving as the container through which healing is held and fostered. Readers are encouraged to reflect on the ways in which they understand the role of relationships in healing, the challenges and dilemmas that can emerge in therapy, and the delicate relational dance that contributes to the healing of children.

In Chapter 34, readers are guided to delve deeply into the interconnectedness of social categorizations and the interdependent systems of oppression, discrimination, marginalization, and disadvantage and how they intersect and compound with exposure to chronic traumatization. Systemic oppression, dismissive approaches, and prejudice toward the child's challenges and symptomatology further aggravate the traumatized child's sense of estrangement, isolation, and disconnection from others. The reluctance to fully acknowledge the social and systemic responsibilities in the healing of developmental and complex trauma in children further alienates this population, perseverating it in future generations. Clinicians working with child complex trauma and dissociation often face ethical and moral dilemmas. They must navigate intricate issues requiring a nuanced approach and moment-to-moment self-exploration and awareness (Chapter 35). We underscore the importance of ongoing consultation and active collaboration to find greater synchrony within the interdisciplinary team so that treatment delivery aligns with the child's needs.

The following chapters are dedicated to the often necessary treatment of caregivers, with Chapter 36 focused on early prevention work in pregnancy with high-risk caregivers through a systemic approach. Chapter 37 focuses on the impact of a caregiver's trauma on a child, its relationship to complex trauma and dissociation, and interventions for addressing this early and throughout treatment in support of the healing of the child and the family system. Chapter 38 offers an exploration into multiple nuanced historical, cultural, and generational differences and viewpoints within the realm of child complex trauma and dissociation, including the challenges and advantages faced by each generation.

Chapter 39 explores the intricacies of therapeutically addressing the multiple shades of shame and guilt, as shame and guilt are emotions intricately linked to complex trauma and dissociation. Often, children hold a deep sense of defectiveness while carrying the responsibilities of their oppressors and abusers. This book offers theoretical perspectives as well as treatment approaches and methodologies that can support such pervasive and challenging trauma-based symptomatology. In the face of overwhelming affect, children's natural rhythms of defense homeostasis are fundamentally altered, perpetuating cycles of defense where the "threat" regulating system dominates (Gilbert, 2022). The active recognition and necessary work to downregulate rigid defensive actions in the presence of safety is thoroughly covered in Chapter 40.

Chapter 41 is dedicated to exploring self-harm and suicidality as it manifests in dissociative children. Chapter 42 follows, addressing the consequences of cumulative trauma, with exposure to ongoing suffering that affects forcibly displaced groups, predominantly refugees, bringing awareness of the challenges of delivering treatment to this population. Medical issues, pain, and physical complaints often accompany complex traumatization and dissociation (Chapter 44), and for some, psychogenic symptomatology and functional neurological symptoms develop (Chapter 43). Chapter 45 focuses on the work with children exposed to abusive mind control and psychological manipulation practices that are systematically inflicted by perpetrators and leave deep cognitive, affective, and somatosensory imprints that lay at the core of their dissociative symptoms. This section ends with Chapter 46, which takes a psychopharmacological approach to reviewing the principles and modalities of the psychiatric treatment of dissociative children.

Conclusion

As we conclude this chapter and our introduction to *The Handbook of Complex Trauma and Dissociation in Children: Theory, Research, and Clinical Applications*, we hope to have offered a panoramic view of the depth and breadth of the content of this compendium. This volume presents theory, research, and clinical applications, with case examples offered throughout, to highlight practical and case-related considerations that arise as clinicians operationalize knowledge into practice.

We hope this book makes it to you at just the right time, whether you are a student, an experienced clinician, a researcher, or simply a lifelong learner like us. While our goal for this book has been to expand the research and stimulate interest in continuing to build our knowledge and practice base, we earnestly hope that it serves as a catalyst for change and transformation in the field. We hope the message of this book resonates across disciplines, driving collective efforts and systemic shifts that prioritize the healing of children exposed to complex trauma and presenting with dissociation. We aspire for this book to equip professionals to deliver culturally responsive and attuned treatments that consider the role of trauma and dissociation from the outset, improve health and wellness outcomes for the next generations, and inspire hope for healing and posttraumatic growth.

References

Arvidson, J., Kinniburgh, K., Howard, K., Spinazzola, J., Strothers, H., Evans, M., Andres, B., Cohen, C., & Blaustein, M. E. (2011). Treatment of complex trauma in young children: Developmental and cultural considerations in application of the ARC intervention model. *Journal of Child & Adolescent Trauma, 4*(1), 34–51. https://doi.org/10.1080/19361521.2011.545046

Bongaerts, H., Van Minnen, A., & de Jongh, A. (2017). Intensive EMDR to treat patients with complex posttraumatic stress disorder: A case series. *Journal of EMDR Practice and Research, 11*(2), 84–95. https://doi.org/10.1891/1933-3196.11.2.84

Brand, B. L., Sar, V., Stavropoulos, P., Krüger, C., Korzekwa, M., Martínez-Taboas, A., & Middleton, W. (2016). Separating fact from fiction: An empirical examination of six myths about dissociative identity disorder. *Harvard Review of Psychiatry, 24*(4), 257–270. https://doi.org/10.1097/HRP.0000000000000100

Braun, B. G. (1984). Towards a theory of multiple personality and other dissociative phenomena. *Psychiatric Clinics of North America, 7*(1), 171–193. https://doi.org/10.1016/S0193-953X(18)30789-5

Braun, B. G. (1988). The BASK model of dissociation. *Dissociation, 1*(1), 4–23. https://hdl.handle.net/1794/1276

Cardeña, E. (1994). The domain of dissociation. In S. L. Lynn & J. W. Rhue (Eds.), *Dissociation: Clinical and theoretical perspectives* (pp. 15–31). Guilford Press.

Cardeña, E. (1997). The etiologies of dissociation. In S. Krippner & S. M. Powers (Eds.), *Broken images, broken selves: Dissociative narratives in clinical practice* (pp. 61–87). Brunner/Mazel.

Carel, H. (2023). Vulnerabilization and de-pathologization: Two philosophical suggestions. *Philosophy, Psychiatry, & Psychology, 30*(1), 73–76. https://doi.org/10.1353/ppp.2023.0013

Chen, R., Gillespie, A., Zhao, Y., Xi, Y., Ren, Y., & McLean, L. (2018). The efficacy of eye movement desensitization and reprocessing in children and adults who have experienced complex childhood trauma: A systematic review of randomized controlled trials. *Frontiers in Psychology, 9*, 534. https://doi.org/10.3389/fpsyg.2018.00534

Cook, A., Spinazzola, J., Ford, J., Lanktree, C., Blaustein, M., Cloitre, M., DeRosa, R., Hubbard, R., Kagan, R., Liautaud, J., Mallah, K., Olafson, E., & van der Kolk, B. (2005). Complex trauma in children and adolescents. *Psychiatric Annals, 35*(5), 390–398. https://doi.org/10.3928/00485713-20050501-05

Correll, C. U., Kratochvil, C. J., & March, J. S. (2011). Developments in pediatric psychopharmacology: Focus on stimulants, antidepressants, and antipsychotics. *The Journal of Clinical Psychiatry, 72*(5), 655–670. https://doi.org/10.4088/JCP.11r07064

Crook, L. (2022). The power of false memory rhetoric. *Journal of Trauma & Dissociation, 23*(2), 148–151. https://doi.org/10.1080/15299732.2022.2028220

Dell, P. F. (2009). The phenomena of pathological dissociation. In P. F. Dell & J. A. O'Neill (Eds.), *Dissociation and the dissociative disorders: DSM-V and beyond* (pp. 225–237). Routledge. https://doi.org/10.4324/9780203893920

Dorahy, M. J., Gold, S. N., & O'Neil, J. A. (Eds.). (2022). *Dissociation and the dissociative disorders: Past, present, future*. Routledge. https://doi.org/10.4324/9781003057314

Dorsey, S., McLaughlin, K. A., Kerns, S. E. U., Harrison, J. P., Lambert, H. K., Briggs, E. C., Revillion Cox, J., & Amaya-Jackson, L. (2017). Evidence base update for psychosocial treatments for children and adolescents exposed to traumatic events. *Journal of Clinical Child & Adolescent Psychology, 46*(3), 303–330. https://doi.org/10.1080/15374416.2016.1220309

Felitti, V. (2012). The adverse childhood events study. *PsycEXTRA Dataset*. https://doi.org/10.1037/e53365 2013-043

Ford, J. D. (2021). Polyvictimization and developmental trauma in childhood. *European Journal of Psychotraumatology, 12*(sup1), 1866394. https://doi.org/10.1080/20008198.2020.1866394

Gabowitz, D., Zucker, M., & Cook, A. (2008). Neuropsychological assessment in clinical evaluation of children and adolescents with complex trauma. *Journal of Child & Adolescent Trauma, 1*(2), 163–178. https://doi.org/10.1080/19361520802003822

Gilbert, P. (2009). *The compassionate mind: A new approach to life's challenges*. Constable.

Gilbert, P. (2022). Introducing and developing CFT functions and competencies. In P. Gilbert & G. Simos (Eds.), *Compassion focused therapy: Clinical practice and applications* (pp. 243–272). Routledge. https://doi.org/10.4324/9781003035879-9

Hébert, M., Daignault, I. V., & Blanchard-Dallaire, C. (2020). Adaptation of trauma-focused cognitive behavioural therapy for cases of complex trauma. *International Journal of Child and Adolescent Resilience, 7*(1), 211–221. https://doi.org/10.7202/1072599ar

Herman, J. L. (1992). Complex PTSD: A syndrome in survivors of prolonged and repeated trauma. *Journal of Traumatic Stress, 5*(3), 377–391. https://doi.org/10.1002/jts.2490050305

Holmes, E. A., Brown, R. J., Mansell, W., Fearon, R. P., Hunter, E. C. M., Frasquilho, F., & Oakley, D. A. (2005). Are there two qualitatively distinct forms of dissociation? A review and some clinical implications. *Clinical Psychology Review, 25*(1), 1–23. https://doi.org/10.1016/j.cpr.2004.08.006

Howell, E. F. (2011). *Understanding and treating dissociative identity disorder: A relational approach*. Routledge. https://doi.org/10.4324/9780203888261

ISSD. (2004). Guidelines for the evaluation and treatment of dissociative symptoms in children and adolescents. *Journal of Trauma & Dissociation, 5*(3), 119–150. https://doi.org/10.1300/J229v05n03_09.

Kisiel, C. L., Torgersen, E., & McClelland, G. (2020). Understanding dissociation in relation to child trauma, mental health needs, and intensity of services in child welfare: A possible missing link. *Journal of Family Trauma, Child Custody & Child Development, 17*(3), 189–218. https://doi.org/10.1080/26904586.2020.1816867

Kliethermes, M., Schacht, M., & Drewry, K. (2014). Complex trauma. *Child and Adolescent Psychiatric Clinics of North America, 23*(2), 339–361. https://doi.org/10.1016/j.chc.2013.12.009

Kluft, R. P. (Ed.). (1985). *Childhood antecedents of multiple personality*. American Psychiatric Press, Inc.

Lawson, D. M., & Quinn, J. (2013). Complex trauma in children and adolescents: Evidence-based practice in clinical settings. *Journal of Clinical Psychology, 69*(5), 497–509. https://doi.org/10.1002/jclp.21990

Lebois, L. A. M., Li, M., Baker, J. T., Wolff, J. D., Wang, D., Lambros, A. M., Grinspoon, E., Winternitz, S., Ren, J., Gönenç, A., Gruber, S. A., Ressler, K. J., Liu, H., & Kaufman, M. L. (2021). Large-scale functional brain network architecture changes associated with trauma-related dissociation. *The American Journal of Psychiatry, 178*(2), 165–173. https://doi.org/10.1176/appi.ajp.2020.19060647

Lichtenstein, A., & Brager, S. (2017). EMDR integrated with relationship therapies for complex traumatized children: An evaluation and two case studies. *Journal of EMDR Practice and Research, 11*(2), 74–83. https://doi.org/10.1891/1933-3196.11.2.74

Liotti, G. (2004). Trauma, dissociation, and disorganized attachment: Three strands of a single braid. *Psychotherapy, 41*(4), 472–486. https://doi.org/10.1037/0033-3204.41.4.472

Loewenstein, R. J. (2018). Dissociation debates: Everything you know is wrong. *Dialogues in Clinical Neuroscience, 20*(3), 229–242. https://doi.org/10.31887/DCNS.2018.20.3/rloewenstein

Ludwig, A. M. (1983). The psychobiological functions of dissociation. *American Journal of Clinical Hypnosis, 26*(2), 93–99. https://doi.org/10.1080/00029157.1983.10404149

Morelli, N. M., & Villodas, M. T. (2022). A systematic review of the validity, reliability, and clinical utility of developmental trauma disorder (DTD) symptom criteria. *Clinical Child and Family Psychology Review, 25*(2), 376–394. https://doi.org/10.1007/s10567-021-00374-0

Nester, M. S., Spicher, B., Pierorazio, N. A., Brand, B. L., & McEwen, L. E. (2024). Coverage of child maltreatment in undergraduate psychopathology textbooks. *Psychological Trauma: Theory, Research, Practice, and Policy.* https://doi.org/10.1037/tra0001683

Norris, F. H., & Slone, L. B. (2007). The epidemiology of trauma and PTSD. In M. J. Friedman, T. M. Keane & P. A. Resick (Eds.), *Handbook of PTSD: Science and practice* (pp. 78–98). Guilford Press.

Novick, A. M., Levandowski, M. L., Laumann, L. E., Philip, N. S., Price, L. H., & Tyrka, A. R. (2018). The effects of early life stress on reward processing. *Journal of Psychiatric Research, 101*, 80–103. https://doi.org/10.1016/j.jpsychires.2018.02.002

Olfson, M., Blanco, C., Wang, S., Laje, G., & Correll, C. U. (2014). National trends in the mental health care of children, adolescents, and adults by office-based physicians. *JAMA Psychiatry, 71*(1), 81–90. https://doi.org/10.1001/jamapsychiatry.2013.3074

Perry, B. D. (2008). Child maltreatment: A neurodevelopmental perspective on the role of trauma and neglect in psychopathology. In T. P. Beauchaine & S. P. Hinshaw (Eds.), *Child and adolescent psychopathology* (pp. 93–128). John Wiley & Sons, Inc.

Perry, B. D., & Pollard, R. (1998). Homeostasis, stress, trauma, and adaptation: A neurodevelopmental view of childhood trauma. *Child and Adolescent Psychiatric Clinics of North America, 7*(1), 33–51. https://doi.org/10.1016/S1056-4993(18)30258-X

Peterson, G. (1991). Children coping with trauma: Diagnosis of "dissociation identity disorder." *Dissociation, 4*(3), 152–164. https://hdl.handle.net/1794/1453

Putnam, F. W. (1997). *Dissociation in children and adolescents: A developmental perspective.* Guilford Press.

Racine, N., Eirich, R., Dimitropoulos, G., Hartwick, C., & Madigan, S. (2020). Development of trauma symptoms following adversity in childhood: The moderating role of protective factors. *Child Abuse & Neglect, 101*, 104375. https://doi.org/10.1016/j.chiabu.2020.104375

Sar, V., Krüger, C., Martínez-Taboas, A., Middleton, W., & Dorahy, M. (2013). Sociocognitive and posttraumatic models of dissociation are not opposed. *The Journal of Nervous and Mental Disease, 201*(5), 439–440. https://doi.org/10.1097/nmd.0b013e31828e112b

Scalabrini, A., Mucci, C., Esposito, R., Damiani, S., & Northoff, G. (2020). Dissociation as a disorder of integration – On the footsteps of Pierre Janet. *Progress in Neuro-Psychopharmacology and Biological Psychiatry, 101*, 109928. https://doi.org/10.1016/j.pnpbp.2020.109928

Schore, A. N. (2003). *Affect regulation and the repair of the self.* Norton Professional Books.

Schore, A. N. (2019). *The development of the unconscious mind.* Norton Professional Books.

Siegel, D. J. (2023). *Intraconnected: Mwe (me + we) as the integration of self, identity, and belonging.* Norton Professional Books.

Silberg, J. L. (2012). *The child survivor: Healing developmental trauma and dissociation* (1st ed.). Routledge. https://doi.org/10.4324/9780203830277

Silberg, J. L. (2021). *The child survivor: Healing developmental trauma and dissociation* (2nd ed.). Routledge.

Sinason, V., & Conway, A. (Eds.). (2021). *Trauma and memory: The science and the silenced.* Routledge.

Solomon, E. P., & Heide, K. M. (1999). Type III trauma: Toward a more effective conceptualization of psychological trauma. *International Journal of Offender Therapy and Comparative Criminology, 43*(2), 202–210. https://doi.org/10.1177/0306624X99432007

Spiegel, D., & Cardeña, E. (1991). Disintegrated experience: The dissociative disorders revisited. *Journal of Abnormal Psychology, 100*(3), 366–378. https://doi.org/10.1037//0021-843x.100.3.366

Spiegel, H. (1963). The dissociation-association continuum. *The Journal of Nervous and Mental Disease, 136*(4), 374–378. https://doi.org/10.1097/00005053-196304000-00008

Spinazzola, J., van der Kolk, B., & Ford, J. D. (2021). Developmental trauma disorder: A legacy of attachment trauma in victimized children. *Journal of Traumatic Stress, 34*(4), 711–720. https://doi.org/10.1002/jts.22697

Terr, L. C. (1991). Childhood traumas: An outline and overview. *The American Journal of Psychiatry, 148*(1), 10–20. https://doi.org/10.1176/ajp.148.1.10

van der Hart, O., & Dorahy, M. J. (2009). History of the concept of dissociation. In P. F. Dell & J. A. O'Neill (Eds.), *Dissociation and the dissociative disorders: DSM-V and beyond* (pp. 3–26). Routledge.

van der Kolk, B. A. (2005). Developmental trauma disorder: Toward a rational diagnosis for children with complex trauma histories. *Psychiatric Annals, 35*(5), 401–408. https://doi.org/10.3928/00485713-20050501-06

van der Kolk, B. A. (2014). *The body keeps the score: Brain, mind, and body in the healing of trauma.* Viking.

van der Kolk, B. A., Pynoos, R. S., Cicchetti, D., Cloitre, M., D'Andrea, W., Ford, J. D., Lieberman, A. F., Putnam, F. W., Saxe, G., Spinazzola, J., Stolbach, B. C., & Teicher, M. (2009). *Proposal to include a developmental trauma disorder diagnosis for children and adolescents in DSM-V* [Unpublished manuscript].

van Dijke, A., Ford, J. D., Frank, L. E., & van der Hart, O. (2015). Association of childhood complex trauma and dissociation with complex posttraumatic stress disorder symptoms in adulthood. *Journal of Trauma & Dissociation, 16*(4), 428–441. https://doi.org/10.1080/15299732.2015.1016253

Vliegen, N., Tang, E., Midgley, N., Luyten, P., & Fonagy, P. (2023). *Therapeutic work for children with complex trauma: A three-track psychodynamic approach.* Routledge. https://doi.org/10.4324/9781003044918

Waters, F. S. (2016). *Healing the fractured child: Diagnosis and treatment of youth with dissociation.* Springer.

Wieland, S. (Ed.). (2011). *Dissociation in traumatized children and adolescents* (1st ed.) Routledge.

Wieland, S. (Ed.). (2015). *Dissociation in traumatized children and adolescents: Theory and clinical interventions* (2nd ed.). Routledge.

Woolard, A., Boutrus, M., Bullman, I., Wickens, N., Gouveia Belinelo, P. d., Solomon, T., & Milroy, H. (2024). Treatment for childhood and adolescent dissociation: A systematic review. *Psychological Trauma: Theory, Research, Practice, and Policy.* Advance online publication. https://doi.org/10.1037/tra0001615

Zilberstein, K. (2022). Trauma in context: An integrative treatment model. *Journal of Child & Adolescent Trauma, 15*(2), 487–500. https://doi.org/10.1007/s40653-021-00416-3

PART 1

Theory, Conceptual Models, and Neurobiology

2
EPIDEMIOLOGY OF DISSOCIATION IN CHILDREN

Colin A. Ross

Introduction

There are no large-scale scientifically designed epidemiological studies of dissociation in children under age 18. There are, however, a number of smaller-scale studies of dissociation in children conducted in clinical populations, and there are published case series, single case reports, and a rich literature on principles of treatment (Gomez, 2013; Putnam, 1997; LaPorta, 1992; Shirar, 1996; Silberg, 2022; Sinason & Marks, 2021; Waters, 2016; Wieland, 2015). Despite this literature, the epidemiology of childhood dissociation in clinical populations, the general population, across cultures, and in different economic, social, and racial subgroups is very poorly understood. Likewise, there is no literature on the rates of dissociation in children with different sexual orientations and gender identities. As a result of this lack of scientific data, only a tentative understanding of the epidemiology of dissociation in children is possible.

Research on dissociation in children is primarily based on the Child Dissociative Checklist (CDC) (Putnam & Peterson, 1994; Putnam et al., 1993; Sim et al., 2005; Zoroglu, Tuzun, et al., 2002) and the Adolescent Dissociative Experiences Scale (A-DES) (Armstrong et al., 1997; Reagor et al., 1992; Zoroglu, Şar, et al., 2002). Although the Structured Clinical Interview for DSM-IV Dissociative Disorders (SCID-D) (Steinberg & Steinberg, 1995) and the Dissociative Disorders Interview Schedule (DDIS) (Ross, 1997) can be used in evaluating adolescents, neither is suitable for children under 12 years of age. Research on the epidemiology of dissociative disorders in children is hampered by the lack of a suitable structured interview.

The Epidemiology of Dissociative Disorders in Adults

An initial estimate of the epidemiology of dissociative disorders in children can be generated from the literature on adults, which includes a large number of studies and replications in many different languages and cultures (Kate et al. 2020). Kate et al. (2020) reviewed 98 studies of dissociation in college students, involving 31,905 students. They found that a dissociative disorder was present in 11.4% of the students overall, including 3.7% with dissociative identity disorder (DID). These authors also reviewed three studies conducted in the general population in Canada (Ross, 1991), the United States (Johnson et al., 2006), and Turkey (Şar et al., 2007). The prevalence of some type of dissociative disorder was 9.0% in Canada, 9.1% in the United States, and 18.3% in Turkey; the prevalence of DID was 1.3% in Canada, 1.5% in the United States, and 1.1% in Turkey. Johnson et al. (2006) conducted clinical interviews with 658 adults in a community sample: they diagnosed a dissociative disorder in 8.9% of the participants, including 1.5% with DID.

DID is the most severe dissociative disorder and, in adults, is almost always related to severe, chronic childhood trauma (Ross, 1997). If we assume that all cases of adult DID began before age 10, then the prevalence of DID among children under 10 in the general population should be 1.1%–1.5%. If we assume that three-quarters of the adult cases began before age 10, then the prevalence in children under 10 would be about 0.8%; and if we assume that half the adult cases began before age 10, then the prevalence in children under 10 would be about 0.4%. Based on the adult clinical literature, the actual figure is likely to be that 1% of children under 10 meet criteria for DID.

Since the 18.3% figure for the prevalence of some type of dissociative disorder in Turkey appears to be a statistical outlier, we can assume that dissociative disorders affect 9.0% of the adult general population. This is close to but lower than the 11.4% rate in college students. This means that the number of children under 10 with a dissociative disorder is 9.0% if all cases begin before age 10, 6.75% if three-quarters begin before age 10, and 4.5% if half begin before age 10. Although no firm conclusions can be drawn from these extrapolations, it is reasonable to conclude that a dissociative disorder affects at least 5% of children under age 10, while DID affects about 1%. Even if these numbers are not exactly accurate, it is unlikely that dissociative disorders are rare in children. Firm conclusions await the results of adequately designed epidemiological research.

Kate et al. (2020) reported that average scores on the Dissociative Experiences Scale (DES) (Bernstein & Putnam, 1986) were lower in North America than in many other countries, which is inconsistent with the socio-cognitive, iatrogenic, suggestion, or contagion models that state that dissociative disorders are an artifact of professional and cultural influence and are most prevalent in North America (Boysen, 2011). These authors also found that average dissociation scores in college students did not increase over a time period of decades with increasing public exposure to dissociative disorders, which is also inconsistent with the contagion or suggestion models.

The Epidemiology of Dissociation in Children

Clinical reports of single cases or small series of DID cases (then called multiple personality disorder or MPD) began to appear in the 1980s (Albini & Pease, 1989; Bowman et al., 1985; Fagan & McMahon, 1984; Kluft, 1984; Malenbaum & Russell, 1987; Riley & Mead, 1988; Weiss et al., 1985). These initial reports were followed by additional papers published in the 1990s (Bowman, 1990; Coons, 1996; Dell & Eisenhower, 1990; Hornstein & Putnam, 1992; Hornstein & Tyson, 1991; Kluft, 1992; Lewis, 1996; Peterson, 1990, 1991; Putnam, 1993; Putnam et al., 1996; Sanders & Giolas, 1991; Silberg, 1998; Snow et al., 1995; Trujillo et al., 1996; Tutkun et al., 1994; Tyson, 1992; Vincent & Pickering, 1988; Yeager & Lewis, 1996; Zoroglu et al., 1997; Zoroglu, Tutkun, Tuzun, & Şar, 1996; Zoroglu, Yargic, Tutkun, Ozturk, & Şar, 1996; Zoroglu, Yargic, Tutkun, Tuzun, & Şar, 1996). After the year 1999, the number of case reports of dissociation in children diminished (Hulette et al., 2008; Macfie et al., 2001a, 2001b; Zoroglu et al., 2000).

In terms of clinical samples slightly larger than the small case series, in an unpublished study my research team in Winnipeg interviewed 45 inpatient adolescents with the DDIS: we found that 44.4% met criteria for a dissociative disorder, including 15.6% with DID (Ross, 1997). In another unpublished study conducted in Winnipeg in the 1980s, we compared 11 adolescents with DID to 166 adults with DID on the DDIS, and only two differences between the two groups were significant, at p <.05: the adolescents reported fewer somatic and amnesia symptoms. During this time period, I diagnosed DID in about 20 children aged 13–17 and in two other children, aged 3 and 8 (Ross, 1996). This experience convinced me that DID is not rare in children, since I was seeing children and adolescents in consultation only, not as part of my primary clinical work with adults.

Waterbury (1991) (as reviewed in Ross, 1996) reported a systematic analysis of 231 children at the Woodbourne Children's Diagnostic. Treatment Center in Baltimore, Maryland. The analysis included extensive clinical interviews, use of a variety of measures, and review of school records. These children were 80% boys and 80% African American. A diagnosis of DID was made in 16 Caucasian and 38 African American children; there were 27 boys and 27 girls with DID. This included 13 children aged 4–8 and 41 aged 9–13. Waterbury reported that many of the children, including many of those under 10 years, had complex personality systems similar to those in adults. In addition to the 54 (23%) children with DID, 76 (33%) met criteria for dissociative disorder not otherwise specified, and a further 40 (17%) met criteria for DID of childhood, a diagnosis that was proposed for but not adopted in the DSM-IV (American Psychiatric Association, 1994).

In another study conducted in Winnipeg in the 1980s (Ross et al., 1989), we administered the adult form of the DES to 168 junior high school students in their classrooms: the average score for the 12-year-old students (N = 59) was 20.2, while the average score for the 14-year-old children (N = 94) was 14.8 ($p < .00001$). In a study of 504 adults in the general population of Winnipeg, interviewed in their homes (Ross, 1991), the average DES score was 10.8. If it is generally true that dissociation scores decline with age in the teens and adulthood, then it is unlikely that dissociative disorders become more common with age; this logic supports the possibility that dissociative disorders are more common in children than they are in adults.

Hulette et al. (2011) administered the CDC to 67 children in foster care and 51 children in a comparison community sample: of the 118 children, 57 were female and their average age was 9.34 years (range: 7.24–12.29 years). Using a cutoff score of 20 on the CDC, the authors found that 20.9% of the children in foster care required further assessment for a dissociative disorder compared to 2% of the control children.

Sanders and Giolas (1991) administered the DES and a set of trauma measures to a sample of 47 children aged 13–17 (35 girls and 17 boys) who were inpatients at private mental hospitals. The average DES score was 19.2 but, notably, the range was 0.44–61.9. Of the 47 children, 11 (23.4%) scored above 31.2 on the DES, indicating a high likelihood of a dissociative disorder. The correlation between the DES scores and the trauma measures in the sample was 0.44.

Endo et al. (2006) made clinical diagnoses and administered the CDC to 39 abused children in Japan with an average age of 10.7 years (16 girls and 23 boys). They made a clinical diagnosis of a dissociative disorder in 59% of the children, including (10.2%) with DID. The children with a dissociative disorder had an average CDC score of 20.4 compared to 7.3 in the children with no dissociative disorder.

Future Research on the Epidemiology of Dissociation in Children

The clinical and treatment literature on children with complex dissociative disorders is well developed (Gomez, 2013; Putnam, 1997; Shirar, 1996; Silberg, 2022; Sinason & Marks, 2021; Wieland, 2015). For conducting treatment outcome studies, it would be helpful if a treatment manual was available so that a standardized but flexible protocol could be adopted. Overall, the treatment of children with dissociative disorders should be shorter than it is for adults; therefore, treatment outcome studies should be less expensive and easier to conduct, assuming that the children have been extricated from their abuse. A first step in this direction would be a naturalistic follow-up study of a group of children in treatment for DID and other specified dissociative disorder (OSDD). The larger the group, the better, but even a small sample would be a start. Ideally, such a study would be prospective in design, as in the landmark study by Trickett et al. (2011), but a retrospective chart review could be a useful contribution.

In terms of epidemiology, as for treatment outcome studies, initial future research will involve relatively small samples of various populations. Besides the time and energy required, a barrier to such studies is having access to a group of children. This could be in an outpatient agency, an inpatient or residential treatment facility, a group practice, a juvenile detention center, or any other setting that provided access to a sample of children. Parental or guardian consent would be required and standardized measures such as the CDC or A-DES would be administered along with other measures such as ones for depression, anxiety, attachment, and trauma. Samples of highly traumatized children, such as those in foster care, gangs, or juvenile detention centers, could be compared to less traumatized children, such as those receiving treatment in a pediatric medical practice.

Besides the intrinsic scientific value of such studies, the resulting data could provide a counter-argument to the view that DID is a contamination artifact occurring in suggestible adults. Having samples from a variety of cultures, languages, and continents would help in this regard. It will be particularly interesting to have data on the variations in presentation and symptomatology of complex dissociation in children across cultures and in subgroups within a given culture. The study by Waterbury (1991) tells us that full DID occurs in boys and girls and in both Caucasian and African American children in the United States.

A challenge faced by the dissociative disorders field is how to interest mainstream researchers in doing studies on dissociation and the dissociative disorders. This could include studies of epidemiology, phenomenology, trauma histories, biology (such as studies of hippocampal volume), environmental and cultural contributors, and a wide range of considerations.

References

Albini, T. K., & Pease, T. E. (1989). Normal and pathological dissociations of early childhood. *Dissociation: Progress in the Dissociative Disorders, 2*(3), 144–150.

American Psychiatric Association (1994). *Diagnostic and statistical manual of mental disorders* (4th ed.). American Psychiatric Association.

Armstrong, J., Putnam, F. W., Carlson, E., Libero, D., & Smith, S. (1997). Development and validation of a measure of adolescent dissociation: The Adolescent Dissociative Experience Scale. *Journal of Nervous & Mental Disease, 185*(8), 491–497. https://doi.org/10.1097/00005053-199708000-00003

Bernstein, E. M., & Putnam, F. W. (1986). Development, reliability, and validity of a dissociation scale. *Journal of Nervous and Mental Disease, 174*(12), 727–735. https://doi.org/10.1097/00005053-198612000-00004

Bowman, E. S. (1990). Adolescent multiple personality disorder in the nineteenth and early twentieth centuries. *Dissociation: Progress in the Dissociative Disorders, 3*(4), 179–187.

Bowman, E. S., Blix, S., & Coons, P. M. (1985). Multiple personality in adolescence: Relationship to incestual experiences. *Journal of the American Academy of Child Psychiatry, 24*(1), 109–114. https://doi.org/10.1016/s0002-7138(09)60418-0

Boysen, G. A. (2011). The scientific status of childhood dissociative identity disorder: A review of published research. *Psychotherapy and Psychosomatics, 80*(6), 329–334. https://doi.org/10.1159/000323403

Coons, P. M. (1996). Clinical phenomenology of 25 children and adolescents with dissociative disorders. *Child and Adolescent Psychiatric Clinics of North America, 5*(2), 361–374. https://doi.org/10.1016/S1056-4993(18)30371-7

Dell, P. F., & Eisenhower, J. W. (1990). Adolescent multiple personality disorder: A preliminary study of eleven cases. *Journal of the American Academy of Child and Adolescent Psychiatry, 29*(3), 359–366. https://doi.org/10.1097/00004583-199005000-00005

Endo, T., Sugiyama, T., & Someya, T. (2006). Attention deficit/hyperactivity disorder and dissociative disorder among abused children. *Psychiatry and Clinical Neuroscience, 60*(4), 434–438. https://doi.org/10.1111/j.1440-1819.2006.01528.x

Fagan, J., & McMahon, P. P. (1984). Incipient multiple personality in children: Four cases. *Journal of Nervous and Mental Disease, 172*(1), 26–36. https://doi.org/10.1097/00005053-198401000-00007

Gomez, A. (2013). *EMDR therapy and adjunct approaches with children: Complex trauma, attachment, and dissociation*. Springer.

Hornstein, N. L., & Putnam, F. W. (1992). Clinical phenomenology of child and adolescent multiple personality disorders. *Journal of the American Academy of Child and Adolescent Psychiatry, 31*(6), 1077–1085. https://doi.org/10.1097/00004583-199211000-00013

Hornstein, N. L., & Tyson, S. (1991). Inpatient treatment of children with multiple personality disorder/dissociative disorders and their families. *Psychiatric Clinics of North America, 14*(3), 631–648.

Hulette, A. C., Fisher, P. A., Kim, H. K., Ganger, W., & Landsverk, J. L. (2008). Dissociation in foster preschoolers: A replication and assessment study. *Journal of Trauma and Dissociation, 9*(2), 173–190. https://doi.org/10.1080/15299730802045914

Hulette, A. C., Freyd, J. J., & Fisher, P. A. (2011). Dissociation in middle childhood among foster children with early maltreatment experiences. *Child Abuse and Neglect, 35*, 123–126.

Johnson, J. G., Cohen, P., Kasen, S., & Brook, J. S. (2006). Dissociative disorders among adults in the community, impaired functioning, and axis I and II comorbidity. *Journal of Psychiatric Research, 40*(2), 131–140. https://doi.org/10.1016/j.jpsychires.2005.03.003

Kate, M. A., Hopwood, T., & Jamieson, G. (2020). The prevalence of dissociative disorders and dissociative experiences in college populations: A meta-analysis of 98 studies. *Journal of Trauma and Dissociation, 21*, 16–61.

Kluft, R. P. (1984). Multiple personality in childhood. *Psychiatric Clinics of North America, 7*(1), 121–134.

Kluft, R. P. (1992). Editorial: Dissociative disorders in childhood and adolescence: New frontiers. *Dissociation: Progress in the Dissociative Disorders, 5*(1), 2–3.

LaPorta, L. D. (1992). Childhood trauma and multiple personality disorder: The case of a 9-year-old girl. *Child Abuse and Neglect, 16*(4), 615–620. https://doi.org/10.1016/0145-2134(92)90076-4

Lewis, D. O. (1996). Diagnostic evaluation of the child with dissociative identity disorder/multiple personality disorder. *Child and Adolescent Psychiatric Clinics of North America, 5*(2), 303–331. https://doi.org/10.1016/S1056-4993(18)30368-7

Macfie, J., Cicchetti, D., & Toth, S. (2001a). The development of dissociation in maltreated preschool-aged children. *Development and Psychopathology, 13*(2), 233–254. https://doi.org/10.1017/s0954579401002036

Macfie, J., Cicchetti, D., & Toth, S. (2001b). Dissociation in maltreated versus normal treated preschooler-aged children. *Child Abuse and Neglect, 25*(9), 1253–1267. https://doi.org/10.1016/s0145-2134(01)00266-6

Malenbaum, R., & Russell, A. T. (1987). Multiple personality disorder in an 11-year-old boy and his mother. *Journal of the American Academy of Child and Adolescent Psychiatry, 26*(3), 436–439. https://doi.org/10.1097/00004583-198705000-00028

Peterson, G. (1990). Diagnosis of childhood multiple personality. *Dissociation: Progress in the Dissociative Disorders, 3*(1), 3–9.

Peterson, G. (1991). Children coping with trauma: Diagnosis of "dissociation identity disorder." *Dissociation: Progress in the Dissociative Disorders, 4*(3), 152–164.

Putnam, F. W. (1993). Dissociative disorders in children: Behavioral profiles and problems. *Child Abuse and Neglect, 17*(1), 39–45. https://doi.org/10.1016/0145-2134(93)90006-q

Putnam, F. W. (1997). *Dissociation in children and adolescents: A developmental perspective.* Guilford Press.

Putnam, F. W., Helmers, K., & Trickett, P. K. (1993). Development, reliability, and validity of a child dissociation scale. *Child Abuse and Neglect, 17*(6), 731–741. https://doi.org/10.1016/s0145-2134(08)80004-x

Putnam, F. W., Hornstein, N., & Peterson, G. (1996). Clinical phenomenology of child and adolescent dissociative disorders: Gender and age effects. *Child and Adolescent Psychiatric Clinics of North America, 5*(2), 351–360.

Putnam, F. W., & Peterson, G. (1994). Further validation of the Child Dissociative Checklist. *Dissociation: Progress in the Dissociative Disorders, 7*(4), 204–211.

Reagor, P. A., Kasten, J. D., & Morelli, N. (1992). A checklist for screening dissociative disorders in children and adolescents. *Dissociation: Progress in the Dissociative Disorders, 5*(1), 4–19.

Riley, R. L., & Mead, J. (1988). The development of symptoms of multiple personality disorder in a child of three. *Dissociation: Progress in the Dissociative Disorders, 1*(3), 41–46.

Ross, C. A. (1991). Epidemiology of multiple personality disorder and dissociation. *Psychiatric Clinics of North America, 14*(3), 503–517.

Ross, C. A. (1996). Epidemiology of dissociation in children and adolescents. *Child and Adolescent Psychiatric Clinics of North America, 5*(2), 273–284.

Ross, C. A. (1997). *Dissociative identity disorder. Diagnosis, clinical features, and treatment of multiple personality* (2nd ed.). Wiley.

Ross, C. A., Ryan, L., Ross, D., & Hardy, L. (1989). Dissociative experiences in adolescents and college students. *Dissociation: Progress in Dissociative Disorders, 2*(4), 239–242.

Sanders, B., & Giolas, M. H. (1991). Dissociation and childhood trauma in psychologically disturbed adolescents. *American Journal of Psychiatry, 148*(1), 50–54. https://doi.org/10.1176/ajp.148.3.A50

Şar, V., Akyüz, G., & Doğan, O. (2007). Prevalence of dissociative disorders among women in the general population. *Psychiatry Research, 149*(1–3), 169–176. https://doi.org/10.1016/j.psychres.2006.01.005

Shirar, L. (1996). *Dissociative children: Bridging the inner and outer worlds.* Book News.

Silberg, J. L. (1998). Dissociative symptomatology in children and adolescents as displayed on psychological testing. *Journal of Personality Assessment, 71*(3), 421–439. https://doi.org/10.1207/s15327752jpa7103_10

Silberg, J. L. (2022). *The child survivor: Healing developmental trauma and dissociation* (2nd ed.). Routledge.

Sim, L., Friedrich, W. N., Davies, W. H., Trentham, B., Lengua, L., & Pithers, W. (2005). The Child Behavior Checklist as an indicator of posttraumatic stress disorder and dissociation in normative, psychiatric, and sexually abused children. *Journal of Traumatic Stress, 18*(6), 697–705. https://doi.org/10.1002/jts.20078

Sinason, V., & Marks, R. T. (2021). *Treating children with dissociative disorders*. Routledge.

Snow, M. S., White, J., Pilkington, L., & Beckman, D. (1995). Dissociative identity disorder revealed through play therapy: A case study of a four year-old. *Dissociation: Progress in Dissociative Disorders, 8*(2), 120–123.

Steinberg, A., & Steinberg, M. (1995). Systematic assessment of dissociative identity disorder in an adolescent who is blind. *Dissociation: Progress in Dissociative Disorders, 7*(2), 117–128.

Steinberg, M., & Steinberg, A. (1995). Using the SCID-D to assess dissociative identity disorder in adolescents: Three case studies. *Bulletin of the Menninger Clinic, 59*(2), 221–231.

Trickett P. K., Noll J. G., & Putnam F. W. (2011). The impact of sexual abuse on female development: Lessons from a multigenerational, longitudinal research study. *Development and Psychopathology, 23*(2), 453–476.

Trujillo, K., Lewis, D. O., Yeager, C. A., & Gidlow, B. (1996). Imaginary companions of school boys and boys with dissociative identity disorder/multiple personality disorder: A normal to pathologic continuum. *Child and Adolescent Psychiatric Clinics of North America, 5*(2), 375–391. https://doi.org/10.1016/S1056-4993(18)30372-9

Tutkun, H., Yargic, I., & Şar, V. (1994). Adölesans döneminde bir cogul kişilik bozuklugu vakası (A case of multiple personality disorder in adolescence). *Psikiyatri Psikoloji Psikofarmakoloji Dergisi, 2*(3), 261–266.

Tyson, G. M. (1992). Childhood MPD/dissociation identity disorder: Applying and extending current diagnostic checklists. *Dissociation: Progress in Dissociative Disorders, 5*, 20–27.

Vincent, M., & Pickering, M. R. (1988). Multiple personality disorder in childhood. *Canadian Journal of Psychiatry, 33*(6), 524–529.

Waterbury, M. (1991). Abuse histories and prior diagnoses in 123 inner city children with dissociative disorders. In B. G. Braun (Ed.), *Proceedings of the eighth international conference on multiple personality/dissociative states* (p. 111). Rush-Presbyterian-St. Luke's Medical Center.

Waters, F. S. (2016). *Healing the fractured child: Diagnosis and treatment of youth with dissociation*. New York: Springer.

Weiss, M., Sutton, P. J., & Utecht, A. J. (1985). Multiple personality in a 10-year-old girl. *Journal of American of Academy Children Psychiatry, 24*(4), 495–501. https://doi.org/10.1016/S0002-7138(09)60571-9

Wieland, S. (2015), *Dissociation in children and adolescents: Theory and clinical intervention*. New York: Routledge.

Yeager, C. A., & Lewis, D. O. (1996). The intergenerational transmission of violence and dissociation. *Child and Adolescent Psychiatric Clinics of North America, 5*(2), 393–430. https://doi.org/10.1016/S1056-4993(18)30373-0

Zoroglu, S. S., Şar, V., Tuzun, U., Tutkun, H., & Savas, H. A. (2002). Reliability and validity of the Turkish Adolescent Dissociative Experiences Scale. *Psychiatry and Clinical Neuroscience, 56*(5), 551–556. https://doi.org/10.1046/j.1440-1819.2002.01053.x

Zoroglu, S. S., Şar, V., & Yargic, I. (1997). Ergen dönemde iki disosiyatif kimlik bozuklugu olgusu (Two cases of dissociative identity disorder in adolescence). *Psikiyatri Psikoloji Psikofarmakoloji Dergisi, 5*(1), 43–53.

Zoroglu, S. S., Tutkun, H., Tuzun, U., & Şar, V. (1996). Cocuk yasta cogul kisilik bozuklugu: Bir olgu sunumu (Multiple personality disorder in childhood: A case presentation). *Cocuk Ve Genclik Ruh Sagligi Dergisi, 3*, 98–113.

Zoroglu, S. S, Tuzun, U., Ozturk, M., & Şar, V. (2000). Cocuk ve ergenlerde dissosiyatif bozukluk: 36 olgunun gözden gecirilmesi (Dissociative disorder in children and adolescents: A review of 36 cases). *Anadolu Psikiyatri Dergisi, 1*(4), 197–206.

Zoroglu, S. S., Tuzun, U., Ozturk, M., & Şar, V. (2002). Reliability and validity of the Turkish version of the Child Dissociation Checklist. *Journal of Trauma and Dissociation, 3*(1), 37–49. https://doi.org/10.1300/J229v03n01_04

Zoroglu, S. S., Yargic, I., Tutkun, H., Ozturk, M., & Şar, V. (1996). Dissociative identity disorder in childhood: Five Turkish cases. *Dissociation: Progress in Dissociative Disorders, 9*(4), 253–260.

Zoroglu, S. S., Yargic, I., Tutkun, H., Tuzun, U., & Şar, V. (1996). Adölesan yasta 17 disosiyatif kimlik bozukluğu olgusunun sosyodemografik, klinik özelliklerive travmatik yasanti.yküleri (Sociodemographic and clinical features and childhood trauma histories of 17 cases of dissociative identity disorder in adolescence). *Düsünen Adam, 9*(2), 9–16.

3
THE DISCRETE BEHAVIORAL STATES/STATES OF BEING MODEL

John Lovern

The Discrete Behavioral States/States of Being Model

When Frank W. Putnam formulated his Discrete Behavioral States/States of Being Model, he laid the foundation for a revolution in how human behavior, development, psychopathology, and personality can and ought to be conceptualized. The model is both intuitively satisfying and practically useful. Familiarity with it should be a basic requirement for every behavioral scientist and mental health clinician.

Origins and Evolution of the Model

With characteristic humility, Putnam declined to claim credit for the model, attributing it to William James instead (personal communication, January 8, 2023). Indeed, James did speak and write about states, notably in a series of lectures that were compiled into a book on religious conversion experiences (James, 1982). But others might also be recognized as pioneers in the field of states of consciousness—for example, early users of hypnosis such as Franz Anton Mesmer and Jean-Martin Charcot (Hammond, 2013); Carl Jung, who endeavored to evoke "vital spiritual experiences" in his patients (Lovern, 1991); and later researchers of hypnosis and other altered states of consciousness, such as Ernest Hilgard (1977), Milton Erickson (Rossi et al., 2010), Charles Tart (1975), and William Miller (Miller & C'de Baca, 2001). But it was Putnam who consolidated historical, clinical, cognitive, developmental, and psychophysiological data and theories into a coherent and comprehensive state model.

Putnam's model has changed and matured over time, beginning in the period between 1976 and 1979, when he learned about the effects of trauma during his psychiatric residency where one of his supervisors was a Vietnam veteran and an expert on the effects of combat trauma. In 1988, Putnam published a landmark study on the switch process in dissociative identity disorder (DID) in which he coined the term "state change disorders." Later, his work with traumatized and dissociative children led to the publication of *Dissociation in Children and Adolescents: A Developmental Perspective* (1997), in which a chapter was devoted to the "Discrete Behavioral States Model." The most comprehensive version of his model, the States of Being Model, may be found in his book *The Way We Are: How States of Mind Influence Our Identities, Personality and Potential for Change* (2016), and the most recent summary of the model may be found in a chapter by Loewenstein and Putnam (2022).

Putnam (1988) coined the term "state change disorders" and explained how many psychiatric disorders may be understood in terms of dysfunctional states and disordered state switching. Examples include a profound disturbance of sense of self, as in DID; being stuck in a dysfunctional state, as in depression; having a disturbed switch mechanism, as in bipolar disorder; switching into states that are distressing and too easily triggered, as in post-traumatic stress disorder (PTSD); and secondary problems caused by individuals' efforts to control or modulate their switches, as in substance-use disorders.

Basic Concepts of the State Model

Merriam-Webster (n.d.) defines a state as "a mode or condition of being," "a condition of mind or temperament," or "a condition or stage in the physical being of something." Putnam (2016) defined states *of being* as "transient, organized patterns of mind, body, and brain variables" (p. 333). By *transient*, he meant that each state stays active for a finite period every time it is activated and stays active until it becomes inactive or is dislodged by another state. By *organized*, he meant that each state consists of or contains a particular set of variables that are organized and function in a distinctive way, and that states are self-organizing, possess emergent properties, and behave as nonlinear dynamical systems. State *variables* can include "perception, cognition, memory, motivation, core values, interpersonal interactions, physiology and a host of other domains and functions" (Putnam, 2016, p. 334). Adults "have multiple identities that they activate in specific life contexts, e.g., work, parenting, intimacy, recreation, religious practice, etc" (Putnam, 2016, p. 335). An especially important variable that many states possess is a sense of self or personal identity. And identity states can possess an entire subjective reality that is distinct and separate from the distinct realities of other identity states, which led Kluft (1996, p. 344) to describe DID as "multiple *reality* disorder" (emphasis added).

Types of States

States exist at many levels in animals and humans, from the cellular level to the level of complex mental and behavioral processes. Neurons have been found to operate in three states: disabled, enabled, and firing (Kepecs & Raghavachari, 2001). Brain microstates, which have been called "atoms of thought" (Tait & Zhang, 2021), are very brief and last between 90 and 160 milliseconds. Switches between global behavioral states such as between wakefulness and sleep or between inattention and vigilance are associated with whole-brain states. States that operate at a level that can influence or drive complex behavior and conscious awareness, such as mental states, states of consciousness, identity states, or states of being (SoB), are many and varied, including emotional, playful, aggressive, hungry, painful, sexual, drugged, hypnotic, meditative, and more. Loewenstein and Putnam (2022) stated, *Each distinct SoB uniquely (state-dependently) influences perception, cognition, memory, emotion, motivation, values, psychophysiology, and interpersonal interactions* (p. 281, original emphasis). There are pathological states, such as post-traumatic flashbacks, depression, and psychosis. And there are innumerable situation-specific or task-specific states, likely because the brain conserves energy and gains efficiency by organizing sets of variables into states and activating them automatically when environmental cues signal that a particular set of thoughts, feelings, and behavioral tendencies is appropriate to a particular situation.

State-Space

States can be depicted pictorially or mapped in a graph with three (or more) axes. The result is a visual representation of multidimensional state-space, in which each axis is a state variable of interest.

The Discrete Behavioral States/States of Being Model

The locations of states in the graph represent their locations in state-space. Imagine a graph drawn with three axes: level of arousal, degree of discomfort, and time. When a state is placed in that simple three-dimensional space, the result is a visual depiction of its level of arousal, degree of discomfort, and duration. When two or more states are placed there, it is possible to see how they relate to one another by looking at where they are located relative to each other in state-space. For example, calm and secure emotional states would be located close to each other in state-space, while a terrified state would be located a distance away, or remote in state-space. Lines with arrows can be drawn between states in state-space to depict the directional pathways between them that occur as they transition from one state to the next. Putnam (2016) stated:

> States exist as discrete regions within a much larger, multidimensional state-space that can be mapped at many scales of scientific analysis. There are isomorphic axes that connect these levels, theoretically allowing descriptions of mechanistic linkages that span the molecular level to gross behavior.
>
> *(p. 334)*

Figure 3.1 shows a rough depiction of state-space in which three calm, pleasant states may be seen switching from one to the next, and an aroused, painful, or terrified state can be seen some distance away.

State-Dependence

State-dependent learning and memory (SDLM) is a key contributor to dissociative phenomena. SDLM is the phenomenon that causes events that take place when a child is in one state to be better remembered when the child is in the same state again; and less well remembered—or not remembered

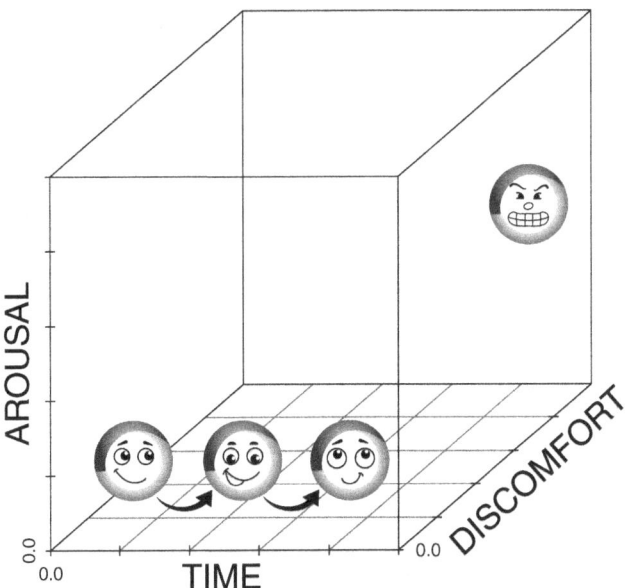

Figure 3.1 A Visual Depiction of Three-Dimensional State-Space with Arousal, Time, and Discomfort as the Variables (Figure Belongs to Author).

at all—when the child is in a different state. SDLM has been found to operate throughout development, from infants (Seehagen et al., 2020) to younger and older adults (Schramke & Bauer, 1997). All of the variables constituting a state can be state-dependent, including, importantly, autobiographical memory. According to Loewenstein and Putnam (2022), "autobiographical memory is most affected by SDLM" (p. 290), and "dissociative amnesia (DA) manifests when some self-states recount experiences as first-hand autobiographical memory whilst others deny recall of these events and may insist, they did not occur" (p. 282). Wilson and Ross (2003) pointed out that "autobiographical memory plays an important role in the construction of personal identity" (p. 137), and that once one's personal identity is established, it then influences both what one remembers about one's past and how one remembers it. Understanding these processes makes it easy to see how states that are generated by traumatic events can develop personal identities with unique personal histories, given that these states tend to be remote in state-space from other states and isolated from those states by SDLM. When certain traumatic events or types of traumatic events are repeated over and over, it is even more likely that traumatic states will develop unique identities and personal histories. The clearly defined identity states seen in adolescents and adults with DID are examples of entire assemblages of state variables that are so state-dependent that they resemble distinct personalities that can seem to be different ages, have different behavior patterns, genders, or even species, and can be completely unaware of the existence of other identity states.

Switches

Transitions between states, or switches, occur when a new state is activated and the previously active state recedes or becomes inactive. Switches take place at every level, from the cellular level to the level of identity states. Some switches take place voluntarily, some automatically and unconsciously, and some are triggered by situational variables. Some take place slowly and gradually, some rapidly or almost instantly. Putnam (1988) noticed that order effects often occur; for example, "transitions from state A to state B may follow a different pathway than transitions from state B to state A" (p. 28). The directionality of switches gave rise to the concept of pathways between states in state-space. More than one state may be active at a time at one level, such as in DID when one identity state is talking and others are listening or co-conscious; and multiple states may be active at different levels, such as when a microstate, an emotional state, and an identity state are all active simultaneously. When parents interact with babies and young children in healthy ways, they can help them gain a degree of control over their state switches and learn to modulate their states. Finally, chaos theory may be useful in the study of the switch process because states and the switches among and between them "fit well with a branch of mathematics, non-linear dynamical systems theory, which quantifies the operation of many complex phenomena that are impervious to more traditional mathematical approaches" (Putnam, 2016, p. 87).

Animal and Brain Network Research

Numerous studies have been conducted examining discrete behavioral states in animals. For example, Chen et al. (2023) studied how ascending neurons encode behavioral states in fruit flies; Marques et al. (2020) studied behavioral states of zebrafish larvae using tracking microscopy to monitor whole-brain neuronal activity; Flavell et al. (2022) reviewed studies of internal states and state transitions in mice, roundworms, and fruit flies and described "advances in the classification of internal states, the insights from studying brain-wide populations, and some of the many biological mechanisms through which neuromodulators can influence states" (p. 16); and Madlon-Kay et al. (2017) used a machine learning model to identify behavioral states in free-ranging macaques.

The Discrete Behavioral States/States of Being Model

Using technology such as functional magnetic resonance imaging (fMRI), electroencephalography (EEG), and magnetoencephalography (MEG), numerous researchers have been studying large-scale brain network activity and its correlation with behavioral states. In their review of recent research on variations in the waking states of mice and humans and how these variations are generated in the brain, McCormick et al. (2020) stated:

> The activity of the brain is constantly varying, wandering between states, and profoundly affecting not only our neural responses to sensory inputs but also our ability to process this influx of information, make decisions, and take appropriate action. Indeed, our entire inner world, both cognitively and emotionally, is in a constant state of flux, flittering from state to state, thought to thought.
>
> *(p. 392)*

Kringelach and Deco (2020) have studied brain states and transitions using computational neuroscience. And Xu et al. (2023) found that "vortex- or spiral-like, rotational wave patterns, which are organized around phase singularities, play a role in organizing complex spatiotemporal brain dynamics" (p. 2), that these spirals "are task relevant and can be used to classify different cognitive tasks" (p. 1), and that reversing the direction of brain spirals "has the potential to control large-scale switching of task-specific activity flows in response to task demands" (p. 11). In other words, switches in the direction of brain spirals may correlate with task-specific state switches.

Normal, Healthy Development from a States Perspective

States Present at Birth, New States, and New Pathways

Putnam (2016) listed six basic states that Wolff (1987) and others—the "baby watchers"—observed taking place in recurring cycles in healthy newborns: State I, Regular Sleep; State II, Irregular Sleep; State III, Alert Inactivity; State IV, Waking Activity; State V, Crying; and State VI, Alert Activity. Then, "as time goes on, additional distinct states appear, adding to the child's growing behavioral complexity" (Putnam, 2016, p. 33). It is likely that new task- or situation-specific behavioral states come into being when clusters of state variables that are active in a given situation are recorded in memory along with contextual cues that link the state variables with that situation. Hahamy, Dubossarsky, and Behrens (2023) found that "humans reactivate neural representations of past events" and that "these reactivations occur in the hippocampus and default mode network, where reactivations are selective to relevant past events" (p. 1080). States created in this way can be reactivated when environmental cues indicate that the same situations, or similar ones, are taking place again. Situation- or task-specific states provide children with an ever-growing repertoire of ready-made response tendencies that can be activated as needed, quickly and automatically. Children's behavioral complexity and flexibility are enhanced by "the evolution and elaboration of existing states," "the development of new pathways between existing states," and "the incorporation of new and existing states into branching behavioral loops" (Putnam, 1997, p. 10).

Modulation of Behavioral States

Beginning in infancy, children attempt to gain some control over their behavioral states—for example, by self-soothing and self-stimulation behaviors such as sucking on pacifiers or rhythmic rocking. But it is the parent/caretaker who has the dominant role in modulating infants' behavioral states, by intervening to distract, comfort, or feed them when they appear distressed, or by encouraging positive affective states by smiling, cooing, or playing peekaboo with them. It is important for healthy development that parents teach their children a variety of methods for modulating their states, and for children to gradually learn to modulate their states on their own. The ability to modulate affective and behavioral states is a critical aspect of both emotion regulation and social behavior, enabling children to function successfully in interactions with peers and adults outside of the home, and ultimately in the complex interpersonal interactions that they will have to navigate as adolescents and adults.

Metacognitive and Executive Functions

As described earlier, SDLM have been found to exist in infants, and they continue to exist through childhood and into adulthood. The ability to integrate information and behavior across different and distinct states relies on the presence of certain cognitive abilities—metacognitive and executive functions—that develop gradually during childhood. Putnam (1997) suggested that these abilities likely overlap with others, such as "source monitoring, visual perspective taking, conceptual perspective taking, seriation, and transitivity" (p. 162). These abilities appear between the ages of 1 and 5 and take many more years to develop as the brain's prefrontal cortex matures.

Parental State-Altering Behaviors and Parent-Child State Interactions

Putnam (1997) noted: "States are contagious: They can be transmitted from parent to child, and most certainly vice versa ... Such sharing of states—be they positive or negative—is a powerful component of 'bonding' between individuals" (p. 162). In addition, if one assumes that imitation is the primary mechanism by which such state sharing takes place, then states can be conceptualized as *memes*, and therefore as modes of cultural transmission (Blackmore, 1999).

Parents and children also "recurrently alter each other's states of consciousness—often deliberately!" (Putnam, 1997). Most parents are sensitive to their infants' states and tend to switch states themselves in order to respond appropriately to their infants' states. For example, an infant in a crying state tends to switch a parent into an attentive state, during which the parent may engage in behaviors designed to switch the infant's state—for example, by feeding or rocking or distracting the infant, or by changing the infant's diaper. Once the infant switches from the crying state into a calmer state, the parent's attentive state can recede.

Culturally mediated child-rearing techniques provide parents with a supply of methods that have been effective in previous generations, and then, through trial and error, parents learn which of these methods are most effective in modulating or switching their own children's states. Meanwhile, children are learning which behaviors on their parts will modulate or switch their parents' states. This process changes and grows more complex as children's repertoires of states grow, as their parents' complementary states increase in number, and as children's needs and abilities change. Putnam put it this way: "The family state game is about power, influence, and control (i.e., the usual human stakes)" (p. 167). As children learn to engage in mutual state switching with siblings, other children, and adults outside the family, and when they learn to communicate using language and continue to improve their language-using abilities, the process becomes even more complex.

As children mature, their ability to recognize states in others improves—an aspect of theory of mind (Sabbagh & Bowman, 2018)—and they become skillful at influencing those states. The ability to recognize and influence the mental states of others is an important social skill, and viewing interactions between people in terms of how they attempt to influence each other's states and state switches is a promising way to understand and study interpersonal and social interactions.

Development and Integration of the Sense of Self and Personal Identity

A biological basis exists for the ability to recognize the difference between self and other, common to virtually all organisms, "from bacteria to higher animals." All these organisms possess "recognition systems that allow them to discriminate between self and nonself" and "effector mechanisms to defend themselves from nonself" (Gonzalez et al., 2011, p. 19). Young infants have been found to possess a rudimentary sense of self as demonstrated by the finding that they root toward an external tactile stimulation more often when touched on the cheek by another person than when touched by themselves (Rochat & Striano, 2000). By 15–24 months of age, most children respond to images of themselves in a mirror by touching a mark on their foreheads that is visible in their reflection (Anderson, 1984), similar to the reactions of chimpanzees (but not monkeys) who demonstrated their ability to recognize themselves in a mirror by touching a mark on their foreheads (Gallup, 1970).

Subsequently, through play and experiences with parents, siblings, peers, and other adults, and with the advent of language, children assume many new roles and add to their repertoires of identity, emotional, and contextual states. One might ask how all these states are consolidated into a coherent, unified self. Putnam (2016) wrote: "In the state model, this consolidating requires assuming a psychological mechanism that bridges the many different identities and emotional states attached to all of our social roles" (p. 180). The mechanism has been called different things: "psychotherapists call this function the observing ego. Cognitive psychologists speak of metacognition. And developmental psychologists refer to these processes as executive functions" (p. 181). These metacognitive and executive functions make it possible for the sense of personal identity to be less state-dependent and to generalize across numerous states, allowing children and ultimately adults to feel, under normal circumstances, like they are the same person as they switch from state to state—that is, to have a unique personality.

State-Related Effects of Child Maltreatment

Creation of Traumatic States

Putnam (1997) noted that trauma has "potent state-generating properties." States created during terrifying maltreatment experiences, called "trauma-related altered states of consciousness" (TRASC) by Lanius (2015), are remote in state-space from everyday states and consist of cognitive, emotional, and physiological variables. Cognitive variables may include confusion and inability to concentrate; thoughts or conclusions that children form about their traumatic experiences, themselves, or their abusers; and thoughts and beliefs that abusers instill in them by what they say or do while abusing them. Emotional variables may include overwhelming terror, helplessness, shame, and disgust; emotions influenced by children's thoughts and beliefs such as guilt and self-blame; and emotions that they have not yet developed language skills to name. Physiological variables may include physical pain, sights, sounds, smells, and other sensations; fight-or-flight physiological hyperarousal; or freezing, numbing, and physiological shutdown. Subsequent reactivations of any of these states may constitute flashbacks, which may be triggered by cues reminiscent of the trauma. "The mental effort that a traumatized child must expend while trying to ignore and suppress these traumatic intrusions disrupts concentration, saps energy, and frays mood" (Putnam, 2016, p. 219).

Traumatic Alterations of the Architecture of State Pathways

The addition of traumatic states to a child's repertoire of states can affect the other states and the pathways between them, leading to altered behavioral sequences and making flashbacks increasingly likely to occur. When flashbacks take place, they may be understood as activations of traumatic states rather than as intrusive memories, thus accounting for the subjective sense that they are being relived rather than merely recalled. Orders of state switches may be altered; comfortable and safe states may be blocked due to order effects of switches; and dysphoric and traumatic states may predominate because their life-or-death quality makes them extremely salient.

Disruption of Metacognitive and Executive Functions and Capacities for Behavioral State Modulation

In their research, Teicher et al. (2016) reported: "Consistent evidence has emerged for maltreatment-associated structural deficits in the adult hippocampus, corpus callosum, ACC [anterior cingulate cortex], OFC [orbitofrontal cortex] and dorsolateral PFC [dorsolateral prefrontal cortex, DLPFC]" (p. 662). The ACC, OFC, and DLPFC are all associated with metacognitive and executive functions and their development (Ardila, 2013). In addition, researchers have documented evidence that child maltreatment disrupts the development of metacognitive abilities (see, for example, Myers & Wells, 2015) and executive functions (see, for example, Mothes et al., 2015). Thus, it is likely that maltreatment-influenced deficits in these brain areas are associated with adverse effects on children's ability to modulate and control their behavioral states.

Disorganized Attachment

Maltreatment and neglect can interfere with parent-child interactions by preventing state-sharing between children and parents and hindering the teaching of state-modulating methods by parents. When infants and children do not receive and participate in these state-related interactions, attachment problems are likely to result. One possible result is Type D attachment, an "insecure, disorganized/disoriented category of infant-parent attachment" that was discovered by Main and Solomon (1986). They observed infants in the Strange Situation Procedure (Ainsworth et al., 2015) behaving in unusual, contradictory ways when reunited with a parent after a period of separation. For example, while some infants appeared to be physically comfortable with the parent, they were simultaneously avoidant and fearful or "dazed," with "an unfocused, 'dead' stare, mouth and chin limp, body stilled" (p. 120). This form of attachment in infants has been thought to predispose them to ultimately develop a dissociative disorder (Liotti, 2004).

Maladaptive Attempts at Self-Modulation of States

Beset by extremely dysphoric states and lacking the ability to adequately modulate those states, maltreated children and adolescents may resort to harmful or extreme state-change and state-control methods. For example, alcohol and other drugs provide one sure way to switch away from unpleasant states, but their use comes with a high price, one that is especially high because of the chemicals' effects on children's developing brains. Squeglia et al. (2009) reported that "exposure to alcohol and drugs during a period of critical neurological development may interrupt the natural course of brain maturation and key processes of brain development." Their review found that alcohol and cannabis can have adverse effects on both brain structure (hippocampal volume, prefrontal cortex volume, white matter volume, quality of white matter, and brain blood flow) and brain functioning (spatial working memory, verbal encoding, inhibition, and cue reactivity). And of course, substance use during childhood and adolescence carries a high risk of developing a substance-use disorder.

Other harmful or extreme state-change strategies maltreated children and adolescents may adopt that can have lifelong implications include disordered eating, cutting and other forms of self-mutilation, sexual acting out, suicidal behavior, aggressive behavior, and criminal behavior such as shoplifting and gang membership. The ACE Study (Felitti et al., 1998) found that

> persons who had experienced four or more categories of childhood exposure, compared to those who had experienced none, had 4-to-12-fold increased health risks for alcoholism, drug abuse, depression, and suicide attempt; a 2-to-4-fold increase in smoking, poor self-rated health, ≥ 50 sexual intercourse partners, and sexually transmitted disease; and a 1.4-to-1.6-fold increase in physical inactivity and severe obesity
>
> *(p. 245)*

as well as significantly greater risk of developing medical conditions that are "leading causes of death in adults" (p. 246).

Identity Disruption

The findings described above regarding the disruptive effects of child maltreatment on the development of the brain and of metacognitive and executive functions pertain to children's ability to not only modulate and control behavioral states but also bridge identity and emotional states to create a unified sense of identity. For example, in a study of college students, Truskauskaite-Kuneviciene et al. (2020) found that "specific severe traumatic experiences, such as sexual abuse, may increase the probability of the development of a more diffused identity" (p. 5).

Traumatic Identity States

Children's imaginative play often involves altering their senses of identity, imputing identity to toys or animals, or creating imaginary places. For example, they may imagine themselves as cowboys, nurses, doctors, animals, or heroes or heroines of fairy tales, movies, or made-up stories. They may name and create imagined identities for their stuffed animals, action figures, or pets. And their own imagined identities and those of their imagined companions may interact in imaginary worlds.

Children's imaginative capacities, and the fluidity with which they are able to create and alter their own and others' identities, are accompanied by an ability to believe convincingly in the reality of imagined entities such as Santa Claus or the Tooth Fairy, which is present during much of early childhood, until it begins to decline in the elementary school years (Boerger et al., 2009). Children can spontaneously shift into a mode of information processing in which they are able to "alter ... their experience of body, self, actions, and world" (Dell, 2017, p. 162), an ability that Dell (2017) defined as "the essence of hypnosis" (from the title of his journal article). These abilities provide young children with a way to protect themselves if they are subjected to abuse and trauma when it is impossible for them to escape or avoid these experiences.

Children whose lives have been marked by repeated abuse and trauma are less likely than others to bridge their states to create a unified identity for two reasons: first, trauma is likely to have disrupted the development of their metacognitive and executive functions that make that bridging possible, and, second, they are likely to have little incentive to bridge the state-dependent separations among their states because those separations are protecting them from emotional and physical pain.

Dissociative Disorders in Children

While the processes described above can help explain the existence of DID in adults, DID's origins in childhood suggest that the disorder is likely also to be present in children but manifesting differently due to developmental differences at different ages and stages. Having recognized this fact, Putnam and a colleague created a profile of what they thought a child with DID would be like, and the profile became the basis for the development of the Child Dissociative Checklist (Bernstein & Putnam, 1986). Several years later, the Adolescent Dissociative Experiences Scale was developed (Armstrong et al., 1997). Dissociation in children "may be seen as a malleable developmental phenomenon that may accompany a wide variety of childhood presentations" (International Society for the Study of Dissociation [ISSD], Task Force on Children and Adolescents, 2004, p. 120). Young children with dissociative disorders will present differently from older children and adolescents, and it is important to avoid false positive diagnoses such as might occur, for example, with a child who has an especially vivid imaginary playmate.

Types of Maltreatment That Can Result in Dissociative Disorders

Briere and Scott (2006) argued that the word trauma "should be reserved for major events that are psychologically overwhelming for an individual" (p. 6), such as child sexual and physical abuse. However, trauma defined in this way is not the only kind of childhood experience that can lead to dissociative pathology. Severe neglect and early attachment disturbance are also important factors. Dorahy et al. (2016) found that emotional abuse contributes to dissociation, and a study by Sar et al. (2006) found that the presence of emotional neglect during childhood differentiated college students with dissociative disorders from those without. Sar (2020) suggested that "disturbances of early interpersonal attachment with caregivers" (p. 5) can lead an infant to develop multiple internal representations of self and attachment figures that surface later in response to abuse and neglect or following exposure to "an overtly or covertly dysfunctional family" (p. 6). Similarly, Lyons-Ruth (2003) summarized two longitudinal studies that found that disorganized attachment behaviors and dysfunctional parent-infant affective communication can leave children vulnerable to developing dissociative symptoms if they are subsequently exposed to abuse.

How a State Model Explains the Effects of Child Maltreatment

Children are born with a handful of discrete behavioral states, and in the course of normal development, they acquire increasing numbers of new states, beginning with a dance in which parents and children create and alter each other's states and parents help children form secure attachments. Complex and interconnected pathways develop between states, defining directions of switches and interactions among states; and state variables, including autobiographical memory and sense of self, develop varying but moderate degrees of state-dependence. An effectively functioning state system and a unified sense of self are facilitated by the development of metacognitive and executive functions. If all goes well through childhood and adolescence, the result is normal, healthy adults.

However, if traumatic events or child maltreatment or severe neglect take place, this developmental process is distorted, and the effect is greater the earlier in development the adverse events occur. The mutual state creation and alteration process between parents and children falters, and children form insecure or disorganized attachments. Variables comprising new states differ and include dysphoric affects, and some new states are traumatic. Pathways between states are altered, and numerous state variables, including autobiographical memory and sense of self, become more state-dependent as children try to defend themselves against the dysphoric feelings that traumatic states contain. Metacognitive and executive functions fail to develop properly, preventing a coherent sense of self from developing and causing the state system to operate in a more haphazard fashion. Traumatic states are triggered, causing flashbacks; thus, children and adolescents often try to defend themselves against activation of traumatic states in maladaptive ways, such as excessive substance use, disordered eating, or self-mutilation, and those behaviors create new problems of their own and may leave children and adolescents vulnerable to new episodes of maltreatment and trauma. Trauma-related mental disorders, including PTSD and dissociative disorders, become more and more likely to occur.

Implications of a States Model for Treatment

Putnam's (2016) description of a state-based approach to therapy applies to both adults and children:

> A state model of therapy should seek to coordinate a range of therapeutic interventions designed to stabilize and optimize an individual's state-space and to integrate different identity and emotional states into a coherent and flexible healthy sense of self. It would seek to reduce the time an individual spends in dysfunctional and dysphoric states and eliminate or redirect maladaptive efforts to suppress painful and destructive states of mind. In cases in which an individual is triggered by some internal or external cue such as a traumatic reminder and rapidly switches into an inappropriate state it may be possible to create new pathways that lead to more temperate reactions.
>
> *(p. 361)*

Several of the therapeutic approaches that Putnam (1997) recommends for children include principles and interventions that are not necessarily state-related, such as keeping children safe, understanding their perspective, recognizing the importance of the therapeutic space, helping them with logical binds, intervening in implicit versus explicit ways, having to be a "hardass" at times, and focusing on themes related to grief and loss and guilt and self-blame. These are explored in more detail below.

It should go without saying that keeping children safe must be a top priority. No amount of therapy can be helpful if, after a session, the child is returned to an unsafe, abusive environment. How can a therapeutic alliance or trust develop if, by failing to stop the abuse, a therapist appears to be colluding with a child's abusers?

A child's perspective, his or her subjective world, is very different from that of adults. Children are small, the world is big, and the human-made world is scaled for adults and adult physical and mental abilities, leaving children often having to struggle with things that adults handle with little thought or effort. Children's experience of time is very different from that of adults. Young children do not operate on a clock model, and an hour of boredom or a few seconds of pain may seem to them like an eternity. Compared to adults, children have little power, and what they do have power over is very different from that of adults. Children's mental equipment for construing and understanding reality is also quite different from that of adults. The distance between real and imagined is much shorter for them, and their developing capacity for rational thought may not yet allow them to think their way out of problems and dilemmas.

Putnam (1997) noted that "children are exquisitely sensitive to the space around them" (p. 273). Therefore, the space, the place in which therapy with children is conducted needs to be "a special place with strength, structure, and stability—a place that can be utilized and internalized as an alternative to the chaotic and unstable world many children inhabit" (p. 273).

"Logical binds originate in the intense need of children to understand and make sense of how things happen" (p. 270). Binds may occur as the result of vague spoken language; fictitious explanations children are given; and inconsistencies and contradictions between words and facial expressions, tone of voice, or context, or between what they are told and what they see. Logical binds can create "powerful behavioral responses in children" (p. 271), and therapists should be attuned to identifying them and helping children clarify and resolve them. One type of logical bind that has been studied extensively is the double-bind, which was originally conceptualized by Bateson et al. (1956) as a form of communication that transmits conflicting messages where one message negates the other, leaving the recipient confused and defeated. This form of bind resembles the Strange Situation studied by Main and Solomon (1986, described earlier) that can give rise to disorganized attachment and subsequent maladjustment. Ceberio and Losada (2014) found a relationship between double-bind communication in childhood and the later development of eating disorders, and Carr and McAlister (2016) noted that institutions communicate in a double-binding fashion that increases the likelihood that adolescents will wind up in the criminal justice system.

In explaining the need to intervene in implicit versus explicit ways, Putnam (1997) maintained that an adult approach to therapy, in which efforts are made to bring unconscious thoughts and motivations into conscious awareness, is counterproductive with children. They may lack the self-monitoring capacity needed for such an approach, and they may not be psychologically minded enough for such approaches to make sense. "With children and many adolescents, much therapeutic work takes place in nonverbal ways" (p. 272), and therapists need to be comfortable "operating in the implicit and 'unconscious' domains" where "magical" interventions and ceremonies may be the most efficacious approach.

Putnam (1997) also stated that sometimes taking "a position that sets firm boundaries with strong and definitive consequences for transgression" (p. 283) can be helpful as an intervention in therapeutic approaches. He called this being a "hardass," though admitted he did not know of a rule for when or how to be one, only that he believed it to be sometimes necessary and possibly therapeutic.

Maltreated children may experience significant losses—for example, the loss of a parent due to death, incarceration, or custody arrangements. "For maltreated children, the issues of loss, grief, and bereavement are complicated and often atypical" (p. 289). For example, they may find themselves idealizing a missing parent in ways that conflict with memories of abuse. They may feel abandoned by, miss, or long for a caregiver and have to listen to adults vilify that person. One approach Putnam recommended for grief is to provide symbolic or ritual acts such as funerals, memorials, or testimonials.

Feelings of guilt, shame, and self-blame are common among victims of abuse, and they are often kept secret and "become sources of private torment that nullify positive accomplishments" (p. 289). These feelings are tenacious and deeply rooted, "and they do not yield to mere logic alone" (p. 290) especially in children, who may lack the capacity to logically analyze their feelings. The feelings may arise because their abusers have blamed them for the abuse, or children may blame themselves because they may have "cooperated" with the abuse. "Specific feelings of guilt are treated with therapeutic clarification and sometimes with cleansing rituals" (p. 290). Clarifications should be offered in a developmentally appropriate manner.

Putnam's state-related recommendations for therapy with children include facilitating self-modulation of states, developing metacognitive functions, and eroding and diffusing dissociative states. He recommended against interventions that could "encourage further differentiation or separation" (p. 294)—for example, by interacting with states as separate, crystallized selves, unless it is clear that they are fully crystallized, and even then, engaging with great care. It is clear that working with traumatized and dissociative children needs to be very different from therapy with adults who have DID.

Play therapy is strongly recommended for work with young children because of their developing verbal skills. Some cognitive-behavioral approaches have been helpful with adolescents due to their proficiency with language. Cognitive-behavioral approaches may be understood from a states-of-being point of view as attempts to modify states by modifying the cognitive state variables comprising them. Regardless of which treatment modality a therapist employs, it is important for them to be continuously aware of their patients' states and state switches, and of the conditions preceding and following patients' switches. In addition, they should monitor their own states and state switches, including those that they initiate intentionally and those that are involuntarily triggered by a patient's states and state switches. Therapy in general should strive to gradually bring children back as closely as possible to the developmental paths that they would and should have been on if maltreatment, trauma, and neglect had never taken place.

The Value of a State Model

The Discrete Behavioral States/States of Being Model's explanatory power is impressive. It simplifies and clarifies. Once one begins thinking in terms of states and observing states and state switches operating in oneself and others, it is as though a veil has been lifted and an entirely new paradigm has been uncovered. Applying the model to understand and predict adult behavior is easier in some ways than applying it to the behavior of children because adult state systems and patterns of state interactions and switches are relatively crystallized and static, whereas those of children are fluid and plastic, varying as they mature through stages of brain and interpersonal development. Nevertheless, the model can be usefully applied to children's behaviors, including—especially—the behaviors of complexly traumatized children, such as aggressiveness, self-mutilation, pathological self-soothing behaviors, and so on.

References

Ainsworth, M. D. S., Blehar, M. C., Waters, E., & Wall, S. N. (2015). *Patterns of attachment: A psychological study of the strange situation*. Routledge.

Anderson, J. R. (1984). The development of self-recognition: A review. *Developmental Psychobiology, 17*(1), 35–49. https://doi.org/10.1002/dev.420170104

Ardila, A. (2013). Development of metacognitive and emotional executive functions in children. *Applied Neuropsychology: Child, 2*(2), 82–97. https://doi.org/10.1080/21622965.2013.748388

Armstrong, J. G., Putnam, F. W., Carlson, E. B., Libero, D. Z., & Smith, S. R. (1997). Development and validation of a measure of adolescent dissociation: The Adolescent Dissociative Experiences Scale. *Journal of Nervous and Mental Disease, 185*(8), 491–497. https://doi.org/10.1097/00005053-199708000-00003

Bateson, G., Jackson, D. D., Haley, J., & Weakland, J. (1956). Toward a theory of schizophrenia. *Behavioral Science, 1*(4), 251–254.

Bernstein, E. M., & Putnam, F. W. (1986). Development, reliability, and validity of a dissociation scale. *Journal of Nervous and Mental Disease, 174*(12), 727–735. https://doi.org/10.1097/00005053-198612000-00004

Blackmore, S. (1999). *The meme machine*. Oxford University Press.

Boerger, E. A., Ansley Tullos, A., & Woolley, J. D. (2009). Return of the candy witch: Individual differences in acceptance and stability of belief in a novel fantastical being. *British Journal of Developmental Psychology, 27*(4), 953–970. https://doi.org/10.1348/026151008x398557

Briere, J. N., & Scott, C. (2006). *Principles of trauma therapy: A guide to symptoms, evaluation, and treatment*. Sage.

Carr, N., & McAlister, S. (2016). The double-bind – Looked after children, care leavers and criminal justice. In P. Mendes & P. Snow (Eds.), *Young people transitioning from care: International research, policy and practice* (pp. 3–21). Palgrave.

Ceberio, M. R., & Losada, A. V. (2014). Double bind, child sexual abuse and speeches. Interlink *Continental Journal of Medicine & Medical Sciences. 1*(1), 16–234. https://transconpublishers.org/icjmms/index.php

Chen, C., Aymanns, F., Minegishi, R., Matsuda, V. D. V., Talabot, N., Günell, S., Dickson, B. J., & Ramdya, P. (2023). Ascending neurons convey behavioral state to integrative sensory and action selection brain regions. *Nature Neuroscience, 26*, 682–695. https://doi.org/10.1038/s41593-023-01281-z

Dell, P. F. (2017). What is the essence of hypnosis? *International Journal of Clinical and Experimental Hypnosis, 65*(2), 162–168. https://doi.org/10.1080/00207144.2017.1276360

Dorahy, M. J., Middleton, W., Seager, L., Williams, M., & Chambers, R. (2016). Child abuse and neglect in complex dissociative disorder, abuse-related chronic PTSD, and mixed psychiatric samples. *Journal of Trauma & Dissociation, 17*, 223–236. https://doi.org/10.1080/15299732.2015.1077916

Felitti, V. J., Anda, R. F., Nordenberg, D., Williamson, D. F., Spitz, A. M., Edwards, V., Koss, M. P., & Marks, J. S. (1998). Relationship of childhood abuse and household dysfunction to many of the leading causes of death in adults: The Adverse Childhood Experiences (ACE) study. *American Journal of Preventive Medicine, 14*(4), 245–258. https://doi.org/10.1016/S0749-3797(98)00017-8

Flavell, S. W., Gogolla, N., Lovett-Barron, M., & Zelikowsky, M. (2022). The emergence and influence of internal states. *Neuron, 110*, https://doi.org/10.1016/j.neuron.2022.04.030.

Gallup, G. (1970). Chimpanzees: Self-recognition. *Science, 167*(3914), 8–87. https://doi.org/10.1126/science.167.3914.86

Gonzalez, S., González-Rodríguez, A. P., Suárez-Álvarez, B., López-Soto, A., Huergo-Zapico, L., & Lopez-Larrea, C. (2011). Conceptual aspects of self and nonself discrimination. *Self/Nonself, 2*(1), 19–25. https://doi.org/10.4161/self.2.1.15094

Hahamy, A., Dubossarsky, H., & Behrens, T. E. J. (2023). The human brain reactivates contest- specific past information at event boundaries of naturalistic experiences. *Nature Neuroscience, 26*, 1–10. https://doi.org/10.1038/s41593-023-01331-6

Hammond, D. C. (2013). A review of the history of hypnosis through the late 19th century. *American Journal of Clinical Hypnosis, 56*(2), 174–191. https://doi.org/10.1080/00029157.2013.826172

Hilgard, E. R. (1977). *Divided consciousness: Multiple controls in human thought and action.* Wiley.

International Society for the Study of Dissociation, Task Force on Children and Adolescents (2004). Guidelines for the evaluation and treatment of dissociative symptoms in children and adolescents. *Journal of Trauma & Dissociation, 5*(3), 119–150. https://doi.org/10.1300/J229v05n03_09

James, W. (1982). *The varieties of religious experience: A study in human nature.* Penguin Books.

Kepecs, A., & Raghavachari, S. (2001). 3 State neurons for contextual processing. In T. G. Dietterich, S. Becker & Z. Ghahramani (Eds.), *Advances in neural information processing systems 14* (pp. 229–236). MIT Press.

Kluft, R. P. (1996). Dissociative identity disorder. In L. K. Michelson & W. J. Ray (Eds.), *Handbook of dissociation: Theoretical, empirical, and clinical perspectives* (pp. 337–366). Plenum Press.

Kringelach, M. L., & Deco, G. (2020). Brain states and transitions: Insights from computational neuroscience. *Cell Reports, 32*, https://doi.org/10.1016/j.celrep.2020.108128

Lanius, R. (2015). Trauma-related dissociation and altered states of consciousness: A call for clinical, treatment, and neuroscience research. *European Journal of Psychotraumatology, 6*(1), Article 27905. https://doi.org/10.3402/ejpt.v6.27905

Liotti, G. (2004). Trauma, dissociation, and disorganized attachment: Three strands of a single braid. *Psychotherapy Theory Research Practice Training, 41*(4), 472–486. https://doi.org/10.1037/0033-3204.41.4.472

Loewenstein, R. J., & Putnam, F. W. (2022). Discrete behavioral states theory. In M. J. Dorahy, S. N. Gold & J. A. O'Neil (Eds.), *Dissociation and the dissociative disorders: Past, present, future* (281–296). Routledge.

Lovern, J. D. (1991). *Pathways to reality: Erickson-inspired treatment approaches to chemical dependency.* Routledge.

Lyons-Ruth, K. (2003). Dissociation and the parent-infant dialogue: A longitudinal perspective from attachment research. *Journal of the American Psychoanalytic Association, 51*(3), 883–911. https://doi.org/10.1177/00030651030510031501

Madlon-Kay, S., Brent, L. J. N., Montague, M. J., Heller, K. A., & Platt, M. L. (2017). Using machine learning to discover latent social phenotypes in free-ranging macaques. *Brain Sciences, 7*(7), 91. https://doi.org/10.3390/brainsci7070091

Main, M., & Solomon, J. (1986). Discovery of an insecure-disorganized/disoriented attachment pattern: Procedures, findings and implications for the classification of behavior. In T. B. Brazelton & M. Yogman (Eds.), *Affective development in infancy* (pp. 95–124). Ablex.

Marques, J. C., Li, M., Schaak, D., Robson, D. N., & Li, J. M. (2020). Internal state dynamics shape brainwide activity and foraging behaviour. *Nature, 577*, 239–243. https://doi.org/10.1038/s41586-019-1858-z.

Merriam-Webster (n.d.). State. In Merriam-Webster.com dictionary. Retrieved [[TK]], from merriam-webster.com/dictionary/state.

McCormick, D. A., Nestvogel, D. B., & He, B. J. (2020). Neuromodulation of brain state and behavior. *Annual Review of Neuroscience, 43*, 391–415. https://doi.org/10.1146/annurev-neuro-100219-105424

Miller, W. R., & C'de Baca, J. (2001). *Quantum change: When epiphanies and sudden insights transform ordinary lives.* Guilford Press.

Mothes, L., Kristensen, C. H., Grassi-Oliveira, R., Paz Fonseca, R., Iracema de Lima Argimon, I., & Quarti Irigaray, T. (2015). Childhood maltreatment and executive functions in adolescents. *Child and Adolescent Mental Health, 20*(1), 56–62. https://doi.org/10.1111/camh.12068

Myers, S. G., & Wells, A. (2015). Early trauma, negative affect, and anxious attachment: The role of metacognition. *Anxiety, Stress, & Coping, 28*(6), 634–649. https://doi.org/10.1080/10615806.2015.1009832

Putnam, F. W. (1988). The switch process in multiple personality disorder and other state-change disorders. *Dissociation: Progress in the Dissociative Disorders, 1*(1), 24–32.

Putnam, F. W. (1997). *Dissociation in children and adolescents: A developmental perspective.* Guilford Press.

Putnam, F. W. (2016). *The way we are: How states of mind influence our identities, personality and potential for change.* International Psychoanalytic Books.

Rochat, P., & Striano, T. (2000). Perceived self in infancy. *Infant Behavior and Development, 23*(3–4), 513–530. https://doi.org/10.1016/S0163-6383(01)00055-8

Rossi, E., Erickson-Klein, R., & Rossi, K. (Eds.). (2010). *The collected works of Milton H. Erickson.* Milton H. Erickson Foundation Press.

Sabbagh, M. A., & Bowman, L. C. (2018). Theory of mind. In J. Wixted (Ed.), *Stevens' handbook of experimental psychology and cognitive neuroscience* (4th ed., Vol. 4, pp.1–34). Wiley.

Sar, V. (2020). Childhood trauma and dissociative disorders. In G. Spalletta, D. Janiri, F. Piras & G. Sani (Eds.), *Childhood trauma in mental disorders: A comprehensive approach* (pp. 333–365) Springer.

Sar, V., Kundakci, T., Kiziltan, E., Yargic, I. L., Tutkun, H., Bakim, B., Bozkurt, O., Özpulat, T., Keser, V., & Özdemir, Ö. (2006). Axis I dissociative disorder comorbidity of borderline personality disorder among psychiatric outpatients. *Journal of Trauma & Dissociation, 4*, 490–506.

Schramke, C. J., & Bauer, R. M. (1997). State-dependent learning in older and younger adults. *Psychology and Aging, 12*(2), 255–262. https://doi.org/10.1037//0882-7974.12.2.255

Seehagen, S., Schneider, S., Sommer, K., & Konrad, C. (2020). *Child development.* https://doi.org/10.1111/cdev.13444

Squeglia, L. M., Jacobus, J., & Tapert, S. F. (2009). The influence of substance use on adolescent brain development. *Clinical EEG and Neuroscience, 40*(1), 31–38. https://doi.org/10.1177/155005940904000110

Tait, L., & Zhang, J. (2021). MEG cortical microstates: Spaciotemporal characteristics, dynamic functional connectivity and stimulus-evoked responses. *NeuroImage, 251*, Article 119006. https://doi.org/10.1016/j.neuroimage.2022.119006

Tart, C. T. (1975). *States of consciousness.* E.P. Dutton & Co.

Teicher, M. H., Samson, J. A., Anderson, C. M., & Ohashi, K. (2016). The effects of childhood maltreatment on brain structure, function and connectivity. *Nature Reviews Neuroscience, 17*(10), 652–666. https://doi.org/10.1038/nrn.2016.111. PMID: 27640984

Truskauskaite-Kuneviciene, I., Brailovskaia, J., Kamite, Y., Petrauskaite, G., Margraf, J., & Kazlauskas, E. (2020). Does trauma shape identity? Exploring the links between lifetime trauma exposure and identity status in emerging adulthood. *Frontiers in Psychology, 15*(11). https://doi.org/10.3389/fpsyg.2020.570644

Wilson, A. E., & Ross, M. (2003). The identity function of autobiographical memory: Time is on our side. *Memory, 11*(2), 137–149. https://doi.org/10.1080/741938210

Wolff, P. H. (1987). *The development of behavioral states and the expression of emotions in early infancy.* University of Chicago Press.

Xu, Y., Long, X, Feng, J., & Gong, P. (2023). Interacting spiral wave patterns underlie complex brain dynamics and are related to cognitive processing. *Nature Human Behavior.* https://doi.org/10.1038/s41562-023-01626-5

4
TRAUMATIC ATTACHMENT
Clinical Reasoning for Attachment Trauma

Benedetto Farina and Adriano Schimmenti

Introduction

The locution "attachment trauma" indicates a severe and prolonged failure of the protective and caring role of parents or other caregivers. Attachment trauma is recognized as one of the major risk factors for mental disorders, worsening clinical picture, prognosis, and response to treatment, regardless of the specific diagnosis and the therapeutic method employed (Farina et al., 2019; Isobel et al., 2019; Lippard & Nemeroff, 2020; McCrory et al., 2017; Schore, 2009). However, despite its crucial role in clinical psychology and psychiatry, attachment trauma is often overlooked by mental health professionals. As described by Jonathan Franzen in the novel *Purity* "The mother had three or four years to fuck with your head before your hippocampus began recording lasting memories. You'd been talking to your mom since you were one year old and listening to her for even longer, but you couldn't remember a single word of what you or she had said before your hippocampus kicked into gear." (2015, p. 116). Indeed, attachment trauma often leaves no traces in autobiographical memory; rather, it remains in the form of a psychopathological vulnerability that constitutes an obstacle to the treatment of some patients. This chapter is devoted to the description of attachment trauma and its clinical signs to facilitate its recognition and appropriate treatment.

From Child Maltreatment to Attachment Trauma: Unveiling the Impact

Child maltreatment has received significant attention in recent decades, shattering the long-standing denial surrounding this issue and fueling a surge in scientific research (Fonagy et al., 2023). This explosion of research has shed light on crucial elements that we can now reliably understand. These elements are summarized below:

a **Widespread nature of child maltreatment.** Approximately one in four children experiences some form of child maltreatment (Lippard & Nemeroff, 2020). However, it is reassuring to note that not all maltreated children will develop psychopathological problems. According to a large-scale study conducted by Green and colleagues (2010) and involving approximately 5,700 individuals, child maltreatment is associated with 44% of psychopathology that emerges during development and roughly 30% of psychopathology that manifests in adult life. We can reliably estimate that around one-third of adult patients will exhibit varying degrees of psychopathological consequences and treatment challenges stemming from child maltreatment (White et al., 2020).

b **Dimensional impact of child maltreatment.** Recent research findings have revealed that the effects of child maltreatment extend beyond specific disorders such as dissociative disorders, borderline personality disorder (BPD), or complex post-traumatic stress disorder (CPTSD). It permeates as a risk factor, contributing to increased psychopathological severity and resistance to treatment across almost all psychiatric disorders, regardless of the therapeutic approaches employed (Farina et al., 2019; Lippard & Nemeroff, 2020; Teicher et al., 2016). This important revelation compels clinicians involved in case formulation and therapy to adopt a dimensional perspective, considering the clinical manifestations and underlying pathogenetic processes, rather than solely relying on traditional diagnostic categories. By acknowledging the wide prevalence and far-reaching implications of child maltreatment, clinicians can better grasp its complex interplay with psychopathology. This understanding prompts the development of more effective treatment approaches tailored to the unique needs of individuals affected by child maltreatment and enhances the overall quality of care provided.

c **In the majority of cases, child maltreatment is represented by attachment trauma.** An essential insight gleaned from decades of scientific literature is that traumatic attachment is the predominant form of child maltreatment (Fonagy et al., 2023; Massullo et al., 2023). A defining characteristic of child maltreatment, as highlighted in recent research, is the severe and prolonged failure of primary attachment relationships, where parents are unable to fulfill their protective and nurturing roles, thereby hindering proper individual development (Schimmenti, 2021; Schimmenti & Caretti, 2010, 2016). In fact, different forms of child maltreatment exist—for example, emotional and physical neglect, and emotional, physical, and sexual abuse). Actually, child maltreatment entails "acts of commission and omission by parents or caregivers that result in harm to the child" (Krug et al., 2002, p. 59). Reliable studies have demonstrated that different forms of child maltreatment rarely occur in isolation (U.S. Department of Health and Human Services, 2016). Instead, there is clear evidence that they tend to co-occur (Bifulco & Schimmenti, 2019), leading to overlapping vulnerabilities in psychopathology (Vachon et al., 2015). Neglect, accounting for approximately 75% of cases, emerges as the most prevalent form of child maltreatment. Neglect is defined as the deprivation of "a stable, sensitive, and responsive caregiver, which is a species-expectant experience. Caregivers are necessary to ensure survival in early human development by providing nutrition and ensuring safety from threats" (McLaughlin et al., 2017, p. 463). Some scholars argue that neglect should be included as an integral component of any definition of child maltreatment, as any form of ongoing abuse where a lack of parental protection and care is observed is unlikely to occur without neglect (Allen, 2003; Massullo et al., 2023). Also, epidemiological data consistently reveal that over 90% of cases of abuse are perpetrated by parents (U.S. Department of Health and Human Services, 2016). In other words, more than 90% of child maltreatment is represented by attachment trauma.

Therefore, understanding the central role of attachment trauma in child maltreatment provides vital insights for clinicians and researchers. It underscores the critical need to address the relational and attachment difficulties in individuals affected by child maltreatment, fostering interventions and support systems that promote healing and healthy attachment relationships. By recognizing the multifaceted nature of child maltreatment and its deleterious impact, we can work toward improving the well-being and outcomes for those who have experienced attachment trauma.

Toward an Operational Definition of Attachment Trauma

Over the past three decades, the concept of attachment trauma (Allen, 2003; Purcell, 1996) has gained significant recognition. Attachment trauma refers to the condition in which a child perceives their primary caregiver as abusive, neglectful, or emotionally unavailable (Isobel et al., 2019). This condition can arise from various circumstances, including parental death, early adoption, severe disruptions in early childhood attachment, or even when parents are frightened or emotionally dysregulated during interactions with their child (Becker-Weidman, 2006; Leerkes et al., 2017). These negative childhood experiences have been variously defined as early relational trauma, interpersonal trauma, developmental trauma, complex trauma, cumulative trauma, or attachment trauma. Isobel and colleagues (2019) attempted to clarify the similarities and variations of these different conceptualizations of psychological trauma occurring within the parent-child relationships: their study shows that most of them refer to a common element, namely, the caregivers' alteration, violation, and/or abdication concerning the crucial roles in the proper development of the child. For this reason, it has been proposed by some scholars to use the concept of *attachment trauma* or *traumatic attachment* (Albasi, 2006; Allen, 2003; Liotti, 2017; Massullo et al., 2023; Schore, 2003).

Childhood is a stage of life during which individuals are entirely dependent on their parents. They rely on them not only for survival through protection, nutrition, and basic care but also for proper physiological and socio-emotional development (Bowlby, 1969/1982; Harlow & Zimmerman, 1959; Lorenz, 1949; Luyten, Campbell & Fonagy, 2020). Humans, similar to most mammals, require a diverse range of environmental experiences (especially those of a relational nature) provided by caregivers, especially during sensitive periods of development, in order to thrive and develop optimally (McLaughlin et al., 2017). When these expected environmental inputs are absent or inadequate due to parental neglect or abandonment of their protective, caring, and regulatory roles, it compromises the child's psychobiological development and creates a threatening situation from which the child cannot escape; these altered attachment experiences can thus be considered traumatic (Farina et al., 2019; Schimmenti, 2022). Drawing on Bromberg's work (2013a, 2013b), Schimmenti and Caretti (2016) defined this type of trauma as "a lack of emotional reciprocity and a disavowal of the child's affective needs" (p. 4). Extensive research has shown that even prolonged periods of cognitive, affective, and neurovegetative disharmony with a dysregulated or unresponsive caregiver, stemming from reasons such as grief or coping with significant life challenges like illness or marital conflicts, pose pervasive and inescapable threat factors that can lead to lasting changes and compromise emotional, cognitive, and social development (Farina et al., 2019; Fonagy et al., 2023; Guérin-Marion et al., 2020; Liotti, 2004; Luyten, Campbell & Fonagy, 2020; McLaughlin et al., 2017; Schimmenti & Caretti, 2016; Schore, 2009). Allen (2003) points out that attachment trauma is characterized by a peculiar dual pathogenic effect: on the one hand, it activates stress and threat response mechanisms, while on the other hand, it prevents the proper development of self-regulation and defense processes.

It is crucial to clarify that the construct of attachment trauma is transnosographic—that is, it represents a psychopathological risk condition that can create challenges in therapy, rather than being the sole cause of a specific disorder. However, it is evident that some clinical presentations, such as CPTSD, BPD, or dissociative disorders, are strongly characterized by a history of attachment trauma. It should also be pointed out that the construct of attachment trauma does not coincide with the construct of attachment disorganization or the other forms of insecure attachment detected by the Strange Situation or the Adult Attachment Interview, as these are constructs and categorizations born and developed in precise experimental contexts, and it would be improper to apply them directly in clinical practice (Granqvist et al., 2017). However, despite this substantial difference, empirical studies on disorganized or insecure attachment are very useful for the understanding of the pathogenetic processes supposedly triggered by attachment trauma (Schimmenti, 2022), which will be described in the next sections.

Before delving into the intricate psychopathogenesis of attachment trauma, it is essential to highlight that the relationship between attachment trauma and psychopathological vulnerability is not a straightforward, linear one. Instead, it is influenced by a multitude of mediating factors that interact in complex ways. These factors include genetic predisposition and its interaction with the environment, the individual's temperamental characteristics, subsequent developmental experiences (both negative and positive), and other existential or contextual circumstances, such as economic difficulties, social problems, or environments lacking in cultural and affective stimuli (Luyten, Campbell & Fonagy, 2020).

The Hidden Trauma

As just mentioned, despite its widespread prevalence and its "devastating" developmental effects (van der Kolk, 2016, p. 267), many clinicians will find it difficult to retrieve biographical elements in their patients' histories that can testify to attachment trauma. This is one of the reasons that child maltreatment and attachment trauma, despite their high prevalence and clinical importance, have been glaringly neglected for decades, deserving the appellation of a *hidden epidemic* (Lanius et al., 2020). We have already observed that most forms of attachment trauma are due to neglect—a condition of significant and enduring inadequacy of care or correct emotional and cognitive attunement that often cannot be spontaneously reported by patients, as it is an experience of absence that may go unrecognized and therefore not reported in clinical dialogue (McLaughlin et al., 2017; Stoltenborgh et al., 2013). In addition, it should be considered that about a quarter of attachment trauma experiences occur before the age of 3—that is, before the formation of autobiographical episodic memory that can be collected in the medical history (U.S. Department of Health and Human Services, 2016). Consider, for example, a mother facing a period of personal difficulties (bereavement, separation, illness) or suffering from untreated depressive episodes, who, after the child's first two or three years of life, regains her equilibrium: of the painful and traumatic experience, nothing will remain in the children's autobiographical memory (especially if the negative events are then hushed up), but its traces will remain in their implicit memories and in the incomplete and defective development of the mental functions that depend most on the attachment relationship (Farina et al., 2019; Luyten, Campbell & Fonagy, 2020; McLaughlin et al., 2017; Schore, 2009). And even when biographical elements can be remembered, there are some forms of maltreatment that are not recognized as such. For instance, recent developments in the study of early caregiving relationships indicate that parents' excessive preoccupation during interactions with their offspring (typical of attachment trauma) may manifest in alarmed overprotection behaviors that can, sometimes, go so far as to produce effects comparable to active maltreatment and neglect (Farber et al., 2019; Farina et al., 2021; Vergara-Lopez et al., 2016). Adding to this, it is often difficult to recognize the presence of attachment trauma in the developmental history of adult patients. Self-administered questionnaires on child maltreatment have the advantage of being quick and inexpensive but not very effective in detecting less evident manifestations of attachment trauma (Imperatori et al., 2022); and even gold-standard, behavioral-based interviews such as the Childhood Experiences of Care and Abuse (Bifulco et al., 1994; Bifulco & Schimmenti, 2019), which has demonstrated good reliability and validity, including independent corroboration of memories of child neglect and abuse (Bifulco et al., 1997), come with some limitations concerning preverbal, forgotten, or otherwise biased childhood memories.

Therefore, the difficulty of obtaining evidence of the inadequate caregiving directly from the patient makes it necessary to subvert the diagnostic process and the clinical reasoning: sometimes, it is necessary to *infer* the presence of attachment trauma in the patient's history, by deriving it from the psychopathological manifestations that concur to characterize the clinical picture in a dimensional way, and from the relative therapeutic difficulties. Both these clinical issues derive from the pathogenetic processes activated by parental failures: therefore, in the following paragraphs we will deal with the pathogenetic processes, the resulting psychopathology, and the related therapeutic difficulties characterizing the attachment trauma. For ease of exposition, these pathogenetic processes will be described separately. It should be pointed out, however, that they are closely interrelated and mutually reinforcing in determining psychopathological vulnerability.

Alterations in Biological Regulatory Systems

Alterations in biological regulatory systems are critical consequences of attachment trauma. The primary attachment relationship plays a vital role in promoting the harmonious development of biological regulatory systems, enabling individuals to adapt to changing environmental circumstances, and particularly to distressing situations (Gunnar & Quevedo, 2007). It is important to acknowledge that the attachment motivational system facilitates stress hormone modulation and restoration of vegetative balance through renewed closeness to a protective and attuned caregiver during stressful or threatening situations (Leerkes et al., 2017). However, when a parent—either because of preoccupation, depression, illness, or active abuse—fails to provide affective, cognitive, and neurovegetative attunement, or when they are emotionally or vegetatively dysregulated, this hampers the restoration of vegetative balance in the child. This can compromise the development of effective self-regulatory responses and disrupt physiological and somatic development (Guerin-Marion et al., 2020; Leerkes et al., 2017; McLaughlin et al., 2017).

Alterations in biological regulatory systems resulting from attachment trauma have been associated with an increased risk of various health conditions, including autoimmune diseases, coronary artery disease, metabolic syndromes, obesity, hypertension, and certain typologies of cancers (Troisi, 2020). Additionally, the well-established relationship between attachment trauma and the occurrence of somatoform disorders, such as sexual and urinary dysfunctions, pain syndromes, tinnitus, colitis, parasomnias, and pseudoneurological syndromes, has been extensively documented (Le et al., 2021; Mysliwiec et al., 2018; Romeo et al., 2022; Sar et al., 2004; Weber & Wetter, 2022; van der Kolk et al., 1996). These somatic manifestations can have a devastating impact on patients' lives, impairing their quality of life and reinforcing relational difficulties and pathogenic beliefs.

Another critical consequence of dysregulation of biological systems that has the greatest impact on psychotherapy outcomes is arousal dysregulation. Altered vegetative balance not only affects sleep, mood, and other regulatory functions but also exacerbates the already impaired regulation of emotions and impulses in individuals affected by attachment trauma. This circularly compromises their relational abilities and undermines the effectiveness of therapies (Leerkes et al., 2017).

Empirical studies have revealed that insecure or disorganized attachment relationships disrupt a child's regulation of arousal (Leerkes et al., 2017). For instance, Oosterman and colleagues (2010) examined measures of arousal in 60 children during the Strange Situation Procedure (Ainsworth et al., 1978) and found that children with experiences of neglect and disorganized attachment exhibited pathological overactivity of the adrenergic system in response to stress and environmental challenges.

Thus, when caregivers are unable to effectively modulate physiological arousal, even in the face of moderate stress, this might lead to deficient or disproportionate activation of the stress-response system and neurovegetative reactions, with significant implications for the development of emotional, behavioral, and cognitive dysregulation, as well as for the onset of detachment and compartmentalization responses (see below in the next sections). Notably, these responses might be particularly activated within relational contexts, including the therapeutic relationship where the attachment system (and the internal working models of attachment trauma) is activated toward the therapist. In a study by Farina and colleagues (2015), it was indeed observed that adults with disorganized attachment showed no significant differences compared to a control group in a baseline situation. However, after discussing their attachment experiences during the Adult Attachment Interview, the disorganized attachment group displayed clear signs of arousal dysregulation, indicating a heightened response triggered by the retrieval of childhood attachment experiences. As a result, clinical conditions may worsen, and the response to treatment can be compromised (Lyons-Ruth et al., 2006; Leerkes et al., 2017). Increased vegetative arousal is known to inhibit cognitive and metacognitive regulation abilities (Young et al., 2017). When this occurs within the therapeutic relationship due to the activation of attachment and its implicit relational memories (Internal Working Models [IWMs]), it further impairs the already compromised cognitive and mentalization functions of patients who were exposed to attachment trauma, making treatment more complex (Farina & Meares, 2022).

Dysregulation of Mental Functions and Self-States

There is a strong consensus among experts regarding dysregulation as the central factor in the psychopathological consequences of attachment trauma. Dysregulation extends beyond arousal and biological systems to encompass higher mental functions (Cicchetti & Toth, 2005; D'Andrea et al., 2012; Luyten, Campbell & Fonagy, 2020; Spinazzola et al., 2018). Primary attachment relationships have a crucial role in nurturing the development of higher mental functions, including executive control, emotional and behavioral regulation, memory and attention, mentalization, and continuity of self-consciousness. This developmental process involves a dynamic bioecological integration, where the biology of mental structures continuously interacts with the environment (Carlson et al., 2009; Fonagy & Target, 1997; Luyten, Campbell & Fonagy, 2020; Linde-Krieger et al., 2022; Schimmenti, 2022; Winnicott, 1962, Chapter 4, pp. 56–63). Indeed, integration is not a predetermined biological outcome; rather, it emerges from a developmental process that initiates at birth (Putnam, 1997). This process is dependent on the presence of suitable relational provisions characterized by connectedness and affective and cognitive synchronization. The culmination of this process results in a hierarchically organized self-system which comprised successive "layers" of mental functioning, each contributing to the individual's experience of self. These "layers" progressively gain coordination and synchronization, and each one involves a "higher" or more refined system of inhibition that regulates the earlier ones (Farina & Meares, 2022).

Biologically, a failure to achieve this evolutionary task seems to be associated with the inadequate formation of brain networks responsible for integrative capacities and their hierarchical and heterarchical organization, which are foundational for higher mental functions (Farina & Meares, 2022; Teicher et al., 2016). The mind is an intricately interconnected and dynamic system that bridges segregated systems, comprising distinct functional modules and mental contents. This integration relies on brain connectivity facilitated by local and global neural networks, enabling not only global information processing but also optimal modulation of functions through inhibitory actions (Deco et al., 2015; Gordon et al., 2018; Lord & Ashworth, 2017; Park & Friston, 2013). Secure attachment relationships, characterized by stable, sensitive, and responsive caregivers, promote brain connectivity and network formation at the biological level (Fitter et al., 2022; Rifkin-Graboi et al., 2015). Furthermore, at the psychological level, secure attachment fosters the integration of mental states and the appropriate development of reflective functions (Blizard, 2003; Lauren et al., 2022; Luyten, Campbell & Fonagy, 2020; Santoro et al., 2021; Winnicott, 1962, Chapter 4, pp. 56–63).

In cases of attachment trauma, where the caregiver lacks sensitivity and responsiveness, the development of higher mental functions that rely on integration is impaired. From a biological perspective, this impairment results in deficits in brain connectivity, as well as failures in integration, coordination, and inhibition processes (Adenzato et al., 2019; Carbone et al., 2022; Massullo et al., 2022; Teicher et al., 2016; Terpou et al., 2020), hindering the harmonious development of these functions (Meares, 2012; Scalabrini et al., 2022).

The disintegrative effect of attachment trauma, termed *traumatic disintegration*, is intricately linked with other pathogenetic processes, which will be further described later. Traumatic disintegration can be considered the most characteristic pathogenetic process of attachment trauma and the main cause of trauma-based psychological dysregulation, which can manifest itself in diverse psychopathological forms, depending on the specific impaired mental functions. Mental functions that rely heavily on high levels of integration, coordination, and inhibition, and develop through interaction with the environment, particularly interpersonal interactions, are more susceptible to traumatic disintegration (Farina & Meares, 2022).

The broad range of symptoms associated with the disintegrative process challenges strict categorical nosology, which classifies symptoms based on the alteration of individual mental functions to define diagnostic profiles. Instead, it is more appropriate to characterize psychopathological manifestations by understanding the collective impact of altered functions, focusing on the primary mechanism that compromises their hierarchical organization and normal reciprocal interactions.

The concept of traumatic disintegration, as recently reformulated (Farina & Meares, 2022), has historical roots. In the early 1900s, Pierre Janet proposed that a central process in post-traumatic psychopathology involved a reduction of "integrative capacity" caused by the intense, prolonged, and long-lasting negative emotions generated by trauma (Janet, 1907, p. 332). Janet suggested that these emotions exert their disintegrative effects by affecting the reflexive and continuity functions of self-experience, which he referred to as personal synthesis (van der Hart & Dorahy, 2009). Janet derived the concept of traumatic disintegration from the theoretical framework of Hughlings Jackson, who, in the late 19th century, hypothesized that a portion of psychopathology resulted from the disruption of the hierarchical and integrated order of mental functions. This hypothesis has been further explored by various scholars throughout the 20th century (Farina et al., 2005).

An increasing body of evidence demonstrates that traumatic disintegration (which is distinct from dissociation proper, see next paragraphs) is influenced by both biological and psychological factors. Biological factors include the activation of stress hormones and inflammatory processes triggered by constant threatening experiences, which can damage brain connectivity (Farina & Meares, 2022; Teicher et al., 2016). Psychological factors encompass the absence of caregiver regulation and mirroring mechanisms, as well as the formation of implicit traumatic memories. These factors collectively contribute to alterations in emotion processing and regulation, overgeneralization of threatening stimuli, difficulties in executive control of behavior, impulsivity, fragmentation of self-identity, feelings of emptiness, and challenges in self-referential processes such as agency. Traumatic disintegration also impacts the state of consciousness and autobiographical memory, and produces deficits in social cognition and disruptions of mentalization (Farina & Meares, 2022; Krause-Utz et al., 2017; Lanius et al., 2020; Luyten, Campbell & Fonagy, 2020; Scalabrini et al., 2022; Schimmenti & Caretti, 2016; Teicher et al., 2016).

Clinical observation and empirical evidence suggest that traumatic disintegration can manifest as both a trait vulnerability and a propensity for momentary and transient failures of integrative or inhibitory functioning. Trait vulnerability refers to a weakness in integrative and inhibitory brain structures that becomes a relatively stable feature of an individual's personality, such as a tendency toward incoherent fragmentation of the experience of self (Liotti & Farina, 2016; Meares, 2012). Momentary and transient failures of integrative or inhibitory functioning, however, are characterized by sudden losses of emotional or behavioral control or the sudden and uncontrolled emergence of traumatic memories. These two aspects are not mutually exclusive; rather, they are closely intertwined. Trait vulnerability may become apparent only in response to specific triggers, often involving the reactivation of interpersonal patterns and implicit relational memories from traumatic attachment experiences, with their disorganized internal working models of attachment (Adenzato et al., 2019; Farina & Meares, 2022; Farina et al., 2014; Schimmenti, 2022).

Disintegrated or disorganized mental states typically arise in response to circumstances that trigger representations of the self as being in danger, threatened, defenseless, or neglected. At the time, the caregiver is perceived as abusive, abandoning, helpless, or frightened. In individuals with attachment trauma histories, this process is particularly evident in intimate interpersonal contexts, such as family relationships, romantic relationships, and even within the therapeutic relationship (Farina et al., 2019; Luyten, Campbell & Fonagy, 2020; Schimmenti, 2022).

The activation of these implicit, traumatic relational memories, coupled with a state of heightened vegetative arousal and trait disintegration, leads to state-dependent disintegration. This state is characterized by impairments in self-continuity, emotional and behavioral control, and metacognitive monitoring abilities. It often manifests as loss of impulse control, dysregulated emotional states dominated by fear or anger (or both), feelings of emptiness and fragmentation of self-identity, compensatory behaviors (such as substance use or self-injury), and collapse of mentalization. These manifestations have a negative impact on relational contexts, reinforcing maladaptive interpersonal patterns that confirm fears of abandonment or mistreatment and support pathogenic beliefs of shame, unworthiness, guilt, and victimization (Liotti & Farina, 2016; Farina & Meares, 2022; Schimmenti, 2013, 2014).

States of Detachment and Dissociation

Disintegrative vulnerability is often erroneously conflated with psychopathological manifestations attributed to other pathogenetic processes commonly categorized as dissociative symptoms (Farina & Meares, 2022). *Detachment states*, which encompass experiences of derealization, depersonalization, and emotional numbing, correspond to altered states of consciousness, likely triggered by an adaptive yet passive defense mechanism that evolved to minimize the potentially debilitating effects of pain and extreme emotional states in situations of inescapable threat (Brown, 2006; Holmes et al., 2005; Salami et al., 2020). These passive responses are believed to have also evolved to simulate death, evoking predator disgust and the instinct of not consuming prey that does not resist because it might be already deceased and thus potentially harmful (Kearney & Lanius, 2022; Kozlowska et al., 2015; Terpou et al., 2019). While detachment reactions serve an adaptive purpose, they can become dysfunctional. Many scholars propose that the persistent state of inescapable threat associated with attachment trauma leads to an ongoing reliance on these defensive reactions throughout development. As a result, detachment symptoms, as observed in panic attacks or other anxiety disorders, may manifest in adulthood even under non-extreme conditions of vulnerability (Frewen et al., 2015; Kearney & Lanius, 2022; Lyons-Ruth et al., 2006; van der Hart, 2021). Subjective experiences induced by detached states of self-consciousness can bear resemblance to those triggered by traumatic disintegration of the state of consciousness. Moreover, it is plausible that these two pathogenetic processes can be simultaneously activated in threatening conditions, with potentially overlapping effects. However, it is important to note that detachment symptoms differ from other manifestations, usually classified in terms of compartmentalization, as supported by clinical and neuroscientific research (Butler et al., 2019; Ellickson-Larew et al., 2020; Steele et al., 2022).

Compartmentalization, also defined in terms of *structural dissociation*, is recognized by experts as a pathological condition, in which parts of the self are isolated from the rest of mental functioning and are inaccessible to awareness. It typically emerges under specific triggering conditions (Nijenhuis & van der Hart, 2011; Şar, 2017; Schimmenti, 2022). Unlike traumatic disintegration, structural dissociation is not simply the result of temporarily nonintegrated self-states or mental contents, but rather the reorganization of these elements, following disintegration, into pathologically over-segregated and enduring parallel structures (Nijenhuis, 2019; Şar, 2017; Steele et al., 2022).

These over-segregated self-states manifest as distinct entities comprising a diverse array of memory types, including episodic, semantic, and procedural memories (e.g., sensorimotor schemas). Additionally, they may incorporate implicit relational schemas (referred to as IWMs) or even more intricate self-states that interweave memories, emotional states, and motivations (Farina & Meares, 2022). These distinct self-states, though rudimentary, possess their own first-person perspective and can eventually develop into multiple identities (Nijenhuis & van der Hart, 2011). The precise mechanisms underlying structural dissociation are still the subject of ongoing debate and span different chapters of this book. However, studies in developmental psychopathology suggest that this type of dissociation arises from the combined effects of several pathogenic processes involved in attachment trauma. These include exposure to maltreatment and to highly inconsistent and contradictory experiences within the traumatic interpersonal environment, together with the lack of the organizing influence of self-experience that is typically fostered by affective and cognitive coordination and attunement with a sensitive, reflective, and empathic caregiver (Amos et al., 2011; Liotti, 2017; Nijenhuis, 2019; Schimmenti, 2022). In this respect, Liotti (1992, 2017) put forth the hypothesis that the simultaneous or rapidly alternating activation of conflicting motivational systems, such as the drive for closeness to the caregiver (attachment motivation) and the urge to escape from the threats the caregiver poses (defense motivation) overwhelms the child's underdeveloped integrative capacities. This leads to the formation of mutually incompatible and incoherent implicit IWMs, which promote the compartmentalization of the experience of self and, in some cases, the pathological segregation of its parts (Amos et al., 2011; Corrigan et al., 2022; Liotti, 1992, 2017; Schimmenti, 2022).

Others argue that the exclusion of painful or discordant aspects of experience may be driven by the defensive need to protect oneself from pain, preserve positive caregiver and self-representations, or maintain a consistent self-identity (Bromberg, 2009; Corrigan & Hull, 2022; Linde-Krieger et al., 2022; Radulovic et al., 2018; Schimmenti, 2022). Nevertheless, there is agreement among scholars regarding the over-segregation and compartmentalization symptoms of dissociation, which can manifest as dissociative amnesias, flashbacks, sensorimotor patterns, and bodily memories, described by some as somatoform dissociation (Nijenhuis, 2009) or conversion symptoms. It can also manifest as nonintegrated self-states or multiple identities (American Psychiatric Association, 2013; Lauren et al., 2022).

Relational Dysregulation

It is worth noting that the clinical presentations typically associated with attachment trauma are characterized by difficulties in forming and maintaining affective relationships (Luyten, Campbell & Fonagy, 2020; Schimmenti & Caretti, 2016). The relational dynamics between the child and the caregiver involved in attachment trauma, frequently including a plethora of disturbing negative feelings continuously experienced by the child, such as confusion, fear, anger, and shame, tend to generate failures in mentalization and the emotion regulation process (Santoro et al., 2021; Schimmenti, 2017). These failures result in lack of trust about the possibility of interpersonal reparation for the early relational damage and in negative expectations toward subsequent attachment relationships. In a study on 352 adults, Midolo and colleagues (2020) highlighted the strong interrelations among the domains of childhood traumatic experiences, adult attachment attitudes, and clinical symptoms: in their sample, childhood experiences of emotional neglect and abuse were linked to insecure relational styles, suggesting that children with emotionally abusing, intrusive, or neglecting caregivers are more prone to develop severely insecure relational patterns in adulthood. Indeed, attachment trauma may shape negative representations of self, others, and relationship between self and others, which can disrupt the sense of trust and security in close relationships.

Moreover, in a vicious cycle, the negative relational expectations deriving from attachment trauma further impair the capacity for mentalization, limiting the possibility to represent the emotional meaning of experiences, and thus to learn from new and potentially more benevolent relational experiences. Santoro and colleagues (2021) suggested that the ready activation of the attachment system may inhibit mentalization by generating uncertainty about the evaluation of one's own and others' relational attitudes and behaviors, thus increasing attachment insecurity and vulnerability to mental disorders.

Such dysregulation in relational attitudes and exchanges is well known among clinicians who treat individuals suffering from attachment trauma. Van der Hart and colleagues (2005) observed that these individuals frequently show an attachment phobia, so that their desire to repair the early relational trauma is blocked by fears of abuse, betrayal, rejection, abandonment, and so on. Schimmenti and Caretti (2016) noted that these fears frequently derive from implicit memories of maltreatment and likely replicate what people with attachment trauma once experienced in their early interactions with caregivers.

Rather than the capacity for intersubjectivity, which is preserved in most cases, it is thus the actual experience of intersubjectivity that is frequently altered or damaged among individuals with attachment trauma, who might perceive the interactions in close relationships as unpredictable and potentially dangerous. This gives rise to challenges when treating these individuals, including ruptures in the therapeutic alliance, negative therapeutic reactions, and, in some cases, even premature termination of therapy (Liotti & Farina, 2016; Schimmenti & Caretti, 2016).

Mentalization Failures

Compromised mentalization is a prominent feature of attachment trauma that significantly impacts personality development and hinders effective therapeutic interventions. In normal development, individuals possess the capacity to continuously and flexibly reassess their sense of self, interpersonal relationships, and the external world. However, attachment trauma may inhibit the development of mentalizing abilities and the capacity to think about oneself and others in terms of internal states—for example, beliefs, desires, feelings, and intentions (Ensink et al., 2014, 2015). Furthermore, attachment trauma might limit the development of capacities related to theory of mind—that is, the ability to attribute and interpret mental state (Nazarov et al., 2014; Pears & Fisher, 2005; Schimmenti, 2017).

Thus, attachment trauma disrupts mentalizing capacities, rendering them rigid and impairing optimal metacognitive monitoring (Fonagy et al., 2023). Some researchers have referred to this cognitive inflexibility as "epistemic freezing," suggesting its defensive function in response to the contradictory nature of attachment trauma experiences (Luyten, Campbell, Allison & Fonagy, 2020). The challenge lies in the difficulty of modifying meaning structures through corrective emotional experiences, due to the presence of epistemic distrust, characterized by a reluctance to perceive others as reliable sources of information. Furthermore, the alterations in mentalization abilities, which are fundamental to the effectiveness of psychotherapy, exacerbate resistance to treatment, regardless of the therapeutic approach or the specific clinical presentation (Farina et al., 2019).

Recognizing the impact of compromised mentalization is crucial for therapists working with individuals affected by attachment trauma. It underscores the importance of creating a therapeutic environment that fosters trust, allows for exploration and correction of maladaptive beliefs, and supports the development of mentalizing abilities. By addressing these barriers, therapists can help individuals with attachment trauma enhance their cognitive flexibility, strengthen their capacity for self-reflectivity, and promote more adaptive ways of relating to themselves and others.

Pathogenic Beliefs

The early attachment to neglectful or maltreating caregivers leads to the construction of meaningful structures, including beliefs and expectations, that allow children to adapt to the unfavorable conditions of their relational environment. However, these meaning structures often transform into dysfunctional beliefs in later stages of development. An essential function of the attachment relationship is to shape meaning structures—which encompass beliefs and expectations about oneself, others, and the dynamics of relationships—guiding individuals toward evolutionarily determined goals and partially defining their personality (Bretherton & Munholland, 2016).

It is widely documented that individuals with a history of attachment trauma commonly develop pathogenic beliefs and dysfunctional interpersonal circularities. Negative alterations in self-perception and personal meanings are prevalent features among disorders related to traumatic experiences. In the case of attachment trauma, the need to adapt to relationships with frightened, neglectful caregivers and within an abusive interpersonal context, from which escape is impossible, inevitably gives rise to beliefs of vulnerability, helplessness, worthlessness, guilt, inauthenticity, and irreparable damage. These beliefs foster pervasive feelings of guilt and shame that become stable personality traits negatively impacting the individual's life (Schimmenti, 2012, 2021; Spinazzola et al., 2014). The adaptation to attachment relationships with frightened, neglectful caregivers and within a mistreating interpersonal context generates expectations of rejection and abandonment that contribute to the relational difficulties characteristic of attachment trauma (Liotti & Farina, 2016).

Attachment trauma also predisposes individuals to other interpersonal trauma, as it has been hypothesized and supported by empirical research conducted by numerous scholars (D'Andrea et al., 2012; Fowler et al., 2013; Liotti, 2017; Schimmenti, 2018; Schore, 2009). In essence, the profound and prolonged failure of primary caregivers to provide protective and nurturing care does not facilitate the development of skills to protect oneself from both impersonal and interpersonal dangers and increases susceptibility to subsequent childhood interpersonal traumatic experiences beyond the primary attachment relationships. Such experiences may involve other family members, acquaintances, or even individuals in caregiving roles outside the immediate family, such as teachers or foster caregivers. This heightened exposure to further traumatization correlates with an elevated risk of developing psychopathology (Luyten, Campbell & Fonagy, 2020; Midolo et al., 2020; Schimmenti, 2018). Moreover, the typical pathogenic beliefs reinforce and expose attachment trauma individuals to new traumas both in childhood and adulthood, and both within and outside the family context (American Psychiatric Association [APA], 2013; Isobel et al., 2019; World Health Organization, 2006; Cook et al., 2005). For example, having the conviction of being unworthy and having adapted to abusive relationships will foster the possibility of maintaining abusive relationships also in adult life. Indeed, women with attachment trauma have been found to be predisposed to domestic violence or dysfunctional partnerships (Speranza et al., 2022).

Understanding the interplay between traumatic attachment and subsequent interpersonal trauma sheds light on the complex trajectory of psychopathological development. It underscores the importance of comprehensive assessments and targeted interventions to address both the effects of early attachment trauma and the potential impact of subsequent traumatic experiences. By recognizing and addressing these interconnected factors, therapeutic approaches can better target the underlying mechanisms and provide individuals with the necessary support to heal, recover, and develop resilience in the face of traumatic events.

Pathogenic beliefs and dysfunctional interpersonal patterns and cycles pose significant challenges to effective psychotherapy. Beliefs centered on powerlessness, helplessness, and unworthiness can subtly erode the therapeutic alliance. Moreover, as observed in the previous section, the activation of implicit memories of attachment trauma often elicits negative expectations of neglect, abandonment, or mistreatment within the therapeutic relationship. These negative expectations can lead to mistrust of the therapist and, in some cases, premature termination of treatment (Liotti & Farina, 2016). Addressing and working through these pathogenic beliefs and negative expectations is crucial for the success of psychotherapy. It requires establishing a secure and attuned therapeutic alliance, where the therapist creates a safe space for the individual to explore and challenge these beliefs, providing experiences that contradict and gradually replace them with more adaptive and empowering beliefs. Therapeutic interventions aimed at fostering self-worth, agency, and trust can help individuals with attachment trauma overcome their pathogenic beliefs, modify dysfunctional patterns, and develop healthier ways of relating to themselves and others.

Conclusion

Almost 20 years have passed since Cook and colleagues (2005) published their seminal article on complex trauma in children and adolescents. They already traced a virtuous path for operationalizing the concept of attachment trauma, by detecting seven major domains of impairment in children who are exposed to it, namely, attachment, biology, affect regulation, dissociation, behavioral control, cognition, and self-concept.

Following this path, in this chapter, we aimed to integrate such diagnostic wisdom deriving from decades of research on child maltreatment with further clinical and research insights that support an operational definition of attachment trauma for clinical practice with children who have histories of complex trauma and dissociative symptoms. We have highlighted the interrelated psychopathogenetic processes implied in attachment trauma in the hope that this might serve clinicians to better recognize its indicators and understand the individuals suffering from them. As we have discussed, attachment trauma likely represents a hidden epidemic. For individuals struggling with its consequences, meeting a clinician who wears epistemic glasses that are able to detect it can make a great difference.

References

Adenzato, M., Imperatori, C., Ardito, R. B., Valenti, E. M., Marca, G. D., D'Ari, S., Palmiero, L., Penso, J. S., & Farina, B. (2019). Activating attachment memories affects default mode network in a non-clinical sample with perceived dysfunctional parenting: An EEG functional connectivity study. *Behavioural Brain Research, 372*, Article 112059. https://doi.org/10.1016/j.bbr.2019.112059

Ainsworth, M. D. S., Blehar, M. C., Waters, E., & Wall, S. (1978). *Patterns of attachment: A psychological study of the Strange Situation*. Erlbaum.

Albasi, C. (2006). *Attaccamenti traumatici: I modelli operativi interni dissociati* (1st ed.). UTET università.

Allen, J. G. (2003). Challenges in treating post-traumatic stress disorder and attachment trauma. *Current Women's Health Reports, 3*(3), 213–220.

American Psychiatric Association (APA) (2013). *Diagnostic and statistical manual of mental disorders* (5th ed.). APA.

Amos, J., Furber, G., & Segal, L. (2011). Understanding maltreating mothers: A synthesis of relational trauma, attachment disorganization, structural dissociation of the personality, and experiential avoidance. *Journal of Trauma & Dissociation, 12*(5), 495–509. https://doi.org/10.1080/15299732.2011.593259

Becker-Weidman, A. (2006). Treatment for children with trauma-attachment disorders: Dyadic developmental psychotherapy. *Child and Adolescent Social Work Journal, 23*(2), 147–171. https://doi.org/10.1007/s10560-005-0039-0

Bifulco, A., Brown, G. W., & Harris, T. O. (1994). Childhood experience of care and abuse (CECA): A retrospective interview measure. *Journal of Child Psychology and Psychiatry, and Allied Disciplines, 35*(8), 1419–1435. https://doi.org/10.1111/j.1469-7610.1994.tb01284.x

Bifulco, A., Brown, G. W., Lillie, A., & Jarvis, J. (1997). Memories of childhood neglect and abuse: Corroboration in a series of sisters. *Journal of Child Psychology and Psychiatry, 38*(3), 365–374. https://doi.org/10.1111/j.1469-7610.1997.tb01520.x

Bifulco, A., & Schimmenti, A. (2019). Assessing child abuse: "We need to talk!". *Child Abuse & Neglect, 98*, Article 104236. https://doi.org/10.1016/j.chiabu.2019.104236

Blizard, R. A. (2003). Disorganized attachment, development of dissociated self states, and a relational approach to treatment. *Journal of Trauma & Dissociation, 4*(3), 27–50. https://doi.org/10.1300/J229v04n03_03

Bowlby, J. (1969/1982). *Attachment and loss: Vol. 1. Attachment*. Basic Books.

Bretherton, I., & Munholland, K. A. (2016). The internal working model construct in light of contemporary neuroimaging research. In J. Cassidy & P. R., Shaver (Eds.), *Handbook of attachment: Theory, research, and clinical applications* (3rd ed., pp. 63–88). Guilford Press.

Bromberg, P. M. (2009). Multiple self-states, the relational mind, and dissociation: A psychoanalytic perspective. In P. F. Dell & J. A. O'Neil (Eds.), *Dissociation and the dissociative disorders: DSM-V and beyond* (pp. 637–652). Routledge.

Bromberg, P. M. (2013a). *Awakening the dreamer: Clinical journeys*. Routledge.

Bromberg, P. M. (2013b). Prefazione [Foreword]. In V. Caretti, G. Craparo & A. Schimmenti (Eds.), *Memorie traumatiche e mentalizzazione. Teoria, ricerca e clinica* (pp. 7–12). Astrolabio Ubaldini.

Brown, R. J. (2006). Different types of "dissociation" have different psychological mechanisms. *Journal of Trauma & Dissociation: The Official Journal of the International Society for the Study of Dissociation (ISSD), 7*(4), 7–28. https://doi.org/10.1300/J229v07n04_02

Butler, C., Dorahy, M. J., & Middleton, W. (2019). The detachment and compartmentalization inventory (DCI): An assessment tool for two potentially distinct forms of dissociation. *Journal of Trauma & Dissociation: The Official Journal of the International Society for the Study of Dissociation (ISSD), 20*(5), 526–547. https://doi.org/10.1080/15299732.2019.1597809

Carbone, G. A., Imperatori, C., Bersani, F. S., Massullo, C., Orlando, E. M., & Farina, B. (2022). Dissociative-traumatic dimension and triple network: An EEG functional connectivity study in a sample of university students. *Psychopathology, 55*(1), 28–36. https://doi.org/10.1159/000519563

Carlson, E. A., Yates, T. M., & Sroufe L. A. (2009). Dissociation and the development of the self. In P. Dell & J. A. O'Neil (Eds.), *Dissociation and dissociative disorders: DSM-V and beyond* (pp. 39–52). Routledge.

Cicchetti, D., & Toth, S. L. (2005). Child maltreatment. *Annual Review of Clinical Psychology, 1*, 409–438. https://doi.org/10.1146/annurev.clinpsy.1.102803.144029

Cook, A., Spinazzola, J., Ford, J., Lanktree, C., Blaustein, M., Cloitre, M., DeRosa, R., Hubbard, R., Kagan, R., Liautaud, J., Mallah, K., Olafson, E., & van der Kolk, B. (2005). Complex trauma in children and adolescents. *Psychiatric Annals, 35*(5), 390–398. https://doi.org/10.3928/00485713-20050501-05

Corrigan, F. M., & Hull, A. (2022). The shadow costs of dissociative identity disorder. *The British Journal of Psychiatry, 220*(2), 98–98. https://doi.org/10.1192/bjp.2021.73

Corrigan, F. M., Lanius, U. F., & Kaschor, B. (2022). The defense cascade, traumatic dissociation and the self: A neuroscientific model. In M. J. Dorahy, S. N. Gold & J. A., O'Neil (Eds.), *Dissociation and the dissociative disorder: Past, present, future* (pp. 587–601). Routledge. https://doi.org/10.4324/9781003057314

D'Andrea, W., Ford, J., Stolbach, B., Spinazzola, J., & van der Kolk, B. A. (2012). Understanding interpersonal trauma in children: Why we need a developmentally appropriate trauma diagnosis. *American Journal of Orthopsychiatry, 82*(2), 187–200. https://doi.org/10.1111/j.1939-0025.2012.01154.x

Deco, G., Tononi, G., Boly, M., & Kringelbach, M. L. (2015). Rethinking segregation and integration: Contributions of whole-brain modelling. *Nature Reviews Neuroscience, 16*(7), 430–439. https://doi.org/10.1038/nrn3963

Ellickson-Larew, S., Stasik-O'Brien, S. M., Stanton, K., & Watson, D. (2020). Dissociation as a multidimensional transdiagnostic symptom. *Psychology of Consciousness: Theory, Research, and Practice, 7*(2), 126–150. https://doi.org/10.1037/cns0000218

Ensink, K., Berthelot, N., Bernazzani, O., Normandin, L., & Fonagy, P. (2014). Another step closer to measuring the ghosts in the nursery: Preliminary validation of the trauma reflective functioning scale. *Frontiers in Psychology, 5*, Article 1471. https://doi.org/10.3389/fpsyg.2014.01471

Ensink, K., Normandin, L., Target, M., Fonagy, P., Sabourin, S., & Berthelot, N. (2015). Mentalization in children and mothers in the context of trauma: An initial study of the validity of the child reflective functioning scale. *The British Journal of Developmental Psychology, 33*(2), 203–217. https://doi.org/10.1111/bjdp.12074

Farber, M. J., Kim, M. J., Knodt, A. R., & Hariri, A. R. (2019). Maternal overprotection in childhood is associated with amygdala reactivity and structural connectivity in adulthood. *Developmental Cognitive Neuroscience, 40*, Article 100711. https://doi.org/10.1016/j.dcn.2019.100711

Farina, B., Ceccarelli, M., & Di Giannantonio, M. (2005). Henri Ey's neojacksonism and the psychopathology of disintegrated mind. *Psychopathology, 38*(5), pp. 285–290.

Farina, B., Imperatori, C., Adenzato, M., & Ardito, R. B. (2021). Perceived parental over-protection in non clinical young adults is associated with affective vulnerability: A cross-sectional study. *Journal of Affective Disorders, 292*, 496–499. https://doi.org/10.1016/j.jad.2021.05.071

Farina, B., Liotti, M., & Imperatori, C. (2019). The role of attachment trauma and disintegrative pathogenic processes in the traumatic-dissociative dimension. *Frontiers in Psychology, 10*, 933. https://doi.org/10.3389/fpsyg.2019.00933

Farina, B., & Meares, R. (2022). The traumatic disintegration dimension. In M. J. Dorahy, S. N. Gold & J. A. O'Neil (Eds.), *Dissociation and the dissociative disorder: Past, present, future* (pp. 50–65). Routledge. https://doi.org/10.4324/9781003057314

Farina, B., Speranza, A. M., Dittoni, S., Gnoni, V., Trentini, C., Vergano, C. M., Liotti, G., Brunetti, R., Testani, E., & Della Marca, G. (2014). Memories of attachment hamper EEG cortical connectivity in dissociative patients. *European Archives of Psychiatry and Clinical Neuroscience, 264*(5), 449–458. https://doi.org/10.1007/s00406-013-0461-9

Farina, B., Speranza, A. M., Imperatori, C., Quintiliani, M. I., & Della Marca, G. (2015). Change in heart rate variability after the adult attachment interview in dissociative patients. *Journal of Trauma & Dissociation:*

The Official Journal of the International Society for the Study of Dissociation (ISSD), 16(2), 170–180. https://doi.org/10.1080/15299732.2014.975309

Fitter, M. H., Stern, J. A., Straske, M. D., Allard, T., Cassidy, J., & Riggins, T. (2022). Mothers' attachment representations and children's brain structure. *Frontiers in Human Neuroscience, 16*, Article 740195. https://doi.org/10.3389/fnhum.2022.740195

Fonagy, P., Campbell, C., & Luyten, P. (2023). Attachment, mentalizing and trauma: Then (1992) and now (2022). *Brain Sciences, 13*(3), 459. https://doi.org/10.3390/brainsci13030459

Fonagy, P., & Target, M. (1997). Attachment and reflective function: Their role in self-organization. *Development and Psychopathology, 9*(4), 679–700. https://doi.org/10.1017/s0954579497001399

Fowler, J. C., Allen, J. G., Oldham, J. M., & Frueh, B. C. (2013). Exposure to interpersonal trauma, attachment insecurity, and depression severity. *Journal of Affective Disorders, 149*(1–3), 313–318. https://doi.org/10.1016/j.jad.2013.01.045

Franzen, J. (2015). *Purity*. Farrar, Straus and Giroux.

Frewen, P., Hegadoren, K., Coupland, N. J., Rowe, B. H., Neufeld, R. W., & Lanius, R. (2015). Trauma-related altered states of consciousness (TRASC) and functional impairment I: Prospective study in acutely traumatized persons. *Journal of Trauma & Dissociation: The Official Journal of the International Society for the Study of Dissociation (ISSD), 16*(5), 500–519. https://doi.org/10.1080/15299732.2015.1022925

Gordon, B. R., McDowell, C. P., Hallgren, M., Meyer, J. D., Lyons, M., & Herring, M. P. (2018). Association of efficacy of resistance exercise training with depressive symptoms: Meta-analysis and meta-regression analysis of randomized clinical trials. *JAMA Psychiatry, 75*(6), 566–576. https://doi.org/10.1001/jamapsychiatry.2018.0572

Granqvist, P., Sroufe, L. A., Dozier, M., Hesse, E., Steele, M., van Ijzendoorn, M., Solomon, J., Schuengel, C., Fearon, P., Bakermans-Kranenburg, M., Steele, H., Cassidy, J., Carlson, E., Madigan, S., Jacobvitz, D., Foster, S., Behrens, K., Rifkin-Graboi, A., Gribneau, N., Spangler, G.,..., & Duschinsky, R. (2017). Disorganized attachment in infancy: A review of the phenomenon and its implications for clinicians and policy-makers. *Attachment & Human Development, 19*(6), 534–558. https://doi.org/10.1080/14616734.2017.1354040

Green, J. G., McLaughlin, K. A., Berglund, P. A., Gruber, M. J., Sampson, N. A., Zaslavsky, A. M., & Kessler, R. C. (2010). Childhood adversities and adult psychiatric disorders in the national comorbidity survey replication I: Associations with first onset of DSM-IV disorders. *Archives of General Psychiatry, 67*(2), 113–123. https://doi.org/10.1001/archgenpsychiatry.2009.186

Guérin-Marion, C., Sezlik, S., & Bureau, J. F. (2020). Developmental and attachment-based perspectives on dissociation: Beyond the effects of maltreatment. *European Journal of Psychotraumatology, 11*(1), Article 1802908. https://doi.org/10.1080/20008198.2020.1802908

Gunnar, M., & Quevedo, K. (2007). The neurobiology of stress and development. *Annual Review of Psychology, 58*, 145–173. https://doi.org/10.1146/annurev.psych.58.110405.085605

Harlow, H. F., & Zimmerman, R. R. (1959). Affectional responses in the infant monkey: Orphaned baby monkeys develop a strong and persistent attachment to inanimate surrogate mothers. *Science, 130*(3373), 421–432. https://doi.org/10.1126/science.130.3373.421

Holmes, E. A., Brown, R. J., Mansell, W., Fearon, R. P., Hunter, E. C., Frasquilho, F., & Oakley, D. A. (2005). Are there two qualitatively distinct forms of dissociation? A review and some clinical implications. *Clinical Psychology Review, 25*(1), 1–23. https://doi.org/10.1016/j.cpr.2004.08.006

Imperatori, C., Adenzato, M., Palmiero, L., Farina, B., & Ardito, R. B. (2022). Assessment of unresolved/disorganized state of mind in relation to attachment: A ROC curve study using the adult attachment interview and the measure of parental style. *Clinical Neuropsychiatry, 19*(4), 197–205. https://doi.org/10.36131/cnfioritieditore20220402

Isobel, S., Goodyear, M., & Foster, K. (2019). Psychological trauma in the context of familial relationships: A concept analysis. *Trauma, Violence & Abuse, 20*(4), 549–559. https://doi.org/10.1177/1524838017726424

Janet, P. (1907). *The major symptoms of hysteria*. London/New York: Macmillan. Second edition with new matter: 1920. Reprint of 1920-edition: New York: Hafner, 1965.

Kearney, B. E., & Lanius, R. A. (2022). The brain-body disconnect: A somatic sensory basis for trauma-related disorders. *Frontiers in Neuroscience, 16*, Article 1015749. https://doi.org/10.3389/fnins.2022.1015749

Kozlowska, K., Walker, P., McLean, L., & Carrive, P. (2015). Fear and the defense cascade: Clinical implications and management. *Harvard Review of Psychiatry, 23*(4), 263–287. https://doi.org/10.1097/HRP.0000000000000065

Krause-Utz, A., Frost, R., Winter, D., & Elzinga, B. M. (2017). Dissociation and alterations in brain function and structure: Implications for borderline personality disorder. *Current Psychiatry Reports, 19*(1), 6. https://doi.org/10.1007/s11920-017-0757-y

Krug, E. G., Mercy, J. A., Dahlberg, L. L., & Zwi, A. B. (2002). The world report on violence and health. *Lancet, 360*(9339), 1083–1088. https://doi.org/10.1016/S0140-6736(02)11133-0

Lanius, R. A., Terpou, B. A., & McKinnon, M. C. (2020). The sense of self in the aftermath of trauma: Lessons from the default mode network in posttraumatic stress disorder. *European Journal of Psychotraumatology, 11*(1), 1807703. https://doi.org/10.1080/20008198.2020.1807703

Lauren, A. M., Lebois, L. A., Kaplan, C. S., Palermo, C. A., Pan, X., & Kaufman, M. L. (2022). A grounded theory of dissociative identity disorder: Placing DID in mind, brain, and body. In M. J. Dorahy, S. N. Gold & J. A. O'Neil (Eds.), *Dissociation and the dissociative disorder: Past, present, future* (pp. 392–408). Routledge. https://doi.org/10.4324/9781003057314

Le, T. L., Geist, R., Bearss, E., & Maunder, R. G. (2021). Childhood adversity and attachment anxiety predict adult symptom severity and health anxiety. *Child Abuse & Neglect, 120*, Article 105216. https://doi.org/10.1016/j.chiabu.2021.105216

Leerkes, E. M., Su, J., Calkins, S. D., O'Brien, M., & Supple, A. J. (2017). Maternal physiological dysregulation while parenting poses risk for infant attachment disorganization and behavior problems. *Development and Psychopathology, 29*(1), 245–257. https://doi.org/10.1017/S0954579416000122

Linde-Krieger, L. B., Yates, T. M., & Carlson, E. A. (2022). A developmental pathways model of dissociation. In M. J. Dorahy, S. N. Gold & J. A. O'Neil (Eds,), *Dissociation and the dissociative disorder: Past, present, future* (pp. 149–160). Routledge. https://doi.org/10.4324/9781003057314

Liotti, G. (1992). Disorganized/disoriented attachment in the etiology of the dissociative disorders. *Dissociation: Progress in the Dissociative Disorders, 5*(4), 196–204.

Liotti, G. (2004). Trauma, dissociation, and disorganized attachment: Three strands of a single braid. *Psychotherapy: Theory, Research, Practice, Training, 41*(4), 472–486. https://doi.org/10.1037/0033-3204.41.4.472

Liotti, G. (2017). The multimotivational approach to attachment-informed psychotherapy: A clinical illustration. *Psychoanalytic Inquiry, 37*(5), 319–331. https://doi.org/10.1080/07351690.2017.1322426

Liotti, G., & Farina, B. (2016). Painful incoherence: The self in borderline personality disorder. In M. Kyrios, R. Moulding, G. Doron, S. S. Bhar, M. Nedeljkovic & M. Mikulincer (Eds.), *The self in understanding and treating psychological disorders* (pp. 169–178). Cambridge University Press. https://doi.org/10.1017/CBO9781139941297.018

Lippard, E. T. C., & Nemeroff, C. B. (2020). The devastating clinical consequences of child abuse and neglect: Increased disease vulnerability and poor treatment response in mood disorders. *American Journal of Psychiatry, 177*(1), 20–36. https://doi.org/10.1176/appi.ajp.2019.19010020

Lord, C. J., & Ashworth, A. (2017). PARP inhibitors: Synthetic lethality in the clinic. *Science, 355*(6330), 1152–1158. https://doi.org/10.1126/science.aam7344

Lorenz, K. (1949). *Er redete mit dem Vieh, den Vögeln und un den Fishen*. Dr. Borotha-Schoeler Verlag.

Luyten, P., Campbell, C., Allison, E., & Fonagy, P. (2020). The mentalizing approach to psychopathology: State of the art and future directions. *Annual Review of Clinical Psychology, 16*, 297–325. https://doi.org/10.1146/annurev-clinpsy-071919-015355

Luyten, P., Campbell, C., & Fonagy, P. (2020). Borderline personality disorder, complex trauma, and problems with self and identity: A social-communicative approach. *Journal of Personality, 88*(1), 88–105. https://doi.org/10.1111/jopy.12483

Lyons-Ruth, K., Dutra, L., Schuder, M. R., & Bianchi, I. (2006). From infant attachment disorganization to adult dissociation: Relational adaptations or traumatic experiences? *The Psychiatric Clinics of North America, 29*(1), 63–viii. https://doi.org/10.1016/j.psc.2005.10.011

Massullo, C., De Rossi, E., Carbone, G. A., Imperatori, C., Ardito, R. B., Adenzato, M., & Farina, B. (2023). Child maltreatment, abuse, and neglect: An umbrella review of their prevalence and definitions. *Clinical Neuropsychiatry, 20*(2), 72–99. https://doi.org/10.36131/cnfioritieditore20230201

Massullo, C., Imperatori, C., De Vico Fallani, F., Ardito, R. B., Adenzato, M., Palmiero, L., Carbone, G. A., & Farina, B. (2022). Decreased brain network global efficiency after attachment memories retrieval in individuals with unresolved/disorganized attachment-related state of mind. *Scientific Reports, 12*(1), Article 4725. https://doi.org/10.1038/s41598-022-08685-0

McCrory, E. J., Gerin, M. I., & Viding, E. (2017). Annual research review: Childhood maltreatment, latent vulnerability, and the shift to preventative psychiatry – The contribution of functional brain imaging. *Journal of Child Psychology and Psychiatry, and Allied Disciplines, 58*(4), 338–357. https://doi.org/10.1111/jcpp.12713

McLaughlin, K. A., Sheridan, M. A., & Nelson, C. A. (2017). Neglect as a violation of species-expectant experience: Neurodevelopmental consequences. *Biological Psychiatry, 82*(7), 462–471. https://doi.org/10.1016/j.biopsych.2017.02.1096

Meares, R. (2012). *A dissociation model of borderline personality disorder*. W. W. Norton.
Midolo, L. R., Santoro, G., Ferrante, E., Pellegriti, P., Russo, S., Costanzo, A., & Schimmenti, A. (2020). Childhood trauma, attachment and psychopathology: A correlation network approach. *Mediterranean Journal of Clinical Psychology, 8*(2). https://doi.org/10.6092/2282-1619/mjcp-2418
Mysliwiec, V., Brock, M. S., Creamer, J. L., O'Reilly, B. M., Germain, A., & Roth, B. J. (2018). Trauma associated sleep disorder: A parasomnia induced by trauma. *Sleep Medicine Reviews, 37*, 94–104. https://doi.org/10.1016/j.smrv.2017.01.004
Nazarov, A., Frewen, P., Parlar, M., Oremus, C., MacQueen, G., McKinnon, M., & Lanius, R. (2014). Theory of mind performance in women with posttraumatic stress disorder related to childhood abuse. *Acta Psychiatrica Scandinavica, 129*(3), 193–201. https://doi.org/10.1111/acps.12142
Nijenhuis, E. R. (2009). Somatoform dissociation and somatoform dissociative disorders. In P. Dell & J. O. O'Neil (Eds), *Dissociation and dissociative disorders* (pp. 259–275). Routledge. https://doi.org/10.4324/9781003057314
Nijenhuis, E. R. (2019). Multiple first-person perspectives in PTSD. *Constructivist Foundations, 14*(2), 218–221. constructivist.info/14/2/218.
Nijenhuis, E. R., & van der Hart, O. (2011). Dissociation in trauma: A new definition and comparison with previous formulations. *Journal of Trauma & Dissociation: The Official Journal of the International Society for the Study of Dissociation (ISSD), 12*(4), 416–445. https://doi.org/10.1080/15299732.2011.570592
Oosterman, M., De Schipper, J. C., Fisher, P., Dozier, M., & Schuengel, C. (2010). Autonomic reactivity in relation to attachment and early adversity among foster children. *Development and Psychopathology, 22*(1), 109–118. https://doi.org/10.1017/S0954579409990290
Park, H. J., & Friston, K. (2013). Structural and functional brain networks: From connections to cognition. *Science, 342*(6158), Article 1238411. https://doi.org/10.1126/science.1238411
Pears, K. C., & Fisher, P. A. (2005). Emotion understanding and theory of mind among maltreated children in foster care: Evidence of deficits. *Development and Psychopathology, 17*(01). https://doi.org/10.1017/S0954579405050030
Purcell, J. (1996). Book reviews. *Work, Employment and Society, 10*(1), 191–193. https://doi.org/10.1177/0950017096101018
Putnam, F. W. (1997). *Dissociation in children and adolescents: A developmental perspective*. Guilford Press.
Radulovic, J., Lee, R., & Ortony, A. (2018). State-dependent memory: Neurobiological advances and prospects for translation to dissociative amnesia. *Frontiers in Behavioral Neuroscience, 12*, 259. https://doi.org/10.3389/fnbeh.2018.00259
Rifkin-Graboi, A., Kong, L., Sim, L. W., Sanmugam, S., Broekman, B. F., Chen, H., Wong, E., Kwek, K., Saw, S. M., Chong, Y. S., Gluckman, P. D., Fortier, M. V., Pederson, D., Meaney, M. J., & Qiu, A. (2015). Maternal sensitivity, infant limbic structure volume and functional connectivity: A preliminary study. *Translational Psychiatry, 5*(10), e668. https://doi.org/10.1038/tp.2015.133
Romeo, A., Tesio, V., Ghiggia, A., Di Tella, M., Geminiani, G. C., Farina, B., & Castelli, L. (2022). Traumatic experiences and somatoform dissociation in women with fibromyalgia. *Psychological Trauma: Theory, Research, Practice and Policy, 14*(1), 116–123. https://doi.org/10.1037/tra0000907
Salami, A., Andreu-Perez, J., & Gillmeister, H. (2020). Symptoms of depersonalisation/derealisation disorder as measured by brain electrical activity: A systematic review. *Neuroscience and Biobehavioral Reviews, 118*, 524–537. https://doi.org/10.1016/j.neubiorev.2020.08.011
Santoro, G., Midolo, L. R., Costanzo, A., & Schimmenti, A. (2021). The vulnerability of insecure minds: The mediating role of mentalization in the relationship between attachment styles and psychopathology. *Bulletin of the Menninger Clinic, 85*(4), 358–384. https://doi.org/10.1521/bumc.2021.85.4.358
Şar, V. (2017). Parallel-distinct structures of internal world and external reality: Disavowing and re-claiming the self-identity in the aftermath of trauma-generated dissociation. *Frontiers in Psychology, 8*, 216. https://doi.org/10.3389/fpsyg.2017.00216
Sar, V., Akyüz, G., Kundakçi, T., Kiziltan, E., & Dogan, O. (2004). Childhood trauma, dissociation, and psychiatric comorbidity in patients with conversion disorder. *The American Journal of Psychiatry, 161*(12), 2271–2276. https://doi.org/10.1176/appi.ajp.161.12.2271
Scalabrini, A., Mucci, C., & Northoff, G. (2022). The nested hierarchy of self and its trauma: In search for a synchronic dynamic and topographical re-organization. *Frontiers in Human Neuroscience, 16*, Article 980353. https://doi.org/10.3389/fnhum.2022.980353
Schimmenti, A. (2012). Unveiling the hidden self: Developmental trauma and pathological shame. *Psychodynamic Practice: Individuals, Groups and Organisations, 18*(2), 195–211. https://doi.org/10.1080/14753634.2012.664873

Schimmenti, A. (2013). Trauma evolutivo: origini e conseguenze dell'abuso e della trascuratezza nell'infanzia [Developmental trauma: On the origins and consequences of child abuse and neglect]. In V. Caretti, G. Craparo & A. Schimmenti (Eds.), *Memorie traumatiche e mentalizzazione. Teoria, ricerca e clinica* (pp. 17–36). Astrolabio Ubaldini.

Schimmenti, A. (2014). Il trauma evolutivo e la ricerca dell'intimità: una prospettiva relazionale [Developmental trauma and the search for intimacy: A relational purview]. *Ricerca Psicoanalitica, 5*(1), 31–53. https://doi.org/10.3280/RPR2014-001004

Schimmenti, A. (2017). The developmental roots of dissociation: A multiple mediation analysis. *Psychoanalytic Psychology, 34*(1), 96–105. https://doi.org/10.1037/pap0000084

Schimmenti, A. (2018). The trauma factor: Examining the relationships among different types of trauma, dissociation, and psychopathology. *Journal of Trauma & Dissociation: The Official Journal of the International Society for the Study of Dissociation (ISSD), 19*(5), 552–571. https://doi.org/10.1080/15299732.2017.1402400

Schimmenti, A. (2021). The aggressor within. In O. B. Epstein (Ed.), *Shame matters* (pp. 114–132). Routledge. https://doi.org/10.4324/9781003175612-8

Schimmenti, A. (2022). The relationship between attachment and dissociation: Theory, research, and clinical implications. In M. J. Dorahy, S. N. Gold & J. A. O'Neil (Eds.), *Dissociation and the dissociative disorder: Past, present, future* (pp. 161–176). Routledge.

Schimmenti, A., & Caretti, V. (2010). Psychic retreats or psychic pits? Unbearable states of mind and technological addiction. *Psychoanalytic Psychology, 27*(2), 115–132. https://doi.org/10.1037/a0019414

Schimmenti, A., & Caretti, V., (2016). Linking the overwhelming with the unbearable: Developmental trauma, dissociation, and the disconnected self. *Psychoanalytic Psychology, 33*(1), 106–128. https://doi.org/10.1037/a0038019

Schore, A. N. (2003). *Affect regulation & the repair of the self.* W. W. Norton.

Schore, A. N. (2009). Attachment trauma and the developing right brain: Origins of pathological dissociation. In P. F. Dell & J. A. O'Neil (Eds.), *Dissociation and the dissociative disorders: DSM-V and beyond* (pp. 107–141). Routledge.

Speranza, A. M., Farina, B., Bossa, C., Fortunato, A., Maggiora Vergano, C., Palmiero, L., Quintigliano, M., & Liotti, M. (2022). The role of complex trauma and attachment patterns in intimate partner violence. *Frontiers in Psychology, 12*, Article 769584. https://doi.org/10.3389/fpsyg.2021.769584

Spinazzola, J., Hodgdon, H., Liang, L.-J., Ford, J. D., Layne, C. M., Pynoos, R., Briggs, E. C., Stolbach, B., & Kisiel, C. (2014). Unseen wounds: The contribution of psychological maltreatment to child and adolescent mental health and risk outcomes. *Psychological Trauma: Theory, Research, Practice, and Policy, 6*(Suppl. 1), S18–S28. https://doi.org/10.1037/a0037766

Spinazzola, J., van der Kolk, B., & Ford, J. D. (2018). When nowhere is safe: Interpersonal trauma and attachment adversity as antecedents of posttraumatic stress disorder and developmental trauma disorder. *Journal of Traumatic Stress, 31*(5), 631–642. https://doi.org/10.1002/jts.22320

Steele, K., Dorahy, M., & van der Hart, O. (2022) Dissociation versus alterations in consciousness: Related but different concepts. In M. J. Dorahy, S. N. Gold & J. A. O'Neil (Eds.), *Dissociation and the dissociative disorder: Past, present, future* (pp. 66–80). Routledge.

Stoltenborgh, M., Bakermans-Kranenburg, M. J., & van Ijzendoorn, M. H. (2013). The neglect of child neglect: A meta-analytic review of the prevalence of neglect. *Social Psychiatry and Psychiatric Epidemiology, 48*(3), 345–355. https://doi.org/10.1007/s00127-012-0549-y

Teicher, M. H., Samson, J. A., Anderson, C. M., & Ohashi, K. (2016). The effects of childhood maltreatment on brain structure, function and connectivity. *Nature Reviews Neuroscience, 17*(10), 652–666. https://doi.org/10.1038/nrn.2016.111

Terpou, A., Papadaki, A., Lappa, I. K., Kachrimanidou, V., Bosnea, L. A., & Kopsahelis, N. (2019). Probiotics in food systems: Significance and emerging strategies towards improved viability and delivery of enhanced beneficial value. *Nutrients, 11*(7), 1591. https://doi.org/10.3390/nu11071591

Terpou, B. A., Densmore, M., Théberge, J., Frewen, P., McKinnon, M. C., Nicholson, A. A., & Lanius, R. A. (2020). The hijacked self: Disrupted functional connectivity between the periaqueductal gray and the default mode network in posttraumatic stress disorder using dynamic causal modeling. *NeuroImage: Clinical, 27*, Article 102345. https://doi.org/10.1016/j.nicl.2020.102345

Troisi, A. (2020). Childhood trauma, attachment patterns, and psychopathology: An evolutionary analysis. In G. Spalletta, D. Janiri, F. Piras & G. Sani (Eds.), *Childhood trauma in mental disorders* (pp. 125–142). Springer International Publishing. https://doi.org/10.1007/978-3-030-49414-8_7

U.S. Department of Health and Human Services, Administration on Children, Youth and Families, Children's Bureau (2016). *Child Maltreatment Report 2015.* Retrieved from acf.hhs.gov/programs/cb/research-data-technology/statistics-research/child-maltreatment

Vachon, D. D., Krueger, R. F., Rogosch, F. A., & Cicchetti, D. (2015). Assessment of the harmful psychiatric and behavioral effects of different forms of child maltreatment. *JAMA Psychiatry, 72*(11), 1135–1142. https://doi.org/10.1001/jamapsychiatry.2015.1792

van der Hart, O. (2021). Trauma-related dissociation: An analysis of two conflicting models. *European Journal of Trauma & Dissociation, 5*(4), Article 100210. https://doi.org/10.1016/j.ejtd.2021.100210

van der Hart, O., & Dorahy, M. (2009). History of the concept of dissociation. In P. F. Dell & J. A. O'Neil (Eds.), *Dissociation and the dissociative disorders: DSM-V and beyond* (pp. 3–26). Routledge. https://doi.org/10.4324/9780203893920

van der Hart, O., Nijenhuis, E. R., & Steele, K. (2005). Dissociation: An insufficiently recognized major feature of complex posttraumatic stress disorder. *Journal of Traumatic Stress, 18*(5), 413–423. https://doi.org/10.1002/jts.20049

van der Kolk, B. A. (2016). Commentary: The devastating effects of ignoring child maltreatment in psychiatry—A commentary on Teicher and Samson 2016. *Journal of Child Psychology and Psychiatry and Allied Disciplines, 57*(3), 267–270. https://doi.org/10.1111/jcpp.12540

van der Kolk, B. A., Pelcovitz, D., Roth, S., Mandel, F. S., McFarlane, A., & Herman, J. L. (1996). Dissociation, somatization, and affect dysregulation: The complexity of adaptation of trauma. *American Journal of Psychiatry, 153*(Suppl 7), 83–93. https://doi.org/10.1176/ajp.153.7.83

Vergara-Lopez, C., Chaudoir, S., Bublitz, M., O'Reilly Treter, M., & Stroud, L. (2016). The influence of maternal care and overprotection on youth adrenocortical stress response: A multiphase growth curve analysis. *Stress, 19*(6), 567–575. https://doi.org/10.1080/10253890.2016.1222608

Weber, F. C., & Wetter, T. C. (2022). The many faces of sleep disorders in post-traumatic stress disorder: An update on clinical features and treatment. *Neuropsychobiology, 81*(2), 85–97.

White, L. O., Schulz, C. C., Schoett, M. J. S., Kungl, M. T., Keil, J., Borelli, J. L., & Vrtička, P. (2020). Conceptual analysis: A social neuroscience to interpersonal interaction in the context of disruption and disorganization of attachment (NAMDA). *Frontiers in Psychiatry, 11*, Article 517372. https://doi.org/10.3389/fpsyt.2020.517372

Winnicott, D. W. (1962). *The maturational process and the facilitating environment*. Routledge.

World Health Organization (WHO) (2006). *Preventing child maltreatment: A guide to taking action and generating evidence*. WHO.

Young, C. B., Raz, G., Everaerd, D., Beckmann, C. F., Tendolkar, I., Hendler, T., Fernández, G., & Hermans, E. J. (2017 Jan 11). Dynamic shifts in large-scale brain network balance as a function of arousal. *Journal of Neuroscience, 37*(2), 281–290.

5
AFFECT REGULATION, ATTACHMENT, AND THE DEVELOPING SOCIAL BRAIN

Implications for Assessment and Treatment of Dissociative Disorders

Richard M. Cross

Introduction

There has been a paradigm shift in child mental health to ensure that understanding the impacts of trauma and adversity is now embedded into many systems and approaches seeking to be trauma informed (APA, 2019). This knowledge has been lost and found for centuries. The harm inflicted in childhood is now seen as a fundamental source of much human suffering and a significant public health concern. No longer is this knowledge being pushed away from consciousness or dissociated by groups and societies. However, there is much more to be done.

We have seen a move away from pathologizing children's emotional and behavioral difficulties to seeing them within the context of evolutionary responses to survival and the ability to hold in our minds what may have occurred to make them feel the way they do. It is advantageous to hold this mindset as mental health professionals and organizational systems that seek to heal the harm caused by others. Humans can create the most hurtful, dark experiences that befall children, families, communities, and whole societies. The acknowledgment of this painful fact is immortalized by Robert Burn's (1784) line in his poem "Man Was Made to Mourn: A Dirge": "Man's inhumanity to man/ Makes countless thousands mourn!" The phrase has been used to describe a wide range of human atrocities, from war and genocide to everyday forms of cruelty and oppression.

The care, protection, and provision of nourishing experiences to help a developing infant are core tasks for adult primary caregivers. We now know the potential developmental impacts of the response's caregivers provide, which can be a power for good or bad. One only needs to look at an infant as young as three months old encountering a "still, non-expressional face" or response to their cues. The infant strives to make a connection, exhibits proximity-seeking behavior, and looks for the multitude of micro-expressions and gestures of caregivers (Tronick et al., 1978). Infants are very responsive to the experiences around them; it is hard-wired in their autonomic nervous system to seek connection. The importance of the earliest stages of development—often referred to as the first 1,000 days—cannot be understated (Shonkoff, 2016). Experiencing relational nourishment creates the building blocks for maintaining and sustaining intimate relationships; the skills of healthy attachment are to "seek care, give care, feel comfortable with an autonomous self, and negotiate" (Cassidy, 2001).

The children who enter our consulting rooms are often referred to us because of problematic behavior in relationships and the world around them, or toward themselves—for example, in the form of self-harm. Many times, these referrals come from educators, social workers, or concerned family members seeking to make a difference in the lives of the children. Often, behaviors can mask the underlying needs of the child. Therefore, care needs to be taken to understand what is being communicated by the child both verbally and nonverbally. The following information provides a framework for understanding what may be observed and felt within the consulting room with regard to attachment, affect regulation, and the developing social brain.

A key aim is to bring to life active ingredients that can aid our work in harnessing knowledge about attachment, affect regulation, trauma, and dissociation. The very antidote to these hurtful experiences is the creation of potent experiences for children that use empathy, patience, consistency, self-awareness, and playfulness, to name a few. I encourage you to consider harnessing some of these ideas in your clinical practice.

Social Beings

"The social and emotional world of children is just as important as their physical world" (Gopnik, 2010). Human beings are not inanimate objects; we are social beings, intrinsically connected, and shaped by the stimulus and experiences we have, particularly early in our development. The social brain of a child undergoes significant development during early childhood, and we are the only animal born with an extended period of absolute dependence on others for our care and protection. This learning is much more than acquiring knowledge. At its core, it is about learning how to be a person, and is shaped by the child's environment and relationships with others.

The social brain refers to the network of neural circuits involved in processing social information and regulating social behavior. These circuits include regions of the prefrontal cortex, amygdala, and other brain structures, and undergo significant development during early childhood, shaped by the child's environment and relationships with others. As early as 42 minutes after birth, infants can mimic the facial gestures of the adult. If the adult sticks out their tongue, the infant will stick out theirs: "It sticks out its tongue, in reply to the same action by the other, before it has even realized that it has a tongue, thereby demonstrating a lived sense of corporeal equivalences" (Crossley, 1996, p. 51).

Colwyn Trevarthen (1979) first coined the term "primary intersubjectivity," which was described as communication between infant and adult made up of sounds and facial and body language, which can build into a meaningful exchange. This supports the notion of the infant being *active* in the interaction with the caregiver, and the significance of early preverbal exchanges that build the internalized structures for subsequent communications based on the quality of relating experiences by the infant. This concept emphasizes that the nature of these exchanges become meaningful for the infant, in this respect their quality begins to shape the internal structures which influence future communication and engagement in relationships. I recommend this be held in mind when we consider the potential developmental trajectory of infants who experience communication that is filled with fear and dread and who are left without responsive love and care.

Attachment Theory

Our understanding of how trauma affects children began in the events surrounding the Second World War; this backdrop provided increased awareness of the impact of early experiences on children's psychological development. Two seminal studies by Anna Freud and Dorothy Burlingham (1943) and Rene Spitz (1945) highlighted the crucial role of caregivers' responses in shaping children's reactions to stress events, the effects of parental trauma on children's emotional and cognitive development, and the importance of attachment to and separation from primary caregivers for healthy psychological development.

In contrast, parents' inconsistent, dismissive, or neglectful responses were associated with maladaptive coping strategies and long-term emotional and behavioral difficulties. Parental trauma profoundly impacts the parent-child relationship, with traumatized parents struggling to provide their children with the emotional support and stability necessary for healthy development. Rene Spitz (1945) found that infants placed in hospital care without their mothers experienced emotional withdrawal, decreased responsiveness to social cues, and diminished cognitive abilities. The severity of these effects was related to the length of separation from the mother, indicating the importance of maintaining close contact between infants and their primary caregivers for healthy psychological development.

Together, these studies provide important insights into the impact of early experiences on children's psychological development. They highlight the crucial role of caregivers in promoting healthy development, the effects of parental trauma on children's emotional and cognitive development, and the significance of attachment to and separation from primary caregivers for healthy psychological development. This research set the stage for what has become one of the most essential frameworks for understanding human development: attachment theory.

Mikulincer and Shaver (2016) stated that "attachment theory has emerged as one of the most important frameworks for understanding human development, personality, and psychopathology" (p. 3).

John Bowlby was a British psychoanalyst who drew on his psychoanalysis training to develop his attachment theory. He was influenced by the work of Melanie Klein, his supervisor during his analytical training, and her focus on the importance of early relationships with caregivers in shaping the developing psyche (Bowlby, 1951). However, he broke new ground by moving away from the intrapsychic fantasy-filled world of the infant to an approach that placed at its center the intrapersonal nature of our relationships and how this shapes our inner world.

Bowlby's theory of attachment was also informed by his observations of children and their caregivers. He conducted extensive interviews with children who had been separated from their parents and noted the profound emotional distress they experienced (1958). His work with emotionally disturbed youth also influenced his attachment theory. He observed that many of these children had experienced early disruptions in their attachment relationships, which he believed contributed to their emotional difficulties (1952).

It is essential to understand the experiences of Bowlby and what lay behind the importance he placed on real-life events for children. He worked in a child guidance clinic, with two social workers, which brought into sharp focus the importance and reality of what was happening with their clients. His work led him to pioneer the view that compounding adversity can impact the developing child.

In 1973, Bowlby wrote:

> When the high incidence of such threats in the lives of children is borne in mind, along with the cumulative effects of actual separations, of threats of separation, of unstable substitute care, and of unstable family life, the fact that many children grow up to be anxiously attached becomes explicable. In the light of these findings, moreover, a number of clinical syndromes can be better understood.
>
> *(p. 274)*

Bowlby's observation highlights what we now know: that adverse childhood experiences (ACEs) can compound difficulties over time, leading to an increased risk of mental health problems and difficulties with relationships and other aspects of life in adulthood. Bowlby believed that early experiences with attachment figures, particularly the mother, were crucial in shaping a child's development at a biological level.

This understanding is similarly embraced by the ACEs study that emerged from the clinical observations of Dr. Vincent Felitti et al. (1998), a medical epidemiologist at the Centers for Disease Control and Prevention (CDC). Dr. Felitti noticed that many of his patients at a weight loss clinic he ran had experienced childhood trauma, such as physical or sexual abuse, which led to their dropping out of the program or regaining weight after initial success. These observations led to the ACEs study investigating the relationship between ACEs and various health outcomes.

However, one key point I would like to make here is that it is not enough to simply use an ACEs score: we must understand the "relational environment" the developing child is in and the level of harshness and unresponsiveness that characterizes the child's daily care experiences. These experiences impact the developing infant at a biological level as they try to develop neurobiological structures to cope with unpredictability, overwhelming anxiety, and a lack of meaning.

Bowlby theorized that every child has an evolved behavioral system activated by fear. His work was heavily influenced by that of ethologists such as Konrad Lorenz and Nikolaas Tinbergen (Lorenz, 1935; Tinbergen et al., 1970), who studied the instinctive behavior of animals in their natural environments. Importantly, this behavior aided in the survival of the species. The offspring of animals were evolutionarily programmed to imprint on and seek to maintain proximity to the adult. The mother-infant interactions become imprinted as interiorized actions, a repertoire of automated ways of acting and being with the attachment figure. Bowlby referred to this attachment behavioral system as the internal working model (IWM). It is viewed as part of our survival system, including fight-flight-freeze reactions. His theory of attachment has also been influenced by a large body of empirical research on attachment, including studies of attachment behaviors in infants and young children and research on the impact of early attachment experiences on later development (Ainsworth et al., 1978).

Proximity Seeking and the Survival System

When an immature primate goes off exploring and finds itself too far from its mother's side, it becomes afraid. With the onset of fear, the *exploration system* is deactivated, and the attachment system is activated (Abbott & Hearn, 1978). The young primate first looks for its mother and assesses whether she is paying attention and if she is alarmed by reading her facial expressions or the nature of the call if given (Andrew, 1963). The mother then performs a "safe haven" function by welcoming the return of the infant. If the infant is reassured of safety by referencing nonverbal communication from the mother's face and posture, the mother is performing a secure base function (note the importance of hearing what is not said from a distance).

In this way, the attachment system aims to restore a sense of "felt security," which allows the child to explore. The function of the attachment figure is to help return the frightened child to a regulated state. Mary Main (1996) stated that the infant will "(a) continually monitor the accessibility of one or an few protective, older "attachment figures" (usually but not necessarily biological relatives) and to (b) flee to these individuals as a haven of safety in times of alarm" (p. 237). When the child cannot feel safe because the parent is consistently unavailable, unpredictable, or frightening, the basic conditions that promote early mental health are severely undermined (Lieberman & Van Horn, 2008). It is hoped that the responses to the child by the caregiver can be conceptualized as "good enough care" (Winnicott, 1956). Donald Winnicott (1896–1971) made significant contributions to the field of child development and psychoanalysis. He is best known for his theories on the importance of mother-infant interactions and the concept of the "good enough mother."

This means that caregivers should be able to meet their child's basic needs most of the time, provide emotional support, and create a dependable and safe environment, by recognizing and then responding to their child's emotional and physical needs, allowing the child to gradually develop a sense of independence and a feeling of being valued.

Clinical Example

A caregiver hears the infant crying and receives and interprets this communication that is signaling distress or discomfort. A good enough mother will then respond to her baby's cry, providing comfort and trying to understand the baby's needs: "Oh, I hear you. Are you too hot? Are you hungry or wet?" This might involve holding the baby, soothing them with a soft voice or gentle touch, or addressing any physical discomfort (such as hunger or a wet diaper). By consistently responding to the infant's needs, the mother helps the baby feel secure and develop trust in their environment.

This is not about being "perfect." Rupture and repair provide opportunities for the "good enough" caregiver and infant. For example, the mother might be a little delayed in responding due to missing the communication or having to respond to another infant, for example. Occasional failures or breaks in the mother's responsiveness are necessary for the child's growth. These breaks allow the child to experience frustration, develop coping skills, and gradually recognize that their mother is a separate individual with her limitations. This understanding is essential for the child's development of a separate sense of self.

This highlights the importance of a nurturing, responsive, and consistent caregiving environment for a child's healthy development. The developing child needs enough nourishment and comfort from the caregiver at times of stress or threat, and a sense of being secure enough in their care to be able to explore the environment and return in times of need. The child's expectations of how the attachment figure will respond guide the attachment system; it is an unconscious process, and the child does not have time to reflect on their responses to the adult. The secure child's attachment interactions are dominated by the attachment figure's reliable accessibility, interest, and sensitive responsiveness. Expectations based on such experiences establish trust in attachment figures' intentions and emotional competency.

Fear and Danger

There is a complex relationship between fear and attachment. Fear is a fundamental aspect of the human experience, linked to the activation of our limbic system, especially when it comes to survival. Early experiences with caregivers shape our ability to regulate emotions and respond to threats. Infants who receive consistent, sensitive care are more likely to develop a secure attachment style, which enables them to feel safe in the face of potential danger. By contrast, infants who experience inconsistent or insensitive care are more likely to develop insecure attachment styles, leading to difficulties regulating fear and anxiety.

Slade (2014) examined the psychic experience of fear, arguing that fear is not simply a physiological response to a threat but a complex and multifaceted phenomenon that involves cognitive, emotional, and relational processes. Fear is linked to unconscious desires and conflicts and shapes our sense of self and our relationships with others—highlighting the complex interplay between attachment, threat, and psychic experience in the development of fear.

Holding a position of curiosity and "unknowing" in trauma and dissociation work allows for the unfolding in greater detail of the child's world, so we can meet the child or young person where they are. We must take great care not to allow our assumptions and beliefs prevent us from creating a culture of curiosity and inquiry with the child. Children who have experienced trauma have great difficulty knowing themselves and elements of their lives, such as the double bind of acknowledging the abusive betrayal of the primary caregiver.

In the child psychotherapeutic process, we harness what we know about the child's external world and continually hold the position of making sense of the child's inner world. We do not use a blunt instrument in this process, but develop an understanding through keeping in mind the large array of observations that can be made in the consultation room, which will allow the identification of patterns and meanings. How does the child regulate affect, in terms of both self-regulation and when another person is available to provide inter-relational regulation? What do we see and experience? This can provide rich qualitative insight that moves beyond that of psychometric measures; being able to experience the child's response within a relational context can illuminate the child's ideas about self, others, and the world. Over time, this provides a series of observations and interpretations that should be cross-validating in terms of also harnessing information from psychometrics and interviews with caregivers.

Case Example[1]

John was a five-year-old boy who had been removed from his family of origin due to chronic neglect, harm, and abuse. On entering the room for his first session, he quickly ran over to me and attempted to almost climb up my body, as though it were a tree. He then noticed the sand tray (sand play) and he leapt from my body to go play in it. At first, he was laughing, but his play became more and more chaotic. Sand from the tray ended up on the floor as his movements became increasingly frantic. I was opposite him by this point, and I took a deep breath to slow my breathing. He looked at me, his eyes wide with fear, and said, "I made a mess, I am bad." I smiled and paused. Then I said, "We are going to have fun putting all the sand back in the tray together later. We can do that at the end." John giggled, his movements slowed, and he relaxed. He began to use the sand tray to explore a situation of adults being angry at children for being "naughty."

Attachment Styles

Attachment styles refer to the emotional bond between infants and their primary caregivers. This bond is crucial, as it influences the child's emotional, social, and cognitive development. Mary Ainsworth (1978) initially identified three main attachment styles: secure, insecure-avoidant, insecure-anxious/ambivalent, and then in later research, disorganized/disoriented (Main & Solomon, 1990b). Secure attachment is characterized by infants who use their caregiver as a secure base for exploration and seek comfort from them when distressed. This style embodies the ability to self-regulate, but when resources feel scarce, there is also the ability to reach out within the dyadic for inter-relational regulation.

Insecure-avoidant attachment is characterized by children who avoid their caregiver when distressed and do not seek comfort from them. Insecure-anxious/ambivalent attachment is characterized by children who are clingy and anxious with their caregiver but also have an inconsistent response to their caregiver's comforting responses. Disorganized attachment is considered the most problematic attachment style. It is associated with various adverse outcomes, including behavioral problems, emotional dysregulation, problems in social relationships (Liotti, 2004), and interpersonal difficulties (Carlson et al., 1989). Children with disorganized attachment exhibit odd, contradictory, and disoriented behaviors in the presence of their caregivers. For instance, they may approach their caregiver while looking away, or freeze, have dazed facial expressions, or exhibit contradictory behavior toward their caregiver.

Disorganized attachment is illustrated by the child who is in a conflicted position of wanting to seek proximity to the carer but also wanting to avoid them (Main & Solomon, 1990b). I characterize this as a situation of fear that cannot be resolved, as the child cannot develop a consistent strategy for coping with the unpredictable caregiving behavior. This often creates a situation where the polarities of frightened or frightening behavior can be experienced. Infant disorganized attachment is significant due to its impact on childhood psychopathology and dissociation (Beebe et al., 2012).

When the child cannot feel safe because the parent is consistently unavailable, unpredictable, or frightening, the primary conditions that promote early mental health are severely undermined (Lieberman & Van Horn, 2008). This is most likely to occur when the caregiver is either frightened or frightening the "attachment figure … is at once the source of and solution to its alarm" (Main & Hesse, 1990, p. 163). Another area that needs to be kept in mind is what the caregiver brings the relationship with respect to projections and attributions, which become the child's (Lieberman & Zeanah, 1999), these being the internal representations of the caregivers which can become part of the child's internal sense of self, others and the world around them. These are sometimes referred to as "ghosts in the nursery" (Fraiberg et al., 1975), which begin to define the child's sense of reality and self.

In my work with foster caregivers, residential care, and adopted families, bringing the unspeakable to life and addressing these underlying transference positions of fear without solution is crucial to ensure "containment" (Bion, 1962; Main & Solomon, 1990a) of the system around the child to ensure emotional holding is possible (Winnicott, 1965). According to Bion (1962), it is through the process of containment that the infant's most unmanageable feelings and deepest anxieties are "projected" onto the parent so that, initially at least, the parent can feel them for him or her, before handing them back in a more manageable form. This is directly connected to development over time of reflective functioning and being able to think and feel. This early thinking, by Wilfred Bion, describes this process as the transformation of raw or concrete material states ("beta-elements") into more tolerable thinkable experiences ("alpha-functions"); the caregiver "digests" the beta-element and then gives them back to the child in a milder form. If this process does not occur, then the child's anxieties are unprocessed, and become that which has been termed "nameless dread." According to Bion (1962),

> it depends for its efficacy on the mother's capacity for reverie [the capacity to make sense of what's going on in the infant]. If the mother fails, then the burden is thrown on the infant's capacity for toleration of frustration for now its capacity for toleration of thought itself is tested.
>
> (p. 37)

Unresolved attachment is a subtype of disorganized attachment that occurs when infants experience traumatic or unresolved experiences, such as parental loss or abuse. Infants with unresolved attachment show a disorganized pattern of behavior, like those with disorganized attachment; however, they also display signs of distress or confusion when discussing their attachment experiences in later life (Hesse & Main, 2000). Unresolved attachment is linked to various adverse outcomes, including personality disorders, dissociative symptoms, and self-harm behaviors (Lyons-Ruth & Jacobvitz, 2008).

Disrupted attachment relationships in infancy have been correlated to higher dissociative symptoms in adulthood, such as dissociative behaviors, altered states of consciousness, and self-harm behaviors, compared to infants with secure attachment relationships (Lyons-Ruth et al., 1998). Similarly, those who had experienced traumatic events in infancy, such as physical abuse or neglect, showed higher dissociative symptoms, such as numbing, derealization, and depersonalization, compared to non-traumatized infants (Carlson et al., 1989).

The Beginning: Attachment, Self, and Others

Before proceeding, it must be emphasized that attachment begins in the uterus before the infant is born into the world (please see the chapter on the Calming Womb Family Therapy Model for more information). Klaus and Kennell (1976) wrote: "Attachment begins in the womb, where the child spends nine months intimately attached to the mother." The emotional bond between a woman and her unborn baby is formed during pregnancy and plays a vital role in the development of the mother-child relationship as well as significantly impacting the health and well-being of both the mother and the baby. According to Winnicott (1992, Original work published, 1964), "there is no such thing as a baby, there is a baby and someone" (p. 8).

Prenatal attachment has been linked to several positive outcomes for the mother and baby. For the mother, prenatal attachment has been associated with lower levels of anxiety and depression during pregnancy (Alhusen et al., 2012). It has also been shown to be a protective factor against postpartum depression (Mercer, 2004). For the baby, prenatal attachment has been linked to better fetal development and improved outcomes in infancy and childhood (Brandon et al., 2009).

Case Example

Sarah is 26 years old and 20 weeks pregnant with her first child. She is married and in a stable relationship with a supportive partner. Her early developmental history is characterized by adversity, her parents were neglectful and emotionally unavailable to Sarah.

She is attending psychotherapy due to her experiences of anxiety. Sarah's therapist, who has experience in prenatal attachment work, has noticed that she is struggling since she disclosed the news of her pregnancy. Sarah expresses that she feels disconnected from her pregnancy and unborn baby. She reports feeling guilty for not feeling more attached and worries that this lack of attachment means she will not be a good mother.

Sarah requires reassurance that her feelings are normal and that she can work on developing a stronger bond with her baby; prenatal attachment can be fostered through various activities, such as talking to the baby, singing, reading stories, and even imagining what the baby will look like. Over the subsequent few sessions, the work with Sarah focuses on developing strategies for fostering prenatal attachment. Sarah practices guided imagery exercises during which she imagines holding and cuddling her baby. Sarah begins to talk to her baby and share her hopes and dreams for their future together. She and the therapist also discuss ways to reduce Sarah's anxiety, such as breathing exercises and mindfulness practices.

After several weeks of therapy, Sarah reports feeling more connected to her baby. She has even started reading children's books to her unborn baby and describes automatically relating to the baby through talk and caringly holding her stomach. This illustrates that the development of an infant is closely intertwined with the social and cultural context in which they are raised, and that it is impossible to fully grasp the nature of an infant without considering their relationships with others. It is essential to see the developing child not as being separate entity from those around them, and to understand the innate responsiveness of the child is to seek to adapt to the responses of the caregiver to maximize the proximity which is regardless of the levels of maternal stimulation and maternal responsiveness.

Affect Regulation

It should come as no surprise that affect regulation is a crucial aspect of human development and that early experiences with caregivers play a critical role in shaping this development. The importance of early caregiving experiences in shaping emotional development, with secure attachment and positive caregiving experiences, promotes healthy affect regulation and resilience. Effective affect regulation allows individuals to navigate the ups and downs of life and maintain stable relationships with others.

In contrast, insecure attachment and negative caregiving experiences can lead to difficulties regulating emotions and increased vulnerability to psychopathology. In infancy, maternal withdrawal is a predictor of both borderline symptoms and suicidality/self-injury in late adolescence (Lyons-Ruth et al., 2013). This withdrawal response by the caregiver is also connected to the child adapting and utilizing strategies of disorganized, controlling behavior. As early as age 8 this caregiver response is seen as contributed independently to the prediction of borderline symptoms. Strikingly, this research identified that such early toxic experiences of disturbed interactions at as early as 18 months old can set the foundation for suicidality and self-harm in adulthood.

As Schore (1994) states:

> The core of self lies in patterns of affect regulation that integrate a sense of self across state transitions, thereby allowing for a continuity of inner experience. Dyadic failures of affect regulation result in the developmental psychopathology that underlies various forms of later forming psychiatric disorders.
>
> *(p. 33)*

Case Example

Imagine a scenario where a caregiver interacts with their five-month-old infant who becomes fussy, irritable, and distressed. By noticing micro nonverbal communication, the adult sees that the infant is starting to become upset, and responds in a way that to develop the infant's affect regulation skills. The caregiver calmly connects to the infant, makes eye contact, and begins to speak in a soothing and reassuring tone of voice, using simple phrases like, "Oh… it is okay, it is okay… I am here" and "You're feeling upset, aren't you… we will make it better." The caregiver picks up the infant and holds them close, rocking them gently back and forth (inter-regulatory soothing and calming).

As the adult continues calming the infant, they may introduce new sensory experiences to help distract the baby from their distress. Maybe they use a soft, plush toy to stroke the baby's cheek or introduce a musical toy to play a soothing melody. Often children develop a particular connection to a favorite toy for soothing. Throughout this interaction, the caregiver remains calm and consistent, which helps the infant feel safe and secure. Over time, the infant learns to associate this type of interaction with comfort and stability, which leads to the development of affect regulation skills.

By responding in this way, caregivers provide the infant with the tools necessary to regulate their emotions and develop a healthy and secure to them.

At this point, it can be helpful to reflect, as the reader, on the responses you may have to a child in the therapeutic space who becomes distressed. How may you act to provide co-regulation and what may hinder this?

The development of the emotion regulation involves a complex interplay between the brain and the body, with the prefrontal cortex, limbic system, and autonomic nervous system all playing essential roles (Panksepp, 1998; Panksepp & Biven, 2012). Panksepp's (1998) research on affect regulation has contributed significantly to our understanding of how emotions are processed and regulated in the brain. He proposed that seven basic emotional systems in the brain are responsible for affect regulation: seeking, rage, fear, lust, care, panic/grief, and play. These emotional systems are thought to have evolved to help animals navigate their environments and respond to different threats and opportunities. Early attachment experiences such as the one in the case example above demonstrate how attunement with caregivers provides the foundation for developing these systems and regulatory capacities for use later in life.

The Importance of Affect Regulation

Supporting affect regulation is particularly important in children, as they are still developing the cognitive and emotional skills to manage their emotions effectively. Effective affect regulation is critical for healthy child development. Children who struggle to manage their emotions are at risk of various adverse outcomes, including anxiety, depression, behavioral problems, and academic difficulties (Eisenberg et al., 2010). In addition, they may have difficulty forming and maintaining positive relationships with others, which can have long-lasting effects on their social development (Thompson & Meyer, 2007). Effective affect regulation, however, is associated with a range of positive outcomes, including greater academic achievement, better social skills, and fewer behavior problems (Denham et al., 2014).

The work of Schore (2012) has influenced our understanding of the importance of early experiences in emotional development and the role of the brain and body in affect regulation. His work has also informed therapeutic approaches in promoting healthy emotional regulation and addressing emotional dysregulation in various psychological disorders. Affect regulation involves the conscious and voluntary control processes that influence our emotions and how we express them behaviorally. Recent data suggests that unconscious affect regulation may be even more crucial for human survival than conscious emotion regulation (Schore, 2016).

The development of knowledge around trauma and dissociation has highlighted the crucial role of the autonomic nervous system (ANS) in regulating emotional responses to stress. Early relational trauma can disrupt ANS functioning and lead to chronic dysregulation of affect and arousal, contributing to dissociative disorders, as we have read in previous chapters. As mental health professionals, we must expand our training to incorporate a sound foundation of neurobiology, the natural and normal body responses, including the range of hormones released during traumatic situations such as sexual abuse (De Bellis et al., 2014), while also keeping in mind the adaptions that occur when our bodies are in a fight, flight, or freeze state for prolonged periods.

Polyvagal theory supports an understanding of affect regulation that suggests that individuals with a well-functioning ventral vagus nerve can better regulate their emotions and engage in social behaviors. However, those with a poorly functioning ventral vagus nerve may struggle with affect regulation and social engagement. Studies have found that interventions designed to improve vagal tone can improve emotional regulation and social behavior (Porges, 2011). Please see the chapter on polyvagal theory for more information.

Putting the Pieces Together: Attachment, Adversity, and Affect Regulation

Attachment theory, as we have seen, illustrates that early experiences with caregivers shape an individual's IWMs of self and others, influencing emotional regulation and responses to stressors throughout life. Secure attachment and adaptive affect regulation can serve as protective factors against the harmful effects of adversity (Bowlby, 1969). Research has shown that individuals with secure attachment styles and adaptive affect regulation strategies are less likely to develop mental health problems in response to stressors (Cicchetti & Toth, 2005; Mikulincer & Shaver, 2016).

However, maladaptive affect regulation strategies, such as emotional suppression or avoidance, can exacerbate negative emotions and increase the risk of mental health problems (Aldao et al., 2010; McLaughlin et al., 2011). Children who are cared for by foster parents or in group care who are disorganized and who have suffered trauma or maltreatment are at high risk of pathological dissociation, perhaps especially those who have experienced sexual abuse. Dissociation should therefore be at the forefront of clinicians' minds when working with this vulnerable population (Martin et al., 2022).

The interplay between adversity, attachment, and affect regulation is complex and multifaceted. Adversity can disrupt the development of secure attachment and lead to maladaptive affect regulation strategies, which increase the risk of mental health problems. Understanding the interplay between these factors is essential for developing interventions for children and young people who have experienced adversity and may have challenges around the impacts of the interpersonal nature of traumatic experiences.

Assessment: Attachment, Affect Regulation, and Dissociation

The assessment of attachment, affect regulation, and dissociation in children is an essential aspect of clinical practice due to its impact on child development and mental health outcomes and the ability to provide early interventions. We have advocated for a standardized assessment of attachment, trauma, and dissociation for children in high-risk groups such as those in foster care or residential group living homes (Cross, 2012) due to the level of difficulties assessed in pre-intake assessments for children who had been removed from their primary caregivers due to abuse, trauma, and neglect. While the following chapters in the book will speak to dissociation-specific assessment, the following sections will speak to the importance of engaging in assessment processes that explore attachment and regulatory capacities.

Attachment-Based Assessment

Given the importance of the early parent-child relationship, it is paramount to have effective and efficient ways to identify caregivers who may benefit from support and interventions. For instance, the Adult Attachment Interview (AAI) is a semi-structured interview and, as with all assessments, those administrating should have undertaken training and be in supervision with regard to its use (Main & Goldwyn, 1984). The AAI is used to categorize an adult's state of mind with respect to attachments. The classifications are secure-autonomous (F), dismissing (D), preoccupied (E), and disoriented/disorganized (U/d). The interview consists of 20 questions focusing on early relationships with parents and the family environment and takes between 45 and 90 minutes to administer.

Other approaches to screening for difficulties exist to aid in the identification of needs, and numerous parental report screening measures have been developed to assess both antenatal and postnatal attachment-oriented responses of the mother. Caregivers must be willing to disclose that things are difficult. When deciding to utilize an assessment measure, mental health professionals should scrutinize it to see that it meets the desired purpose, and then ensure the psychometric validity of each measure.

For example, the Maternal–Fetal Attachment Scale (MFAS), which was the first self-report questionnaire on antenatal maternal feelings toward the unborn baby (Cranley, 1981), has been researched, and attempts have been made to increase the psychometric properties (Busonera et al., 2016) of the original 24-item scale. The Postpartum Bonding Questionnaire (PBQ), which is designed to screen for difficulties in the mother-infant relationship, has been extensively used as a self-report questionnaire (Brockington et al., 2006) and has been adapted to several countries. This is a 25-item scale that is responded to on a six-point scale, so it can be completed in a timely manner by parents. The scale measures four factors: (1) general emotional factor, (2) anger toward and rejection of the baby, (3) infant focus anxiety, and (4) risk of abuse.

The most widely used measure of attachment in children is the Strange Situation Procedure (SSP), developed by Mary Ainsworth in the 1970s (Ainsworth et al., 1978). In this procedure, the child and caregiver are placed in a room with toys, and then the caregiver leaves the room, leaving the child alone with a stranger. The caregiver then returns to the room, and the stranger leaves. Finally, the caregiver leaves again, leaving the child alone. The procedure is designed to assess the child's attachment style based on their behavior during the different stages of the procedure. Securely attached children use the caregiver as a secure base from which to explore their environment, display distress when the caregiver leaves, and seek comfort from the caregiver when they return. Insecure-avoidant children do not seek comfort from the caregiver when they return, and may even avoid them. Insecure-resistant children show ambivalent behavior toward the caregiver, simultaneously seeking comfort and resisting it.

A child with disorganized attachment may display various confusing and contradictory behaviors. These children may seem overwhelmed and disoriented by the separation and reunion experiences in the Strange Situation and may display a lack of coherent attachment strategies. Some common behaviors displayed by children with disorganized attachment include:

- *Freezing or remaining motionless*: These children may appear stuck or unable to move, even when their caregiver leaves or returns.
- *Contradictory behaviors:* These children may show a mix of clinging and avoidant behaviors when their caregiver is present, indicating confusion about how to approach the caregiver.
- *Dazed or dissociated behavior*: These children may appear in a daze or dissociate from their surroundings, showing a lack of emotional regulation in response to separation and reunion experiences.
- *Fear or apprehension*: These children may show signs of fear or apprehension when their caregiver returns, even though they may have been seeking proximity to the caregiver moments before.

Another measure of attachment is the Attachment Q-Set (Waters & Deane, 1987), which involves observing the child in a naturalistic setting and rating their attachment-related behaviors. The Q-Set consists of 90 cards with statements describing attachment behaviors, and the observer sorts the cards into nine piles based on how well they describe the child's behavior. The resulting profile is used to assess the child's attachment style.

Attachment Assessment in Practice

The Story Stem Assessment Profile (SSAP) is a tool used to assess attachment in children between three and nine years old (Hodges et al., 2000). The SSAP is particularly useful in identifying attachment difficulties in children who have experienced early trauma or disruption in their caregiving relationships. It involves presenting the child with a set of story stems, which are incomplete stories that the child is encouraged to finish using a set of provided characters. The child's responses to the story stem are then analyzed and coded to assess their held "internal representations" of self and key relational figures. By identifying attachment difficulties early on, interventions can be implemented to promote healthy attachment relationships and improve outcomes for children.

The SSAP activity has demonstrated validity in identifying children's needs within the clinical population. For example, Hillman et al. (2020) reported that children in foster care displayed more disorganized, avoidant, and negative representations while at the same time having significantly fewer representations characteristic of "secure" attachment. Furthermore, the assessment also helps clinicians understand significant themes presented by children who have experienced trauma. For example, in a group of children who had experienced sexual abuse, three key themes emerged: blurred boundaries, a sense of threat, and a focus on sound (Mackin et al., 2022), though no direct projection of sexual abuse was evident in the assessment.

Using the SSAP assessment with children over time showed that *security* representations significantly increased, and *defensive-avoidance* ones decreased as the outcome of attachment-focused care. The SSAP helps demonstrate how secure representations can be developed in new caregiving relationships, which helps guide more reliable caregiving. However, the insecure and disorganized attachment might be more challenging and slower to modify, pointing ultimately to the importance of stability in care arrangements and the longer-term nature of therapeutic support (Hillman et al., 2022). In situations where caregivers were offered consultation which involves helping the caregiver to understand their own affective neurobiological responses and to ensure reflective capacity during their interactions. Over time, the gradual impact of the dyadic interactions illustrates significant improvement for many children and observes in the areas of both internalizing and externalizing behaviors, such as acts of anger, harmful behavior toward self, others, or the world around them.

Affect Regulation Assessment

A commonly used measure of affect regulation in children is the Emotion Regulation Checklist (ERC) (Shields & Cicchetti, 1995, 1997). The ERC is a 24-item caregiver report inventory that assesses the child's ability to regulate emotions and behavior in response to different situations. The items on the ERC are grouped into three subscales: lability/negativity, emotion regulation, and emotion expression. The lability/negativity subscale assesses the child's tendency to experience negative emotions and the intensity of their emotional responses. The emotion regulation subscale assesses the child's ability to regulate emotions in response to different situations. The emotion expression subscale assesses the child's ability to express their emotions in an appropriate and socially acceptable way.

Another measure of affect regulation is the Difficulties in Emotion Regulation Scale (DERS) (Gratz & Roemer, 2004). The DERS is a 36-item self-report inventory that assesses different aspects of emotion regulation, including awareness and understanding of emotions, acceptance of emotions, and strategies for emotion regulation. As a mental health professional, however, it is crucial to learn from the observational process and to follow the child's affective states and make sense of what they bring into the consultation room. We must utilize our sensitivity to assess the child's affective state; doing so will ensure our attunement is communicated. This shifts away from what could become affective contagion that could mirror the child's emotional state; professionals must ensure they harness these experiences for good purposeful, known understanding.

Creating Change

Schore's (2012) work has significantly contributed to the treatment of attachment, trauma, and dissociative disorders. He has argued that effective treatment requires a focus on both the cognitive and emotional aspects of the therapeutic relationship and an understanding of the neurobiological mechanisms underlying these disorders (the therapeutic relationship will be further expanded on in a later chapter). There are many techniques to aid the provision of support, which can at times feel like an alphabet soup of abbreviations. However, we will focus on some of the active ingredients that make treatment successful:

1 The relationship: the capacity to provide a healing experience and alternative working model of attachment
2 The ability to create affect tolerance and emotional management (self- and inter-regulation)
3 A therapeutic relationship to increase affect tolerance and build dual awareness for reprocessing traumatic material

One active ingredient continually stands out in treating complex trauma, namely, the ability to create a therapeutic relationship (whether between child and psychotherapist or between caregiver and child in dyadic approaches with young children) that can provide the necessary footbridge to increase internal connection and integration, focusing on the use of the interpersonal relationship to improve emotional regulation and self-soothing. Research has shown that a solid therapeutic relationship is associated with positive outcomes in treating trauma and dissociation in children and adolescents (Gil, 2010; Nuñez et al., 2022).

The ability to create safety and stabilization is critical to any intervention for children with histories of complex trauma and dissociative symptoms. To state the obvious, one must remember that this also includes the present external environment. Professionals often seek effective intervention for children but are often still grappling with the fact that the child is living within a "trauma-organized" system (Bentovim, 1992) where their survival strategies are still needed. Safety stabilization interventions focus on building skills for emotion regulation, mindfulness, and self-soothing, and providing education and support for families and caregivers. Despite the challenges that some children may face in regulating their emotions, various strategies can promote healthy affect regulation. One approach is to provide children with opportunities to engage in activities that promote emotional awareness and expression, such as art, music, or play therapy. These activities can help children identify and express their emotions in a safe and supportive environment, which can facilitate the development of effective affect regulation skills. Later chapters will focus specifically on the use of these modalities.

Another approach is to teach children specific strategies for managing their emotions, such as deep breathing, progressive muscle relaxation, or cognitive restructuring (Denham et al., 2014). These strategies can help children to regulate their emotions in the present moment and can also help build their overall affect regulation skills over time. However, it is essential to note that these strategies may not be effective for all children and may need to be adapted to meet the unique needs of individual children. It's important that adults begin to model and demonstrate affect regulation strategies to children and young people—for example, "I am going to slow things down a little; I am going to feel my feet on the floor and drink my cold water." We might be initially met with dismissal, but in future sessions, I often observe the child or adolescent utilizing the strategies practiced.

In addition to providing children with opportunities to engage in emotional expression and teaching specific affect regulation strategies, creating a supportive and nurturing environment for children involves consistent and responsive caregiving, and setting clear and consistent boundaries is crucial. In providing these, caregivers and professionals can help children develop the skills and resources necessary for healthy affect regulation. There is a need to ensure that during all stages of the therapeutic process, there are efforts to maintain therapeutic support to the child. Care should be taken to avoid destabilizing the child's environment, such as moving them away to another foster placement, such that the psychotherapy process would be interrupted or could not be completed.

Whenever possible, the healthy caregiving system should be mobilized, and at these times, the interactional dyadic should be between the child and the caregiver. Attachment-based interventions should focus on improving the relationship between the caregiver and the child. These interventions may involve teaching the caregiver to be more sensitive to the child's needs and emotions, promoting positive interactions between the caregiver and child, and helping the caregiver develop more consistent and predictable behavior patterns (Lyons-Ruth et al., 1990).

Conclusion

Affect regulation and attachment are critical factors in the development of the social brain, and disruptions in these processes can lead to a range of difficulties, such as disorganized attachment, affect regulation issues, and dissociative disorders. Assessment of affect regulation, attachment, and social development in children with complex trauma requires a comprehensive understanding of these processes and their interplay. Treatment approaches should target the underlying mechanisms of affect regulation and attachment, as well as promote the development of healthy social connections. Psychotherapy, particularly attachment-based therapy, has shown promising results in treating dissociative disorders. Overall, a greater emphasis on affect regulation and attachment in assessment and treatment can help improve outcomes.

Note

1 Case examples in this chapter are compilations of hypothetical cases.

References

Abbott, D. H., & Hearn, J. P. (1978). Physical, hormonal and behavioral aspects of sexual development in the marmoset monkey, *Callithrix jacchus. Journal of Reproduction and Fertility, 53*(1), 155–166. https://doi.org/10.1530/jrf.0.0530155

Ainsworth, M. D. S., Blehar, M. C., Waters, E., & Wall, S. (1978). *Patterns of attachment: A psychological study of the strange situation.* Lawrence Erlbaum.

Aldao, A., Nolen-Hoeksema, S., & Schweizer, S. (2010). Emotion-regulation strategies across psychopathology: A meta-analytic review. *Clinical Psychology Review, 30*(2), 217–237. https://doi.org/10.1016/j.cpr.2009.11.004

Alhusen, J. L., Gross, D., Hayat, M. J., Woods, A. B., & Sharps, P. (2012). The role of mental health on maternal-fetal attachment in low-income women. *Journal of Obstetric, Gynecologic, & Neonatal Nursing, 41*(6), E71–81. https://doi.org/10.1111/j.1552-6909.2012.01385.x

American Psychological Association (APA). (2019). *APA handbook of trauma psychology: Vol. 1. Foundations in knowledge.* APA Publishing.

Andrew, R. J. (1963). The origin and evolution of the calls and facial expressions of the primates. *Behaviour, 20*(1/2), 1–109. https://www.jstor.org/stable/4533025

Beebe, B., Lachmann, F., Markese, S., & Bahrick, L. (2012). On the origins of disorganized attachment and internal working models: Paper I. A dyadic systems approach. *Psychoanalytic Dialogues, 22*(2), 253–272. https://doi.org/10.1080/10481885.2012.666147

Bentovim, A. (1992). *Trauma-organized systems: Physical and sexual abuse in families* (1st ed.). Routledge.

Bion, W. R. (1962). *Learning from experience.* Karnac Books.

Bowlby, J. (1951). Maternal care and mental health. *Bulletin of the World Health Organization, 3,* 355–533.

Bowlby, J. (1952). Some pathological processes set in train by early mother–child separation. *Journal of Mental Science, 99*(415), 265–272. https://doi.org/10.1192/bjp.99.415.265

Bowlby, J. (1958). The nature of the child's tie to his mother. *International Journal of Psychoanalysis, 39,* 350–373.

Bowlby, J. (1969). *Attachment and loss: Vol. 1.* Attachment. Basic Books.

Bowlby, J. (1973). *Attachment and loss: Vol. 2.* Separation: Anxiety and anger. Basic Books.

Brandon, A. R., Pitts, S., Denton, W. H., Stringer, C. A., & Evans, H. M. (2009). A history of the theory of prenatal attachment. *Journal of Prenatal & Perinatal Psychology & Health, 23*(4), 201–222.

Brockington, I. F., Fraser, C., & Wilson, D. (2006). The postpartum bonding questionnaire: A validation. *Archives of Women's Mental Health, 9*(5), 233–242. https://doi.org/10.1007/s00737-006-0132-1

Busonera, A., Cataudella, S., Lampis, J., Tommasi, M., & Zavattini, G. C. (2016). Psychometric properties of a 20-item version of the Maternal–Fetal Attachment Scale in a sample of Italian expectant women. *Midwifery, 34,* 79–87. https://doi.org/10.1016/j.midw.2015.12.012

Carlson, V., Cicchetti, D., Barnett, D., & Braunwald, K. G. (1989). Finding order in disorganization: Lessons from research on maltreated infants' attachments to their caregivers. In D. Cicchetti & V. Carlson (Eds.), *Child maltreatment: Theory and research on the causes and consequences of child abuse and neglect* (pp. 494–528). Cambridge University Press.

Cassidy, J. (2001). Truth, lies, and intimacy: An attachment perspective. *Attachment & Human Development, 3*(2), 121–155. https://doi.org/10.1080/14616730110058999

Cicchetti, D., & Toth, S. L. (2005). Child maltreatment. *Annual Review of Clinical Psychology, 1,* 409–438. https://doi.org/10.1146/annurev.clinpsy.1.102803.144029

Cranley, M. S. (1981). Development of a tool for the measurement of maternal attachment during pregnancy. *Nursing Research, 30*(5), 281–284.

Cross, R. (2012). Interpersonal childhood trauma and the use of the therapeutic community in recovery. *Therapeutic Communities: The International Journal of Therapeutic Communities, 33*(1), 39–53. https://doi.org/10.1108/09641861211286311

Crossley, N. (1996). *Intersubjectivity.* Sage Publications.

De Bellis, M. D., Spratt, E. G., & Hooper, S. R. (2014). Neurodevelopmental biology associated with childhood sexual abuse. *Journal of Child Sexual Abuse, 23*(1), 74–93.

Denham, S. A., Bassett, H. H., & Wyatt, T. M. (2014). The socialization of emotional competence. In J. E. Grusec & P. D. Hastings (Eds.), Handbook of socialization: Theory and research (2nd ed., pp. 590–613). The Guilford Press.

Eisenberg, N., Spinrad, T. L., & Eggum, N. D. (2010). Emotion-related self-regulation and its relation to children's maladjustment. *Annual Review of Clinical Psychology, 6*, 495–525. https://doi.org/10.1146/annurev.clinpsy.121208.131208

Felitti, V. J., Anda, R. F., Nordenberg, D., Williamson, D. F., Spitz, A. M., Edwards, V., Koss, M. P., & Marks, J. S. (1998). Relationship of childhood abuse and household dysfunction to many of the leading causes of death in adults. The Adverse Childhood Experiences (ACE) Study. *American Journal of Preventive Medicine, 14*(4), 245–258. https://doi.org/10.1016/s0749-3797(98)00017-8

Fraiberg, S., Adelson, E., & Shapiro, V. (1975). Ghosts in the nursery: A psychoanalytic approach to the problems of impaired infant-mother relationships. *Journal of the American Academy of Child & Adolescent Psychiatry, 14*(3), 387–421. https://doi.org/10.1016/s0002-7138(09)61442-4

Freud, A., 1895–1982 & Burlingham, D. T. (1943). *War and children/by Anna Freud and Dorothy T. Burlingham*. Medical War Books.

Gil, E. (Ed.). (2010). *Working with children to heal interpersonal trauma: The power of play*. Guilford Press.

Gopnik, A. (2010). *The philosophical baby: What children's minds tell us about truth, love, and the meaning of life*. Farrar, Straus and Giroux.

Gratz, K. L., & Roemer, L. (2004). Multidimensional assessment of emotion regulation and dysregulation: Development, factor structure, and initial validation of the difficulties in emotion regulation scale. *Journal of Psychopathology and Behavioral Assessment, 26*(1), 41–54. https://doi.org/10.1177/0145445514566504

Hesse, E., & Main, M. (2000). Disorganized infant, child, and adult attachment: Collapse in behavioral and attentional strategies. *Journal of the American Psychoanalytic Association, 48*(4), 1097–1127. https://doi.org/10.1177/00030651000480041101

Hillman, S., Cross, R., & Anderson, K. (2020). Exploring attachment and internal representations in looked-after children. *Frontiers in Psychology, 11*. https://doi.org/10.3389/fpsyg.2020.00464

Hillman, S., Villegas, C., Anderson, K., Kerr-Davis, A., & Cross, R. (2022). Internal representations of attachment in story stems: Changes in the narratives of foster care children. *Journal of Child Psychotherapy, 48*(2), 261–289. https://doi.org/10.1080/0075417X.2022.2088824

Hodges, J., Hillman, S., & Steele, M. (2000). *Story stem assessment profile*. Anna Freud Centre.

Klaus, M. H., & Kennell, J. H. (1976). *Maternal-infant bonding*. C. V. Mosby.

Lieberman, A. F., & Van Horn, P. (2008). *Psychotherapy with infants and young children: Repairing the effects of stress and trauma on early attachment*. Guilford Press.

Lieberman, A. F., & Zeanah, C. H. (1999). Contributions of attachment theory to infant–parent psychotherapy and other interventions with infants and young children. In J. Cassidy & P. R. Shaver (Eds.), *Handbook of attachment: Theory, research, and clinical applications* (pp. 555–574). Guilford Press.

Liotti, G. (2004). Trauma, dissociation, and disorganized attachment: Three strands of a single braid. *Psychotherapy: Theory, Research, Practice, Training, 41*(4), 472–486.

Lorenz K. (1935). Der kumpan in der umwelt des vogels. *Journal für Ornithologie, 83*, 137–213. https://doi.org/10.1007/BF01905355

Lyons-Ruth, K., Bureau, J. F., Holmes, B., Easterbrooks, M. A., & Brooks, N. H. (2013). Borderline symptoms and suicidality/self-injury in late adolescence: Prospectively observed relationship correlates in infancy and childhood. *Psychiatry Research, 206*(2–3), 273–281. https://doi.org/10.1016/j.psychres.2012.09.030

Lyons-Ruth, K., Connell, D. B., Grunebaum, H. U., & Botein, S. (1990). Infants at social risk: Maternal depression and family support services as mediators of infant development and security of attachment. *Child Development, 61*(1), 85–98. https://doi.org/10.1111/j.1467-8624.1990.tb02762.x

Lyons-Ruth, K., Dutra, L., Schuder, M. R., & Bianchi, I. (1998). From infant attachment disorganization to adult dissociation: Relational adaptations or traumatic experiences? *Psychiatric Clinics of North America, 21*(1), 1–24. https://doi.org/10.1016/j.psc.2005.10.011

Lyons-Ruth, K., & Jacobvitz, D. (2008). Attachment disorganization: Genetic factors, parenting contexts, and developmental transformation from infancy to adulthood. In J. Cassidy & P. R. Shaver (Eds.), *Handbook of attachment: Theory, research, and clinical applications* (pp. 666–697). Guilford Press.

Mackin, J., Hillman, S., Cross, R., & Anderson, K. (2022). The internal worlds of sexually abused looked-after children. *The Psychoanalytic Study of the Child, 75*(1), 278–298. https://doi.org/10.1080/00797308.2021.2022413

Main, M. (1996). Introduction to the special section on attachment and psychopathology: 2. Overview of the field of attachment. *Journal of Consulting and Clinical Psychology, 64*(2), 237–243. https://doi.org/10.1037//0022-006x.64.2.237

Main, M., & Hesse, E. (1990). Parents' unresolved traumatic experiences are related to infant disorganized attachment status. In M. T Greenberg, D. Cicchetti & E. M. Cummings (Eds.), *Attachment in the preschool years* (pp. 161–181). University of Chicago Press.

Main, M., & Solomon, J. (1990a). Parents' unresolved traumatic experiences are related to infant disorganized attachment status: Is frightened and/or frightening parental behavior the linking mechanism? In M. Greenberg, D. Cicchetti & E. M. Cummings (Eds.), *Attachment in preschool years: Theory, research, and intervention* (pp. 161–182). University of Chicago Press.

Main, M., & Solomon, J. (1990b). Procedures for identifying infants as disorganized/disoriented during the Ainsworth Strange Situation. In M. T. Greenberg, D. Cicchetti & E. M. Cummings (Eds.), *Attachment in the preschool years: Theory, research, and intervention* (pp. 121–160). University of Chicago Press.

Martin, H., Hillman, S., Cross, R., & Anderson, K. (2022). The manifestations and correlates of dissociation amongst looked-after children in middle childhood. *European Journal of Trauma & Dissociation, 6*(1), Article 100232. https://doi.org/10.1016/j.ejtd.2021.100232

McLaughlin, K. A., Hatzenbuehler, M. L., Mennin, D. S., & Nolen-Hoeksema, S. (2011). Emotion dysregulation and adolescent psychopathology: A prospective study. *Behaviour Research and Therapy, 49*(9), 544–554. https://doi.org/10.1016/j.brat.2011.06.003

Mercer, R. T. (2004). Becoming a mother versus maternal role attainment. *Journal of Nursing Scholarship, 36*(3), 226–232. https://doi.org/10.1111/j.1547-5069.2004.04042.x

Mikulincer, M., & Shaver, P. R. (Eds.). (2016). *Attachment in adulthood: Structure, dynamics, and change* (2nd ed.). Guilford Press.

Nuñez, L., Fernández, S., Alamo, N., Midgley, N., Capella, C., & Krause, M. (2022). The therapeutic relationship and change processes in child psychotherapy: A qualitative, longitudinal study of the views of children, parents, and therapists. *Research in Psychotherapy, 25*(1), Article 556. https://doi.org/10.4081/ripppo.2022.556

Panksepp, J. (1998). *Affective neuroscience: The foundations of human and animal emotions*. Oxford University Press.

Panksepp, J., & Biven, L. (2012). *The archaeology of mind: Neuroevolutionary origins of human emotions*. W. W. Norton.

Porges, S. W. (2011). *The polyvagal theory: Neurophysiological foundations of emotions, attachment, communication, and self-regulation*. W W Norton.

Schore, A. N. (1994). *Affect regulation and the origin of the self: The neurobiology of emotional development*. Lawrence Erlbaum Associates, Inc.

Schore, A. N. (2012). *The science of the art of psychotherapy*. W. W. Norton.

Schore, A. N. (2016). *The development of the unconscious mind*. W. W. Norton.

Shields, A. M., & Cicchetti, D. (1995). *The development of an emotion regulation assessment battery: Reliability and validity among at-risk grade-school children*. Poster session presented at the biennial meeting of the Society for Research in Child Development, Indianapolis, IN.

Shields, A. M., & Cicchetti, D. (1997). Emotion regulation among school-age children: The development and validation of a new criterion Q-sort scale. *Developmental Psychology, 33*(6), 906–916. https://doi.org/10.1037//0012-1649.33.6.906

Shonkoff, J. P. (2016). Capitalizing on advances in science to reduce the health consequences of early childhood adversity. *JAMA Pediatrics, 170*(10), 1003–1007. https://doi.org/10.1001/jamapediatrics.2016.1559

Slade, A. (2014). Imagining fear: Attachment, threat, and psychic experience. *Psychoanalytic Dialogues, 24*(3), 253–256. https://doi.org/10.1080/10481885.2014.911608

Spitz, R. A. (1945). Hospitalism: An inquiry into the genesis of psychiatric conditions in early childhood. *Psychoanalytic Study of the Child, 1*, 53–74.

Thompson, R. A., & Meyer, S. (2007). Socialization of emotion regulation in the family. In J. Gross (Ed.), *Handbook of emotion regulation* (pp. 249–268). Guilford Press.

Tinbergen, N., Falkus, H., & Ennion, E. (1970). *Signals for survival*. Clarendon Press.

Trevarthen, C. (1979). Communication and cooperation in early infancy. A description of primary intersubjectivity. In M. Bullara (Ed.), *Before speech: The beginning of human communication* (pp. 321–347). Cambridge University Press.

Tronick, E., Als, H., Adamson, L., Wise, S., & Brazelton, T. B. (1978). The infant's response to entrapment between contradictory messages in face-to-face interaction. *Journal of the American Academy of Child Psychiatry, 17*(1), 1–13. https://doi.org/10.1016/s0002-7138(09)62273-1

Waters, E., & Deane, K. E. (1987). *Attachment Q-set* [Database record]. APA PsycTests.

Winnicott, D. W. (1965). *The maturational processes and the facilitating environment: Studies in the theory of emotional development*. International Universities Press.

Winnicott, D. W. (1992). *The child, the family, and the outside world*. Da Capo Press. (Original work published 1964.)

6
STRUCTURAL DISSOCIATION
Developmental Pathways and Treatment Implications

Kathy Steele

Introduction

Structural dissociation is not a specific therapy, but rather a theory that informs an integrative treatment approach primarily for severe trauma-related disorders. While the major focus on structural dissociation has been on the treatment of adults, it is innately a developmental model with implications for the treatment of children and adolescents, consistent with the large body of literature on the developmental origins of dissociation, including neglect and trauma, discrete mental states, theory of mind, emotion regulation, and attachment (Farina et al., 2019; Ford & Courtois, 2015; Gomez, 2012; Linde-Krieger et al., 2023; Liotti, 1992, 2009, 2021; Loewenstein & Putnam, 2023; Paetzold & Rholes, 2021; Putnam, 1997, 2016; Schimmenti, 2017, 2020; Silberg, 2021; Sinason & Potgieter Marks, 2021; Waters, 2016; Wieland, 2015).

The first step in understanding structural dissociation is to distinguish it from the much broader definitions of dissociation as a symptom, as various "types" of dissociation require different treatment approaches (Steele et al., 2023).

Types of Dissociation: Distinguishing Structural Dissociation from Other Dissociative Symptoms

Over many decades, more symptoms and phenomena have been included under a broad rubric of dissociation characterized by the individual's general failure to integrate or be aware of different elements of psychological experience or the environment that are important for adaptive functioning. It is important to realize that not all integrative failures are dissociative (Farina & Meares, 2023; Mosquera & Steele, 2017). For example, a very normal grieving process takes time and implies a lack of full integration (realization) of loss for some time, but we would not consider that a dissociative symptom or problem. An avoidant person may have only vague recollections of important relational moments and lack rich and emotional narratives, not due to dissociation proper but to a more general inhibitory defensive avoidance. Individuals with serious personality disorders do not function in well-integrated ways across domains of experience, but may not have underlying dissociation. In fact, integration as a process is never complete, but rather is an ongoing series of mental and behavioral actions that involves continual reorganization of experience (and sense of self) as new information is encountered.

The broad category of dissociation includes a wide range of experiences and symptoms, including (1) cognitive and attentional problems such as mental absorption, spaciness or detachment, daydreaming, and imaginative involvement; (2) disturbances in perception (depersonalization and derealization); (3) trauma-related physiological hypo-arousal ("faint" or collapse; Porges, 2011); and (4) structural dissociation, a division or fragmentation of the personality and sense of self (Van der Hart et al., 2006; Van der Hart & Steele, 2019). Each of these symptoms exists on a continuum from normal to pathological, the latter implying they interfere with functioning. The first three types can exist with or without structural dissociation as an underlying problem, so it is imperative to accurately assess for structural dissociation in addition to "general" dissociation.

It seems economical to understand dissociation along two dimensions: the first being general dissociative symptoms that range from normal to pathological and which are also found in many mental disorders. The second is a continuum from normal ego states to structural dissociation, the latter of which is found only in the more severe trauma-related disorders. Ego states are normal phenomena present in all people. It is likely that dissociative parts in structural dissociation are elaborations of ego states, but there are significant differences between the two phenomena that impact treatment. This will be discussed briefly below (see Table 6.1).

While general dissociative symptoms are necessary for the development of structural dissociation, they are not sufficient. For example, spaciness by itself does not lead to divisions in the self, even when it is severely pathological. Below, more will be discussed about how structural dissociation occurs, along what lines and for what reasons.

Dissociation as Alterations in Attention and Awareness

Alterations in attention and awareness are experienced by everyone, particularly when fatigued, stressed, or ill. These include spaciness, absorption, trance-like states, daydreaming, and other experiences that imply difficulty staying focused on the present moment. They are also found in more severe forms in virtually every mental disorder (e.g., spacing out in depression or anxiety), and thus are not specific to trauma or structural dissociation, although they are always found in highly traumatized individuals. In children, these rudimentary states may form the foundation for more visible structural dissociation.

The treatment of all types of alterations in conscious awareness, such as spaciness, absorption, and maladaptive daydreaming primarily requires the stabilizing trifecta of mindfulness, mentalizing, and emotion regulation (Steele et al., 2023). Of course, these should be facilitated within the context of secure attachment.

Dissociation as Alterations in Perception: Depersonalization and Derealization

Symptoms of depersonalization and derealization are not specific to any particular disorder unless they are severe and persistent enough to quality for depersonalization disorder. Virtually anyone may experience transient symptoms of depersonalization and derealization under conditions of stress, illness, or severe fatigue. They are also found in many mental disorders; for example, depersonalization is pervasive and can be severe in panic disorder and schizophrenia. Only when these symptoms are the prominent mental health concern in the absence of other comorbidities and significantly interfere with functioning do we consider a diagnosis of depersonalization disorder.

A wide variety of symptoms are included in depersonalization and derealization, all involving perceptual difficulties connecting to and experiencing oneself and the world. Symptoms involving sense of self include feeling unreal, feeling as though one is acting instead of living, feeling as if one is in a dream, feeling like an automaton, or feeling one-dimensional. Some individuals experience body distortions, such one's hands or tongue feeling too large, or one's entire body feeling distorted. A sense of being outside oneself or floating and observing oneself (out-of-body experience) is common. In addition, the world may seem distorted, with a sense of being down a tunnel so that vision and hearing are distorted, or colors or shapes are warped. Finally, many individuals experience distortions of time sense, such that time feels faster or slower than normal.

Treatment of depersonalization begins with fourth-generation cognitive-behavioral therapy (CBT) (Simeon & Abugel, 2023). Other forms of psychotherapy may follow if CBT is not successful. For many clients, treatment also includes the triple skills of mindfulness, mentalizing, and emotion tolerance, plus psychoeducation about the symptoms. Medication has proved helpful for a substantial minority of patients (Simeon & Abugel, 2023). Newer approaches include the use of transcranial magnetic stimulation (TMS) at the temporoparietal junction (Orrù et al., 2021).

Dissociation as Dorsal Vagal Activation

Dissociation is also more recently described in the literature as a physiological shutdown or extreme hypo-arousal due to parasympathetic activation (Porges, 2011, 2021; Schore, 2012). This is an innate, primitive physical reaction to neurocepted life threat that results in rapid loss of energy and movement ("flag") and ultimately in total collapse or "faint" (Porges, 2011, 2021; Schauer & Elbert, 2010; Steele et al., 2017; Van der Hart et al., 2006). It does involve a disconnect from the present moment, which is why it is called dissociation, but first and foremost it is a physiological defense and only secondarily a psychological one once it becomes habituated in traumatized individuals.

It is interesting that we consider severe hypo-arousal to be dissociative, but not severe hyper-arousal, which also includes many symptoms of dissociation. In neither condition is the client fully present with self, others, and the world. For example, flashbacks are considered dissociative and typically involve high hyper-arousal states (American Psychiatric Association, 2013; Steele et al., 2017). So, we might consider that when the client is significantly outside the window of tolerance, whether high or low, general dissociative symptoms (not necessarily structural dissociation) will be present.

Treatment of the dorsal vagal response involves activation of the ventral vagal system, which regulates both the sympathetic and parasympathetic nervous systems. There are many ways to activate the ventral vagal system that are beyond the scope of this chapter (see Dana, 2018, 2023). Activation of the ventral vagal system is an excellent treatment for the moment of shutdown, but it is essential to explore reasons why the client is dropping into hypo-arousal. Usually, these reasons include difficulties with mentalizing and emotion regulation, so the stabilization trifecta skills are also appropriate treatments.

Structural Dissociation

The three "types" of dissociation described above are limited to certain domains of experience. For example, spaciness and absorption are primarily cognitive and attentional problems; depersonalization is a perceptual problem. Structural dissociation is much more encompassing of all domains of experience: cognition and attention, emotion, sensorimotor, perception, prediction, goal-orientation, and systems of meaning, memory, and identity. The most distinctive feature of structural dissociation is the subjective experience of different parts of self that feel separate to a greater or lesser degree (Steele et al., 2017, 2023; Van der Hart et al., 2006). Structural dissociation is a particular organization of the personality and self that includes a lack of voluntary awareness and control over various mental and behavioral actions. In children, these are likely to be less rigid and separate, following developmental pathways to greater rigidity and dissociative separateness only over time. The "parts" of children are based on the same principles of organization as those of adults, but may not be experienced as so separate.

Structural Dissociation versus Ego States

As noted above, it is likely that dissociative parts are more elaborated and separate forms of normal ego states that progress over some time in the development of the traumatized child. But significant differences between the two phenomena require somewhat different treatment approaches. What is the difference between an ego state and a dissociative part? First, everyone has ego states, but only individuals with serious trauma-related disorders have dissociative parts. Such individuals have experiences that those with ego states do not have. Typically, clients with dissociative parts have serious amnesia of the past and also the present. Children can present with a variety of memory difficulties and lack of memory for either certain aspects or complete episodes of abuse. Developmentally, this compartmentalization occurs primarily due to the need to attach to caregivers who may be abusive. The child cannot contain the affects and memories of abuse when the need for attachment is also necessary. In structural dissociation, there may be a lack of voluntary awareness and control over parts. For example, the child may be accused of lying because they do not recall something they have done, or they may blame "Superman" or "The Bad Cat" for doing something they feel they did not have control over doing. Of course, this type of behavior must be differentiated from the very normal "projection of blame" that is developmentally appropriate in children who cannot yet mentalize and own all of their behaviors and motivations.

Clients may also have a subjective sense of "not me" when confronted with dissociative parts. Different dissociative parts often have different autobiographical material, unlike ego states. Dissociative parts may have a more elaborated sense of self and experience themselves as separate from the individual; however, in young children, this is less likely. Generally, dissociative clients have a serious phobic avoidance of dissociative parts, much more severe than is typical of ego states. Table 6.1 summarizes these contrasts.

Table 6.1 Differences between Ego States and Structural Dissociation

Ego States	Dissociative Parts (Structural Dissociation)
Normal, found in everyone	Observed only in more severe trauma-related disorders (complex developmental trauma disorder, dissociative identity, other specified dissociative disorder)
A general sense of ego states belonging to self ("That is me, even if I don't like it")	A range of "not me" experiences (e.g., "That part is not me")
Awareness of ego states	A range of amnesia for dissociative parts
Share same autobiography	Various parts may have different autobiographies
Permeable boundaries between ego states	Relatively rigid boundaries between dissociative parts
Less phobic avoidance among ego states for each other	Typically more extreme phobic avoidance of dissociative parts for each other
Generally less intense defenses to engaging with ego states	Generally stronger defenses against engaging with dissociative parts
A range of experiences; not necessarily traumatized	More severe, chronic, and pervasive trauma
Reasonable degree of voluntary control over ego states	Significant lack of voluntary control over dissociative parts
Ego states are relatively simple (e.g., the little girl; "me" as a child)	Dissociative parts may be much more elaborated (e.g., "Mary," age 3, who likes ice cream and is scared of loud sounds, freezes, has short black hair, red shoes, and a dirty shirt; versus "Molly," age 5, who loves to draw, feels sad but never afraid, does not like ice cream, has long golden hair, and is dressed like a princess)

Structural Dissociation

Structural Dissociation as Deficit and Defense

The theory of structural dissociation supports the idea that not only is dissociation a defense against intolerable experiences and emotions, but also it arises out of deficits in the child's capacity to mentalize, regulate emotions, and develop a cohesive and coherent sense of self across time and situations. The research literature notes that dissociation is correlated with impairment in mentalizing and reflective functioning (Liotti & Gilbert, 2011; Liotti & Intreccialagli 1998; Mitchell & Steele, 2021), emotion regulation (Brand & Lanius, 2014; Cavicchioli et al., 2021; Paetzold & Rholes, 2021; Schore, 2003; Van Dijke et al., 2018), and the ability to organize a coherent and cohesive autobiographical memory and sense of self across time and contexts (Chiu et al., 2019; Steele et al., 2017; Van der Hart et al., 2006). Absence or limitations in these capacities may lead to chronic experiential avoidance (Bishop et al., 2018; Hayes-Skelton & Eustis, 2020; Orcutt et al., 2020). We have called this a "trauma-related phobia of inner experience" (Steele et al., 2017; Van der Hart et al., 2006). Treatment that supports development of these capacities improves symptoms (Farina et al., 2019; Schlumpf et al., 2019).

Specific Symptoms of Structural Dissociation

While general dissociative symptoms may or may not be trauma-related, structural dissociation appears to occur only under conditions of severe trauma and neglect and typically begins in childhood. Structural dissociation is the only condition that includes dissociative parts of the self. Symptoms in structural dissociation include

- amnesia of the past and present,
- Schneiderian symptoms in clients who otherwise exhibit no indications of psychosis (e.g., hearing voices),
- alternations in sense of self,
- puzzling symptoms of temporary functional losses (e.g., sensation, movement, vision, and skills), and
- jarring intrusions (e.g., voices and behaviors of dissociative parts).

These symptoms are not found in clients with normal ego states, or in those who only experience absorption, physiological shutdown, or depersonalization: they are exclusive to structural dissociation and the more severe trauma-related disorders.

Table 6.2 lists the differences in symptoms and treatments between the four types of dissociation.

Developmental Pathways to Structural Dissociation

Normal integration of self and personality is a developmental achievement over time, not something we are inherently born with. Both temperament and other genetic contributions and our social world combine to shape who we are. But self and identity are not static experiences; they require consistent updating and adaptation in continuous cycles of organization, disorganization, and reorganization (Damasio, 1999, 2012; Schore, 2003). Incorporating new experiences and reevaluating old ones provides regular opportunities to expand and update our views of self, others, and the world and thus adapt more efficiently to the present moment. This ongoing process involves both stability of self (what remains the same about me across time and situations) and flexibility of self (what is different about me across time and situations).

Table 6.2 Types of Dissociation and Treatment Differences

Type of Dissociation	Affected Domains of Experience	Symptoms	Treatment
Alterations in attention and awareness	Cognition and consciousness	Spaciness, absorption, daydreaming, thinking of nothing, trance-like behaviors	Mindfulness Emotion regulation Mentalizing plus secure attachment Potential trauma processing Play therapy Sensory and somatic-based approaches Child-friendly EMDR approaches Somatic and sensory approaches to grounding and orienting
Depersonalization and derealization	Perception	Feeling unreal or as if in a dream, feeling like an automaton, out-of-body experiences, distortions of reality and the body: vision, hearing, sensation, etc.	Fourth-generation cognitive-behavioral therapy involving acceptance Medication Emotion regulation Mentalizing plus secure attachment Child-friendly EMDR approaches Play therapy Grounding exercises in play therapy Somatic and sensory-based approaches Potential trauma processing
Dorsal vagal activation	Hypo-arousal involving attention, awareness, somatics, and perception	Sense of being completely "gone," immobility, difficulty, or inability to speak and respond, in extreme cases, loss of consciousness	Provision of safety Activation of ventral vagal system using sensory and somatic-based approaches Secondarily, focus on reasons why client's dorsal vagal system is activated
Structural dissociation	All domains of experience can be affected, including sense of self/identity Various parts may have different sense of self, perceptions, predictions, goals, systems of meaning, memories, somatic experiences, etc.	All symptoms above, plus jarring intrusions (voice hearing, somatic sensations, flashbacks) and functional losses (amnesia, temporary loss of skills) Multiple and contradictory senses of self	Mindfulness (may need to start with external rather than internal focus) Emotion regulation Mentalizing Plus secure attachment Exploration of dissociative parts Improving awareness, communication, and cooperation among parts Play therapy Child-friendly EMDR approaches Facilitating integration of parts Trauma processing

In an individual with structural dissociation, this continual adaption becomes stalled in childhood, leaving the child with discrete states that may not progress sufficiently into more fluid and flexible ones that operate in harmony. Eventually, these discrete states become more solidified into dissociative parts of self, each organized around relatively fixed and limited ways of thinking, feeling, perceiving, predicting, and behaving, somewhat impervious to the normal integration that supports adaptive growth and development. Internal working models of self and others remain relatively separated and not sufficiently updated. Structural dissociation is thus a complex developmental deficit in which traumatized children have been unable to adequately integrate their personality and sense of self into a cohesive organization that is stable across time and situations.

Dissociation is based on normative developmental foundations. In other words, symptomatic expressions of structural and other types of dissociation have normal and adaptive origins. Early childhood involves naturally occurring predispositions to dissociation. These include (1) naturally isolated affective experiences, so called "discrete states;" (2) developmental reliance on others to soothe, organize experience, and make meaning; (3) natural childhood fantasy proneness, including confusion between internal and external realities; (4) a delicate emerging sense of self that is still highly subject to discrete state switches, the vagaries of a caregiver's state of mind, and overwhelming environmental stressors; (5) higher levels of hypnotizability, which are associated with dissociation (Butler et al., 1996; Cleveland et al., 2020; Dell, 2019, 2023); and (6) only the most nascent capacities for integrating overwhelming, conflicted, or highly complex experiences.

It makes sense to use a diathesis-stress model to understand the development of structural dissociation. In addition to the normal conditions that naturally predispose young children to dissociation, we can also add the individual's innate temperament and other genetic contributions to either greater vulnerability or more resilience in general. A variety of external stressors may stretch the vulnerable child beyond capacity, such as unavailability of caregivers, severe isolation, serious neglect and/or abuse, medical trauma, and other overwhelming and pervasive experiences such as extreme poverty, war, racism, or cultural oppression.

Research has shown that pathological dissociation (not necessarily structural dissociation) can occur under a variety of stressful conditions, not only overt trauma (Cavicchioli et al., 2021; Dell, 2023; Farina et al., 2019; Gold, 2020; Paetzold & Rholes, 2021; Schimmenti, 2017, 2020). These conditions include neglect; severe attachment disruptions; the presence of disorganized attachment; the state of mind of the caregiver, particularly helpless states of mind; and the (physical or emotional) unavailability of caregivers.

Unfortunately, the research does not distinguish between pathological forms of dissociative symptoms in general and the presence of dissociative parts in structural dissociation, so we cannot be certain how much these studies can reliably apply to clients with structural dissociation. What we do know is that individuals with complex dissociative disorders such as dissociative identity disorder (DID) report the highest levels of severe and chronic relational trauma, including emotional, physical, and sexual abuse (Ellason et al., 1996; Swica et al., 1996), and neurobiological studies indicate that DID is a severe form of post-traumatic stress disorder (Reinders & Veltman, 2021).

Motivational Systems in Structural Dissociation

In addition to naturally occurring conditions that are fertile soil for pathological dissociation, a primitive set of neural networks called motivational systems also likely provide a pathway for development of structural dissociation. The theory of structural dissociation proposes these systems may be the basic fault lines along which structural dissociation can occur (Nijenhuis, 2015; Steele, 2021; Steele et al., 2017; Van der Hart et al., 2006).

Evolutionary-prepared motivational systems organize experience via basic affects and direct us either toward attractive goals that support surviving and thriving or toward avoidance of threat. The systems we are most familiar with are attachment and defense (fight, flight, freeze, faint), but there are others. Each system not only organizes but also limits our perceptions, predictions, emotional range, and behaviors to focus on and achieve certain goals. Thus, they ultimately impact our sense of self and state of mind. Because they limit our focus and goals, they seriously affect mentalizing functions (Liotti & Prunetti, 2010; Mitchell & Steele, 2021; Steele, 2021). Since mentalizing is one of the basic stabilization capacities, it is essential to understand the role of motivational systems in facilitating or inhibiting mentalizing. Treatment that supports the client's shift from a less adaptive to a more adaptive motivational system for the situation will support better mentalizing.

Motivational systems include three broad categories: (1) primitive systems that organize basic seeking and energy regulation; (2) a defense system involving threat-related states of flight, fight, freeze, and faint; (3) and more evolved prosocial or interpersonal systems that organize interpersonal strategies, including (a) attachment, (b) collaboration, (c) caregiving, (d) competition/ranking, (e) play, and (f) sexuality involving relational strategies (Cortina & Liotti, 2010; Feeny & Woodhouse, 2016; Gilbert, 2014; Lichtenberg et al., 2017; Liotti, 2011, 2017a, 2017b, 2018, 2021; Liotti & Intreccialagli, 1998; Panksepp, 1998; Panksepp & Biven, 2012; Steele, 2021; Steele et al., 2017; Van der Hart et al., 2006).

Motivational systems may complement or inhibit each other, depending on their goals and physiological states. The most common example of incompatible motivational systems in structural dissociation is the conflict between the attachment system and the threat-related system in disorganized attachment. The child needs to simultaneously attach and defend against the same caregiver. Not only are the goals and affects of these systems in direct opposition to each other, but also their physiological states are incompatible (ventral vagal states in attachment versus high sympathetic or parasympathetic states in defense). Also, when safety is not an option, the attachment system will naturally be inhibited by the defense system. This insoluble conflict may result in profound dissociation, not only of cognition or emotion or behavior, but also of the entire sense of self. In fact, several authors have noted that disorganized attachment is actually a kind of dissociative organization (Barach, 1991; Liotti, 1992, 2009, 2021; Steele, 2021; Steele et al., 2017; Van der Hart et al., 2006). This is the most basic division in structural dissociation—between a sense of self organized around attachment goals and a sense of self organized by the animal defenses of flight, fight, freeze, and faint (Nijenhuis, 2015; Steele et al., 2017; Van der Hart & Steele, 2023; Van der Hart et al., 2006). Further dissociation along the lines of other motivational systems can occur, as we will explore below.

The theory of structural dissociation distinguishes between dissociative parts that primarily have social/relational functions in the present versus those that continue to react to threat with flight, fight, freeze, or faint. Of course, parts that have relational functions may engage animal defenses, as well as psychological/relational defenses. Thus, we include in treatment not only the animal defenses, but also the psychological and relational ones as well (Steele et al., 2017; Steele, 2021).

The focus on which motivational systems organize a given dissociative part is important because the systems related to interpersonal functioning and those related to defense are diverse in physiology, predictions, emotions, perceptions, mentalizing functions, meaning, identity and memory. This leads to natural conflicts among dissociative parts, which can be partly resolved by the therapist understanding the different goals of various motivational systems (Steele, 2021). Treatment approaches will vary slightly according to the motivational systems and goals of each part.

Each dissociative part develops a kind of psychobiological profile, organized by motivational systems of threat or interpersonal and daily life functioning, which limits awareness, adaptation, and integration. Dissociative parts stuck in trauma are often disoriented to time, place, and even person, which involves a profound lack of realization. Not only do these parts not know the trauma is over, but they also often have trouble accurately perceiving the present. This "stuckness" results in parts that remain forever frightened or angry or ashamed, as they still feel they are in the traumatic experience of the past.

Collaborative Motivational System

The collaborative system involves explicit understanding and sharing, allowing us to work on mutually shared goals (Cortina & Liotti, 2010; Lichtenberg et al, 2017; Trevarthen & Aitken, 1994). Collaboration commences in nascent form when we neurocept safety or danger with another person. Neuroception is a prelanguage function at a somatic, implicit, neural level. But once safety is detected, we can collaborate on a more nuanced intersubjective—implicit—level, and then can begin to use language for explicit sharing and cooperation. We have a need to understand ourselves and our own minds—what we think and feel and why we do what we do—and then to understand others in a similar manner. Thus, the collaboration system involves mentalizing and reflective functioning, and attention to intersubjective communication. The collaborative system is separate from other interpersonal motivational systems, but likely operates simultaneously with them.

In treatment, the collaborative system can be activated by a focus on mutually shared therapeutic goals and by supporting a curious, compassionate egalitarian relationship that is not overly caretaking. This allows attachment—a highly cathected and conflicted system for clients who have been traumatized—to operate more quietly in the background to avoid over-activation in the therapeutic relationship. In a positive feedback loop, cooperation supports and strengthens social engagement, which allows for the eventual possibility of the client feeling able to engage safely with attachment.

Caregiving Motivational System

Caregiving is an innate drive to protect and care for others in distress, particularly the vulnerable young. Caregiving is present even in very young children, so it is readily available for traumatized individuals to use as a relational strategy when attachment fails them.

Many clients have over-activated caregiving systems. They strive to please, care for, and serve others in order to be accepted. When a parent is persistently frightened, depressed, or dependent, the child may develop *controlling caregiving* strategies that emerge from the caregiving system, as the parent views the child as the "stronger, wiser" one. While appeasing (submissive) behaviors may appear similar to actual caregiving behaviors in the *controlling caregiving* strategy, it is important to determine whether the individual is operating from the caregiving or competition system, as they involve different emotions and dynamics to be worked through in psychotherapy.

The Separation Cry: The Panic and Loss Motivational System

The separation cry is part of the motivational system associated with panic and loss (Panksepp, 1998), and the attachment system. It is activated by the absence of a caregiver and directs the individual to frantically seek out a (stronger, wiser) person who will provide help and comfort. The separation cry is organized by several primary affects: *panic* at separation, *sadness* at loss, and *joy* at reunion. The genuine unmet needs of the child in the absence of a responsive caregiver can lead to a vulnerability to intense activation of the separation cry, particularly in situations where the child feels distressed. Research indicates that trauma survivors have higher levels of dependency than other populations (Hill et al., 2000), leaving them vulnerable to becoming overwhelmed and desperate for connection and help.

The intense negative affects of separation cry can become chronic or inhibited in traumatized individuals, preventing the harmonious completion of this cycle (Steele, 2018). The client may become stuck in panic, or in sadness and despair that prevents the resolution of grief, unable to experience the joy and safety of connection.

When frantic attachment-seeking (the separation cry) is activated in the traumatized client, the interpersonal motivational systems are temporarily deactivated, along with mentalizing and reflective functioning. Thus, regulatory implicit communication is inhibited. The singular goal of the client becomes gaining proximity to and caregiving by the therapist or another person, limiting the client's ability to explore, enjoy, and engage with the world.

Maladaptive dependency involves a chronically activated separation cry (Steele et al., 2017; Steele, 2021). Because the separation cry involves a profound sense of helplessness and vulnerability, it can also activate traumatic memories. In many cases, activation of the separation cry is followed by shame. Shame functions as an inhibitory attempt to quash the intense attachment need but has the overall effect of increasing it in a negative feedback loop (Steele et al., 2017; Steele, 2018, 2021).

It is imperative that the therapist recognize the separation cry in clients—for example, in those who consistently have difficulty leaving sessions due to dysregulation, or who (or whose caregivers) make frequent requests or demands for contact outside of session or for additional sessions. The content of these requests may be quite real—for example, needing help with flashbacks and suicidal crises—but the underlying goal of the separation cry to gain proximity to and caregiving by the therapist must always be acknowledged and worked with.

When the separation cry and maladaptive dependency are chronic and intense, the therapist may become increasingly distressed and concerned about the safety and well-being of the highly dysregulated client, resulting in what Solomon and George have terms "helpless caregiving" (George & Solomon, 2011; Solomon & George, 1999). This can result in strong rescue efforts ("I must do something, anything!") or withdrawal from the client ("There is nothing I can do!"). In either case, the therapist feels helpless and has difficulty tolerating the distress of the client (and of their caregivers), often resulting in mutually escalating over-arousal (Beebe, 2005). The therapist's distress decreases reflective capacities, leaving the therapist ever more reliant on action rather than reflection and process orientation. A meta-approach, often with the help of consultation, can support the therapist in recognizing that the caregiving system has become over-activated and is part of the problem, not the solution. In these cases, a cooperative approach focused on specific and mutually shared therapeutic goals can be reparative (Steele et al., 2017).

The goal of therapy is not to prevent the client from experiencing loss and abandonment feelings, but to create a holding environment in which those can be accepted compassionately, validated, and effectively grieved.

Competition/Ranking Motivational System

The competition/ranking system evolved from the need to compete within a social group for resources. Mammalian social structures are typically hierarchical, requiring group members to abide by social codes involving dominance and submission. Competitive behaviors in humans can be either dominant or submissive. In disorganized attachment, the child reorganizes by generally engaging in two types of controlling behavior that can emerge from the dominant and submissive components of the competitive system: *controlling punitive* and *controlling caregiving strategies* (Main & Cassidy, 1988).

Submission

Children may learn to appease or engage in fawning behaviors with frightening, abusive caregivers. These controlling caregiving behaviors are submissive and fear-based and emerge from the competitive/ranking system. The controlling caregiving strategies linked to the *caregiving* system are based on guilt, not fear. Fearful (appeasing) strategies are geared toward creating safety, while guilty caregiving strategies are directed to care for others who are distressed. The latter can create a sense of moral injury in clients. ("I have not done what I should have done; therefore, I am bad."). While the behavior is similar in both cases, the child's goals and emotions are different.

Dominance

Dominance in the competitive system can be understood as a *controlling punitive* strategy that emerges in children following the collapse of attachment strategies. Competitive aggression is concerned with achieving a goal: *"You have something I want, and I am going to hurt or punish you in order to get what I want or need."* The goal is not to physically or emotional hurt or injure, but to apply enough pain to obtain the desired object or experience (food, love, care, attention, etc.). The aggression will cease as soon as the goal has been achieved.

Competitive aggression is different from defensive aggression (*fight;* Liotti, 2019). Defensive aggression is an attempt to deal with danger, with the goal of safety. Competitive aggression is directed to get what is wanted or needed. Understanding the goal of aggression is important in treatment. A shift to cooperative work on shared goals is often the best option and makes controlling strategies unnecessary (Liotti, 2011, 2017b; Liotti & Gilbert, 2011).

Sexual Motivational System

Maladaptive sexual behaviors in traumatized individuals emerge from the sexual motivational system (Liotti, 2017a; Steele, 2021). Traumatized children may utilize sexual behaviors with or without attachment, play, or competitive components. There is often confusion between love and sex; thus, the goals of attachment and the sexual system are confounded. Other clients may separate the attachment and sexual systems, viewing others only as objects of sexual gratification, without meaningful emotional connection. This may become a compulsive activity that wards off painful emotions or conflicts, avoiding the possibility of attachment and love.

Play Motivational System

Play, including sense of humor, is a form of social learning and experiencing social limits. Through play, children practice skills, develop bonds with others, and learn the parameters of what is fun and enjoyable versus what is not acceptable. Play is an important component of interpersonal relationships and can be used from time to time when attachment is too fraught to promote connection and emotion regulation. Like attachment and collaboration it does activate the ventral vagal system.

Dissociative Parts and Motivational Systems

Each dissociative part may be organized by specific motivational systems. Often, they have an internal organization much like the abusive family: victim, abuser, rescuer, and neglectful bystander (Liotti, 2017; Steele et al., 2017). These roles can be understood as being organized by various motivational systems. For example, victim parts are often organized by animal defenses or controlling caregiving strategies (caregiving or competitive systems). Internal abusers are typically dominant, organized by the competitive ranking system, concerned with power and control. Internal neglectful bystanders mimic the helpless strategies of overwhelmed caregivers. Sexualized parts may be more of a victim or an abuser paradigm, depending on whether they are seeking love or power and control through sexual behavior.

Of course, motivational systems are rudimentary; there are also much more sophisticated psychological defenses that accompany them. For example, clients who operate more from a competitive/ranking system may have an idealized, narcissistic fantasy of self and a devalued fantasy of others, which fits with their need to rank higher than others. Victim parts may have rescue fantasies that keep them dependent and passive. In children, these variations in sense of self can appear in a wide range of behaviors. With more dominant behaviors, some children may be unable to tolerate making a mistake and become rigidly perfectionistic in an effort to be seen as perfect. Some may insist on being seen as more special than others. Some may bully other children or be excessively jealous and angry when attention is directed to other children. With more submissive behaviors, children can be extremely passive in asking for what they want or need. Some may demand that caregivers treat them as babies, doing everything for them. Others become more passive with peers, leading to being bullied or influenced to engage in problematic behaviors.

Treatment Implications

The theory of structural dissociation draws upon the many accepted treatment methods that address psychodynamic, relational, cognitive, emotional, somatic, and autohypnotic issues in the context of working with ego states and dissociative parts in children, adolescents, and adults. The basic principles of the theory support a tailored and organized treatment regardless of the preferred therapy approach(es) of the therapist. With children, there should be an additional focus on working with caregivers to provide an emotionally stable environment for the child, in which further adaptive development can occur.

The focus of treatment is first on eliminating deficits in adaptive cognitive, emotional, somatic, and relational capacities according to the developmental level of the individual. In the case of very young children, the focus of treatment is on supporting caregivers to offer adequate emotional regulation and mentalizing strategies that help children with developmentally appropriate levels of emotional and mentalizing skills. Once a reasonable degree of developmentally appropriate capacity is present, including a sufficiently stable living environment, treatment systematically addresses a paced reduction of the client's experiential avoidance as it manifests in structural dissociation, including avoidance of dissociative parts of the self. It is common for dissociation to also be accompanied by a range of significant other psychological and relational defenses as well as habituated threat reactions. Strategies to promote a naturalistic integration of self and experiential acceptance across time and contexts is encouraged in each session, according to the client's capabilities. In addition, work to prevent further solidification of dissociative parts in children is part of the treatment plan; this is an advantage of early childhood treatment over therapy in later life, when dissociative parts are more fixed and rigid. While the treatment of traumatic memory is an important element of the work, it is equally essential to support clients in improving limited developmental capacities, particularly mentalizing and emotion regulation functions (Gold, 2020; Steele et al., 2017).

The theory of structural dissociation recommends the therapist take a collaborative rather than caretaking approach to avoid undue activation of the client's attachment system. This includes identifying and working on mutually shared treatment goals (caregivers must be included when working with children). Excessive warmth and caretaking can evoke unbearable dependency needs, which, in turn, activate helplessness and shame in the client (and more caretaking or withdrawal from the therapist). The therapist is encouraged to be warm, but not "too" warm, compassionate but not caretaking, and guiding but not leading. The therapist provides consistent and predictable—not constant—availability to children and their caregiving systems, with limited access between sessions, and attempts relational repair when there is a rupture.

The therapist is also encouraged to focus on process rather than content, as with any good psychotherapy. The therapist's and client's attention should primarily be directed to intrapsychic and relational experiences in the moment during therapy, which is supported by the intersubjective focus of the collaborative system. Excessive focus on content and crisis tends to activate the therapist's caregiving system and the child's and often the caregiver's separation cry.

The therapist should make sustained efforts to treat all dissociative parts equally and as aspects of one person. Children generally have not yet developed strongly solidified dissociative parts. The therapist can facilitate their understanding and acceptance of parts as aspects of self. The therapist should employ a sequenced, integrative approach that focuses on improving the dynamic relationships among all dissociative parts within the client as a whole individual.

Trauma-Related Phobias

Structural dissociation typically involves an extensive range of phobic avoidance that exacerbates and maintains dissociation and restricts adaptation. They include the phobias of (1) inner experience as a central avoidance of one's own experience—that is, emotions, thoughts, memories, body sensations, movements, needs, wishes, dreams and fantasies; (2) dissociative parts, based on fear and/or shame; (3) attachment and attachment loss (rejection or abandonment); (4) traumatic memory; and (5) change and healthy risk-taking (Van der Hart et al., 2006). These trauma-related phobias developed from skills deficits in mentalizing and emotion regulation, and thus need an early and strong focus on skills building.

In a stepwise manner, the therapist begins to first address the overarching phobia of inner experience, the sine qua non without which therapy cannot proceed. Using titrated experiences with the client's window of tolerance, additional phobias can be addressed gradually. Often, there is simultaneous piecemeal work on several phobias at once. For example, a child may be afraid to attend school, so the therapist works on phobic avoidance of new experiences and change. Simultaneously, the child may engage in disorganized attachment behaviors, so the therapist shuttles between dealing with the fear of closeness and the fear of loss. Perhaps the child hears voices, and the therapist will be attempting to normalize and reduce the fear and shame of having dissociative parts. In a careful spiral manner, each phobia is addressed, opening the child to more curiosity and less suffering.

Conclusion

This chapter has offered a brief overview of the theory of structural dissociation and the developmental pathways to it. We have briefly explored how structural dissociation may look different in children. It is vital to differentiate between structural dissociation and other forms or types of dissociation, as treatment differs significantly. Likewise, it is essential to distinguish between normal ego states and dissociative parts that are present in only the most serious trauma-related disorders. An emphasis on motivational systems as the faulty lines of structural dissociation is explored, with brief descriptions of each system and its manifestations in structural dissociation. Finally, a few implications for treatment are discussed, with encouragement of the therapist to use their own preferred methods and modalities of treatment with some modifications.

References

American Psychiatric Association (2013). *Diagnostic and statistical manual of mental disorders* (5th ed.). American Psychiatric Publishing.

Barach, P. M. (1991). Multiple personality disorder as an attachment disorder. *Dissociation: Progress in the Dissociative Disorders, 4*(3), 117–123.

Beebe, B. (2005). Mother-infant research informs mother-infant treatment. *Psychoanalytic Study of the Child, 60*(1), 7–46. https://doi.org/10.1080/00797308.2005.11800745

Bishop, L. S., Ameral, V. E., & Palm Reed, K. M. (2018). The impact of experiential avoidance and event centrality in trauma-related rumination and posttraumatic stress. *Behavior Modification, 42*(6), 815–837. https://doi.org/10.1177/0145445517747287

Brand, B. L., & Lanius, R. A. (2014). Chronic complex dissociative disorders and borderline personality disorder: Disorders of emotion dysregulation? *Borderline Personality Disorder and Emotion Dysregulation, 1*(1), 1–13. https://doi.org//10.1186/2051-6673-1-13

Butler, L. D., Duran, R. E. F., Jasiukaitus, P., Koopman, C., & Spiegel, D. (1996). Hypnotizability and traumatic experience: A diathesis-stress model of dissociative symptomatology. *American Journal of Psychiatry, 153*, 42–63. https://doi.org/10.1176/ajp.153.8.A42

Cavicchioli, M., Scalabrini, A., Northoff, G., Mucci, C., Ogliari, A., & Maffei, C. (2021). Dissociation and emotion regulation strategies: A meta-analytic review. *Journal of Psychiatric Research, 143*, 370–387. https://doi.org/10.1016/j.jpsychires.2021.09.011

Chiu, C. D., Tollenaar, M. S., Yang, C. T., Elzinga, B. M., Zhang, T. Y., & Ho, H. L. (2019). The loss of the self in memory: Self-referential memory, childhood relational trauma, and dissociation. *Clinical Psychological Science, 7*(2), 265–282. https://doi.org/10.1177/2167702618804794

Cleveland, J. M., Reuther, B. J., & Gold, S. N. (2020). The varied relationship between hypnosis and dissociative phenomena: Implications for traumatology. *American Journal of Hypnosis, 63*(2), 139–149. https://doi:10.1080/00029157.2020.1789545

Cortina, M., & Liotti, G. (2010). Attachment is about safety and protection, intersubjectivity is about sharing and social understanding: The relationships between attachment and intersubjectivity. *Psychoanalytic Psychology, 27*, 410–444. https://doi.org/10.1037/a0019510

Damasio, A. (1999). *The feeling of what happens: Body and emotion in the making of consciousness*. Houghton, Mifflin, Harcourt.

Damasio, A. (2012). *Self comes to mind: Constructing the conscious brain*. Vintage.

Dana, D. (2018). *The polyvagal theory in therapy: Engaging the rhythms of regulation*. W. W. Norton.

Dana, D. (2023). *Polyvagal practices: Anchoring the self in safety*. W. W. Norton.

Dell, P. F. (2019). Reconsidering the autohypnotic model of the dissociative disorders. *Journal of Trauma & Dissociation, 18*, 58–87. https://doi.org/10.1080/15299732.2018.1451806

Dell, P. F. (2023). Clarifying the etiology of the dissociative disorders: It's not all about trauma. In M. J. Dorahy, S. N. Gold & J. A. O'Neil (Eds.), *Dissociation and the dissociative disorders: Past, present, future* (2nd ed., pp. 238–260). Routledge.

Ellason, J. W., Ross, C. A., & Fuchs, D. (1996). Lifetime Axis I and II comorbidity and childhood trauma history in dissociative identity disorder. *Psychiatry, 59*(3), 255–266. https://doi.org/10.1080/00332747.1996.11024766

Farina, B., Liotti, G., & Imperatori, C. (2019). The role of attachment trauma and disintegrative pathogenic processes in the traumatic-dissociative dimension. *Frontiers in Psychology, 10*, https://doi.org/10.3389/fpsyg.2019.00933

Farina, B., & Meares, D. (2023). The traumatic disintegration dimension. In M. J. Dorahy, S. N. Gold & J. A. O'Neil (Eds.), *Dissociation and the dissociative disorders: Past, present, future* (2nd ed., pp. 50–65). Routledge.

Feeny, B. C., & Woodhouse, S. S. (2016). Caregiving. In J. Cassidy & P. R. Shaver (Eds.), *Handbook of attachment: Theory, research and clinical applications* (3rd ed., pp. 827–851). Guilford Press.

Ford, J. D., & Courtois, C. A. (Eds.). (2015). *Treating complex traumatic stress disorders in children and adolescents: Scientific models and therapeutic approaches*. Guilford Press.

George, C., & Solomon, J. (2011). Helpless caregiving: The development of a screening measure. In J. Solomon & C. George (Eds.), *Disorganized attachment and caregiving* (pp. 133–166). Guilford Press.

Gilbert, P. (2014). The origins and nature of compassion focused therapy. *British Journal of Clinical Psychology, 53*(1), 6–41. https://doi.org/10.1111/bjc.12043

Gold, S. N. (2020). *Contextual trauma therapy: Overcoming traumatization and reaching full potential*. American Psychological Association.

Gomez, A. (2012). *EMDR therapy and adjunctive approaches with children: Complex trauma, attachment, and dissociation*. Springer.

Hayes-Skelton, S. A., & Eustis, E. H. (2020). Experiential avoidance. In J. S. Abramowitz & S. M. Blakey (Eds.), *Clinical handbook of fear and anxiety: Maintenance processes and treatment mechanisms* (pp. 115–131). American Psychological Association. https://doi.org/10.1037/0000150-007

Hill, E. L., Gold, S. N., & Bornstein, R. F. (2000). Interpersonal dependency among adult survivors of childhood sexual abuse in therapy. *Journal of Child Sexual Abuse, 9*(2), 71–86. https://doi.org/10.1300/J070v09n02_05

Lichtenberg, J. D., Lachmann, F. M., & Fosshage, J. L. (2017). *Self and motivational systems: A theory of psychoanalytic technique*. Routledge.

Linde-Krieger, L. B., Tuppett, M. Y., & Carlson, E. A. (2023). A developmental pathways model of dissociation. In M. J. Dorahy, S. N. Gold & J. A. O'Neil (Eds.), *Dissociation and the dissociative disorders: Past, present, future* (2nd ed., pp. 149–160). Routledge.

Liotti, G. (1992). Disorganized/disoriented attachment in the etiology of dissociative disorders. *Dissociation, 5*(4), 196–204.

Liotti, G. (2009). Attachment and dissociation. In P. F. Dell & J. A. O'Neil (Eds.), *Dissociation and the dissociative disorders: DSM-V and beyond* (pp. 53–65). Routledge.

Liotti, G. (2011). Attachment disorganization and the controlling strategies: An illustration of the contributions of attachment theory to developmental psychopathology and to psychotherapy integration. *Journal of Psychotherapy Integration, 21*(3), 232–252. https://doi.org/10.1037/a0025422

Liotti, G. (2017a). Conflicts between motivational systems related to attachment trauma: Key to understanding the intra-family relationship between abused children and their abusers. *Journal of Trauma and Dissociation, 18*(3), 304–318. https://doi.org/10.1080/15299732.2017.1295392

Liotti, G. (2017b). The multimotivational approach to attachment-informed psychotherapy: A clinical illustration. *Psychoanalytic Inquiry, 37*(5), 319–331. https://doi.org/10.1080/07351690.2017.1322426

Liotti, G. (2019). Conflicts in motivational systems related to attachment trauma: Key to understanding the intra-family relationship between abused children and their abusers. In W. Middleton, A. Sachs & M. Dorahy (Eds.), *The abused and the abuser: Victim-perpetrator dynamics* (pp. 62–76). Routledge.

Liotti, G. (2021). Infant attachment and dissociative psychopathology: An approach based on the evolutionary theory of multiple motivational systems. In V. Sinason & R. Potgieter Marks (Eds.), *Treating children with dissociative disorders: Attachment, trauma, theory and practice* (pp. 10–26). Routledge.

Liotti, G., & Gilbert, P. (2011). Mentalizing, motivation, and social mentalities: Theoretical considerations and implications for psychotherapy. *Psychology and Psychotherapy: Theory, Research and Practice, 84*(1), 9–25. https://doi.org/10.1348/147608310X520094

Liotti, G., & Intreccialagli, B. (1998). Metacognition and motivational systems in psychotherapy: A cognitive–evolutionary approach to the treatment of difficult patients. In C. Perris & P. D. McGorry (Eds.), *Cognitive psychotherapy of psychotic and personality disorders: Handbook of theory and practice* (pp. 333–349). Wiley.

Liotti, G., & Prunetti, E. (2010). Metacognitive deficits in trauma related disorders: Contingent on interpersonal motivational contexts? In G. DiMaggio & P. Lysaker (Eds.), *Metacognition and severe adult mental disorders: From basic research to treatment* (pp. 196–214). Routledge.

Loewenstein, R. J., & Putnam, F. W. (2023). Discrete behavioral states theory. In M. J. Dorahy, S. N. Gold & J. A. O'Neil (Eds.), *Dissociation and the dissociative disorders: Past, present, future* (2nd ed., pp. 281–296). Routledge.

Main, M., & Cassidy, J. (1988). Categories of response to reunion with the parent at age six: Predictable from infant attachment classifications and stable over a 1-month period. *Developmental Psychology, 24*, 415–526. https://doi.org/10.1037/0012-1649.24.3.415

Mitchell, S., & Steele, K. (2021). Mentalising in complex trauma and dissociative disorders. *European Journal of Trauma & Dissociation, 5*(3), Article 100168. https://doi.org/10.1016/j.ejtd.2020.100168

Mosquera, D., & Steele, K. (2017). Complex trauma, dissociation and borderline personality disorder: Working with integrative failures. *European Journal of Trauma and Dissociation, 1*(1), 63–71. https://doi.org/10.1016/j.ejtd.2017.01.010

Nijenhuis, E. R. S. (2015). *The trinity of trauma: Ignorance, fragility and control* (Vol. 1). Vandenhoeck & Ruprecht.

Orcutt, H. K., Reffi, A. N., & Ellis, R. A. (2020). Experiential avoidance and PTSD. In M. T. Tull & N. A. Kimbrel (Eds.), *Emotion in posttraumatic stress disorder* (pp. 409–436). Academic Press.

Orrù, G., Cesari, V., Conversano, C., & Gemignani, A. (2021). Targeting temporal parietal junction for assessing and treating disembodiment phenomena: A systematic review of TMS effect on depersonalization and derealization disorders (DPD) and body illusions. *AIMS Neurosciense, 8*(2), 181–194. https://doi.org/10.3934/Neuroscience.2021009

Paetzold, R. L., & Rholes, S. (2021). The link from child abuse to dissociation: The roles of adult disorganized attachment, self-concept clarity, and reflective functioning. *Journal of Trauma and Dissociation, 22*(5), 615–635. https://doi.org/10.1080/15299732.2020.1869654

Panksepp, J. (1998). *Affective neuroscience: The foundations of human and animal emotions*. Oxford University Press.

Panksepp, J., & Biven, L. (2012). *The archaeology of mind: Neuroevolutionary origins of human emotions*. W. W. Norton.

Porges, S. W. (2011). *The polyvagal theory: Neurophysiological foundations of emotions, attachment, communication, and self-regulation*. W. W. Norton

Porges, S. W. (2021). *Polyvagal safety: Attachment, communication, self-regulation.* W. W. Norton.

Putnam, F. W. (1997). *Dissociation in children and adolescents: A developmental perspective.* Guilford Press.

Putnam, F. W. (2016). *The way we are: How states of mind influence our identities, personality and potential for change.* IPBooks.

Reinders, A., & Veltman, D. (2021). Dissociative identity disorder: Out of the shadows at last? *British Journal of Psychiatry, 219*(2), 413–414. https://doi.org/10.1192/bjp.2020.168

Schauer, M., & Elbert, T. (2010). Dissociation following traumatic stress. *Zeitschrift für Psychologie [Journal of Psychology], 218*(2), 109–127. https://doi.org/10.1027/0044-3409/a000018

Schimmenti, A. (2017). The developmental roots of dissociation: A multiple mediation analysis. *Psychoanalytic Psychology, 34*, 96–105. https://doi.org/10.1037/pap0000084

Schimmenti, A. (2020). Can dissociative symptoms exist without underlying dissociation of the personality? Yes! *European Journal of Trauma and Dissociation, 6*(2), Article 100243. https://doi.org/10.1016/j.ejtd.2021.100243

Schlumpf, Y. R., Nijenhuis, E. R. S., Klein, C., Jäncke, L., & Bachmann, S. (2019). Functional reorganization of neural networks involved in emotion regulation following trauma therapy for complex trauma disorders. *NeuroImage: Clinical, 23*, Article 101807. https://doi.org/10.1016/j.nicl.2019.101807

Schore, A. N. (2003). *Affect regulation and the development of the self.* W. W. Norton.

Schore, A. N. (2012). *The science of the art of psychotherapy.* W. W. Norton.

Silberg, J. (2021). *The child survivor: Healing developmental trauma and dissociation* (2nd ed.). Routledge.

Simeon, D., & Abugel, D. (2023). *Feeling unreal: Depersonalization and the loss of the self* (2nd ed.). Oxford University Press.

Sinason, V., & Potgieter Marks, R. (Eds.). (2021). *Treating children with dissociative disorders: Attachment, trauma, theory and practice.* Routledge.

Solomon, J., & George, C. (1999). Attachment and caregiving: The caregiving behavioral system. In J. Cassidy & P. R. Shaver (Eds.), *Handbook of attachment: Theory, research, and clinical applications* (pp. 649–670). Guilford Press.

Steele, K. (2018). Dependency in the psychotherapy of chronically traumatized individuals: Using motivational systems to guide effective treatment. *Cognitivismo Clinico, 15*(2), 221–226. apc.it/wp-content/uploads/2013/03/18_Steele_CC18-2-2.pdf

Steele, K. (2021). Beyond attachment: Understanding motivational systems in complex trauma and dissociation. In D. Siegel, A. Schore & L. Cozolino (Eds.), *Interpersonal neurobiology and clinical practice* (pp. 85–112). W. W. Norton.

Steele, K., Boon, S., & Van der Hart, O. (2017). *Treating trauma-related dissociation: A practical integrative approach.* W. W. Norton.

Steele, K., Van der Hart, O., & Dorahy, M. J. (2023). Dissociation versus alterations in consciousness: Different but related concepts. In M. J. Dorahy, S. N. Gold & J. A. O'Neil (Eds.), *Dissociation and the dissociative disorders: Past, present, future* (2nd ed., pp. 66–80). Routledge.

Swica, Y., Lewis, D. O., & Lewis, M. (1996). Child abuse and dissociative identity disorder/multiple personality disorder: The documentation of childhood maltreatment and the corroboration of symptoms. *Child and Adolescent Psychiatric Clinics of North America, 5*(2), 431–447. https://doi.org/10.1016/S1056-4993(18)30374-2

Trevarthen, C., & Aitken, K. J. (1994). Brain development, infant communication, and empathy disorders: Intrinsic factors in child mental health. *Development and Psychopathology, 6*, 597–633. https://doi.org/10.1017/S0954579400004703

Van der Hart, O., Nijenhuis, E. R. S., & Steele, K. (2006). *The haunted self: Stuctural dissociation of the personality and treatment of chronic traumatization.* Norton.

Steele, K., & Van der Hart, O. (2019). Assessing and treating complex dissociative disorders. In C. A. Courtois & J. A. Ford (Eds.), *Treating complex traumatic stress disorders in adults: Scientific foundations and therapeutic models* (2nd ed., pp. 149–167). Guilford.

Van Dijke, A., Hopman, J. A., & Ford, J. D. (2018). Affect dysregulation, psychoform dissociation, and adult relational fears mediate the relationship between childhood trauma and complex posttraumatic stress disorder independent of the symptoms of borderline personality disorder. *European Journal of Psychotraumatology, 9*(1), 1400878.

Waters, F. (2016). *Healing the fractured child: Diagnosis and treatment of youth with dissociation.* Springer.

Wieland, S. (2015). *Dissociation in traumatized children and adolescents.* Routledge.

7
THE AUTOHYPNOTIC MODEL OF DISSOCIATION

D. Michael Coy

Introduction

It has been known since at least the time of Charcot (1878/1991) that dissociative features and hypnotic phenomena overlap. More contemporary research has indicated that persons with dissociative disorders are highly hypnotizable (Bliss, 1983; Frischholz et al., 1992). Putnam (1997) considered the "autohypnotic model" of dissociation—which, broadly speaking, posits that higher hypnotizability and hypnotic capacities play a central role in the development and maintenance of dissociative disorders—to be the foremost theory of dissociation.

Despite the model's alleged dominance, the value to clinicians of developing a basic understanding of hypnotizability in service of treating traumagenic dissociation seems to have been obscured by both continuing controversies surrounding the existence of dissociative disorders and concerns that clinical hypnosis contributes to iatrogenic treatment outcomes (Brand et al., 2016; Goodwin, 1985; Kluft, 1992; Loewenstein, 2018). Dell (2019, 2023a) suggested that the centrality of hypnotizability in dissociative disorders has been sidelined by erroneous research conclusions, resulting in a wholesale dismissal of an autohypnotic model. With that, we have seen widespread acceptance of more explicitly trauma-centric conceptualizations of dissociation, which derive from the work of Pierre Janet and others, such as the trauma model (Ross, 2007) and the structural model (see Chapter 6; van der Hart et al., 2006). These often seem to be accepted, at least generally, as incontrovertible fact. However, different models of dissociation each reflect only isolated facets of the entire domain of dissociation (Lebois et al., 2023). Despite the almost exclusive focus on traumagenesis in most current models of dissociation, the assertion that trauma is the sole catalyst for the development of pathological dissociation remains arguable (Ganaway, 1995; Kluft, 1985a). Dell (2023a) highlighted an inadequate correlation between reported trauma and a dissociative diagnosis, leading him to the conclusion that "trauma cannot be the sole determinant—or even the primary determinant?—of dissociation" (p. 238). Dell (2023a) characterized the limited attention given to overlaps between hypnotizability and dissociation since the 1990s as "the road not taken" (p. 239). Even with renewed, if localized, attention to the autohypnotic model since 2009 (courtesy of Paul Dell, mostly), there remain many unexplored avenues. Before we discuss the autohypnotic model itself, let us first establish some common ground by examining hypnosis, hypnotizability, and dissociation.

Hypnosis and Hypnotizability

Hypnosis

The American Psychological Association (2014) defines hypnosis as "[a] state of consciousness involving focused attention and reduced peripheral awareness characterized by an enhanced capacity for response to suggestion" (Definition and description of hypnosis section, para. 1). The term "hypnosis" is sometimes used to describe both the state itself, also referred to as a "trance" or a state of heightened suggestibility, and the method for achieving this state. Traditionally, trance is understood to be elicited in one of three ways:

1. through the use of a hypnotic "induction" by another person (heterohypnosis)
2. by one's own conscious, intentional use of an induction (self-hypnosis)
3. spontaneously, without one realizing that they have entered such a state (autohypnosis; see Bliss, 1986).

Typically, a trance state is achieved via focused attention such as absorption in an external task or internal preoccupation of some sort or a sudden, emotionally jarring experience such as surprise, shock, or confusion (Terhune & Cardeña, 2016). The American Psychological Association's (APA's) (2014) definition of hypnosis describes a person's ability to respond to suggestions, which squarely points to heterohypnosis—that is, formal trance induction by another person—as the sole route for achieving hypnotic trance (Kirsch et al., 2007). Dell (2021) said this assumes one must be "hypnotized" for the effects of a hypnotic suggestion to be realized. Kirsch and Braffman (2001) asserted that "hypnotizability is an inaccurate and misleading name for a very important trait, ability, or propensity that has little to do with the induction of hypnosis" (p. 58). This viewpoint is amply supported in findings with adults and children alike (Milling et al., 2005; Morgan & Hilgard, 1978; Tellegen & Atkinson, 1974; Vandenberg, 1998).

Dell (2021) has dismissed hypnosis as "a Western, culture-bound ritual" (p. 17) and instead proposed that *"hypnotizability reflects an ability to alter experience that is inherent, to various degrees, in all humans, and has nothing to do with hypnosis (or even with suggestions)"* (p. 19, emphasis in original). Dell (2023b) has recently extended his deconstruction of the hypnotist-subject paradigm by contending that hypnosis itself is not real. He countered that it is instead a cultural myth or illusion, and that a person's aptitude for altering different dimensions of their experience is similar, in its way, to someone's natural aptitude for athletic or musical ability. This echoes Bliss (1983), who cited evidence from other cultures that heightened hypnotic ability can be cultivated, "just as learning can influence many other genetic behavioral traits" (p. 118).

Hypnotizability

The American Psychological Association (2014) characterizes hypnotizability as "[a]n individual's ability to experience *suggested* [emphasis added] alterations in physiology, sensations, emotions, thoughts, or behavior during hypnosis" (Definition and description of hypnosis section, para. 3). Whatever we call it, the ability to alter one's experience via "hypnotic" means, to maintain hyperfocused attention, to become more deeply absorbed—whether with the assistance of someone else or by oneself, intentionally or not—appears to have a genetic basis (Gialluisi, 2016; Morgan, 1973; Szekely et al., 2010). Hypnotizability is typically evaluated via testing of different, objectively measurable skills in response to heterohypnosis. This sort of testing, courtesy of a handful of validated instruments, has suggested that most adults are hypnotically responsive to a greater or lesser degree, and the trait of hypnotizability for adults appears to be relatively stable over time (Piccione et al., 1989). Research has indicated three broad categories of hypnotizability: low, medium, and high. It is important to keep in mind that these classifications are based on a person's behavioral responsivity to *heterohypnotic* suggestions, following a formal hypnotic induction, according to standardized measures. Most adults have been found to be in the lower range of hypnotizability, with comparatively fewer in the high-hypnotizable range, with the uppermost range of highs (5%–10% of the population) termed "virtuosos," who possess the widest range of hypnotic abilities (Kihlstrom, 2004; Register & Kihlstrom, 1986). Both clinical experience and research suggest that the more highly hypnotizable (i.e., suggestible and trance-prone) a person is, the more intense their hypnotic experience and broader their repertoire of hypnotic abilities are. Such abilities include, but are not limited to, (1) involuntary eye closure; (2) postural sway (more on this below); (3) experiences of amnesia—that is, an absence of knowledge/awareness, both naturally occurring while in a deeper trance and suggested by another as a post-hypnotic experience; (4) perceptual distortions, including auditory and visual hallucinations—that is, hearing or seeing something that *is not* there (positive hallucinations) and *not* hearing/seeing something that *is* there (negative hallucinations); (5) arm rigidity; (6) full-body immobilization (i.e., tonic immobility); (7) verbal inhibition; (8) age regression; and (9) post-hypnotic suggestions (e.g., an experience that will manifest even after the person has been re-alerted), among others (Bliss, 1986; Hilgard, 1986; Kohen & Olness, 2011). (Notably, all of these phenomena can manifest, without conscious involvement and absent a formal hypnotic induction or suggestion, for persons with a dissociative disorder.)

Although significant, sex-based differences in hypnotizability have been difficult to quantify (Kihlstrom, 2008; Kohen & Olness, 2011), age-based differences have been observed. Children in general have been found to be more highly responsive to suggestion than adults. As with adults, however, not all children are equally suggestible (Page & Green, 2007; Morgan & Hilgard, 1973). Owing to developmental limitations imposed by cognitive capacity and language development—as well as continuing debate about the nature of hypnosis itself—it has been difficult to study hypnotizability in infants and pre-age three toddlers using standardized measures (Vandenberg, 1998). Gardner (1977) observed that infants and toddlers are responsive to soothing, repetitive stimuli that may or may not result in sleep (see also Kohen & Olness, 2011). In general, the lowest degree of hypnotic responsiveness via language-based trance elicitation has been observed in four- to five-year-olds, followed by a sharp increase for those aged 8–12, then a decline in responsiveness into adolescence (see Vandenberg, 2002). It has been noted, however, that research-based generalizations such as these obscure important, individual differences in responsiveness. For example, some four- to five-year-olds demonstrate greater suggestibility than is the norm even for slightly older, typically more hypnotically responsive, children (Kohen & Olness, 2011).

Research has also indicated that relational factors influence children's susceptibility to formal hypnotic induction. Perhaps the most central of these is the child's attitude toward the person engaging them, e.g., their experience of the (adult) hypnotist as safe. Another factor is the child's actual motivation to engage hypnotically (Kohen & Olness, 2011; London & Cooper, 1969; Vandenberg, 2002), which would seemingly be reinforced over time by a positive outcome (e.g., relief of distress, not being harmed while in a less cognitively alert state). Speaking to the challenge of understanding how children respond to heterohypnotic engagement, Vandenberg (1998) surmised that

> the challenge [...] is not to determine [the] 'absolute value' [of hypnotizability] in young childhood and compare it to older ages. Rather, what must be examined is the comparative contextual ecology of responding: better or worse, in what ways, and under what conditions?
>
> *(p. 241)*

additionally noting that the use of standardized measures "will not illuminate the developmental characteristics of hypnotic responsivity" (p. 242).

Perhaps most notably for a discussion of hypnosis and dissociation, research by Morgan and Hilgard (1978) found that children under seven years old were significantly more responsive to hypnotic engagement via imagination (i.e., fantasy) than through relaxation-based (e.g., eye closure-focused) elicitations. Vandenberg (1998) also suggested an infant's natural, imitative mirroring of their caregiver as a foundation for the development of heightened hypnotic susceptibility later in life—a bit like exercising a (hypnotic) muscle over thousands of interactions. We could imagine that, since some individuals have a greater innate capacity for trance-like experiences than others, some infants may "benefit" more from this kind of "exercise." This would be within the realm of hypnotic abilities that inform healthy, if variably deep, absorption in play, creative endeavors, and other engaging, task-based activities.

London and Cooper (1969) compared hypnotic abilities of children to those of adults, as evidenced by the difficulty of the suggestion given. Among 12 different tasks, children were more responsive than adults to suggestions for auditory hallucinations and postural sway and slightly less responsive than adults for the experience of amnesia. The postural sway, which is both a test of hypnotic susceptibility and a more advanced trance elicitation technique, essentially engages someone's fear of falling and their efforts to avoid it. As described by Watkins (1987), a hypnotic subject is invited to imagine that their feet are hinged to the floor, while at the same time recognizing the inevitability of falling (onto a soft chair, etc.). Watkins (1987) observed that some "patients will become so cataleptic throughout their entire body that they fall backward completely rigid, like a board" (p. 138).

Conversely, Jacobs and Jacobs's (1966) study of 64 children and adolescents revealed factors that may *impede* a child's susceptibility to heterohypnosis. Here, suggestibility was indicated by the child's capacity to "enter a trance state and achieve visual and auditory recall hallucinations" (p. 271). Children who were low/non-hypnotizable had not developed a left/right eye, hand, or foot preference, reportedly due to un(der)developed hemispheric dominance (per EEG results) and/or exhibited poor attention span, engaged in temper tantrums, and had "lower academic achievement, often in spite of average or above average intelligence" (p. 273). The EEG results correlated with intellectual delays, though the children with "minimal brain damage" notably were labeled as such due to "poor coordination, poor mobility patterns and the failure to establish laterality [left/right] preferences, by hyperactivity, perseveration, distractibility, perceptual difficulties and reading difficulties" (p. 272).

Notably, the children in the Jacobs and Jacobs (1966) study who were most *readily* able to enter a trance state were those with "emotional problems" without any evidence of neurological issues (92%), those diagnosed with "childhood schizophrenia" (80%), and those with minimal brain damage (66%). Of the children with emotional problems, 92% were able to achieve visual hallucinations, and 66% achieved auditory hallucinations. For children diagnosed with schizophrenia, those percentages were 100% (visual) and 33% (auditory), and for those with "minimal brain damage," they were 83% (visual) and 17% (auditory). The study reported that children with the highest IQs (115 to 130+) were the most responsive overall. Jacobs and Jacobs (1966) did not mention factors such as the children's attachment history, exposure to adverse experiences, or trauma-related symptoms. Additionally, the possibility of dissociation appears to have been entirely overlooked. This seems unsurprising considering the long, fraught history of persons with dissociative disorders being misdiagnosed or underdiagnosed in favor of schizophrenia (see Kluft, 1987). On a darker note, the research discussed here is based on formal studies of children and do not consider salient, yet even today, often-ignored issues such as the possible misuse of a child's natural hypnotic (and possibly dissociative) capacities and hypnotic techniques by those with ill intent. With all these hypnosis-related considerations in mind, let us shift our gaze more explicitly toward dissociation.

Dissociation

The *DSM-5-TR* (American Psychiatric Association, 2022) describes dissociation as the "disruption of and/or discontinuity in the normal integration of consciousness, memory, identity, emotion, perception, body representation, motor control, and behavior" (p. 329), with somatosensory hallucinations experienced by dissociative individuals due to "*autohypnotic* [emphasis added] posttraumatic, and dissociative" factors (p. 336). Silberg and Dallam (2023), however, emphasize that the *DSM* definition of dissociation is less helpful in understanding dissociation in children, as it suggests a retrospective disruption—one that has already occurred—rather than an unfolding, *in vivo* process still in its early stages. Loewenstein (2023, p. 744) observed that,

> ...childhood DID typically is less elaborated than in most adults (Silberg, 2013), with self-states manifesting more as independently acting, autonomous imaginary companions operating through influence/intrusion, less by state shifting (Silberg & Dallam, 2023). [It is only] [i]n adolescence, where issues of sexuality, separation and individuation are central, [that] self-states may become more elaborated and manifest more concretized forms of internal conflict.

A more in-depth discussion of manifestations of dissociation in children and related diagnostic considerations may be found in Chapters 12 and 13 of this volume, respectively. Here, it should suffice to enumerate the features of pathological dissociation in children that seem most obviously hypnotic in nature. These include amnesia (an absence of explicit knowledge, for both past and day-to-day experiences); deeper, trance-like states (e.g., staring off into space without conscious awareness of the present moment); a higher capacity for absorption in fantasy and engagement with "imaginary friends" that is more immersive and/or pervasive than in typical play scenarios; developmental issues/delays; functional neurological issues (e.g., somatic numbing, paralysis, seizures, pain, temporary loss of sight, and hearing) that defy medical explanation; and hallucinations (e.g., auditory and visual) (Otnow Lewis, 1996; Peterson, 1991, 1998; Silberg, 2013; Silberg & Dallam, 2023; Waters, 2016). This leads us directly to the autohypnotic model of dissociation.

The Autohypnotic Model: Context and a Brief Overview

Coy and Madere (2022) suggested that there are three different types of theories of dissociation:

1 *Explanatory* models posit etiological factors that precipitate dissociation (e.g., the trauma model; Ross, 2007).
2 *Descriptive* models elaborate the symptom features of dissociation without explicit regard for etiology—e.g., Dell's (2006) subjective-phenomenological model.
3 *Explanatory/descriptive* models both posit etiological factors and elaborate symptom features—for example, the theory of structural dissociation of the personality (van der Hart et al., 2006) and Putnam's discrete behavioral states theory (Loewenstein & Putnam, 2023).

At the surface, the autohypnotic model is explanatory, with a clear focus on etiology. However, if hypnotic abilities are foundational to and interwoven with the development of what eventually become dissociative symptoms and disorders, then the autohypnotic model can be considered both explanatory and descriptive. Whether and how hypnotizability may be facilitative of dissociation remains largely in the realm of conceptual speculation and debate, though plenty of existing evidence indicates significant overlap (see Dell, 2023a, for deeper exploration).

A more formal autohypnotic model of dissociation has its roots in the work of Charcot (1878/1991) and Breuer and Freud (1893/1956), though hypnosis was much more of interest to Breuer than to Freud. Kluft (2018a, 2018b, 2019) discussed in depth how Freud's dismissal of the therapeutic value of hypnosis, despite his early collaboration with Breuer, served as a "nail in the coffin" for widespread acceptance and serious examination of overlaps between hypnosis and dissociation. Although

Janet, like his mentor Charcot, viewed hypnotizability as a sign of psychopathology (Janet, 1907; Dell, 2023a), his observational understanding of dissociation yielded the concept of *automatisms*, or "behaviors and reactions that occur automatically, 'on their own,' without being directed by the conscious mind or by the stimuli of the environment" (Dell, 2009, p. 770).

Sidis and Goodhart (1904/1968) authored an early volume on "multiple personality" in which hypnotic phenomena and dissociation via hypnotic means are discussed throughout, including a chapter dedicated specifically to hypnoid states as they relate to dissociation. The work of Morton Prince, in both his monographs and his founding editorship of the *Journal of Abnormal Psychology* (1906–1929), continued investigation in this area. T. W. Mitchell (1921) both critiqued Janet's stance that hypnotic capacity was but a by-product of hysteria—or hysterical neurosis, a prototype for the modern somatoform and dissociative disorders, with a distinctly misogynistic flavor (see Tasca et al., 2012)—and attempted to parse out normative and pathological varieties of hypnotic susceptibility and phenomena. Shepherd Ivory Franz (1933) documented his hypnosis-informed treatment of a World War I veteran presenting with "multiple personalities." John G. Watkins (1949), who presented case studies that included his first encounter with a veteran of World War II who initially presented with "battle neurosis" (now PTSD), but whom Watkins came to discover was struggling with far more internal complexity. This was apparently Watkins's first knowing encounter with a person with MPD/DID, which predated his co-development of Ego State Therapy (Watkins & Watkins, 1997).

In the modern era, we can look to Henri Ellenberger (1970), whose comprehensive history of the early years of dynamic psychiatry, including the study of dissociation, contributed to rejuvenating interest in this topic. Eugene Bliss's (1986) exploration of hypnosis and dissociative disorders offers a deep dive into autohypnotic phenomena and remains the only volume of its kind. Paul F. Dell, who has written extensively about and perhaps single-handedly revived interest in the autohypnotic model over the past 15 years, has taken successive "road trips" looking at the existing literature and returned each time with a wealth of both conceptual and practical considerations.

Dell (2019) looks to Kluft's (1985a) Four Factor theory of dissociative disorders as a framework for contextualizing the role of hypnotizability in the development of pathological dissociation. Kluft posits four conditions that must be present for DID to develop:

1 dissociative capacity.
2 exposure to overwhelming experiences that usually include abuse of some kind.
3 a variety of underlying qualities and characteristics that inform the development of a diverse array of dissociative self-states; and
4 a lack of support from caregivers and other important figures in both helping the child make sense of what has happened and protecting the child from further harm.

Dell has employed this framework with a minor modification. While Kluft, in Dell's view, focuses on the child's experience of helplessness in the development of a dissociative disorder, Dell (2019) emphasizes the necessity for "the active, motivated use of autohypnotic coping mechanisms (to escape intolerable circumstances)" (p. 60). He notes that a highly hypnotizable individual, if not faced with Kluft's second, third, and fourth factors, may also not be spurred to mentally escape the physically inescapable, and, in turn, will not discover their ability to flee via innate, autohypnotically-driven means. These means of escape include any of a variety of autohypnotic abilities, all of which reflect an underlying capacity for initially spontaneous and, later, intentional alteration of one's own relationship to their self and the world around them (Dell, 2010, 2021). (To understand the evolution of Dell's thinking on this topic, refer to Dell, 2009, 2010, 2017a, 2017b, 2019, 2021, 2023a, 2023b.)

Notably, Silberg (2013) briefly describes a similar hypothesis for the autohypnotically motivated development of a dissociative disorder, though without discussing mechanisms specific to hypnosis and hypnotizability that may facilitate this. In any case, there is ample evidence that the foundations of pathological dissociation are laid in childhood (Coons, 1994; Hornstein & Putnam, 1992; Kluft, 1985a, 1985b) and solid support for the assertion that humans can organically alter their experience, both voluntarily and involuntarily, in the face of overwhelm (Dell, 2009, 2010, 2021). However, despite Dell's recent efforts to (re)establish hypnotic capacity as the essential catalyst for the development of a dissociative disorder, little attention has been given to the actual, concrete capacities of infants and children within this context.

Deepening into the Autohypnotic Model

Pathological or Normative Dissociation?

Barabasz and Watkins (2005, p. 67) offer that,

> Orne (1959) held that the essence of hypnosis, and that which distinguishes truly hypnotized individuals from simulators, is the ability of hypnotized participants to freely mix perceptions derived from reality with those that stem from […] imagination. This characteristic tolerance of logical inconsistencies Orne termed *trance logic* [emphasis in original]. Trance logic is closely related to the concrete thinking or primary process that characterizes […] dissociative reactions […] and children.

So, then, is this phenomenon pathological, normative, or both? Recall Charcot's and Janet's belief that hypnotizability is itself a sign of pathology. Sidis and Goodhart (1904/1968) contrastingly viewed *all* hypnoid states as essentially dissociative in nature, while clarifying that "hypnoid or coexistent dissociated states may be cultivated by healthy individuals with some success" (pp. 327–328). Along a similar line, Ernest Hilgard (1984) demonstrated what Sidis and Goodhart described, in his accidental (re)discovery(?) of the "hidden observer" phenomenon, which he characterized as a metaphorical construct for this temporary presence *within a subset of highly hypnotizable individuals*. This seeming observer has direct access to and the ability to report on experience outside conscious awareness (e.g., pain and knowledge)—without the "central executive" being aware of that observer, from a place of dissociated control. Hilgard (1986) stressed both that this state is "temporary" and that his conceptualization (and demonstration of the phenomenon) were not intended to suggest the more pronounced and abiding division seen in persons with dissociative disorders. He described this temporary state as "an organized cognitive structure of recent information acquired covertly [i.e., outside conscious awareness] that could be made available only through special [hypnotic] procedures (Hilgard, 1984)" (p. 299). It was from these and other observations that Hilgard (1986) developed his neodissociation theory of hypnosis. This model posits different levels of executive control, most of which exist outside conscious awareness (as they are hypothesized to be separated by naturally occurring amnesia barriers), but which may be accessed via formal hypnosis. (This description is reminiscent of hypnotic phenomena described by Watkins & Watkins (1997) in the context of Ego State Therapy.)

There is something of automaticity implied here, i.e., "it's just happening on its own"—at least from the point of view of a "central executive." However, there is also the possibility of dissociated control at play—that is, a different level of executive control outside conscious intentionality, but also not experienced by the "central executive" as jarring or intrusive, suggesting it is not necessarily pathological (Dell, 2006). Kihlstrom (1992) argued that "the experience of automaticity, like so much else about hypnosis, is illusory" (p. 308), suggesting that there is always *some* level of executive control of actions, even if it is not obvious. Both Woody and Bowers (1994) and Dell (2010), however, took at least partial exception to this. Dell (2010) explored in meticulous detail the overlaps among the kinds of "involuntariness" (aka automaticity) observed in hypnotic responding, dissociative phenomena, and other areas of human functioning. He cited neuroimaging studies strongly suggesting that "involuntariness in hypnotic responding and in dissociative symptoms (and a variety of related experimental situations) share a common neural underpinning—increased activity of the inferior parietal cortex (i.e., angular gyrus and supramarginal gyrus; BA 39 and 40, respectively)" (p. 12). What, though, might "prime the pump" for this seemingly natural involuntariness to become problematic and, ultimately, pathological?

Attachment, Tonic Immobility, and Shock

Barach (1991) first suggested that dissociative disorders are, etiologically speaking, rooted in attachment-related harm. Liotti (1992, 1999a, 1999b) subsequently suggested that disorganized attachment is a correlate for the development of dissociative disorders. Discussing the insecure-disorganized/disoriented attachment pattern seen in 12-month-olds as part of the "Strange Situation" studies (Main & Solomon, 1986), Schore (2001) reflected on their "uniquely disturbing behaviors," noting that

> these episodes of interruptions of organized behavior and low stress tolerance are often brief, frequently lasting 10–30 seconds, yet they are highly significant. *For example, they show a simultaneous display of contradictory behavior patterns, such as 'backing' towards the parent rather than approaching face to face.*
>
> *(emphasis added, p. 215)*

Hesse et al. (2003) observed more specifically of this disorganized/disoriented behavior that "the infant may freeze with a *trancelike expression* [emphasis added], hands in air; may rise at parent's entry then fall prone and huddled on the floor; or may cling while crying hard and leaning away with gaze aversion" (p. 74).

The "sudden immobilized postures" seen in the Strange Situation may refer to tonic immobility (TI), an animal defensive response observed in a variety of species, including humans. Abrams et al. (2009) described TI as a "temporary behavioral state of motor inhibition thought to occur in response to situations involving intense fear, such as sexual assault, or for animals, encounters with predators" (p. 550). This state manifests as a "stuporous catatonic-like immobility with muscular hyper- or hypo-tonicity, odd postures, suppression of vocalization, intermittent eye closure, and Parkinsonian-like tremors" and "typically terminates abruptly with either dramatic flight or defensive attack" (pp. 550–551).

Simonov and Paikin (1969) suggested that "motor inhibition in animals and the state of hypnotic trance in man (sic) appear to be genetically interrelated, have a similar adaptive significance and, in all probability, possess certain neurophysiological mechanisms" (p. 67). Putnam (2016) observed an overlap between the phenomenon of tonic immobility and altered states of consciousness seen during clinical hypnosis. Charcot (1878/1991, p. 335) described hypnotically induced paralysis in two patients:

> Nervous shock is produced by some strong emotion, a fright, a feeling of terror determined by an accident, especially when this accident menaces life […]. […] On these occasions a peculiar mental condition is often developed, […], *which is very intimately connected, in my judgment, with the hypnotic state.*
>
> *(emphasis added)*

Tonic immobility could be a precipitant and/or sign of both peritraumatic dissociation (Rocha-Rego et al., 2009) and pathological (traumagenic) dissociation more generally (Kearney & Lanius, 2022; Nijenhuis et al., 1998). However, Dell (2023a) pointed out that "there is little research [...] on the question of whether humans undergo a spontaneous, temporary increase in their ability to manage pain (1) during moments of severe injury and imminent threat to life, and (2) during recuperation from injury" (p. 254).

A landmark study investigated the impact of early, enduring exposure to traumatic overwhelm stemming from medical/surgical intervention, its sequelae, and their relationship to dissociation in adolescence and adulthood. Diseth (2006) reported that, as part of post-operative treatment for a subset of cases in the study, "*short-term, nonrepetitive restraint of the child was reported* [emphasis added] by parents to be unpleasant for the child and parents alike, *but no significant dissociative problems were reported as adolescents or adults*" [emphasis added] (p. 244). This subset of children were treated only by medical professionals, with their parents being witnesses to the treatment. Caregivers were offered guidance on how to comfort their child post-procedure.

Another portion of the study sample, due to a differing but similar medical condition, were forced by circumstance to endure

> repeated unpleasant, painful, stressful, and traumatic medical treatment procedures, as well as a relationship-type trauma owing to the fact that it involves a treatment procedure [that involved repetitive restraint and anal dilation at home] 'inflicted' by the primary caregivers on their child.
>
> *(Diseth, 2006, p. 245)*

This group subsequently developed dissociative features. All the children in this study were exposed to the conditions noted above before the age of 5, spanning back, for some, to infancy. Brand et al. (2012) noted the "similarities between animal defensive responses including freezing responses, tonic immobility, analgesia, and dissociative states in humans [...]," adding that "psychometrically measured tonic immobility has been shown to correlate positively with dissociative symptoms" (p. 18).

Among all the factors studied, Diseth (2006) noted that "the only significant predictor of the adolescents' dissociative problems ten years post-treatment was the duration of anal dilation" (p. 242). Duration, here, refers to the span of time over which the treatment was necessary rather than per-episode time—in other words, the higher frequency of invasive procedures over a longer span of time, the more acute the dissociative issues. Speaking to the question of whether intentionality matters, Diseth (2006) observed that "depending on the child's cognitive level, it may not matter whether the perpetrator is truly helping the child or deliberately causing harm and pain" (p. 247). This statement suggests that perception of the problem of being held down has some bearing. This invites the question of how one might solve the problem like inescapable pain.

It was mentioned earlier in this discussion that it is possible to elicit a trance state via a sudden, emotionally jarring experience such as surprise, shock, or confusion (Terhune & Cardeña, 2016), and later that there appears to be some kind of relationship between shock and tonic immobilities. Corrigan and Christie-Sands (2020) described a phenomenon they called *attachment shock*, which they suggested occurs as a result of "those experiences which were suddenly and unpredictably unpleasant and which carried a high-energy impact" (p. 2). They delineated two different manifestations. The first, called pre-affective shock, is "high-energy impact shock which occurs before the affective response." The second "occurs with sudden and overwhelming affect and is hypothesized to be mediated by the structures of the defensive system, the PAG [periaqueductal grey] and hypothalamus, and may be the precursor to neurochemical dissociation" (p. 6). Neurochemical dissociation involves the release of endogenous cannabinoids and opioids. These neurochemicals are connected to experiences of depersonalization, derealization, tonic immobility, and collapsed immobility (for more information on this process, please see Chapter 11).

Corrigan (2023) cited Campagner et al. (2023) in describing what the latter characterized as a specialized "escape" circuit in many species, including humans, which helps facilitate a rapid flight toward shelter in the face of existential threat. In essence, this makes it possible for us to find a "safe place"—whether that is a person, place, or thing. What if there is no safe, external resource in that moment? What if that moment is sustained or repetitious? Dell's (2019) position is that the development of a dissociative disorder requires "active, motivated use of autohypnotic coping mechanisms (to escape intolerable circumstances)" (p. 60), which can occur only for persons who are highly hypnotizable (Dell, 2023b). If shock of this kind can incite peritraumatic dissociation, what are the implications for the development of pathological dissociation? And, what additional factors have we not yet considered?

Genetic, Epigenetic, and Neurobiological Correlates

Lebois et al. (2023) pointed out that, to date, there is no research on genetic and/or epigenetic aspects of the dissociative disorders specifically. Both genetic and neurobiological correlates linking hypnotizability and dissociative disorders *do* appear to exist, though most studies have occurred separately in the hypnosis and dissociative disorders fields. Definitive genetic evidence for a connection between the two phenomena remains elusive (Rajkumar, 2022). However, the COMT gene, which appears to be implicated in the experience of absorption, hypnotizability, the perception of time, and the release of endogenous opioids in the face of extreme stress, has been named as a compelling focus for further study (Savitz et al., 2008). We do know that trauma, broadly speaking, has an impact on gene expression, particularly related to cortisol release (Yehuda & Lehrner, 2018). Thus, it makes sense that epigenetic factors could also exert an effect on the traits of hypnotizability and dissociation—perhaps even within an individual over time.

From the field of hypnosis, Barnier et al. (2022, p. 131) noted the work of Josephine Hilgard and Arlene Morgan, who "explored childhood pathways to hypnotic ability and its genetic underpinnings suggesting, for instance, that imaginative involvement (whether through play, storytelling, or perspective-taking) both develops and potentially preserves hypnotizability (Morgan & Hilgard, 1973)." With this being the case, and considering other elements of this discussion, it seems at least possible that the *maladaptive* employment of each of these might also preserve dissociation—especially if one's "safe place," as noted above, is to be found only within.

Contemporary Phenomenological Data

Butler et al. (1996) offered up a "diathesis-stress" model of hypnotic and traumagenic dissociative phenomena based on a comprehensive exploration of the overlaps between the two domains; in summary, the model indicates that available evidence suggested that "the interaction of hypnotizability and traumagenic experience is, in most cases, a necessary and sometimes sufficient condition for such [dissociative] pathology" (p. 60).

With a slightly different "take," Cleveland et al. (2015) and Cleveland et al. (2020) examined relationships between hypnotic capacity and state (rather than trait) dissociation. Ultimately, their work, particularly the latter study, strongly suggested that dissociation occurs along a continuum. Specific to traumagenic dissociation, Cleveland et al. (2020) noted:

> While it is clear that hypnotic susceptibility and dissociative capacity are not, in fact, the same construct, a number of their components do appear to overlap, namely: amnesia, derealization, depersonalization, and somatoform dissociation [...]. Our study also suggests that three putative

components of dissociation that may not be involved in hypnosis include hypermnesia [acute recall], identity disturbance, and identity alteration. The lack of a relationship between hypnosis and the latter two components seems to intuitively make sense when considering that such manifestations tend to characterize pathological variants, such as dissociative multiplicity, which are widely thought to represent the most extreme types of dissociative, trauma-rooted pathology.

(pp. 145–146)

Based on their findings, Cleveland et al. (2020) advocated for transitioning to more evolved ways of understanding and languaging dissociation, citing Barlow and Freyd's (2009) conceptualization of "Branch A" and "Branch B" forms of dissociation, with "B" being traumagenic in nature. "Branch A" would encompass experiences of non-traumagenic, but pervasive and potentially problematic, imaginative involvement and absorption in fantasy, one manifestation of which is maladaptive daydreaming, which Soffer-Dudek and Somer (2023) asserted is a dissociative disorder. Though further discussion of this is outside the scope of this chapter, these phenomena may hold particular relevance for the experiences of older children, adolescents, and young adults who interact with social media and who may identify has having DID, but who do not meet current clinical criteria for any dissociative disorder (see also Soffer-Dudek et al., in press).

Potential Links Derived from Functional Neuroimaging

Technological limitations made it difficult for the field of psychoanalysis to establish scientific evidence validating the interpersonal phenomena observed in treatment settings (Cieri & Esposito, 2019). However, advances in computing and high-resolution scans over the past 35 years have provided means for clarifying that psychodynamics such as transference and countertransference may have neurobiological correlates (Gallese, 2009).

Similarly, more recent functional brain research has demonstrated not only that dissociative disorders exist in observable ways (Reinders et al., 2012; Schlumpf et al., 2014; Staniloiu et al., 2012) and can be distinguished as such (Dorahy et al., 2014), but also that different diagnostic features of dissociation appear to be associated with distinct brain activity "signatures" (Lebois et al., 2022). (For those interested in digging deeper, Lebois et al. [2023] offered a concise overview of the current state of research into the dissociative disorders.) Likewise in the hypnosis field, careful investigation has provided insight into the mechanisms of action involved in hypnosis (Jensen et al., 2015). Following on from previous foundational examination of hypnotic susceptibility (Spiegel, 1974), apparent neurobiological distinctions between low- and high-hypnotizable individuals have also been identified (Hoeft et al., 2012; Jiang et al., 2017).

Dell (2023a) urges asserted that to clarify the role of hypnotic phenomena in severe dissociative disorders, "more research on the hypnotizability of DID and other dissociative disorder patients is needed," with a particular focus on "the hypnotizability of trauma patients who report episodes of extreme dissociative detachment" (p. 253). Although there is no single study with such a focus, the Hoeft et al. (2012) and Jiang et al. (2017) studies of hypnosis and the Lebois et al. (2022) study of pathological dissociation share common ground, as all three studied neurobiological correlates of each phenomenon through the lens of the triple network model of psychopathology (Menon, 2011). According to Menon (2018):

the triple network model of psychopathology posits that aberrant functional organization of the salience network (SN), frontoparietal network (FPN) [also Central Executive Network (CEN) or Executive Central Network (ECN)], and default mode network (DMN) and their dynamic cross-network interactions underlie a wide range of psychopathologies […].

(p. 236)

Buckner (2013) explained that the default mode network is "a set of regions more active during passive tasks than tasks demanding focused external attention. One hypothesis is that the default network contributes to internal modes of cognition used when remembering, thinking about the future, and mind wandering." He added that "several observations suggest that disruption in executive control processes may impact the function of the default network and contribute to disturbances of thought" (p. 355). The "functional architecture" underlying this network is present at birth and undergoes significant change in childhood and adolescence during the process of cognitive, emotional, and social maturation (Fan et al., 2021, citing Bhana, 2010). Menon (2018) noted that the salience network "integrates sensory, emotional, and cognitive information and acts as an interface between" the default mode network and the frontoparietal network, "balance[ing] internal mental processes with external stimulus–driven cognitive and affective processes" (p. 236). Marek and Dosenback (2018, p. 133) described the frontoparietal/central executive network as "critical for our ability to coordinate behavior in a rapid, accurate, and flexible goal-driven manner," and that which "demonstrates a large degree of connectivity to many diverse brain networks, meaning that the frontoparietal network is a functional hub both globally and specifically in terms of distributed connectivity" (p. 135).

These studies suggest several commonalities/overlaps between brain activity for persons with DID and highly hypnotizable individuals based on both intra- and inter-network activities, which presently are not possible to explore in detail. There appear to be aspects of brain activity unique to each cohort, as well, though it seems possible that these could be attributable to factors related to differences between "Branch A" and "Branch B" dissociators. In any case, an intentional exploration of the commonalities and differences in brain network connectivity would surely be of value, in children and adults, for the sake of both better clarifying the role of hypnosis in dissociation and better understanding the full domain of dissociation in general.

Conclusion

With so many potential implications arising from our shared exploration of this autohypnotic "road less traveled," it may be of value to consider the bottom line via a series of "what ifs":

1 What if serial experiences of shock and the release of anesthetic-like neurochemicals were enough to activate a highly hypnotizable child's heightened ability to distance from and alter their subjective experience?
2 What if that child's need to escape intolerable pain leads them to a temporary shelter within their own developing mind?
3 What if the child is forced back to that place again and again through repetitive threat?
4 What if the child begins to capitalize on this initially reflexive use of hypnotic distancing/escape maneuvers, leading them down any number of paths, unique to them, in search of shelter in the (comparatively) safe recesses of their own mind?
5 What if, alongside their efforts to alter their own somatosensory experience to dull/avoid seemingly inescapable pain, they also become increasingly absorbed in their developing internal world—first, spontaneously, and later, as a consciously discovered and intentionally employed ability—simply because they visit so often?
6 What if this, over time and as the result of the serial disruption of the brain's normal processing of experience, also disrupts that child's development of a unified sense of self, eventually resulting in discrete behavioral states or schemas indicative of structural dissociation?

In instances when a child's daily functioning is fit to purpose, aligned with how they learned to get their needs met—whatever that looks like—and the demands of an unhealthful environment they cannot voluntarily escape, it seems likely that symptoms could be even more challenging to identify because the child's coping is ego-syntonic. The child's symptoms would likely not be experienced by them as such, in the same way that many adults do not think of their symptoms as anything outside the norm—it is their norm, after all, even if it is intolerable—until someone else recognizes and highlights them. It would be imperative that someone besides the child be aware and interested enough to notice that something of a dissociative nature is happening and thus to seek support for the child. This makes it even more important for mental health practitioners, including those who work with children, to consider dissociation as part of their initial and ongoing evaluation process.

Additionally, the discerning clinician is well-advised to obtain training in clinical hypnosis and develop an understanding of the overlaps between hypnosis and dissociation. It then becomes possible to explore the literature and engage in training to better understand how children respond to, experience, and use hypnosis differently from adolescents and adults. Practitioners might consider exactly how susceptible to trance states their young clients are, and whether they endured experiences of early life suffering that could have motivated them to rely and capitalize on auto- and self-hypnosis to cope. Our clients may not tell us because they may not realize it themselves.

More practically, hypnotic techniques, when employed by knowledgeable and experienced practitioners, can be very effective in the treatment of dissociative disorders, including with children (Gold & Quiñones, 2020; Kluft, 1985b, 2012; Ross & Norton, 1989; Williams & Velazquez, 1996). As I learned in my very first hypnosis training, it is likely that you are already engaging your clients' natural hypnotic capacities, regardless of the treatment modalities you employ, even when you do not realize it. Other chapters in this volume discuss the variety of options for conceptualizing childhood dissociation and engaging children and their families in effective healing work to transcend that dissociation. I hope you will walk away from *this* chapter feeling that a door has opened. I invite you to walk through it, bringing with you a deeper and abiding curiosity about hypnotic phenomena as a more central consideration in your work with children of all ages, both within and beyond the context of dissociation and the dissociative disorders.

References

Abrams, M. P., Carleton, R. N., Taylor, S., & Asmundson, G. J. (2009). Human tonic immobility: Measurement and correlates. *Depression and Anxiety, 26*(6), 550–556. https://doi.org/10.1002/da.20462

American Psychological Association (2014). *About the society of psychological hypnosis.* https://www.apadivisions.org/division-30/about

American Psychiatric Association (2022). *DSM-5-TR – Diagnostic and statistical manual of mental disorders* (5th ed.). American Psychiatric Publishing.

Barabasz, A., & Watkins, J. G. (2005). *Hypnotherapeutic techniques* (2nd ed.). Brunner-Routledge.

Barach, P. M. (1991). Multiple personality disorder as an attachment disorder. *Dissociation, 4*(3), 117–123. scholarsbank.uoregon.edu/xmlui/handle/1794/1448

Barlow, M. R., & Freyd, J. J. (2009). Adaptive dissociation: Information processing and response to betrayal. In P. F. Dell & J. A. O'Neil (Eds.), *Dissociation and the dissociation disorders: DSM-V and beyond* (pp. 93–105). Routledge.

Barnier, A. J., Terhune, D. B., Polito, V., & Woody, E. Z. (2022). A componential approach to individual differences in hypnotizability. *Psychology of Consciousness: Theory, Research, and Practice, 9*(2), 130–140. https://doi.org/10.1037/cns0000267

Bhana, A. (2010). *Middle childhood and pre-adolescence.* HSRC Press.

Bliss, E. L. (1983). Multiple personalities, related disorders, and hypnosis. *American Journal of Clinical Hypnosis, 26*(2), 114–123. https://doi.org/10.1080/00029157.1983.10404151

Bliss, E. L. (1986). *Multiple personality, allied disorders and hypnosis.* Oxford University Press.

Brand, B. L., Lanius, R., Vermetten, E., Loewenstein, R. J., & Spiegel, D. (2012). Where are we going? An update on assessment, treatment, and neurobiological research in dissociative disorders as we move toward the DSM-5. *Journal of Trauma & Dissociation, 13*(1), 9–31. https://doi.org/10.1080/15299732.2011.620687

Brand, B. L., Sar, V., Stavropoulos, P., Krüger, C., Korzekwa, M., Martínez-Taboas, A., & Middleton, W. (2016). Separating fact from fiction: An empirical examination of six myths about dissociative identity disorder. *Harvard Review of Psychiatry, 24*(4), 257–270. https://doi.org/10.1097/HRP.0000000000000100

Breuer, J., & Freud, S. (1893/1956). *Studies in hysteria.* Hogarth Press.

Buckner, R. L. (2013). The brain's default network: Origins and implications for the study of psychosis. *Dialogues in Clinical Neuroscience, 15*(3), 351–358. https://doi.org/10.31887/DCNS.2013.15.3/rbuckner

Butler, L. D., Duran, R. E. F., Jasiukaitis, P., Koopman, C., & Spiegel, D. (1996). Hypnotizability and traumatic experience: A diathesis-stress model of dissociative symptoms. *American Journal of Psychiatry, 153*(7, Festschrift Supplement), 42–63. https://doi.org/10.1176/ajp.153.8.A42

Campagner, D., Vale, R., Tan, Y. L., Iordanidou, P., Pavón Arocas, O., Claudi, F., Stempel, A. V., Keshavarzi, S., Petersen, R. S., Margrie, T. W., & Branco, T. (2023). A cortico-collicular circuit for orienting to shelter during escape. *Nature, 613*(7942), 111–119. https://doi.org/10.1038/s41586-022-05553-9

Charcot, J.-M. (1878/1991). *Clinical lectures on diseases of the nervous system* (R. Harris, Ed.). Tavistock/Routledge.

Cieri, F., & Esposito, R. (2019). Psychoanalysis and neuroscience: The bridge between mind and brain. *Frontiers in Psychology, 10*, Article 1790. https://doi.org/10.3389/fpsyg.2019.01983

Cleveland, J. M., Korman, B. M., & Gold, S. N. (2015). Are hypnosis and dissociation related? New evidence for a connection. *International Journal of Clinical and Experimental Hypnosis, 63*(2), 198–214. https://doi.org/10.1080/00207144.2015.1002691

Cleveland, J. M., Reuther, B. T., & Gold, S. N. (2020). The varied relationship between hypnosis and dissociative phenomena: Implications for traumatology. *American Journal of Clinical Hypnosis, 63*(2), 139–149. https://doi.org/10.1080/00029157.2020.1789545

Coons, P. M. (1994). Confirmation of childhood abuse in child and adolescent cases of multiple personality disorder and dissociative disorder not otherwise specified. *The Journal of Nervous and Mental Disease, 182*(8), 461–464. https://doi.org/10.1097/00005053-199408000-00007

Corrigan, F. M. (2023, October 29). *Deep brain reorienting (DBR) in complex trauma disorders: The pain of disconnection – And the dissociation from that pain* [Plenary presentation]. International Society for the Study of Trauma and Dissociation 2023 Virtual Conference.

Corrigan, F. M., & Christie-Sands, J. (2020). An innate brainstem self-other system involving orienting, affective responding, and polyvalent relational seeking: Some clinical implications for a "deep brain reorienting" trauma psychotherapy approach. *Medical Hypotheses, 136,* Article 109502. https://doi.org/10.1016/j.mehy.2019.109502

Coy, D. M., & Madere, J. A. (2022, December 9). *An introduction to dissociation and the MID – Definitions and foundations for assessment* [Webinar]. D & JAM Trainings. https://trainings.dandjam.com/courses/introduction-to-the-MID

Dell, P. F. (2006). A new model of dissociative identity disorder. *Psychiatric Clinics of North America, 29*(1), 1–26. https://doi.org/10.1016/j.psc.2005.10.013

Dell, P. F. (2009). Understanding dissociation. In P. F. Dell & J. A. O'Neil (Eds.), *Dissociation and the dissociative disorders: DSM-V and beyond* (pp. 709–825). Routledge.

Dell, P. F. (2010). Involuntariness in hypnotic responding and dissociative symptoms. *Journal of Trauma & Dissociation, 11*(1), 1–18. https://doi.org/10.1080/15299730903317964

Dell, P. F. (2017a). Is high hypnotizability a necessary diathesis for pathological dissociation? *Journal of Trauma & Dissociation, 18*(1), 58–87. https://doi.org/10.1080/15299732.2016.1191579

Dell, P. F. (2017b). What is the essence of hypnosis? *International Journal of Clinical and Experimental Hypnosis, 65*(2), 162–168. https://doi.org/10.1080/00207144.2017.1276360

Dell, P. F. (2019). Reconsidering the autohypnotic model of the dissociative disorders. *Journal of Trauma & Dissociation, 20*(1), 48–78. https://doi.org/10.1080/15299732.2018.1451806

Dell, P. F. (2021). Hypnotizability and the natural human ability to alter experience. *International Journal of Clinical and Experimental Hypnosis, 69*(1), 7–26. https://doi.org/10.1080/00207144.2021.1834859

Dell, P. F. (2023a). Clarifying the etiology of the dissociative disorders: It's not all about trauma. In M. J. Dorahy, S. N. Gold & J. A. O'Neil (Eds.), *Dissociation and the dissociative disorders: Past, present, future* (2nd ed., pp. 238–260). Routledge.

Dell, P. F. (2023b). What is the source of hypnotic responses? *International Journal of Clinical and Experimental Hypnosis,* 1–20. Advance online publication. https://doi.org/10.1080/00207144.2023.2276846

Diseth, T. H. (2006). Dissociation following traumatic medical treatment procedures in childhood: A longitudinal follow-up. *Development and Psychopathology, 18*(1), 233–251. https://doi.org/10.1017/s0954579406060135

Dorahy, M. J., Brand, B. L., Sar, V., Krüger, C., Stavropoulos, P., Martínez-Taboas, A., Lewis-Fernández, R., & Middleton, W. (2014). Dissociative identity disorder: An empirical overview. *Australian and New Zealand Journal of Psychiatry, 48*(5), 402–417. https://doi.org/10.1177/0004867414527523

Ellenberger, H. F. (1970). *The discovery of the unconscious: The history and evolution of dynamic psychiatry.* Basic Books.

Fan, F., Liao, X., Lei, T., Zhao, T., Xia, M., Men, W., Wang, Y., Hu, M., Liu, J., Qin, S., Tan, S., Gao, J. H., Dong, Q., Tao, S., & He, Y. (2021). Development of the default-mode network during childhood and adolescence: A longitudinal resting-state fMRI study. *NeuroImage, 226*, Article 117581. https://doi.org/10.1016/j.neuroimage.2020.117581

Franz, S. I. (1933). *Persons one and three: A study in multiple personality.* Whittlesey House.

Frischholz, E. J., Lipman, L. S., Braun, B. G., & Sachs, R. G. (1992). Psychopathology, hypnotizability, and dissociation. *American Journal of Psychiatry, 149*(11), 1521–1525. https://doi.org/10.1176/ajp.149.11.1521

Gallese, V. (2009). Mirror neurons, embodied simulation, and the neural basis of social identification. *Psychoanalytic Dialogues, 19*(5), 519–536. https://doi.org/10.1080/10481880903231910

Ganaway, G. K. (1995). Hypnosis, childhood trauma, and dissociative identity disorder: Toward an integrative theory. *International Journal of Clinical and Experimental Hypnosis, 43*(2), 127–144. https://doi.org/10.1080/00207149508409957

Gardner, G. G. (1977). Hypnosis with infants and preschool children. *American Journal of Clinical Hypnosis, 19*(3), 158–162. https://doi.org/10.1080/00029157.1977.10403864

Gialluisi, A. (2016). Hypnotizability and polymorphisms of the COMT gene: An association study [Doctoral thesis, Radboud University Nijmegen]. ResearchGate, researchgate.net/publication/298612420_Hypnotizability_and_Polymorphisms_of_the_COMT_gene_an_association_study

Gold, S. N., & Quiñones, M. (2020). Applicability of hypnosis to the treatment of complex PTSD and dissociation. *American Journal of Clinical Hypnosis, 63*(2), 78–94. https://doi.org/10.1080/00029157.2020.1789546

Goodwin, J. (1985). Credibility problems in multiple personality disorder patients and abused children. In R. P. Kluft (Ed.), *Childhood antecedents of multiple personality* (pp. 1–20). American Psychiatric Press.

Hesse, E., Main, M., Abrams, K. Y., & Rifkin, A. (2003). Unresolved states regarding loss or abuse can have "second generation" effects: Disorganization, role inversion, and frightening ideation on the offspring of traumatized, non-maltreating parents. In M. F. Solomon & D. J. Siegel (Eds.), *Healing trauma: Attachment, mind, body, and brain* (pp. 1–56). W. W. Norton.

Hilgard, E. R. (1984). The hidden observer and multiple personality. *International Journal of Clinical and Experimental Hypnosis, 32*(2), 248–253. https://doi.org/10.1080/00207148408416014

Hilgard, E. R. (1986). *Divided consciousness: Multiple controls in thought and action* (Exp. ed.). Wiley-Interscience.

Hoeft, F., Gabrieli, J. D., Whitfield-Gabrieli, S., Haas, B. W., Bammer, R., Menon, V., & Spiegel, D. (2012). Functional brain basis of hypnotizability. *Archives of General Psychiatry, 69*(10), 1064–1072. https://doi.org/10.1001/archgenpsychiatry.2011.2190

Hornstein, N. L., & Putnam, F. W. (1992). Clinical phenomenology of child and adolescent dissociative disorders. *Journal of the American Academy of Child and Adolescent Psychiatry, 31*(6), 1077–1085. https://doi.org/10.1097/00004583-199211000-00013

Jacobs, L., & Jacobs, J. (1966). Hypnotizability of children as related to hemispheric reference and neurological organization. *American Journal of Clinical Hypnosis, 8*(4), 269–274. https://doi.org/10.1080/00029157.1966.10402505

Janet, P. (1907). *The major symptoms of hysteria.* MacMillan.

Jensen, M. P., Adachi, T., Tomé-Pires, C., Lee, J., Osman, Z. J., & Miró, J. (2015). Mechanisms of hypnosis: Toward the development of a biopsychosocial model. *International Journal of Clinical and Experimental Hypnosis, 63*(1), 34–75. https://doi.org/10.1080/00207144.2014.961875

Jiang, H., White, M. P., Greicius, M. D., Waelde, L. C., & Spiegel, D. (2017). Brain activity and functional connectivity associated with hypnosis. *Cerebral Cortex, 27*(8), 4083–4093. https://doi.org/10.1093/cercor/bhw220

Kearney, B. E., & Lanius, R. A. (2022). The brain-body disconnect: A somatic sensory basis for trauma-related disorders. *Frontiers in Neuroscience, 16*, Article 1015749. https://doi.org/10.3389/fnins.2022.1015749

Kihlstrom, J. F. (1992). Hypnosis: A sesquicentennial essay. *International Journal of Clinical and Experimental Hypnosis, 40*(4), 301–314. https://doi.org/10.1080/00207149208409663

Kihlstrom, J. F. (2004). Hypnosis. In C. Spielberger (Ed.), *Encyclopedia of applied psychology* (pp. 243–248). Elsevier/Academic Press.

Kihlstrom, J. F. (2008). The domain of hypnosis, revisited. In M. R. Nash & A. J. Barnier (Eds.), *The Oxford handbook of hypnosis: Theory, research, and practice* (pp. 21–52). Oxford University Press.

Kirsch, I., & Braffman, W. (2001). Imaginative suggestibility and hypnotizability. *Current Directions in Psychological Science, 10*(2), 57–61. https://doi.org/10.1111/1467-8721.00115

Kirsch, I., Mazzoni, G., & Montgomery, G. (2007). Remembrance of hypnosis past. *American Journal of Clinical Hypnosis, 49*(3), 171–178. https://doi.org/10.1080/00029157.2007.10401574

Kluft, R. P. (1985a). Childhood multiple personality disorder: Predictors, clinical findings, and treatment results. In R. P. Kluft (Ed.), *Childhood antecedents of multiple personality* (pp. 167–196). American Psychiatric Press.

Kluft, R. P. (1985b). The natural history of multiple personality disorder. In R. P. Kluft (Ed.), *Childhood antecedents of multiple personality* (pp. 197–238). American Psychiatric Press.

Kluft, R. P. (1987). First-rank symptoms as a diagnostic clue to multiple personality disorder. *American Journal of Psychiatry, 144*(3), 293–298. https://doi.org/10.1176/ajp.144.3.293

Kluft, R. P. (1992). The use of hypnosis with dissociative disorders. *Psychiatric Medicine, 10*(4), 31–46.

Kluft, R. P. (2012). Hypnosis in the treatment of dissociative identity disorder and allied states: An overview and case study. *South African Journal of Psychology, 42*(2), 146–155. https://doi.org/10.1177/008124631204200202

Kluft, R. P. (2018a). Freud's rejection of hypnosis, Part I: The genesis of a rift. *American Journal of Clinical Hypnosis, 60*(4), 307–323. https://doi.org/10.1080/00029157.2018.1426321

Kluft, R. P. (2018b). Freud's rejection of hypnosis, Part II: The perpetuation of a rift. *American Journal of Clinical Hypnosis, 60*(4), 324–347. https://doi.org/10.1080/00029157.2018.1426326

Kluft, R. P. (2019). Freud's rejection of hypnosis: Perspectives old and new: Part III of III — Toward healing the rift: Enriching both hypnosis and psychoanalysis. *American Journal of Clinical Hypnosis, 61*(3), 208–226. https://doi.org/10.1080/00029157.2018.1544432

Kohen, D. P., & Olness, K. (2011). *Hypnosis and hypnotherapy with children* (4th ed). Routledge.

Lebois, L. A. M., Kaplan, C. S., Palermo, C. A., Xi, P., & Kaufman, M. L. (2023). A grounded theory of dissociative identity disorder: Placing DID in mind, brain, and body. In M. J. Dorahy, S. N. Gold & J. A. O'Neil (Eds.), *Dissociation and the dissociative disorders: Past, present, future* (2nd ed., pp. 392–407). Routledge.

Lebois, L. A. M., Kumar, P., Palermo, C. A., Lambros, A. M., O'Connor, L., Wolff, J. D., Baker, J. T., Gruber, S. A., Lewis-Schroeder, N., Ressler, K. J., Robinson, M. A., Winternitz, S., Nickerson, L. D., & Kaufman, M. L. (2022). Deconstructing dissociation: A triple network model of trauma-related dissociation and its subtypes. *Neuropsychopharmacology, 47*(13), 2261–2270. https://doi.org/10.1038/s41386-022-01468-1

Liotti, G. (1992). Disorganized/disoriented attachment in the etiology of the dissociative disorders. *Dissociation, 5*(4), 196–204. scholarsbank.uoregon.edu/xmlui/handle/1794/1722

Liotti, G. (1999a). Disorganization of attachment as a model of understanding dissociative psychopathology. In J. Soloman & C. George (Eds.), *Attachment disorganization* (pp. 291–317). Guilford Press.

Liotti, G. (1999b). Understanding the dissociative processes: The contribution of attachment theory. *Psychoanalytic Inquiry, 19*(5), 757–783. https://doi.org/10.1080/07351699909534275Loewenstein, R. J. (2018). Dissociation debates: Everything you know is wrong. *Dialogues in Clinical Neuroscience, 20*(3), 229–242. https://doi.org/10.31887/DCNS.2018.20.3/rloewenstein

Loewenstein, R. J. (2023). Conceptual foundations for long-term psychotherapy of dissociative identity disorder. In M. J. Dorahy, S. N. Gold & J. A. O'Neil (Eds.), *Dissociation and the dissociative disorders: Past, present, future* (2nd ed., pp. 770–790). Routledge.

Loewenstein, R. J., & Putnam, F. W. (2023). Discrete behavioral states theory. In M. J. Dorahy, S. N. Gold & J. A. O'Neil (Eds.), *Dissociation and the dissociative disorders: Past, present, future* (2nd ed., pp. 281–296). Routledge.

London, P., & Cooper, L. M. (1969). Norms of hypnotic susceptibility in children. *Developmental Psychology, 1*(2), 113–124. https://doi.org/10.1037/h0027002

Main, M., & Solomon, J. (1986). Discovery of an insecure-disorganized/disoriented attachment pattern: Procedures, findings and implications for the classification of behavior. In T. B. Brazelton & M. W. Yogman (Eds.), *Affective development in infancy* (pp. 95–124). Ablex.

Marek, S., & Dosenbach, N. U. F. (2018). The frontoparietal network: Function, electrophysiology, and importance of individual precision mapping. *Dialogues in Clinical Neuroscience, 20*(2), 133–140. https://doi.org/10.31887/DCNS.2018.20.2/smarek

Menon, V. (2011). Large-scale brain networks and psychopathology: A unifying triple network model. *Trends in Cognitive Sciences, 15*, 483–506. https://doi.org/10.1016/j.tics.2011.08.003

Menon, V. (2018). A triple network model, insight, and large-scale brain organization in autism. *Biological Psychiatry, 84*(4), 236–238. https://doi.org/10.1016/j.biopsych.2018.06.012

Milling, L. S., Kirsch, I., Allen, G. J., & Reutenauer, E. L. (2005). The effects of hypnotic and nonhypnotic imaginative suggestion on pain. *Annals of Behavioral Medicine, 29*(2), 116–127. https://doi.org/10.1207/s15324796abm2902_6

Mitchell, T. W. (1921). *The psychology of medicine.* Methuen & Co.

Morgan, A. H. (1973). The heritability of hypnotic susceptibility in twins. *Journal of Abnormal Psychology, 82*(1), 55–61. https://doi.org/10.1037/h0034854

Morgan, A. H., & Hilgard, E. R. (1973). Age differences in susceptibility to hypnosis. *International Journal of Clinical and Experimental Hypnosis, 21*(2), 78–85. https://doi.org/10.1080/00207147308409308

Morgan, A. H., & Hilgard, J. R. (1978). The Stanford hypnotic clinical scale for children. *American Journal of Clinical Hypnosis, 21*(23), 148–169. https://doi.org/10.1080/00029157.1978.10403969

Nijenhuis, E. R., Vanderlinden, J., & Spinhoven, P. (1998). Animal defensive reactions as a model for trauma-induced dissociative reactions. *Journal of Traumatic Stress, 11*(2), 243–260. https://doi.org/10.1023/A:1024447003022

Orne, M. (1959). The nature of hypnosis: Artifact and essence. *Journal of Abnormal and Social Psychology, 58*(3), 277–299. https://doi.org/10.1037/h0046128

Otnow Lewis, D. (1996). Diagnostic evaluation of the child with dissociative identity disorder/multiple personality disorder. *Child and Adolescent Psychiatric Clinics of North America, 5*(2), 303–331. https://doi.org/10.1016/S1056-4993(18)30368-7

Page, R. A., & Green, J. P. (2007). An update on age, hypnotic suggestibility, and gender: A brief report. *American Journal of Clinical Hypnosis, 49*(4), 283–287. https://doi.org/10.1080/00029157.2007.10524505

Peterson, G. (1991). Children coping with trauma: Diagnosis of "dissociation identity disorder." *Dissociation, 4*(3), 152–164. scholarsbank.uoregon.edu/xmlui/handle/1794/1453

Peterson, G. (1998). Diagnostic taxonomy: Past to future. In J. L. Silberg (Ed.), *The dissociative child: Diagnosis, treatment, and management* (2nd ed., pp. 3–26). Sidran Press.

Piccione, C., Hilgard, E. R., & Zimbardo, P. G. (1989). On the degree of stability of measured hypnotizability over a 25-year period. *Journal of Personality and Social Psychology, 56*(2), 289–295. https://doi.org/10.1037//0022-3514.56.2.289

Putnam, F. W. (1997). *Dissociation in children and adolescents.* Guilford Press.

Putnam, F. W. (2016). *The way we are: How states of mind influence our identities, personality and potential for change.* International Psychoanalytic Books.

Rajkumar, R. P. (2022). The molecular genetics of dissociative symptomatology: A transdiagnostic literature review. *Genes, 13*(5), Article 843. https://doi.org/10.3390/genes13050843

Register, P. A., & Kihlstrom, J. F. (1986). Finding the hypnotic virtuoso. *International Journal of Clinical and Experimental Hypnosis, 34*(2), 84–97. https://doi.org/10.1080/00207148608406974

Reinders, A. A. T. S., Willemsen, A. T., Vos, H. P., den Boer, J. A., & Nijenhuis, E. R. (2012). Fact or factitious? A psychobiological study of authentic and simulated dissociative identity states. *PLoS One, 7*(6), Article e39279. https://doi.org/10.1371/journal.pone.0039279

Rocha-Rego, V., Fiszman, A., Portugal, L. C., Garcia Pereira, M., de Oliveira, L., Mendlowicz, M. V., Marques-Portella, C., Berger, W., Freire Coutinho, E. S., Mari, J. J., Figueira, I., & Volchan, E. (2009). Is tonic immobility the core sign among conventional peritraumatic signs and symptoms listed for PTSD? *Journal of Affective Disorders, 115*(1–2), 269–273. https://doi.org/10.1016/j.jad.2008.09.005

Ross, C. A. (2007). *The trauma model: A solution to the problem of comorbidity in psychiatry* (2nd ed.). Manitou Communications.

Ross, C. A., & Norton, G. R. (1989). Effects of hypnosis on the features of multiple personality disorder. *American Journal of Clinical Hypnosis, 32*(2), 99–106. https://doi.org/10.1080/00029157.1989.10402807

Savitz, J. B., van der Merwe, L., Newman, T. K., Solms, M., Stein, D. J., & Ramesar, R. S. (2008). The relationship between childhood abuse and dissociation. Is it influenced by catechol-O-methyltransferase (COMT) activity? *International Journal of Neuropsychopharmacology, 11*(2), 149–161. https://doi.org/10.1017/S1461145707007900

Schlumpf, Y. R., Reinders, A. A., Nijenhuis, E. R., Luechinger, R., van Osch, M. J., & Jäncke, L. (2014). Dissociative part-dependent resting-state activity in dissociative identity disorder: A controlled fMRI perfusion study. *PLoS One, 9*(6), Article e98795. https://doi.org/10.1371/journal.pone.0098795

Schore, A. N. (2001). The effects of early relational trauma on right brain development, affect regulation, and infant mental health. *Infant Mental Health Journal, 22*(1–2), 201–269. https://doi.org/10.1002/1097-0355(200101/04)22:1<201::AID-IMHJ8>3.0.CO;2-9

Sidis, B., & Goodhart, S. P. (1904/1968). *Multiple personality: An experimental investigation into the nature of human individuality.* D. Appleton and Co./Greenwood.

Silberg, J. (2013). *The child survivor: Healing developmental trauma and dissociation.* Routledge.
Silberg, J., & Dallam, S. (2023). Dissociative disorders in children and adolescents. In M. J. Dorahy, S. N. Gold & J. A. O'Neil (Eds.), *Dissociation and the dissociative disorders: Past, present, future* (2nd ed., pp. 433–448). Routledge.
Simonov, P. V., & Paikin, D. (1969). The role of emotional stress in the hypnotization of animals. In L. Chertok (Ed.), *Psychophysiological mechanisms of hypnosis* (pp. 67–87). Springer-Verlag.
Soffer-Dudek, N., & Somer, E. (2023). Maladaptive daydreaming is a dissociative disorder: Supporting evidence and theory. In M. J. Dorahy, S. J. Gold & J. A. O'Neil (Eds.), *Dissociation and the dissociative disorders: Past, present, future* (2nd ed., pp. 547–563). Routledge.
Soffer-Dudek, N., Somer, E., Spiegel, D., Chefetz, R., O'Neil, J., Dorahy, M. J., Cardeña, E., Mamah, D., Schimmenti, A., Musetti, A., Boon, S., van Dijke, A., Ross, C., Nijenhuis, E., Krause-Utz, A., Dell, P., Gold, S., Pietkiewicz, I., Silberg, J., Steele, K., Moskowitz, A., Draijer, N., Thomson, P., Barach, P., Kinsler, P., Maves, P., Şar, V., Kruger, C., & Middleton, W. (in press). Maladaptive daydreaming should be included as a dissociative disorder in psychiatric manuals: A position paper. *British Journal of Psychiatry.*
Spiegel, H. (1974). The Grade 5 syndrome: The highly hypnotizable person. *International Journal of Clinical and Experimental Hypnosis, 22*(4), 303–319. https://doi.org/10.1080/00207147408413010
Staniloiu, A., Vitcu, I., & Markowitsch, H. J. (2012). Neuroimaging and dissociative disorders. In V. Chaudhary (Ed.), *Advances in brain imaging* (pp. 11–34). InTech.
Szekely, A., Kovacs-Nagy, R., Bányai, E. I., Gosi-Greguss, A. C., Varga, K., Halmai, Z., Ronai, Z., & Sasvari-Szekely, M. (2010). Association between hypnotizability and the catechol-O-methyltransferase (COMT) polymorphism. *International Journal of Clinical and Experimental Hypnosis, 58*(3), 301–315. https://doi.org/10.1080/00207141003760827
Tasca, C., Rapetti, M., Carta, M. G., & Fadda, B. (2012). Women and hysteria in the history of mental health. *Clinical Practice and Epidemiology in Mental Health, 8*(1), 110–119. https://doi.org/10.2174/1745017901208010110
Tellegen, A., & Atkinson, G. (1974). Openness to absorbing and self-altering experiences ("absorption"), a trait related to hypnotic susceptibility. *Journal of Abnormal Psychology, 83*(3), 268–277. https://doi.org/10.1037/h0036681
Terhune, D. B., & Cardeña, E. (2016). Nuances and uncertainties regarding hypnotic inductions: Toward a theoretically informed praxis. *American Journal of Clinical Hypnosis, 59*(2), 155–174. https://doi.org/10.1080/00029157.2016.1201454
Vandenberg, B. (1998). Infant communication and the development of hypnotic responsivity. *International Journal of Clinical and Experimental Hypnosis, 46*(4), 334–350. https://doi.org/10.1080/00207149808410013
Vandenberg, B. (2002). Hypnotic responsivity from a developmental perspective: Insights from young children. *International Journal of Clinical and Experimental Hypnosis, 50*(3), 229–247. https://doi.org/10.1080/00207140208410101
van der Hart, O., Nijenhuis, E. R. S., and Steele, K. (2006). *The haunted self: Structural dissociation and the treatment of chronic traumatization.* W. W. Norton.
Waters, F. S. (2016). *Healing the fractured child: Diagnosis and treatment of youth with dissociation.* Springer.
Watkins, H. H., & Watkins, J. G. (1997). *Ego states: Theory and therapy.* W. W. Norton.
Watkins, J. G. (1949). *Hypnotherapy of war neuroses: A clinical psychologist's casebook.* Ronald Press Company.
Watkins, J. G. (1987). *Hypnotherapeutic techniques, Volume I: The practice of clinical hypnosis.* Irvington Publishers.
Williams, D. T., & Velazquez, L. (1996). The use of hypnosis in children with dissociative disorders. *Child and Adolescent Psychiatric Clinics of North America, 5*(2), 495–508. https://doi.org/10.1016/S1056-4993(18)30377-8
Woody, E. Z., & Bowers, K. S. (1994). A frontal assault on dissociated control. In S. J. Lynn & J. W. Rhue (Eds.), *Dissociation: Clinical and theoretical perspectives* (pp. 52–79). Guilford Press.
Yehuda, R., & Lehrner, A. (2018). Intergenerational transmission of trauma effects: Putative role of epigenetic mechanisms. *World Psychiatry, 17*(3), 243–257. https://doi.org/10.1002/wps.20568

8

KNOWLEDGE ISOLATION, PROTECTIVE ADAPTATION, AND LONG-TERM IMPACTS

Betrayal Trauma Theory's Contribution to Our Understanding of Complex Trauma and Dissociation in Childhood[1]

Laura K. Noll

Introduction

Children rely on their caregivers to meet their most basic needs for physical safety, human connection, and a secure base from which to explore the world (Bowlby, 1969/1982; Bowlby, 1980; Bernstein & Freyd, 2014). As such, childhood abandonment, neglect, or abuse perpetrated against children by parents or other adult custodians responsible for their welfare represent forms of betrayal trauma insofar as these acts significantly violate the trust implicit in the child-caregiver relationship and harm the developing child's well-being (Freyd, 1996). When maltreatment by caregivers occurs at an early age, repeatedly, and/or escalates over time, both the trauma itself and the reactions it generates are often "complex," affecting multiple domains of the developing child's mind and body (Courtois, 2004; Ford & Courtois, 2013), including cognitive strategies for engaging in knowledge isolation of past and ongoing abuse (e.g., traumatic amnesia and dissociation). The purpose of this chapter is to provide an overview of betrayal trauma theory (BTT) (Freyd 1994, 1996, 2001) as a framework that helps situate complex childhood trauma and knowledge isolation in the interpersonal (Freyd 1994, 1996; Freyd & Birrell, 2013), familial (Delker et al., 2018), institutional (Smith & Freyd, 2014), and cultural (Gómez, 2019, 2023; Gómez & Gobin, 2020) contexts in which child maltreatment occurs. In the sections that follow, I first provide an overview of BTT and a summary of the history of its development as a framework to explain knowledge isolation in the context of childhood sexual abuse, its dimensional approach to conceptualizing trauma along social betrayal and fear/terror-inducing axes, and the recent expansion of BTT across interpersonal contexts. Second, I describe what is known about the prevalence of betrayal trauma in childhood and the complexity of its impact on child development, with an emphasis on knowledge isolation as a means of preserving attachment relationships. Focusing on dissociation as one mechanism by which knowledge isolation may occur, I summarize empirical research on dissociation in adult survivors of childhood betrayal trauma and the growing literature documenting dissociation in child survivors of betrayal trauma. Third, I discuss the implications of BTT for clinicians and researchers working with high betrayal trauma in children, highlighting three principles with utility across contexts. Lastly, I discuss several promising future directions for research on betrayal trauma, with an emphasis on methodological approaches that may help advance our understanding of individual differences in betrayal trauma outcomes in a world where traumatized children and their families are increasingly at the epicenter of dramatic social and environmental change.

Betrayal Trauma Theory: Overview and Historical Context

BTT (Freyd 1994, 1996, 2001) conceptualizes betrayal by a trusted other as an interpersonally toxic dimension of trauma that significantly impacts the way negative events are processed and remembered (Sivers et al., 2002). Underlying BTT are two core premises: first, consistent with Bowlby and Ainsworth's attachment theory (Bowlby, 1980, 1969/1982; for historical overview of attachment theory see Bretherton, 1992) and the earlier security theory (Blatz, 1940), BTT assumes that humans have evolved to have strong motivation to maintain bonds with close others (Bernstein & Freyd, 2014). One correlate of this is that children rely on their caregivers for survival, and the human attachment system helps children interact with their caregivers in ways that elicit physical and emotional care. Second, drawing from premises entailed by social exchange theory (Cosmides, 1989; Cosmides & Tooby, 1992), BTT emphasizes that humans have the capacity to detect violations of trust (i.e., "cheating") in close relationships (Freyd, 1996). Importantly, it is in the interaction between the attachment and cheater-detection systems that the core predictions of BTT arise (i.e., when a child's need to maintain an important attachment bond conflicts with their betrayal detection).

In the context of high betrayal events, such as child maltreatment by a caregiver or other individual responsible for a child's welfare (e.g., sexual, physical, or emotional abuse; emotional or physical neglect), BTT provides an explanatory framework for *knowledge isolation* (including but not limited to childhood dissociation) as an adaptive response to interpersonal trauma—thus complementing and differentiating it from fear- and shattered assumptions-based theories (Adams-Clark et al., 2021). Specifically, under conditions of childhood abuse and neglect, maintaining *betrayal blindness* (i.e., unawareness or lack of memory of betrayal) via cognitive mechanisms such as repression, amnesia, and/or dissociation may help the child preserve their attachment relationship with their caregiver (Freyd, 1996), upon whom they depend for food, shelter, safety, and emotional care. This, by extension, has evolutionary benefits for child survival vis-à-vis social exchange. Said more simply, BTT proposes that traumatized children may need to remain unaware they have been betrayed to function in the relationships they need for survival. Although BTT provides a conceptual and scientific rationale to explain motivations for trauma unawareness, independent of the mechanism(s) for knowledge isolation (DePrince et al., 2012), this idea is consistent with Bowlby's earlier discussions of children's defensive processing and exclusion of information that is at odds with internal working models of close others (Bowlby, 1980).

While perhaps intuitive to trauma-informed clinicians and scholars today, the adaptive benefits of knowledge isolation for betrayal were not widely recognized when BTT was introduced into the literature three decades ago. As Freyd explained in her seminal text *Betrayal Trauma: The Logic of Forgetting Childhood Abuse* (1996), she began developing BTT early in 1991 to explicate the phenomenon of forgetting and remembering child sexual abuse (CSA). In stark contrast to today, a lack of information about CSA (e.g., prevalence in families) and its long-term consequences prevailed. Fortunately, in large part due to the explosion of research on CSA initiated by the introduction of BTT to the literature,[2] alongside other efforts to document the consequences of child maltreatment on long-term health outcomes (e.g., the foundational Adverse Childhood Experiences Study; Anda et al., 2006; Felitti et al., 1998; longitudinal studies of CSA, Trickett et al., 2011), we now know much more about how significant violations of the trust in a caregiver-child relationship deleteriously impact children across the lifespan. Although many questions remain regarding the exact mechanism(s) by which high betrayal trauma impacts children across diverse interpersonal contexts, one thing is clear: violations of trust in a relationship on which a child depends for survival have a profound negative impact on development.

Conceptualizing Betrayal as a Separable Dimension of Complex Childhood Trauma

One of BTT's key contributions to the field was conceptually separating social betrayal and fear/terror-inducing dimensions of trauma—an innovation that has informed the design of research studies investigating the mechanisms by which relational trauma in childhood impacts self-referential memory (Chiu et al., 2019) and helped clinicians conceptualize and name the unique impacts of betrayal by caregivers on traumatized children. As shown below, Freyd's (1996) two-dimensional model for traumatic events categorizes events along two orthogonal axes: low-to-high levels of social betrayal and low-to-high levels of terror/fear-inducing (see Figure 8.1). While events that are low on both axes are not generally traumatic, events that are low on social betrayal but high on the fear/terror-inducing axis (e.g., natural disasters and auto accidents) represent traumatic events with no-to-low levels of interpersonal/social betrayal. Such traumas may produce adverse outcomes (e.g., post-traumatic stress disorder) but are less likely to include outcomes specific to interpersonal trauma (e.g., betrayal blindness via knowledge isolation). Along the continuum of high betrayal interpersonal trauma, fear/terror-inducing events may range from low to high. BTT posits that some "genuinely traumatic" events (for in-depth discussion of how CSA has or has not been historically treated as traumatic, see Freyd et al., 2007) need not be fear-inducing (and, indeed, are often not) to be highly traumatic, and, moreover, the absence of fear-inducing/terror dimensions of trauma may have its own implications for traumatic memory and recovery processes (Freyd, 2001). Specifically, BTT proposes that survivors of trauma are more likely to experience knowledge isolation for high betrayal traumas compared to those involving fear/terror, although the two may co-occur (Freyd, 1996). Here, it is also important to note that, in contrast to theoretical frameworks that define trauma as an intrapsychic phenomenon (e.g., a psychological injury and a stress reaction), within the BTT

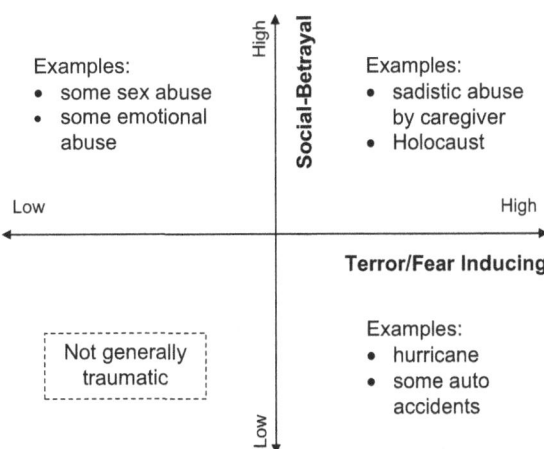

Figure 8.1 Freyd's Two-Dimensional Model for Traumatic Events. Copyright Jennifer J. Freyd, 1996. Reprinted with permission.

framework betrayal trauma is, by definition, the social dimension of trauma, regardless of an individual's reaction to the trauma (Freyd, 1994, 1996; Freyd et al., 2007).

Expansion of Betrayal Trauma Theory across Interpersonal Contexts

Since its introduction into the literature in the early 1990s to address knowledge isolation relating to CSA, BTT has been applied to contexts involving the trauma of interpersonal betrayal by a trusted individual (e.g., childhood abuse or neglect by a caregiver and infidelity of a partner) (Freyd, 1994, 1996, 2001; Freyd & Birrell, 2013), family system (Delker et al., 2018), institution (Smith & Freyd, 2014), or culture (Gómez & Gobin, 2020; Gómez, 2023). Notably, recent BTT scholarship has also focused on the observation that high betrayal events in childhood may transact with betrayal experiences in other interpersonal contexts, thereby complicating post-traumatic outcomes for child survivors of betrayal trauma. For example, in *The Cultural Betrayal of Black Women and Girls* (2023), which is grounded in Black liberation theory and intersectional feminism, Gómez describes the complexities of sexual trauma for Black survivors of cultural betrayal whose abuse was perpetrated by a member of the culture group. For clinicians and researchers working with betrayal trauma, attunement to the intersectional dimensions of childhood betrayal trauma is especially critical, particularly when conceptualizing the impact of high betrayal events on traumatized children.

Prevalence and Risk of High Betrayal Trauma Exposure in Childhood

A proliferation of terminology in the research literature documenting the prevalence of early trauma exposure combined with measurement challenges makes it difficult to accurately estimate how many children experience high betrayal events in childhood. Complementary and sometimes conflicting conceptualizations of trauma—(e.g., defining trauma as a stressful event external to the child verses an internal reaction a child has to an external event), research design issues (e.g., sampling techniques), and other measurement challenges (e.g., reliance on self-report for phenomena that are, by definition, subject to denial and underreporting)—have resulted in a wide range of prevalence estimates for high betrayal trauma exposure in childhood. While it is now widely recognized that at least one in four children experiences some form of child abuse or neglect, most events go unreported (Lippard & Nemeroff, 2020). Moreover, the different age groups, methods, and instruments used to gather data on the epidemiology of child abuse and neglect make it difficult to compare results across studies (Massullo et al., 2023).

Regarding the minority of events that come to the attention of child protective services, the U.S. Department of Health and Human Services (USDHHS) has documented a rate of at least 8.1 victims of child abuse and neglect for every 1,000 children. While not being representative of all abused children, examination of the perpetrator-victim relationship in substantiated cases of child maltreatment sheds light on the high betrayal dimension of child abuse and neglect. For example, in 2021, 90.6% of child victims who were the subject of a substantiated report to child protective services were abused and/or neglected by one or both parents (U.S. Department of Health & Human Services [USDHHS], 2023). In other words, most cases of child maltreatment (at least those measured by government agencies) *are by definition* high betrayal traumas. In this vein, it is worth noting that, in contrast to the broader literature on childhood adversity (which includes stressful life events such as growing up in poverty or experiencing bullying at school), harm by a someone who has responsibility for the child is often included in definitions of child maltreatment (e.g., those offered by the Center for Disease Control or American Psychological Association) (Massullo et al., 2023). While epidemiological studies that use these definitions do not allow scholars of betrayal trauma to parse the specific impact of betrayal on child development per se (over and above other elements of complex child trauma), they do indicate that high betrayal trauma is relatively common in the general population.

Studies that assess betrayal trauma using the BTT framework often administer the Brief Betrayal Trauma Survey (Goldberg & Freyd, 2006) and ask adult respondents to report retrospectively on their experiences of high betrayal events in childhood alongside other types of traumatic events. Consistent with the epidemiological literature on child maltreatment, such studies also suggest that lifetime betrayal trauma exposure is relatively high. For example, in their study of the relationship between childhood betrayal trauma exposure and subsequent revictimization in a sample of college students, Gobin and Freyd (2009) found that 30% of respondents experienced at least one type of betrayal trauma before age 12 and that childhood betrayal trauma exposure was significantly associated with experiencing high betrayal trauma during adolescence. Betrayal trauma exposure risk appears to vary by demographics (e.g., gender, ethnicity, and socioeconomic status), with some studies reporting higher rates for women compared to men (DePrince & Freyd, 2002; Goldberg & Freyd, 2006; Martin et al., 2013; Tang & Freyd, 2012), ethnic minorities, and individuals from lower socioeconomic class (Klest et al., 2013). That said, the barriers to acknowledgment and disclosure of trauma at individual, familial, institutional, and cultural levels are many. As such, intersectional work that more closely examines risk of experiencing betrayal trauma and post-traumatic outcomes within frameworks well-suited to documenting the complexity of risk (e.g., those provided by cultural BTT; Gómez, 2023) are still needed.

Impact of High Betrayal Trauma on Children

Ample empirical literature documents the profound impact of high betrayal trauma (e.g., child abuse and neglect by caregivers) on development across physical, mental, and social domains (Adams-Clark et al., 2021; Cook et al., 2005; Fisher et al., 2016; Fisher, 2017; Lippard & Nemeroff, 2020). For example, in research studies examining the physical correlates of early trauma, child maltreatment has been associated with biomarkers of cellular aging (e.g., shorter leukocyte telomere length; Edmonds et al., 2016; Woo et al., 2022), elevated risk for physical complaints (Freyd et al., 2005), regional cortical thinning and gray matter volume reductions in the brain (Yang et al., 2023), lower functional health (Edwards et al., 2012), and sleep disturbances (Klest et al., 2013). Equally significant, mental and behavioral health problems associated with high betrayal trauma in childhood include higher rates of substance use problems (Delker & Freyd, 2014), borderline tendencies (Kaehler & Freyd, 2012), hallucinations (Edwards et al., 2012), dissociation (Dalenberg et al., 2012; Freyd et al., 2005; Klest et al., 2013; Vonderlin et al., 2018), suicidality (Edwards et al., 2012), persistent post-traumatic stress disorder (Trickett et al., 2011), and emotional problems, including increased rates of alexithymia, depression, anxiety, and panic (Edwards et al., 2012; Goldsmith et al., 2009, 2012; Liu et al., 2023; Nelson et al., 2017), among others. Impacts on relational health include lower general and relational trust (Gobin & Freyd, 2014) and revictimization for trauma (Gobin & Freyd, 2009). Regarding the latter, Gobin and Freyd (2009) quantified risk for experiencing revictimization following high betrayal trauma in childhood: high childhood betrayal survivors in childhood were 4.31 times more likely to be abused again in adolescence and 5.44 times more likely to be victimized in adulthood. Notably, in this study, dissociation was significantly associated with revictimization. Severe impacts of childhood relational trauma on self-referential memory (Chiu et al., 2019), structural dissociation of the personality (Fisher, 2017), and self-concept (Delker & Freyd, 2017) may result in the development of serious mental illnesses, including borderline personality disorder (Yalch & Levendosky, 2019) or dissociative identity disorder (Şar et al., 2017). Since one of BTT's most important contributions to our understanding of complex trauma has been to provide theoretical and empirical evidence for adaptive knowledge isolation as a means of preserving attachment relationships, in the sections that follow, I focus on what is known about the relationship between high betrayal trauma and knowledge isolation in the context of complex childhood trauma.

Isolating Knowledge of Betrayal Trauma to Preserve Attachment Relationships in Childhood

As mentioned previously, BTT posits that *knowledge isolation* is one mechanism by which an individual may maintain unawareness of information (e.g., knowledge of abuse) that could threaten a relationship on which they depend for emotional and/or physical survival (Barlow & Freyd, 2009; Freyd, 1996). Said differently, BTT proposes that, due to the threat that awareness of betrayal poses to needed attachment relationships, traumas that are most likely to be forgotten are not those that are most painful or terrifying, although high betrayal events may also have these characteristics (Freyd, 1996). Rather, early relational traumas in which betrayal is a core element are most likely to elicit knowledge isolation. Freyd (1996) explained:

> The concept of knowledge isolation encompasses a range of phenomena, motivations, and mechanisms implied by the varying uses of words like "repression," "amnesia," and "dissociation." This concept is useful specifically because it does not assume particular motivations, mechanisms, or resulting phenomena.
>
> *(p. 27)*

In the context of BTT, knowledge isolation is often used interchangeably with the most neutral of these terms: dissociation.

To briefly clarify the subtle yet important difference between these key terms, in psychoanalytic theory, repression is regarded as a universal mental process that blocks impulses or desires from entering consciousness, thus representing one mechanism by which thoughts, images, and/or memories that are unacceptable to a child's ego may be kept at bay (see Laplanche & Pontalis, 1973/1988). In the context of clinical work, repressed material may find expression in the symptoms of illness and reconciliation in the process of treatment. While no doubt relevant to discussions of knowledge isolation in the context of BTT, the terms "repression" and "repressed memories" frequently have been mobilized by trauma skeptics to support erroneous and ironic claims that memories of recovered childhood sexual abuse are fantasies (Ross, 2022), thereby generating substantial confusion for lay audiences regarding the meaning of these terms in psychoanalytic discourse. By contrast, amnesia (i.e., the lack of memory for some or all aspects of a past event) may have organic and/or psychological causes and is, thus, a broader concept that is leveraged to describe one outcome of traumatic events.

Within this context, the term "dissociative amnesia" is "an inability to recall important autobiographical information, usually of a traumatic or stressful nature, that is inconsistent with ordinary forgetting" (American Psychiatric Association, 2022, p. 329). When used without reference to amnesia, the term "dissociation" is used to describe partial or full lack of awareness in the current situation, indexing a wide range of experiences ranging from mild emotional detachment to severe fragmentation of the personality (e.g., disconnection of parts of self from one another, as seen in dissociative identity disorder). As a form of knowledge isolation, dissociation in childhood may be adaptive insofar as it helps the child preserve their bond with a maltreating caregiver on whom they depend even though they are also the source of great harm (Adams-Clark et al., 2023). Research studies with adult and child survivors of child abuse focusing on links between childhood relational trauma and dissociation provide empirical support for this notion (Dalenberg et al., 2012; Vonderlin et al., 2018). However, mixed results in the literature and methodological issues (e.g., not consistently examining the strength of relationship between victim and perpetrator; not assessing biological and cognitive predispositions that might act as moderators of dissociation proneness) raise important questions about the mechanisms by which childhood relational trauma impacts self-referential memory (Chiu et al., 2019). This is particularly important, as some studies have found that intrafamilial abuse (in contrast to extrafamilial abuse) is associated with dissociation in youth (Plattner et al., 2003) and symptom profiles for high betrayal traumas differ when trauma type, level of betrayal, and frequency are considered (Gamache Martin et al., 2016), thus highlighting the importance of considering the interpersonal context in which childhood trauma occurs. These caveats notwithstanding, extant literature indicates that cognitive responses that help a child adapt to traumatic events, while preserving needed attachment relationships, are likely to occur in the context of complex trauma.

Research on Dissociation in Adult Survivors of Childhood Betrayal Trauma

In current diagnostic nosology, dissociative disorders are characterized by "a disruption of and/or discontinuity in the normal integration of consciousness, memory, identity, perception, body representation, motor control, and behavior" (American Psychiatric Association, 2022, p. 329). In adult populations, a history of high betrayal trauma (e.g., abuse by caregivers) during childhood has been shown to impact attention and memory, thus increasing risk for dissociation in adulthood (Dalenberg et al., 2012; Vonderlin et al., 2018). This is true even when individual variations in fantasy proneness are controlled for (for an evaluation of the evidence comparing trauma and fantasy models of dissociation, see Dalenberg et al., 2012). For clinicians treating traumatized children, this is important to know, in part because of documented links between a parent's own history of betrayal trauma in childhood, parental dissociation, and children's presentation of trauma (see Chu & DePrince, 2006; Hulette et al., 2011).

Importantly, recent work has also examined the cross-cultural relevance of betrayal trauma as a framework for understanding traumatic dissociation stemming from childhood trauma. For example, Fung and colleagues (2023) found that compared to childhood non-betrayal trauma, childhood betrayal trauma was significantly associated with dissociative amnesia (DA) and identity dissociation (ID) in two convenience samples of English and Chinese speakers seeking web-based educational interventions for dissociation. That said, cultural variability in betrayal trauma processes likely exists, as recent research with understudied minority groups (e.g., Latinx women) points toward variables such as enculturation as key moderators in the link between childhood betrayal trauma exposure and post-traumatic outcomes. For example, Wills and colleagues (2022) recently reported that there was a stronger relationship between childhood family-perpetrated victimization and anxiety in adulthood for highly enculturated Latinx women compared to low-enculturated women. Additional cross-cultural work is needed to further examine how cultural and institutional contexts transact with family dynamics in the context of complex trauma, particularly regarding dissociation and other mechanisms that facilitate knowledge isolation. Taken together, at this point, there is a large and growing body of literature documenting links between high betrayal trauma in childhood and dissociation in adulthood across a variety of populations and contexts. However, disparities in the strength of associations between early childhood relational trauma and dissociation proneness in adulthood have generated controversy regarding the exact mechanisms by which early betrayal trauma results in knowledge isolation (Chiu et al., 2019), highlighting the importance of examining moderating variables that impact linkages between high betrayal trauma exposure and post-traumatic sequelae.

Research indicates that variables such as greater trauma severity (Carlson et al., 2012), higher trauma frequency (Vonderlin et al., 2018), and earlier age of trauma exposure (Vonderlin et al., 2018) increase a child's risk for developing a dissociative disorder as a result of betrayal trauma. For example, using a meta-analytic approach, Vonderlin and colleagues (2018) examined the relationship between childhood interpersonal maltreatment and dissociation (as measured by the Dissociative Experiences Scale, DES) in 65 studies with 7,352 abused or neglected individuals. Results indicated that victims of childhood abuse and neglect (especially those reporting sexual and physical abuse) had higher levels of dissociation compared to non-abused controls. Additionally, earlier age of onset, longer duration of abuse, and parental abuse all significantly predicted higher dissociation scores, thus highlighting the role high betrayal events play in the etiology of complex trauma. That said, more research focusing on other possible risk factors, moderators, and mediators for the relationship between high betrayal trauma exposure in childhood and adult dissociation is still needed (Chiu et al., 2019; Dalenberg et al., 2012).

In this vein, one promising avenue for further investigation focuses on the mechanisms by which high betrayal traumas impact self-referential memory processes across development. Although systematic descriptions of childhood and adult dissociation vary considerably in the literature, dating back to Pierre Janet's first book on the transformation of traumatic experiences into psychopathology (1889/1973), dissociation arising from cumulative childhood trauma by caregivers may be roughly divided into positive (i.e., transient and intrusive) symptoms such as unexplained pain, voices, emotions that seem to come out of nowhere, or intrusive thoughts; and negative (i.e., the absence or loss of function) symptoms such as numbness, loss of motor function, or unexplained fluctuation in skills such as driving—both of which may occur across cognitive, affective, and sensorimotor domains (Steele et al., 2017). Within contemporary structural dissociation theory, the functional significance of positive and negative symptoms of dissociation may be understood in the context of dissociative "parts" of the personality and their relationship to evolutionary action systems (e.g., fight, flight, freeze, flag, collapse, cry for help, and social engagement) that are activated in the context of threat. Thus, from a developmental perspective, complex trauma stemming from maltreatment perpetrated by caregivers during childhood (i.e., high betrayal trauma) may result in the *structural dissociation of the personality* (van der Hart et al., 2006), which is accompanied by alterations in attention and consciousness that may be differentiated from other forms of normative dissociation and compartmentalization (Fisher, 2017). This possibility is consistent with literature stating that the activation of knowledge isolation may vary according to attentional and environmental contexts (Gómez et al., 2023; Becker-Blease et al., 2004) and recent work demonstrating that low accessibility to self-referential representations moderates the link between childhood relational trauma and dissociation proneness in adults (Chiu et al., 2019).

Research on Dissociation in Child Survivors of Betrayal Trauma

Compared to research with adult survivors of betrayal trauma, the number of studies documenting associations between betrayal trauma in childhood and dissociation using child samples is smaller. It fits within a broad literature base documenting the impact of childhood adversity on children's executive functions, including cognitive control, attention, working memory, and threat detection (for review, see Fisher et al., 2016). Notably, research with abused and non-abused young children supports the idea that traumatized children use divided attention to remain unaware of threatening information, placing them at elevated risk for dissociation (Becker-Blease et al., 2004; Hulette et al., 2008a, 2008b; Modrowski & Kerig, 2017). For example, using a divided attention memory task, Becker-Blease and colleagues (2004) found that abused preschool-aged children remembered fewer charged pictures compared to non-abused children. This pattern was also observed when comparing abused children with high dissociation scores to non-abused children with low dissociation scores. Complementing these findings, Hulette and colleagues (2008a, 2008b) found that compared to their non-maltreated peers, maltreated preschool age children in foster care had higher average levels of dissociation. Taken together, these studies with traumatized children suggest that under certain conditions, some children use divided attention to keep threatening information out of their conscious awareness.

Unsurprisingly, given that betrayal trauma often occurs within a familial context (Delker et al., 2018), intergenerational associations between betrayal trauma and dissociation have also been observed in studies examining caregiver-child dyads. For example, one study of 72 mother-child dyads found that both mothers' and children's betrayal trauma history was associated with children's dissociation (Chu & DePrince, 2006)—suggesting, among other things, that the caregiver's history of maltreatment represents a risk factor for child dissociation, alongside more proximate sources of trauma in the home. Consistent with this, in a study examining the short- and long-term consequences of betrayal trauma in a sample of 67 mother-child dyads, Hulette and colleagues (2011) found that high betrayal trauma was associated with higher levels of dissociation in both mothers and children. Furthermore, maternal revictimization was related to child interpersonal trauma history—a finding that highlights the possibility that maternal betrayal blindness and dissociation may play key roles in shaping caregivers' awareness of interpersonal threats to the child in the family environment.

Given the limitations of cross-sectional research designs (e.g., the inability to examine causal links between variables of interest), prospective longitudinal designs are needed to further assess caregiver dissociation as a risk factor for children's exposure to potentially traumatic events and, importantly, to unpack the intergenerational mechanisms by which a caregiver's betrayal trauma history may increase a child's risk of experiencing complex trauma and dissociation. Although most studies have not examined the closeness of relationship between child victims and their abusers, some prospective studies have documented severe outcomes in children abused by their biological parents. For example, findings from one 23-year longitudinal study examining the impact of intrafamily sexual abuse on female development found that girls abused by their biological fathers had the most severe post-traumatic sequelae compared to subgroups of girls abused by other father figures (e.g., stepfather and mother's boyfriend) or relatives (Trickett et al., 2011). Taken together, while our understanding of betrayal trauma and its impact on children has increased significantly over the past three decades, many questions regarding the exact mechanism(s) by which high betrayal trauma in childhood impacts children across the lifespan remain. Research designs that allow for causal inferences to be made regarding the relationships between key variables, especially with respect to knowledge isolation and dissociation or other mechanisms of action, are still needed.

Implications for Clinicians and Researchers Working with High Betrayal Trauma in Children

Principle 1: Childhood Dissociation Stemming from High Betrayal Trauma May Be Adaptive and Serving an Important Function in the Family System

By situating dissociation in an interpersonal context, BTT provides an explanatory framework for the adaptive role that knowledge isolation may play in a family system characterized by complex trauma (Adams-Clark et al., 2023). Consistent with strength-based approaches for treating trauma in pediatric populations, the BTT framework may be especially helpful for clinicians engaging in case conceptualization for children who have experienced high betrayal events, especially but not limited to those low on the fear/terror-inducing dimension of Freyd's (1996) two-dimensional model for trauma (e.g., CSA and some emotional abuse). When engaging in case conceptualization and treatment planning, useful questions to consider may include: To what extent might interrupting or treating adaptive dissociation impact the short- or mid-term benefits conferred by the child's knowledge isolation with respect to their experience of psychological or physical dependency on the perpetrator of abuse? Is the child safe enough from ongoing abuse and/or familial denial of past abuse to begin treating dissociation or other forms of knowledge isolation that may be helping them preserve a needed relationship? What is at stake for the child in knowing or not knowing certain information about abuse or neglect perpetrated by caregivers? What might the child need to tolerate the information about the family system that is being kept at bay by dissociation in the here and now? How are other family members (siblings, non-abusive family members, non-helping caregivers) likely to react to the treatment of dissociation in a child protecting themselves from information about high betrayal trauma? Who else is engaging in knowledge isolation of a child's betrayal trauma?

In contrast to empowered adults for whom trust is violated by an important other, where confrontation or withdrawal may be effective responses to betrayal (Adams-Clark et al., 2023), children who acknowledge abuse may face dire consequences that threaten their survival. Yet, ongoing adaptation to abuse via knowledge isolation may also confer deleterious impacts of long-term physical and mental health. This places clinicians in a profound clinical dilemma—one that may be interwoven with significant ethical and legal considerations (Haverkamp & Daniluk, 1993). On the one hand, a clinician who helps the child directly or indirectly acknowledge their betrayal trauma may therapeutically counter the toxic impacts of high betrayal on child development. On the other, doing so may increase their short- or mid-term risk for adverse outcomes within the family system. Lawson and Akay-Sullivan (2020) noted in their discussion of childhood betrayal trauma stemming from incest that social acknowledgment of abuse within the family system may elicit a variety of harmful responses, including rejection of the abused child by the non-abusing family member(s) and withdrawal of support and protection. Even non-offending parents who believe the abuse happened may exhibit ambivalent responses to a child who discloses maltreatment (Elliott & Carnes, 2001), which may impact the child's own knowledge isolation processes. Within BTT, denying high betrayal abuse, attacking the abused child, and assuming the role of victim to the child's accusations is a well-documented pattern of behavior that perpetrators and non-helping observers of abuse utilize (consciously and unconsciously) to avoid responsibility (Freyd, 1997, 2018). Termed "DARVO," which stands for "deny, attack, and reverse victim and offender," this pattern of behavior has been the subject of recent research examining the impact of DARVO on victim self-blame (Harsey et al., 2017) and perceived perpetrator and victim credibility (Harsey & Freyd, 2020). How does a clinician treating a child victim of high betrayal trauma navigate these complex realities and the thorny ethical dilemmas associated with treating betrayal trauma? As a starting point, conceptualizing the intrapsychic and intrafamilial operation of knowledge isolation for betrayal trauma during case conceptualization and treatment planning may help clinicians deepen their understanding of a child's adaptation and resilience in relation to complex trauma and anticipate possible changes in family dynamics during treatment. This theoretical understanding is necessary but insufficient for decision-making that intersects with legal statutes and professional codes of conduct for helping professionals. As such, adequate training, a team-based approach to treatment that offers protection against burnout, peer consultation, and continuing education for resolving confusion ethical dilemmas that may arise when treating children who have experienced and/or are currently experiencing betrayal trauma may help professionals navigate the complexities associated with treating high betrayal trauma in children.

Principle 2: Recovery from High Betrayal Trauma Is Unlikely to Be Linear and Knowledge Isolation May Fluctuate in Response to Changing Internal and External Conditions

Human beings have evolved via natural selection to detect betrayal (i.e., cheating) in interpersonal relationships (Cosmides, 1989; Cosmides & Tooby, 1992; Freyd, 1996). However, awareness of betrayal that poses a threat to a relationship that a child depends on for survival represents a survival threat that adaptive knowledge isolation may mitigate. As Freyd aptly observed:

"Humans can be exquisitely sensitive detectors of betrayal or cheating. But they can also be remarkably blind to betrayal or cheating that may seem obvious to an outside observer" (1996, p. 63). This is particularly true for children who are most dependent on adult caregivers for survival. For this reason, awareness of high betrayal trauma may not fully emerge (if at all) until the child is no longer fully dependent on their caregiver for emotional and physical care (i.e., in adulthood). Even so, the path to knowing one has been betrayed by a trusted other in childhood is far from linear (Gómez et al., 2023) and knowledge of betrayal may change significantly as one engages in other close relationships across the course of development. Consistently recognizing and acknowledging the importance of relational processes in healing is critical and may help well-meaning helping professionals avoid inadvertently localizing the pathology of trauma within the traumatized child, rather than within the perpetrator(s) of harm and/or social contexts in which abuse occurred (Gómez et al., 2016). Taken together, since both true and false memories of abuse are possible (Freyd, 2001) and a child's awareness of betrayal may fluctuate (Gómez et al., 2023), it is imperative that clinicians and scholars not automatically assume that allegations of child maltreatment by a caregiver are false (Freyd, 2001). This is especially true when children recant, deny, or alter prior disclosures of abuse and, equally, when adult survivors of betrayal trauma seek professional help.

Principle 3: In Addressing High Betrayal Trauma in Children, Monitor Your Own Knowledge Isolation and Maintain Connections to Healthy Supports

At the heart of childhood high betrayal trauma is disconnection—from the self, from others, and from safety—which is partially why trauma is contagious (Herman, 1992/1997). To help someone who has experienced childhood trauma establish stability and integrate their experiences of disconnection, helping professionals must maintain active and ongoing connection to safe professional and personal supports. Although much less discussed in the context of academic research, the same is true for the betrayal trauma researcher. Just as traumatic experiences from childhood may be activated when an individual becomes a caregiver themselves (Fraiberg et al., 1975), a clinician's or researcher's own experiences of trauma by caregivers may rise to the surface while bearing witness to traumatic dissociation stemming from complex childhood trauma—a phenomenon that can become overwhelming and isolating. Left unaddressed, such traumatic countertransference or vicarious traumatization (McCann & Pearlman, 1990) may result in dissociation and other symptoms of post-traumatic stress, which pose a threat to everyone involved and to the integrity of the work itself. No matter how experienced a practitioner or researcher is, engaging in trauma treatment or research in isolation is not only poor modeling for reconnection but a recipe for burnout. As Goldsmith and colleagues (2004) aptly noted, awareness of trauma is complex for the helping professional, involving multiple levels of analysis to navigate knowing and not knowing about abuse. Within this context, professional awareness of betrayal trauma and attitudes toward interpersonal violence are both likely to impact the behavior of clinicians treating traumatized children. Supervision, regular peer consultation groups, lab or project meetings, personal therapy, support groups, reading groups, and trauma-related continuing education activities all represent important sites of connection that can help providers sustain a healthy relationship to the difficult but highly rewarding work of treating and learning from individuals who have experienced high betrayal trauma in childhood. Importantly, this is true not only for clinicians but for researchers as well. As Herman cogently argued in *Truth and Repair: How Trauma Survivors Envision Justice* (2023), "Never work alone. If you are going to witness the worst of what human beings are capable of, you will need to surround yourself with people who exemplify the best. Otherwise, you will eventually give in to despair" (p. 236).

Emerging Directions for Research on Childhood Betrayal Trauma

As Herman (1992/1997) aptly noted, the history of psychological trauma research is "one of episodic amnesia" (p. 7). Today, we are arguably in a period of integration and remembering, such that research documenting the impact of complex childhood trauma on developmental outcomes is burgeoning, and efforts to construct a more coherent and comprehensive diagnostic nosology are gaining unmistakable traction. Although there are many unanswered questions to be addressed by trauma research, we have never understood dissociation and complex trauma arising from high betrayal trauma in childhood more than we do today. As such, the frontiers of childhood trauma research are full of exciting possibilities. Many unanswered questions remain and deserve attention.

Since dissociation arising from trauma by caregivers may be particularly pronounced when the trauma occurs at times when the developing brain is especially susceptible to environmental influences, such as in infancy, early childhood, and adolescence (Fisher et al., 2016), research that advances our understanding of how positive and negative symptoms of dissociation emerge across development represents an important future direction for prevention science. Thus far, the longitudinal study of dissociation stemming from betrayal trauma in childhood remains limited (with some notable exceptions; see Trickett et al., 2011) and the logistical barriers to conducting such work are many. Despite this, in clinical settings, adolescents and adults are often able to recall when they first experienced various positive and negative symptoms of dissociation. As such, retrospective studies with youth that map the developmental trajectories of dissociative parts alongside the individual's changing contextual risk and protective factors (e.g., the reactions of non-offending caregivers) may help advance our understanding of how dissociative states develop over time, thereby advancing BTT. Additionally, research that combines self-report measures and clinical accounts of dissociation with validated bio-behavior measures (e.g., implicit measure of physical reactions to betrayal trauma) may help bridge the gap between extant neurophysiological work documenting both the deleterious impact of childhood trauma on the body and observations from clinical practice. To accomplish this task, innovative collaborations between academic researchers, community partners, and individuals undertaking the courageous work of healing from childhood trauma are needed.

Alongside the logistical barriers to conducting rigorous prospective and multimodal studies of betrayal trauma impacts across development, measurement issues also hinder our understanding of post-traumatic sequalae in traumatized children. Knowledge isolation and betrayal blindness are, by definition, hard to measure via self-report, and doing so with children is even more difficult. Efforts to address this in adult populations include adaptation of the implicit association task (IAT) to measure identification with a betrayed/traumatized self-concept (Delker & Freyd, 2017) and, recently, the development of the Betrayal Blindness Questionnaires (Gómez et al., 2023), which include items designed to measure one's fluctuating awareness of high betrayal experiences. However, fewer innovations have been developed to measure betrayal trauma processes in children. To date, experimental studies with children have often relied on laboratory tasks designed to measure attention to and recall of threatening information (Becker-Blease et al., 2004) in a controlled setting. By comparing differences between groups of children (e.g., traumatized versus non-traumatized; high versus low dissociation), such studies allow for the study of attention and memory processes hypothesized to underly knowledge isolation. While important, additional work is needed to advance our understanding of how and under what conditions adaptive knowledge isolation operates in the context of complex trauma. Regarding the latter, some efforts have been made to measure intergenerational associations for betrayal trauma across parent-child dyads (Hulette et al., 2011) and identify moderators that help account for variability in outcomes for families experiencing high betrayal trauma (e.g., emotional skills; Gagnon et al., 2016). Complementing this, further research that examines the interplay between children's dyadic, familial, and institutional/cultural betrayal experiences is especially crucial for understanding the intersection between experiences of marginalization or oppression and complex trauma experienced within a child's family context (for discussion, see Adams-Clark et al., 2023).

Conclusion

The core ideas of BTT are inextricably interwoven with descriptions of complex trauma and dissociation in children and epidemiological approaches to studying child maltreatment across disciplines. Three decades of betrayal trauma scholarship document robust links between exposure to high betrayal events in childhood and deleterious outcomes across the lifespan. Yet, additional research is needed to advance our understanding of adaptive knowledge isolation in the context of betrayal by a close other in childhood. Given that BTT conceptualizes betrayal as a socially harmful dimension of childhood trauma that predicts the ways in which traumatic events are processed and remembered (Sivers et al., 2002), novel methodologies are crucial for examining the mechanisms underlying knowledge isolation. Equally important, clinically informed scholarship that explores individual- and community-based processes for healing and meaning-making may be particularly powerful. Finally, in a rapidly changing world marked especially by climate crisis and growing economic inequality, betrayal trauma research must examine the interplay between these forces while continuing to develop novel interventions that respond to complex traumas across individual, familial, institutional, and cultural levels.

Notes

1 The author wishes to acknowledge Dr. Jennifer Freyd for her support, Kayla Larsen for her assistance reviewing recent literature on high betrayal trauma in pediatric populations, and Dr. Ira Allen for his reading and feedback on the chapter.
2 Readers interested in learning more about the backlash against BTT and "memory wars" of the 1990s may be interested in this popular article, by Katie Heaney, describing the personal circumstances surrounding Dr. Freyd's disclosure of sexual abuse: "The memory war," *The Cut*, January 6, 2021, thecut.com/article/false-memory-syndrome-controversy.html.

References

Adams-Clark, A. A., Gómez, J. M., & Barlow, M. R. (2023). Adaptive dissociation: A response to interpersonal, institutional, and cultural betrayal. In M. Dorahy, S. Gold & J. A. O'Neil (Eds.), *Dissociation and the dissociative disorders: Past, present, future* (2nd ed., pp. 98–110). Taylor & Francis Group. https://doi.org/10.4324/9781003057314-9

Adams-Clark, A. A., Gómez, J. M., Gobin, R. L., Noll, L. K., & Delker, B. C. (2021). Impact of interpersonal, family, cultural, and institutional betrayal on adult survivors of abuse. In R. Geffner, J. W. White, L. K. Hamberger, A. Rosenbaum, V. Vaughan-Eden & V. I. Vieth, (Eds.), *Handbook of interpersonal violence and abuse across the lifespan: A project of the national partnership to end interpersonal violence across the lifespan (NPEIV)* (pp. 4275–4301). Springer International Publishing. https://doi.org/10.1007/978-3-319-62122-7_310-1

American Psychiatric Association. (2022). *Diagnostic and statistical manual of mental disorders* (5th ed., text rev.). https://doi.org.10.1176/appi.books.97808904

Anda, R. F., Felitti, V. J., Bremner, J. D., Walker, J. D., Whitfield, C. H., Perry, B. D., Dube, S. R., & Giles, W. H. (2006). The enduring effects of abuse and related adverse experiences in childhood. *European Archives of Psychiatry and Clinical Neuroscience, 256*(3), 174–186. https://doi.org/10.1007/s00406-005-0624-4

Barlow, M. R., & Freyd, J. J. (2009). Adaptive dissociation: Information processing and response to betrayal. In P. F. Dell & J. A. O'Neil (Eds.), *Dissociation and the dissociative disorders: DSM-V and beyond* (pp. 93–105). Routledge/Taylor & Francis Group.

Becker-Blease, K. A., Freyd, J. J., & Pears, K. C. (2004). Preschoolers' memory for threatening information depends on trauma history and attentional context: Implications for the development of dissociation. *Journal of Trauma & Dissociation, 5*(1), 113–131. https://doi.org/10.1300/J229v05n01_07

Bernstein, R. E., & Freyd, J. J. (2014). Trauma at home: How betrayal trauma and attachment theories understand the human response to abuse by an attachment figure. *Attachment: New Directions in Psychotherapy and Relational Psychoanalysis, 8,* 18–41.

Blatz, W. (1940). *Hostages to peace: Parents and the children of democracy.* William Morrow.

Bowlby, J. (1969/1982). *Attachment and loss, Vol. 1:* Attachment. Basic Books.

Bowlby, J. (1980). *Attachment and loss, Vol. 3:* Loss: Sadness and depression. Basic Books.

Bretherton, I. (1992). The origins of attachment theory: John Bowlby and Mary Ainsworth. *Developmental Psychology, 28*(5), 759–775. https://doi.org/10.1037/0012-1649.28.5.759

Carlson, E. B., Dalenberg, C., & McDade-Montez, E. (2012). Dissociation in posttraumatic stress disorder part I: Definitions and review of research. *Psychological Trauma: Theory, Research, Practice, and Policy, 4*(5), 479–489. https://doi.org/10.1037/a0027748

Chiu, C.-D., Tollenaar, M. S., Yang, C.-T., Elzinga, B. M., Zhang, T.-Y., & Ho, H. L. (2019). The loss of the self in memory: Self-referential memory, childhood relational trauma, and dissociation. *Clinical Psychological Science, 7,* 265–282. https://doi.org/10.1177/2167702618804794

Chu, A., & DePrince, A. P. (2006). Development of dissociation: Examining the relationship between parenting, maternal trauma and child dissociation. *Journal of Trauma & Dissociation, 7*(4), 75–89. https://doi.org/10.1300/J229v07n04_05

Cook, A., Spinazzola, J., Ford, J., Lanktree, C., Blaustein, M., Cloitre, M., DeRosa, R., Hubbard, R., Kagan, R., Liautaud, J., Mallah, K., Olafson, E., & van der Kolk, B. (2005). Complex trauma in children and adolescents. *Psychiatric Annals, 35*(5), 390–398. https://doi.org/10.3928/00485713-20050501-05

Cosmides, L. (1989). The logic of social exchange: Has natural selection shaped how humans reason? Studies with the Wason selection task. *Cognition, 31*(3), 187–276. https://doi.org/10.1016/0010-0277(89)90023-1

Cosmides, L., & Tooby, J. (1992). Cognitive adaptations for social exchange. In J. H. Barkow, L. Cosmides & J. Tooby (Eds.), *The adapted mind: Evolutionary psychology and the generation of culture* (pp. 163–228). Oxford University Press.

Courtois, C. A. (2004). Complex trauma, complex reactions: Assessment and treatment. *Psychotherapy: Theory, Research, Practice, Training, 41*(4), 412–425. https://doi.org/10.1037/0033-3204.41.4.412

Dalenberg, C. J., Brand, B. L., Gleaves, D. H., Dorahy, M. J., Loewenstein, R. J., Cardeña, E., Frewen, P. A., Carlson, E. B., & Spiegel, D. (2012). Evaluation of the evidence for the trauma and fantasy models of dissociation. *Psychological Bulletin, 138*(3), 550–588. https://doi.org/10.1037/a0027447

Delker, B. C., & Freyd, J. J. (2014). From betrayal to the bottle: Investigating possible pathways from trauma to problematic substance use. *Journal of Traumatic Stress, 27,* 576–584. https://doi.org/10.1002/jts.21959

Delker, B. C., & Freyd, J. J. (2017). Betrayed? That's me: Implicit and explicit betrayed self-concept in young adults abused as children. *Journal of Aggression, Maltreatment, & Trauma, 26,* 701–716. https://doi.org/10.1080/10926771.2017.1308982

Delker, B. C., Smith, C. P., Rosenthal, M. N., Bernstein, R. E., & Freyd, J. J. (2018). When home is where the harm is: Family betrayal and posttraumatic outcomes in young adulthood. *Journal of Aggression, Maltreatment & Trauma, 27*(7), 720–743. https://doi.org/10.1080/10926771.2017.1382639

DePrince, A. P., Brown, L. S., Cheit, R. E., Freyd, J. J., Gold, S. N., Pezdek, K., & Quina, K. (2012). Motivated forgetting and misremembering: Perspectives from betrayal trauma theory. In R. F. Belli (Ed.), *True and false recovered memories: Toward a reconciliation of the debate* (pp. 193–242). https://doi.org/10.1007/978-1-4614-1195-6_7

DePrince, A. P., & Freyd, J. J. (2002). The intersection of gender and betrayal in trauma. In R. Kimerling, P. C. Ouimette & J. Wolfe (Eds.), *Gender and PTSD* (pp. 98–113). Guilford Press.

Edmonds, G. W., Hampson, S. E., Côté, H. F., Hill, P. L., & Klest, B. (2016). Childhood personality, betrayal trauma, and leukocyte telomere length in adulthood: A lifespan perspective on conscientiousness and betrayal traumas as predictors of a biomarker of cellular aging. *European Journal of Personality, 30*(5), 426–437. https://doi.org/10.1002/per.2051

Edwards, V. J., Freyd, J. J., Dube, S. R., Anda, R. F., & Felitti, V. J. (2012). Health outcomes by closeness of sexual abuse perpetrator: A test of betrayal trauma theory. *Journal of Aggression, Maltreatment & Trauma, 21*(2), 133–148. https://doi.org/10.1080/10926771.2012.648100

Elliott, A. N., & Carnes, C. N. (2001). Reactions of the nonoffending parents to the sexual abuse of their child: A review of the literature. *Child Maltreatment, 6*(4), 314–324. https://doi.org/10.1177/1077559501006004005

Felitti, V. J., Anda, R. F., Nordenberg, D., Williamson, D. F., Spitz, A. M., Edwards, V., Koss, M. P., & Marks, J. S. (1998). Relationship of childhood abuse and household dysfunction to many of the leading causes of death in adults: The Adverse Childhood Experiences (ACE) Study. *American Journal of Preventive Medicine, 14,* 245–258. https://doi.org/10.1016/s0749-3797(98)00017-8

Fisher, J. (2017). *Healing the fragmented selves of trauma survivors: Overcoming internal self-alienation.* Routledge.

Fisher, P. A., Beauchamp, K. G., Roos, L. E., Noll, L. K., Flannery, J., & Delker, B. C. (2016). The neurobiology of intervention and prevention in early adversity. *Annual Review of Clinical Psychology, 12,* 331–357. https://doi.org/10.1146/annurev-clinpsy-032814-112855

Ford, J. D., & Courtois, C. A., (Eds.). (2013). *Treating complex traumatic stress disorders in children and adolescents: Scientific foundations and therapeutic models.* Guilford Press.

Fraiberg, S., Adelson, E., & Shapiro, V. (1975). Ghosts in the nursery: A psychoanalytic approach to the problems of impaired infant-mother relationships. *Journal of the American Academy of Child Psychiatry, 14*(3), 387–421. https://doi.org/10.1016/s0002-7138(09)61442-4

Freyd, J. J. (1994). Betrayal trauma: Traumatic amnesia as an adaptive response to childhood abuse. *Ethics & Behavior, 4,* 307–329. https://doi.org/10.1207/s15327019eb0404_1

Freyd, J. J. (1996). *Betrayal trauma: The logic of forgetting childhood abuse.* Harvard University Press.

Freyd, J. J. (1997) Violations of power, adaptive blindness and betrayal trauma theory. *Feminism & Psychology, 7*(1), 22–32. https://doi.org/10.1177/0959353597071004

Freyd, J. J. (2001). Memory and dimensions of trauma: Terror may be "all-too-well remembered" and betrayal buried. In J. R. Conte (Ed.), *Critical issues in child sexual abuse: Historical, legal, and psychological perspectives* (pp. 139–173). Sage Publications.

Freyd, J. (2018). What is DARVO? Retrieved July 1, 2023, from pages.uoregon.edu/dynamic/jjf/defineDARVO.html

Freyd, J. J., & Birrell, P. J. (2013). *Blind to betrayal: Why we fool ourselves we aren't being fooled.* John Wiley & Sons.

Freyd, J. J., DePrince, A. P., & Gleaves, D. H. (2007). The state of betrayal trauma theory: Reply to McNally—Conceptual issues, and future directions. *Memory, 15*(3), 295–311. https://doi.org/10.1080/09658210701256514

Freyd, J. J., Klest, B., & Allard, C. B. (2005). Betrayal trauma: Relationship to physical health, psychological distress, and a written disclosure intervention. *Journal of Trauma & Dissociation, 6*(3), 83–104. https://doi.org/10.1300/J229v06n03_04

Fung, H. W., Chien, W. T., Chan, C., & Ross, C. A. (2023). A cross-cultural investigation of the association between betrayal trauma and dissociative features. *Journal of Interpersonal Violence, 38*(1–2), NP1630–NP1653. https://doi.org/10.1177/08862605221090568

Gagnon, K. L., DePrince, A. P., Chu, A. T., Gorman, M., & Saylor, M. M. (2016). Betrayal trauma and child symptoms: The role of emotion. *Journal of Trauma & Dissociation, 17*(2), 207–222. https://doi.org/10.1080/15299732.2015.1077915

Gamache Martin, C., Van Ryzin, M. J., & Dishion, T. J. (2016). Profiles of childhood trauma: Betrayal, frequency, and psychological distress in late adolescence. *Psychological Trauma: Theory, Research, Practice, and Policy, 8*(2), 206–213. https://doi.org/10.1037/tra0000095

Gobin, R. L., & Freyd, J. J. (2009). Betrayal and revictimization: Preliminary findings. *Psychological Trauma: Theory, Research, Practice, and Policy, 1*(3), 242–257. https://doi.org/10.1037/a0017469

Gobin, R. L., & Freyd, J. J. (2014). The impact of betrayal trauma on the tendency to trust. *Psychological Trauma: Theory, Research, Practice, and Policy, 6*(5), 505–511. https://doi.org/10.1037/a0032452

Goldberg, L. R., & Freyd, J. J. (2006). Self-reports of potentially traumatic experiences in an adult community sample: Gender differences and test-retest stabilities of the items in a brief betrayal-trauma survey. *Journal of Trauma & Dissociation, 7*(3), 39–63. https://doi.org/10.1300/J229v07n03_04

Goldsmith, R. E., Barlow, M. R., & Freyd, J. J. (2004). Knowing and not knowing about trauma: Implications for therapy. *Psychotherapy: Theory, Research, Practice, Training, 41*(4), 448–463. https://doi.org/10.1037/0033-3204.41.4.448

Goldsmith, R. E., Freyd, J. J., & DePrince, A. P. (2009). To add insight to injury: Childhood abuse, abuse perceptions, and the emotional and physical health of young adults. *Journal of Aggression, Maltreatment & Trauma, 18*(4), 350–366. https://doi.org/10.1080/10926770902901527

Goldsmith, R. E., Freyd, J. J., & DePrince, A. P. (2012) Betrayal trauma: Associations with psychological and physical symptoms in young adults. *Journal of Interpersonal Violence, 27*(3), 547–567. https://doi.org/10.1177/0886260511421672

Gómez, J. M. (2019). Isn't it all about victimization? (Intra)cultural pressure and cultural betrayal trauma in ethnic minority college women. *Violence against Women, 25*(10), 1211–1225. https://doi.org/10.1177/1077801218811682

Gómez, J. M. (2023). *The cultural betrayal of Black women and girls: A Black feminist approach to healing from sexual abuse.* American Psychological Association.

Gómez, J. M., & Gobin, R. L. (2020). Black women and girls & #MeToo: Rape, cultural betrayal, & healing. *Sex Roles: A Journal of Research, 82*, 1–12. https://doi.org/10.1007/s11199-019-01040-0

Gómez, J. M., Lewis, J. K., Noll, L. K., Smidt, A. M., & Birrell, P. J. (2016). Shifting the focus: Nonpathologizing approaches to healing from betrayal trauma through an emphasis on relational care. *Journal of Trauma & Dissociation, 17*(2), 165–185. https://doi.org/10.1080/15299732.2016.1103104

Gómez, J. M., Zounlome, N. O., & Noll, L. K. (2023). Development and initial validation of the Betrayal Blindness Questionnaires (BBQs). *Journal of Aggression, Maltreatment & Trauma, 32*(3), 449–466. https://doi.org/10.1080/10926771.2022.2112339

Harsey, S. J., & Freyd, J. J. (2020). Deny, attack, and reverse victim and offender (DARVO): What is the influence on perceived perpetrator and victim credibility? *Journal of Aggression, Maltreatment & Trauma, 29*(8), 897–916. https://doi.org/10.1080/10926771.2020.1774695

Harsey, S. J., Zurbriggen, E. L., & Freyd, J. J. (2017). Perpetrator responses to victim confrontation: DARVO and victim self-blame. *Journal of Aggression, Maltreatment & Trauma, 26*(6), 644–663. https://doi.org/10.1080/10926771.2017.1320777

Haverkamp, B., & Daniluk, J. C. (1993). Child sexual abuse: Ethical issues for the family therapist. *Family Relations: An Interdisciplinary Journal of Applied Family Studies, 42*(2), 134–139. https://doi.org/10.2307/585445

Herman, J. L. (1992/1997). *Trauma and recovery: The aftermath of violence—From domestic abuse to political terror.* Basic Books.

Herman, J. L. (2023). *Truth and repair: How trauma survivors envision justice.* Basic Books.

Hulette, A. C., Fisher, P. A., Kim, H. K., Ganger, W., & Landsverk, J. L. (2008a). Dissociation in foster preschoolers: A replication and assessment study. *Journal of Trauma and Dissociation, 9*(2), 173–190. https://doi.org/10.1080/15299730802045914

Hulette, A. C., Freyd, J. J., Pears, K. C., Kim, H. K., Fisher, P. A., & Becker-Blease, K. A. (2008b). Dissociation and post-traumatic symptomatology in maltreated preschool children. *Journal of Child and Adolescent Trauma, 1*(2), 93–108. https://doi.org/10.1080/19361520802083980

Hulette, A. C., Kaehler, L., & Freyd, J. (2011). Intergenerational associations between trauma and dissociation. *Journal of Family Violence, 26*(3), 217–225. https://doi.org/10.1007/s10896-011-9357-5

Janet, P. (1889/1973). *L'automatisme psychologique: essai de psychologie expérimentale sur les forms inférieures de l'activité humaine.* Félix Alcan/Societé Pierre Janet/Payot.

Kaehler, L. A., & Freyd, J. J. (2012). Betrayal trauma and borderline personality characteristics: Gender differences. *Psychological Trauma: Theory, Research, Practice, and Policy, 4*(4), 379–385. https://doi.org/10.1037/a0024928

Klest, B., Freyd, J. J., & Foynes, M. M. (2013). Trauma exposure and posttraumatic symptoms in Hawaii: Gender, ethnicity, and social context. *Psychological Trauma: Theory, Research, Practice, and Policy, 5*(5), 409–416. https://doi.org/10.1037/a0029336

Laplanche, J., & Pontalis, J. (1988). *The language of psychoanalysis.* Karnac Books (Original work published 1973).

Lawson, D. M., & Akay-Sullivan, S. (2020). Considerations of dissociation, betrayal trauma, and complex trauma in the treatment of incest. *Journal of Child Sexual Abuse, 29*(6), 677–696. https://doi.org/10.1080/10538712.2020.1751369

Lippard, E. T., & Nemeroff, C. B. (2020). The devastating clinical consequences of child abuse and neglect: Increased disease vulnerability and poor treatment response in mood disorders. *American Journal of Psychiatry, 177*(1), 20–36. https://doi.org/10.1176/appi.ajp.2019.19010020

Liu, J., Deng, J., Zhang, H., & Tang, X. (2023). The relationship between child maltreatment and social anxiety: A meta-analysis. *Journal of Affective Disorders, 329*, 157–167. https://doi.org/10.1016/j.jad.2023.02.081

Martin, C. G., Cromer, L. D., DePrince, A. D., & Freyd, J. J. (2013). The role of cumulative trauma, betrayal, and appraisals in understanding trauma symptomatology. *Psychological Trauma: Theory, Research, Practice and Policy, 5*(2), 110–118. https://doi.org/10.1037/a0025686

Massullo, C., De Rossi, E., Carbone, G. A., Imperatori, C., Ardito, R. B., Adenzato, M., & Farina, B. (2023). Child maltreatment, abuse, and neglect: An umbrella review of their prevalence and definitions. *Clinical Neuropsychiatry, 20*(2), 72–99. https://doi.org/10.36131/cnfioritieditore20230201

McCann, I. L., & Pearlman, L. A. (1990). Vicarious traumatization: A framework for understanding the psychological effects of working with victims. *Journal of Traumatic Stress, 3*(1), 131–149. https://doi.org/10.1007/BF00975140

Modrowski, C., & Kerig, P. (2017). Investigating factors associated with PTSD dissociative subtype membership in a sample of traumatized justice-involved youth. *Journal of Child & Adolescent Trauma, 10*(4), 343–351. https://doi.org/10.1007/s40653-017-0153-0

Nelson, J., Klumparendt, A., Doebler, P., & Ehring, T. (2017). Childhood maltreatment and characteristics of adult depression: Meta-analysis. *British Journal of Psychiatry, 210*(2), 96–104. https://doi.org/10.1192/bjp.bp.115.180752

Plattner, B., Silvermann, M. A., Redlich, A. D., Carrion, V. G., Feucht, M., Friedrich, M. H., & Steiner, H. (2003). Pathways to dissociation: Intrafamilial versus extrafamilial trauma in juvenile delinquents. *Journal of Nervous and Mental Disease, 191*(12), 781–788. https://doi.org/10.1097/01.nmd.0000105372.88982.54

Ross, C. (2022). False memory researchers misunderstand repression, dissociation and Freud. *Journal of Child Sexual Abuse, 31*(4), 488–502. https://doi.org/10.1080/10538712.2022.2067095

Şar, V., Dorahy, M. J., & Krüger, C. (2017). Revisiting the etiological aspects of dissociative identity disorder: A biopsychosocial perspective. *Psychology Research and Behavior Management, 10*, 137–146. https://doi.org/10.2147/PRBM.S113743

Sivers, H., Schooler, J., & Freyd, J. J. (2002). Recovered memories. In V. S. Ramachandran (Ed.), *Encyclopedia of the human brain* (Volume 4, pp 169–184). Academic Press.

Smith, C. P., & Freyd, J. J. (2014). Institutional betrayal. *American Psychologist, 69*(6), 575–587. https://doi.org/10.1037/a0037564

Steele, K., Boon, S., & van der Hart, O. (2017). *Treating trauma-related dissociation: A practical, integrative approach*. Norton.

Tang, S. S. S., & Freyd, J. J. (2012). Betrayal trauma and gender differences in posttraumatic stress. *Psychological Trauma: Theory, Research, Practice, and Policy, 4*(5), 469–478. https://doi.org/10.1037/a0025765

Trickett, P. K., Noll, J. G., & Putnam, F. W. (2011). The impact of sexual abuse on female development: Lessons from a multigenerational, longitudinal research study. *Development and Psychopathology, 23*(2), 453–476. https://doi.org/10.1017/S0954579411000174

USDHHS (U.S. Department of Health & Human Services). (2023). *Child Maltreatment 2021*. Administration for Children & Families, Administration on Children, Youth and Families, Children's Bureau. acf.hhs.gov/cb/data-research/child-maltreatment

van der Hart, O., Nijenhuis, E. R., & Steele, K. (2006). *The haunted self: Structural dissociation and the treatment of chronic traumatization*. W. W. Norton.

Vonderlin, R., Kleindienst, N., Alpers, G. W., Bohus, M., Lyssenko, L., & Schmahl, C. (2018). Dissociation in victims of childhood abuse or neglect: A meta-analytic review. *Psychological Medicine, 48*(15), 2467–2476. https://doi.org/10.1017/S0033291718000740

Wills, C., Cuevas, C. A., & Sabina, C. (2022). The role of the victim–offender relationship on psychological distress among Latinx women: A betrayal trauma perspective. *Psychological Trauma: Theory, Research, Practice, and Policy, 14*(1), 20–28. https://doi.org/10.1037/tra0000923

Woo, J. M., Parks, C. G., Hyde, E. E., Auer, P. L., Simanek, A. M., Konkel, R. H., Taylor, J., Sandler, D. P., & Meier, H. C. (2022). Early life trauma and adult leucocyte telomere length. *Psychoneuroendocrinology, 144*, Article 105876. https://doi.org/10.1016/j.psyneuen.2022.105876

Yalch, M. M., & Levendosky, A. A. (2019). Influence of betrayal trauma on borderline personality disorder traits. *Journal of Trauma & Dissociation, 20*(4), 392–401. https://doi.org/10.1080/15299732.2019.1572042

Yang, W., Jin, S., Duan, W., Yu, H., Ping, L., Shen, Z., Cheng, Y., Xu, X., & Zhou, C. (2023). The effects of childhood maltreatment on cortical thickness and gray matter volume: A coordinate-based meta-analysis. *Psychological Medicine, 53*(5), 1681–1699. https://doi.org/10.1017/S0033291723000661

9
INTERPERSONAL NEUROBIOLOGY

Robyn Gobbel

Introduction

Jayme baffled me. She had bright eyes and a wide smile, and exhibited cheerful exuberance. I half-expected her to burst through my office door with jazz hands, trailing a spray of peacock feathers, she was that bright and shiny. But I didn't resonate with her; I didn't feel connected to her. Jayme wasn't even close to the most disruptive or out-of-control child I'd ever worked with, but still, I did not like her.

When I imagine you reading those words, I notice a flash of shame. Uh oh. Will you immediately reject me? Will you judge me for feeling that way? Will you dismiss me as unfit to be a child therapist? Or will you resonate with my vulnerability and allow it to soothe a part of you who sometimes doesn't like the children who come to your office? Will you notice any curiosity arise in you about why I didn't like this bright-eyed, lively little one?

Curiosity toward ourselves and our clients is a core tenet of interpersonal neurobiology (IPNB). Curiosity both invites and emerges from an integrated state of mind. I imagine you and I feel similarly about children: we love them! Since I was 15 years old, I've devoted my life to being with children. Especially the ones whom others find the most difficult. In my world, and maybe yours too, these are the kids smearing feces, urinating behind their beds, or hurting the family pet. These are the kids we all want to refer out to our colleagues. We know that otherwise we'll have to clean up every single one of the sandtray miniatures from the middle of the room, rub antiseptic on the bite marks on our forearms, or hide a spare set of keys outside for the inevitable moment when a child locks us out of our office. Again. I love those kids the most. That's probably why I became the therapist with a practice full of them—the kids nobody else could or wanted to handle.

But Jayme was different. Despite her history of extreme neglect, she was academically gifted and bubbly, with big, brown puppy dog eyes that should have won me over. She never spit on me, threw things at me, or broke my toys on purpose. But from the moment I met Jayme, I did not like her or how I felt around her—edgy, unsettled, and irritated. And that confused me. Jayme and her not-that-bad behavior baffled me.

By the time Jayme came to my office for the first time, my therapeutic work had been grounded in IPNB for over a decade, and I knew that feelings of dislike for a client had deeper meaning. Instead of judging or shaming myself for these feelings or deciding that Jayme was just an unlikeable little girl, I was able to notice these sensations arise and consider them more deeply.

Bonnie Badenoch (2008), an IPNB expert and my primary mentor, wrote that it's important for mental health practitioners to "become aware of our own implicit vulnerabilities so that we can notice when we are being impacted by our clients' struggles" (p. 155). I understood that my feelings about Jayme reflected the way I was *impacted by her struggle*; most likely these feelings of dislike were similar to feelings she held toward herself or perhaps feelings an attachment figure held toward her. From the moment we met, Jayme allowed me to know her story, even the parts of her that were too overwhelming for her to know herself. And even still, because I'm just as human as anyone else, it was very hard to spend a lot of time with a child I did not like. Every week, I had to remind myself that these uncomfortable sensations, sensations that tried to trick me into believing Jayme was an unlikeable child, were a gift. Every week, when I heard Jayme climb out of her parent's station wagon, slamming the door behind her, I noticed my initial experience of dread. Then I took a breath and connected to gratitude:

> Thank you, Jayme. Thank you for trusting me to see and hold this part of you. I will hold it here with me until you and I can hold it together.

As you'll learn in this chapter on IPNB and complex trauma and dissociation, IPNB doesn't offer clinicians a toolbox full of things to do with their clients. Instead, the approach offers a theoretical foundation that informs clinical reasoning, inviting us to use, with humble confidence, the various clinical tools and interventions we hold in our toolbox. Because IPNB is a human development theory as opposed to a clinical theory, it allows clinicians to use clinical interventions intuitively instead of rigidly following a protocol. Even more importantly, IPNB suggests a road map for a way of being with our clients, as well as a road map for a way of being with ourselves.

Interpersonal Neurobiology

My own discovery of IPNB came not as a mental health clinician but as a new mom. While studying reactive attachment disorder in grad school, I'd learned that a child's attachment style was largely predicted by "parent state of mind with regard to attachment" (van IJzendoorn, 1995). But when I had my own child, I realized I had no idea what that meant. I knew that secure attachment was good, and I also knew that if my child was securely attached, then I was too. I decided that having a securely attached child would mean I was a good mom, and my kid would be fine. So, I went searching for the secure attachment checklist. I had read *The Baby Book* by Sears and Sears (2003), and although it kind of had a checklist, I wanted clear, step-by-step instructions on how to not "screw up my kid."

In case it's not clear, none of my new-mom conclusions about secure attachment are true. But my sleep-deprived brain and limited understanding of attachment had me convinced I needed a checklist for secure attachment. Feeling sorely let down by Sears's checklist of baby-wearing, breastfeeding, and co-sleeping (check, check, and check), I kept searching. I was grateful Sears gave me tasks I could achieve, but something about it still didn't sit quite right.

Parenting From the Inside Out by Siegel and Hartzell (2004) was a little harder to read than *The Baby Book*, but it was my first glance into parenting without a checklist. Siegel and Hartzell were describing a way of *being*, not a way of *doing*. It was both frustrating and relieving. It wasn't until many years later, when I began working full-time again after several years mostly at home with my son, that I understood Siegel didn't just write a complicated parenting book; he created a completely new field of study: IPNB.

A colleague lent me a burned audio CD of Siegel's plenary session at the 2010 Eye Movement Desensitization and Reprocessing International Association (EMDRIA) Conference. There was a lot

I didn't understand. The way he used words like *coherence*, *complexity*, and *integration* didn't make any sense to me. This didn't matter; I was hooked. What the CD offered me was hope: hope that the behaviors of the kids in my office made sense, and hope that I could help them.

IPNB isn't a treatment approach. It's an interdisciplinary theory of human development that weaves together contributions from diverse fields of study, including anthropology, biology, computer science, mathematics, physics, psychology, sociology, and systems theory. IPNB considers how the mind, brain, and relationships come together to create who we are. This triangle of well-being (the mind, the brain, and relationships) is continuously shifting and changing in response to how the individual pieces of the triangle shift and change (Siegel, 2020).

Complex Systems

The mind, the brain, and relationships are all complex systems. In *Pocket Guide to Interpersonal Neurobiology*, Siegel (2012) wrote that a complex system is

> a collection of elements that (a) is open to influences from outside of itself, (b) changes in a nonlinear way such that small inputs lead to large and unpredictable long-term changes, and (c) is capable of entering chaotic states. Complex systems can be influenced by an emergent, self-organizing process that recursively shapes the flow of the system as it changes across time.
>
> *(p. 325)*

Think about a musical ensemble. That ensemble, whether it's the Foo Fighters or the New York Philharmonic, is open to influences from outside of itself. Once, I saw a video from when the Foo invited a young audience member to jam with them onstage. Talk about an influence from outside itself! The kid was amazing, and the crowd went wild! He was up there only for a few minutes, but his unexpected skill and confidence changed the energy in the whole arena—and the band! Ensembles like the Foo Fighters and the New York Philharmonic are skilled at quickly moving back into coherence, but not all complex systems are that stable. Have you ever been to a sixth-grade band concert? Chaos easily emerges from that complex system, indeed.

Integration

IPNB defines integration as the linkage of differentiated parts (Siegel, 2020). If we stay with our music ensemble example, the New York Philharmonic shows the world their integrated state. The French horns, flutes, and violins are different and unique instruments. When they come together in an ensemble, they maintain their differentiated selves. If I listen closely with a discerning ear, I can identify those individual parts. In the ensemble, their differentiated parts become linked, and their unique linkage creates something that doesn't exist anywhere else: the New York Philharmonic.

The brain comprises structures that are differentiated yet linked. The hippocampus is differentiated from the amygdala and from the middle prefrontal cortex. In the developmental trajectory of integration, differentiation occurs first, linkage second. When integrated, the hippocampus, amygdala, and prefrontal cortex (among other structures) are linked together as neuronal connections become more numerous and complex. Siegel (2020) uses the acronym FACES to describe what makes an integrated system: flexible, adaptive, coherent, energized, and stable.

Let's reconsider the New York Philharmonic as an integrated complex system. There is flexibility (F) within the system in that it can bend and shift slightly without completely breaking and falling apart. It's adaptive (A) in that it can change, as needed, due to conditions. If the conductor was out ill, the ensemble would adjust to the substitute. When the ensemble is coherent (C), it makes sense. The chords line up and the music doesn't feel confusing to the listener. The music is energized (E), exciting and full of vitality as opposed to flat, boring, or overwhelming. And finally, the ensemble is stable (S). The New York Philharmonic can withstand a significant impact before falling apart. Likewise, an integrated mind is flexible, adaptive, coherent, energized, and stable.

Chaos and Rigidity

Impaired integration moves a complex system toward either chaos or rigidity. A chaotic system is highly unpredictable and frequently changing, whereas a rigid system is the opposite; highly predictable and unchanging (Siegel, 2012). For example, due to the strength of both the differentiation and the linkage among musicians, the New York Philharmonic is a relatively stable complex system and mostly remains in an integrated state. That sixth-grade band, however, is much less integrated and can more easily move toward either chaos or rigidity. Because the individual, differentiated musicians are less skilled and the linkage between the parts is still tenuous and immature, that sixth-grade ensemble has less flexibility, adaptability, coherence, energy, and stability.

An ensemble moving toward chaos leaves the listener feeling uncomfortable. Where's the beat? Who's in charge? Chords no longer line up, and it sounds like noise, not music. However, an ensemble that errs toward rigidity might have the chords and the tempo all lined up but feel flat due to the lack of energy and resonance. As complex systems, humans have the capacity to move toward both chaos and rigidity; this is a normal part of the human experience. From an IPNB perspective, mental health symptoms (and *DSM* diagnoses) emerge when the chaos and/or rigidity negatively impacts the individual's relationships and functioning (Siegel, 2020).

Nine Domains of Integration

The theory of IPNB proposes nine domains of integration that I will list out briefly here. For further exploration, I'll refer you to the many resources authored by Siegel.

1 *Integration of consciousness* allows us "look at" an experience without *becoming* the experience, whether it's another's experience or our own. When we can simply *be* with whatever is arising, we can stay out of judgment of it.
2 *Interpersonal integration* invites the co-creation of a "we" by offering a *dynamically awake* (Badenoch, 2017) way of being that allows others to feel seen, felt, and known. Our resonance circuits, including the mirror neuron system, allow us to remain connected to our own deep inner experience while also connecting with the deep inner experience of another. Impaired interpersonal integration may be experienced as a felt sense of all-aloneness.
3 *Vertical integration* can be interpreted in two ways:
   a Brain/body: the conscious mind allows awareness of energy and sensation in the body. Poor integration may lead to being "cut off" from sensations in our body or flooded by sensations without the ability to either monitor or modify them.
   b Neurosequential: connection between the brain stem, limbic, and cortical regions of the brain, which then allows for connection between sensations, feelings, and cognition.
4 *Horizontal integration* refers to the integration between the right and left hemispheres of the brain. Lack of horizontal integration can result in difficulty labeling or describing the sensations or physical experience of emotion, either due to too much linkage (a flooding of sensation and emotion) or too much differentiation (limited access to the felt sensation of emotion).

5 *Memory integration* allows for the ability to recall a memory in an embodied way while also having the felt sense that the experience happened in the past and is *not* happening now. Memory integration is related to both horizontal and narrative integration.
6 *Narrative integration* creates an autobiographical story that is both coherent and cohesive. It invites awareness of the memory while also making sense of the memory—for example, where I came from and how those experiences impact me. Lack of narrative integration leaves an individual with limited awareness as to how their past has contributed to their present.
7 *State integration* leads to flexibility to move between our different parts of self, while also having compassion and curiosity for those different parts of self. Different states or parts of self naturally emerge because multiple neural networks are always online, processing information in different ways and attempting to support the best possible functioning of the system.
8 *Temporal integration* leads to an acceptance of and ease with the inevitable uncertainty of life. Temporal integration allows us to hold in mind that change is constant, without trying to stop it. Lack of temporal integration can look like obsessive compulsive symptoms, anxiety, and existential challenges such as a preoccupation with the purpose or meaning of life.
9 *Transpirational integration* was coined by Siegel (2009). Transpire means "to breathe across." Transpirational integration is an awareness of being a part of a larger whole, our connections to others and the earth, emerging from the other domains of integration.

Complex trauma impacts all nine domains of integration. However, for this chapter's exploration of complex trauma and dissociation in children, we will look most closely at *integration of consciousness, interpersonal integration, vertical integration,* and *state integration*.

Characteristics of Integration

In his book *Pocket Guide to Interpersonal Neurobiology*, Siegel (2012) identifies the following nine characteristics of integration.

1 Body regulation: Keeping the organs of the body and the autonomic nervous system coordinated and balanced.
2 Attuned communication: Tuning in to the internal state of another.
3 Emotional balance: Enabling internal states to be optimally activated: not too aroused, not too deflated.
4 Response flexibility: Pausing before acting to reflect on available options of response.
5 Fear modulation: Reducing fear.
6 Insight: self-knowing awareness that links past, present, and future. This is a mindsight map of "me." ("Mindsight" is Siegel's term for the ability to perceive the internal world, and not just observable behaviors, of ourselves and others.)
7 Empathy: Imagining what it is like to be another person, to see from another's perspective. This is a mindsight map of "you."
8 Morality: Imagining, reasoning, and behaving from the perspective of the larger good. This is a mindsight map of "we."
9 Intuition: A non-logical knowing.

When we are in an integrated state, meaning when we are flexible, adaptive, coherent, energized, and stable, these characteristics emerge. IPNB defines mental wellness as integration.

Interpersonal Neurobiology

The Development of Integration

Integration is a journey, not a destination. Children have less integration across all domains than adults simply due to their chronological age. It's important to have a solid understanding of child development when considering if a child's emotional balance, for example, is as flexible, adaptive, coherent, energized, and stable as we would expect from a typical peer, or if the child appears to have impaired integration that would benefit from support.

Integration isn't something to achieve or master, and no one has an integrated mind or brain, or integrated relationships, all the time—most certainly not a still-developing child. An integrated adult has the capacity to create a relational experience that invites integration *between* the child and the adult and *within* the child's own brain, mind, and nervous system. In their book *The Power of Showing Up* (2020), Siegel and Payne Bryson described how children need experiences of being safe, seen, and soothed in order to feel secure. Felt security invites integration. In her chapter "Becoming a Therapeutic Presence in the Counseling Room and the World in IPNB and Clinical Practice," Badenoch (2021), referencing Siegel (2020), wrote, "The brain is a complex system with natural co-organizing ability. While the capacity for neural integration is built into our system, it requires the presence of another to emerge" (p. 120). This is true in both the caregiver-child relationship and the therapist-client relationship.

Attachment, Disorganization, Complex Trauma, and Dissociation

If Integration Unfolds in the Presence of Another, What Happens When No One Is Present?

Although I immediately noticed my dislike for Jayme, her unlikableness isn't what brought her to therapy. Jayme was born to a mother who tried her best but had extremely limited resources. As I pieced together the sparse documentation, the picture I created of Jayme's first 12 months of life involved her spending a lot of time strapped into her car seat, even when she was home with her mother. Jayme received the calories she needed and probably had her diapers changed regularly. Most likely, her care ended there.

When Jayme was hospitalized for respiratory syncytial virus (RSV) at ten months old, she and her mother were brought to the attention of the local child protective services (CPS). Hospital staff had noticed that Jayme was delayed in meeting developmental milestones and presented with a flat, disconnected affect. Most concerning was the lack of interaction or reciprocity observed between Jayme and her mother. There was no reading picture books together or snuggling under Jayme's Winnie-the-Pooh blanket. CPS provided support services for Jayme and her mother when they went home, but those were unsuccessful, and Jayme was placed in foster care right around her first birthday.

For 18 months, social services worked to unify Jayme with her mother or place her with a member of her extended family. Neither of these options proved viable. Ultimately, Jayme's foster family became her adoptive family. At first, Jayme thrived. She caught up quickly, meeting or exceeding developmental milestones and soon surpassing her peers academically. When I met Jayme at age 6, her parents told me there'd been occasional unusual behavior, but nothing frequent enough to warrant services. Until now. Despite being fully toilet-trained since age 2, Jayme would occasionally urinate and defecate in inappropriate places, like the middle of her parents' bed. Although they couldn't explain why, Jayme's parents agreed those instances always felt oddly personal, as if in retaliation for something.

Jayme's mother also acknowledged, sheepishly, that she once suspected Jayme of luring the cat into her bedroom only to purposefully hurt the cat. No one quite knew what happened, but the cat screamed a "horrible scream," and Jayme was left with scratches on her face and abdomen.

She cried so hysterically that all the focus was on Jayme's injuries, and nobody investigated what had caused the usually docile cat to react in such an unexpected way. Jayme's mother felt guilty that she suspected Jayme of hurting the cat on purpose, especially since she couldn't really explain why she thought that.

Up to the end of her kindergarten year, Jayme was a well-behaved child who was doted on by other adults. But her transition to first grade had been fraught with difficulty. The day before Jayme's parents emailed me, Jayme had been sent to the principal's office for biting the child sitting next to her at story time. The teacher didn't notice anything amiss until the child screamed, and blood was pooling on her forearm. When asked what happened, Jayme said calmly that the child was sitting too close to her.

As we sat in my office, Jayme's parents told me about their life with her. At home, she was mostly compliant and cooperative, doing her chores and playing with the neighbor kids in the cul-de-sac. But about once a month, Jayme had a giant meltdown, usually preceded by a seemingly small frustration: not finding a library book she wanted or learning that someone had eaten the last cookie. Then, for an hour or more, Jayme would scream like she was possessed, yanking the drawers out of her dresser, dumping out buckets of building blocks, and hurling shoes and books at the walls. Most concerning, she would hit herself in the forehead with her fists. Occasionally, Jayme's dad would hold her down to keep her from hitting herself. At some point, and they could never predict when, the episode would just be over, as if a switch had been flipped. Jayme would collapse into shame, apologizing profusely and sobbing that she was bad and didn't deserve to be loved. After reassurance and a snuggle with her mom or dad, Jayme could move on. She would pop up and ask for a snack or to play a game. But her parents would be reeling, sometimes for hours.

While other adults described Jayme as adorable, precocious, sweet, and charming, Jayme's parents used words like whiplashed, confused, and shocked to describe how they felt with her. I myself was stunned by how quickly Jayme could shift from extreme dysregulation to ready to play. I began to wonder about these different states. How much disconnection or dissociation existed between them? I understood that Jayme had impairment in nearly all nine domains of integration, but I didn't yet understand the frequency, intensity, or severity of her impairment.

Attachment

John Bowlby, considered by many to be the father of attachment theory, proposed that a child's early experience with their caregiver is critical to their social-emotional development. Eventually, Bowlby and two of his colleagues, Mary Ainsworth and Mary Main, articulated four distinct categories of attachment: secure, insecure anxious, insecure avoidant, and insecure disorganized (Bowlby, 1969; Ainsworth et al., 1978; Main & Solomon, 1986; Wallin, 2007). This chapter will briefly examine the difference between secure and insecure disorganized attachment patterns as related to IPNB, complex trauma, and dissociation. For a more in-depth exploration of attachment through an IPNB lens, read *The Developing Mind* (2020) by Daniel Siegel or *Being a Brain Wise Therapist* (2008) by Bonnie Badenoch.

As other chapters that focus on attachment share, the way a child attaches to their primary caregiver becomes their mental model—their how-to guide—for all relationships that follow. Children considered to have a secure attachment style had caregiver experiences that let them feel safe, seen, soothed, and secure (Siegel & Payne Bryson, 2020). That doesn't mean they had perfect parents. In fact, attachment theory is clear that *imperfection* is the soil in which secure attachment blooms. These imperfect caregivers sometimes got it wrong, but they noticed and attuned to the ruptures in the relationship. Furthermore, these caregivers were themselves distressed by the rupture, which motivated them to make a repair.

Interpersonal Neurobiology

A child with a mental model of secure attachment has learned that ruptures and misattunements can be repaired and that their caregiver sees them as good, even through distress and occasional "bad" behavior. They have learned to trust that their caregiver will dependably keep them safe. Children with secure attachment also understand that they are separate from their caregivers. They learn to be comfortable with both independence and intimacy. From an IPNB perspective, children with secure attachment grow to be adults who demonstrate the nine characteristics of integration and mental wellness. Secure attachment is well established as a resilience factor in both physical and mental health.

Attachment Behaviors

To understand how complex trauma can lead to disintegration and dissociation in the child's mind, we need to briefly consider Bowlby's (1969) description of the three attachment-seeking behaviors:

1. **Stay Close!** One of the primary jobs of the attachment system is to keep babies close to their caregivers. This keeps them safe and alive. Babies fuss and cry to keep their caregivers close. As they grow and develop, they begin to crawl or run toward their caregiver. Even just being cute is an attachment behavior—it keeps their caregivers engaged.
2. **Be curious and explore!** Once a baby feels confident in the closeness and dependability of their caregiver, the next attachment behavior is to be less close. When babies and eventually toddlers, preschoolers, and older kids and adults feel confident that they have a dependable attachment figure, they feel safe enough to let their curiosity bring them out into the world to explore.
3. **Feel Better!** Going out and exploring the world will inevitably lead to some big feelings. Excitement, surprise, and fear are just some of the feelings that will overwhelm babies and young children. The next attachment behavior is to use the attachment figure to feel better. When an infant feels unsafe, alone, overwhelmed, or just in need of some connection, their attachment system propels them toward their caregiver so they can be safe, seen, soothed, and secure.

A Biological Paradox: Disorganized Attachment

As we have learned in other chapters in this book, when the nervous system detects a threat, it mobilizes the body to either flee or fight that danger. Next, the attachment system activates and propels us toward our primary attachment figure, for both physical safety and emotional soothing. What happens when a child's attachment system propels them toward their caregiver, but the caregiver is the same person who activated their threat-response system? And what happens when this occurs repeatedly?

If there is no one available to provide that safe soothing, or if that caregiver causes more fright, a child is left in what attachment researchers refer to as a *biological paradox* (Siegel, 2012). Danger? From their attachment figure? This is fright without solution (Hesse & Main, 1999) Eventually, the child's mind has no choice but to keep these two experiences disconnected. The part of their mind that holds the fright stays dissociated from the part of their mind that holds safety, connection, and attachment. While not specifically related to IPNB, the Circle of Security paradigm (Powell et al., 2016) offers clear and concise descriptors for the types of caregivers whose parenting leads to disorganization: mean, weak, or gone, which are described as follows.

- **Mean** describes the caregiver that we typically consider abusive. Their behavior is terrifying.
- **Weak** describes the caregiver who isn't overtly abusive but is so terrified themselves that they cannot offer their child experiences of being safe, seen, soothed, or secure.
- **Gone** describes the caregiver who is either physically or energetically "gone." This caregiver might regularly leave their child alone—literally. This also could be a caregiver who, due to their

own trauma history, leaves a child alone figuratively. Their own internal disconnection leaves them unavailable to their child, who is left vulnerable and distraught.

Based on the little information we had about Jayme's first year of life, my best guess was that she had experienced a caregiver who was frequently gone. She had likely missed out on thousands of micro-moments of being cooed at, fussed over, and generally adored. She had likely not been picked up or soothed, but rather left alone to cry. In interviews with CPS, Jayme's mother described roommates who engaged in a lot of drinking and physical fighting. She coped by putting on headphones and playing video games. Jayme probably heard it all, alone in her car seat. For an infant, that amount of aloneness is terrifying. It's a threat! So, their nervous system mobilizes, their attachment system activates... and nothing changes. Eventually, the nervous system tries another tactic: it disconnects the mind from the body to protect itself from the experience of pain and terror, of fright without solution. Over time, this disconnected state just becomes the default.

Dissociation through an IPNB Lens

The word *dissociation* is commonly used by both clinicians and non-clinicians to describe the floaty, hazy, detached state that is a protective mechanism against life threat. Along with other kinds of terrifying situations, prolonged traumatic experiences that are not co-regulated by a safe and attuned caregiver are interpreted by the nervous system as life threat.

As the heart rate slows, endorphins and opioids are released, and the terrified person is brought into a state of collapse, feigning death (Badenoch, 2017). It is the body's wise last attempt at survival, as often a predator will abandon prey that appears dead. If the predator doesn't lose interest and continues its attack, the dissociated response decreases, or even eliminates, pain and allows the person to disengage from the experience. If the person survives, the dissociative experience may prevent them from having explicit recall of the trauma, another protective mechanism.

By its very definition, dissociation causes the mind to disconnect, separate, and do anything but "be with" an overwhelming or terrifying experience. This disconnection impairs integration. Therefore, a treatment approach grounded in the theory of IPNB invites integration across the nine domains.

From an IPNB perspective, dissociation simply means disconnection. It is the opposite of integration. Dissociation can exist between and among all nine domains of integration and on a wide continuum. Dissociation can refer to the disconnect between the brain and body (vertical integration) or the disconnect between parts of self (state integration). The impact of vertical dissociation can occur on a wide continuum from mild, presenting as a decrease in interoception, to extensive, presenting as symptoms of depersonalization disorder. Similarly, the impact of state dissociation can also exist on the wide continuum between mild, perhaps causing an individual to feel as though they shift between different states of themselves quickly or without much warning, all the way to extensive, presenting as symptoms of dissociative identity disorder (DID).

Repeated experiences of terror that cause an individual to disconnect or dissociate from themselves can have profound impacts on integration of consciousness, which impacts all other domains of integration. Integration of consciousness involves having the mindful attention to "be with" an experience as it unfolds. The impact of dissociation of consciousness can also exist on a continuum. Mild dissociation of consciousness may present simply as a need for extra support within a safe relationship (e.g., with a therapist) to notice or be with an experience. More extensive dissociation of consciousness may present as an inability to demonstrate any mindful attention to one's present experience.

Assessment is essential, and IPNB approaches assessment through the nine domains of integration. Familiarity and understanding of the nine domains, including symptoms and characteristics associated with each, held in a developmental context, is required. As mentioned previously, IPNB is a theory of human development, not a clinical theory. Therefore, clinicians can utilize their clinical training, including in assessment, while contextualizing their assessment through the lens of IPNB. It's also important to note that while many clinical theories consider the assessment phase to occur at the beginning of treatment, IPNB considers assessment to be an ongoing process, occurring throughout treatment. As you'll see in my work with Jayme, the level of disconnection and dissociation in the four of the nine domains that I write about in this chapter is continuously assessed, and assumed to be continuously shifting. An important tenet of IPNB is that the clinicians remain in a state of curiosity, trusting the client to bring exactly what is needed in that moment.

A Paradox of Impossible

Except for in our first few sessions, the Jayme that others described as precious and adorable existed only until she crossed the threshold of my office. She'd greet me in the waiting room with a warm smile and a bright "hello!" Sometimes she'd even pull something out of her backpack to enthusiastically share with me. Together, we would head around the corner to my bright, polka-dotted office, and the moment the door was closed, she'd shrug off her backpack and turn toward me with a glare.

"What stupid things are we going to do today?" she would ask, and the taunting would begin. Jayme would tell me I was dumb, therapy was for babies, and she couldn't believe her mom actually paid me money.

"It feels like we're doing baby things here," I would carefully reflect back.

"Are you stupid? That's what I just said."

"It feels like I'm stupid," I would say.

"I can't believe you're calling me stupid!" Jayme would shout, in feigned outrage.

And for the next 45 minutes, we would dance in the paradox of impossible. She would sneer at every curious statement I offered about what she might be feeling. Sometimes I would articulate my own feelings—stuck, confused, adrift. Sometimes I said nothing.

My attempts at attunement were always rejected. She would tell me I was wrong, that I was ridiculous, an idiot. She would defend herself against things I never said. When I stayed quiet, she would roll her eyes and pointedly look at the clock: *Will this ever end?*

In the game of serve and return, I would serve, and she'd chuck it back in my face. Jayme invited me into her disorganization, and I didn't like it. I felt stuck, helpless, angry, and powerless. In other words, I probably felt exactly the way Jayme felt when she was a baby. Though it's difficult to be certain, and I always work to stay in a state of curiosity, my own implicit memory likely left me vulnerable to resonating with Jayme's implicit memory. This bidirectional resonance is why Badenoch teaches and writes so emphatically about the importance of the therapist becoming aware of their own implicit vulnerabilities, as described in the next section.

It was the most excruciating hour of my week. I doubted myself. I doubted the process. I doubted my skills. I wondered if Jayme needed a different therapist. Jayme's behaviors did not improve in my office; in fact, she only escalated as the weeks went on. In contrast, Jayme's behaviors did slowly and steadily improve both with her family and at school.

At the end of our hour together, Jayme would gather her belongings and put her shoes on. She would take a breath, smile brightly, and say, "Miss Robyn, you are the best therapist ever! I wish I could come here every day!"

I would smile gently—always easier at the end of the hour—and say, "This is a place you get to bring all your feelings, even the confusing and overwhelming ones. All your feelings get to come here. It's my job to hold them." She would look at me then with confusion and desperation—the most excruciating hour of my week ended with the most heartbreaking two minutes. Artifice dropped away and Jayme was just a baby, tiny and defenseless, strapped into her car seat and trapped in chaos and longing. I would stand silently, feeling equal parts tenderness and despair for her. As soon as she moved, I would open the door and she walked back out to her parents' station wagon.

Interpersonal Integration

IPNB asserts that our role as therapists is to collaborate with our clients in a way that liberates their natural drive toward integration. We do this through our own interpersonal integration, which allows us to remain dynamically awake in relationship (Badenoch, 2017), connecting (linking) with our clients in a resonant way while also maintaining our autonomous, separate selves (differentiating).

Interpersonal integration isn't terribly difficult with others in an integrated state themselves (flexible, adaptive, coherence, energetic, and stable). But maintaining connection and resonance with someone in a disintegrated state is much more difficult. As the other moves into chaos or rigidity, our own vulnerabilities may shift us into that same state. Once there, we risk either merging (too much interpersonal linkage) or disconnecting (too much interpersonal differentiation).

Badenoch (2008) described three steps on a therapist's journey toward maintaining our own integration while connecting with our clients' disintegration.

- Heal what we can, widening our window of tolerance.
- Become conscious of our unique implicit vulnerabilities and release any expectations that we can or must be perfect containers will, or should, always be able to remain in an integrated state.
- Develop sufficient mindfulness so we can become aware in the moment when we are activated by our patients' struggles (p. 155).

Badenoch's steps were crucial in my work with Jayme. They became a road map for me to tend to my own integration—which I hoped would eventually help Jayme learn to tend to hers. I worked to heal what I could inside myself, which helped me tolerate the discomfort of being with Jayme in her most challenging moments. From an IPNB perspective, our resonance circuitries leave us vulnerable for implicit awakenings when our client's implicit world offers us a mirror. I worked to become conscious of and release my own vulnerabilities, like wanting to be a "good" therapist, or wanting to claim "success" with a tough case. I learned to maintain a sense of curiosity and compassion toward myself, which helped me maintain curiosity and compassion toward Jayme. Although it wasn't easy, I worked to release myself from the expectation of being a perfect container for Jayme. I learned to accept that I couldn't and shouldn't remain in a place of integration and resonance at all moments. I worked to stay mindfully present with the sensations that arose within me during our time together. IPNB helped me see my feelings of dislike for Jayme simply as information that I was leaving an integrated state and decreasing the possibility of resonance between Jayme and me.

A Way to Be With

One of the hardest parts about working with Jayme was that because we were chronically stuck in an enactment of disorganization, I could never offer her any information to help her make sense of her behavior. She would ignore or insult me for an hour and then collapse into shame, shifting into a part of herself that used appeasement and flattery to maintain our relationship. Her collapse into shame felt palpable. My own heart would sink, I would feel a wave of nausea in my belly, and tears would sting my eyes. I was following Jayme into the dissociative collapse of her infancy while also feeling the shame she held now about the intensity and confusion of her behavior.

Using Siegel's (2012) metaphor of the Wheel of Awareness in these moments, I recognized that Jayme was stuck on her rim. She could shift between rim points but rarely returned to her hub. I knew that if we were ever going to bring any integration to her dissociated parts, Jayme would need to find her way to her hub and stay there while connecting with these parts of herself with compassion and curiosity. Before that would ever be possible, I needed to find a way for her to see these parts of herself, to *be with* them, instead of disappearing into them.

One day, Jayme disappeared behind the curtain that hid a giant white board. She wrote me a note that I discovered later. "I love Miss Robyn" with hearts and flowers all around it.

This gave me an idea. What if Jayme and I could write to each other? Would she be better able to receive the compassion and curiosity I held about her behavior this way? I asked Jayme's mom's permission to write to her. I selected a three-ring binder just for Jayme, filled it with lined paper, and wrote her a note.

Dear Jayme,

I wondered if you might like to write me a note each week. I'll write back.
You can write about whatever you want.

Robyn

Jayme loved the idea. "You got this for me?" she asked with some incredulousness. She immediately took the binder to the waiting room and sat down to write. This began many weeks of back-and-forth communication, exchanged through the binder. Jayme told me about a fight she had with her friends. Another time she told me about yelling at her parents. I'd write back about her friend's watchdog brain (my playful term for the protective and energized part of the nervous system), how her friend's mean words probably made Jayme's watchdog brain want to be mean too. I told her that sometimes my own watchdog brain would take over and it was like I wasn't even me anymore. I told her that sometimes I confused myself but knew that even if it didn't make any sense, my watchdog brain was working so, so hard to protect me. I told her I knew she had a watchdog brain too, and even though her watchdog brain probably confused her, I was very grateful that it worked so hard to keep her safe. Even when her watchdog brain was mean to me. But Jayme was never mean in her writings. She was brave and honest and surprisingly articulate, especially in contrast to the words she usually yelled at me.

During these weeks and months when we wrote back and forth to each other, our sessions didn't change. After we exchanged the binder, our sessions would unfold as usual. She would huff and puff, call me names, and tell me how mad she was about things I never said. Then, at the end, she'd put on her big smile and tell me what a great therapist I was. I would tell her she didn't need to compliment me, that it was okay to leave without saying something extra-nice. I would remind her that all of her feelings were allowed to come to my office, and she was doing exactly what she needed to do. One day, she didn't apologize. She just smiled and waved goodbye.

The next session, she skipped into my office, shrugged off her backpack, and reached up toward the aerial hammock that hung down from my ceiling in a tidy knot. With one swift tug, she freed all nine feet of teal fabric, turned toward me as she spread it open wide, and asked, "Can I sit here?"

Integration of Consciousness

Siegel (2009) developed the metaphor of the Wheel of Awareness to describe integration of consciousness. When we are in the hub of the mind, we can use our attention to travel down the spokes to various rim points. Rim points are anything that draws our attention and can include thoughts, feelings, sensations, perceptions, sensory experiences, or even parts of the self. When we remain in the hub of our mind, we can see the various rim points with flexibility, as options. From our hub, we can be with what is happening instead of becoming what is happening. It is this awareness that invites the possibility of change.

One way to assess a child's integration of consciousness is by noticing how quickly they are able to be with their own mental processes through play. While always taking into consideration the child's chronological age, we can observe a child's integration of consciousness by considering the ease with which they engage in symbolic or projective play. Children with more mild presentations of dissociation come to therapy with some capacity to be with their parts of self and other mental processes through play. The safety of the therapy space and the therapist's own integration invite the child to strengthen the hub of their mind and increase their integration of consciousness, often without any specific intervention or technique.

Jayme was clearly stuck on her rim and out of her hub. Not only that, but she worked hard to pull me out of my hub too. Jayme's history of disorganized attachment meant that to her, connection was equivalent to terror. Therefore, she was preoccupied with doing anything she could to prevent me from creating a connection with her. Unfortunately, this strategy left Jayme stuck bouncing between chaos and rigidity. Any attempt I made to help her see her behavior instead of being consumed by her behavior was met with increased dysregulation. I desperately wanted to help Jayme develop a sense of understanding and even compassion toward these overwhelming, confusing, and chaotic parts of herself, and I was devastated that I couldn't find a way to do so. Sometimes I joined her on the rim with my own feelings of helplessness and hopelessness.

Communicating through the binder meant that Jayme could take in information about her behavior without being triggered by the intimacy of our relationship. It allowed her the possibility of making new meaning out of her behavior. It wasn't that she was a bad kid; it was that her watchdog brain was overactive. This decreased her shame just enough that she could begin to risk staying in the hub of her mind just a little bit longer. Ever so slowly, she began to experience an increase in her integration of consciousness and a decrease in dissociation.

Throughout this stage of our work together, my time with Jayme did not get any more comfortable. I was regularly and intensely swept away by my own implicit vulnerabilities and would then find myself stranded on my own rim. To find my way back, I relied on my professional consultations with Bonnie Badenoch, peer consultation with a group of colleagues grounded in IPNB, and personal therapy. These deeply resonant spaces increased my capacity to remain flexible, adaptive, coherent, energetic, and stable while also resonating with the chaotic and dissociated energy Jayme brought with her to my office. Over time, I could notice the rim points of my overwhelm and helplessness while remaining in my hub. This did not make my time with Jayme any more comfortable, but it did create more safety for Jayme.

Connecting Mind and Body

Jayme's dramatic shift in how she entered the session and pulled down the hammock in my office shouldn't have shocked me. The rigidity with which she shifted states was congruent with the level of dissociation and disorganization I understood was present in her neurobiology. Even so, I felt a little whiplashed and had to take a moment to reorient. In retrospect, I continue to marvel at how in almost every moment Jayme was showing me a map of her inner world.

"Of course, you can sit there," I said, then paused, uncertain. *Should I offer to show her how to sit in the hammock or let her experiment with it on her own?* I carried the whisper of fear in my body with Jayme, never sure what the right next step was and feeling as though any misstep would be harshly punished.

Again. How committed she was to showing me a map of her inner world.

The pause allowed for the path to present itself when Jayme asked, "Can you show me how?" It wasn't until later that I was able to appreciate the gravity of this moment. In that short little sentence, Jayme offered me something she hadn't yet offered in session: trust.

"Of course," I said. I took hold of the hammock and positioned it in a way that made sitting both easy and comfortably. I sank my bottom down into the fabric, sitting in it like a swing about two feet off the ground.

Jayme smiled and stepped toward me, my cue to step out of the hammock. She easily maneuvered the fabric to create a comfortable, nest-like swing. Jayme kept her feet on the ground and seemed reluctant to relax her body fully into the fabric. She continued to hold her own body without relying on the fabric to hold her.

I tightened my body slightly by flexing the muscles in my back and thighs, wanting to mirror the tension that remained in Jayme's body. Then I took a quiet breath, exhaled softly, and allowed all the tension in my muscles to release. So did Jayme. Her spine softened as she rested into the fabric, allowing the hammock to hold her. With this, we stepped into a new and unexpected phase of treatment.

For about six weeks, my sessions with Jayme involved only the hammock. She came into the office, pulled the hammock down, kicked off her shoes, and climbed in. Slowly, she became less tenuous and more trusting of the fabric. She would pull her feet into the fabric and use a kicking motion to open it up underneath her. The nine feet of fabric easily allowed her to lie back fully, suspended in midair. I watched her roll around in the fabric, punch it out with her fists and push with her feet. At times, I felt like I was watching an unborn baby exploring the safe confines of the womb. This wasn't regressive therapy, though. Jayme was safely exploring her somatosensory system while also being safely held in relationship.

I got braver and bolder with my role in our relationship, no longer afraid everything I said would cause a flareup of dysregulation, and I would offer reflections like, "You're moving your hand," or "I see your five fingers up against the fabric," or "Oh! You rolled over!" Since Jayme was cocooned inside the fabric, obstructing eye contact, this seemed to allow her to titrate the intimacy so that my comments didn't cause dysregulation.

"Would you like to know how to hang upside down?" I asked one afternoon. This was the first time I attempted to initiate the dance of our relationship.

"Like what?" Jayme asked, curious yet wary. I took the hammock into my hands, sat down, and slowly inverted, my legs coming above my head and wrapping around the fabric. We locked eyes; me upside down and Jayme right side up. A slight nod from her told me she was ready to try. First, she attempted to fling her feet up over her head with such force she essentially ricocheted back to sitting. She did this a few times, growing frustrated. I took a big breath, exhaled, and reflected, "Notice the muscles in your legs." Coming back to a seated position, Jayme paused to sit squarely in the hammock. She took a breath, exhaled, and moved smoothly into a fully inverted position.

At around the six-week mark, Jayme once again shifted her play. After spending about 20 minutes in the hammock, she hopped out and moved to the previously untouched sand tray. She continued to use the hammock weekly for many months, growing in her skills, confidence, and body awareness, while also integrating sand tray work into her sessions.

Vertical Integration

The brain develops from the bottom up and the inside out. The brainstem, which sits at the very bottom of the brain and connects the brain to the spinal column, begins to develop in utero. Responsible for autonomic functions such as heart rate, respiration, and energy and arousal in the autonomic nervous system, the fetal brainstem develops in connection with the rhythms of the pregnant person's brainstem and autonomic nervous system. At birth, a healthy, full-term infant has a brainstem that allows them to breathe on their own and express distress through crying. Newborn babies don't know what the different sensations of distress mean—they just know there is distress.

Ideally, a present and regulated caregiver soothes the baby and alleviates the distress. Not only does this begin to strengthen the developing baby's regulatory circuits, but also the co-regulation allows the baby to tolerate and make sense of internal sensations. Caregivers try different things to soothe a baby, like offering a warm bottle of milk, covering with a blanket, rocking or singing. Over time, they make connections between the baby's behavior and the type of distress they are experiencing. This, in turn, allows the baby to make sense of their own distress. Certain sensations are soothed with a bottle, others with a diaper change. The baby learns there is a solution to their distress and that they will not be alone in it. They learn that they can stay present with their own distress because it's tolerable and it will end. These are the building blocks for vertical integration and ultimately interoceptive awareness. You may be noticing that the experiences that support integration also support the development of secure attachment.

When the developing baby is not soothed, does not receive the co-regulation and presence that allow them to tolerate their stress and understand that it will end, or has distressing sensations caused by the person who is supposed to help them feel safe, vertical integration is impaired. This impairment doesn't prevent uncomfortable sensations from happening in the body, but it prevents the brain from noticing and being aware of the uncomfortable sensations. This is brilliantly protective for an infant who has been left alone with intolerable distress, but this adaptation also has significant costs.

Dampening awareness of uncomfortable sensations inadvertently dampens awareness of pleasant ones too, such as sensations of connection. This leads to an impairment in what we could consider internal resonance—the individual's capacity to be with themselves. When internal resonance is impaired, the development of interpersonal resonance—empathy—is also impaired. Impaired vertical integration leaves the mind dissociated from the body. Older children and adults articulate this experience with words like "I don't know who I am" or "Sometimes I don't even feel like I have a body." This dissociation from the body can contribute to injuries due to increased pain tolerance, or enuresis and encopresis due to inability to feel the sensations of needing to void. Sometimes this mind-body dissociation contributes to over- or under-nourishing our bodies with food and calories.

In play therapy, kids may demonstrate this disconnect from their body through play that is either very chaotic or rigid. I've had kids destroy the room, dump toys, and overturn the sandbox in a dysregulated and disembodied manner. I've also had kids on the opposite end of the spectrum who come into the playroom and do nothing. They sit and stare, sink into the couch and say nothing for the entire 50-minute session.

Jayme missed crucial experiences that would have created connections between her cortex and the lower regions of her brain and body. Although she didn't have any difficulty with things like toileting, feeding, modulating temperature, or being over- or under-responsive to pain, her history and current difficulty with emotion regulation led me to suspect that she had poor vertical integration. I interpreted Jayme's curiosity in the hammock as her natural drive for integration, facilitated by experiencing enough safety in her relationship with me that she could risk noticing her body. Slowly, she began to experience a linkage between previously disconnected and dissociated parts.

Welcoming All Parts

Jayme pulled the lid off my sand tray and silently stared.

"It's not big enough," she said without looking at me.

"It feels too small," I agreed. Jayme turned to look at me, her eyes expecting me to know what to do next.

And actually, I did.

An image came to mind of a session I'd had with my own therapist, some years before, when I had said something similar. The sand tray in her office was simply too small. It could never convey the vastness of my empty inner world. She'd grabbed a stack of 8.5-by-14-inch manila paper and spread several sheets across the floor. That's how big I needed the sand tray to be.

"What if," I suggested to Jayme, "we cover the whole floor in sand-colored paper and pretend the whole office is a sand tray. Would it be big enough?"

She shrugged. The contrast between the Jayme who seemed to barely have enough energy to respond and the Jayme who could confidently flip upside down in the aerial hammock was striking—another reminder of the disconnect and dissociation between her different parts of self.

"How about I lay the paper down, and you can decide," I suggested.

Again, she silently shrugged, and it was starting to feel as though she was becoming more and more disconnected from me and probably from herself. I grabbed the paper and slowly covered the floor of my office, just as my therapist had once done for me.

"Does this feel done?" I asked, when it seemed as if I'd covered every inch of floor. She shrugged. Jayme sat crisscross applesauce on the couch while I had essentially painted myself into a corner at the other side of the office. She quietly walked to my sand tray shelves, selected a tiny mouse, and placed it in the middle of the room. She returned to her spot on the couch and tucked her legs underneath her, and we sat in silence for the rest of our time together. We did this for weeks.

In some ways, this stage of our work together was more uncomfortable than when we were stuck together in the paradox of impossible. There was a sense of nothingness in the office that caused the minutes to tick away like hours. I found myself feeling bored, irritated, and distracted. I detailed out long to-do lists in my head and fantasized about what I would do when the session was over. I realized that by drifting away with my thoughts, I was being with Jayme in exactly the way she expected: without any resonant presence at all. I shifted my focus in our sessions away from my grocery list and worked instead on staying present with her nothingness, her lack of resonance. I needed to stay in my hub while Jayme was stuck on a rim point of nothingness. I worked to hold that space open for as long as she needed, with an invitation for resonance and connection, but without any agenda for her to change or do something different.

The little mouse sat all alone in the middle of my room, week after excruciating week. The discrepancy between the size of the tiny, vulnerable mouse and the vast nothingness that surrounded it seemed to be Jayme's way of attempting to externalize how big and overwhelming her state of nothingness felt. I wondered if she felt utterly alone in a desert that was otherwise void of anything. No resonance, no connection. Nothing.

Then, one day, after meticulously covering my floor with manila paper and placing the little mouse in the middle, Jayme brought me a tiny squirrel. "You can be the tree where the squirrel lives," she said. She had me hold my hands in front of me and she carefully placed the squirrel on my open palm, directly facing the mouse. For half an hour my arms shook as I held that position, unwilling to falter after having been trusted to care for this watchful squirrel. Jayme went back to the sand tray shelves and began to build a home for the mouse.

This stage of treatment unfolded for more than nine months. Some weeks Jayme would build a safe home for the mouse. Some weeks, there would be chaos and danger surrounding the mouse while Jayme created stories of unpredictability and danger. Every week, she placed the squirrel in my palms and told me I was the tree. Sometimes, I would offer up a reflection like, "Wow, the mouse must feel so scared," and she'd remind me that trees do not talk. Sometimes, the mouse would simply exist in the middle of chaos that would end as abruptly as it started. When she was finished with the mouse and the sand tray the size of my office, Jayme would abandon the figures and climb into the hammock. By now, she had grown quite skilled in the hammock and was accomplishing many complex poses.

State Integration

What is a state? Neurobiologically speaking, a state is "composed of a cluster of neural firing patterns that embed within them certain behaviors, a feeling tone, and access to particular memories" (Siegel, 2009, p. 262). Different states of mind help the brain work more efficiently and are both normal and adaptive. We all have different states. I have my mom state, my social worker state, and my aerial silks state. My aerial silks state comes alive as I head to the studio, and that state helps me safely hang upside down by quickly lighting up the neural patterns that have previously fired in class. The feeling of pleasure that is encoded into that state helps me with the frustration tolerance needed to learn new skills; it all awakens together.

Siegel (2009) wrote about a proverbial "neural glue" that links these feelings, sensations, thoughts, and behavior patterns together into different states. Some states have glue that allows for a lot of flexibility. The state is open and receptive to new information and new ways of being. For example, the flexibility allows me to take a skill I learned on the silks and build on it to learn similar yet new and more difficult skills. Sometimes states aren't as flexible, keeping us locked into old neural patterns without being open and receptive to new information. This lack of receptivity leaves us reacting to situations largely out of our past learning instead of combining our past learning with the newness of the unfolding experience.

In addition to identity-based states (like my mom, social worker, and aerialist states), we can develop states around different sensory and feeling experiences, like shame, humiliation, rage, and even nothingness. When the neural glue holding those states together is flexible, we can take in new information such as, "This feeling of shame is from the past, but it's not right; I wasn't shameful then, and I'm not shameful now." When the neural glue holding the state together is not flexible, it is very difficult to update those states to reflect the present experience.

The less flexibility there is within a state, the less flexibility there is between states. This results in what can feel like unexpected state shifts, and often, the person doesn't seem to realize how quickly they are shifting or the impact this could have on others. Disintegration or dissociation between states exists on a broad spectrum. It can range from a lack of flexibility that leads to fast and unpredictable shifts between states, all the way to a disruption in consciousness, which can look like disconnection from self or reality. At its most disintegrated and dissociated, state disintegration can lead to DID.

Jayme's "neural glue" seemed inflexible, but I did not suspect DID. Although she shifted between parts of self quickly and abruptly, she didn't present with distinct personality states. If she had, the phase of treatment that focuses on interpersonal integration would likely have been much longer. I may also have expanded my treatment team and potentially increased her level of care, depending on her symptoms.

Individuals with poor state integration don't usually have a very strong hub. It is difficult for them to be with what's happening on the rim without shifting completely to that rim point, losing mindsight and awareness of other states. When Jayme trusted me to care for the tiny squirrel, I wondered if she was asking me to hold her observing self—herself in her hub. Badenoch (2017) wrote about how clients and therapists can co-create a joint window of tolerance. Through interpersonal resonance, our clients borrow from our window of tolerance so they can be with their own dysregulation in a way that is almost impossible otherwise. Our weekly repeated experience eventually led to Jayme embedding our relationship of safety, presence, and co-regulation into her neurobiology.

Conclusion: Reflections on the Journey toward Integration

To write a coherent chapter, I've written about some of the different domains of integration as if they exist in a silo, with treatment progressing neatly from one domain of integration to the next. As you synthesize the ideas I've shared, I hope you will recognize that although the information has been presented in a linear way for organizational purposes, treatment does not follow a straight path from one domain of integration to the next.

Jayme's lack of state integration was clear from the beginning, based on how her parents described her versus how other people experienced her. The rapid shifts in her affect and behavior suggested significant disconnection and dissociation between her parts, though not to the extent of DID. Jayme eventually had periods of treatment where it seemed as though state integration was the primary shift taking place. Actually, state integration was happening from our first moments together when she experienced that all parts of her were welcome.

While only Jayme can truly know what was happening for her at the different stages of treatment, here is my best guess. At the beginning of our work together, my invitation for interpersonal integration and resonance was too threatening, as it would have opened up more access to states that she worked tirelessly to avoid re-experiencing, including her state of nothingness. Jayme initially relied on a state that was focused on rejecting all connection and intimacy. She would switch quickly to a state of fawning at the end of our sessions in an attempt to avoid being rejected by me. Outside the office, she relied on a state that others described as precious and adorable. All of these state shifts were part of her brilliant and effective strategy to avoid awakening the nothingness that I later learned felt so consuming for her. No wonder she worked so hard to avoid it.

When we started using the binder to communicate with each other outside of sessions, we began strengthening the hub of Jayme's mind. This was new for her, and it reduced her shame just enough that she began to risk being with herself, even in hard moments. I gave her some language to describe the shifts in her state with compassion, not judgment. Strengthening the hub of her mind with compassion invited the possibility of beginning to increase flexibility between states. Jayme's work in the sand tray emerged when the hub of her mind could hold seeing her different states without becoming flooded by them. Strengthening her vertical integration through the work she did in the aerial hammock likely contributed to her increased body regulation. By the time we progressed to the sand tray, Jayme was beginning to experience the safety of our interpersonal connection, which allowed her to borrow, in a way, from my own integration while she risked staying present with herself even as uncomfortable states came forward.

Because her earliest experiences had left her all alone, without co-regulation or connection, Jayme had very little experience in a safe "we" space. I pictured my work with her resting on a bed of my own integration. In order for Jayme to ever begin to experience interpersonal integration, I had to stay steadfast in my commitment to remaining integrated in the face of her rejection and attempts to humiliate me. Over the course of our work together, Jayme brought me many of her parts, just as I told her she could. She brought her parts that rejected connection by being mean and taunting, as well as her part that held a desperate need to appease. She brought the parts of her that were disconnected from herself and just beginning to feel and explore her body.

And then she brought her nothingness and bravely asked me to also be with that. At first, we would both fall down the pathway of dissociation. As she sat on my couch, disconnected, I could feel myself disconnecting too. Over time, as I learned to stay available and meet Jayme in her nothingness without any attempts to rescue her from it. Jayme risked bringing in the parts of herself that held the chaos and the danger. Together, we witnessed her multiple parts of self. She had the wisdom to place me in the role of quiet observer while possibly also entrusting me to care for her own observing self.

Throughout our two years of treatment, I used a variety of therapeutic tools, including play therapy, sand tray therapy, and body-based somatic therapy. The tools simply provided a vehicle for Jayme and me to travel on a journey toward integration. Throughout our time together, I worked tenaciously to remain as integrated (flexible, adaptive, coherent, energetic, and stable) as possible while also increasing my awareness of when I was moving toward chaos or rigidity.

Due to her history of complex trauma, Jayme's dissociation was present between and among all the domains of integration. This dissociation was adaptive, even lifesaving, and Jayme didn't need to be fixed. But the dissociation was not without cost, impacting her relationships with others, but most importantly, with herself. In order to truly extend an invitation toward integration, I released myself from any agenda to change or fix Jayme, and any agenda to be a good therapist. With the support of my mentors, colleagues, and therapist, I remained anchored in IPNB theory, trusting that all complex systems move toward integration when they are met by the presence of another.

References

Ainsworth, M. D. S., Blehar, M., Waters, E., & Wall, S. (1978). *Patterns of attachment: A psychological study of the strange situation.* Erlbaum.

Badenoch, B. (2008). *Being a brain-wise therapist: A practical guide to interpersonal neurobiology.* W. W. Norton.

Badenoch, B. (2017). *Heart of trauma.* W. W. Norton.

Badenoch, B. (2021). Becoming a therapeutic presence in the counseling room and the world. In D. Siegel, A. Schore & L. Cozolino (Eds.), *Interpersonal neurobiology and clinical practice* (pp. 113–133). W. W. Norton.

Bowlby, J. (1969). *Attachment and loss: Vol. 1.* Attachment. Basic Books.

Hesse, E., & Main, M. (1999). Second-generation effects of unresolved trauma in nonmaltreating parents: Dissociated, frightened, and threatening parental behavior. *Psychoanalytic Inquiry: A Topical Journal for Mental Health Professionals, 19*(4), 481–540. https://doi.org/10.1080/07351699909534265

Main, M., & Solomon, J. (1986). Discovery of an insecure-disorganized/disoriented attachment pattern. In T. B. Brazelton & M. W. Yogman (Eds.), *Affective development in infancy* (pp. 95–124). Ablex Publishing.

Powell, B., Cooper, G., Hoffman, K., & Marvin, B. (2016). *The circle of security intervention* (Reprint). Guilford Press.

Sears, W., & Sears, M. (2003). *The baby book: Everything you need to know about your baby from birth to age two* (Revised ed.). Little, Brown & Company.

Siegel, D. (2009). *Mindsight: The new science of personal transformation.* Bantam Books.

Siegel, D. (2010, August 28). Mindsight and the power of neural integration in healing [Plenary session]. EMDRIA 2010 International Conference, Phoenix, AZ.

Siegel, D. (2012). *Pocket guide to interpersonal neurobiology.* W. W. Norton.

Siegel, D. (2020). *The developing mind.* W. W. Norton.

Siegel, D., & Hartzell, M. (2004). *Parenting from the inside out: How a deeper self-understanding can help you raise children who thrive.* Tarcher Perigee.

Siegel, D., & Payne Bryson, T. (2020). *The power of showing up: How parental presence shapes who our kids become and how their brains get wired.* Ballantine Books.

van IJzendoorn, M. (1995). Adult attachment representations, parental responsiveness, and infant attachment: A meta-analysis on the predictive validity of the Adult Attachment Interview. *Psychological Bulletin, 117*(3), 387–403.

Wallin, D. (2007). *Attachment in psychotherapy.* Guilford Press.

10
POLYVAGAL THEORY AND THE AUTONOMIC NERVOUS SYSTEM

George S. Thompson[1]

Introduction

The substitute teacher asked a 9-year-old fourth grader to put away their paper because it was time for a social studies lesson. When the student kept drawing, the teacher called out loudly, "Luca! I don't want to tell you more than once. Put that drawing away!" Luca slammed their pencil box on the desk, ripped up the drawing, and glared at the teacher, their face red and chest heaving from breathing hard. When the teacher put their hands on their hips and said, "Now you're in trouble," Luca jumped up and ran out of the classroom, slamming the door behind them.

How can we make sense of Luca's unforeseen and explosive behavior? If we learn that Luca has experienced physical abuse and was recently placed in foster care, we can hazard a guess: the teacher's request triggered a fight-or-flight reaction. Luca's heart beat faster, breathing became shallow, pupils widened, and blood flow to the big muscles increased. Such a reaction is mediated by the autonomic nervous system (ANS)—specifically, the sympathetic nervous system. But how does the ANS get triggered, and what returns it to a more regulated state?

As we sort through these questions in this chapter, we will learn about the role of the ANS in regulating the body's organs and responding to threats. We will also learn about Polyvagal Theory, which links the ANS to threat surveillance, emotional co-regulation, defensive states, and social engagement. Polyvagal Theory makes sense of Luca's behavior and provides helpful guidance to people who live and work with traumatized children. In addition, Polyvagal Theory offers us a deep and compassionate understanding of the experience of trauma along with an opportunity to embody a neurophysiologic presence with the capacity to heal.

The Autonomic Nervous System and Polyvagal Theory

The Autonomic Nervous System

The ANS maintains our physical well-being by paying close attention to both internal and external signals and adjusting our organs' physiological functions to meet the challenges we encounter. Autonomic means "acting or occurring involuntarily" (Merriam-Webster, n.d.) and refers to the fact that these processes require neither our voluntary control nor our conscious awareness to continue operating. When things are going well, our hearts beat at a healthy rate, we breathe enough oxygen to keep our tissues functioning, and we digest the food we have consumed. Behind the scenes, autonomic feedback circuits provide near-instantaneous functional adjustments in response to changing conditions and circumstances, which seemingly all proceed of their own accord.

For example, when we stand up, cardiovascular dynamics suddenly change and more blood flows into our legs due to the combined effect of gravity and change in position. Blood flow to our brain immediately decreases as a result, putting us in danger of passing out. Fortunately, there are stretch receptors in the aorta and carotid arteries that sense the change in blood pressure, and these receptors send quick messages to the brainstem. Nerve centers in the brainstem, in turn, send signals back to the heart and blood vessels, to increase heart rate, the force of heart contractions, and the amount of blood the heart is pumping.

This entire process, which is called the baroreflex (Karemaker & Wesseling, 2008), occurs within a couple of heartbeats to maintain cardiovascular equilibrium. In fact, the neural circuit itself likely makes its adjustments in as little as one-quarter of a second (0.25 seconds). The vagus nerve, which is the parasympathetic part of the ANS, sends signals from the stretch receptors in the aorta and carotid, then back to the sinoatrial node in the heart, which regulates heartbeat. Please note that 80% of the vagus nerve's fibers are afferent, carrying information about the viscera to the brainstem in what is largely a bottom up process. These afferent neurons form the basis of interoception, an awareness of our visceral states.

The characteristics of the baroreflex are:

- A moment-to-moment monitoring system
- "Interpretation" of signals
- Responses that utilize both vagal and sympathetic pathways
- Rapidity of response
- Protection of organs and the organism as a whole
- Afferent feedback from organs and top-down influence from cortical areas to influence brainstem areas

We all know we can't live long if our heart stops beating. But how many of us give much consideration to this exquisite regulation that results in moment-to-moment adaptation to our changing circumstances? I clearly remember the awe I felt in my medical school physiology class when I first learned about the elegantly intricate self-regulation systems that keep cardiopulmonary, gastrointestinal, and renal systems operating well. You can sense a similar state of wonder in the young researcher we will meet next.

Stephen Porges, Heart Rate Variability, and the Roots of Polyvagal Theory

Stephen Porges, developer of Polyvagal Theory, didn't start out with a plan to develop a theory with profound implications for understanding and treating trauma. He is a neuroscientist specializing in psychophysiology, which aims to understand human thinking, emotion, and behavior by measuring physiological responses under diverse conditions. Porges's earliest work explored the relationship between sustained attention and the ANS (Porges & Raskin, 1969). While working on his master's thesis, he was first to notice that cognitive stress caused a decrease in his subjects' heart rate variability (HRV), the beat-to-beat responsiveness we discussed above (Porges, 2022).

The focus of Porges's work across seven decades has been a particular pattern of HRV called respiratory sinus arrhythmia (RSA), the speeding of the heart during in-breath and slowing during exhalation (2022). It turns out that the same branch of the vagus that participates in the baroreflex also creates RSA. Over these decades, research has shown a variable heart rate is a measure of health and resilience. For instance, increased HRV may be correlated with cardiovascular health (Kleiger et al., 2005) and resilience to stress (Perna et al., 2020; Porges, 1992) and may be improved with mindfulness meditation (Krick et al., 2021), yoga (Tyagi & Cohen, 2016), and exercise (Graessler et al., 2021). Still, a letter Porges received from a neonatologist in 1992 raised a perplexing question about HRV known as the vagal paradox (Porges & Winn, 2021).

The Vagal Paradox

Porges's research on HRV, including in fetuses and newborn babies, had shown that increased HRV was a measure of increased vagal tone in babies and associated with their resilience (Porges, 1992). However, vagal activity had also been associated with sudden and potentially lethal drops in newborn's heart rate, known as bradycardia. The observation that the vagus could cause resilience in some instances and death in others was known as *the vagal paradox* (Porges, 1995, 2021, 2023).

On October 8, 1994, in Atlanta, Georgia, Porges gave the presidential address to the Society for Psychophysiological Research in which he described Polyvagal Theory, which resolved the vagal paradox by proposing that rather than having one branch that causes two opposite responses, the vagus nerve has different branches that can do different things (1995). He described evidence that one of those branches of the vagus could be an indicator of health, while another could threaten a newborn's life.

The Polyvagal Theory

Polyvagal Theory emerged from this idea of a multibranched vagus, which is the origin of the term *polyvagal*. In a recent clarification, Porges identified five principles that summarize the theory, reflecting both its scientific basis and its usefulness to patients and clinicians (2021, 2023). We will present these principles here in an order that makes sense for this chapter.

The first principle of Polyvagal Theory we will discuss presupposes that there is a neural mechanism for monitoring signs of safety and threat a person is exposed to, which Porges called *neuroception* (2018, 2021). Moreover, just as the baroreflex can trigger near-instantaneous changes in cardiac physiology, neuroception can trigger near-instantaneous changes in our neurophysiologic state to put us in an optimal position to handle what is in front of us (or inside us). The next principle, referred to as a *hierarchy of autonomic response*, describes three neurophysiological states that neuroception can trigger, depending on whether conditions are sensed as safe, dangerous, or life-threatening.

In another principle, Porges detailed the circuit that enables mammals to communicate with and co-regulate other members of their own species (Porges, 2021, 2023). This circuit forms the foundation of what Porges called the *social engagement system*, which provides the safety and trust we need to collaborate with others and succeed in our human endeavors. When the neurophysiologic state we are in doesn't provide the safety we need for survival, another state takes over, in reverse evolutionary order: a process known as *dissolution*. The last principle, that *autonomic state is an intervening variable* between stimulus and response, describes how our neurophysiologic state prepares us to meet the challenges we face.

First Polyvagal Principle: Neuroception

Polyvagal Theory postulates that *neuroception* is a surveillance system for risk that operates automatically, continually, and outside our moment-to-moment awareness, making rapid adjustments in our physiology as needed for survival and health (Porges, 2021, 2023). Porges hypothesized that neuroception circuits may include areas in or around the temporal cortex that evaluate whether movements of the face, head, hands, and body, and inanimate objects, represent a threat (2018).

As I typed this, I was watching a group of five tweens eating pizza on a restaurant patio. A glass was accidentally knocked over, spilling liquid on one boy in particular. They all jumped up, he looked angry, and I held my breath in anticipation. Shortly, he started to laugh, and the others joined in, causing me to exhale in relief. Neuroception was involved in how quickly they leapt to stay dry as well as in the friendly resolution. The boy who was soaked likely neurocepted in that moment more safety than danger: his neuroception circuits weighed the familiar faces of his friends, their looks of surprise, friendly tones of their voice, and their smiling expressions against the movement of a drink pouring into his lap. Conclusion: this was a mistake made by companions who wished him no harm, and the danger is now over. Neuroception also caused me to hold my breath and then to let it go.

This situation might have gone differently for several reasons:

1 Neuroception is presumed to go through a process of programming. If the boy had a big brother who spilled things on him on purpose, he would have been more likely to neurocept this spill as a deliberate and hostile act. As an aside, this process of programming neuroception is a way we unconsciously pass implicit bias from one generation to the next.
2 The state we are in orients our neuroception. If we are already in a state of alarm, we are more likely to neurocept people, animals, objects, or circumstances as risky and threatening. Since they were enjoying each other, they were primed to accurately neurocept whatever signs of safety were present.
3 If one of the other young people had gone into fight-or-flight themself, their state could have tipped the balance in the direction of danger for all of them.
4 One or more of the teenagers might have had a trauma history, like Luca from our opening scenario.

What are the cues of risk that neuroception senses and evaluates? When facial expression and vocal tone are animated, according to Polyvagal Theory, that signals safety. When they are unexpressive and flat, that usually signals that the person is threatening. We are constantly sending signals of the state we are in, and we are constantly neurocepting signals broadcasted by others' states. Furthermore, according to Polyvagal Theory, safety is not simply the absence of danger. Neuroception must detect sufficient signals of safety in order to cause the shift into social engagement.

Neuroception characteristics are:

- A continuous, automatically reflexive, out-of-awareness process
- Particularly attuned to facial expression, tone of voice, and head and hand gestures
- Reflexively induces rapid shifts in physiologic state to address the neurocepted survival needs
- Not always accurate. There can be a mismatch between actual and neurocepted threats (or safety).

Neuroception often errs on the side of interpreting ambiguous phenomena as dangerous, playing out "better safe than sorry," even under the best of circumstances. When I was 12, I came around the corner of my house at a pace and suddenly found myself in the air. As I was coming back down, I realized I thought I had seen a snake, but it was actually a coiled garden hose. I leapt without conscious awareness of having seen something. This is the difference between neuroception and perception. Neuroception happens prior to awareness. From a survival standpoint, it's better to leap a hundred times, even if it turns out to be a poisonous snake only once out of the hundred. There is good evidence that we interpret ambiguous stimuli as dangerous (Baylin & Hughes, 2016), or as polyvagal trainer Dr. Liz Charles put it, "For the nervous system, the unfamiliar is unsafe" (personal communication, January 17, 2023).

Second Polyvagal Principle: Hierarchy of Response

Polyvagal Theory hypothesizes three neurophysiological states addressing three broad conditions: a safe setting, a circumstance of imminent danger, and a life-threatening situation (see Table 10.1).

1. Polyvagal Theory refers to the *social engagement system*, elicited by neurocepted safety, as a *ventral vagal state*, since the branch of the vagus associated with that response originates in the nucleus ambiguus on the ventral side of the brainstem.
2. The *fight-or-flight* response is mediated by the sympathetic nervous system; therefore, it is also known as a *sympathetic state*.
3. The *shutdown response* is also known as *dorsal vagal collapse*, in reference to the unmyelinated vagus, which originates on the dorsal side of the brainstem.

Let's look at these three states, starting with the oldest in evolution, the dorsal vagus.

LIFE THREAT AND COLLAPSE

Under conditions of neurocepted life threat, the unmyelinated dorsal vagus pathway can initiate several responses, ranging from mild dizziness to fainting and collapse. This response is familiar to us as death feigning in mammals, sometimes known as "playing possum," which is a misnomer because there is no pretending involved. In life-threatening situations, such as when attacked by a predator, the possum actually becomes catatonic as a result of a dramatic vagally mediated slowing of heart rate and drop in blood pressure (Gabrielsen & Smith, 1985), the same bradycardia that is life-threatening in preterm human infants. Fright-induced urination and defecation is another dorsal vagal response known to occur in life-threatening situations. Death feigning has been hypothesized to increase an animal's survival because a predator will not need to continue to attack or subdue its prey once it's immobilized (Humphreys & Ruxton, 2018).

Each of the three states produces a range of effects. The dorsal vagal state is virtually synonymous with dissociation. A person in a milder dorsal vagal state may feel spacy, emotionally numb, or that they have brain fog. It's hard to think and impossible to make a decision. Children who self-cut often report a disturbing sense of disconnection from themself or their body, describing that they cut because they "just need to feel something." The shutdown state can make it feel hard to move, like they're walking through mud or that someone suddenly turned up the dial on gravity. If frightened and restrained, the person may then feel paralyzed, helpless, and hopeless. Porges (2017) pointed out

Table 10.1 Polyvagal Theory and Three Autonomic Responses

Neuroception	Life Threat	Danger	Safety
Physiologic state	Shutdown, collapse	Fight-or-flight	Social engagement
Nerve/system	Unmyelinated dorsal vagus	Sympathetic	Myelinated ventral vagus
Evolution	500 million years ago	400 million years ago	200 million years ago
Embryology	16 weeks	20 weeks	30+ weeks
Purpose	Nonprovocation, conservation of energy	Vigorous defense or escape	Cooperation, growth, healing, restoration
Psychological response	Dissociation: emotional numbing, depersonalization, derealization	Anxiety, irritability, anger, aggression	Connection, communication, reflection, flexible thinking

that though these dissociative symptoms cause distress, a human's ability to dissociate under threat is a valuable way of managing an overwhelming experience.

If a person has some ability to move, they may feel either frustrated with the state they find themself in or self-critical. After a period of dorsal collapse in the face of assault, the victim often feels shame that they didn't fight back or stand up for themselves. Defense attorneys take advantage of this dynamic in sexual assault cases, saying, "If it was so terrible, why didn't you try to run away? Why did you just lie there?" Since the person may have had these same doubts and criticisms themself, they may say, "I have no good answer. I ask myself the same thing." The attorney's attack on their experience can exacerbate any feeling that they were unacknowledged, unimportant, and unseen. However, if they have learned that being restrained under terrifying circumstances causes the neurophysiologic response of tonic immobility, then their reaction becomes evidence *that* they were assaulted, rather than evidence against it.

DANGER AND THE FIGHT-OR-FLIGHT RESPONSE

Neurocepting danger activates the sympathetic nervous system. This is the well-coordinated, sudden fight-or-flight response, the autonomic response usually most familiar to those of us who work with traumatized children. In fight-or-flight, the heart beats faster and stronger, bronchi in the lungs dilate to take in more oxygen, the liver releases more glucose into the bloodstream, and blood vessels to the large muscles dilate. By immediately increasing oxygen- and glucose-rich blood flow, these physiologic responses deliver increased energy to power our ability to run or fight, which improves our odds of surviving dangerous situations.

The sympathetic nervous system consists of neurons that emerge from the thoracic and lumbar sections of the spinal cord and travel to most organs in the body, including the medullary part of the adrenal gland, where they stimulate the release of epinephrine (adrenaline) (see Wehrwein et al., 2016). This sympathetic adrenal medullary (SAM) axis causes responses so immediate that your brain doesn't process the stimulus that caused your fright until after you have responded. In the scenario I mentioned earlier, I probably neurocepted the snake-like form in under 100 milliseconds, less than the blink of an eye, but didn't visually process it until a second or two later (Potter et al., 2014).

A slower system takes over after this initial burst of energy, through the hypothalamic-pituitary-adrenal (HPA) axis, causing the release of cortisol from the adrenal cortex (see Smith & Vale, 2022). Cortisol, another fight-or-flight hormone, also increases blood sugar and blood pressure, which aids survival, and suppresses digestion, the immune system, growth and reproductive function, and memory and cognitive function, none of which are needed in the moments it takes to deal with danger.

What does a child in fight-or-flight experience? Their heart is pounding, and their breathing is fast and shallow. They feel shaky and like they need to do something, anything, *now*. Their hands feel clammy, sweaty, and cold. They may be angry or enraged; they may feel anxious, scared, or terrified. If you observe them, you see that their chest is heaving, and veins may bulge in their neck and arms. Their eyes are open wide with pupils filling most of the iris, and they make darting glances this way and that. Their skin could be either pale or flushed and have goosebumps. Their muscles are trembling and tense and their shoulders raised. They are quite restless.

We sense our environments differently in each of the three states. When the sympathetic nervous system is activated, the adrenaline can sharpen the senses. However, a child in fight-or-flight may not seem to see or hear you, and indeed, research shows that this state can also cause visual limitations such as tunnel vision or loss of depth perception, night vision, and the ability to change focus effectively. Sympathetic activation can cause auditory changes such as stress-induced deafness, called auditory exclusion, as well.

Furthermore, Polyvagal Theory notes that in a state of fight-or-flight, middle ear muscles, which tune the middle ear to the human voice in a ventral vagal state, will tune toward frequencies of predators or distress and away from those of the human voice (Kolacz et al., 2018). Sympathetic output literally causes the child (or adult) to tune you out. Moreover, sympathetic output also changes how we read faces, and a face that looks neutral during calmer times can look threatening when we are in fight-or-flight (Dana, 2018; Porges, 2006).

Many people have heard of the "freeze response" and use the term to mean a dorsal vagal shutdown, as described above. Ruth Lanius and colleagues (2018) elucidated an orienting freeze response in an animal model of defense cascade, which may have correlates in human behavior. When the animal is first threatened, it halts to locate and examine the threat, like "a deer in headlights." As it processes what it is sensing, it may go into fight-or-flight or a shutdown state, depending on the level of threat sensed.

SAFETY AND THE SOCIAL ENGAGEMENT SYSTEM

Neurocepting safety evokes the social engagement system, which is mediated by the ventral myelinated branch of the vagus nerve, originating in the nucleus ambiguus, on the ventral side of the brainstem. The ventral vagus is also responsible for sending signals to the heart's sinoatrial node as part of the baroreflex and creating HRV. Polyvagal Theory presumes that the ventral vagus down-regulates threat reactivity, allowing mammals of the same species to approach each other without triggering a fight-or-flight response.

A child in ventral vagal may feel held, safe, sheltered, and shielded, in which case they may experience comfort and care. When we see this child in their caregiver's arms, they are at peace and relaxed. Ventral vagal may range from calm security to being brave and adventurous. A child's vitality affect (Stern, 2010) is boosted by the ventral vagal state as well, allowing them to feel fully and vigorously alive. In dorsal vagal, they may feel dead and lifeless, while sympathetic activation lies in between—more energetic, but with a quality of fighting for one's life.

Third Polyvagal Principle: The Ventral Vagal Complex Is a Communication and Co-Regulation Circuit

In this third principle, Polyvagal Theory speculates that the social engagement system is formed by an integration of the ventral vagal nucleus ambiguus with other brain stem nuclei, which give rise to the special visceral efferent pathways that innervate the striated muscles of the head and face. Porges (2018) explained, "Functionally, the social engagement system emerges from a face-heart connection that coordinates the heart with the muscles of the face and head" (p. 54). The neural circuitry connecting head and heart allows us to read the facial expressions and vocalizations of our fellow humans and to display our state in our face and voice as well. In addition, the social engagement system receives "top down" input from higher brain centers and "bottom up" input from the vagal afferent neurons responsible for interoception (Porges, 2018).

The social engagement face-heart circuitry also plays a role in dampening sympathetic activation, enabling mammals to approach other members of their species and cooperate (Porges, 2017, 2018, 2023). Safe cooperation, which Porges (2017) called a "biological imperative" for health and well-being, allows for mating, child rearing, play, and coordinating efforts to acquire resources and defend against threats. Each of these activities increases survival potential for a mammalian species. However, the role that social engagement plays in child development may be its most important.

At birth, children cannot care for themselves; they rely on their caregivers for food, drink, shelter and warmth, and cleanliness. Nevertheless, even if provided with these resources, without a caring connection, they will fail to thrive. There are few, if any, developmental processes that can fulfill their function except when there is a present and attuned caregiver who sends signals of safety to their child. Children are born wired to connect, to recognize their mothers, find delight in faces, and seek and expect safety from their caregivers. When things go well, in thousands and thousands of interactions, the child communicates a need that is then met well enough by good enough parenting. This has a profound and beneficial effect on the child's development.

When parent and child relationships are anchored in a loving ventral vagal state, they can share experiences with each other, venturing into each other's worlds or looking together at something they both see. These intersubjective experiences form the basis of a child's ability to regulate their emotions, direct their attention, and align their intentions in collaborative efforts (Baylin & Hughes, 2016). Through these same means, social engagement likely forms a neurophysiological platform for development of secure attachment too (Porges, 2006).

Parents co-regulate their child's affect through their calm and competent presence that conveys, "I've got this" and by demonstrating that they understand the child's state, conveying, "I get you." Deb Dana (2018), the leading translator of Polyvagal Theory into therapy settings, defined co-regulation as a "reciprocal regulation of our autonomic states that [allows us to] feel safe to move into connection and create trusting relationships" (p. 4). Caregivers are not always attuned or accurate in their attunement, nor do they need to be as long they repair misattunements as a form of both co-regulation and neural exercise (Porges, 2017), which builds the child's faith in the relationship (Baylin & Hughes, 2016; Dana, 2020a). As Dana pointed out (2020a), we learn from research that Winnicott's concept of "good enough mothering" was correct (1960): paying attention around 30% of the time is sufficient to convey safety and connection (Ostlund et al., 2017; Tronick & Gianino, 1986).

It is important to note that children need co-regulation before they develop any ability to engage in self-regulation. We wouldn't tell a baby, "Use your coping skills" (Sanders & Thompson, 2022). Additionally, humans likely require co-regulation throughout their lifespan (Porges & Furman, 2011). Caregivers need to regulate themselves to co-regulate their child, as it's not possible to co-regulate another from a state of fight-or-flight or shutdown (Porges & Carter, 2017). One's dysregulation sends signals of danger to the other person's nervous system.

Social engagement can be paired or blended with another state in order to exercise the ANS and allow for activities that might not otherwise be possible. Porges (2018) said that playful activities, like peekaboo, serve as a form of neural exercise by bringing the child into a mild state of sympathetic activation and then co-regulating the heightened energy to bring the child back into social engagement. Play thus increases the child's ability to tolerate sympathetic activation and stay connected without devolving into aggression. Therapy can serve a similar function as the therapist co-regulates the client's defensive state and brings them back into a ventral vagal connection (Porges, 2018). Likewise, intimacy pairs a dorsal vagal state with co-regulating social engagement, allowing for a couple to be still together without immobilization triggering shutdown (Figure 10.1).

Fourth Polyvagal Principle: Dissolution

Polyvagal Theory observes that the three autonomic states likely arose during three different periods in our evolutionary or phylogenetic history: first the dorsal vagal, then the sympathetic, and most recently the ventral vagal. In medical school, we learned that *ontogeny recapitulates phylogeny*, meaning that events in fetal development occur in the same order as they did in evolutionary history. Indeed, the three autonomic systems appear in the same sequence during in utero development as they did in evolution (Sanders & Thompson, 2022) (see Table 10.1).

The fourth principle of Polyvagal Theory hypothesizes that if the newest autonomic circuit does not handle a threat successfully, then the next newer system is activated to address it. Porges (2009)

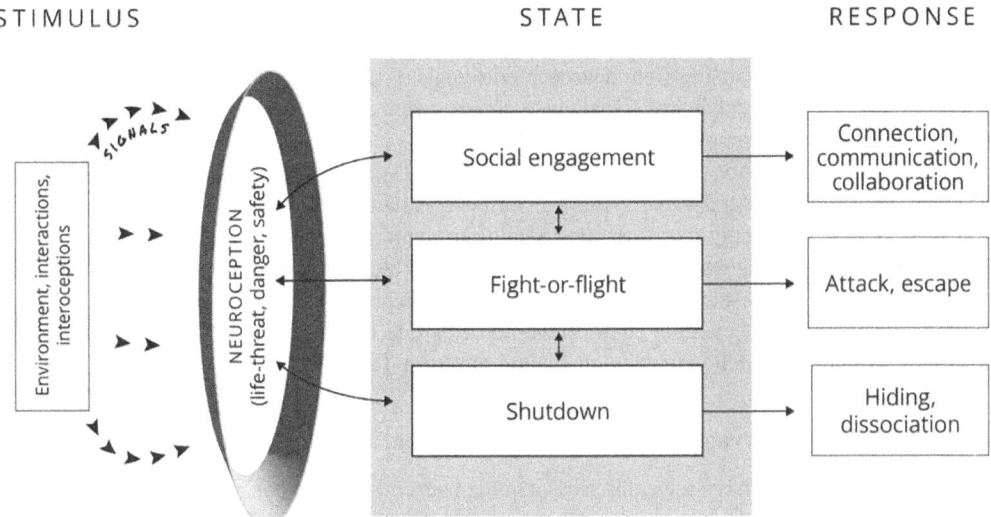

Figure 10.1 State Determines Response and Orients Neuroception.

Note: We see in Figure 10.1 major elements of the Polyvagal Theory. Through the out-of-awareness process of neuroception, the nervous system monitors our internal, external, and relational environments and evaluates them for risk. The balance of risk neurocepted at any given time is presumed to be sorted into categories of safety, danger, and life threat, evoking a state of social engagement, fight-or-flight, or shutdown. The state is presumed to be an intervening variable between stimulus and response, and therefore the state a person is in shapes and ultimately determines their behaviors. The state also influences the quality of neuroception.

aligned this process with Jacksonian dissolution, which presumes that newer brain circuits inhibit older circuits. Porges explained that in Jacksonian dissolution, if something interrupts a newer circuit's functioning, the older circuits are activated, since they are no longer inhibited. In Polyvagal Theory, this looks like using our newest circuit first—social engagement. If our ability to connect and collaborate isn't sufficient in keeping us safe, the next newer system, fight-or-flight, comes into play. When that isn't sufficient, then the oldest system, dorsal vagal collapse, begins operating. When we discuss trauma, we will see the disastrous effect of losing our ability to connect and collaborate.

Fifth Polyvagal Principle: Autonomic State Is an Intervening Variable

Porges (2018) pointed out that while our behavioral response to a situation emerges from the neurophysiological state the situation has evoked, this is not a simple stimulus-response pattern: the autonomic state is an intervening variable between stimulus and response that prepares us physiologically to respond to conditions of safety, danger, and life threat. Our behavioral responses, as well as our perceptions, experiences, and narratives, emerge from our physiological state. A child in a state of shutdown will respond to a particular situation one way, while a child in a state of social engagement will respond differently. Since behavior emerges from state, it is more important to attend to the child's state and the neuroceptions that evoked it, than it is to try to change their behavior. Changing what the child is neurocepting will change their state, and their behavior will follow close behind.

This fifth principle demonstrates the integrative nature of Polyvagal Theory. It captures a broader perspective about the functioning of our nervous system. As we saw with the baroreflex, the ANS is a dynamic, moment-to-moment system for monitoring and responding to the challenge in front of us. With interoceptive input from our viscera, sensory input from our environment, and input from our higher brain centers, it operates by changing our physiological state, which provides us the resources needed to survive and thrive.

A felt sense of safety, arising from neurocepted signals of safe people and a safe environment, activates the evolutionarily advanced social engagement system, which serves as a neural platform for a host of development-promoting, relational, and integrative processes. Secure attachment, emotional regulation, intersubjectivity, executive functioning, and resilience in the face of stress all depend on a well-functioning ventral vagal system. Even beyond that, children need a healthy hierarchy of response: to have the energy that fuels their vitality to explore and respond when challenged, to be able to shut down and rest when appropriate, and to access blended states, such as play and stillness. It would be hard to overestimate the importance of neurocepted and felt safety for the future of our children's well-being (Tucci et al., 2018). It would be hard to overestimate the devastating impact of trauma in disrupting this felt safety and the neural platform it supports.

Polyvagal Theory, Complex Trauma, and Dissociation

Polyvagal Theory, as we have seen, describes a human nervous system constantly monitoring for signals of safety and threat, and that can precipitate rapid shifts in physiological state to meet the needs of the moment. For children experiencing complex relational trauma, the effects can be disastrous, both during the traumatic events and on an ongoing basis. Peter Levine recognizes that Polyvagal Theory provides a trustworthy guide to both the effects of trauma and its treatment. He says "just as maps are useful in finding particular parts of a city, maps of the human organism are useful in navigating the landscape of trauma and informing its healing. It is here that Porges's groundbreaking work provides an eloquent, well-reasoned, and broadly supported treasure map of the psychophysiological systems that implicitly govern traumatic states. The same systems also mediate core feelings of safety, goodness, and belonging" (Levine, 2018, p. 14).

Trauma Resets the Nervous System

Complex trauma upends a child's development. To speak plainly, when an adult abuses a child, it terrifies the child. Their system immediately neurocepts the danger and evokes a fight-or-flight response or a shutdown. To recover from what happened, the child needs a trustworthy and non-traumatized adult who listens to their experience and validates what they have gone through to regulate the intense neurophysiological and emotional states that come as predictable aftershocks. For example, Daniel Hughes writes that

> for young children, the central purpose of developing attachments is to ensure their safety. Once safety is guaranteed, other aspects of childhood can proceed. The mind works best under conditions of perceived safety. Without safety, the mind's almost exclusive function is to reduce threat and create safety through variations of fight, flight, or freeze.
>
> *(2017, pp. 3–4)*

But as van der Kolk (2005) reminded us, "most trauma begins at home; the vast majority of people (about 80%) responsible for child maltreatment are children's own parents" (p. 402). When a caregiver attacks or exploits a child, the child's world is turned upside down. The person who is supposed to love them floods them with disgust, rage, or lust. This is the same adult to whom the child would turn to recover from their destabilizing experience. In this upside-down world, they have experienced danger where they should have found safety and protection. This kind of experience has a serious impact on their nervous system's functioning in the months and years to come.

Polyvagal Theory and the Autonomic Nervous System

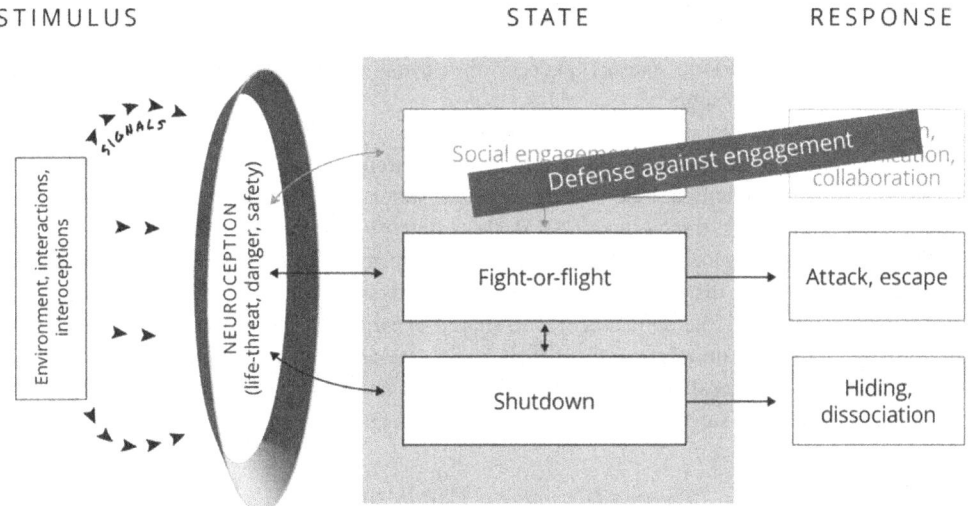

Figure 10.2 Complex Trauma Makes Social Engagement Largely Unavailable.

Note: In Figure 10.2, we note that complex trauma has had a profound effect on the child's nervous system. Relationships and adults are neurocepted as dangerous and/or life-threatening. Instead of a beloved and trusted caregiver toward whom the child is oriented, the child must protect themself from abusive adults. Attempts to engage with such a child can elicit states of both fight-or-flight and shutdown, with their resulting behavioral responses of attack and escape as well as hiding and dissociation, respectively. The state of social engagement is largely unavailable, and this makes connection, communication, and cooperation much more difficult.

No longer does the nervous system learn that safety, comfort, and care come from adults. Instead, it registers the message that suffering is unpredictable, uncontrollable, and relentless. Not only is no one coming to save them, but their so-called caregivers are the ones torturing them. Consequently, the traumatized nervous system reorients and neurocepts people and relationships as dangerous. Routes to evoking a state of social engagement are blocked or severely limited.[2]

We can understand how devastating developmental trauma is if we consider that it *turns off* the social engagement system (see Figure 10.2). The child loses social engagement and all that goes with it: connection, comfort, communication, and collaboration. Baylin and Hughes (2016) describe in disquieting neurobiological and psychological detail trauma's ability to shut down longings for care and affiliation and to block the child's ability to form trusting relationships. Indeed, a number of traumatized children become anxious if things are going well and so create chaos or turmoil that spoils any emerging social engagement and relational safety.

If people and relationships are dangerous and social engagement is restricted, where does safety come from? Porges said, "The body is stuck in a state of defense" (Porges & Winn, 2021, p. 238). In fact, when relationships are neurocepted as dangerous, people's approach triggers defensive reactions. Not only can the child not seek shelter *in* relationships, but now they must seek shelter *from* relationships.

This reset can confuse adults who raise, educate, or treat traumatized children. Teachers, coaches, and scout leaders may ask why a child would attack, hide from, or shut down in the presence of a trustworthy adult. If they are unaware that the child neurocepts relationships as dangerous, they may have an automatic urge to make sense of it by saying, "Something is wrong with the child." When parents adopt a traumatized child, adoptive aunts, uncles, and grandparents may tell the adoptive parents, "That child is nothing but trouble," and advise them to send the child away. Trauma has turned off the child's social engagement and removed the neurophysiological foundation that allows for civil relations. But that is not the end of the story. This confusing reset is also an opportunity to explain how trauma affects autonomic states. If successful, it usually deepens the person's compassion for what the child is going through.

When we look at official descriptions of trauma symptoms through a polyvagal lens, we can see how symptoms emerge from this pattern: traumatized children need to defend against a state of social engagement, relying on sympathetic and dorsal vagal states to protect themselves. As we will see in Ana Gomez's chapter in this volume (2025), these defensive responses are responsible for PTSD symptoms such as avoidance, emotional numbness, dissociation, and anger. Likewise, oppositional defiant disorder, conduct disorder, and disruptive mood dysregulation disorder arise when trauma physiologically constrains the child's access to shared experiences and empathy for others, making them look like they have no remorse for their harmful actions. If we are concerned about a traumatized child's lack of cooperation, it will be better to work on eliciting a state of social engagement, which requires signals of safety and trustworthiness to emerge.

Trauma Disrupts the Child's Integration

When trauma turns off social engagement, it disrupts integration, which Dan Siegel postulated is "the central mechanism by which health is created in mind, brain, body, and relationships" (2012, p. 336). He said that for integration to occur, the child must experience connection, communication, care, and compassion, qualities that emerge when caregiver and child are in (or returning to) a state of ventral vagal social engagement. Siegel describes integration as a process of differentiation and linkage that occurs across nine functions or domains, including domains of narrative, memory, state, and consciousness.

Trauma disrupts integration during at least three time periods (see Beutler et al., 2022): (1) peritraumatically, at the time it occurs; (2) post-traumatically, when the child becomes acutely dysregulated, for example, due to post-traumatic reminders; and (3) chronically, when defensive states replace social engagement. The following are some of the phenomena that may be observed in each of the three states:

- In dorsal vagal shutdown, disruption of integration produces:

  - Peritraumatic dissociative disconnections of consciousness, like emotional numbing, depersonalization, and derealization; as well as analgesia, immobility, and fainting. These disconnections interfere with the creation of memory.
  - Dissociation may also occur during periods of dysregulation—that is, acute post-traumatic dissociation.
  - In addition, as Beutler and colleagues pointed out, when dissociation occurs frequently, it can become the predominant mode of operating. It is then called "trait dissociation" (2022, p. 4). Extrapolating from Polyvagal Theory provides an additional explanation for trait dissociation; it occurs when trauma has made social engagement unavailable.

- In sympathetic fight-or-flight, disruption of integration produces:

  - Perceptual distortions discussed above, such as tunnel vision, changes in hearing, slowing of time, etc.
  - The changes can occur at the time of the trauma and when the child is dysregulated afterward.
  - When a sympathetic state becomes chronic, it appears similar to disruptive mood dysregulation disorder, with continuous irritability and anger, along with frequent, severe rage episodes.

- Clinicians frequently observe that traumatized children appear unresponsive during a temper outburst. We may suppose that perceptual changes in a sympathetic state differ from those of dorsal vagal dissociation. While dorsal dissociation disconnects the child from themselves and their surroundings, a sympathetic state appears to focus the child on the threat (van der Kolk & Fisler, 1995). The child may not remember what happened because the context was excluded from their focus. They may also experience "speechless terror," which interrupts the formation of explicit memory of the event.
- In addition, during a rageful fight response, activity is reduced in prefrontal/thinking brain areas (Lanius et al., 2018).

- In contrast, ventral vagal social engagement promotes the child's integration, and domains of narrative, memory, state, and consciousness function within an expected range for the child's developmental level.

We see in practice that trauma hinders multiple developmental processes that depend on trustworthy relationships with a caring adult for their healthy unfolding. In a paper outlining the effects of complex trauma in childhood, Cook and colleagues (2005) detailed seven domains of impairment: attachment, biology, affect regulation, dissociation, behavioral control, cognition, and self-concept. Like Siegel (2012), they recognized that trauma disrupts the development of core capacities like language, abstract reasoning, problem-solving, and emotional regulation.

Trauma causes sympathetic activation and dorsal vagal shutdown, which prioritize deploying rapid action response circuits over the slower prefrontal reflection circuits. Moreover, when a child lives mostly in defensive states, their mental energies are focused on protection. They don't get the space and freedom from danger to be curious about their world and engage in joyful play and intriguing explorations that further nurture development (Siegel, 2012).

Through these constraints, trauma's impact spreads outward in widening circles, impeding progress in school and social learning with friends, on teams, or in community groups. The traumatized child, whose nervous system has been focused on identifying threats, operates from internal working models based on where trouble lies and how it can be avoided (see Bowlby, 1969). Because the child hasn't explored details of the people and places around them, their maps lack the nuance that scaffolds other children's ability to navigate their worlds of home, school, friends, and community.

Traumatized children often look serious, as they are occupied with the serious work of survival. Their lives lack spontaneity and joy as well as connection, communication, and collaboration. There's no one with whom to connect, ask questions, or compare notes. As Peter Levine (2018) said above, there are no "feelings of safety, goodness, and belonging" (p. 14). Figure 10.3 conveys how bleak this existence can be by examining how the characteristics of five elements of human functioning appear in each of the three physiological states. *Consciousness*, the ability to stay present and attend to what's important, emerges fully in social engagement and can fade to black in dorsal vagal collapse. The child's sense of *vitality* blooms when they are safe and connected, and withers under states of life threat. *Agency*, sense of *self*, and *hope* are similarly affected by change in autonomic state.

It is important to acknowledge that Figure 10.3 depicts the dorsal vagal and sympathetic states under terrifying and threatening conditions. As we discussed above, both sympathetic and dorsal states can be paired or blended with ventral vagal energy. Ogden (2018) said that pairing ventral and *sympathetic* states supports high energy activities, like "sports, dance, [and] energizing debates" (p. 39). She went on to explain that a blend of ventral and *dorsal* states allows a person to enjoy low-arousal emotions and activities, like relaxation or restful repose.

As trauma disrupts a child's development and integration, their emotional and behavioral dysregulation can disrupt the lives of their families. Traumatized children, in order to defend against potential

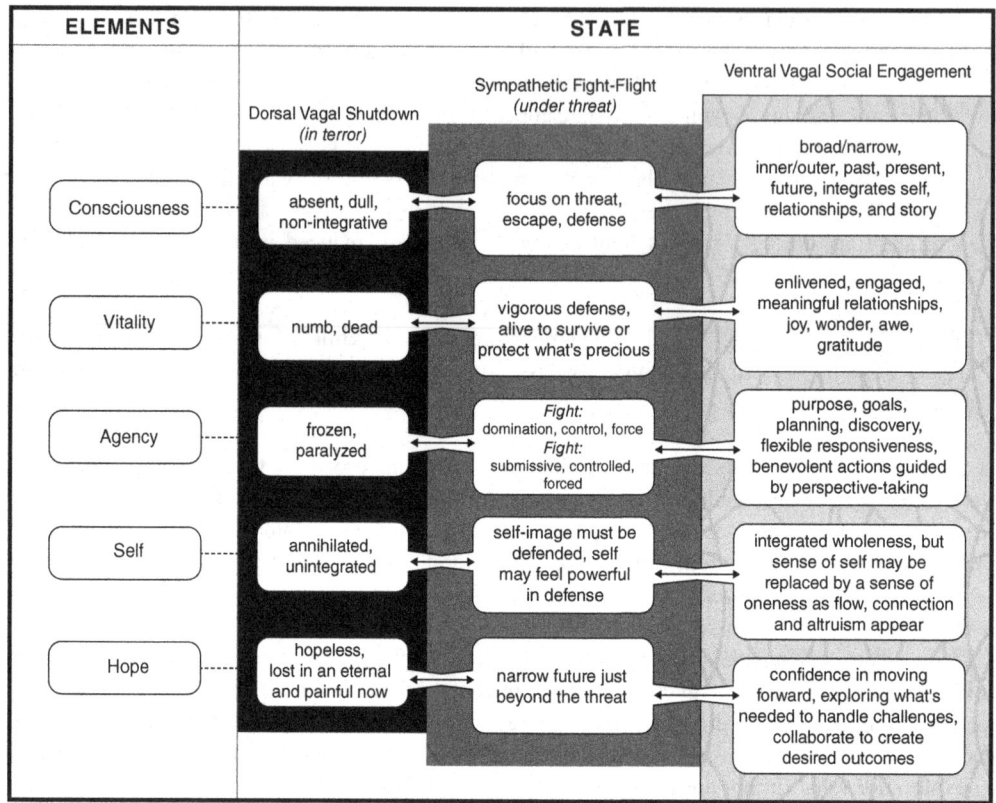

Figure 10.3 How State Affects Elements of Human Functioning (in the Context of Fear).

Note: In Figure 10.3, we see how a shift in autonomic state differentially affects five elements of human functioning. Note that the chart shows dorsal vagal and sympathetic states when the child is under threat and in terror. A number of things can be discovered from the chart, such as the richness of experience that emerges as we move from dorsal to sympathetic to ventral states. The reader is encouraged to explore the chart by comparing it to their own experience, putting it in their own words, introducing additional elements, etc.

harm from adults, ignore or attack their caregiver's care. Over time, these assaults can turn off the adult's social engagement system in the same way that trauma turns off the child's (Tucci et al., 2018). It is no longer safe for the adult to be connected with the child in social engagement, which is required for them to attune to and co-regulate the child. This can be especially devastating when the adult has made significant changes to their life to provide the child with the care they need, such as occurs with foster or adoptive parents or with kinship placements. Dan Hughes and Jon Baylin call the parents' withdrawal of social engagement "blocked care," and their book *Brain-Based Parenting* (2012) is a good resource for parents and therapists alike.

Fragmentation and Structural Dissociation

Trauma sets the stage for what Kathy Steele (2025) described as structural dissociation in her chapter in this handbook, which includes fragmentation of self, ego states, and autobiographical narrative. Fragmentation occurs when a child experiences horrifying trauma that elicits intense states of flight, flight, and shutdown and when the absence of social engagement blocks integrative functioning.

Polyvagal Theory has the potential to inform the development, perpetuation, and healing from structural dissociation.

Not everyone who experiences a frightening or threatening event develops PTSD (Ozer & Weiss, 2004). A recent study by Feiler and colleagues (2023) noted that benevolent childhood experiences, including "perceived safety, security, and support" and "having a safe caregiver," moderated university students' development of PTSD symptoms (p. 274). As we have seen, a safe caregiver will provide a child who has experienced potential trauma with co-regulation and social buffering that dampens the intensity of what they have experienced to a manageable level. A safe caregiver also helps the child make sense of the frightening experience, integrating the event into a sensible narrative of their life and a coherent sense of themselves as a person. In other words, they *integrate* the frightening event through affect regulation and meaning-making, both of which occur during ventral vagal social engagement.

However, we have been discussing severe early childhood trauma, especially by caregivers, that violates the biological expectation that they will provide their child with care and security (Tucci et al., 2018). This violation often causes both terror and shame in great measure. When a child is treated as disgusting, contemptible, or malevolent, the resulting shame and terror destabilizes their sense of self, their emotions, and their ability to organize their actions. The presence of this sort of destabilization prevents any hope of integration, as the child's social engagement system is largely unavailable, and the child is left with intense experiences they don't have the basic physiologic resources to manage.

Without the hope of comforting co-regulation, clarifying meaning-making, and the prospect of integrated wholeness, how does the child manage the trauma they have experienced? Let's explore two possibilities. First, we may note that the self fragments into parts that are associated with intensely dysphoric ego states (van der Kolk & Fisler, 1995; Nijenhuis et al., 2010). To cope with an out-of-control inner world, sometimes these children attempt to control the people and events in their lives, while simultaneously concealing any sign that they need help from others, in what can be thought of as a disorganized controlling attachment pattern (Grant et al., 2024). In the most severe cases, there is no integrated self to regulate and make sense of these agonizing ego states, which flood the child in what we may call a "feeling flashback"—intense affect that comes out of nowhere, devoid of context (van der Kolk & Fisler, 1995). The child attempts to make sense by generating a plausible story, in a largely unconscious process that is similar to confabulation in people who have dementia. To make matters worse, the instability of this system is self-perpetuating or, as the literature on borderline personality disorder puts it, "stably unstable" (Greene & Ugarriza, 1995, p. 26). In trying to control the adults in their life to regulate their own dysregulation, fragmentation, and shame, the child often provokes them to respond with punishment or abandonment, further exacerbating the child's dysregulation, fragmentation, and shame.

Another pattern of structural dissociation that we can also consider stably unstable was described by Nijenhuis et al. (2010) as arising from two emotional operating systems or personalities within the child, one that defensively detaches from trauma and the other that reactively re-experiences it. The defensive system detaches from traumatic memories in order to function on a daily basis and to reproduce and care for young. The reactive system is subjected to unpredictable eruptions of frightful and agonizing states, with or without memories of past traumatic events. Nijenhuis and colleagues cited Myers (1940), who referred to the defensive system as the *apparently normal personality* (ANP) and the reactive system as the *emotional personality* (EP). Nijenhuis et al. (2010) went on to say that the blow that cleaved the child's consciousness into these two systems—a process called "primary structural dissociation"—was a catastrophic level of perilous terror. In polyvagal terms, under this level of threat, the only way to preserve any access to the ventral vagal state and its life-sustaining emergent properties is to wall off, as best as possible, the ANP from contamination by the EP's reactive system. However, because the ANP can remain relatively safe only by being as unaware and unaffected by the EP as possible, there's no way for the ANP to use its ventral vagal social engagement to facilitate integration of the traumatic memories and experiences held by the EP, so this pattern is stably unstable as well.

Studies have explored the relationships between trauma, dissociation, and the ANS, and by extension, Polyvagal Theory. Reinders and colleagues in the Netherlands (2006) studied physiological characteristics across two dissociative identity states analogous to the ANP and EP, finding that "these [states] exhibit different regional cerebral blood flow patterns as well as autonomic and subjective reactions when exposed to identical trauma-related stimuli" (p. 739). A take home message: not only do individuals have unique variations in neuroception and autonomic states, but each of the ego states or emotional operating systems in structural dissociation do too. Karaosmanoğlu and colleagues (2022) studied the relationship between schema modes and three autonomic states described by the Polyvagal Theory. Ruth Lanius and her group (2018) studied a number of phenomena related to trauma, threat, dissociation, and brain functions and networks, such as the release of endogenous opioids in dorsal shutdown, which is associated with emotional numbness, decreased awareness of surroundings, and depersonalization. Finally, Lebois and colleagues (2022) described changes in the central executive, salience, and default mode networks produced by trauma and associated with dissociation.

For a child to heal from the devastation of structural dissociation, they need care from an adult who can tolerate the child's fragmented self and chaotically agitated states while staying connected to the child (or returning to connection). This requires the adult to mentalize the child's condition—how they got there, what it means, and what will be helpful. Adults who do so will learn to increasingly tolerate the child's rejection, as they understand it as representing the child's fear of connection, rather than an indictment of the adult's care and love. By providing continued relentless connection—like an accepting, curious, and empathic attitude (Hughes, 2017)—until the child learns to allow them to co-regulate their emotions, adults can help the child grow trust, connection, and opportunities for co-regulation. In turn, the child's nervous system can neurocept enough safety to enter social engagement in small doses (Tucci et al., 2018). The caregiver must do these heroic tasks in and of themselves, and in addition provide structure, limits, and the natural and logical consequences that all children need, even knowing the child is likely to react negatively at first.

Now that we have reached a conclusion in our polyvagal understanding of structural dissociation, it may be helpful to review a polyvagal-informed hierarchy of dissociation that parallels the four types of dissociation that Steele (2025) discusses in her chapter in this handbook.

Mild problems with attention may arise when a person neurocepts danger and begins to drop into sympathetic activation via dissolution. A sudden noise, a worry, or a pain can be the source of this danger signal. Because the amygdala often interprets an unfamiliar stimulus as threatening, unfamiliar sensations within the body, an unfamiliar scent in the environment, or an unfamiliar tone or behavior in a loved one can also trigger the beginnings of a sympathetic response. The person orients to what caught the attention of their nervous system and goes through a process of appraising its actual level of threat. Assuming the stimulus is assessed as benign, they return to social engagement, and attention is freed up from its temporary protective duty.

Moderate problems occur when sympathetic or dorsal vagal states are activated. Sympathetic anxiety reactions demand more full attention for longer periods. Dorsal vagal states can cause emotional numbness or a split between the experiencing self and the observing self, such as in depersonalization or derealization.

More severe problems arise when the sympathetic and dorsal vagal systems are more fully engaged, shifting brain activity away from the neocortex. Full flight can appear as a panic attack that turns off cortical areas required for thoughtful reflection and generating flexible responses. It can also appear as blind rage that turns off cortical areas. Either full flight or fight may appear as a flashback of a traumatic event as well. Full shutdown results in fainting or the level of dissociation that completely disconnects a person from their body and surroundings.

Finally, structural dissociation and fragmentation of self occurs when events are so extreme that they immediately cause disorganization of self, emotions, and behavior. Siegel (2012) stated that these disorganizing states arise when there is strong activation of both sympathetic and dorsal vagal systems. However, Porges proposes another possible mechanism for these disorganizing states: perhaps they represent "an oscillation between sympathetic aggressor states and dorsal vagal victim states, in which the sympathetic nervous system 'rescues' the child from slipping into 'the great abyss' of dorsal collapse and total loss of purpose" (personal communication, November 18, 2023). Chronic replacement of social engagement with defensive states prevents integration, and the fragmentation and dissociation of parts of self and experiences continues. In any case, there is often no caregiver available to provide co-regulation to buffer that state, even if the child were receptive.

Autonomic Patterns in Complex Trauma and Dissociation

There are several other patterns that can be observed in autonomic responses of a traumatized child:

- *Stuck in dorsal vagal, afraid of sympathetic:* A traumatized child has often learned that acting from a fight-or-flight state is dangerous; any sign that they are threatening their abuser, such as acting defiant, disobedient, or disrespectful, will cause the abuser to harm them more. Dorsal vagal collapse keeps them immediately safer, but as they come out of this state and into sympathetic activation, neurocepting that energy as dangerous can throw them back into the dorsal state. Dana calls this and like patterns being "stuck in an autonomic cycle" (2020b, p. 13).
- *Stuck in sympathetic, afraid of dorsal vagal:* Some children feel more at risk in dorsal vagal, leading them to find safety in sympathetic arousal. These children are unable to back down from a fight but feel uneasy and troubled if either they or things around them get too calm. They often will provoke conflict to create a comfortably chaotic environment.
- *Prolonged sympathetic irritability when a child moves out of dorsal vagal:* Some children have been stuck in dorsal vagal disconnection for so long that their emergence from that state can be prolonged as well, manifesting in an irritable mood that can last for months, confusing caregivers, clinicians, and managed care reviewers. This irritability may look like a regression, but it is actually a sign of progress. They are now in contact with a world that in the past was too painful to experience. If they are supported to keep building their capacity for ventral vagal connection, they eventually move through this period to a more easeful yet present demeanor.
- *High levels of sympathetic and dorsal vagal:* Dan Siegel (2012) hypothesized that when a parent rages at their child, it causes a flood of both sympathetic and dorsal vagal output, and the child is abandoned to terror and confusion. This is a pattern of disorganized attachment, and the child learns that dissociating back into the chaotic emotional state is one way to self-regulate.

Trauma Treatment Fails without Addressing Social Engagement

Many believe treatment requires a therapeutic alliance to be effective but haven't yet seen that a child with complex trauma does not have access to social engagement and instead sees such treatment as dangerous. We may feel that defensive children are "treatment resistant," but the problem is that the child is unable to muster enough safety on their own to down-regulate defensive states. As Jon Baylin said, "They're not treatment resistant; they're relationship resistant" (personal communication, July 2, 2023). Self-protection is the only safety strategy in their repertoire. Peter Levine (2018) points to the helpfulness of Porges's theory in clarifying "why certain common approaches to trauma therapy frequently fail" and how "it illuminates the pathways for integration, recovery, and transformation (Porges, 2021)" (p. 14).

When a child has experienced complex relational trauma, bringing the social engagement system back online is a foundational objective. This applies to psychotherapies, educational approaches, coping skills, and medication. As a psychiatrist, I am acutely aware that the patient must have some degree of trust in the doctor to receive the full benefit of a psychotropic medication. I've seen children fight against beneficial effects of medicine, just as they have fought all other attempts to help them. Again, not treatment resistant, but resistant to any form of relationship.

Moreover, because our thinking brains work best when we are in a state of social engagement, treatments that rely on cognitive interventions alone won't be effective until the child regains the ability to enter into a ventral vagal state. Cognitive interventions are top down processes, but turning on social engagement needs a bottom up approach, one that can get signals of safety to the child's brainstem.

(Re)Awakening the Social Engagement System

He takes a deep breath. The journey the two of them embark on together must begin with love, Rune thinks. To love the sick—isn't that always the first step?

He gives Digby's forearms a meaningful and sustained squeeze while looking him in the eye. The young man is startled. He's like a wild animal, Rune thinks; his instinct is to snarl, to pull back... but Rune holds his gaze and his forearms. He hopes this man will see in Rune's eyes not pity but recognition, warriors fighting shoulder to shoulder, against a common foe (2023, pp. 254–255).

—Abraham Verghese, *Covenant of Water*

Complex trauma challenges clinicians to coax a child into social engagement when they are likely to neurocept even that intention as dangerous. We must find the ANS equivalent of restarting a computer in "safe mode." Two treatment approaches described in this handbook, Somatic Experiencing and Dyadic Developmental Psychotherapy (DDP), each present strategies to help a child reorient toward relationships when traumatic experiences have oriented them solely toward danger.

Passive and Active Pathways Regulating the Social Engagement System

Porges (2018) described two pathways, one passive and the other active, that both evoke the social engagement system. While the passive pathway works nonconsciously through neuroception, requiring nothing from the child, the active pathway recruits the child's knowing participation in neural exercises to change their own neurophysiological state. These are often referred to as "coping skills." Here are some examples of each:

Passive pathway to social engagement

- *Nonverbal signals*: Vocal prosody, animated facial expressions and gestures, which impinge upon the child's outside-of-awareness neuroception.
- *Environmental cues*: Colors, images, objects, textures, and sounds designed to convey comfort, care, and safety.
- *Structured routines and rituals*: Predictability is usually neurocepted as safety, while a lack of structure broadcasts an "anything could go wrong" sense of danger.
- *Discipline that cultivates relationship*: For example, DDP's "two hands of parenting" (Grant et al., 2024). The parent establishes the supervision, structure, and boundaries the child needs for successful development (first hand) but within the context of a warm relationship that regulates the child's emotional state and explores their experience with interest and understanding (second hand). This is also called "correction with connection."

Polyvagal Theory and the Autonomic Nervous System

- *Defined and safe culture*: It is possible to develop an explicit culture (for an organization, educational facility, or family) that serves as a predicable standard for behavior and attitudes. For instance, KidsTLC, a child behavioral health organization, created a constitution to guide them in their work (see kidstlc.org/about-kidstlc/why-kidstlc/).

Active pathway to social engagement

- Breathing exercises: in particular, when exhale is longer than inhale.
- Singing in groups: a social breathing exercise.
- Hands on heart, self-hug: several postures tend to move people in the direction of regulation.
- Yoga poses.
- There are many active pathway strategies described in this book.

Porges (2018) stated, "Access to the client's active pathway is dependent on the passive pathway effectively triggering a state of safety in the client" (p. 66). But how do you know when to switch from the passive pathway to an active pathway? You read the child's nonverbal communication, the nonverbal expression of their ANS, to watch for signs that they have begun to relax. Relaxation, which you may think of as the child "letting down their neurobiological guard," is a sign they are entering a ventral vagal state. Their shoulders drop an inch or two, they make better eye contact, and they let out a sigh, as if they have been holding their breath for quite some time. You may think of the passive pathway as building safety and trust with the child's nervous system, and at the point that they let down their neurobiological guard, you have crossed a hypothetical "threshold of mistrust" (see Figure 10.4). This is the point when the child's neuroception has concluded, "I guess you're okay."

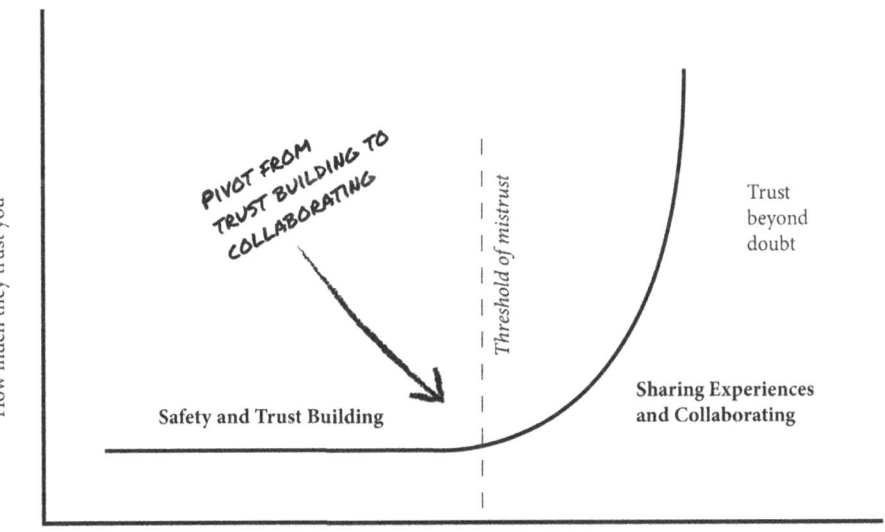

Figure 10.4 Turning on the Social Engagement System: The Trust Building Sequence.

Note: To coax a traumatized child into a state of social engagement, one must send sufficient signals of safety. Demonstrating understanding of the child's experience, such as through acceptance, curiosity, and empathy, which are part of DDP's PACE attitude, conveys authentic interest and trustworthiness. Trust tends to happen suddenly, when the balance of safe neuroceptions cross the child's hypothetical "threshold of mistrust." At that point, one can collaborate with the child—for example, engaging in active pathway self-regulating activities.

This usually happens suddenly and is accompanied by a simultaneous relaxation in the therapist's nervous system as well.

As mentioned, before the child's nervous system crosses the threshold of mistrust, it neurocepts active pathway coping skills and neural exercises as dangerous. Efforts to help, like advice, problem-solving, information, and even encouragement, are also neurocepted as dangerous. A helpful reminder in this situation is that *a nervous system focused on danger can't focus on solutions. It first needs to know that it is safe.* This safety comes through passive pathways that builds the gestalt of a concerned adult who understands the child's experience of alarm, and fights shoulder to shoulder as the child's ally against whatever imperils them. When a child's nervous system crosses the threshold of mistrust, they often spontaneously start thinking of solutions themselves. At this point, the child is open to collaboration. A child who up to that point in treatment may have resisted anything that focused on their behavior, may actually ask for a "sticker chart," to get a colorful sticker each time they brush their teeth, put away their socks, or take out the trash.

In harmony with the child's ventral vagal willingness to engage, the therapist relaxes into ventral vagal safety too. Bonnie Badenoch (2018) described the implications of this shift in the therapist:

> All the protocols and interventions we have learned now have the potential to become a rich storehouse of supplies we can draw on in the moment in response to our patients' emerging needs… rather than a set of instructions about how to undo certain symptoms.
>
> *(p. 82)*

The therapist embodies their polyvagal understanding, and their ventral vagal state becomes their biggest ally. They also come to trust the child and caregiver's nervous system to help guide treatment. They may ask, for example, "How would your nervous system feel about learning some calm-down activities (taking some medication, filling out a feelings sheet) now?"

A Polyvagal-Informed Treatment of Complex Childhood Trauma and Dissociation

Therapists and caregivers support the child to neurocept enough safety through passive pathways to evoke their social engagement system, then move into self-agency and carry out an active pathway strategy. With each round of trust building and collaboration, the child learns to recognize their states and move from one state to another in a process Dana calls "autonomic navigation" (2018, p. 205). As this process continues, the child gains confidence in the adult's intentions, skills, and trustworthiness (Tucci et al., 2018). As described above, this doesn't have to be a perfect process. The adult will have many chances to repair their misattunements to the child's states or needs. Each turn through the cycle of relating, experiencing a rupture in relating, and then repairing the rupture shows the child that this is a relationship they can count on. Growing confidence in themself, the adult, and the relationship cultivates their stability in social engagement, the leading goal for treating the devastating effect of complex trauma on the nervous system.

At this point, we can ask, what are the clinical lessons we can distill from our exploration? The elements in the following list are each important in creating a felt (neurocepted) sense of safety that coaxes a child to allow enough connection to reawaken their social engagement system:

Principles of polyvagal-informed treatment of complex trauma

1. The therapist or caregiver themself is in a state of social engagement.
2. From an embodiment of safety, the therapist or caregiver expresses signals that emerge from social engagement—that is, prosody, animated face, etc.

3 The setting and context also communicate safety, through soothing physical qualities, predictable structure, and compassionate limit setting.
4 The therapist or caregiver demonstrates that they understand and can make sense of the child's inner experience:

   a Carefully tracking the child's changes in autonomic state, with warmth and curiosity, rather than defensively reacting to the state, and making their observations explicit when appropriate (Somatic Experience) (please see Maggie Kline's chapter on Somatic Experiencing (2025) for further details).
   b Repeatedly attuning to the child's experience through PACE—a playful, accepting, curious, and empathic attitude (DDP) (please see Kim Golding's chapter on Dyadic Developmental Psychotherapy [2025] for further details).

5 The therapist or caregiver skillfully and repeatedly guides the child to experience defensive and mistrusting states and persistently assists them to move out of defensiveness back into states of opening and trust.
6 The therapist and caregiver attend to the times they are misattuned to the child's state or needs, and through reattunement and co-regulation, circle through the relate, rupture, and repair cycle again.
7 After crossing the threshold of mistrust, the therapist or caregiver helps the patient learn activities that are emotionally regulating.
8 The therapist and caregiver continue to provide heartfelt connection and attunement to the child until the child is more stable in their ability to return to social engagement each time circumstances evoke a sympathetic fight-or-flight or dorsal vagal collapse state.

If these recommendations seem daunting, please remember that treating complex trauma usually *is* a formidable proposition, requiring adequate support and resources for its success that also offers adults involved opportunities for meaningful growth. Additionally, residential treatment may provide the resources needed to follow these recommendations. Grant, Thompson, and Golding (2024) have proposed that a child whose whole environment has traumatized them may need a whole new and therapeutic environment to counter trauma's disastrous effects. They acknowledge that, while residential treatment is often seen as a failure of outpatient treatment, for children who have experienced complex trauma, it may be more appropriate to view residential care as an expected intervention that can even shorten the child's overall treatment timeline.

Conclusion

Complex trauma turns the safe harbor of relationships into a minefield through which a child dare not tread. Without connection to a safe and trusted caregiver, the child has no viable path into ventral vagal social engagement. The ventral vagal state is the neural platform that supports the child's healthy development, physically, mentally, and relationally. Without access to the ventral vagal state, the child is left in a harsh and dangerous world, and their lessons all involve threat and protection. Polyvagal Theory offers a way to make sense of what has happened to the child and suggests a path out that involves coaxing the child back into relationship by incremental offers of safe connection. Using polyvagal-informed models like Somatic Experiencing and Dyadic Developmental Psychotherapy, we have seen children whose trauma was considered to have made them unreachable begin to trust again. Little by little, the child trusts their skilled companions who know how to reawaken social engagement; then they learn to trust themselves. Both child and companion develop a deeply respectful understanding of what the nervous system has been through, how it has tried to adapt, and ways to support its healing going forward. From the stable platform of a warm and relational social engagement, the child can venture out into the world, exploring with wonder and awe, perhaps for the first time. As Dylan Thomas so aptly put it, "Children in wonder watching the stars, / is the aim and the end" (2003, p. 33).

Notes

1 The author would like to thank the book's editors, Ana Gomez and Jill Hosey, for their support in writing this chapter, and Stephen Porges, Jon Baylin, Brandon Mock, Belinda Hoole, and Julia Fishman, for reading the chapter and making helpful suggestions.
2 Note: while this chapter tends to paint some situations in absolute terms, such as when it says social engagement is blocked, in most of these situations there can be a partial expression of the dynamic. For instance, when trauma is less consistent or support is more available, access to social engagement may not be blocked in all situations. This caveat applies to other situations that the chapter paints in absolute terms as well.

References

Badenoch, B. (2018). Safety is the treatment. In S. W. Porges & D. Dana (Eds.), *Clinical applications of the polyvagal theory: The emergence of polyvagal-informed therapies* (pp. 73–88). W. W. Norton.
Baylin, J., & Hughes, D. A. (2016). *The neurobiology of attachment-focused therapy: Enhancing connection and trust in the treatment of children and adolescents.* W. W. Norton.
Beutler, S., Mertens, Y. L., Ladner, L., Schellong, J., Croy, I., & Daniels, J. K. (2022). Trauma-related dissociation and the autonomic nervous system: A systematic literature review of psychophysiological correlates of dissociative experiencing in PTSD patients. *European Journal of Psychotraumatology, 13*(2), 1–25. https://doi.org/10.1080/20008066.2022.2132599
Bowlby, J. (1969). *Attachment and loss: Vol. 1.* Attachment. Basic Books.
Cook, A., Spinazzola, J., Ford, J., Lanktree, C., Blaustein, M., Cloitre, M., DeRosa, R., Hubbard, R., Kagan, R., Liautaud, J., Mallah, K., Olafson, E., & van der Kolk, B. (2005). Complex trauma in children and adolescents. *Psychiatric Annals, 35*(5), 390–398. https://doi.org/10.3928/00485713-20050501-05
Dana, D. (2018). *Polyvagal theory in therapy: Engaging the rhythm of regulation.* W. W. Norton.
Dana, D. (2020a). *Polyvagal exercises for safety and connection: 50 Client-centered practices.* W. W. Norton.
Dana, D. (2020b). *Polyvagal flip chart: Understanding the science of safety.* W. W. Norton.
Feiler, T., Vanacore, S., & Dolbier, C. (2023). Relationships among adverse and benevolent childhood experiences, emotion dysregulation, and psychopathology symptoms. *Adversity and Resilience Science, 4,* 273–289. https://doi.org/10.1007/s42844-023-00094-0
Gabrielsen, G. W., & Smith, E. N. (1985). Physiological responses associated with feigned death in the American opossum. *Acta Physiologica Scandinavica, 123*(4), 393–398. https://doi.org/10.1111/j.1748-1716.1985.tb07605.x
Golding, K. S. (2025). Dyadic developmental psychotherapy. In A. Gomez & J. Hosey (Eds.), *The handbook of complex trauma and dissociation in children: Theory, research, and clinical applications* (pp. 328–344). Routledge.
Gomez, A. M. (2025). The trauma-formed defense and self-protective system. In A. Gomez & J. Hosey (Eds.), *The handbook of complex trauma and dissociation in children: Theory, research, and clinical applications* (pp. 752–773). Routledge.
Graessler, B., Thielmann, B., Boeckelmann, I., & Hoekelmann, A. (2021). Effects of different training interventions on heart rate variability and cardiovascular health and risk factors in young and middle-aged adults: A systematic review. *Frontiers in Physiology, 12,* Article 657274. https://doi.org/10.3389/fphys.2021.657274
Grant, E. M., Thompson, G. S., & Golding, K. S. (2024). *Working with relational trauma in children's residential care: A guide to using dyadic developmental practice.* Jessica Kingsley Publishers.
Greene, H., & Ugarriza, D. N. (1995). The 'stably unstable' borderline personality disorder: History, theory, and nursing intervention. *Journal of Psychosocial Nursing and Mental Health Services, 33*(12), 26–30.
Hughes, D. A. (2017). *Building the bonds of attachment: Awakening love in deeply traumatized children* (3rd ed.). Rowman & Littlefield.
Hughes, D. A., & Baylin, J. (2012). *Brain-based parenting: The neuroscience of caregiving for healthy attachment.* W. W. Norton.

Humphreys, R. K., & Ruxton, G. D. (2018). A review of thanatosis (death feigning) as an anti-predator behaviour. *Behavioral Ecology and Sociobiology, 72,* 1–16. https://doi.org/10.1007/s00265-017-2436-8

Karaosmanoğlu, H. A., Ateş, N., Köse Karaca, B., & Aytaç, M. (2022). A new viewpoint to schema modes and mode domains through polyvagal theory: Could schema modes be just a way of coping? *Current Psychology, 42*(24), 1–14. https://doi.org/10.1007/s12144-022-03176-x

Karemaker, J. M., & Wesseling, K. H. (2008). Variability in cardiovascular control: The baroreflex reconsidered. *Cardiovascular Engineering, 8*(1), 23–29. https://doi.org/10.1007/s10558-007-9046-4

Kleiger, R. E., Stein, P. K., & Bigger Jr., J. T. (2005). Heart rate variability: Measurement and clinical utility. *Annals of Noninvasive Electrocardiology, 10*(1), 88–101. https://doi.org/10.1111/j.1542-474X.2005.10101.x

Kline, M. (2025). Somatic experiencing. In A. Gomez & J. Hosey (Eds.), *The handbook of complex trauma and dissociation in children: Theory, research, and clinical applications* (pp. 441–459). Routledge.

Kolacz, J., Lewis, G. F., & Porges, S. W. (2018). The integration of vocal communication and biobehavioral state regulation in mammals: A polyvagal hypothesis. In S. M. Brudzynski (Ed.), *Handbook of ultrasonic vocalization: A window into the emotional brain* (pp. 23–34). Elsevier Academic Press. https://doi.org/10.1016/B978-0-12-809600-0.00003-2

Krick, A., Felfe, J., & Klug, K. (2021). Building resilience: Trajectories of heart rate variability during a mindfulness-based intervention and the role of individual and social characteristics. *International Journal of Stress Management, 28*(3), 220–231. https://doi.org/10.1037/str0000227

Lanius, R. A., Boyd, J. E., McKinnon, M. C., Nicholson, A. A., Frewen, P., Vermetten, E., Jetly, R., & Spiegel, D. (2018). A review of the neurobiological basis of trauma-related dissociation and its relation to cannabinoid- and opioid-mediated stress response: A transdiagnostic, translational approach. *Current Psychiatry Reports, 20,* 1–14. https://doi.org/10.1007/s11920-018-0983-y

Lebois, L. A., Kumar, P., Palermo, C. A., Lambros, A. M., O'Connor, L., Wolff, J. D., Baker, J. T., Gruber, S. A., Lewis-Schroeder, N., Ressler, K. J., Robinson, M. A., Winternitz, S., Nickerson, L. D., & Kaufman, M. L. (2022). Deconstructing dissociation: A triple network model of trauma-related dissociation and its subtypes. *Neuropsychopharmacology, 47*(13), 2261–2270. https://doi.org/10.1038/s41386-022-01468-1

Levine, P. A. (2018). Polyvagal theory and trauma. In S. W. Porges & D. Dana (Eds.), *Clinical applications of the polyvagal theory: The emergence of polyvagal-informed therapies* (pp. 3–25). W. W. Norton.

Merriam-Webster. (n.d.). Autonomic. In Merriam-Webster.com dictionary. Retrieved July 8, 2023, from merriam-webster.com/dictionary/autonomic

Nijenhuis, E., van der Hart, O., & Steele, K. (2010). Trauma-related structural dissociation of the personality. *Activitas Nervosa Superior, 52,* 1–23.

Ogden, P. (2018). Polyvagal theory and sensorimotor psychotherapy. In S. W. Porges & D. Dana (Eds.), *Clinical applications of the polyvagal theory: The emergence of polyvagal-informed therapies* (pp. 34–49). W. W. Norton.

Ostlund, B. D., Measelle, J. R., Laurent, H. K., Conradt, E., & Ablow, J. C. (2017). Shaping emotion regulation: Attunement, symptomatology, and stress recovery within mother-infant dyads. *Developmental Psychobiology, 59*(1), 15–25. https://doi:10.1002/dev.21448

Ozer, E. J., & Weiss, D. S. (2004). Who develops posttraumatic stress disorder? *Current Directions in Psychological Science, 13*(4), 169–172. jstor.org/stable/20182942

Perna, G., Riva, A., Defillo, A., Sangiorgio, E., Nobile, M., & Caldirola, D. (2020). Heart rate variability: Can it serve as a marker of mental health resilience? Special Section on "Translational and Neuroscience Studies in Affective Disorders," Section Editor, Maria Nobile MD, PhD. *Journal of Affective Disorders, 263,* 754–761. https://doi.org/10.1016/j.jad.2019.10.017

Porges, S. W. (1992). Vagal tone: A physiologic marker of stress vulnerability. *Pediatrics, 90*(3), 498–504.

Porges, S. W. (1995). Orienting in a defensive world: Mammalian modifications of our evolutionary heritage. A polyvagal theory. *Psychophysiology, 32*(4), 301–318. https://doi.org/10.1111/j.1469-8986.1995.tb01213.x

Porges, S. W. (2006). The role of social engagement in attachment and bonding: A phylogenetic perspective. In C. S. Carter, L. Ahnert, K. E. Grossman, S. B. Hrdy, M. E. Lamb, S. W. Porges & N. Sachser (Eds.), *Attachment and bonding: A new synthesis* (pp. 33–54). MIT Press.

Porges, S. W. (2009). The polyvagal theory: New insights into adaptive reactions of the autonomic nervous system. *Cleveland Clinic Journal of Medicine, 76*(Suppl 2), S86–S90. https://doi.org/10.3949/ccjm.76.s2.17

Porges, S. W. (2017). *The pocket guide to the polyvagal theory: The transformative power of feeling safe.* W. W. Norton.

Porges, S. W. (2018). Polyvagal theory: A primer. In S. W. Porges & D. Dana (Eds.), *Clinical applications of the polyvagal theory: The emergence of polyvagal-informed therapies* (pp. 50–72). W. W. Norton.

Porges, S. W. (2021). *Polyvagal safety: Attachment, communication, self-regulation.* W. W. Norton.

Porges, S. W. (2022). Heart rate variability: A personal journey. *Applied Psychophysiology and Biofeedback, 47*(4), 259–271. https://doi.org/10.1007/s10484-022-09559-x

Porges, S. W. (2023). The vagal paradox: A polyvagal solution. *Comprehensive Psychoneuroendocrinology, 16*, Article 100200. https://doi.org/10.1016/j.cpnec.2023.100200

Porges, S. W., & Carter, C. S. (2017). Polyvagal theory and the social engagement system. In P. L. Gerbarg, P. R. Muskin & R. P. Brown (Eds.), *Complementary and integrative treatments in psychiatric practice* (pp. 221–241). American Psychiatric Association Publishing.

Porges, S. W., & Furman, S. A. (2011). The early development of the autonomic nervous system provides a neural platform for social behaviour: A polyvagal perspective. *Infant and Child Development, 20*(1), 106–118. https://doi.org/10.1002/icd.688

Porges, S. W., & Raskin, D. C. (1969). Respiratory and heart rate components of attention. *Journal of Experimental Psychology, 81*(3), 497–503. https://doi.org/10.1037/h0027921

Porges, S. W., & Winn, D. (2021). The significance of stillness. In S. W. Porges (Ed.), *Polyvagal safety: Attachment, communication, self-regulation* (pp. 231–245). W. W. Norton.

Potter, M. C., Wyble, B., Hagmann, C. E., & McCourt, E. S. (2014). Detecting meaning in RSVP at 13 ms per picture. *Attention, Perception, & Psychophysics, 76*, 270–279. https://doi.org/10.3758/s13414-013-0605-z

Reinders, A. S., Nijenhuis, E. R., Quak, J., Korf, J., Haaksma, J., Paans, A. M., Willemsen, A. T., & den Boer, J. A. (2006). Psychobiological characteristics of dissociative identity disorder: a symptom provocation study. *Biological Psychiatry, 60*(7), 730–740. https://doi.org/10.1016/j.biopsych.2005.12.019

Sanders, M. R., & Thompson, G. S. (2022). *Polyvagal theory and the developing child: Systems of care for strengthening kids, families, and communities.* W. W. Norton.

Siegel, D. J. (2012). *The developing mind: How relationships and the brain interact to shape who we are* (2nd ed.). Guilford Press.

Smith, S. M., & Vale, W. W. (2022). The role of the hypothalamic-pituitary-adrenal axis in neuroendocrine responses to stress. *Dialogues in Clinical Neuroscience, 8*(4), 383–395. https://doi.org/10.31887/DCNS.2006.8.4/ssmith

Steele, K. (2025). Structural dissociation: Developmental pathways and treatment implications. In A. Gomez & J. Hosey (Eds.), *The handbook of complex trauma and dissociation in children: Theory, research, and clinical applications* (pp. 73–88). Routledge.

Stern, D. N. (2010). *Forms of vitality: Exploring dynamic experience in psychology, the arts, psychotherapy, and development.* Oxford University Press.

Thomas, D. (2003). Being but men. In D. Jones (Ed.), *The poems of Dylan Thomas* (p. 33). New Directions.

Tronick, E. Z., & Gianino, A. (1986). Interactive mismatch and repair: Challenges to the coping infant. *Zero to Three, 6*(3), 1–6.

Tucci, J., Weller, A., & Mitchell, J. (2018). Realizing "deep" safety for children who have experienced abuse: Application of polyvagal theory in therapeutic work with traumatized children and young people. In S. W. Porges & D. Dana (Eds.), *Clinical applications of the polyvagal theory: The emergence of polyvagal-informed therapies* (pp. 89–105). W. W. Norton.

Tyagi, A., & Cohen, M. (2016). Yoga and heart rate variability: A comprehensive review of the literature. *International Journal of Yoga, 9*(2), 97–113. https://doi.org/10.4103/0973-6131.183712

van der Kolk, B. A. (2005). Developmental trauma disorder: Toward a rational diagnosis for children with complex trauma histories. *Psychiatric Annals, 35*(5), 401–408. https://doi.org/10.3928/00485713-20050501-06

van der Kolk, B. A., & Fisler, R. (1995). Dissociation and the fragmentary nature of traumatic memories: Overview and exploratory study. *Journal of Traumatic Stress, 8*(4), 505–525.

Wehrwein, E. A., Orer, H. S., & Barman, S. M. (2016). Overview of the anatomy, physiology, and pharmacology of the autonomic nervous system. *Comprehensive Physiology, 6*(3), 1239–1278. https://doi.org/10.1002/cphy.c150037

Winnicott, D. W. (1960). The theory of the parent-infant relationship. *International Journal of Psychoanalysis, 41*, 585–595.

11
THE INNATE CONNECTION SYSTEM AND SENSORY-AFFECTIVE ORIENTING

Relevance to Deep Brain Reorienting (DBR)

Jessica Christie-Sands and Frank Corrigan

Introduction

Deep Brain Reorienting (DBR) is a neurobiologically respectful and developmentally sensitive approach to working with early-life adversity, trauma, and neglect-related shock states. The neural architecture mapped out in this therapeutic approach foregrounds the "deep brain" (brainstem) systems and emphasizes the importance of tracking a distinctive brainstem-mediated neurophysiological sequence that is consonant with the evolutionary process of the developing brain and nervous system. One of the unique features of DBR as a trauma therapy is the linking of the functional organization of midbrain systems with a developmentally sensitive therapeutic practice. While this approach is currently being developed to work with children, the theoretical framework of this model is grounded in the neurobiology of emerging early-life processes. The neural structures underpinning the evolution of connection and attachment, which are brainstem-based, are already emerging during embryonic development (Mai & Paxinos, 1990). This is one of the key reasons we propose that DBR has promising clinical applications for therapeutic work with children.

In this chapter, we propose that attachment has its origin in what we describe as the "innate connection system" (ICS). We argue that *before* we can form attachment, there is a more basic need for connection through sensory-affective orienting. The ICS is thereby seen as a pivotal neural substrate for priming orienting toward and/or away from connection *before* the emergence of attachment. The ICS is envisaged as a mechanism for priming sensory-affective orienting during early prenatal development and it thereby provides the innate neural scaffolding for bonding and attachment postnatally. We describe the prenate as having a primordial emotional life, one that shows an evolving capacity for *relationally* organizing experience in womb space through an array of sensory-affective communications. These pre-reflective *orienting* interactions can be seen through the different ways in which the prenate is *moved to move toward or away from* maternal and placental tissues as well as through sensory-affective touch. Thus, from early beginnings, the prenate is exhibiting primary forms of sensorimotor intentionality, directionality, and transformation.

We suggest that the prenate is primed to *seek the felt experience of connection* and that sensory-affective orienting is the vehicle through which this is achieved. Early-life disruptions in neural circuits linked to the functional organization of the ICS may lead to hyperactivation of the "innate defensive system" (IDS) and the "innate alarm system" (IAS); our use of these terms will be described presently. We wish to emphasize three key points: (1) these primary neural pathways are laid down early in utero, (2) they are fundamental to initial sensory-affective orienting responses, and (3) they share the same basic templates for connection and disconnection essential for the neonate. We propose that the basic need for connection and the pain of disconnection register below affective and defensive responses at the level of the brainstem. This means that early-life shock can interrupt fluid orienting, lead to core disturbances in primary affective and defensive responses, and create enhanced states of vigilance, all of which constitute what we describe as *pre-attachment wounding*.

It is important to emphasize that the clinical application of DBR for children remains in the early stages of development. Our primary aim here is to provide a theoretical overview, from a brainstem-based perspective, of traumatic dissociation and how it might be manifested in children. We suggest an alternative way of understanding dissociation and introduce the idea of supracortical dissociation, which is unique to the DBR perspective on the brainstem. We argue that supracortical dissociation arises from a profound sense of core aloneness—a pain so intense and utterly unbearable that it is impossible to turn toward at the level of the midbrain. When a neonate or infant experiences a fundamental *absence of connection*, the core wound may be to their felt experience of being. It is this loss in the vitality of connection, an absence that is so wounding, that we suggest foreshadows the inability to turn toward. How do we turn toward the shock of being unwanted, the absence of felt belonging, or the horror of being relinquished? How do we turn toward the painful ambiguity between presence and absence so characteristic of neglect-related shock, an absence that may remain painfully present throughout life? It is this core wound of aloneness that closes off the possibility of turning toward and is central to what we describe as supracortical dissociation.

In DBR, we describe the superior colliculus (SC) and the periaqueductal gray (PAG) as the twin structures that underpin the ICS and the IDS. We build on the idea that *before* we can form attachments, we need to have basic connections, which are rooted in brainstem systems mediating primary affective and defensive responses. The SC forms a multisensorial "superhub" (Merker, 2007) that provides a moment-by-moment, sensorimotor navigational mapping of the body, while the PAG has its own "unique hub for primal emotional tone" (Pfaff, 2019, p. 51). While the locus coeruleus (LC), in the pons is known to have a modulatory role in attention and arousal (see Pfaff, 2019, for an extended discussion), we also consider it to be highly activated by the SC in traumatic shock states; interaction between the LC and SC then promotes shock-induced states of vigilance. The SC-PAG pathway mediates prototypical affective and defensive responses, while interactions between the LC and PAG contribute to the intensification of primary affective states. Additionally, we suggest that the dorsal raphe nucleus (DRN) is one of the structures underpinning core aloneness pain. Thus, the SC–PAG–DRN pathway may be crucial to understanding what we describe as supracortical dissociation. These deep brain structures form a refined representational body map of sensory-affective experience beginning in utero. However, when the functional integrity of these networks is compromised by early-life shock (SC–LC) and pre-attachment wounding (SC–PAG), or by the painful absence of connection (SC-PAG-DRN), this may lead to shock-induced surges in vigilance and/or neurochemical overwhelm, thereby altering the regulation of physiological stability prenatally and postnatally (Arancibia et al., 2023; Feldman et al., 2019; Gotlieb et al., 2022; Weinstein, 2016). By pre-attachment wounding, we are referring specifically to disruptions in connection, the pain of disconnection, or the fundamental absence of connection leaving an imprint of core aloneness pain.

The notion of co-embodiment (the idea that we emerge into life *within* the body of another) is a critically overlooked aspect of early-life affective experience (Ciaunica et al., 2021a). Yet, from the moment of conception, we begin life sharing biological resources in a co-embodied or "amphoteronomic" (Trevarthen et al., 2006) womb space. In just a few days, both the embryo and endometrial tissues of the mother are sharing resources to support the bidirectional coordination of early state-dependent regulatory processes. This is an important point, as alterations in the balance between cortisol and oxytocin prenatally have been implicated in the development of disorganized attachment postnatally (see Arancibia et al.'s seminal review of the literature, 2023). With this sharing of biological resources, the prenate is also *relationally* organizing their experience *within* the body of another. Thus, from the onset, there is arguably a co-embodied sense of *two*, not *one*, that forms the "background orientation" (Ratcliffe, 2008) and "background feeling" (Damasio, 1994) and signals a felt sense of *co-presence*. Therefore, early disruptions in the ICS may not only register as a loss of co-embodiment and co-presence, but also as a loss of connection with the surrounding space. This may create disruptions in sensorimotor directionality (*where I am in time and space?*) and contribute to the experience of a loss in self-location. Furthermore, the idea of co-embodiment provides an important context for us to explore how the developing sense of connection in utero is mediated through sensory-affective orienting. This allows us to suggest that there is already an innate scaffold for connection that intersects with an innate mechanism for orienting.

Considering the experience of connection through a bottom-up developmental lens is not subverting the critical importance of attachment in early life. We wish to show that the ICS is the scaffold upon which our capacity for attachment is built. We argue that to understand the roots of attachment, we must also consider how basic forms of *connection* are organized in utero—from the nascent development of cells *orienting* to their preferred destinations, to the building of a human body *within* the body of another. While our intention is to show that DBR offers a new perspective on the brainstem origins of connection and attachment, we also wish to emphasize how early-life disruptions in the ICS may underpin the developing trajectory of trauma-related dissociation. Thus, in DBR we pay close attention to felt experience of *connection* and the *pain of its absence*. The painful absence of connection in early life may register as shock and thereby have persisting impacts on the body's affective and defensive systems throughout life. Exploring the co-embodied roots of connection may therefore offer fresh insights into the developmental implications of early-life shock and pre-attachment wounding and provide an important context for understanding the emergence of different forms of trauma-related dissociation after birth.

We propose that early sensory-affective experience is foundational to building a body-self, not only an embodied sense of *who* we are, but also *where* we are in time and space. This developing sense of self-location provides an anchor to sensory-affective experience of connection *before* birth. The scent, taste, touch, sound, and spatiotemporal aspects of womb space offer the prenate a visceral connection to *where they are* and *where they want to be* (Lee, 2005). Intriguingly, early sensory-affective orienting actions, which contribute to sensorimotor body maps, enable the prenate to *feel* the space around them as well as feel their body moving in space (Ahmed et al., 2020; Fagard et al., 2018). The capacity to map womb space is developed through multisensory experience in olfactory, tactile, and proprioceptive interactions. This emerging sense of self-location unfolds *before* face and gaze attachment communications ground the feeling of where we are in space and time in a postnatal world. Thus, we consider the dual implications of early-life shock and pre-attachment wounding on pre-reflective states of co-embodiment and our developing sense of self-location both prenatally and postnatally.

Background Orientation and Background Feeling

The idea of "background orientation" is borrowed from Ratcliffe's (2008) phenomenological perspective on the embodied self as forming an existential background orientation to *all* experience, including early-life sensory experiences (scent, touch, and sound) *within* the body of another. As Ciaunica et al. (2021a) explained:

> Precisely because sensory proximal inputs are ubiquitous, they tend to be "transparently" processed "in the background," typically unnoticed and taken for granted. Yet they constitute the

fundamental "invisible" roots of our sense of self and sense of presence in the world [Rarcliffe, 2008, p. 3]" and are blended to form a "tactic background existential orientation."

While early-life olfactory and tactile sensory inputs tend to be processed in the "background," they nevertheless form an important sensory channel for scaffolding a primordial sense of self and the vitality of connection. The idea of existential bodily "background feelings" is taken from Damasio (1994):

> I am postulating another variety of feeling which I suspect preceded the others in evolution. I call it *background feeling* [emphasis added] because it originates in the "background" body states rather than in emotional states ... *emerging from* [emphasis added] the tone and beat of life itself, the sense of being ... The background feeling is our image of the body landscape when it is not shaken by emotion ... I submit that without them the very core of your representation of the self would be broken.
>
> *(pp. 150–151)*

Since background feelings *precede* emotion and correspond directly to core body states, it seems plausible to consider them naturally coalescing with background orientation to form a bodily background of connection, one that originates in our core experience of *being* and *being with*. Thus, we can envisage these twin sources of being as having roots in brainstem pathways for background orientation and background feelings. The term "sensory-affective orienting" has its lineage in the biological beginnings of life and in the evolutionary principles underpinning affective neuroscience. Orienting first emerges within the co-embodied experience of being *moved to turn toward or away from* some aspect of experience at any given moment. Sensory-affective orienting may therefore be considered foundational to the development of a co-embodied sense of connection in utero (examples of such will be provided later in this chapter).

While attachment research has historically focused on the more observable and measurable aspects of attachment *behavior*, the integration of studies linked to neurobiology underpinning specific attachment behaviors is growing (see Abraham & Feldman, 2018; Arancibia et al., 2023; Feldman, 2021; and Reijman et al., 2018 for reviews). Some research considers the prenatal roots of attachment loosely within a neurobiological context of "fetal programming" (see Verdult, 2021), but little is written on the prenate's experience of womb life (see Verny, 2021; Weinstein, 2016, for a review) or on the possibility of an emerging "phenomenal consciousness" (see Ciaunica & Crucianelli, 2019; Ciaunica et al., 2021a; Merker, 2007; Trevarthen et al., 2006) in early life. The focus on minimal forms of embodied consciousness offers a context for exploring how background orientation and background feelings provide a relational bridge for *connection* and a nascent sense of self emerging firstly *within* the body of another. Thus, the primary focus of this chapter is on the emergence of orienting to connection as an organizing principle of early development and its sensory-affective bodily roots.

Sensory-Affective Orienting and the Innate Connection System

During early embryogenesis, whole body movements (sideways bending of head/body) are often characterized by their fluency, variation, and rhythm (Piontelli, 2010; Reissland et al., 2014). Such preorganized rhythmic movements not only serve to register the *motoric presence* of the embryo but may also be indicative of early forms of sensorimotor *directionality* (Delafield-Butt & Gangopadhyay, 2013). At only seven weeks old and no bigger than a coffee bean, the embryo begins to *orient toward* the multisensory aspects of womb space *before* sensory pathways are functionally organized. These nascent orienting gestures appear to be primed to seek tactile sources of sensory feedback through self-directed micro-rotational movements of whole head/body, which also often show preferential right-sided body orientations (Delafield-Butt & Gangopadhyay, 2013; Fagard, et al., 2018; Piontelli, 2010; Trevarthen, 1985). If we accept, as some of the literature suggests, that our basic sense of self arises from a dynamic interplay between multisensorial and sensorimotor experiences in utero (Ciaunica & Crucianelli, 2019; Ciaunica et al., 2021a; Quintero & De Jaegher, 2020), then it seems plausible to suggest that disruptions in brainstem-based pathways due to early-life shock (SC–LC) and pre-attachment wounding (SC–PAG) may lead to profound alterations in the self, notably in terms of an inchoate sense of distaste toward the self.

Sophisticated forms of sensorimotor orienting actions, designed to seek connection, emerge far earlier than previously assumed. These allow the embryo/prenate to develop a felt sense of the space around it and to feel its own body touching and being touched by maternal and placental tissues. The continuous sense of touching and being touched (the location of which tactile contact registers in the intermediate layers of the SC), may also be a way for the prenate to map the spatiotemporal features of womb space to enhance a felt sense of where they are moment by moment. Thus, sensory-affective touch may contribute to an evolving sense of self-location within the body of another. However, the prenate moves with purpose and intention, seeking connection through self-directed sensorimotor gestures (Buil et al., 2022; Delafield-Butt & Gangopadhyay, 2013; Piontelli, 2010; Trevarthen et al., 2006). Some aspects of this dynamic feedback flow, influenced by the qualities of background orientation and background feeling, provide the scaffolding for an emerging sense of self, primed to seek connection, in a shared biological space (Ciaunica & Crucianelli, 2019; Ciaunica et al., 2021a). While we do not foreground the molecular and neurobiological implications of maternal stress during early life on developing hormonal systems (cortisol and oxytocin), we recognize that these systems play a critical role neurodevelopmentally (see Arancibia et al., 2023, for an excellent discussion on the neurobiology of disorganized attachment).

From the moment of conception, cells are primed to orient toward their preferred direction—that is, embryonic body or placental body (see Mukherjee, 2022; Zernicka-Goetz & Highfield, 2020). Thus, cell signaling forms the background orientation for the molecular scaffolding required to build a human body. Similarly, our first sensorial experiences (notably olfactory and tactile as well as proprioceptive and interoceptive) form the background orientation needed to sense the sensory presence of *connection* in utero. This is mediated through the affective tone of sensory input, which is continuously processed in the background (Ciaunica et al., 2021a). Thus, early olfactory and tactile interactions can be seen as forming a basic "experiential background" that registers the *sensory presence* and *sensory vitality* of connection for the prenate and neonate.

The emergence of early forms of movement with a rudimentary degree of sensorimotor control begins during embryonic development (Piontelli, 2010; Trevarthen & Delafield-Butt, 2017). The notion of "sensorimotor intentionality" that is brainstem-based has been foregrounded by Delafield-Butt and Gangopadhyay (2013):

> Our account of a developing sensorimotor intentionality ... aligns with the centrencephalic theory of consciousness (Merker, 2007) that proposes the functional role of conscious experience is to integrate sensory information; the brainstem and midbrain are identified as the "core central control system" ... This primary sensorimotor intentionality that develops ... during ontogenesis, but remains fundamentally unchanged and continuous throughout life.
>
> *(p. 401)*

Intriguingly, they argue that from the early beginnings of life, brain activity has a certain vitality, a movement or action. Brainstem nuclei that are functional long before birth arguably provide the neural substrates for the development of connection in utero:

Brainstem territories include the necessary functional characteristics for enabling a primary form of consciousness as "acting with knowing"—an embodied and prospective agentive experience. Somatotopic mapping giving access to proprioceptive body-space and tactile information that is preserved in [the] brainstem.

(Delafield-Butt & Gangopadhyay, 2013, p. 408)

Additionally, the idea of sensorimotor intentionality also intersects with the notion of sensorimotor directionality, an early form of *motoric presence* that registers in the background and primes the basic need for connection. The prenate has acquired a knowledge of womb space and can anticipate some sensory-affective outcomes, suggesting that minimal forms of bodily awareness are present long before birth. Early prospective orienting actions may be primed by a dual source of vitality linking background orientation and background feeling to the prenate's inchoate sense of being moved to move toward and/or away from multisensorial experience. For example, even simple self-directed orienting actions such as micro-rotations of the head/body or soft touch of tiny finger buds to forehead allows the emerging prenate to move from where it is now to where it wants to be (Lee, 2005). Thus, the foundational template for prospective awareness of movement and of spatiotemporal mapping of womb space is emergent in the most rudimentary sensorimotor actions of the embryo. This may be indicative of a more complex geographical mapping of self-location arising from the dynamic interplay of sensory-affective (olfactory and tactile) signals that form a sense of co-embodiment. The basic templates for mapping self-location—that is, where we are in space and time—may already be laid down during embryonic development as the primordial axial body planes (cranio-caudal, ventral, and dorsal) are forming (Zernicka-Goetz & Highfield, 2020).

Alessandra Piontelli's (2002) observations of twins in utero showed the complex and sophisticated forms of affectionate tactile communication between twins seeking to connect with each other, each touching, pushing, and sucking the nose, chin, and fingers of the other twin. Significantly, differential touch patterns are evident in tactile interactions with both maternal tissues (umbilical cord, placental wall, or uterine wall) and co-twin (Piontelli, 2002, 2010). Other studies exploring tactile communication between twins (14–18 weeks of gestational age) found evidence of affectionate touching (head-to-head, head to arm, head to leg, arm to arm, leg to head, cheek to cheek and nose to nose but not their eyes) with varying degrees of other-sensitivity (Castiello et al., 2010; Hata et al., 2015). The controlled timing and sequencing of touch shown in these studies suggests not only that early forms of "other-awareness" are present at as early as 14–16 weeks, but also that the prenate is *seeking connection with feeling*. Indeed, there is a wide body of research showing that the ability to seek connection and communicate with purpose and intention does not simply unfold after birth (see Castiello et al, 2010; Marx & Nagy, 2017; Piontelli, 2015 Reissland & Kisilevsky, 2016). This suggests that the prenate may be primed to seek connection through olfactory and tactile interactions (registering in brainstem-mediated pathways) far earlier than previously assumed. This fits with our proposal that the innate scaffolding for connection is the foundational template upon which attachment is built after birth.

Touch is perhaps one of the most unique aspects of early multisensorial experience; when we touch, we are simultaneously being touched. The basic experience of touching and being touched in utero may therefore be considered the primary relational bridge to connection. Touch may also be envisaged as the sensorial interface for mapping the surrounding space and building a primary sense of self-location *before* birth:

> Our first sensorial experiences provide us with information about our own body and the surrounding environment arise in the womb. In these early sensory-*affective* [emphasis added] interactions, touch is possibly the first route by which the developing body receives inputs

from the external world ... Thus, affective touch constitutes a fundamental aspect of bodily self-consciousness from the very first *embryonic* [emphasis added] stages of human life.

(Crucianelli & Filippetti, 2020, pp. 575–576)

The prenate is held and rocked by the amniotic fluids and can sense touching maternal tissues and simultaneously being touched by them. Even as early as six gestational weeks, the embryo exhibits withdrawal movements from light touching of lips with tiny finger buds (Hata et al., 2015; Montague, 1986). The evolution of different touch patterns varies in pressure and direction depending on where the prenate is touching—its own body or twin, maternal tissues, placenta, or umbilical cord. Whether the prenate is exploring their own body or their surrounding womb space, each movement appears to be made with purpose and intention, showing proprioceptive and tactile awareness. However, it is important to emphasize that when the prenate is *moved* to move toward or away from the softness or wetness of sensorial womb space, they are not simply seeking sensory feedback, but rather seeking connection through delicately timed tactile gestures with strong communicative intent (Marx & Nagy, 2017). Perhaps we can envisage *orienting to connection* as a primary relational scaffold at the level of the brainstem and mediated prenatally through senses such as olfaction and touch (first and second trimester) and later sound (third trimester).

There is a nascent form of sensorimotor intentionality and directionality in orienting toward connection through touching and being touched, either sequentially or simultaneously. By the second trimester, the prenate appears to be developing a felt sense of touching and being touched (Paterson, 2007; Piontelli, 2002, 2010). Intriguingly, the prenate is moved to orient toward the feeling of touching and being touched with an innate sense of "other-awareness" and "other-sensitivity" (Crucianelli & Filippetti, 2020; Marx & Nagy, 2015; Trevarthen, 2017). In a remarkable series of studies using 4D ultrasound videos, researchers at the University of Dundee, Scotland (Marx & Nagy, 2015, 2017), found that the prenate exhibits a distinct preference for maternal touch of the abdomen over maternal voice. Furthermore, the prenate was more likely to reach out and touch the uterine wall when their mother touched the abdomen. The timing of these tactile communications also appeared to synchronize with the mother's touch. Curiously, there was an increase in head movements during the maternal touch of the abdomen, although the precise direction was not specified. However, differential responses (in arm, head, and mouth movements) were evident depending on who was touching—that is, mother, father, or stranger. Similar differences were found in a later study (Nagy et al., 2021) designed to explore "communication readiness" of the prenate. Interestingly, 4D illustrations showing rotational head movements do appear to indicate that the head was turning toward the uterine wall in the direction of the hand resting on the abdomen, perhaps in anticipation of connection with the felt experience of touching and being touched. Thus, the moment the prenate *turns toward* the felt experience of connection—and is received through touch—a greater sense of *co-presence* may simultaneously register.

What these studies show is that the primary relational scaffolding for orienting toward connection synchronizes the feeling of being moved to seek connection through touching (maternal tissues) and being touched (maternal stroking of abdomen). This draws our attention to an important but often overlooked aspect of the prenate's experience—that is, they are primed to orient to connection with not only purpose and intention but also feeling. As Trevarthen (2017) highlights,

> during the second and third trimester, the prenate is ready to coordinate movements of face, voice, and hands to express a pattern of expressions that seek to take part in consciousness of a delicately timed dialogue with a responsive adult. They share "vitality dynamics" with "affective attunement."

(p. 5)

What Trevarthen may be alluding to here is the *vitality of connection* mediated through sensory-affective communications. This is more akin to Feldman's (2017) descriptions of biological synchrony that form dynamic expressions of other-awareness and other-sensitivity through touch before birth. Orienting to touch plays a pivotal role in shaping connection (bodily and affective) with maternal and placental tissues (Quintero & De Jaegher, 2020). The skin mediates a sensory-affective matrix of signals through touch, pain, and temperature, all of which are present before birth. Sensory-affective touch also provides a multisensory scaffold for early forms of *relational orienting* that underpin the development of primary forms of connection and consciousness (Merker, 2007) emerging first in utero and continuing after birth. As previously noted, the innate scaffolding for connection and the innate mechanism for orienting arise at the level of the brainstem and are laid down in the first few weeks of life. However, if we accept, as some of the above studies indicate, that primary forms of embodied awareness are present during early life, then it seems feasible to envisage that orienting to connection prenatally is a precursor to the development of attachment postnatally.

In the introduction to this chapter, we proposed that the neural pathways underpinning attachment are embedded in the midbrain ICS and that early life disruptions in the functional organization of the ICS can lead to hyperactivation of the innate defense system (IDS), which has its roots in the PAG but is separated, in our usage, from the innate alarm system (IAS), involving the LC. These brainstem-based pathways may offer a new perspective on different forms of traumatic dissociation we see emerging in children with early life experiences of developmental trauma.

Early-Life Shock and Pre-Attachment Wounding

We have argued that brainstem systems play a major role in understanding the developing capacity for connection and attachment (Arancibia et al., 2023; Cassidy & Shaver, 2018; Feldman, 2017; Reijman et al., 2018) and in the neuromodulation of core affective and defensive states (Delafield-Butt & Trevarthen 2017; Delafield-Butt et al., 2021; Panksepp, 1998; Panksepp & Biven, 2012). A midbrain-based model therefore offers a more nuanced understanding of the complex state-based modulatory difficulties arising from shock-induced traumatic experience. When the basic templates for connection have been disrupted by an early-life absence of connection (which may be characterized by multiple separation shocks after birth) or the painful ambiguity between presence and absence (arising from neglect-related shock), this registers at a brainstem level and leaves a powerful imprint of pre-attachment wounding. Separation shock at birth, for example, may lead to a lack of differentiation between presence and absence; a dark wound to an infant's core sense of being. Additionally, the loss of the sensory presence of the other may lead to shock-induced alterations in multisensory experience from birth onward.

Chronic disruptions in the early integration of multisensory experience not only lead to profound disturbances in affect regulation (see Joseph et al., 2021; Kearney & Lanius, 2022; Panksepp & Northoff, 2009; Perry, 2006; Yochman & Pat-Horenczyk, 2019), but also have significant impacts on the development of an embodied sense of self (Delafield-Butt & Trevarthen, 2017; Ciaunica & Crucianelli, 2019; Ciaunica et al., 2021a, 2021b; Rabellino et al., 2019; Tsakiris, 2010, 2017). Some of the critical alterations in multisensory experience arising from disturbances in embodiment are expressed through dissociative symptomatology (see Kearney & Lanius, 2022). To capture this complexity within the theoretical context of DBR, our definition of clinically relevant dissociation has been expanded to incorporate intracortical or shock-induced derealization and depersonalization, and neurochemical, structural, and supracortical dissociation. We will briefly consider each aspect of our suggested definition, in turn, but our purpose is to provide the reader with a rudimentary framework for understanding traumatic dissociation within the context of DBR.

1. **Shock-induced derealization and depersonalization** are hypothesized to result from overwhelming activation of the ascending noradrenergic projections from the pontine LC, which disturbs the balance of cortical activity and thereby leads to *alterations in the subjective experience of self*. We consider derealization and depersonalization to be epiphenomena of the physiological impact of emotional shock. Shock-induced states of depersonalization and derealization may arise from early-life experiences of repeated separation shock. The painful ambiguity between presence and absence may be mediated through an equally painful loss of embodiment (depersonalization) and loss of self-location in the surrounding space (derealization). Shock-induced depersonalization may be accompanied by uncanny bodily sensations (face/arm/leg may feel separate or not belong to the body) and a loss in sensory presence and sensory resonance due to alterations in the multisensorial experience of self (loss of bodily presence and sense of being unreal).
2. **Neurochemical dissociation** in DBR is understood to be part of a more nuanced matrix of *defensive responses* mediated by the midbrain PAG. The PAG elicits changes in muscle tension appropriate to defensive responses (fight or flight) and initiates relevant autonomic nervous system (ANS) changes. The PAG has mechanisms for stress-induced analgesia and is a significant structure in pain modulation. Its analgesic chemicals include endogenous cannabinoids and endogenous opioids, which can cap extreme activations of dorsal (cannabinoids) and ventrolateral (opioids) PAG. The putative endocannabinoid capping of fear, rage, grief, or shame is often experienced as numbing with high muscle tone, whereas the endogenous opioid experience may be one more of warmth and drowsiness with loss of muscle tone.
3. **Structural dissociation** is a term we borrowed from the work of van der Hart et al. (2006). We propose that separated emotional and apparently normal parts of the traumatized personality are based in the separation of cortico-striato-thalamo-cortical loops, which can command executive functioning networks, thereby leading to the emergence of different self-states. We postulate that endogenous opioids, probably in the anterior cingulate cortex, are instrumental in the traumatic separation of cortical and subcortical loops.
4. **Supracortical dissociation** is perhaps the most difficult to fit into existing models of dissociation, as it arises directly from the DBR perspective on the supracortical decision-making capacity of the SC (as described by Merker, 2007). With supracortical dissociation, it is the SC that initiates orienting away from what is too unbearable to turn toward. Thus, we are proposing that the midbrain has a capacity to orient toward or away from something in conscious awareness, thereby engaging an involuntary disconnection from what registers as intolerable. However, turning away from a painful loss in connection may have ontological impacts on the self. It may be too painful to turn toward the self who holds the imprint of core aloneness pain but equally painful to be disconnected from any sense of self.

As previously noted in the introduction, we are proposing an alternative way of understanding dissociation, one that is developmentally sensitive in its theoretical application to early-life shock and trauma. We map out below the neural pathways (SC–PAG and SC–LC as well as SC–PAG–DRN) linked to pre-affective shock with an emphasis on how absence of connection may leave an imprint of profound shock-induced pain. Can disruptions in connection or an absence of connection be experienced as painful by the neonate and infant? Can the sudden shock of disconnection have a cascading impact via subcortical anatomical pathways for pain? Is it possible to envisage the *experience of pain* arising from a more visceral sense of *being in pain* with the immediate body-based apprehension as the sensory-affective conduit. While we already have remarkably refined theoretical and clinical approaches to traumatic dissociation in children, the impact of shock on the functional organization of brainstem-based pathways is absent in the literature. Similarly, while the unfolding neurodevelopmental implications of early-life neglect, for example, is a central theme in attachment discourse, the significance of core aloneness pain is equally absent in current conceptualizations on the strategic organization of attachment in children. Thus, the model for dissociation we use in DBR is based on pre-affective shock and PAG-mediated affective and defensive states.

As noted above, we suggest that supracortical dissociation arises from a fundamental inability to turn toward the pain of core aloneness. If we consider, for example, an infant's journey into care, shock may form an epicenter, but core aloneness pain will be the emanating source. If an infant is relinquished at birth, the sensory shock (a core aspect of pre-attachment wounding) may be so great that it leads to shock-induced alterations in multisensory experiences and thereby enhances the inability to turn toward the absence of felt belonging throughout a child's life. With separation shock, we have the SC-PAG-DRN interacting in response to a sudden loss of the *sensory presence* of connection and all its associated sensory resonance. When there is no touch, holding, or warmth, how is the loss in the sensory presence of the other registered in the neonate or infant? When there is an absence of sensory resonance (scent, touch, and sound) that mediates the sensory presence of connection, how does an infant turn toward this more basic sense of not-thereness or goneness at the heart of core aloneness? The retrosplenial cortex and the SC together form a circuit for orienting to safety and shelter in animal models (Campagner et al., 2023)—an embodied map for knowing *where* safety and shelter are. For the neonate, this is primarily mapped through the sensory presence of connection. When the loss in sensory presence is disrupted by a sudden disconnection or separation shock, how does an infant map where safety is if there is a complete absence in the sensory resonance of connection? If an infant can no longer map where safety and shelter are, the only possibility may be for the retrosplenial cortex to promote dissociation. Moreover, when there is no sensory resonance of affective warmth and all defensive responses fail, the infant or young child may also exhibit prototypical freeze states corresponding to tonic or collapsed immobility.

We argue for two distinctive ways in which early-life adversity can disrupt and modify arousal levels through pathways in the midbrain. The first pathway is through what we describe as pre-affective shock, in which deeply horrifying experiences elicit widespread activation of the brain and body through systems ascending and descending from the brainstem. The deep layers of the SC, in response to incoming information, activate the LC in the upper pons of the brainstem. The engagement of the innate alarm system (IAS) is often part of a shock response, even when rapid detection of threat or an intensely disturbing and frightening experience is registered below the threshold of consciousness (Rabellino et al., 2019). Sustained exposure to shock may lead to enhanced states of shock-induced vigilance, which can manifest as a deep sense of "stillness," which can easily be mistaken for a state of composure. Similarly, shock-induced vigilance may be expressed through musculoskeletal rigidity. It is, however, important to differentiate pre-affective shock states from generically described freeze states. We suggest that there is increased network connectivity within the IAS involving the SC and LC that can generate pre-affective shock and lead to states of shock-induced vigilance. However, with shock, there are projections from the LC that elicit shock-related body sensations—for example, a shiver or shudder. While the idea of shock-induced vigilance is based on animal models of LC sensitization (Li et al., 2018), we suggest that the SC–LC and SC–PAG pathways may become sensitized by early-life adversity (Corrigan & Christie-Sands, 2019).

The second midbrain pathway, linked to primary affective and defensive responses arising from the PAG, sets the priorities for strategic action. The PAG orchestrates defensive actions (active and/or passive) related to survival need. There may be a physiological need for high arousal capping of intense affects by endogenous cannabinoids and low arousal capping by endogenous opioids. The PAG exerts complex modulatory responses, which we see in mixed states of arousal arising from the coactivation of different columnar circuits. The dorsal PAG (DPAG) engages active defensive responses (fight or flight), with their ANS circuitry and increased muscle tension requirements, while the ventrolateral PAG (VLPAG) is associated with passive defensive responding, sympathetic nervous system withdrawal, loss of muscle tone, and opioid mediated analgesia. Tonic immobility is a state in which there is coactivation of both dorsal and ventrolateral columns of the PAG and should be distinguished from collapsed immobility as well as from states of compliance and obedience. Pain modulation by the PAG is achieved, in part, through endogenous cannabinoids and opioids. Positive affective states (care and nurture) are also mediated by the PAG and enhanced by sensory-affective touch.

If we use the ANS as our guide, we may miss the opportunity of understanding the more complex responses of PAG-mediated affective and defensive states, notably differential high and low arousal freeze states that arise in children with early developmental trauma. For example, tonic immobility freeze states involve different activations of the PAG (DPAG and VLPAG). A child may exhibit intense active states of anger (DPAG) simultaneously combined with equally intense passive responses (VLPAG) organized primarily around states of utter hopelessness. The infant who is trapped and helpless in a disorganized attachment communication, for example, may exhibit an early form of tonic immobility through PAG-induced patterns of muscular rigidity. With early neglect-related experiences, there is a fundamental ambiguity between presence and absence, which may also underpin the conflicted urges to attach that we see in young infants exhibiting disorganized attachment behaviors. With conflicted orienting patterns, being moved to move toward *and* away from can simultaneously be the expression of the urge to both attach and defend. Thus, the impulse to approach may arise in parallel with the impulse to pull away from. Such neurophysiological paradoxes cannot be fully captured within the context of ANS responses. This is why it is important to consider the PAG as a model for understanding the complex nuances of affective and defensive responses as well as for differentiating freeze states.

It is important to note that within the context of DBR, all basic affects are arising, at least in part, from the dorsal PAG, and activate the sympathetic nervous system. We cannot, therefore, rely on ANS profiles to distinguish whether PAG-mediated affects are positively or negatively valenced. A simple dichotomy between high and low arousal ignores the intermediate arousal states we commonly see arising from early-life traumatic experiences (Corrigan & Christie-Sands, 2019; Hambrick et al., 2018a, 2018b; Perry, 2006, Perry et al., 2018). It also fails to capture more complex states of coactivation in which there may be high levels of internal distress but no visible emotional or behavioral expression of these core pain states. Not only is the PAG a regulatory mechanism in the expression of affect, but it also has a central role in the modulational of emotional and behavioral states (Corrigan, 2014; Kearney & Lanius, 2022; Panksepp, 1998; Panksepp & Biven, 2012; Pfaff, 2019; Solms, 2021; Venkatraman et al., 2017).

The developmental organization of these networks is a complex process both within brain regions and across neural pathways. The capacity for emotional and behavioral regulation is a function of diverse cortical connectivity and functional organization of brainstem-based ascending, descending, and modulatory networks (Kearney & Lanius, 2022; Tau & Peterson, 2010; Teicher et al., 2020; Valizadeh & Madadi Asl, 2023; Venkatraman et al., 2017). We know that the SC–PAG and LC pathways are laid down, albeit in the most rudimentary form, around four to six gestational weeks (Mai & Paxinos, 1990). We also know from some of the studies cited above that this dynamic primary-process network is sufficiently functionally organized during the second-to-third trimester to initiate preferential approach and withdrawal movements that exhibit sensorimotor intentionality and sensorimotor directionality, a sense of other-awareness and other-sensitivity within the body of another. Since the bodily roots of awareness emerge first within the body of another, there is a need to restate the developmental primacy of early sensory-affective experience, notably olfactory, tactile, and interoceptive, as the primary vehicle for mediating connection. Thus, the mechanism for orienting contributes to a co-embodied state of *co-presence*, a sense of *two* rather than *one*. It is important to emphasize that while these basic templates for initiating orienting are already established in utero, they are also fundamental to connection and attachment for the neonate and young infant.

While the developmental maturation of these brainstem and midbrain circuits continues post-birth, they generate neuromodulatory signals for priming both valence (positive or negative) and salience (level of importance) long before birth. Of course, the *timing* of early-life experiences of adversity is critically important when considering how the signatures of these differing affectively charged primary process systems impact directly on functional organization (Arancibia et al., 2023; Fuller, 2022; Hodel, 2018). While these midbrain pathways are functionally organizing during the second and third trimester, they are not functionally mature until at least six months after birth and therefore remain especially vulnerable to early life sensitization. There is already a large body of literature that suggests the developmental implications of early attachment disruptions are manifested through altered neurobiological functioning (see Cassidy & Shaver, 2018; Feldman et al., 2016; Feldman, 2021; Hesse et al., 2003; Reijman et al., 2018; Schore, 2003; Tronick, 2007, for a comprehensive overview and Arancibia et al., 2023 for more recent reviews). Indeed, some recent research has shown that critical alterations in hormonal systems during pregnancy, notably increases in cortisol and decreases in oxytocin, due to maternal stress, may be linked to the development of disorganized attachment in infants (Arancibia et al., 2023). However, what remains elusive is an understanding of the acute impacts of early life shock and pre-attachment wounding.

In DBR, as previously noted, the model for traumatic dissociation is based on pre-affective shock and PAG-mediated affective and defensive responses. Therefore, shock is broadly defined as a bodily reaction, arising primarily from the brainstem, that can precede any affective, emotional, behavioral, or cognitive response—hence the term "pre-affective shock." While the term "shock" is commonly used to describe responses to more obviously catastrophic events, such as a natural disaster, the horror of war, or a violent and terrifying assault, we are focusing on the cascading neurophysiological impacts of shock on the child. For example, a momentary surge of shock can break through in an attachment interaction that is experienced as suddenly and unexpectedly horrifying. Similarly, it can arise from a relational communication where a painfully harsh tone of voice momentarily extinguishes the feeling of connection. Shock may register in the body as a barely perceptible diffuse wave of high-energy sensations. For example, a sudden surge of activation may not have the sustained visceral quality of strong affects, although the visceral charge may be equally powerful. While it is not possible for us to be definitive, we envisage that the shock cascade may follow a relatively similar body-based trajectory in children.

We proposed that early-life shock interrupts the dynamic bidirectional flow of multisensory information (olfactory, tactile, auditory, and proprioceptive) from within and outside of the body. These sensory modalities play a key role in maintaining bodily integrity within the body of another and in developing a coherent and stable sense of self in connection with others. We also suggested that early life shock interrupts fluid orienting (SC), leads to core disturbances in affective and defensive responses (PAG), creates enhanced states of vigilance (LC–SC), and, when there is sudden loss of connection, can contribute to core aloneness pain (SC–PAG–DRN). When an infant is exposed to pervasive early-life neglect, the experience of connection may be mediated through a painful relational ambiguity between presence and absence. Similarly, where the basic experience of connection is channeled through an aloneness pain too unbearable to turn toward, this may lead to what we described earlier as supracortical dissociation. The imprint of shock may subsequently become the fulcrum of how an infant's attachment system relationally organizes. If we accept that connection precedes attachment, then it follows that shock-related disturbances in orienting to connection may underpin the strategic organization of insecure and disorganized patterns of attachment from early infancy onward. We have suggested that the basic experience of connection and disconnection registers before basic affective and defensive responses. If we already have a basic primordial need for connection, then the basic experience of disconnection must be painful at this deepest level.

Consider the infant who is repeatedly exposed to the still face of their mother or caregiver—this can register as painfully shocking. The literature on the still-face paradigm exemplifies this, although shock is not included as a key component of the infant's experience (see Tronick, 2007, for an extensive review of the empirical research). Similarly, Fisher's (2014) seminal research on the application of neurofeedback in the treatment of developmental trauma foregrounds the absence of connection (in the mother's inability to turn toward) as key to emerging disturbances in core arousal states (please see Chapter 24 for related information). Fisher revealed important insights into how the early loss in the vitality of connection leads to shock-related disturbances in rhythmicity: "Shock alters brains waves. Shock in childhood disorganizes brain rhythms, and enduring shock reinforces disorganization" (2014, p. 267). Furthermore, Fisher's description of the "enduring catastrophe of the child whose mother has turned away" (p. 3) brings into sharp focus the potential intergenerational lineage of supracortical dissociation.

It is possible that a loss in the sensory presence of connection in early life disrupts rhythmicity in ways that fundamentally alter the background orientation and background feeling required to sustain the ability to turn toward connection. From some of the studies already described, we can see that the prenate is moved to move toward the scent, touch, and sound of womb space, thereby enhancing the sensory vitality of connection. These early multisensorial experiences of connection provide a co-embodied sense of co-presence, a sense of two, not one. Similarly, for the neonate or young infant, the sensory presence of connection supports scaffolding embodiment postnatally. Thus, the sensory resonance and sensory depth of co-embodied experiences in utero may be more akin to a primordial sense of "being with," which also serves to enhance the sensory presence of connection for the neonate. When there is a loss in the vitality of connection, the pain of disconnection may have a deep visceral resonance throughout the entire body. In view of this, we consider the basic primordial need for connection and the absence of any vitality of connection as an existential wound to beingness.

Conclusion

In this chapter, we set out to provide a theoretical framework that offers a new approach to understanding early-life shock and pre-attachment wounding. We proposed that the foundational templates of attachment have their origins in the ICS, and that before we can form attachment, there is a more basic need for connection. More specifically, we suggested that the innate scaffold for connection intersects with a primary mechanism for orienting, and that together they form a multisensorial bodily background to an emerging sense of self. We argued that the templates for connection and disconnection are brainstem-based, and the painful absence of connection registers *below* affective and defensive responses. Our emphasis on prenatal experience was to bring into focus the view that the templates for orienting to connection develop first in utero and are functionally organized after birth; that the neural pathways that underpin the emergence of prototypical affective and defensive states in the infant are based in the midbrain; and that this model for traumatic dissociation is based on pre-affective shock (a concept unique to DBR) and PAG-mediated affective and defensive responses. This led us to consider the unfolding developmental implications of a sudden loss in the vitality of connection or a fundamental absence of connection: most notably, that an absence of connection (registered at the level of the brainstem) resonates in core aloneness pain and may remain present throughout life. Our primary aim was to highlight that shock-induced and absence-induced core aloneness states can contribute to the development of different forms of traumatic dissociation in children. As a model for early-life shock and pre-attachment wounding, DBR allows us to think through the larger implications of the brainstem as a potential source of transformational healing. While DBR is currently being adapted to work with children, our hope is that the light this new theoretical perspective sheds on traumatic experience is the light you can use to inform your clinical practice.

References

Abraham, E., & Feldman, R. (2018). The neurobiology of human allomaternal care; implications for fathering, coparenting, and children's social development. *Physiology & Behavior, 193*, 25–34. https://doi.org/10.1016/j.physbeh.2017.12.034

Ahmed, E., El Khoribi, R. A., Darwish, D., Muzy, A., & Bernot, G. (2020). Modeling of the development of the fetus cognitive map from the sensorimotor system. *Egyptian Informatics Journal, 21*(4), 191–199. https://doi.org/10.1016/j.eij.2020.01.002

Arancibia, M., Lutz, M., Ardiles, A., & Fuentes, C. (2023). Neurobiology of disorganized attachment: A review of primary studies on human beings. *Neuroscience Insights, 18*, 1–10. https://doi.org/10.1177/26331055221145681

Buil, A., Sankey, C., Caeymaex, L., Gratier, M., Apter, G., Vitte, L., & Devouche, E. (2022). Skin-to-skin SDF positioning: The key to intersubjective intimacy between mother and very preterm newborn: A pilot matched-pair, case-control study. *Frontiers in Psychology, 13*, Article 790313. https://doi.org/10.3389/fpsyg.2022.790313

Campagner, D., Vale, R., Tan, Y. L., Iordanidou, P., Pavón Arocas, O., Claudi, F., Stempel, A. V., Keshavarzi, S., Petersen, R. S., Margrie, T. W., & Branco, T. (2023). A cortico-collicular circuit for orienting to shelter during escape. *Nature, 613*(7942), 111–119. https://doi.org/10.1038/s41586-022-05553-9

Cassidy, J., & Shaver, P. R. (2018). *Handbook of attachment: Theory, research, and clinical applications.* (3rd ed.). Guilford Press.

Castiello, U., Becchio, C., Zoia, S., Nelini, C., Sartori, L., Blason, L., D'Ottavio, G., Bulgheroni, M., & Gallese, V. (2010). Wired to be social: The ontogeny of human interaction. *PLoS One, 5*(10), e13199. https://doi.org/10.1371/journal.pone.0013199

Ciaunica, A., Constant, A., & Preissl, H. (2021a) The first prior: From co-embodiment to co-homeostasis in early life. *Conscious Cognition, 91*, Article 103117. https://doi.org/10.1016/j.concog.2021.103117

Ciaunica, A., & Crucianelli, L. (2019). Minimal self-awareness: From within a developmental perspective. *Journal of Consciousness Studies, 26* (3–4): 207–226.

Ciaunica, A., Roepstrorff, A., Fotopoulou, K., & Petreca, B. (2021b). Whatever next and close to my self—The transparent senses and the "second skin': Implications for the case of depersonalization. *Frontiers in Psychology, 12*, Article 613587. https://doi.org/10.3389/fpsyg.2021.613587

Corrigan, F. M. (2014). Defense responses: Frozen, suppressed, truncated, obstructed, and malfunctioning. In U. F. Lanius, S. L. Paulsen, & F. M. Corrigan (Eds.), *Neurobiology and the treatment of traumatic dissociation: Towards an embodied self* (pp. 131–152). Springer.

Corrigan, F. M., & Chrisite-Sands, A. J. (2019). An innate brainstem self-other system involving orienting, affective responding, and polyvalent relational seeking: Some clinical implications for a "Deep Brain Reorienting" trauma psychotherapy approach. *Medical Hypotheses, 136*, 109502. https://doi.org/10.1016/j.mehy.2019.109502

Crucianelli, L., & Filippetti, M. L. (2020). Developmental perspectives on interpersonal affective touch. *Topoi, 39*, 575–586. https://doi.org/10.1007/s11245-018-9565-1

Damasio, A. (1994). *Descartes' error: Emotion, reason, and the human brain.* G. P. Putnam's Sons.

Delafield-Butt, J. T., Dunbar, P., & Trevarthen, C. (2021). Disruption to the core self in autism and its care. *Psychoanalytic Inquiry, 42*(1), 53–75. https://doi.org/10.1080/07351690.2022.2007031

Delafield-Butt, J. T., & Gangopadhyay, N. (2013). Sensorimotor intentionality: The origins of intentionality in prospective agent action. *Developmental Review, 33*(4), 399–425. https://doi.org/10.1016/j.dr.2013.09.001

Delafield-Butt, J. T., & Trevarthen, C. (2017). On the brainstem origin of autism: Disruption to movements of the primary self. In E. Torres & C. Whyatt (Eds.), *Autism: The movement sensing perspective* (pp. 1–41). CRC Press.

Fagard, J., Esseily, R., Jacquey, L., O'Regan, K., & Somogyi, E. (2018). Fetal origin of sensorimotor behavior. *Frontiers in Neurorobotics, 12*(23), 1–7. https://doi.org/10.3389/fnbot.2018.00023

Feldman, R. (2017). The neurobiology of human attachments. *Trends in Cognitive Sciences, 21*(2), 80–99. https://doi.org/10.1016/j.tics.2016.11.007

Feldman, R. (2021). The neurobiology of human attachments. *Trends in Cognitive Science, 21*(2), 80–99.

Feldman, R., Braun, K., & Champagne, F.A. (2019). The neural mechanisms and consequences of maternal caregiving. *Nature Reviews: Neuroscience, 20*, 205–224. https://doi.org/10.1038/s41583-019-0124-6

Feldman, R., Monakhov, M., Pratt, M., & Ebstein, R. P. (2016). Oxytocin pathway genes: Evolutionary ancient system impacting on human affiliation, sociality, and psychopathology. *Biological Psychiatry, 79*, 174–184. https://doi.org/10.1016/j.biopsych.2015.08.008

Fisher, S. F. (2014). *Neurofeedback in the treatment of developmental trauma: Calming the fear-driven brain.* New York: Norton.

Fuller, M. A. (2022). *Being biological: Human meaning in the age of neuroscience.* Lightening Source.

Gotlieb, N., Wilsterman, K., Finn, S. L., Brown, M. F., Bever, S. R., Iwakoshi-Ukena, E., Ukena, K., Bentley, G. E., & Kriegsfeld, L. J. (2022). Impact of chronic prenatal stress on maternal neuroendocrine function and embryo and placental development during early-to-mid pregnancy in mice. *Frontiers in Physiology, 13*, 1–15. https://doi.org/10.3389/fphys.2022.886298

Hambrick, E. P., Brawner, T. W., & Perry, B. D. (2018a). Examining developmental adversity and connectedness in child welfare-involved children. *Children Australia, 43*(2), 105–115. https://doi.org/10.1017/cha.2018.21.

Hambrick, E. P., Brawner, T. W., Perry, B. D., Brandt, K., Hofmeister, C., & Collins, J. O. (2018b). Beyond the ACE score: Examining relationships between timing of developmental adversity, relational health, and developmental outcomes in children. *Archives of Psychiatric Nursing, 33*(3), 238–247. https://doi.org/10.1016/j.apnu.2018.11.001

Hata, T., Kanenishi, K., Mostafa AboEllail, M. A., Marumo, G., & Kurjak, A. (2015). Fetal consciousness: Four-dimensional ultrasound study. *Donald School Journal of Ultrasound in Obstetrics and Gynecology, 9*(4), 471–474. https://doi.org/10.5005/jp-journals-10009-1434

Hesse, E., Main, M., Yost-Abrams, K., & Rifken, A. (2003). Unresolved states regarding loss or abuse can have second-generation effects: Disorganization, role inversion, and frightening ideation in the offspring of traumatized, non-maltreating parents. In M. F. Solomon & D. J. Siegal (Eds.), *Healing trauma: Attachment, mind, body, and brain* (pp. 57–106). W. W. Norton.

Hodel, A. S. (2018). Rapid infant prefrontal cortex development and sensitivity to early environmental experience. *Developmental Review, 48*(6), 113–144. https://doi.org/10.1016%2Fj.dr.2018.02.003

Joseph, R. Y., Casteleijn, D., van der Linde, J., & Franzsen, D. (2021). Sensory modulation dysfunction in child victims of trauma: A scoping review. *Journal of Child & Adolescent Trauma, 14*, 455–470. https://doi.org/10.1007/s40653-020-00333-x

Kearney, B. E., & Lanius, R. A. (2022). The brain-body disconnect: A somatic sensory basis for trauma-related disorders. *Frontiers in Neuroscience, 16*, Article 1015749. https://doi.org/10.3389/fnins.2022.1015749

Lee, D. N. (2005). Tau in action in development. In J. J. Rieser, J. J. Lockman, & C. A. Nelson (Eds.), *Action as an organizer of learning and development: Vol. 33 in the Minnesota Symposia on child psychology* (pp. 3–49). Lawrence Erlbaum Associates Publishers.

Li, L., Feng, X., Zhou, Z., Zhang, H., Shi, Q., Lei, Z., Shen, P., Yang, Q., Zhao, B., Chen, S., Li, L., Zhang, Y., Wen, P., Lu, Z., Li, X., Xu, F., & Wang, L. (2018). Stress accelerates defensive responses to looming in mice and involves a locus coeruleus-superior colliculus projection. *Current Biology, 28*(6), 859–871. https://doi.org/10.1016/j.cub.2018.02.005

Mai, J. K., & Paxinos, G. (1990). *The human nervous system* (3rd ed.). Academic Press.

Marx, V., & Nagy, E. (2015). Fetal behavioural responses to maternal voice and touch. *PLoS One, 10*(6), Article e0129118. https://doi.org/10.1371/journal.pone.0129118

Marx, V., & Nagy, E. (2017). Fetal behavioural responses to touch of the mother's abdomen: A frame-by-frame analysis. *Infant Behaviour and Development, 47*, 83–91. https://doi.org/10.1016/j.infbeh.2017.03.005

Merker, B. (2007). Consciousness without a cerebral cortex: A challenge for neuroscience and medicine. *Behavioral & Brain Sciences, 30*(1), 63–81. https://doi.org/10.1017/S0140525X07000891

Montague, A. (1986). *Touching: The human significance of the skin* (3rd ed.). HarperCollins.

Mukherjee, S. M. (2022). *The song of the cell: An exploration of medicine and the new human.* The Bodley Head.

Nagy, E., Thompson, P., Mayor, L., & Doughty, H. (2021). Do foetuses communicate? Foetal responses to interactive versus non-interactive maternal voice and touch: An exploratory analysis. *Infant Behavior and Development, 63*, Article 101562. https://doi/org/10.1016/j.infbeh.2021.101562

Panksepp, J. (1998). *Affective neuroscience: The foundations of human and animal emotions.* Oxford University Press.

Panksepp, J., & Biven, L. (2012). *The archaeology of mind: Neuroevolutionary origins of human emotions.* W. W. Norton.

Panksepp, J., & Northoff, G. (2009). The trans-species core SELF: The emergence of active cultural and neuro-ecological agents through self-related processing within subcortical-cortical midline networks. *Consciousness & Cognition, 18*(1), 193–215. https://doi.org/10.1016/j.concog.2008.03.002

Paterson, M. (2007). *The senses of touch.* Berg Publishers.

Perry, B. D. (2006). The neurosequential model of therapeutics: Applying principles of neuroscience to clinical work with traumatized and maltreated children. In N. Webb (Ed.), *Working with traumatized youth in child welfare* (pp. 27–52). Guilford Press. https://doi.org/10.1007/s10615-006-0072-2

Perry, B. D., Griffin, G., Davis, G., Perry, J. A., & Perry, R. D. (2018). The impact of neglect, trauma, and maltreatment on neurodevelopment: Implications for juvenile justice practice, programs, and policy. In A. R. Beech, A. J. Carter, R. E. Mann, & P. Rothstein (Eds.), *The Wiley Blackwell handbook of forensic neuroscience* (pp. 813–835). John Wiley & Sons Ltd. https://doi.org/10.1002/9781118650868.ch31

Pfaff, D. (2019). *How brain arousal mechanisms work: Paths towards consciousness.* Cambridge University Press.

Piontelli, A. (2002). *Twins: From fetus to child.* Routledge.

Piontelli, A. (2010). *Development of normal fetal movements: The first 25 weeks of gestation.* Springer-Verlag.

Piontelli, A. (2015). *Development of normal fetal movements: The last 15 weeks of gestation.* Springer-Verlag.

Quintero, M. A., & De Jaegher, H. (2020). Pregnant agencies: Movement and participation in maternal–fetal interactions. *Frontiers in Psychology 11*, Article 1977. https://doi.org/10.3389/fpsyg.2020.01977

Rabellino, D., Boyd, J. E., McKinnon, C., & Lanius, R. (2019). The innate alarm system: A translational approach. In G. Fink (Ed.), *Stress: Physiology, biochemistry, and pathology: Handbook of stress* (pp. 197–212). Academic Press.

Ratcliffe, M. (2008). *Feelings of being: Phenomenology, psychiatry, and the sense of reality.* Oxford University Press. https://doi.org/10.1093/med/9780199206469.001.0001

Reijman, S., Foster, S., & Duschinsky, R. (2018). The infant disorganised attachment classification: Patterning within the disturbance of coherence. *Social Science & Medicine, 200*(3), 52–58. https://doi.org/10.1016/j.socscimed.2017.12.034

Reissland, N., Francis, B., Aydin, E., Mason, J., & Schaal, B. (2014). The development of anticipation in the fetus: A longitudinal account of human fetal mouth movements in reaction to and anticipation of touch. *Developmental Psychobiology, 56*, 955–963. https://doi.org/10.1002/dev.21172

Reissland, N., & Kisilevsky, B. S. (Eds.). (2016). *Fetal development: Research on brain and behavior, environmental influences, and emerging technologies.* Springer International.

Schore, A. N. (2003). *Affect regulation and disorders of the self.* W. W. Norton.

Solms, M. (2021). *The hidden spring: A journey to the source of consciousness.* Profile Books Ltd.

Tau, G. Z., & Peterson, B. S. (2010). Normal development of brain circuits. *Neuropsychopharmacology Reviews, 35*, 147–168.

Teicher, M. T., Samson, J. A., Anderson, C. M., & Ohashi, K. (2020). The effects of childhood maltreatment on brain structure, function and connectivity. *Nature Reviews Neuroscience, 17*(9), 652–666. https://doi.org/10.1038/nrn.2016.111

Trevarthen, C. (1985). Neuroembryology and the development of perceptual mechanisms. In F. Faulkner & J. M. Tanner (Eds.), *Human growth* (2nd ed., pp. 301–383). Plenum.

Trevarthen, C. (2017). Maternal voice and communicative musicality: Sharing the meaning of life from before birth. In M. Filippa, P. Kuhn, & B. Westrup (Eds.), *Early vocal contact and preterm infant brain development: Bridging the gaps between research and practice* (pp. 3–23). Springer.

Trevarthen, C., Aitken, K. J., Vandekerckhove, M., Delafield-Butt, J., & Nagy, E. (2006). Collaborative regulations of vitality in early childhood: Stress in intimate relationships and postnatal psychopathology. In D. Cicchetti & D. J. Cohen (Eds.), *Developmental psychopathology: Vol. 2, Developmental neuroscience* (2nd ed., pp. 65–126). Wiley.

Trevarthen, C., & Delafield-Butt, J. T. (2017). Development of consciousness. In B. Hopkins, E. Geangu, & S. Linkenauger (Eds.), *Cambridge encyclopedia of child development* (2nd ed., pp. 821–835). Cambridge University Press.

Tronick, E. (2007). *The neurobehavioral and social-emotional development of infants and children.* W. W. Norton.

Tsakiris, M. (2010). My body in the brain: A neurocognitive model of body-ownership. *Neuropsychologia 48*(3), 703–712. https://doi.org/10.1016/j.neuropsychologia.2009.09.034

Tsakiris, M. (2017). The multisensory basis of the self: From body to identity to others. *Quarterly Journal of Experimental Psychology, 70*, 597–609. https://doi.org/10.1080/17470218.2016.1181768

Valizadeh, A., & Madadi Asl, M. (2023). Synaptic plasticity during brain development: Implications for therapeutic reorganization of neural circuits. In *Encyclopedia of child and adolescent health* (pp. 14–24). Academic Press. https://doi.org/10.1016/B978-0-12-818872-9.00128-X

Van der Hart, O., Nijenhuis, E.R.S., & Steele, K. (2006). *The haunted self: Structural dissociation and the treatment of chronic traumatization.* New York: W. W. Norton.

Venkatraman, A., Edlow, B. L., & Immordino-Yang, M. H. (2017). The brainstem in emotion: A review. *Frontiers in Neuroanatomy, 11*(15), 1–12. https://doi.org/10.3389/fnana.2017.00015

Verdult, R. (2021). Prenatal roots of attachment. In: K. Evertz, L. Janus, & R. Linder (Eds.), *Handbook of prenatal and perinatal psychology*. Cham: Springer. https://doi.org/10.1007/978-3-030-41716-1_14

Verny, T. R. (2021). *The embodied mind: Understanding the mysteries of cellular memory, consciousness, and our bodies*. Pegasus Books.

Weinstein, A. D. (2016). *Prenatal development and parents' lived experience: How early events shape our psychophysiology and relationship*. W. W. Norton.

Yochman, A., & Pat-Horenczyk, R. (2019). Sensory modulation in children exposed to continuous traumatic stress. *Journal of Child and Adolescent Trauma, 13*, 93–102. https://doi.org/10.1007/s40653-019-00254-4

Zernicka-Goetz, M., & Highfield, R. (2020). *The dance of life: Symmetry, cells and how we become human*. Ebury Publishing.

PART 2

Symptomatology, Assessment, and Diagnosis

12
SYMPTOMATOLOGY

Betsy de Thierry

Introduction to Complex Trauma Symptoms

With years of research put into the etiology of trauma, we now know that symptoms of complex trauma manifest as a result of experiencing interpersonal traumatic events that are repetitive and cumulative and often disrupt critical periods of development (Boyer et al., 2022; Draijer & Langeland, 1999; Haferkamp et al., 2015; Herman, 1997; Cook et al., 2003). Complex trauma negatively impacts the child's development of identity and sense of self, disrupts their ability to trust appropriately, and hinders their ability to naturally operate with emotional regulation, which causes them to experience an overactive sympathetic nervous system, frequently leading to risky or impulsive behaviors and self-soothing coping mechanisms. When a child is exposed to terrifying, traumatic experiences with the absence of a positive attachment relationship, they can form an inability to trust others and present with behaviors that are defensive and rooted in self-protection, alongside demonstrating a lack of the intuitive concept of relational safety. Subconscious defense mechanisms may become embedded, due to the repetitive terrifying experiences of powerlessness with adults who should be caring for them. In 2005, the term *developmental trauma disorder* was proposed to be included within the DSM-5 (van der Kolk, 2005) to elucidate the symptoms of complex trauma in childhood that indicated an interruption to the healthy development of the child in their early years. The exposure to traumatic experiences in these early years of rapid growth and development is associated with enduring symptoms that are interrelated with attachment trauma (Liotti, 1992; Schore, 2001).

Introduction to Symptoms of Dissociation

Dissociation is intrinsically connected to complex trauma due to its purpose of providing a way for a child to survive what seems intolerable, overwhelming, or a threat to their life. It is seen as an automatic, primitive, non-conscious defense mechanism and as a characterological adaptation to trauma and inner organization. Researchers "indicate that infants arrive in the world with their behavior organized into a set of half a dozen or so discrete states that cycle around feeding and sleeping," and as they develop, more discrete states are added to create complex "behavioral architecture" (Putnam, 1997, p. 14). If the child finds responsible caregivers who support them in maintaining organization of these discrete states in the face of tension and distress, then later on, the child will be able to participate in the modulation of their own arousal, and the result will be the emergence of a coherent inner organization (Sroufe, 1982). When an infant experiences trauma, then the child can be unable to integrate these states and instead find that they separate themselves psychologically from the experience of terror, shame, and powerlessness in circumstances in which they cannot separate physically. However, the child can subsequently have an automatic dissociative reaction whenever danger is later sensed. Dissociation is a survival mechanism that seems to be little understood or spoken of in the full sense of the definition. Şar (2014) affirmed the lack of research into this specific area of psychological trauma symptoms and saw the impact on adults traumatized as children. He stated that "dissociation is the ultimate form of human response to chronic developmental stress because patients with dissociative disorders report the highest frequency of childhood abuse and neglect among all psychiatric disorders" (p. 171). Dissociation occurs when the child is unable to integrate their experiences and emotional responses, due either to terror or the lack of the adult's ability to naturally support the integration of experience with comfort, co-regulation, and emotional attuned language.

On a continuum of experience and phenomena, dissociation may be understood as mild and not maladaptive—for example, when a child watches TV, has imaginary friends, or enjoys some time gaming online or role playing. "Normative dissociation" may be understood as a child daydreaming in the classroom or staring at the TV without moving when their name is called. It could be when they are lost in their imaginary play and seem irritated about taking off their costume and "coming out of character" to sit for a meal. When the child occasionally zones out, it is not abnormal, particularly when they have had a busy, productive day at preschool or school and need to relax and reduce multiple stimulations. In these circumstances, dissociation is used as the ability to be single-focused and absorbed in one activity, with conscious knowledge and intention. Dissociation becomes problematic, however, when the behavior becomes intrusive, interruptive, and an automatic, unconscious reaction to any threat or perceived threat. The zoned-out, daydreaming child who seems forgetful and sometimes impulsive or erratic may be in a survival state with highly developed automatic mechanisms to avoid feeling emotions or sensations in their body. They may be automatically "switching off" their sight, smell, or hearing or instinctively taking a bird's eye view of what is happening around them. An older child may flop or faint frequently and dramatically for no apparent reason. They may be switching presenting "parts" while they hear loud voices and chaos inside their heads, or they may have partial amnesia, not remembering experiences or sections of their life. The reality is that many children have a highly developed and complex dissociative system of survival; professionals may suggest that they are "in their own world," are being manipulative or lazy, and do not understand the severity of distress their symptoms indicate. More observable symptoms include the child presenting as spaced out or dreamy, or they may be staring with a blank expression. They may be talking to someone who is not there, or they may speak about something that sounds like their own elaborate and detailed imaginary world. In this way, dissociation enables the child to continue, in some way, with the daily routine of life, school, and what is perceived as "normal," including completing many of the tasks expected of them, despite the traumatic experiences that they may be simultaneously enduring. Some can hide their levels of distress and turmoil in a way that is almost completely impossible for them to verbalize. This subsequently enables the child to retain some aspects of their life that they deem vital, such as going to school or playing with toys, because dissociation is hidden from most of the adults and peers behind confusing and slightly strange behaviors that are usually misunderstood or misinterpreted.

Some children find that if they fight back or cry for help when, for example, they are being abused or undergoing a medical intervention, the adult could become angry or violent or hurt them further. This escalating threat and terror could cause them to be further disconnected from the adults whom they feel they so desperately need to stay alive. Similarly, if the child cannot regulate their other trauma symptoms, such as hypervigilance, agitation, or aggression, they learn quickly that dissociation effectively reduces the perceived threat of frightening adult attention. The mechanism of dissociation is frequently hidden from the adults around them due to a lack of understanding of the subtle symptoms of dissociation and its internal subjective experience and mechanisms. The child would rarely be able to articulate their coping mechanisms, and unless asked, they would rarely share what to them is experienced as normal. However, they may be aware that "something is not quite right" and they are usually aware that their experience is often one where they have "feelings of constant conflict and overwhelm, often with no real sense of why, accompanied by many sorts of strange behaviors and memory problems, all because what started as a survival method becomes a dysfunctional division of the self" (de Thierry, 2020, p. 62). The child may not feel safe enough even to begin to contemplate these coping mechanisms unless there are adults around them who have the capacity and strength to both ask about them and support them in their exploration.

The Three Types of Trauma

The research around complex trauma, or developmental trauma, widely acknowledges that "complex traumatic experiences" for a child usually means exposure to two or more of the following forms of trauma exposure: sexual, physical, or emotional abuse, domestic violence, neglect, severe caregiver impairment, and school or community violence (Kisiel et al., 2009, p. 148). It is noted that complex trauma is an ongoing or repeated experience, rather than a one-off experience or short-term traumatic period where there was a degree of emotional support, described as Type I trauma (Terr, 1991). Type 2 trauma is described as chronic traumatic experiences that are prolonged and repeated, leading to further stressors, where symptoms are more hidden or multilayered (Terr, 1991). Solomon and Heide (1999) further developed this categorization to add Type 3 trauma, which is described as experiences that are multiple, pervasive, or violent, which begin at an early age and continue over a long period of time. Type 2 and 3 traumas are considered more complex forms of trauma; Solomon and Heide (1999) described the common symptoms of complex trauma as

> alterations in memory and consciousness, frequently including dissociation; emotional numbing; major developmental deficits; poorly developed, often fragmented, sense of self; a core belief that he or she is fatally flawed and has no right to be alive; a sense of hopelessness and shame; trust issues that interfere with normal relationships; and no concept of a future.
> *(p. 202)*

Children who have experienced complex trauma consistently present with more widespread behavioral difficulties compared with those children who were exposed to traumatic events of less severity, such as those that were non interpersonal or acute traumatic experiences (Wamser-Nanney & Vandenberg, 2013). Though not identified in the DSM-5, complex trauma is now included within the ICD-11 (International Classification of Diseases, 11th revision), defined as:

> arising after exposure to an event or series of events of an extremely threatening or horrific nature, most commonly prolonged or repetitive events from which escape is difficult or impossible (for example, torture, slavery, genocide campaigns, prolonged domestic violence, repeated childhood sexual or physical abuse.
> *(World Health Organization, 2018, Code 6B41)*

Dissociation Continuum

The dissociation continuum illustrates the range of dissociative symptoms, from "normal," adaptive behaviors at one end to the opposite, where the maladaptive mechanisms have increased in their complexity and severity and have an increasingly negative impact on functioning. Dissociative amnesia,

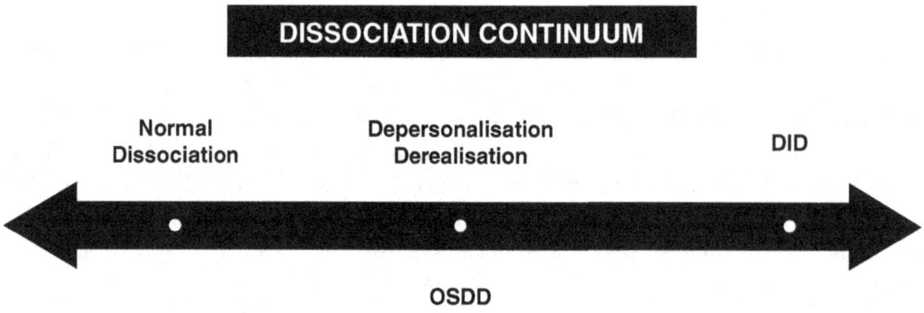

DISSOCIATION CONTINUUM

```
  Normal          Depersonalisation
  Dissociation    Derealisation              DID

  <----------•---------------•---------------•---------->

                       OSDD
```

Figure 12.1 Dissociation Continuum.

depersonalization, derealization, identity confusion, and identity alterations are explored further in this chapter and are core phenomena of dissociative psychopathology, which can be viewed on this spectrum of severity (Figure 12.1).

The continuum enables an exploration of what could be happening for the child internally in response to their external experiences. If they are offered attuned, co-regulating, emotionally nurturing, and soothing relational support that is consistent, the severity of the symptoms could de-escalate back along the continuum as the child is supported and enabled to express, make meaning, and accept their feelings or needs. However, if their distress is left undetected or unattended to and is ongoing and pervasive, the child will remain terrified and in inexpressible overwhelm, and escalate to the furthest end of the continuum, into a further separation of their self into distinct parts that can be necessary to survive the overwhelming experiences that they are enduring.

A child's "disordered experience of self" is due to instinctive survival mechanisms in the presence of attachment terror. It may be considered an adaptive response to maladaptive conditions and experiences. This internal damage to the psyche does not have to lead to long-term turmoil if early signs of distress and dissociation are recognized and intervention is given to enable the child to develop emotional safety and positive, nurturing attachment figures.

In the middle of the continuum are derealization and depersonalization symptoms. Depersonalization is a survival mechanism that enables a child to not have to cope with the feeling of physical pain in abuse, torture, hunger, turmoil, or devastation by disconnecting from mental processes, the self, the body, or the senses via numbing and detachment.

> Derealization enables the child to block out the reality of the here and now and can allow them to escape in their minds to a place where either things are more blurred, more numb or where they don't have to realize how awful their experience is because it would be too much to cope with. The experience doesn't seem real and so can't be happening, so they create some method to be able to survive it without really 'being there'.
>
> *(de Thierry, 2020, p. 52)*

Both these dissociative symptoms are easily misdiagnosed and misunderstood, leaving children unable to move into emotional safety, and will be further explored later in this chapter.

At the furthest end of the dissociative continuum is dissociative identity disorder, which includes the psychological compartmentalization of experience, affect, memory, and emotions outside of conscious memory in different self-states with different roles and identities. This diagnosis was renamed from multiple personality disorder and, despite the media fascination, is evidenced to be an effective subconscious mechanism that has enabled children to survive unbearable turmoil and terror.

Symptomatology

The etiology of dissociation was viewed by Putnam (1997) as a defense mechanism with three major tasks: "a) the automatization of behavior in the face of psychologically overwhelming circumstances; b) compartmentalization of painful affects and memories; and c) estrangement from self in the face of potential annihilation" (pp. 67–75).

Introduction to Symptom Domains

As mentioned earlier, dissociative symptoms cannot be separated from the experience and symptoms of complex trauma. Researchers and practitioners suggest that there are multiple common domains of symptoms that occur in childhood following experiences of complex trauma. Cook et al. (2003) suggested that there are six domains: physiological, behavioral, biological, cognitive, self, and relational dysregulation. In 2005, Cook and colleagues developed symptom sub-groups common to the experience of complex trauma, and notably, two other domains were added: dissociation and attachment. This became eight primary domains of symptomology: attachment, biology, affect regulation, dissociation (i.e., alterations in consciousness), behavioral regulation, cognition, and self-concept (Cook et al., 2005, p. 2). Within these sub-groups, they noted five broader categories. These five domains of symptoms of complex trauma are "(a) self-regulation, attachment, anxiety, and affective disorders in infancy and childhood; (b) addictions, aggression, social helplessness, and eating disorders; (c) dissociative, somatoform, cardiovascular, metabolic, and immunological disorders; (d) sexual disorders in adolescence and adulthood; and (e) revictimization" (Cook et al., 2005, p. 7).

It is vital to remember what is regarded as a normal developmental pathway for a healthy child when reflecting on the symptoms of complex trauma. Children who have not experienced complex trauma travel a developmental pathway that includes the healthy development of one's

> physiology and brain; the ability to identify, tolerate, control and appropriately express emotions, impulses and bodily sensations; to concentrate, learn and engage in goal-directed behavior; to form a positive and cohesive sense of self, meaningful values and hopeful future outlook; to cultivate secure and healthy attachment bonds, sustain intimate relationships, safely negotiate conflict and communicate their needs; and to interpret social cues accurately, set healthy personal boundaries and differentiate safe from threatening situations and interactions with peers and adults.
>
> *(Spinazzola et al., 2013, p. 8)*

Categories of Dissociative Symptoms

As indicated on the dissociative continuum, there is a range of severity of dissociative reactions to trauma. Dissociative symptoms at the entry point of the continuum can occur during an experience of psychological shock as an instinctive survival mechanism. This can then develop and become a habitual reaction when a threat is sensed. If the child has access to positive, nurturing attachment figures, they develop self-regulation skills through repetitive, consistent, and dependable experiences of co-regulation and soothing. Co-regulation may be understood as when an adult is able to attune, validate, and regulate together with a child until the child learns to internalize the process and automatically follows the same pattern independently, and is an essential element to healthy childhood development and the recovery from complex trauma. Consistent care, co-regulation, and attunement from caregiving and attachment figures lead to a reduction of the need for dissociation as a coping mechanism. If the child continues to feel emotionally unsafe and the feelings of shock, terror, and powerlessness remain, the dissociative symptoms that become normalized for them may develop in complexity, moving to the middle of the continuum. When a child experiences prolonged threat and a lack of emotional safety, they can remain in a state of psychological shock, where habitual dissociative reactions can create the pathway for the development of a dissociative disorder. There is agreement that pathological dissociation is thought to begin in childhood, with roots in infancy, usually between the ages of 6 months and 12 years (Putnam, 1991).

Silberg (2012) identified five classes of symptoms related to dissociation, which are

[p]erplexing shifts of consciousness, i.e., 'feeling in a fog,' momentary lapses of consciousness, flashback; [v]ivid hallucinatory experiences, i.e., hearing voices, seeing imaginary entities, or vivid imaginary friends; [m]arked fluctuation in knowledge, moods, or patterns of behavior and relating, i.e., feeling that moods have a 'mind of their own,' and skills and abilities are inconsistent, and the sense of self is divided; [p]erplexing memory lapses for one's own behavior and recently experienced events, i.e., cannot remember behavior, cannot remember assignments; and abnormal somatic experiences, i.e., self-harming behaviors, pain sensitivity, bowel or bladder incontinence.

(p. 36)

Additionally, Choi and colleagues (2018) list the following dissociative symptoms in children within the parent's guide to dissociation in The National Center for Child Trauma Stress Network (Choi et al., 2018):

- Amnesia for important or traumatic events known to have occurred,
- Frequent dazed or trance-like states,
- Perplexing forgetfulness (e.g., the child knows facts or skills one day and not the next),
- Rapid, profound age regression,
- Difficulties deriving cause-and-effect consequences from life experiences,
- Lying or denying responsibility for misbehavior despite obvious evidence to the contrary,
- Repeatedly referring to self in the third person,
- Unexplained injuries/recurrent self-injurious behavior,
- Vivid imaginary companionship that controls the child's behavior (i.e., passive influence experiences),
- Auditory and visual hallucinations,
- Flashbacks.

The various symptom categorizations share common themes of physical and somatoform symptoms, cognitive and psychoform symptoms, confusing behavior symptoms, and symptoms connected to their sense of self. These symptoms can differ in presentation according to the child's age, and this shall be highlighted in the coming pages.

Subtle Symptom Indicators of Dissociation in Children

While some symptoms can be distinguished across ages, there can be overlap across ages depending on the child's experiences and age at which they occurred. In young and preadolescent children, the following symptoms may be observed or identified through screening and assessment.

Young and Preschool-Aged Children

Research regarding dissociative symptoms in preschool and younger children indicates that infants and very young children are more prone to dissociation because they don't have the functional coping

Symptomatology

mechanisms to handle fearful or stressful situations independently (Perry, 2001; Solomon & George, 1999). A positive attachment figure is tasked with reducing the impact of a traumatic or stressful situation, and the absence of one or the presence of a terrifying or terrified attachment figure can escalate the symptoms of terror, rather than support resolution. Waters (2005) asserted that it is vital to understand the role and symptoms of disorganized attachment in dissociative children as "crucial to early detection and intervention of dissociative processes with pre-school children" (p. 2). According to Putnam et al. (1993), the following are understood to be indicators of suspicion of dissociative symptoms in preschool children:

- Staring, spacing out or trance-like states, including inattention
- Amnesia, such as forgetting important past events or conversations
- Extreme fluctuations in emotions and behaviors, including "regressive behaviors"
- Rigid play themes and overcontrolling behaviors
- Dissociative states that are not fully formed and may be understood as transitional identities, which Silberg (2021a, 2021b) states may include "internal voices, referring to themself in the third person and imaginary playmates that go beyond what is normative for young children" (p. 10).

Cintron and colleagues (2018) interviewed parents of young children who had dissociative reactions and adaptations after trauma, to ascertain the symptom presentation. They reported that the children were easily triggered into emotional overwhelm, often observed to be in their own world (i.e., spaced out or shut down), experienced flashbacks during which they seemed to be re-experiencing the traumatic experience (i.e., yelling specific words or having body movements that indicated a past experience was being remembered physically), or were unresponsive.

Case example: *Little Mya would often sit strapped in her pushchair, silently staring at the people in the café while her mom chatted with friends. Occasionally, she would arch her back and scream as if in pain, and a soother was forcefully put in her mouth while she resisted and then flopped again, staring silently.*

School-Aged Children

When asked, children often describe their complex coping mechanisms in simplistic language to adults, who remain unaware that they're describing important trauma and turmoil symptoms. Children often say things like, "In my head, I go to my land where I am in charge," or "When I don't like it, I just switch off that part of my body with my magic switch," or "It's my clever friend who stops bad things happening" when referring to an imaginary friend. In school-aged children, the following symptoms may be observed or identified through screening and assessment:

- Automatic behaviors while being dazed or staring.
- Speaking of a memory and describing watching from the ceiling or outside their body.
- A glazed look or blanking out for periods of time.
- Eyes flickering or fluttering in conversation, with a following change in presentation.
- Reports of hearing voices.
- Communication of visual hallucinations, such as objects changing size or shape.
- The presence of invisible friends or imaginary companions.
- Memory problems of specific experiences or choices/amnesia.
- Sexually inappropriate behavior.
- Speaking about themselves as "we."
- Depersonalization or derealization.

- Emotional dysregulation and mood switches that seem to come from nowhere.
- Physical violence toward those they love and shame following.
- Changes of preference, ability, interest, clothing style, or voice.
- Accusations of lying.
- Regressive behavior, including sudden changes in voice and posture change.
- Denial of outbursts, including ones that have been witnessed/recorded.
- Little long-term progress made with verbal or cognitive therapy or mentoring.
- Saying they don't feel anything, emotionally or physically.
- Saying they don't feel like "themselves."
- A feeling that everything around them is unreal, like they are in a dream.
- Feeling floaty.
- Feeling as if other people are not real or that they are like robots.
- Feeling as if there are different people inside them.
- Speaking about "going up to fly" or "not being there for a bit," despite being physically present.
- Flashbacks.
- Self-destructive behaviors or self-harm.

Client example: *Susan, aged 10, often came to therapy speaking in a voice that made her sound much younger. She would then change her tone of voice and become reflective while using the sand tray. She used insightful, mature words and had an ability to speak about the voices in her head and the landscape where different people who directed her time inhabited different houses and areas. She spoke of the pain in her head when the voices disagreed and the impact on her ability to complete homework in time or move her body to respond to her mom's call for dinner. Susan cried about how she kept getting into trouble and had to lie because she did not know how to explain herself but was stuck and felt hopeless.*

Other Symptom Clusters

According to Fisher (2017),

> [f]eeling helpless, overwhelmed, inadequate, vulnerable, terrified, and alone, the lived experience is that there is nowhere to turn, nowhere to hide, no one to help. The only resources upon which everyone can draw reside in the body: disconnection, numbing, dissociation, neurochemicals such as adrenaline and endorphins, and the animal defense survival responses such as fight, flight, freeze and submit, and attach for survival. These are 'desperate times calling for desperate measures'.
>
> *(p. 126)*

Depersonalization

Depersonalization can present in preschool, young, and school-aged children as being unaware of physical feelings in their bodies. Young children may struggle to learn to use the toilet or seem oblivious to normal physical needs that are apparent to others around them, like messy fingers or very wet socks. Preschool and school-aged children may suddenly rush to use the bathroom; they may injure themselves and not notice the blood or bruise and not show any pain or distress; they may not realize they are hungry or may not notice that they are full and therefore become unwell. They may create drawings of themselves without clearly indicating their skin, outer edges, or firm boundaries of the body. They may describe themselves as not having needs that other children have and shrug their shoulders if they are offered food or drink, and they may be compliant and people-pleasing. School-aged children with depersonalization symptoms may be unfamiliar with their image in a mirror and may not recognize or notice themselves, be surprised by their shadow, or be fascinated by making any marks or imprints with their body, as if it is a surprise. The child can react in this way because their experience may be that of feeling weightless, not in or disconnected from their body, or disorientated in their body, and they may appear to others as clumsy or disorientated. While young children may stare blankly, older children can exhibit trance-like behaviors that include self-harm or compulsive masturbation to check that they still have physical sensations and are alive.

Depersonalization and Self-Harm

When a child has developed depersonalization as a survival mechanism, they can be drawn to cutting, banging their head, picking their skin, and hurting themselves in any way to relieve the experience of numbness or internal turmoil that they feel. A young child may harm themselves when they are in a state of numbness or a trance-like state by banging their head against a wall or throwing themselves on the floor with force. They may harm themselves due to feelings of frustration or anger about what they feel they have done or had done to them, or to feel in control of their body when they have felt powerless over what happens to it. As the child becomes older, they may also self-injure to gain the help, support, or empathy they need when they cannot use words to describe their emotional or invisible agony. These subthemes indicate that self-injury is an attempt to cope with distress by self-soothing or facilitating them back into the window of tolerance from being hyper-aroused due to trauma-related cues or stressors or hypo-aroused due to dissociation. Please see Chapter 41 for more information.

Depersonalization, Feeling Numb, Encopresis, and Enuresis

When asked, children may describe themselves as floaty or spacey and unable to "tie themselves down" to be able to think, despite adults asking them to do so, and often, this can lead them to underperform in education and be labeled as lazy, inattentive, or not trying. They may struggle to complete a task, lose their train of thought, be unaware of their lack of ability to concentrate, and therefore lie and make up reasons to make sense of the behavior to themselves and others. Proper screening and assessment that is done in an age-appropriate manner allows for a deeper understanding of what is happening for the child and discern whether the child is experiencing symptoms of depersonalization. The symptom of depersonalization may occur to manage overwhelm or when the needs of a child are not being met, resulting in them feeling paralyzed by feelings of terror (Simeon et al., 2001). For example, if we use the polyvagal theory to understand the behavior of an infant who is in a state of hyper-arousal and danger is neurocepted, we know that the sympathetic nervous system edges its limit with no escape in sight. Threat to life may then be neurocepted, with a child suddenly becoming silent, staring blankly, and stopping all movement as they shift into a parasympathetic dorsal vagal state, where they feel "scared to death." The lack of available help brings a child to the peak of terror, which becomes too overwhelming, and consequently, the child dissociates from their surroundings to survive. This instinctive dissociation from their body and inner sensations causes the child to overlook external cues such as the voice or movement of a caregiver, because their survival energy is internalized and focused on staying alive. This leads to an automatic series of somatic functions slowing down to keep the body alive, such as breathing, heart rate, and body moving to a low metabolic state.

When a child of any age is experiencing significant terror, powerlessness, and overwhelm, they may be unable to feel those powerful emotions within their smaller frame without a sense of implosion.

This can lead to a disconnection from inner experiences and sensations so they can continue with their daily activities, engaging somewhat of an "automatic pilot" and moving through experiences without any conscious thought or feeling. Waters (2016) explained that during these moments, "the child is not fully aware of what she is really experiencing and may become numb and depersonalized" (p. 9). When the child cannot feel or connect to their body, they are less aware of their primitive bodily functions, such as the need for the toilet, and consequently can experience encopresis and enuresis. They may bump into others or objects, pick their skin, and not be aware of bleeding, bruises, or physical pain. They may feel as if they have a part of their body missing, present as mute or deaf, grow stiff or faint, have strong reactions to smell and taste, or display conversive symptoms such as psychogenic non-epileptic seizures (please see Chapter 43). Parents or caregivers may report a need to take spare clothes with them when they go out in case their school-aged child has a wetting or soiling accident, despite them being fully capable of age-appropriate toilet use most of the time.

Case example: *John was 9 years old when he told adults around him that he didn't need to feel scared of the pain that bullies caused anymore and demonstrated this with a sense of pride by banging his head against the wall and not feeling anything. He was unable to control his bladder and bowels, and the pediatrician found no physiological explanation for this.*

Depersonalization and Eating Behaviors

Depersonalization can also impact eating, with children of all ages potentially being unable to easily swallow, taste, or chew their food due to not feeling their bodily sensations and feeling disorientated about the task. They may not experience the feeling of being full or hungry and may demonstrate confusion about appropriate quantities and times to eat. This sensitivity may be viewed as fussy eating or develop into eating disorders. Waller and colleagues (2003) found that dissociative symptoms are more common in individuals with an eating disorder. Nilsson et al. (2020) researched the correlation between eating disorders and dissociation and found that participants with eating disorders reported a greater extent of both psychoform and somatoform dissociation compared with the non-clinical sample. Analyses also showed a correlation between the degree of dissociation and the severity of eating disorder symptoms. Some researchers argue that high levels of dissociation seem to be linked to more severe eating symptoms (Nilsson et al., 2020).

Derealization

Derealization may be described as an automatic subconscious response whereby the world feels unreal, or the person may experience "the sense of loss of reality of the immediate environment" (Putnam, 1997, p. 86).

It is a disconnection from the world around oneself, and a child may appear dazed or zoned out or struggle to articulate their experience of being unaware that they have "gone somewhere" but may use words such as "I'm back now—I'm not sure where I went." When asked, children may report that they find that the world looks foggy, blurry, far away, or as if seen through glasses that are misty. Some people describe seeing the world as if they are detached or as if they were watching a movie (Steinberg & Steinberg, 1995). As a result, children may struggle with concentration, how and where they fit in the world, and how others view them.

Derealization may be understood as a distressing experience characterized by a kind of separation from the external world, or the child's sense of place in their world. A preschool child who has derealization symptoms may persistently play alone and either resist or look confused at other children who are full of energy, but also may move suddenly from staring or looking blank in a frozen bodily state to exhibiting tantrums or behavior that seems disproportionate to the environment or surroundings.

Symptomatology

A young child may be observed to stare blankly, even with adults moving around them, and be described as a "good" infant or baby because they seem to be compliant, make little fuss, or seem undisturbed by the chaos around them. A school-aged child may display similar symptoms alongside being called *dysregulated, volatile, or in their own world* (emphasis added by author).

Depersonalization and Derealization in Self-Perception

The self-perception or self-experience of children struggling with symptoms of depersonalization and/or derealization is altered, leading to a profound disruption in self-awareness and self-consciousness. Liu et al. (2022) found that implicit self-esteem was impaired, and stated:

> When they evaluated themselves, they did not think it was their own evaluation but that of a bystander, leading to abnormal self-cognition. They lack the ability to perceive themselves accurately, which promotes their negative evaluation of themselves. They may feel estranged from one's own image when looking in the mirror and present with a strong sense of self-separation. The ability to identify oneself and distinguish between 'self' and 'not-self' is critical to many higher-order cognitive abilities, such as self-awareness and theory of mind.
>
> (p. 8)

Young children may seem to be confused about who they are in relation to others due to struggling to integrate both the experiences of themselves with friends and adults alongside memories of previous experiences, positive or negative. Older children may describe their life feeling like it is moving in slow motion, as though they are walking through fog every day and their energy is taken up trying to survive, just so they tolerate the lack of clarity and firmness in the world around them and how they fit within it. This can lead them to be isolated or to struggle with relationships.

Depersonalization seems to be more commonly represented in research and papers, while derealization is less discussed as an individual symptom. Depersonalization disorder and depersonalization/derealization disorder (DPDR) are now considered synonymous. Childhood interpersonal trauma, particularly emotional abuse, may play a role in the pathogenesis of depersonalization/derealization disorder (Simeon et al., 2001). Based on two-factor data analyses from large samples of persons with depersonalization disorder (Sierra, 2009), as cited in Dell (2011), argues that depersonalization disorder has four clusters of symptoms: first, anomalous body experiences, such as hallucinations or strange behavior that is beyond an age-appropriate imagination. Second, emotional numbing, where the child may have flat affect and seem unaffected by positive or negative experiences. Third, anomalous subjective recall, where the child may be describing something alarming but shows little appropriate emotional response to the words. Fourth, alienation from surroundings, where the child seems detached from their environment and unfamiliar with what is actually a familiar setting. Sierra (2009) also states that depersonalization is rarely diagnosed, and "the average person with DPDR spends 12 years in the mental health system before receiving the correct diagnosis" (p. 401). Research indicates that trauma, specifically emotional maltreatment, is the most frequent predisposing factor and trigger (O'Laoide et al., 2018; Simeon et al., 2001). Children can additionally experience depersonalization or derealization due to sudden stress or shock without it becoming a disorder, lending to why thorough assessment of symptoms is so important.

Dissociative Amnesia or Memory Confusion

Amnesia refers to the frightening experience of not remembering an event or a situation in time. It is a lack of ability to recall important information, often a specific time period, such as when a child attended a certain school, lived in a particular area, went on a trip, or regularly visited a relative each week. Amnesia exists on a continuum, ranging from the loss of a memory of minutes, days, weeks, or years of one's life, often of a specific experience of abuse or terror, and can develop into significant memory confusion. It is disconcerting and can cause anxiety and confusion and feels different from normal memory loss regarding a specific fact or conversation. Amnesia, or loss of time, may cause a child to suddenly look blank, confused, and disorientated about where they are or what may be happening. Children of all ages may find themselves trying to cover up for their lack of memory or confusion about what has happened. Older children can "lose time" in school and get into trouble for not being in the right place at the right time.

Case example: *"When taking her out, she would be walking quite nicely with me and would then suddenly run at strangers, growling, and screaming. During one outing, we were in a shop when she suddenly started to grab all the items off a shelf and throw them on the floor. When I asked her to stop, she didn't seem to hear me. There was no defiance. She just didn't seem to be there. When she did 'come back,' she denied that it was her that had put all the things on the floor, and she ran off."*

Memory challenges can also occur due to the impact of threats of harm and resulting terror, leading children to urgently push experiences and affect away from conscious awareness to continue with daily life and maintain a good enough image of their caregiving system. The child's primitive need for attachment leads to an unsolvable inner dilemma, as each memory of abuse or terror threatens the ability to ensure such basic needs are met. Outside of conscious awareness, children instinctually learn to survive terrifying and threatening experiences in order to not be alone and without their attachment figures. If they hold the traumatic memories in their daily life, they may find daily life intolerable and relationships with adults too terrifying. Silberg (2012) suggested that "over time, children whose minds are basically practicing forgetting may display sporadic memory for many recently experienced events, leading them to forget their homework or even plans made with friends" (p. 45).

Children can get into trouble when they seem to have lost time, and the assumption is often made that they were not concentrating or they are lying, which leads to the symptom being less noted by those who come into contact with complexly traumatized children. Children with dissociative amnesia may try to hide or minimize their memory loss due to feelings of shame, leading them to think there is something wrong with them. Sometimes children with dissociative amnesia are found to be exhibiting symptoms of dissociative identity disorder.

Dissociative Identity Disorder (DID)

The International Society for the Study of Trauma and Dissociation (ISSTD, 2009) describes the etiology of DID as being interconnected with a child's sense of safety, as in order to feel safe, a child must separate trauma-derived emotions, physical sensations, or experiences completely from awareness into compartments of self that hold the disavowed emotions, sensations, or experiences. While symptoms of dissociation remain as invisible internal mechanisms to survive, they can quickly become visible when the child is triggered by sensory stimuli that serve as implicit or explicit reminders of the past, leading to sudden changes in emotion, behavior, abilities, and preferences. Children may suddenly change from being quiet to acting angry and aggressive, or from presenting as their biological age to regressing to a baby-like state needing comfort or becoming too old for their age. They may shift from being passionate about an interest to hating it and displaying no memory of enjoyment or skill in the activity or interest. They may engage in sexually inappropriate behavior and have no memory of it or be observed to crawl around like an animal but deny any memory of it.

Symptomatology

The sudden shift in behaviors and the lack of memory of some challenging behaviors can be the most perplexing and stressful symptoms of dissociation for most caregivers and professionals working with complexly traumatized children.

Shifts in behavior can be subtle and easy to miss in school-aged children and even harder to notice in preschool and young children due to the normative child developmental processes and the natural volatility of emotional expression in young children. However, distinctly erratic behaviors may be due to a mechanism that separates the self into different parts or states to contain different overwhelming experiences and affect. This separation of the self causes confusion, internal busyness, often with voices in their head, big feelings of shame about conflicting ways of being, a vague awareness of different presentations of ages, and an internal feeling of chaos. DID is at the most severe end of the dissociation continuum and may include all five of the dissociative symptom domains: amnesia and memory confusion, depersonalization and derealization, identity alternation with changes of presentation, and identity confusion that can become apparent as they grow from preschool to school age (Steinberg, 1994), though likely not enduring in pattern and thus not meeting the criteria for the adult DSM-5 diagnosis (Silberg, 2021 a, 2021b).

Every individual part or self-state has a specific purpose and was created to fulfill a need for the child to survive. Some states act as protectors and work hard to stop adults around them from knowing about their internal survival mechanism, so they protect "the internal team" and act either silly or angry to cause those wanting to help to stay at a safer distance. Some states are more skilled at being relational, and others present at different ages when a traumatic experience occurred. Those states may contain memories and emotions outside of conscious awareness to enable the child to continue to go through the daily routine. Sometimes a child finds comfort in a pet or a computer game character in the midst of the terror and develops a self-state that internalizes that familiar, comforting person or animal to find comfort. Research suggests that young children and preschool children are more likely to have cuddly toys that act as imaginary friends who become a separate state of the child and can engage in conversation with them (ISSTD, 2020). While it can seem hard to distinguish the difference between a young child and their age-appropriate fantasy play with soft toys, it is evident that the relationship of a dissociative child who needs their other self-states to survive can manifest terror or anger if there is any threat of the soft toy being removed.

Case example: *Joe, aged 7, was keen to explore his "inside family" in the therapy room, which included a pet dog who had been by the door while he was being sexually abused but was now part of his internal dissociative invisible world. He would frequently start to present as a dog in school and especially in times when he felt anxious, such as large gatherings of children. He would often begin growling and would then bite anything that he could see while falling to his knees to crawl. He would often have no memory of being in the dog state and would look blankly if there were any questions about it happening.*

When a child experiences relentless and terrifying situations without enough adult comfort, they can be unable to naturally integrate the normal "discrete states" of their mind, and they remain internally disconnected (please refer back to Chapter 3 on the Theory of Discrete Behavioral States). Alternatively, further separation develops into more distinct unintegrated parts, or states, in order to survive. While this compartmentalization enables survival, it may become problematic to functioning long term, adding to the sense of powerlessness and overwhelm as one aspect of them gets on with daily life with no obvious memory of the horrors they have seen and experienced, while other parts of them hold the details of the trauma, and the core organizers of the traumatic experiences. Dissociation and dissociative compartmentalization can be understood as ways to feel protected from the horrors of the trauma and the emotions, sensations, thoughts, and images that are connected to the trauma, though long term, they cause confusion (de Thierry, 2020).

Perpetrator Introjects

An internal, subconscious dissociative system or internal team is ultimately about surviving that which is intolerable. In order to survive, children of all ages who experience the horrors of abuse may non-consciously internalize their perpetrator's behaviors, feelings, or personality traits in a separate dissociative state called a *perpetrator introject*. This may be understood to be another attempt to reduce a sense of powerlessness by creating a part of them that can defend in the way they have learned through their own horrific experiences. These dissociative states hold the sensory and emotional memories of the abuse, but cause children to behave in ways that may lead others to see them as perpetrators rather than victims when complex dissociation is not fully understood. Waters (2016) explained that

> these states which are present within the dissociation system of the child are often those who hold the worst memories of abuse and turmoil. This state or states can be violent or aggressive or sexually inappropriate, often re-enacting experiences that have happened to them.
>
> (p. 180)

Sexually Inappropriate Behavior

The presence of perpetrator introjects may cause child victims to engage in concerning sexualized behaviors, which may have been normalized through abuse experiences. Children may report experiencing powerful but ambivalent feelings of relief about being touched and seen with a simultaneous, conflicting horror of it being through abuse. This may lead to compulsive masturbation as a means of self-soothing. Concerning sexualized behaviors in children are not a norm in childhood unless there has been the influence of inappropriate or abusive behavior from adults.

Sleep Difficulties

Protective avoidance and disconnection from memories of abuse can lead to sleep disruptions, with subconscious attempts of the mind to process the distressing experiences. Children may have terrifying nightmares that feel very vivid and may manifest from different dissociative states. Children may struggle with sleep as a result of internal chaos manifesting from different states that may need different times to be heard or to play. A complexly traumatized child may also struggle with sleep due to hyper-arousal, where they struggle to find a sense of calm away from a need for hypervigilance.

Case example: *He would wake up at night screaming in terror while shouting that we had to see the blood on his legs. There wasn't any blood, and yet this was a frequent nightmare, where his level of distress caused the whole house to wake up terrified too.*

Hyperactivity

While hypo-arousal and dissociation are symptoms commonly associated with complex trauma, children of all ages can display symptoms of hyper-arousal due to chronically activated stress hormones, leading to displays of agitation and disruptive behavior, significant startle responses, and difficulties sitting still or focusing. These two opposing symptom groupings vacillate and often take a child outside of their window of tolerance (Siegel, 2020), and may create a chaotic and confusing range of behaviors and emotional reactivity. Children struggle to regulate these big emotions, as they need the support of adults to do so, and, in turn, shift between hyper- and hypo-arousal, which may also be manifesting from different internal states. If the child receives negative attention, which activates increased shame, they may instinctively seek to avoid hyper-arousal behaviors and shift into hypo-aroused behaviors where they present as lethargic, depressed, quiet, withdrawn, floppy, dazed, or with a lack of ability to think or communicate easily.

Imaginary Playmates

Young children with dissociation are more likely to be found to have imaginary playmates that shift beyond what is developmentally normative. Silberg (2012) developed an imaginary companions' questionnaire that has been used by professionals working with distressed children. Through its use, it became evident that children with dissociative symptoms had more invisible companions "who were experienced as annoying, commanded the child and made the child do things the child did not want to do, did bad things and blamed the child, and fought with each other about the child" (p. 43). These children spoke about their imaginary friends as more than just imaginative, instead describing them as preoccupying their minds and wishing that some of them would go away. They reported feeling frustrated, as though they could not control them, and complained that they caused internal conflict (Silberg, 2012). Children who have experienced trauma sometimes speak of not being able to remember misbehaviors that they are accused of and blame them on the imaginary friend. Dissociation theory enables us to view imaginary friends as potentially different states of the personality that have been formed to contain certain traumatic experiences and memories. An invisible child can be invisible or a soft toy or a doll. It is important to make a distinction between an invisible friend and a transitional object, however. According to Huolman and Peltonen (2022),

> [t]ransitional objects and Imaginary Companion [IC] toys might both be important for the child, and they might be of comfort for the child. The child might also talk and listen to both. The distinction between a transitional object and an IC toy is that the child creates a distinct personality for the latter, and they (IC toys) have enduring human-like features.
>
> *(p. 1)*

Silberg (2021a, 2021b) coined the term *transitional identities* to help distinguish between developmentally normative imaginary friends and figures from those who hold the function of holding traumatic content. According to Silberg and Dallam (2022),

> these transitional identities are projected elements of the self to which a child attributes living characteristics and with whom they develop relationships. Some transitional identities may be internalized attachment figures, which provide a cushion of protection against the chaotic relationships experienced with their real caregivers. Other transitional identities may be the personification of feelings like anger and fear, or the internalization of the characteristics of abusive people in their environment, setting the stage for perpetrating self-states seen in older children and adults.
>
> *(p. 436)*

Regressed States and Hearing Voices

Children who operate with an internal dissociative system due to the neurobiological capacity to dissociate in the face of continual terror, helplessness, and threat can demonstrate regressed behaviors. Sometimes the regressed behavior is due to the intuitive understanding that younger children need more nurturing and gentle care, while other children mention that "voices told them to do things they don't want to do." It is recognized that in the case of a dissociative system having the presence of perpetrator introjects or protector parts, children may present with separate internal parts or states that both regress in age-appropriate behavior and present as voices that are often "in my head who can change [my] behavior." A child may be distracted by internal voices and may complain of headaches due to the feeling of internal chaos.

Emotion Regulation

Emotion regulation is a central element of growth and learning during the first decade of a child's life, and this development forms a foundation of emotional literacy and self-regulatory behaviors that enable children to form positive relationships and enjoy learning. Gross and Thompson (2007) viewed emotion regulation as a continuum from conscious, effortful, and controlled regulation to unconscious, effortless, and automatic regulation. Emotion dysregulation is seen as a core symptom of traumatic experiences. Complex trauma is defined as the impact of traumatic experiences that are too overwhelming to process easily, thus causing emotion dysregulation, and the use of dissociation as a survival mechanism and means of regulation. Silberg (2012) explained that "children may substitute one intense feeling state for another in a furtive avoidance dance, like someone walking on hot coals, jumping from one foot to another" (p. 149). Ford (2013) advocated for a vision of dissociation as a biologically based self-regulatory response to extreme emotions and suggests that fostering self-regulation abilities is essential to the treatment of dissociation. Dissociation was also conceptualized as an avoidance strategy used to face emotions that overwhelm internal affect regulation capacities following trauma (Briere et al., 2010). Therefore, while some scholars view dissociation as an emotion regulation strategy, other experts in the field tend to see it as a result of deficits in the ability to effectively self-regulate intense emotions. Hébert et al. (2018) hypothesized that deficits in emotion regulation precede the occurrence of dissociation symptoms. Overcontrolled children are thought to exert excessive control over their emotions and behaviors and are at risk for developing internalizing problems. However, under-controlled children tend to be less able to regulate themselves effortfully and are therefore at risk for developing externalizing problems (Eisenberg et al., 2010). Each symptom needs to be viewed from the perspective of how disruptive it is to the child's daily life and how much they cause them to "deviate from what is characteristic of normal phenomena" (ISSTD, 2003, p. 130).

Psychoform and Somatoform Symptoms

Nijenhuis (2017) introduced the concept of two different categories of dissociative symptoms—psychoform and somatoform—with research showing that dissociation can manifest in both manners (Nilsson et al., 2020). Somatoform dissociation comprises somatic experiences, such as a reduction in sensory perception and loss of the usually integrated functions of the body (i.e., loss of sensation, enuresis, and encopresis). School-aged children may have medically unexplained symptoms that cause distress and pain, resulting in hospital visits due to the severity of the distress, but no physical issue is found. Psychoform dissociation is a separation of the elements of the mind and encompasses dissociative amnesia, depersonalization, derealization, identity confusion, and identity alteration (Kienle et al., 2017).

The Interconnection of Shame

Shame and trauma are interconnected, and while shame can be a protective factor in the aftermath of a horrific traumatic experience, it can become toxic and create a perception of the self that is damaged, deficient, and unlovable. Shame is a subconscious belief that the child caused the terrifying event to occur because of something they did wrong or was wrong about them.

When shame is experienced, it functions as an urgent signal that danger is here: the danger of rejection, failure, exposure and abandonment. It is an experience rooted in interpersonal relationships. It threatens the very basic human experience of being alive and needing to belong, be loved, and be accepted.

(de Thierry, 2019, p. 15)

Shame will be more deeply explored in a separate chapter of this book, as well as the ways in which shame is connected to disorganized attachment as a pathway to dissociation and relational difficulties.

Conclusion

When the adults who work with and support children can grasp even the slightest possible symptom of complex trauma and dissociation, there is hope for the little lives as they develop into adulthood that they will recover from the suffering they have experienced. Noticing the subtle symptoms in a child that hide terrifying distress and overwhelming fear can change the path the child will walk for the rest of their lives. The journey of noticing, reflecting, being curious, and watching for patterns and abnormal reactions can become natural in our quest to help the most traumatized know emotional safety and recover from horrific trauma.

References

Boyer, S. M., Caplan, J. E., & Edwards, L. K. (2022). Trauma-related dissociation and the dissociative disorders: Neglected symptoms with severe public health consequences. *Delaware Journal of Public Health, 8*(2), 78–84. https://doi.org/10.32481/djph.2022.05.010

Briere, J., Hodges, M., & Godbout, N. (2010). Traumatic stress, affect dysregulation, and dysfunctional avoidance: A structural equation model. *Journal of Traumatic Stress, 23*(6), 767–774. https://doi.org/10.1002/jts.20578

Choi, K. R., Seng, J. S., Briggs, E. C., Munro-Kramer, M. L., Graham-Bermann, S. A., Lee, R., & Ford, J. D. (2018). *Dissociation and PTSD: What parents should know.* National Center for Child Traumatic Stress.

Cintron, G., Salloum, A., Blair-Andrews, Z., & Storch, E. A. (2018). Parents' descriptions of young children's dissociative reactions after trauma. *Journal of Trauma & Dissociation: The Official Journal of the International Society for the Study of Dissociation (ISSD), 19*(5), 500–513. https://doi.org/10.1080/15299732.2017.1387886

Cook, A., Blaustein, M., Spinazzola, J., & van der Kolk, B. (2003). Complex trauma in children and adolescents. White paper from the National Child Traumatic Stress Network, Complex Trauma Task Force. nctsn.org/resources/complex-trauma-children-and-adolescents

Cook, A., Spinazzola, J., Ford, J., Lanktree, C., Blaustein, M., Cloitre, M., DeRosa, R., Hubbard, R., Kagan, R., Liautaud, J., Mallah, K., Olafson, E., & van der Kolk, B. (2005). Complex trauma in children and adolescents. *Psychiatric Annals, 35*(5), 390–398. https://doi.org/10.3928/00485713-20050501-05

de Thierry, B. (2015). *Teaching the child on the trauma continuum.* Grosvenor House Publishing Limited.

de Thierry, B. (2019). *The simple guide to understanding shame.* Jessica Kingsley Publishers.

de Thierry, B. (2020). *The simple guide to complex trauma and dissociation.* Jessica Kingsley Publishers.

Dell, P. F. (2011). Review: *Depersonalization: A new look at a neglected syndrome*, by M. Sierra. *Journal of Trauma & Dissociation, 12*(4), 401–403. https://doi.org/10.1080/15299732.2011.573763

Draijer, N., & Langeland, W. (1999). Childhood trauma and perceived parental dysfunction in the etiology of dissociative symptoms in psychiatric inpatients. *American Journal of Psychiatry, 156*(3), 379–385. https://doi.org/10.1176/ajp.156.3.379

Eisenberg, N., Spinrad, T. L., & Eggum, N. D. (2010). Emotion-related self-regulation and its relation to children's maladjustment. *Annual Review of Clinical Psychology, 6*, 495–525. https://doi.org/10.1146/annurev.clinpsy.121208.131208

Fisher, J. (2017). *Healing the fragmented selves of trauma survivors overcoming self-alienation.* Routledge.

Ford, J. D. (2013). How can self-regulation enhance our understanding of trauma and dissociation? *Journal of Trauma & Dissociation, 14*(3), 237–250. https://doi.org/10.1080/15299732.2013.769398

Gross, J. J., & Thompson, R. A. (2007). Emotion regulation: Conceptual foundations. In J. J. Gross (Ed.), *Handbook of emotion regulation* (pp. 3–24). Guilford Press.

Haferkamp, L., Bebermeier, A., Möllering, A., & Neuner, F. (2015). Dissociation is associated with emotional maltreatment in a sample of traumatized women with a history of child abuse. *Journal of Trauma & Dissociation, 16*(1), 86–99. https://doi.org/10.1080/15299732.2014.959149

Hébert, M., Langevin, R., & Oussaïd, E. (2018). Cumulative childhood trauma, emotion regulation, dissociation, and behavior problems in school-aged sexual abuse victims. *Journal of Affective Disorders, 225*, 306–312. https://doi.org/10.1016/j.jad.2017.08.044

Herman, J. (1997). *Trauma and recovery: The aftermath of violence-from domestic abuse to political terror.* Basic Books.

Huolman, M., & Peltonen, K (2022). Dissociative features related to imaginary companions in the assessment of childhood adversity and dissociation: A pilot study. *European Journal of Trauma & Dissociation, 6*(4), Article 100295. https://doi.org/10.1016/j.ejtd.2022.100295

Institute for the Study of Trauma and Dissociation (ISSTD). (2009). FAQs for teachers. Retrieved March 25, 2020, from isst-d.org/resources/faqs-for-teachers

Institute for the Study of Trauma and Dissociation (ISSTD). (2020). Child and adolescent fact sheet for caregivers. Retrieved March 25, 2023, from https://www.isst-d.org/public-resources-home/child-adolescent-fact-sheet-for-caregivers/

Kienle, J., Rockstroh, B., Bohus, M., Fiess, J., Huffziger, S., & Steffen-Klatt, A. (2017). Somatoform dissociation and posttraumatic stress syndrome – Two sides of the same medal? A comparison of symptom profiles, trauma history and altered affect regulation between patients with functional neurological symptoms and patients with PTSD. *BMC Psychiatry, 17*, Article 248. https://doi.org/10.1186/s12888-017-1414-z

Kisiel, C., Fehrenbach, T., Small, L., & Lyons, J. S. (2009). Assessment of complex trauma exposure, responses, and service needs among children and adolescents in child welfare. *Journal of Child & Adolescent Trauma, 2*(3), 143–160. https://doi.org/10.1080/19361520903120467

Liotti, G. (1992). Disorganized/disoriented attachment in the etiology of the dissociative disorders. *Dissociation: Progress in the Dissociative Disorders, 5*(4), 196–204.

Liu, S., Jia, Y., Zheng, S., Feng, S., Zhu, H., Wang, R., & Jia, H. (2022). An experimental study of subliminal self-face processing in depersonalization-derealization disorder. *Brain Sciences, 12*(12), 1598. https://doi.org/10.3390/brainsci12121598

Nijenhuis, E. R. S. (2017). Ten reasons for conceiving and classifying posttraumatic stress disorder as a dissociative disorder. *European Journal of Trauma & Dissociation, 1*(1), 47–61. https://doi.org/10.1016/j.ejtd.2017.01.001

Nilsson, D., Lejonclou, A., & Holmqvist, R. (2020). Psychoform and somatoform dissociation among individuals with eating disorders. *Nordic Journal of Psychiatry, 74*(1), 1–8. https://doi.org/10.1080/08039488.2019.1664631

O'Laoide, A., Egan, J., & Osborn, K. (2018). What was once essential, may become detrimental: The mediating role of depersonalization in the relationship between childhood emotional maltreatment and psychological distress in adults. *Journal of Trauma & Dissociation: The Official Journal of the International Society for the Study of Dissociation (ISSD), 19*(5), 514–534. https://doi.org/10.1080/15299732.2017.1402398

Perry, B. D. (2001). The neurodevelopmental impact of violence in childhood. In D. Schetky & E. P. Benedek (Eds.), *Textbook of child and adolescent forensic psychiatry* (pp. 221–238). American Psychiatric Press.

Putnam, F. W. (1991). Dissociative disorders in children and adolescents. A developmental perspective. *The Psychiatric Clinics of North America, 14*(3), 519–531.

Putnam, F. W. (1997). *Dissociation in children and adolescents: A developmental perspective.* Guildford Press.

Putnam, F. W., Helmers, K., & Trickett, P. K. (1993). Development, reliability, and validity of a child dissociation scale. *Child Abuse & Neglect, 17*(6), 731–741. https://doi.org/10.1016/s0145-2134(08)80004-x

Şar, V. (2014). The many faces of dissociation: Opportunities for innovative research in psychiatry. *Clinical Psychopharmacology and Neuroscience: The Official Scientific Journal of the Korean College of Neuropsychopharmacology, 12*(3), 171–179. https://doi.org/10.9758/cpn.2014.12.3.171

Schore, A. N. (2001). Effects of a secure attachment relationship on right brain development, affect regulation, and infant mental health. *Infant Mental Health Journal, 22*(1–2), 7–66. https://doi.org/10.1002/1097-0355(200101/04)22:1<7::aid-imhj2>3.0.co;2-n

Siegel, D. (2020). *The developing mind: Toward a neurobiology of interpersonal experiences* (3rd ed.). Guilford Press.

Sierra, M. (2009). *Depersonalization: A new look at a neglected syndrome.* Cambridge University Press.

Silberg, J. L. (2012). *The child survivor: Healing developmental trauma and dissociation.* Routledge.

Silberg, J. L. (2021a). *The child survivor: Healing developmental trauma and dissociation* (2nd ed.). Oxford: Routledge.

Silberg, J. L. (2021b). A case series of 70 children exploited by child sexual abuse imagery. In V. Sinason & P. R. Marks (Eds.), *Treating children with dissociative disorders: Attachment trauma, theory and practice* (pp. 49–72). Routledge.

Silberg, J., & Dallam, S. (2022). Dissociative disorders in children and adolescents. In M. J. Dorahy, S. N. Gold, & J. A. O'Neil (Eds.), *Dissociation and the dissociative disorders: Past, present, future*. Taylor & Francis. https://doi.org/10.4324/9781003057314-33

Simeon, D., Guralnik, O., Schmeidler, J., Sirof, B., & Knutelska, M. (2001). The role of childhood interpersonal trauma in depersonalization disorder. *The American Journal of Psychiatry, 158*(7), 1027–1033. https://doi.org/10.1176/appi.ajp.158.7.1027Solomon, E. P., & Heide, K. M. (1999). Type III trauma: Toward a more effective conceptualization of psychological trauma. *International Journal of Offender Therapy and Comparative Criminology, 43*(2), 202–210. https://doi.org/10.1177/0306624X99432007

Solomon, J., & George, C. (1999). The place of disorganization in attachment theory: Linking classic observations with contemporary findings. In J. Solomon & C. George (Eds.), *Attachment disorganization* (pp. 3–32). Guilford Press.

Spinazzola, J., Habib, M., Knoverek, Arvidson, J., Hodgdon, H., Nisenbaum, J., Wentworth, Pond, & Kisiel, C. (2013). The heart of the matter: Complex trauma in child welfare. *CW360 Trauma-Informed Child Welfare Practice, 8–9*, 37.

Sroufe, L. A. (1982). The organization of emotional development. *Psychoanalytic Inquiry, 1*(4), 575–599. https://doi.org/10.1080/07351698209533421

Steinberg, M. (1994). *Structured clinical interview for DSM-IV dissociative disorders-revised (SCID-D-R)*. American Psychiatric Press.

Steinberg, M., & Steinberg, A. (1995). Using the SCID-D to assess dissociative identity disorder in adolescents: Three case studies. *Bulletin of the Menninger Clinic, 59*(2), 221–231.

Terr L. C. (1991). Childhood traumas: An outline and overview. *The American Journal of Psychiatry, 148*(1), 10–20. https://doi.org/10.1176/ajp.148.1.10

van der Kolk, B. A. (2005). Developmental trauma disorder: Toward a rational diagnosis for children with complex trauma histories. *Psychiatric Annals, 35*(5), 401–408. https://doi.org/10.3928/00485713-20050501-06

Waller, G., Babbs, M., Wright, F., Potterton, C., Meyer, C., & Leung, N. (2003). Somatoform dissociation in eating-disordered patients. *Behaviour Research and Therapy, 41*(5), 619–627. https://doi.org/10.1016/s0005-7967(03)00019-6

Wamser-Nanney, R., & Vandenberg, B. R. (2013). Empirical support for the definition of a complex trauma event in children and adolescents. *Journal of Traumatic Stress, 26*(6), 671–678. https://doi.org/10.1002/jts.21857

Waters, F. (July/August 2005). Recognizing dissociative children in preschool children. *The International Society for the Study of Dissociation, 23*(4), 1–2, 4–5. Retrieved from isst-d.org/wp-content/uploads/2019/02/From-the-President-Recognizing-Dissociation-in-Preschool-Children-Waters-2005.pdf

Waters, F. (2016). *Healing the fractured child*. Springer.

World Health Organization. (2018). *International statistical classification of diseases and related health problems* (11th rev.). WHO.

13
CONSIDERATIONS IN SCREENING, ASSESSMENT, AND CLINICAL INTERVIEWING

Alexis Arbuthnott, Billie Jo Bennett, Jillian Hosey, and Patti van Eys

Introduction

The assessment of complex trauma and dissociation in children is an under-researched, broad category that includes the gathering of information about the child's history, observations of the child's functioning across settings, and formal testing (e.g., screening measures such as self-report and caregiver checklists, clinical interviews, and projective techniques) (van Eys & Truss, 2012). Assessment may include clinical impressions as well as standardized measures that are reliable, valid, and evidence-based, and are normed or tested across a target population (American Psychological Association, 2014; Hunsley & Di Giulio, 2001). This chapter begins with an explanation of the rationale and process for assessment of complex trauma and dissociation in children. Next, assessment tools and techniques for use with traumatized children are outlined. Finally, the chapter ends with a clinical case example to demonstrate the assessment process.

Assessment Rationale and Process

Recognition of dissociation and dissociative disorders in children dates back to 1840 when French physician Antoine Despine composed a relatively overlooked monograph about an 11-year-old child named Estelle (Fine, 1988; Wieland, 2015). One hundred and forty years later, reports of children with identity alterations, constellations of self-destructive behaviors, and apparent amnesia were published by Dr. Richard Kluft (1984) and Fagan and McMahon (1984). Numerous articles and a few books were published in the 1990s specific to children with dissociation. Retrospective, longitudinal, and prospective studies flourished in the 1990s, linking disorganized attachment in early childhood with dissociation, along with age of onset, chronicity, and severity of abuse (Silberg & Dallam, 2009). Advancement of screening and assessment measures for dissociation in children modeled after adult measures thus progressed in the 1990s as well (Silberg & Dallam, 2009). The 2000s saw new trauma instruments for children increasingly include dissociation scales, the ongoing development of new diagnostic tools, and dissociative pathology increasingly accepted in journals under the topic of child maltreatment (Silberg & Dallam, 2009). By then, well-established screening measures like the Child Dissociative Checklist (CDC) were more readily being integrated into research. The International Society for the Study of Trauma and Dissociation (ISSTD) released guidelines in 2004 for the assessment and treatment of dissociative symptoms in children (updated guidelines are currently in progress), with the European Society for Trauma and Dissociation (ESTD) releasing similar guidelines in 2017 (Child and Adolescent Committee of the ESTD, 2017). Significant gains have been made over the last several decades in general dissociation research and the field of assessment (Bailey & Brand, 2017), yet empirical information about childhood dissociation continues to evolve more slowly (ISSTD, 2004, in press; Wilkinson & DeJong, 2021).

Experts in the child trauma field advocate for the early detection and treatment of dissociation (Armstrong et al., 1997; Cintron et al., 2018; Somer, 2011), as dissociation can interfere with treatment, impact daily functioning and development, and decrease overall quality of life (Lanius et al., 2012), and is most efficiently addressed when viewed as a primary target for treatment (Hornstein, 1996). Early recognition of dissociation may lead to better treatment outcomes as intervention for dissociation tends to be more rapid and efficient in childhood compared to in adulthood (Kluft, 1984). Early detection of dissociative symptoms also supports diagnosis and allows for effective directed treatment planning (Hornstein, 1996) that can avert years of ineffective treatment, prevent long-term suffering, disrupt the trajectory toward deeply entrenched investment in separateness of self, and reduce long-term societal fiscal costs (Kluft, 1984; Silberg & Wieland, 2013).

Dissociative Symptoms and Disorders in Children

Normative dissociation, or the absence of awareness (e.g., losing track of time, being unable to recall the walk home from school, daydreaming), occurs naturally from time to time for everyone and is common in young children (Bernier et al., 2013). Pathological dissociation, however, emerges as a psychophysiological, instinctual survival strategy to escape awareness of a situation, feelings, or sensations in response to fear, threat, or insecurity (Silberg & Wieland, 2013; Waters, 2016), and is encoded neurologically and within the body (Schore, 2003; van der Kolk, 2005). Dissociation is adaptive at the time of a traumatic event, but becomes problematic (i.e., pathological) when ongoing use of dissociation becomes a means of coping with stressful, but not dangerous, situations. Pathological dissociation is typically characterized by "a disruption of and/or discontinuity in the normal integration of consciousness, memory, identity, emotion, perception, body representation, motor control, and behavior" (American Psychiatric Association, 2022, p. 329). The most severe form of dissociation is the presence of dissociated self-states that take executive control of the body (Waters, 2013). Normative dissociation does not cause fragmentation or division of experience or self (Wieland, 2015). For more detailed information on symptom presentations, please refer to Chapter 12.

While this chapter seeks to explore the use of formal and informal assessment and diagnostic procedures to make sense of the often perplexing symptoms and behaviors that emerge within the context of complex trauma and dissociation in children, there is additional consideration of the ways in which formal assessment and diagnostics are the subject of a more recent movement that seeks to depathologize psychopathology (Taylor & Shrive, 2023; Wasserman & Wasserman, 2016). This movement feels important to name and honor while also clarifying that the use of assessment and diagnostics within the context of this chapter is to support the process of case conceptualization and treatment planning to ensure treatment is attuned to the needs of the child, rather than to determine a label that defines *what is wrong with them*. Moving beyond the notion of "bad behaviors" conceptualizes symptoms as an expression of what has happened to the child and the legacy of trauma they bear. Clinicians are encouraged to hold this in mind as they take in the information and simultaneously remain aligned with their scope of practice and corresponding practice-based ethics and standards, while considering the ways in which formal and informal assessment and diagnostics may impact a child both positively and negatively. The chapter in this volume focused on case conceptualization and treatment planning further incorporates these considerations.

Although research shows dissociative disorders begin in childhood (American Psychiatric Association, 2022; Kluft, 1984), current DSM-5-TR diagnostic categories for dissociative disorders are based heavily on research with adults. These diagnostic categories are dissociative identity disorder, dissociative amnesia, depersonalization/derealization disorder, other specified dissociative disorder, and unspecified dissociative disorder (American Psychiatric Association, 2022). However, dissociation may present uncharacteristically in childhood compared to adulthood (Fagan & McMahon, 1984; Hornstein, 1996; Kluft, 1984; Putnam, 1997; Steinberg, 1995), and these diagnostic categories may not adequately account for the representations of dissociative disorders in children (American Psychiatric Association, 2022; Peterson, 1991; Putnam, 1997; Silberg & Dallam, 2009, 2023; Steinberg, 1995). For example, in reference to dissociative identity disorder in children, Silberg (2022) noted:

> Dissociative features found in children may be in a preliminary form that does not meet adult DSM-5 criteria. DSM-5 criteria require that "two or more distinct identities or personality states are present, each with its own relatively enduring pattern of perceiving, relating to and thinking about the environment and self" (American Psychiatric Association, 2013, p. 292). Instead, the manifestations of dissociation found in children range across a continuum of severity and the differing states the child may present do not always include an "enduring pattern," as they may shift, and in some ways resemble normal developmental processes, such as the phenomenon of vivid imaginary friends in young children. All or nothing labels which view the client as having a rigid disorder are less helpful than a view of dissociative phenomena as existing on a continuum of severity.
>
> *(p. xxv)*

Child-specific diagnostic categories for dissociative disorders that accurately reflect the symptom profiles of dissociative children are direly needed and would assist in early identification and intervention (Silberg & Dallam, 2009). A proposed DSM-5 diagnosis, developmental trauma disorder (DTD) (van der Kolk, 2005), was rejected for DSM-5 inclusion despite ongoing, solid research that continues to show the connection between exposure to chronic early trauma and severe dysregulation across behavior, emotion, perceptual and somatic experiences, and relationships (Ford, 2023). Putnam (1997) purported that dissociative symptoms in children can be divided into two large categories: amnesias/memory symptoms and dissociative processes. Amnesias include losing time, perplexing forgetfulness for basic information, gaps in the continuity of autobiographical memory, amnesia for the source of information, and intrusive memories. Dissociative process symptoms include depersonalization and derealization, passive influence/interference experiences, auditory hallucinations, trance-like states, discrete identity disturbances, and unique alterations in cognitive processing.

However, children with dissociation have a small "window of diagnosability" (Steinberg, 1995, p. 334), and symptom profiles that change over time (Steinberg, 1995). Dissociation in children must be evaluated on a continuum ranging from normative to pathological (Putnam, 1997; Silberg & Wieland, 2013; Wieland, 2015; Waters, 2016; Young, 2022) and can be categorized as mild, moderate, or extreme (Silberg & Wieland, 2013; Wieland, 2015). Determining how disruptions in consciousness, identity, and memory impact the achievement of normative developmental tasks is pertinent when assessing the severity of dissociation in children (ISSTD, 2004). Attention to dissociative symptoms across the continuum of severity is necessary to prevent misdiagnosis (Stolbach, 2005).

Indicators for Screening and Assessment of Dissociation in Children

It is essential for clinicians working with children to familiarize themselves with warning signs that call for the screening and assessment of complex trauma and dissociation in children. A history of childhood trauma and/or conditions of early relational wounding are foundational etiologies of complex trauma and dissociation (Spiegel et al., 2011; Waters, 2016). Physical, sexual, and emotional abuse, neglect, painful medical procedures, natural disasters, witnessing violence, abandonment, and/or exposure to war are traditional examples of childhood trauma (Waters, 2016). Children exposed to overwhelmingly frightening experiences without support, which can also include incongruent affective responses from caregivers, are also risk factors in the development of dissociative processes (Bailey & Brand, 2017; Putnam, 1997; Schore, 2013; Wieland, 2015). A caregiver's own unresolved trauma history is often an invisible threat that leaves the dependent and vulnerable child "caught in a 'biological paradox' between the 'survival reflex' and the 'attachment circuit'" (Kezelman & Stavropoulus, 2020, p. 19). Theory suggests disorganized attachment creates vulnerability and risk toward the development of pathological dissociation (Barach, 1991; Liotti, 1992, 2004; Schimmenti, 2023) and research shows a strong association between persons with disorganized attachment strategies and dissociation (Dutra et al., 2009; Ogawa et al., 1997).

According to Waters (2016), additional warning signs that may point to the presence of dissociative processes include previous multiple and/or changing diagnoses and treatment failures; inadequate progress in treatment despite the child being in a safe, nurturing environment; and symptoms of dissociation themselves (e.g., memory problems or amnesia; extreme behavioral changes in voice, food, handwriting, preferences, and dress; imaginary playmates reported as real that tell the child to do things; referring to the self as "we" or in the third person; regressed behavior; extreme mood switches that appear to be unprovoked or minimally provoked; complaints of a headache before a change in behavior; denial of witnessed behavior; a sense of depersonalization or derealization; glazed look or blanking out; eyes that roll back or flutter; and reports of auditory or visual hallucinations).

Assessment Process: HOT (History, Observation, and Testing) Framework

Referrals to children's mental health agencies are often due to a child's dysregulated behavior and emotions. Complex trauma and dissociation are frequently the root cause of the most perplexing dysregulation. Unfortunately, unless children are systematically and thoroughly assessed by trauma- and dissociation-informed providers, they are often misdiagnosed with common childhood disorders (e.g., ADHD), wrongly assigned adolescent- and adult-oriented labels (e.g., psychosis or bipolar disorder), or only partially understood (e.g., omissions of critical co-occurring conditions such as an eating disorder *and* dissociation). Even if correctly diagnosed with "trauma" (e.g., PTSD), symptoms of dissociation or severe attachment disturbances may be overlooked. Indeed, dissociative disorders have overlapping symptoms with more commonly accepted diagnoses such as attention deficit hyperactivity disorder, oppositional defiant disorder, obsessive compulsive disorder, anxiety disorders, mood disorders, reactive attachment disorder, substance use disorders, neurodevelopmental disorders, and eating disorders (Hornstein, 1996; ISSTD, 2004; Peterson, 1991; Waters, 2016; see Chapter 14). General medical disorders that may mimic dissociative symptoms must also be ruled out and may include seizure disorders, allergy, other neurological conditions, exposure to toxins, and legal or illegal drug effects (ISSTD, 2004).

The full scope of assessing children for dissociation is a comprehensive and complex process; guidance on assessment for dissociation in children beyond the scope of this chapter is available in Silberg (2022), van Eys and Truss (2012), and Waters (2016). Note that although the assessment process is described in a linear fashion throughout this chapter, it is rarely this straightforward when working with traumatized children. The purpose of the assessment may impact how the assessment is delivered. Where the assessment is intended to inform interventions, assessment tools and techniques may be interspersed with preliminary interventions focused on increasing the child's safety and stability, as well as building therapeutic rapport to support the process. In this case, assessment becomes a part of the intervention process. Where the assessment is needed for diagnostic clarification only (e.g., research, forensic settings, formal psychological evaluation), care needs to be taken to develop sufficient rapport and relational safety within the therapeutic relationship that the child is comfortable enough to disclose personal and sensitive information. Children should be informed of the assessment rationale and process in a developmentally appropriate manner, and their assent is essential to commencing the process.

The timing and pace of assessment is determined by the child's affect tolerance, level of environmental safety, and the strength of the therapeutic relationship (Courtois, 2004; Waters, 2016). Asking questions about traumatic experiences or dissociative symptoms has the potential to be destabilizing for children, as it evokes memories and distress of past trauma. Careful pacing is necessary to provide containment throughout the assessment and treatment process (Hornstein, 1996). This may mean informally assessing the child's readiness to address the assessment topics (e.g., assess the child's ability to talk about planning to assess these topics at an upcoming session), titrating assessment tasks (e.g., breaking up tasks across multiple sessions, discontinuing or pausing a task if it becomes too distressing for the child), and responding supportively to a child's increase in distress or in-session dissociation (e.g., shifting to teaching grounding or stabilization techniques).

Some children are not ready or able to disclose dissociative experiences early in the treatment process (Courtois, 2004; Hornstein, 1996; Waters, 2016); alternatively, children's dissociative systems can be surprisingly flexible, and many children disclose and process symptoms more readily than adults. When a child is unable or unwilling to complete an assessment task, it is important to uphold the child's dignity and sense of agency. Attempting to force a child to complete the assessment process removes their autonomy and reenacts the power differentials experienced during maltreatment. A child's disengagement from the assessment process should be viewed as communication that there is insufficient safety within the context of the assessment, which needs to be addressed prior to continuing. This may indicate insufficient rapport with the clinician, topics that feel too distressing to talk about, or ongoing safety or allegiance concerns within the child's home or family environment. Solid assessment is the key to arriving at accurate case formulations and diagnoses, as well as creating effective treatment plans. Effective treatment hinges on an assessment of the *whole child* within each child's unique context. A multi-informant, multi-method assessment of children's symptoms across settings is an ongoing and collaborative process. The HOT (History, Observation, and Testing) framework (van Eys & Truss, 2012) can provide structure for this assessment process, and is outlined below.

(H) History

A complete biopsychosocial history from the prenatal period to the present is gained through interviews and record reviews. Valuable information can be gathered, with appropriate consents for the collection of information, from any significant person or institution who can provide historical information about the child (e.g., past or current caregivers, extended family members, service providers, child protection workers, teachers). The clinician must attend closely to the *child in context*—that is, how the child's environment (e.g., school, home, and community) has influenced their presentation (e.g., symptoms and protective factors) both historically and currently. *Child in context* also includes a thorough exploration of developmental stage and vulnerabilities (e.g., speech and language, disability, and developmental delays), cultural/ethnic identity, current family dynamics (including attachment strength and style), general societal influences (e.g., social media and gun violence), peer culture, school factors, sexual and gender orientation, and health status.

A timeline of the child's life can help piece together child and family adversities and milestones with an emphasis on identifying traumas, losses, successes, and strengths. The timeline documents events within stages of development and clarifies how much developmental time has been impacted by trauma. A timeline helps clinicians develop hypotheses about trauma and loss reminders and accompanying adaptive "survival" responses, as well as protective factors (e.g., an invested adult) and periods of "felt safety" that shielded the child from adversity (see ISSTD, 2004). This timeline can be reviewed and updated throughout the course of assessment and treatment. There are often hidden or unknown pieces of history or experience due to deliberate withholding, the young age of the child at the time of the trauma, or dissociative inaccessibility (see Appendix A for areas to include on a trauma timeline; ISSTD, 2004).

(O) Observation

Clinicians can obtain information about observations of the child both firsthand (i.e., in person) and through collateral information (e.g., interviews and screening checklists) from teachers, caregivers, and other relevant third parties in a child's life. This approach allows the clinician to gather observations of the child across settings. Separate in-person sessions with the caregiver(s), the child, and the child with the caregiver(s) are optimal for observing the child's cognitive, affective, behavioral, somatic, relational, and linguistic domains. Clinicians must be alert to more observable dissociative moments such as zoning out and extreme shifts in behavior, as well as the child's baseline behavior and social relating (clinicians are reminded that many dissociative symptoms are not observable, which is why further testing is necessary as part of the assessment process). Observations of the child in their natural environments also enrich understanding of the child, and can be obtained in person, virtually, or through videos supplied by parents, teachers, or others. Observations of the family provide information about communication patterns, child and caregiver attachment styles, caregiver attunement and reflective capacity, and discipline practices. Observing children and caregivers working together in play or on a clinician-directed task (e.g., making a playdough sculpture) gives opportunity to witness attachment behaviors such as mutual delight and the child's ability to accept assistance.

(T) Testing

Testing, or the use of formal and informal symptom measurement tools, helps clarify or refine emerging clinical impressions gathered in the History and Observation stages. Screening measures filled out by teachers, parents, and/or children may indicate that more in-depth testing is warranted. This further testing may be of a formal nature, such as standardized clinical interviews or projective testing. It may also include testing through other medical and allied health disciplines (e.g., speech and language, medical or genetic testing, and occupational therapy).

For clinicians to fully understand a child's inner experience, the child needs to be able to report on their own dissociative experiences, such as through self-report measures and interviews with the child directly. However, information from caregivers (e.g., parents, teachers, and other adults who know the child well) obtained through observer-report measures and subsequent follow-up clinical interviewing can help clinicians better understand caregiver observations of a child's presenting symptoms, behaviors, and possible triggers across the different environments and contexts they inhabit. According to Cintron et al. (2018),

> to be able to appropriately diagnose young children with PTSD, professionals rely on caregivers to accurately report their child's PTSD symptoms. A better understanding of how parents describe dissociative reactions in young children may help caregivers become better reporters of these occurrences.
>
> *(p. 10)*

Assessment Tools

Clinical tools specific to trauma and dissociation are valuable throughout the entire assessment process. These tools can elicit information essential for understanding the traumatized child's experiences, clarifying diagnoses, and determining the pace of treatment. They may also be used throughout interventions to assess progress (Bailey & Brand, 2017; Cardeña & Weiner, 2004). Clinical tools commonly used in the assessment of trauma and dissociation in children include standardized tools (i.e., screening measures, structured and semi-structured interviews), projective tests, and unstructured interviewing techniques. The role of each of these methods in the assessment of complex trauma and dissociation in children is described throughout the following sections of this chapter.

Standardized tools include valid and reliable screening measures and structured or semi-structured clinical interviews. These tools provide norms, which allow for the child's scores to be meaningfully compared to those of other similar children. It is important to note that the usefulness of standardized assessment tools is dependent on the tool's reliability and validity within the context in which the tool is being used. Reliability refers to the extent to which the responses obtained on the assessment measure or tool are consistent (e.g., if readministered and between reporters), whereas validity refers to the extent to which the measure or tool is assessing what it claims. Validity includes the extent to which the content of the tool covers the range of symptoms it is assessing (i.e., content validity), the extent to which the measured symptoms are unique to dissociation (i.e., discriminant validity), and the performance of the tool in relation to other tools assessing the same symptoms (i.e., convergent validity); strong validity is necessary when using standardized tools to inform differential diagnoses.

Standardized assessment tools determined to be valid with one population of a specific demographic (e.g., age range, language, and culture) cannot be assumed to be valid with a population of a different demographic. The child's maturity level, language abilities, and cultural background can all affect the extent to which the child understands the assessment questions and can accurately report on their experiences. Clinicians are encouraged to use assessment tools with established and adequate psychometric properties for their client population(s). Although extending tools for use with a child outside of the population on which they were normed (e.g., when age and/or culturally appropriate measures do not exist) may provide useful qualitative information about the child's symptoms, it may also introduce unintended biases into the assessment that either miss symptoms of interest or over-pathologize developmentally normative experiences within the context of that population (e.g., age or culture).

In contrast to standardized tools, projective tests can be construed as a form of extended interview that allows clinicians to create hypotheses regarding the child's inner life. Techniques such as drawings, storytelling, completing sentences, or other tasks designed to give a child psychological distance from troubling issues are used to gain insight into the child's perceptions of self and relationship to others. There are no right or wrong answers to projective tasks.

Furthermore, in cases when standardized tools are not available or practical, and where additional information is desired to supplement other information obtained, unstructured interviews can provide rich data to round out the case formulation. As there are no validated standardized clinical interviews for symptoms of complex trauma and dissociation normed with children less than 11 years old, interviews with most children will by default be unstructured. Care needs to be taken to ensure appropriate interviewing techniques when interviewing traumatized children. Specific questions, techniques, and concerns around unstructured interviewing (ISSTD, 2004; Silberg, 2022; Waters, 2016) are discussed in detail later in this chapter.

Note that the context of the administration of these assessment tools and techniques may influence responses. While underreporting and overreporting of symptoms may reflect an intent to deceive the clinician (e.g., malingering), it is more likely that inaccurate responses are communicating something other than what the tool is attempting to assess. For example, during times of acute crises (e.g., inpatient care due to acute safety concerns and change in housing due to placement breakdown), assessment measures may indicate higher levels of dissociative symptoms relative to the child's true baseline. This difference may reflect the child's acute increase in use of dissociative coping as a means of managing the acute stressor. Inflated responses may also indicate an overreporting of symptoms (either intentionally or unintentionally) as a means of communicating distress within the context of other acute stressors. In contrast to overreporting symptoms, children and caregivers may also underreport and minimize symptoms (also either intentionally or unintentionally). Underreporting may reflect a child's or caregiver's denial of the child's difficulties (e.g., to dismiss the need for further assessment or intervention and minimization due to limited resources to deal with the challenges), or a genuine lack of awareness of symptoms (e.g., caregiver is not attuned to child's difficulties, or a child's experiences of trauma and symptoms of dissociation are dissociated from their own awareness). Furthermore, there may be a low correlation between child and caregiver reports of a child's trauma (Skar et al., 2021), indicating that caregivers may not know the entirety of the child's experiences. Thus, information obtained from any single means of assessment needs to be corroborated by other information about the child.

Screening Measures

It is important that screening for complex trauma and dissociation in children is connected back to the etiology of these symptoms—trauma—rather than disconnected from it. As such, screening measures are one method of obtaining information about the child within the larger HOT framework for assessment. Follow-up interviewing around responses on screening measures can provide rich examples of the symptoms endorsed, which can further assist in understanding the *child in context*. Furthermore, clinicians need to be clear on *why* they are using specific screening instruments. When used alongside information about a child's history and clinical observations of the child's behavior (including the more observable dissociative symptoms previously discussed), screening tools can capture children's descriptions of their internal experiences and others' descriptions of their observations of the child. Thus, screening tools inform formulation and need for further diagnostic evaluation, treatment planning, and monitoring of treatment progress.

Screening tools are generally brief and provide data about core indicators that suggest the need for further evaluation around identified concerning symptoms (Bailey & Brand, 2017; ISSTD, 2004; Waters 2016). Screening tools may be an invaluable place to start with children and their caregivers (Waters, 2016), but they are neither essential nor diagnostic (ISSTD, 2004). Screening measures use a dimensional approach to quantify the number and severity of symptoms. While some screening measures of complex trauma or dissociation measure the full range of trauma symptoms and dissociative experiences, others measure only specific subsets of these symptoms. Although some screening measures provide the mean (i.e., average) scores of samples of children with dissociative disorders (and sometimes the mean scores of children with other disorders), no specific score is indicative of a dissociative disorder diagnosis. Similarly, some screening measures provide cutoff scores to distinguish clinically significant levels of symptoms from symptoms that are not generally considered concerning; these cutoff scores are often used as indicators that further assessment is recommended. Indeed, the usefulness of cutoff scores is dependent on a measure's sensitivity (i.e., the extent to which it can correctly identify a child who has a dissociative disorder) and specificity (i.e., the extent to which children who do not have dissociative disorders score in the nonclinical range). Thus, higher scores reflect a need for further assessment toward diagnostic clarification.

No one measure is used universally with all children. Instead, clinicians are called on to consider the purpose of assessment, context and conditions, age of the child and ability to self-report, psychometric rigor of the measure and whether it's been normed, and the cost and accessibility of specific measures (Strand et al., 2005). As such, differences in how screening is carried out will be seen with preschool children, young children, and school-aged children. For example, within infancy and the first years of childhood, dissociation is observed through spontaneous behavioral observations from caregivers, as self-report skills are not yet developed (Cardeña & Weiner, 2004). In preschool children, as other observable indicators of dissociation emerge (see Chapter 12 for more information), more formal observer-report measures can be introduced, and self-report measures may be used depending on the child's self-report capacities. In screening young and school-aged children, assessors can discern more definitive dissociative phenomena (i.e., more differentiated dissociated states and/or identities; Silberg & Dallam, 2009) that may be screened in via observer and self-report measures and/or behavioral checklists; however, this must be carried out and paced according to the child's social, emotional, and developmental capacities.

Screening Measures for Dissociation

There are several screening measures currently in use that are intended to identify dissociative symptoms in children. These measures are outlined below.

ADOLESCENT DISSOCIATIVE EXPERIENCES SCALE (A-DES)

The A-DES (Armstrong et al., 1997) is a 30-item self-report questionnaire for children aged 11–18 years old modeled after the Dissociative Experiences Scale for adults. This measure uses a 10-point ratio scale assessing a child's perspective of the amount of time during which they experience symptoms of dissociation (where 0 is 0% of the time, and 10 is 100% of the time). The A-DES is scored by taking the average of scores across items, such that overall scores range from 0 to 10. Higher scores indicate higher levels of dissociation. The A-DES has good reliability and validity (Armstrong et al., 1997; Farrington et al., 2001; Smith & Carlson, 1996), and research into the A-DES's factor structure using traumatized samples tends to suggest that this scale distinguishes between multiple forms of dissociation: depersonalization and derealization; amnesia; and loss of conscious control (Kerig et al., 2016).

THE CHILD BEHAVIOR CHECKLIST-3 (CDC)

Created by Putnam and colleagues (1993) as both a clinical and research tool, this 20-item caregiver-/observer-report measure for school-aged children (preschool to 12 years old) assesses a caregiver's observations of their child's potential dissociative symptoms over the past 12 months using a three-point Likert scale. The CDC has been shown to have strong internal consistency, interrater reliability, and concurrent and discriminative validity (Putnam & Peterson, 1994; Wherry et al., 1994). As this scale is based on observable manifestations of dissociation, items emphasize observations of amnesia and identity alterations, and no items assess the child's experience of depersonalization or derealization. Higher scores indicate higher levels of dissociation. This measure has been translated into several languages.

CHECKLIST OF INDICATORS OF TRAUMA & DISSOCIATION IN YOUTH (CIT-DY)

The CIT-DY (Waters, 2021) is a relatively new comprehensive trauma and dissociation assessment tool that can be used with caregivers, clinicians, educators, and children/youth aged 3–19 years (both caregiver and youth versions are available). The CIT-DY contains multiple scales assessing the child's history of placements (six items) and treatment (seven items); the child's exposure to a variety of potentially traumatic events (22 items) alongside the age at which these exposures occurred; and a checklist of current dissociative symptoms (17 items measured on a four-point Likert scale). Space is provided alongside each item for additional comments to contextualize responses. Comments can be examined for qualitative information pertaining to the interrelation between treatment history, placement history, trauma history, and dissociative symptoms. Collecting this data on a single measure allows for a comprehensive analysis of a child's history and current symptoms. As the CIT-DY has been found to be clinically useful by many clinicians in the field of child and adolescent dissociation due to the richness of the information elicited, experts in the field have supported its use within clinical settings (Silberg, 2022). Initial research into validating this measure is currently underway (Arbuthnott et al., 2023).

THE CHILDREN'S PERCEPTUAL ALTERATION SCALE (CPAS)

The CPAS (Evers-Szostak & Sanders, 1992) is a 28-item child-appropriate adaptation of the Perceptual Alterations Scale (Sanders, 1986) used to screen for dissociative symptoms in children aged 8–12. Children are asked to rate their experience of symptoms on a four-point Likert scale (where 1 is that the symptom "never happens" and 4 indicates the symptom "almost always happens"). While this measure appears to have adequate reliability (Evers-Szostak & Sanders, 1992), one study has shown low correlation between the CPAS and the CDC, calling into question the CPAS's validity (Eisen et al., 2002).

THE BRIEF DISSOCIATIVE EXPERIENCES SCALE (DES-B)

The DES-B (Dalenberg & Carlson, 2010) is a brief eight-item screening measure developed for DSM-related research with children aged 11–17 years. This measure uses a five-point Likert scale to rate dissociative symptoms across the past seven days. To date, there are limited studies on its use (Naish, 2020) and it does not necessarily index symptoms of pathological dissociation (Kira & Shuwiekh, 2022). It is intended to be used periodically among youth with dissociative disorders to track the severity of the child's dissociative symptoms over time.

CHILD/ADOLESCENT DISSOCIATIVE CHECKLIST (CADC)

The CADC (Reagor et al., 1992) is a 17-item clinician-administered checklist of 13 dissociative index characteristics for use with children aged 3–18 years old. Ten or more "yes" answers call for further diagnostic evaluation of dissociative symptoms. Two validity studies were performed in the late 1980s (Reagor et al., 1992), though these psychometric properties are now considered outdated.

CHILDREN'S DISSOCIATIVE EXPERIENCES SCALE AND POST-TRAUMATIC SYMPTOM INVENTORY (CDES/PTSI)

The CDES/PTSI (Stolbach, 1997) is a clinician-administered self-report scale assessing symptoms of trauma (13 items) and dissociation (21 items) among children. This measure is unique in that it does not ask children to reflect on their symptom severity or frequency in the usual manner. Instead, each item consists of two sentences about the experiences of hypothetical children; the child is asked to indicate which child they are more like, and then whether they are a lot or just a little like that child. This scale also includes social desirability items to assess for response validity. Though this is not a standardized interview, the clinician reads each item out loud to the child to ensure the child's understanding. The measure takes 10–15 minutes to complete. Although information about this measure's psychometric properties is limited and outdated, preliminary assessments indicate that further evaluation is warranted (Stolbach, 1997).

Screening Measures for Trauma Symptoms

Various trauma-specific measures for children exist, including the Center for Youth Wellness Adverse Childhood Experiences Questionnaire (CYW-ACE-Q) (Burke Harris & Renschler, 2015), PTSD in Preschool Aged Children (Levendosky et al., 2002), the UCLS Brief Screen for Child/Adolescent PTSD (Rolon-Arroyo et al., 2020), the Child Stress Disorders Checklist (Saxe et al., 2003), and the Acute Stress Checklist for Children (ASC-K) (Kassam-Adams, 2006). Some of these measures include items assessing dissociative symptoms. The following are other commonly used trauma-screening measures that identify exposure to trauma and trauma-related symptoms, some of which also include subscales assessing dissociation.

INTERNATIONAL TRAUMA QUESTIONNAIRES: CHILD AND ADOLESCENT VERSION (ITQ-CA)

The ITQ-CA (Cloitre et al., 2018) is a 12-item self-report questionnaire using a five-point Likert scale to assess the child's perspective of how much trauma symptoms related to a specific event have bothered them over the past month. Used with children 7–17 years old, the ITQ-CA has two subscales with three symptom clusters in each: PTSD (i.e., re-experiencing, avoidance, sense of threat), and Self-Organization (i.e., affective dysregulation, negative self-concept). Disturbances in self-organization are intended to reflect key symptoms of complex PTSD (C-PTSD). The questionnaire also asks whether these symptoms have interfered with each of five different domains of functioning (i.e., friends, family, schoolwork, other important things, general happiness). Categorical scoring (i.e., endorsement of symptoms across clusters alongside functional impairment) can be used to obtain preliminary impressions for both PTSD and C-PTSD. Dimensional scoring can be used to track symptoms over time, including response to treatment. The ITQ-CA has excellent internal reliability, concurrent and convergent validity, and partial support for discriminant validity (Haselgruber et al., 2020).

THE CHILD AND ADOLESCENT TRAUMA SCREEN (CATS)

CATS (Goldbeck & Berliner, 2014) is a 25-item self-report screening instrument with a clinical guide for identifying trauma events and DSM-5 PTSD criteria in both clinical and research settings. Designed for preschoolers, children, and adolescents, the CATS is available in 11 languages (Akkuş et al., 2021; Nilsson et al., 2021; Sachser et al., 2017). This measure has strong reliability and validity (see Dowdy-Hazlett et al., 2021). Research supports that the CATS has a four-factor structure (i.e., re-experiencing, avoidance, negative alterations in mood and cognitions, hyper-arousal), which align with the underlying DSM-5-TR symptom clusters for PTSD (Dowdy-Hazlett et al., 2021; Sachser et al., 2017). A recently updated version of this measure (i.e., CATS-2; Sachser et al., 2022) has similarly been found to be reliable and valid for use with traumatized youth aged 7–17 and is able to distinguish between the ICD-11 C-PTSD and PTSD diagnoses.

TRAUMA SYMPTOM CHECKLIST FOR CHILDREN (TSCC) AND THE TRAUMA SYMPTOM CHECKLIST FOR YOUNG CHILDREN (TSCYC)

The TSCC (Briere, 1996) and TSCYC (Briere et al., 2001) are complementary measures assessing the effects of childhood trauma via PTSD-related symptoms among young children, children, and adolescents (Briere & Spinazzola, 2005). The TSCC is a 54-item self-report measure for post-traumatic symptoms across six clinical scales (i.e., anxiety, depression, anger, post-traumatic stress, dissociation, and sexual concerns) among youth aged 8–16 years. The TSCYC is a 90-item caretaker report measure assessing post-traumatic symptoms across eight clinical scales (anxiety, depression, anger/aggression, post-traumatic stress intrusions, post-traumatic stress avoidance, post-traumatic stress arousal, dissociation, and sexual concerns) among children aged 3–12 years. The dissociation scale contains two subscales (i.e., overt dissociation, fantasy dissociation) that measure symptoms of derealization, emotional numbing, and memory problems. Higher scores reflect greater symptomatology. Scores on the dissociation scale may signal the need for additional assessment in this area. Both the TSCC and the TSCYC include two validity scales (under response and hyper-response) and provide separate norms for males and females across several age groupings. These measures may be administered individually or in groups and can be completed by the respondent or an interviewer. Both scales have been translated into Spanish. The TSCC has demonstrated strong reliability and validity (Briere, 1996). A systematic review (Stanley & Stanley, 2021) of the psychometric properties of the TSCYS has found strong reliability as well as moderate validity among older (but not necessarily younger) children; thus, the results of the TSCYC may be more clinically useful for assessing trauma symptoms in older children when paired with the TSCC.

Other Screening Tools

Broadband and comprehensive assessment systems can be useful means to quickly identify the presence of dissociation while screening for a wide variety of mental health and behavioral challenges affecting children. These tools provide a snapshot of the child's overall functioning beyond trauma-specific symptoms, which can be valuable in understanding concurrent challenges. Two screening tools in this category are described below.

CHILD BEHAVIOR CHECKLIST (CBCL)

The CBCL (Achenbach & Edelbrock, 1983, 1987) is a broadband measure intended to screen for a wide range of internalizing and externalizing difficulties among children, and it may be particularly useful as a means of rapidly obtaining a general picture of a child's overall emotional and behavioral functioning. This measure contains a few items overlapping with dissociative symptoms. Parent, teacher, and youth self-report versions are available, which can provide rich collateral information about a young person's functioning across settings. Two versions of dissociation scales have been derived from items on the CBCL for use in clinical and research settings. The role of these scales is to quickly identify the potential presence of dissociative processes that warrant further investigation, while also screening for a range of other mental disorders. The scale derived by Ogawa and colleagues (1997) was composed of 12 items on earlier versions of the CBCL that mapped onto items on the CDC. These items assessed both state (i.e., trance) dissociation as well as amnesia and identity alteration. Sim and colleagues (2005) later attempted to use the CBCL to screen children for trauma symptoms and derived three trauma-related scales: the PTSD scale (seven items), the dissociation scale (three items), and the PTSD/dissociation scale (16 items). Here, the dissociation scale taps into only symptoms of dissociative trance and absorption, whereas the PTSD/dissociation scale also includes items related to identity confusion and alteration. This scale has received preliminary validation among neglected children (Milot et al., 2013).

CHILD AND ADOLESCENT NEEDS AND STRENGTHS (CANS)

The CANS is an information integration and systemic communication tool used mostly by non-clinicians (e.g., child welfare and juvenile justice workers) to gather information from family members, current and past caregivers (e.g., foster parents), collateral sources (e.g., teachers), and records to summarize mental health- (including trauma-) related needs and strengths of children, adolescents, and their families (John Praed Foundation, 2021). The clinically anchored scoring system is designed to translate responses into service action levels. Questions span six domains (life-functioning, strengths, cultural factors, caregiver resources and needs, behavioral/emotional needs, and risk behaviors). Items assessing dissociation are included within the measure and have been the topic of recent research regarding the high prevalence of youth with dissociation in residential care (Kisiel et al., 2020). There is much research on the reliability and validity of the CANS as an integrative and multisystemic assessment strategy as it relates to levels of care (see John Praed Foundation, 2021, for a summary). The integrity of the measure's outcomes relies on access to robust information, well-trained assessors, the ability of informers to report accurate observations of a child's symptoms and presentation, and accurate input of information. Data collection can be difficult within the culture of child welfare and juvenile justice due to its crisis-driven nature and frequent family fragmentation.

Standardized Clinical Interviews

Clinical interviews remain the gold standard for diagnosing dissociative disorders. When self-report measures are used to screen for dissociative symptoms or to obtain a diagnostic impression, further interviews are required to better understand the subjective experience of symptoms and the emerging diagnostic impressions, and to confirm the appropriateness of a dissociative disorder diagnosis. Note, however, that interviews should not be used as the sole source of information when making a diagnosis. Interviews allow for the elicitation of rich details and examples pertaining to the reported symptoms, and clinical observations during the interview process can be informative in and of themselves. It should be noted that these tools should be used in combination with other assessment information from the HOT framework to provide a holistic view of the child, their strengths (e.g., protective factors), and their challenges (e.g., co-occurring mental disorders, factors that may be perpetuating symptoms). Where possible, information obtained from clinical interviews should be substantiated through collateral information.

Research supporting the use of standardized structured or semi-structured interviews assessing symptoms of complex trauma and dissociation is lacking among children aged 12 years or younger. Nonetheless, established interviews assessing for PTSD among children may also cover key symptoms of C-PTSD. Similarly, in many cases, interviews assessing for dissociation and dissociative disorders in adolescents and adults may be used with older children (e.g., aged 11 or 12) provided that the child has sufficient developmental maturity and cognitive abilities necessary to understand the questions, self-reflect, and provide accurate responses. Clinicians should have appropriate training prior to administering structured or semi-structured interviews. The following interview tools have been used to assess for complex trauma and dissociation in children.

Standardized Interviews for Trauma

Interviews intended to assess for PTSD among children can serve as a starting point for the assessment of complex trauma and dissociation provided that the clinician initially follows standardized protocols in the administration of the measure prior to branching off into questions about topics beyond those in the structured interview. If the administration of the structured or semi-structured interview is altered from the standardized protocol (e.g., if a clinician chooses to extend the interview to add further questions about complex trauma or dissociation), any scores obtained through the interview should be interpreted with caution.

Screening and Assessment

THE KIDDIE SCHEDULE FOR AFFECTIVE DISORDERS AND SCHIZOPHRENIA—PRESENT AND LIFETIME VERSION (K-SADS-PL)

The K-SADS-PL (Kaufman et al., 1997) is a semi-structured interview used to assess current and past symptoms of a range of mental disorders, including post-traumatic stress disorder, among children 6–18 years old. Both the child and their caregiver report on the child's symptoms. Versions of the K-SADS are available in over 30 languages, making this diagnostic interview widely accessible. The most recent version (K-SADS-PL-DSM5) has been updated to align with the diagnostic criteria outlined in the DSM-5. The interview takes approximately 45–75 minutes to administer and begins with a screening module that uses probes for the child's past and current symptoms as a means of determining which supplemental modules to administer. Although this measure is not intended for the diagnosis of complex trauma or dissociative disorders, specifically, the Trauma-Related Disorders supplement assesses some dissociative symptoms associated with PTSD (e.g., amnesia for parts of the traumatic event; depersonalization and derealization) as well as some cognitive, physiological, affective, and social symptoms that are common in complex trauma. Given that the interview assesses for many mental disorders, the K-SADS can simultaneously be used to identify some (but not all) co-occurring disorders and symptomatology among children with complex trauma. The K-SADS has been validated in both research and clinical settings.

Standardized Interviews for Developmental Trauma

Two promising clinician-administered structured interview tools, the Developmental Trauma Disorder Structured Interview for Child (DTD SI-C) and the Developmental Trauma Disorder Structured Interview for Parent/Caregiver (DTD SI-P/Care), are ready for clinical use due to strong preliminary support for their psychometric properties (Ford et al., 2018; Spinazzola et al., 2018; van der Kolk et al., 2019), and continued validation in field research trials (Ford et al., 2021; Spinazzola et al., 2021). These interviews are designed for administration to children aged 7–10 in the presence of a caregiver, and to adolescents aged 11–18 alone or accompanied by a caregiver as deemed clinically appropriate for a given youth. The DTD Field Trial Study Group maintains a DTD-SI research catalogue showing the DTD construct and its intersection with other diagnoses, risk trajectories, trauma profiles, treatment models, and clinical sequelae associated with complex trauma generally (J. Spinazzola, personal communication, September 9, 2023), and specifically, such as predictive modeling for youth suicidality and self-harm (Hyland et al., 2022).

Standardized Interviews for Dissociation

There is a paucity of diagnostic instruments available for the assessment of dissociation in children. Only one standardized interview has ever been developed specifically for use in children, though this instrument was never adequately validated and is now out of date (Lewis, 1996). Two other instruments, detailed below, were designed for use with adults and have been used to assess dissociation in youth (including children aged 11 or 12), though these diagnostic tools have not yet been empirically validated for use with younger children. Furthermore, while adequate psychometric properties have been found in adolescent and adult samples, there are no norms available specific to children independent of those available for adolescents and adults. Clinicians who choose to use these interviews with older children need to be mindful of the ways in which dissociation in children may present differently than in adults.

SEMI-STRUCTURED CLINICAL INTERVIEW FOR DISSOCIATIVE SYMPTOMS AND DISORDERS (SCID-D)

The SCID-D, updated in 2022 (Steinberg, 2023), assesses dissociation among adults and adolescents. It can be used with children at least 11 years old who can engage in self-report (Kilic et al., 2017; Sar et al., 2014). This semi-structured interview assesses five domains of dissociative symptoms (i.e., amnesia, depersonalization, derealization, identity confusion, and identity alteration) that can be mapped onto DSM-5-TR criteria for dissociative disorders. The interview can take three to five hours to administer and has traditionally been considered the most accurate tool for diagnosing dissociative disorders. A recent meta-analysis (Mychailyszyn et al., 2021) assessing the SCID-D's psychometric properties found strong evidence supporting its use in clinical, research, and forensic settings, with both the overall SCID-D interview score and the scores of each of the five subscales able to differentiate between adults with and without dissociative disorders. The SCID-D is also effective in differentiating between true dissociative disorders and feigned presentations. An earlier version of the SCID-D is available in German, Dutch, and Turkish translations.

MULTIDIMENSIONAL INVENTORY OF DISSOCIATION—ADOLESCENT VERSION (A-MID)

The A-MID (Dell, 2006) combines a self-administered 218-item multi-scale questionnaire with a follow-up interview to clarify responses. The A-MID was developed from the Multidimensional Inventory of Dissociation for adults and includes revised developmentally appropriate language for adolescents. It has been used in research with children as young as 12 years old. The self-administered questionnaire takes about 30–60 minutes to complete, with the follow-up interview taking additional time. A computer-generated analysis report provides scores across 23 dissociative symptoms alongside diagnostic impressions. The results of this report are not valid in the absence of the follow-up interview, and symptoms must be substantiated before conferring diagnoses. Validity and characterological scales flag responses that may reflect over- or underreporting and which may require closer consideration in the follow-up interview. Multiple translations are also available.

BELLEVUE DIAGNOSTIC INTERVIEW FOR DISSOCIATION IN CHILDREN AND ADOLESCENTS (BDID-C)

The BDID-C is the only semi-structured diagnostic interview developed specifically for use with children (see Lewis, 1996). Pilot studies with this instrument found good interrater reliability at the time of its creation (see Cardeña & Weiner, 2004; Putnam, 1997), though further validation is required to support its use. This measure could be carried out in the context of play therapies to specifically explore states of consciousness, memory, mood, imaginative experiences, auditory hallucinations, visual and sensory experiences, fluctuations in temperament (e.g., aggression), disciplinary experiences, medical complaints, sexual behaviors and disturbances, alterations in skills abilities, and identity disturbances and alterations.

Projective Testing

Projective testing assists children in revealing important information about their experiences, allowing them freedom to share their idiosyncratic and subjective reality. Clinicians can hypothesize about a child's inner world and their unique relationship experiences through the child's drawings, reactions to visual images, sentence stem completions, and storytelling. Children "project" their own perceptions through these tasks, thus revealing their values, wishes, worldviews and struggles without a sense of being evaluated. The typically ambiguous stimuli presented in projective testing do not suggest specific responses, and there are no right or wrong answers. The process and results of projective testing are often viewed as a form of extended unstructured interview that illuminates the child's subjective experience. Below are several of the main types of projective testing techniques used in child assessments.

Rorschach Inkblot Method (RIM)

Although most projective tests are not tightly normed or standardized, the RIM (Rorschach, 1941) provides extensive norms and standardization (Exner, 1995; Meyer & Eblin, 2012) and has recent research validation (Mihura et al., 2013; Tuber et al., 2008; Tuber, 2018). The RIM can be used with children with abuse histories to inform differential diagnosis regarding psychosis or a thought disorder (Friedrich, 2002). Furthermore, children may offer idiosyncratic content that leads to hypotheses about their trauma context (van Eys & Truss, 2012), and predicts future functioning (Tuber, 2018) and coping under extreme stress (Donahue & Tuber, 1993).

Projective Storytelling

In projective storytelling, children are asked to tell a story about what is happening in a scene on a card. Some children tell stories that reveal their inner world of relationships, fears, desires, and beliefs. Other children are guarded and provide concrete descriptors of the card content, leading to hypotheses around rigid defenses or neurodivergence. Themes across stories, such as intense anger or a sense of abandonment, facilitate understanding of a child. Frequently used projective storytelling tests are the Roberts Apperception Test (RAT-C) (McArthur & Roberts, 1982), available with gender- and race-specific images, and the race/ethnic ambiguous Tell-Me-A-Story test (TEMAS) (Constantino et al., 1988). Maltreatment-specific projective storytelling tools with more suggestive images, such as Projective Storytelling (PST) (Caruso & Pulcini, 1990) and the Sexual Projective Card Set (SPCS) (Behavioral Technology, 1996), should be used judiciously, as they may be over-activating due to reminders of trauma experiences.

Drawings

Techniques such as the Draw-A-Person (DAP) (Koppitz, 1968), Kinetic Family Drawing (KFD) (Burns, 1970), and the House-Tree-Person (HTP) (Buck & Hammer, 1969) yield rich insight into children's relationships with self and others, as well as fears and desires. More current techniques such as Color-Your-Heart (Goodyear-Brown, 2010) and the Inside-Outside Technique (Baita, 2022) offer methods to capture the nuances of feelings and self-image. Following children's free-flowing description of their pictures, clinicians pose strategic questions to glean more detail and depth within a drawing.

Incomplete Sentences

Incomplete Sentences is a brief, easy-to-administer semi-projective measure (Loevinger & Wessler, 1970) that can be used as an effective warm-up or a break between more intense measures. Children supply a short answer to a sentence stem, such as "I like…" Themes across the answers reveal the concerns and wishes of children, such as issues of loss or inadequacy.

Unstructured Clinical Interviewing

When working with children, clinical interviewing is often unstructured and multisystemic in nature, including initial (e.g., history-gathering) and follow-up (e.g., after administering standardized assessment tools) interviews with children, caregiving systems, and third-party systems that are involved with the child. The purpose of unstructured interviews is to obtain collateral information, gather social-emotional-behavioral observations, support the use and meaning of screening and assessment results, and assist in relationship building with the child and caregivers. It is through the process of clinical interviewing that a clinician "gains entrance into the phenomenological world of the dissociative child" (Silberg & Dallam, 2023, p. 439).

The ISSTD's *Guidelines for the Evaluation and Treatment of Dissociative Symptoms in Children and Adolescents* (2004), Silberg (2022), and Waters (2016) have outlined detailed guidelines for conducting dissociation-specific clinical interviews with children. Unstructured clinical interviews consist of conversations as well as unstandardized but developmentally appropriate methods such as the sand tray, expressive arts, play, books, cards, puppets, movement, illustrations, and charts. Specific methods may vary based on the child's age (e.g., preschool versus school-age) and developmental capacities. During the interview process, clinicians pay close attention to the content of responses, as well as somatic, behavioral, emotional, and play-based shifts in the child. Clinicians are encouraged to be vigilant for any triggering (i.e., acute distress or dysregulation) that may occur during clinical interviewing with children, as careful attention is required to identify what preceded the triggering (Silberg, 2012; Waters, 2013). Within this process, clinicians must also be mindful of both what is observable and verbalized, and what is omitted or avoided. Timing and pacing of the process attends to the child's and caregiving system's level of affect tolerance and self/other-reporting capacities (Gomez, 2013), allowing for greater detail and data to emerge over time.

Domains to explore during clinical interviews include those described in the HOT framework (outlined earlier in this chapter), as well as a more thorough exploration of the child's symptoms and experiences. Topics of interest may include imaginary friends and other transitional objects, auditory and visual hallucinations, perplexing forgetfulness, intrusive thoughts and feelings, numbing, anxiety, nightmares, self-injury, flashbacks, somatic concerns, sexual concerns, depersonalization and derealization, and identity alteration and confusion. Additional exploration of the family environment is essential and includes physical and emotional safety, dysfunctional family patterns, history of psychiatric illness of all family members, family secrets that may impact the child, sources of support outside the immediate family, practices or beliefs that are unusual for the family's culture and ethnicity, and the child's functioning across different settings. Waters (2016) provided a list of questions that are often valuable for clinicians, and Silberg (1998) outlined applicable cautions for conducting these interviews.

Within the context of clinical interviewing, broaching conversations about culture, racism, discrimination, and oppression within assessment and clinical interviewing is essential, as many standard measures fail to consider these as traumatic stressors and experiences (Williams et al., 2021). Furthermore, cultures differ in the extent to which dissociative phenomena are encouraged via sociocultural practices (Rhoades & Şar, 2005). Gaining a greater understanding of the child's and family's unique experiences is essential, as chosen standardized assessment tools may not capture cultural differences in symptom expression (Canino & Alegria, 2008).

Systems and Ethical Issues in Assessment

Assessment of children with symptoms of C-PTSD (with or without dissociation) must be sensitively pursued with an understanding of and appreciation for the systemic context. For example, the use of projective assessment is not yet supported in the context of child sexual abuse evaluations (Murrie et al., 2009). Children and families may be involved with ongoing legal and/or child welfare proceedings that carry weighty consequences for the child and family, including decisions about custody, placement, and criminal and civil charges. Regardless of whether assessments are completed in a forensic (e.g., aiding the court in custody or dependency evaluations) or therapeutic (e.g., assessments to aid treatment planning and delivery) context, clinicians are reminded to adhere to foundational principles of assessment such as conducting informed consent procedures, adhering to "do no harm" (e.g., not conducting parent-child observation that is likely to retraumatize the child), appropriately administering testing, using multiple sources of information (e.g., HOT model), carefully documenting assessment data, monitoring one's confirmation bias, and ethically reporting information arising from assessment regarding danger to self or others and/or suspicion of child abuse not yet reported.

Clinicians should be well-trained in child maltreatment and symptoms of C-PTSD and dissociation. They should have an understanding of the relevant scientific and clinical literature on children's memory and suggestibility, objective child interviewing and disclosure (Saywitz et al., 2018; Wheeler, 2018), and child development, including psychosexual development, family systems, and insecure attachment styles.

Clinical Case Example

The following is a summary of how a complex trauma-informed assessment, using the HOT model, promoted critical steps toward stability and ultimate thriving for an eight-year-old girl (Amber[1]) who had been placed in foster care with her three younger siblings three months prior to the assessment. The children were removed because of neglect, physical abuse, and drug exposure. At a child welfare team meeting prior to the evaluation, Amber was described as "willfully disobedient," and recommendations for "giving her higher consequences for behavior" were endorsed by all involved.

Reason for Referral

Amber was referred for an urgent assessment by her foster care case manager because she was at risk of losing her foster care placement due to her challenging behaviors. Amber had ongoing difficulty with bowel incontinence and was smearing feces at home and school. Medical reasons were ruled out. She displayed regressive behaviors (such as baby talk), especially following visits or phone calls with her birth mother. She had trouble with maintaining hygiene, forgetting to wash her hands and not properly taking care of her toileting accidents. She had sexualized behaviors such as public masturbation. She was defiant. Her foster mother reported that Amber was lying and stealing, hoarding food, had intense outbursts of anger, tended to zone out, was forgetful, and had wide variations in mood and behavior. Amber was described as sometimes aggressive to her siblings; at other times, she was overprotective of them, competing with her foster mother, and stating that she [Amber] was their sole caregiver.

Assessment Process Using the HOT Framework

Assessment of symptoms of trauma and dissociation occurs within the context of a comprehensive assessment of the child's psychological, social, and behavioral functioning. In this case example, current history (H) and caregiver observations (O) provided a helpful initial lens for assessment. Formal testing (T) then clarified the case formulation. Assessment measures beyond those assessing specifically for trauma and dissociation (such as those outlined in this chapter) may be invaluable for case formulation. This case example combines information obtained from trauma- and dissociation-specific measures with additional assessment measures that complement each other to provide a more comprehensive understanding of the child.

Assessment Measures

The following assessment measures were used as part of this assessment:

- Interviews: foster care staff, foster mother, birth mother, guardian ad litem, and child welfare worker
- Kaufman Brief Intelligence Test, second edition (KBIT-2)
- Northshore Trauma History Checklist
- Children's Dissociative Experiences Scale (CDES)
- Child Dissociative Checklist-3 (caregiver) (CDC-3)
- Imaginary Friends Questionnaire
- Child Depression Inventory-2 (CDI-2)
- Child Sexual Behavior Inventory-3 (CSBI)
- Draw-A-Person
- Systematic Touch Inventory

History (H)

Interviews with multiple collateral informants (i.e., foster care staff, foster mother, birth mother, guardian ad litem, child welfare worker) provided important information about Amber's history, including maternal substance use, stress, and poor health during pregnancy with Amber; continued maternal struggle with substance misuse through Amber's childhood; current and multigenerational domestic violence; a series of abusive partners exposed to the children at home and at both grandmothers' homes; long-standing troubles with encopresis (Amber was never fully potty trained); repeated bouts of pneumonia and RSV as an infant that required hospitalizations; and the death a year prior of Amber's paternal grandmother, who was a primary attachment figure. Sexual abuse was consistently denied (though discovered in this evaluation). This history was suggestive of exposure to early pathogenic conditions (i.e., chaotic, abusive, and neglectful early environment; impaired maternal caregiving due to substance use and mental health challenges; stress from intimate partner violence) that are known to contribute to the formation of symptoms of complex trauma and dissociation.

Collateral information also provided evidence for significant behavioral symptoms often arising from abuse and neglect, including hoarding, bowel incontinence, smearing feces, regression, sexualized behaviors, and dissociative symptoms.

Observations (O)

Amber had very controlled and compliant behavior for the first two hours of the assessment. She was perfectionistic in her attention to her drawing, taking her time and taking pride in her work. However, she became agitated after completing the Systematic Touch Inventory (Hewitt, 1999) in which she not only discussed physical abuse, neglect, and domestic violence, but also disclosed sexual abuse for the first time. After that, Amber appeared to change dramatically in her speech and affect: she became guarded and her eyes appeared glazed over. At the end of the session, when the evaluator was talking with Amber and her foster mother together, Amber's behavior regressed, and she began walking in a very strange and clumsy manner to the restroom. Her foster mom stated that she had observed this strange walk on several occasions when Amber seemed to be agitated. The foster mother said that it was as if Amber couldn't fully walk (e.g., "walking like a toddler") and became baby-like (e.g., reverting to baby talk).

Screening and Assessment

These observations provided clues to dissociative processes. Amber exhibited hallmark dysregulation of body systems such as difficulty walking, dysregulation of affect through mood shifts from calm and organized to agitated, zoning out, and dysregulation in behavior such as changes in speech and eye gaze.

Testing (T)

COGNITIVE FUNCTIONING

Amber scored in the Below Average range on a standardized test of intellectual functioning. However, observations of behavior during interviews suggested that she presented at times as higher functioning than her scores ultimately indicated. Since dissociative children display unpredictable shifts in cognitive and developmental levels, even during assessment (Silberg, 2022), it is important to realize that scores on cognitive assessments may fluctuate across time and context. Amber would need to be retested when she was more stable.

DEPRESSIVE SYMPTOMS

Amber scored in the Very Elevated range on the CDI-2, indicating significant depressive symptoms. Depression commonly co-occurs with trauma symptoms (Verlinden et al., 2015).

SEXUALIZED BEHAVIORS

Amber scored in the Clinically Significant range on the CSBI-3 Sexual Abuse Specific Behaviors symptom scale when compared to other girls her age.

TRAUMA EXPOSURE

Trauma- and dissociation-specific screening measures were key to understanding Amber. On a trauma events screener, Amber endorsed: (1) suffering physical abuse by several caregivers that resulted in bruises, (2) being threatened with physical assault, (3) witnessing domestic violence toward her mother and grandmother, and (4) being left alone with her younger siblings "in a dark, ugly house when she was 9 years old." Amber did not endorse sexual abuse on the initial screener (i.e., Northshore) but disclosed it later on the Systematic Touch Inventory, which is a structured measure designed to explore touch in a safe manner through a drawing continuum that gives the child control in the process.

TRAUMA SYMPTOMS

Amber endorsed a significant level of PTSD symptoms on the PTSD (i.e., PTSI) subscore on the CDES. She endorsed symptoms such as intrusive thoughts, hyperstartle response, restlessness/jumpiness, nightmares, poor concentration, unhappiness, and headaches/stomach aches.

DISSOCIATIVE SYMPTOMS

The CDC-3 completed by Amber's foster mother received a score of 20, which was well past the cutoff score of 12 that is considered indicative of clinically significant levels of dissociation. Specifically, Amber's foster mother endorsed that the following items are "very true" of Amber: goes into a daze or trance-like state; shows rapid personality changes; unusually forgetful or confused about things she should have known; shows marked day-to-day or even hour-to-hour variations in her skills, knowledge, food preferences, etc.; shows rapid regressions in age-level behavior; has a difficult time learning from experience; continues to deny misbehavior even when the evidence is obvious; rapidly changing physical complaints; and has two or more distinct and separate personalities that take control over the child's behavior. Items endorsed as "sometimes or somewhat true" included the following: child does not remember or denies traumatic or painful experiences that are known to have occurred; child has a very poor sense of time (e.g., loses track of time, gets confused about morning or afternoon or what day it is, gets confused about when something has happened); and child is unusually sexually precocious.

Amber's CDES self-report was also significant for a number of high-level dissociative symptoms—her score of 31 exceeded the clinical cutoff score of 21. Symptoms endorsed included: derealization (e.g., feeling like she's dreaming when she's awake, getting so involved in her daydreams that she sometimes feels like they are really happening), depersonalization (e.g., not recognizing herself in the mirror; feeling like she's not in her body but instead floating away, feeling like her body is doing things she doesn't want it to do), and disturbances of memory or presence (e.g., hard time remembering things, wondering if she did things or just thought about doing them, wonders if things she remembers really happened or if she just dreamed them, and staring off into space thinking of nothing). Furthermore, the CDES/PTSI measure had a total score of 55; the clinical cutoff score for full PTSD with dissociation is 43.

PROJECTIVE TESTING

A simple projective test was administered in which Amber received the instructions to "draw a person... any person you choose, someone you know or don't know... it's up to you." Amber drew a picture of a beautiful young girl in a long princess dress with a rainbow over her head. She named the girl "Kristi." As this is one of her sibling's names, it was initially assumed by the evaluator that the drawing was an idealized picture of her beautiful little sister, perhaps grown up. Instead, when Amber was asked to "tell about her picture," she indicated that the girl was her imaginary friend. Amber related how "Kristi" had been with her as long as she could remember, she is more assertive than Amber, and she "comes out" sometimes to act for Amber. She stated that Kristi "loved on me," is "the same age as me," and is "worried about other people hurting me." She described Kristi as having a stronger personality and as being the "defiant me."

Amber's discussion about her imaginary friend brought out a sense of yet another "someone" on the inside who was "behind a gate" in her stomach area. The evaluator asked her to close her eyes and concentrate on that part of her body, and Amber said, "I can open the gate." She then discovered a small girl behind the gate who "came out." She did not know this girl, but asked her name, and it was "Eliza." Later, Amber told her therapist that this was the first time Eliza had ever talked with anyone. Eliza is a self-state that is young, scared, vulnerable, and the one who has trouble with pooping. Amber's experience of inside self-states with distinct names and personalities was an important discovery to help her with her healing. It was likely that there were more self-states to discover, though this was not a focus during the assessment process; discovery would happen naturally later in therapy.

IMAGINARY FRIENDS

To further explore imaginary friends, Amber was administered the Imaginary Friends Questionnaire. This 13-question survey asks about imaginary friends, which is a common experience of dissociative children. While imaginary friends are common for young children, they typically disappear by age 6 or 7. However, children with dissociation may have survived their trauma by creating inner self-states, some of which may be experienced as imaginary friends. Amber answered 8 of the 13 questions as "true," as follows: *My imaginary friend* [Kristi] *gives good advice; I have more than one imaginary friend and they disagree* [most likely she disagrees with Eliza; they are fighting on the inside and fighting someone else]; *My imaginary friend tells me to keep secrets; My imaginary friend has skills or abilities that I don't have* ["she has a good arm," "she is stronger in her personality," "she's the defiant me"]; *My imaginary friend does not want others to know about her; My imaginary friend plays with me when I'm lonely; I wish everyone could see my imaginary friend like I do; My imaginary friend helps me when I am afraid.*

Amber endorsed a significant item that differentiates normal imagination from dissociative processes—that is, having imaginary friends who are in conflict (Silberg, 2022). Further, she described that the imaginary friends know things about her past that she did not know. For example, Eliza knows that she had a "disease thing" in her bottom as a baby that is now causing her to poop. Furthermore, Kristi knows when Amber is about to poop and can help her with that problem.

Formulation and Diagnoses

Through the HOT framework, this assessment uncovered the key to Amber's needs. It was evident that she had experienced multiple forms of abuse and neglect, which caused the formation of disorganized attachment and interfered with her early brain's ability to form a coherent sense of self. She clearly laid out a dissociative system that helped her caregivers and future therapist understand Amber's perplexing and challenging behaviors. She gave new disclosures about sexual abuse and extent of domestic violence that were key to the court proceedings and her therapy.

Amber was diagnosed with the following disorders as outlined in the DSM-5-TR:

- Post-traumatic Stress Disorder with dissociation
- Dissociative Identity Disorder (DID)
- Encopresis (without constipation and overflow incontinence)
- Other Specified Depressive Disorder (more significant than just negative mood/thoughts that accompany PTSD, but not full symptom set of major depressive disorder)

Outcomes

Following this assessment, Amber was provided with dissociation-specific therapy. Amber's caregivers were educated and coached on dissociation-specific caregiving skills, and she was moved to a home (i.e., her "forever home") that better met her needs. The court terminated the birth mother's parental rights for all four children, and they were all successfully adopted.

Amber is now in high school and enjoys dancing and cheerleading. She is, not surprisingly, much more intelligent than the initial IQ test showed. She is able to manage school with support, and she functions as an average student. She and her therapist recently celebrated therapy closure after working together for six years and will meet for boosters as needed in the years to come.

Challenges and Limitations to Comprehensive Assessment in Children

There are developmental limitations to consider when assessing for complex trauma and dissociation in children. Child clinicians have the difficult job of working with children in various developmental stages cognitively, verbally, and socio-emotionally (Hornstein, 1996; Yehuda, 2015) when attempting to adapt adult descriptors of dissociative experiences to children in concrete ways (Hornstein, 1996).

Additionally, wide variations in children's normative behavior and imaginative processes in children's play can make it difficult to distinguish what is normative versus pathological dissociation (Haugaard, 2004; Hornstein, 1996; Peterson, 1991). In children younger than school age, dissociation can be recognized, but making the diagnosis of a dissociative disorder is very difficult (Hornstein, 1996).

Dissociative defenses in childhood can be covert, may mimic other conditions (Hornstein, 1996; Somer, 2011), and will be further addressed in a subsequent chapter focused on defenses. Assessment of dissociative symptoms in children is further complicated by high comorbidity of symptoms with more commonly accepted diagnoses such as attention deficit hyperactivity disorder, oppositional defiant disorder, anxiety, depression, reactive attachment disorder, and eating disorders (Waters, 2016; please see "Differential and Co-Occurring Diagnoses, Neurodivergence, & the Complexity of Dissociative Features in Children" in this book). Despite established research on childhood dissociation, symptoms often remain overlooked in trauma assessment and treatment (Briere & Spinazzola, 2005; Steinberg, 1995). Generally, few clinicians receive adequate training in the recognition and diagnosis of dissociative symptoms and disorders in children (Silberg & Dallam, 2009; Wilkinson & DeJong, 2021). Early detection is further impeded by society's overall deficiency in awareness of childhood dissociative presentations, as well as children's unlikely tendency toward self-disclosure of dissociative experiences (Hornstein, 1996; Waters, 2016), both of which impact access to treatment in childhood. All these factors can be barriers to early recognition and comprehensive assessment, and can result in misdiagnosis (Peterson, 1991; Sinason & Potgieter Marks, 2022).

Additionally, sociocultural realities that permeate the child's internal world, external world, and the therapeutic world of the clinician must be considered. Awareness of process themes that emerge related to discrimination, migration, language, skin color, gender, sexual orientation, religion, spirituality, age, identity, roles, responsibilities, stigma, and cultural strengths need to be a part of both assessment and intervention (Bryant-Davis, 2019).

Hope and Areas for Growth

There is hope for the future of children's mental health when clinicians are aware, willing, and able to hear the perspectives and understand the behavioral presentations of dissociative children (Sinason & Potgieter Marks, 2022). The early detection, comprehensive assessment, and directed treatment of dissociative defenses early in life have the potential to interrupt the intensity of symptoms and turn the child toward a healthy developmental trajectory (Silberg, 1998). Dissociative children adapt to their adverse situations and experiences in remarkable ways while attempting to convey their internal experiences through intense complex behaviors and symptoms (Sinason & Potgieter Marks 2022). Clinicians who work with children must become astute at recognizing the behavioral indicators and symptomatic warning signs of dissociative children, as this is the first step toward developing a comprehensive assessment and treatment plan that will honor the internal experiences of the child.

Conclusion

Comprehensive assessments compile information about the child's history, observations of their behaviors and functioning, and testing results to clarify symptoms (i.e., HOT framework). Assessment is a crucial first step in identifying a child's and family's complex trauma reactions, needs, resources, and strengths. The information gained through this process allows early and preventative interventions to be tailored to the child and family (Kisiel et al., 2009), which may have long-standing benefits for the child, family, and society as a whole (Kluft, 1984; Steinberg, 1995; Kisiel et al. 2009). Clearly understanding the child's behavioral presentation and dissociative symptoms promotes accurate diagnosis and treatment (Cintron et al., 2018).

Clinicians are encouraged to consider the purpose of the assessment when deciding which assessment measures to use. Screening tools and diagnostic interviews inform case formulation and the development of an effective treatment plan. The gathered information supports clinical awareness of symptoms and severity, encourages appropriate pacing of interventions, allows clinicians to account for the dissociative phenomena, and empowers clinicians to tailor the treatment plan to each client's unique needs. Accurately targeting the underlying causes of symptomatology will improve treatment outcomes and support post-traumatic growth. The context and conditions surrounding the assessment, the psychometric rigor of the assessment tools being used, and whether the measure has been normed for age (Strand et al., 2005) and culture (Bertule et al., 2021; Canino & Alegria, 2008; Williams et al., 2021) are additional factors to consider when deciding which assessment tools to use.

Appendix A: Checklist of Domains for Consideration on a Trauma Timeline[2]

- Pre-birth circumstances
  - Parental substance use
  - Domestic violence
  - Poor prenatal nutrition
  - Lack of prenatal medical care

- Birth/infant trauma
  - Substance dependence at birth
  - Difficult birth
  - Intrusive medical procedures
  - Limited caregiving at birth (orphanage, foster care)

- Infant difficulty with regulation and possible use of dissociation as infants
- Parental factors
  - Changes in caregivers (past and present)
  - Parental mental illness
  - Parental history of trauma, troubled attachment, legal, financial, medical issues
  - Parental substance use
  - Parental strengths
  - Parents' relationship history

- Interpersonal violence and/or maltreatment of child
  - Neglect
  - Physical, emotional, and/or sexual abuse
  - Lack of a protective adult
  - Witness of interpersonal violence
  - Exposure to environmental or community trauma
  - Community disasters

- Significant attachment separation/disruptions
  - Foster care
  - Adoption
  - Youth inpatient or residential treatment

- Youth arrested, detained, or incarcerated
- Hospitalization or incarceration of caregiver
* Permanent loss or death of parent or significant other
* High-conflict divorce
* Medical trauma, chronic illness, disability
  - Intrusive or painful medical procedures and frequency
  - Availability and effectiveness of caregiver comfort
  - Age of child (younger child is more vulnerable to helplessness and overwhelm)
  - Child's reactions to medical procedures
* Bullying (including cyberbullying)
* Online victimization or human trafficking
* Societal/cultural trauma
  - Mass gun violence
  - Intergenerational trauma
  - Historical or cultural trauma
  - Refugee
  - War
  - Immigration
  - Felt discrimination related to race, gender, sexual orientation, disability or another aspect of identity
* Placement history
* Child and family strengths, resiliencies, and protective factors
* Treatment history
* Medication history

Notes

1 Name and other identifying details are changed in this case compilation.
2 See ISSTD (2004).

References

Achenbach, T. M., & Edelbrock, C. (1983). *Manual for the child behavior checklist and revised child behavior profile*. Burlington, VT: University of Vermont, Department of Psychiatry.

Achenbach, T. M., & Edelbrock, C. (1987). *Manual for the youth self-report and profile*. Burlington, VT: University of Vermont, Department of Psychiatry.

Akkuş, P., Serdaroğlu, E., Kömürlüoğlu, A., Asena, M., Bahadur, E., Özdemir, G., Karahan, S., & Özmert, E. (2021). Screening traumatic life events in preschool aged children: Cultural adaptation of Child and Adolescent Trauma Screen (CATS) caregiver-report 3–6 years version. *Turkish Journal of Pediatrics*, 63(1), 95–101. https://doi.org/10.24953/turkjped.2021.01.011

American Psychiatric Association. (2013). *Diagnostic and statistical manual of mental disorders* (5th ed.). Arlington, VA: Author.

American Psychiatric Association. (2022). *Diagnostic and statistical manual of mental disorders: DSM-5-TR* (5th ed., rev.). Washington, DC: American Psychiatric Association.

American Psychological Association. (2014). *Distinguishing between screening and assessment for mental and behavioral health problems*. American Psychological Association. https://www.apaservices.org/practice/reimbursement/billing/assessment-screening

Arbuthnott, A. E., Peluola, F., & Waters, F. (2023). *A preliminary analysis of the checklist of indicators of trauma and dissociation in youth*. Poster presented at the International Society for the Study and Trauma and Dissociation, Annual Conference, Louisville, KY.

Armstrong, J. G., Putnam, F. W., Carlson, E. B., Libero, D. Z., & Smith, S. R. (1997). Development and validation of a measure of adolescent dissociation: The Adolescent Dissociative Experiences Scale. *Journal of Nervous & Mental Disease, 185*(8), 491–497. https://doi.org/10.1097/00005053-199708000-00003

Bailey, T., & Brand, B. (2017). Traumatic dissociation: Theory, research, and treatment. *Clinical Psychology: Science and Practice, 24*(2), 170–185.

Baita, S. (2022). The inside-outside technique: Exploring dissociation and fostering self-reflection. In V. Sinason & R. Potgieter Marks (Eds.), *Treating children with dissociative disorders: Attachment, trauma, theory and practice* (pp. 155–167). New York: Routledge.

Barach, P. M. (1991). Multiple personality disorder as an attachment disorder. *Dissociation: Progress in the Dissociative Disorders, 4*(3), 117–123.

Behavioral Technology Inc. (1996). *MONARCH sexual projective card set.* Behavioral Technology Inc.

Bernier, M.-J., Heber, M., & Collin-Vezina, D. (2013). Dissociative symptoms over a year in a sample of sexually abused children. *Journal of Trauma and Dissociation, 14*(4), 455–472. https://doi.org/10.1080/15299732.2013.769478

Bertule, M., Sebre, S., & Kolesovs, A. (2021). Childhood abuse experiences, depression and dissociation symptoms in relation to suicide attempts and suicidal ideation. *Journal of Trauma & Dissociation, 22*(5), 598–614. https://doi.org/10.1080/15299732.2020.1869652

Briere, J. (1996). Trauma Symptom Checklist for Children (TSCC), professional manual. Psychological Assessment Resources, 00253-8, Odessa, FL.

Briere, J., Johnson, K., Bissada, A., Damon, L., Crouch, J., Gil, E., Hanson, R. & Ernst, V. (2001). The Trauma Symptom Checklist for Young Children (TSCYC): Reliability and association with abuse exposure in a multi-site study. *Child Abuse & Neglect, 25*(8), 1001–1014.

Briere, J., & Spinazzola, J. (2005). Phenomenology and psychological assessment of complex posttraumatic states. *Journal of Traumatic Stress: Official Publication of the International Society for Traumatic Stress Studies, 18*(5), 401–412. https://doi.org/10.1002/jts.20048

Bryant-Davis, T. (2019). The cultural context of trauma recovery: Considering the posttraumatic stress disorder practice guideline and intersectionality. *Psychotherapy, 56*(3), 400–408. https://doi.org/10.1037/pst0000241

Buck, J. N., & Hammer, E. F. (Eds.). (1969). *Advances in house-tree-person techniques: Variations and applications.* Los Angeles: Western Psychological Services.

Burke Harris, N., & Renschler, T. (2015). ACE-Q user guide for health professionals. Center for Youth Wellness. centerforyouthwellness.org/wp-content/uploads/2018/06/CYW-ACE-Q-USer-Guide-copy.pdf

Burns, R. C. (1970). *Kinetic family drawings (KFD): An introduction to understanding children through kinetic drawings.* New York: Brunner/Mazel.

Canino, G., & Alegria, M. (2008). Psychiatric diagnosis: Is it universal or relative to culture? *Journal of Child Psychology and Psychiatry, 49*(3), 237–250. https://doi.org/10.1111/j.1469-7610.2007.01854.x

Cardeña, E., & Weiner, L. A. (2004). Evaluation of dissociation throughout the lifespan. *Psychotherapy: Theory, Research, Practice, Training, 41*(4), 496–508. https://doi.org/10.1037/0033-3204.41.4.496

Caruso, K. R., & Pulcini, R. J. (1990). *Projective storytelling card interactive assessment and treatment system.* Redding, CA: Northwest Psychological.

Child and Adolescent Committee of the European Society on Trauma and Dissociation. (2017). *Guidelines for the assessment and treatment of children and adolescents with dissociative symptoms and dissociative disorders.* European Society for Trauma and Dissociation. https://estd.org/sites/default/files/files/estd_guidelines_child_and_adolescents_first_update_july_2.pdf

Cintron, G., Salloum, A., Blair-Andrews, Z., & Storch, E. A. (2018). Parents' descriptions of young children's dissociative reactions after trauma. *Journal of Trauma & Dissociation, 19*(5), 500–513. https://doi.org/10.1080/15299732.2017.1387886

Cloitre, M., Shevlin, M., Brewin, C. R., Bisson, J. I., Roberts, N. P., Maercker, A., Karatzias, T., & Hyland, P. (2018). The International Trauma Questionnaire: Development of a self-report measure of ICD-11 PTSD and complex PTSD. *Acta Psychiatrica Scandinavica, 138*(6), 536–546. https://doi.org/10.1111/acps.12956

Constantino, G., Malgady, R. C., & Rogler, L. H. (1988). *TEMAS (tell-me-a-story).* Western Psychological Services.

Courtois, C. A. (2004). Complex trauma, complex reactions: Assessment and treatment. *Psychotherapy: Theory, Research, Practice, and Training, 41*, 412–425. https://doi.org/10.1037/0033-3204.41.4.412

Dalenberg, C., & Carlson, E. (2010, November 4–6). New versions of the Dissociative Experiences Scale: The DES-R (revised) and the DES-B (brief). Annual meeting of the International Society for Traumatic Stress Studies, Montreal, Quebec.

Dell, P. F. (2006). The Multidimensional Inventory of Dissociation (MID): A comprehensive measure of pathological dissociation. *Journal of Trauma & Dissociation, 7*(2), 77–106. https://doi.org/10.1300/J229v07n02_06

Donahue, P., & Tuber, S. (1993). Rorschach adaptive fantasy images and coping in children under severe environmental stress. *Journal of Personality Assessment, 60*(1), 421–434. https://doi.org/10.1207/s15327752jpa6003_1

Dowdy-Hazlett, T., Killian, M., & Woods, M. (2021). Measurement of traumatic experiences of children within survey and intervention research: A systematic review of the Child and Adolescent Trauma Screen. *Child and Youth Services Review, 131*, Article 106259. https://doi.org/10.1016/j.childyouth.2021.106259

Dutra, L., Bureau, J. F., Holmes, B., Lyubchik, A., & Lyons-Ruth, K. (2009). Quality of early care and childhood trauma: A prospective study of developmental pathways to dissociation. *Journal of Nervous and Mental Disease, 197*(6), 383–390. https://doi.org/10.1097/NMD.0b013e3181a653b7

Eisen, M. L., Goodman, G. S., Qin, J. J., & Davis, S. L. (2002). Memory and suggestibility in maltreated children: Age, stress arousal, dissociation, and psychopathology. *Journal of Experimental Child Psychology, 83*(3), 167–212. https://doi.org/10.1016/s0022-0965(02)00126-1

Evers-Szostak, M., & Sanders, S. (1992). The Children's Perceptual Alteration Scale (CPAS): A measure of children's dissociation. *Dissociation: Progress in the Dissociative Disorders, 5*(2), 91–97.

Exner, J.E., (1995). *The Rorschach: A comprehensive system: Vol. 3. Assessing children and adolescents*. Hoboken, NJ: John Wiley & Sons.

Fagan, J., & McMahon, P.P. (1984). Incipient multiple personality in children. *Journal of Nervous & Mental Disease, 172*(1), 26–36. https://doi.org/10.1097/00005053-198401000-00007

Farrington, A., Waller, G., Smerden, J., & Faupel, A. W. (2001). The Adolescent Dissociative Experiences Scale: Psychometric properties and difference in scores across age groups. *Journal of Nervous and Mental Disease, 189*(10), 722–727. https://doi.org/10.1097/00005053-200110000-00010

Fine, C. (1988). The work of Antoine Despine: The first scientific report on the diagnosis and treatment of a child with multiple personality disorder. *American Journal of Clinical Hypnosis, 31*(1), 33–39. https://doi.org/10.1080/00029157.1988.10402765

Ford, J. D. (2023). Why we need a developmentally appropriate trauma diagnosis for children: A 10-year update on developmental trauma disorder. *Journal of Child and Adolescent Trauma, 16*, 403–418. https://doi.org/10.1007/s40653-021-00415-4

Ford, J. D., Spinazzola, J., van der Kolk, B., & Grasso, D. J. (2018). Toward an empirically based developmental trauma disorder diagnosis for children: Factor structure, item characteristics, reliability, and validity of the developmental trauma disorder semi-structured interview. *Journal of Clinical Psychiatry, 79*(5), Article 17m11675. https://doi.org/10.4088/JCP.17m11675

Ford, J. D., van der Kolk, B., and Spinazzola, J. (2021). Psychiatric comorbidity of developmental trauma disorder (DTD) and posttraumatic stress disorder (PTSD): Findings from the DTD field trial replication (DTDFT-R). *European Journal of Psychotraumatology, 12*(1). https://doi.org/10.1080/20008198.2021.1929028

Friedrich, W. N. (2002). *Psychological assessment of sexually abused children and their families*. Thousand Oaks, CA: Sage.

Goldbeck, L., & Berliner, L. (2014). Child And Adolescent Trauma Screen. istss.org/clinical-resources/child-trauma-assessments/child-and-adolescent-trauma-screen-(cats)

Gomez, A. M. (2013). *EMDR therapy and adjunct approaches with children: Complex trauma, attachment, and dissociation*. New York: Springer.

Goodyear-Brown, P. (2010). *Play therapy with traumatized children: A prescriptive approach*. Hoboken, NJ: John Wiley & Sons.

Haselgruber, A., Sölva, K., & Lueger-Schuster, B. (2020). Symptom structure of ICD-11 complex posttraumatic stress disorder (CPTSD) in trauma-exposed foster children: Examining the International Trauma Questionnaire – Child and Adolescent Version (ITQ-CA). *European Journal of Psychotraumatology, 11*(1), Article 1818974. https://doi.org/10.1080/20008198.2020.1818974

Haugaard, J. J. (2004). Recognizing and treating uncommon behavioral and emotional disorders in children and adolescents who have been severely maltreated: Dissociative disorders. *Child Maltreatment, 9*(2), 146–153. https://doi.org/10.1177/1077559504264311

Hewitt, S. K. (1999). *Assessing allegations of sexual abuse in preschool children: Understanding small voices*. Thousand Oaks, CA: Sage.

Hornstein, N. L. (1996). Dissociative disorders in children and adolescents. In L. Michelson & W. Ray (Eds.), *Handbook of dissociation: Theoretical, empirical, and clinical perspectives* (pp. 139–159). New York: Springer.

Hunsley, J., & Di Giulio, G. (2001). Norms, norming, and clinical assessment. *Clinical Psychology: Science and Practice, 8*(3), 378–382. https://doi.org/10.1093/clipsy.8.3.378

Hyland, P., Karatzias, T., Ford, J., Fox, R., & Spinazzola, J. (2022). Psychiatric comorbidity of developmental trauma disorder (DTD) and posttraumatic stress disorder (PTSD): Findings from the DTD field trial replication (DTDFT-R). *European Journal of Psychotraumatology, 12*(1). https://doi.org/10.1080/20008198.2021.1929028

ISSTD (International Society for the Study of Dissociation Taskforce). (2004). Guidelines for the evaluation and treatment of dissociative symptoms in children and adolescents. *Journal of Trauma and Dissociation, 5*(3), 119–150.

John Praed Foundation. (2021). *Child and adolescent needs and strengths: Standard CANS comprehensive 3.0 ages 6 through 20*. Chicago, IL: John Praed Foundation.

Kassam-Adams, N. (2006). The Acute Stress Checklist for children (ASC-Kids): Development of a child self-report measure. *Journal of Traumatic Stress, 19*(1), 129–139.

Kaufman, J., Birmaher, B., Brent, D., & Rao, U. (1997). Affective disorders and schizophrenia for school-age children–present and lifetime version (KSADS-PL): Initial reliability and validity data. *Journal of the American Academy of Child Adolescent Psychiatry,36*(7), 980–988. https://doi.org/10.1097/00004583-199707000-00021

Kerig, P. K., Charak, R., Chaplo, S. D., Bennet, D. C., Armour, C., Modrowski, C. A., & McGee, A. B. (2016). Validation of the factor structure of the Adolescent Dissociative Experiences Scale in a sample of trauma-exposed detained youth. *Psychological Trauma: Theory, Research, Practice, and Policy, 8*(5), 592–600. https://doi.org/10.1037/tra0000140

Kezelman, C. A., & Stavropoulus, P. A. (2020). *Practice guidelines for identifying and treating complex trauma-related dissociation*. Blue Knot Foundation.

Kilic, F., Coskun, M., Bozkurt, H., Kaya, I., & Zoroglu, S. (2017). Self-injury and suicide attempt in relation with trauma and dissociation among adolescents with dissociative and non-dissociative disorders. *Psychiatry Investigation, 14*(2), 172–178. https://doi.org/10.4306/pi.2017.14.2.172

Kira, I. A., & Shuwiekh, H. (2022). Development and validation of the brief pathological dissociation scale PDS(B): Initial psychometrics. *European Journal of Trauma & Dissociation, 6*(4), 100294. https://doi.org/10.1016/j.ejtd.2022.100294

Kisiel, C. L., Fehrenbach, T., Small, L., & Lyons, J. S. (2009). Assessment of complex trauma exposure, responses, and service needs among children and adolescents in child welfare. *Journal of Child & Adolescent Trauma, 2*, 143–160. https://doi.org/10.1080/19361520903120467

Kisiel, C. L., Torgersen, E., & McClelland, G. (2020). Understanding dissociation in relation to child trauma, mental health needs, and intensity of services in child welfare: A possible missing link. *Journal of Family Trauma, Child Custody & Child Development, 17*(3), 189–218. https://doi.org/10.1080/26904586.2020.1816867

Kluft, R. P. (1984). Multiple personality in childhood. *Psychiatric Clinics of North America, 7*, 121–134.

Koppitz, E. M. (1968). *Psychological evaluation of children's human figure drawings*. New York: Psychological Corporation.

Lanius, R. A., Brand, B., Vermetten, E., Frewen, P.A., & Spiegel, D. (2012). The dissociative subtype of posttraumatic stress disorder: Rational, clinical and neurobiological evidence, and implications. *Depression and Anxiety, 29*, 701–708. https://doi.org/10.1002/da.21889

Levendosky, A. A., Huth-Bocks, A. C., Semel, M. A., & Shapiro, D. L. (2002). Trauma symptoms in preschool-age children exposed to domestic violence. *Journal of Interpersonal Violence, 17*(2), 150–164. https://doi.org/10.1177/0886260502017002003

Lewis, D. O. (1996). Diagnostic evaluation of the child with dissociative identity disorder/multiple personality disorder. *Child & Adolescent Psychiatric Clinics of North America, 5*(2), 303–331. https://doi.org/10.1016/S1056-4993(18)30368-7

Liotti, G. (1992). Disorganized/disoriented attachment in the etiology of the dissociative disorders. *Dissociation, 5*(4), 196–204.

Liotti, G. (2004). Trauma, dissociation, and disorganized attachment: Three strands of a single braid. *Psychotherapy: Theory, Research, Practice, Training, 41*(4), 472. https://doi.org/10.1037/0033-3204.41.4.472

Loevinger, J., & Wessler, R. (1970). *Measuring ego development: Vol. 1. Construction and use of a sentence completion test*. St. Louis, MO: Jossey Bass.

McArthur, D. S., & Roberts, G. E. (1982). *Roberts apperception test for children*. Los Angeles: Western Psychological Services.

Meyer, G. J., & Eblin, J. J. (2012). An overview of the Rorschach Performance Assessment System (R-PAS). *Psychological Injury and Law*, *5*(2), 107–121. https://doi.org/10.1007/s12207-012-9130-y

Mihura, J. L., Meyer, G. J., Dumitrascu, N., & Bombel, G. (2013). The validity of individual Rorschach variables: Systematic reviews and meta-analyses of the comprehensive system. *Psychological Bulletin*, *139*(3), 548–605. https://doi.org/10.1037/a0029406

Milot, T., Plamandon, A., Éthier, L. S., Lemelin, J.-P., St-Laurent, D., & Rousseau, M. (2013). Validity of the CBCL-derived PTSD and dissociation scales: Further evidence in a sample of neglected children and adolescents. *Child Maltreatment*, *18*(2), 122–128.https://doi.org/10.1177/1077559513490246

Murrie, D. L., Martindale, D. A., & Epstein, M. E. (2009). Unsupported assessment techniques in child sexual abuse evaluations. In K. Kuchnle & M. Connell (Eds.), *The evaluation of child sexual abuse allegations: A comprehensive guide to assessment and testimony* (pp. 397–420). Hoboken, NJ: John Wiley & Sons.

Mychailyszyn, M., Webermann, A., Brand, B., Sar, V., & Draijer, N. (2021). Differentiating dissociative from non-dissociative disorders: A meta-analysis of the structured clinical interview for DSM dissociative disorders (SCID-D). *Journal of Trauma & Dissociation 22*(1), 19–34. https://doi.org/10.1080/15299732.2020.1760169

Naish, B. L. (2020). *Relative efficacy of the clinician-administered PTSD scale-5, the dissociative subtype of PTSD scale, and the dissociative experiences scales to identify the PTSD dissociative subtype* [Doctoral dissertation, Alliant International University]. Alliant International University ProQuest Dissertations Publishing, 2020. 28023067.

Nilsson, D., Dävelid, I., Ledin, S., & Svedin, C. G. (2021). Psychometric properties of the Child and Adolescent Trauma Screen (CATS) in a sample of Swedish children. *Nordic Journal of Psychiatry*, *75*(4), 247–256. https://doi.org/10.1080/08039488.2020.1840628

Ogawa, J. R., Sroufe, A., Weinfield, N. S., Carlson, E. A., Egeland, B. (1997). Development and the fragmented self: Longitudinal study of dissociative symptomatology in a nonclinical sample. *Developmental Psychopathology*, *9*(4), 855–879. https://doi.org/10.1017/S0954579497001478

Peterson, G. (1991). Children coping with trauma: Diagnosis of "Dissociation Identity Disorder." *Dissociation: Progress in the Dissociative Disorders*, *4*(3), 152–164.

Putnam, F. W. (1997). *Dissociation in children and adolescents: A developmental perspective*. New York: Guilford Press.

Putnam, F. W., Helmers, K., & Trickett, P. K. (1993). Development, reliability, and validity of a child dissociation scale. *Child Abuse & Neglect*, *17*(6), 731–741. https://doi.org/10.1016/S0145-2134(08)80004-X

Putnam, F. W., & Peterson, G. (1994). Further validation of the Child Dissociative Checklist. *Dissociation: Progress in the Dissociative Disorders*, *7*(4), 204–211.

Reagor, P., Kasten, J., & Morelli, N. (1992). A checklist for screening dissociative disorders in children and adolescents. *Dissociation*, *5*(1), 4–19.

Rhoades, G. F., & Şar, V. (2005). *Trauma and dissociation in a cross-cultural perspective: Not just a North American phenomenon*. New York: Hawthorn Press.

Rolon-Arroyo, B., Oosterhoff, B., Layne, C. M., Steinberg, A. M., Pynoos, R. S., & Kaplow, J. B. (2020). The UCLA PTSD reaction index for DSM-5 brief form: A screening tool for trauma-exposed youths. *Journal of the American Academy of Child & Adolescent Psychiatry*, *59*(3), 434–443. https://doi.org/10.1016/j.jaac.2019.06.015

Rorschach, H. (1941). *Psychodiagnostics*. (Hans Huber Verlag, Trans.). Bircher. (Original work published 1921).

Sachser, C., Berliner, L., Holt, T., Jensen, T. K., Jungbluth, N., Risch, E., Rosner, R., & Goldbeck, L. (2017). International development and psychometric properties of the Child and Adolescent Trauma Screen (CATS). *Journal of Affective Disorders*, *210*, 189–195. https://doi.org/10.1016/j.jad.2016.12.040

Sachser, C., Berliner, L., Risch, E., Rosner, R., Birkeland, M. S., Eilers, R., Hafstad, G. S., Pfeiffer, E., Plener, P. L., & Jensen, T. K. (2022). The Child and Adolescent Trauma Screen 2 (CATS-2) – Validation of an instrument to measure DSM-5 and ICD-11 PTSD and complex PTSD in children and adolescents. *European Journal of Psychotraumatology*, *13*(2), 2105580. https://doi.org/10.1080%2F20008066.2022.2105580

Sanders, S. (1986). The perceptual alteration scale: A scale measuring dissociation. *American Journal of Clinical Hypnosis*, *29*(2), 95–102.

Sar, V., Onder, C., Kilincaslan, A., Zoroglu, S. S., & Alyanak, B. (2014). Dissociative identity disorder among adolescents: Prevalence in a university psychiatric outpatient unit. *Journal of Trauma & Dissociation: The Official Journal of the International Society for the Study of Dissociation (ISSD)*, *15*(4), 402–419. https://doi.org/10.1080/15299732.2013.864748

Saxe, G., Chawla, N., Stoddard, F., Kassam-Adams, N., Courtney, D., Cunningham, K., Lopez, C., Hall, E., Sheridan, R., King, D., & King, L. (2003). Child Stress Disorders Checklist: A measure of ASD and PTSD in children. *Journal of the American Academy of Child & Adolescent Psychiatry, 42*(8), 972–978. https://doi.org/10.1097/01.CHI.0000046887.27264.F3

Saywitz, K., Lyons, T., & Goodman, G. (2018). When interviewing children: A review and update. In J. Klika & J. Conte (Eds.), *The APSAC handbook on child maltreatment* (4th ed., pp. 310-329). Thousand Oaks, CA: Sage.

Schimmenti, A. (2023). The relationship between attachment and dissociation: Theory, research, and clinical implications. In M. J. Dorahy, S. N. Gold, & J. A. O'Neil (Eds.), *Dissociation and the dissociative disorders: Past, present, future* (pp. 161–175). New York: Routledge.

Schore, A. N. (2003). *Affect regulation and the repair of the self* (Vol. 2). New York: W. W. Norton.

Schore, A. N. (2013). Relational trauma, brain development, and dissociation. In J. Ford & C. Courtois (Eds.), *Treating complex traumatic stress disorders in children and adolescents: Scientific foundations and therapeutic models* (pp. 3–23). New York: Guilford Press.

Silberg, J. L. (Ed.). (1998). *The dissociative child*. Lutherville, MD: Sidran Press.

Silberg, J. L. (2012). *The child survivor: Healing developmental trauma and dissociation*. New York: Routledge.

Silberg, J. L. (2022). *The child survivor: Healing developmental trauma and dissociation* (2nd ed.). New York: Routledge.

Silberg, J. L., & Dallam, S. (2009). Dissociation in children and adolescents: At the crossroads. In P. F. Dell & J. A. O'Neil (Eds.). *Dissociation and the dissociative disorders: DSM-V and Beyond* (pp. 67–105). New York: Routledge.

Silberg, J. L., & Dallam, S. (2023). Dissociative disorders in children and adolescents. In M. J. Dorahy, S. N. Gold, & J. A. O'Neil (Eds.). *Dissociation and the dissociative disorders: Past, present, future.* (pp. 433–447). New York: Routledge.

Silberg, J. L., & Wieland, S. (2013). Dissociation-focused therapy. In J. Ford & C. Courtois (Eds.), *Treating complex traumatic stress disorders in children and adolescents: Scientific foundations and therapeutic models* (pp. 162–183). New York: Guilford Press.

Sim, L., Friedrich, W. N., Davies, W. H., Trentham, B., Lengua, L., & Pithers, W. (2005). The Child Behavior Checklist as an indicator of posttraumatic stress disorder and dissociation in normative, psychiatric, and sexually abused children. *Journal of Traumatic Stress, 18*(6), 697–705. https://doi.org/10.1002/jts.20078

Sinason, V., & Potgieter Marks, R. (2022). *Treating children with dissociative disorder: Attachment, trauma, theory and practice*. New York: Routledge.

Skar, A. M. S., Jensen, T. K., & Harpviken, A. N. (2021). Who reports what? A comparison of child and caregivers' reports of child trauma exposure and associations to post-traumatic stress symptoms and functional impairment in child and adolescent mental health clinics. *Research on Child and Adolescent Psychopathology, 49*(7), 919–934. https://doi.org/10.1007/s10802-021-00788-y

Smith, S. R., & Carlson, E. B. (1996). Reliability and validity of the Adolescent Dissociative Experiences Scale. *Dissociation, 9*(2), 125–129.

Somer, E. (2011). Dissociation in traumatized children & adolescents. In V. Ardino (Ed.), *Post-traumatic syndromes in childhood and adolescence: A handbook of research and practice*. Hoboken, NJ: Wiley Blackwell.

Spiegel, D., Loewenstein, R. J., Lewis-Fernandez, R., Sar, V., Simeon, D., Vermetten, E., Cardeña, E., & Dell, P. F. (2011). Dissociative disorders in DSM-5. *Depression and Anxiety, 28*, E17–E45. https://doi.org/10.1002/da.20923

Spinazzola, J., van der Kolk, B., & Ford, J. D. (2018). When nowhere is safe: Interpersonal trauma and attachment adversity as antecedents of posttraumatic stress disorder and developmental trauma disorder. *Journal of Traumatic Stress, 31*(5), 631–642. https://doi.org/10.1002/jts.22320

Spinazzola, J., van der Kolk, B., & Ford, J. D. (2021). Developmental trauma disorder: A legacy of attachment trauma in victimized children. *Journal of Traumatic Stress, 34*(4), 711–720. https://doi.org/10.1002/jts.22697

Stanley, L. H. K., & Stanley, C. T. (2021). The Trauma Symptom Checklist for Young Children: A psychometric review. *Journal of Evidence-Informed Social Work, 18*(3), 323–339.

Steinberg, M. (1995). *Handbook for the assessment of dissociation: A clinical guide*. Washington, DC: American Psychiatric Pub.

Steinberg, M. (2023). *The SCID-D interview: Dissociation assessment in therapy, forensics, and research*. Washington, DC: American Psychiatric Pub.

Stolbach, B. C. (1997). *The children's Dissociative Experiences Scale and Posttraumatic Symptom Inventory: Rationale, development, and validation of a self-report measure*. [Doctoral dissertation, University of Colorado at Boulder]. ProQuest Dissertations Publishing, 9725794.

Stolbach, B. C. (2005). Psychotherapy of a dissociative 8-year-old boy burned at age 3. *Psychiatric Annals, 35*(8), 685–694. https://doi.org/10.3928/00485713-20050801-10

Strand, V., Sarmiento, T., & Pasquale, L. (2005). Assessment and screening tools for trauma in children and adolescents: A review. *Trauma Violence Abuse, 6*(1), 55–78. https://doi.org/10.1177/1524838004272559

Taylor, J., & Shrive, J. (2023). *Indicative trauma impact manual: A non-diagnostic, trauma-informed guide to emotion, thought, and behaviour.* VictimFocus.

Tuber, S. (2018). *Using projective methods with children: The selected works of Steve Tuber.* New York: Routledge.

Tuber, S., Goudsmit, N., Ferst, A., Shagrin, S., & Wolitzky, R. (2008). A review of projective tests for children: Recent developments. In C. Coulacoglou (Ed.), *Exploring the child's personality: Developmental, clinical and cross-cultural applications of the Fairy Tale Test* (pp. 5–28). Springfield, IL: Charles C Thomas Publisher.

van der Kolk, B. A. (2005). Developmental Trauma Disorder: Toward a rational diagnosis for children with complex trauma histories. *Psychiatric Annals, 35*(5), 401–408. https://doi.org/10.3928/00485713-20050501-06

van der Kolk, B., Ford, J. D., & Spinazzola, J. (2019). Comorbidity of developmental trauma disorder (DTD) and post-traumatic stress disorder: Findings from the DTD field trial. *European Journal of Psychotraumatology, 10*(1), Article 1562841. https://doi.org/10.1080/20008198.2018.1562841

van Eys, P., & Truss, A. (2012) Comprehensive and therapeutic assessment of child sexual abuse: A bridge to treatment. In P. Goodyear-Brown (Ed.), *Handbook of child sexual abuse* (pp. 143–170).. Hoboken, NJ: John Wiley and Sons.

Verlinden, E., Opmeer, B. C., Van Meijel, E. P., Beer, R., De Roos, C., Bicanic, I. A., Lamers-Winkelman, F., Olff, M., Boer, F., & Lindauer, R. J. (2015). Enhanced screening for posttraumatic stress disorder and co-morbid diagnoses in children and adolescents. *European Journal of Psychotraumatology, 6,* Article 26661. https://doi.org/10.3402/ejpt.v6.26661

Wasserman, T., & Wasserman, L. D. (2016). *Depathologizing psychopathology: The neuroscience of mental illness and its treatment.* Cham: Springer.

Waters, F. S. (2013). Assessing and diagnosing dissociation in children: Beginning the recovery. In A. M. Gomez (Ed.), *EMDR therapy and adjunct approaches with children* (pp. 129–149). New York: Springer.

Waters, F. S. (2016). *Healing the fractured child: Diagnosis and treatment of youth with dissociation.* New York: Springer.

Waters, F. S. (2021). CIT-DY – Checklist of Indicators of Trauma & Dissociation in Youth: A comprehensive checklist to guide assessment & diagnosis of youth with complex trauma. waterscounselingandtraining.com/check-list-for-trauma-assessment

Wheeler, J. (2018). Psychological assessment of the child and family. In J. Klika & J. Conte (Eds.), *The APSAC handbook on child maltreatment* (4th ed., pp. 163–181). Thousand Oaks, CA: Sage.

Wherry, J. N., Jolly, J. B., Feldman, J., Adam, B., & Manjanatha, S. (1994). The child dissociative checklist. *Journal of Child Sexual Abuse, 3*(3), 51–66. https://doi.org/10.1300/J070v03n03_04

Wieland, S. (2015). Dissociation in children and adolescents: What it is, how it presents, and how we can understand it. In S. Wieland (Ed.), *Dissociation in traumatized children and adolescents: Theory and clinical interventions* (pp. 1–39). New York: Routledge.

Wilkinson, S., & DeJong, M. (2021). Dissociative identity disorder: A developmental perspective. *BJPsych Advances, 27*(2), 96–98. https://doi.org/10.1192/bja.2020.35

Williams, M.T., Osman, M., Gran-Ruaz, S., & Lopez, J. (2021). Intersection of racism and PTSD: Assessment and treatment of racial stress and trauma. *Current Treatment Options in Psychiatry, 8,* 167–185. https://doi.org/10.1007/s40501-021-00250-2

Yehuda, N. (2015). *Communicating trauma: Clinical presentations and interventions with traumatized children.* New York: Routledge.

Young, E. (2022). I didn't know where you were: In the play space of treatment with a young dissociative boy. In V. Sinason & R. Potgieter Marks (Eds.), *Treating children with dissociative disorders: Attachment, trauma, theory and practice* (pp. 180–197). New York: Routledge.

14
DIFFERENTIAL AND CO-OCCURRING DIAGNOSES, NEURODIVERGENCE, AND THE COMPLEXITY OF DISSOCIATIVE FEATURES IN CHILDREN

Patti van Eys and Alexis Arbuthnott

Introduction

Symptoms of complex (i.e., developmental) trauma, usually associated with varying degrees of dissociative symptoms, affect multiple domains of child functioning, including dysregulation of relating (i.e., attachment disturbance), biology, affect, behavior, consciousness and cognition, and self-concept (Cook et al., 2005; Ford, 2023). Symptoms of complex/developmental trauma and dissociation overlap considerably with and commonly co-occur alongside symptoms across other mental/behavioral disorders (Ford et al., 2021). Furthermore, disruptions of normative development caused by complex/developmental trauma, particularly neglect, may mimic symptoms of neurodevelopmental disorders. Overlapping, co-occurring, and interacting symptoms, complicated by development itself, can thrust clinicians into a diagnostic labyrinth. Undetected diagnoses and/or misdiagnoses are common (Silberg & Dallam, 2023). Complex/developmental trauma and dissociation may be misdiagnosed as another mental disorder (e.g., oppositional defiant disorder [ODD]), overshadowed by a co-occurring disorder (e.g., bipolar disorder) or atypical neurodevelopment (e.g., autism spectrum disorder [ASD]), or hide a true co-occurring disorder when symptoms are overly attributed to complex/developmental trauma. Despite similarities, symptoms of developmental trauma are distinct from other psychiatric disorders, are clinically useful and significant, and are "not effectively treated by gold-standard therapeutic interventions for post-traumatic stress disorder (PTSD) or any other psychiatric disorder of childhood" (Ford, 2023, p. 407). Unfortunate consequences of inaccurate or missed diagnoses include delayed access to effective treatment, negative side effects of unnecessary treatment (e.g., medication-induced metabolic changes), stigma, shame, disruptions of normative development, and a sense of failure for children and caregivers (Spiegel et al., 2011).

This chapter starts with an overview of diagnostic considerations for children with complex/developmental trauma, including the role of classifications and common co-occurring and differential diagnoses. Given the impact of complex/developmental trauma and dissociation on development, this chapter then explores the overlap and its relationship with neurodivergence. Case examples demonstrate the complexities of dysregulation within this population, with specific attention to dissociative features in children.[1]

Diagnostic Classifications

Diagnoses of mental disorders are conferred following a systematic assessment that ideally includes a review of the child's history, behavioral observations, interviews with the child and key adults, symptom screening, and, when needed, psychological testing (see Chapter 13). This multi-method, multi-informant approach to assessment tracks the child's development and symptoms over time when conceptualizing the child's current difficulties. Both symptoms and diagnoses may evolve as the child develops (Costello et al., 2003). Thus, assessment is ongoing and continuous.

While a thorough assessment is essential for identifying and treating dissociation in children, a formal diagnosis of a dissociative disorder is not. Although formal diagnoses are required in some circumstances (e.g., insurance coverage, research criteria, and location), it may be prudent to defer formal diagnosis while discerning the presence and nature of dissociative symptoms within the broader case conceptualization. A diagnostic label is but one component of case conceptualization used to inform appropriate interventions (see Chapter 15). As stated by Silberg (2022, p. 39), "the label we choose is less important than whether the therapist and client can devise mutually shared constructs that not only describe the problem, but also potentiate healing and growth." To that end, diagnosis requires consideration of the child in context, development, and resiliency.

There are two main systems in use for classifying mental disorders: The International Classification of Diseases (ICD) and the *Diagnostic and Statistical Manual of Mental Disorders (DSM)*. A separate manual exists for infants and toddlers: the *Diagnostic Classification of Mental Health and Developmental Disorders of Infancy and Early Childhood (DC:0–5*; Zero to Three, 2016). The ICD-11 is the current official classification of all diseases worldwide (ICD-11; World Health Organization, 2021). The *DSM-5-TR* is the current official classification system of psychiatric disorders in North America (American Psychiatric Association, 2022), and has been adopted worldwide for psychiatric research (O'Neil, 2023). The ICD and *DSM* are derived from a combination of scientific research and political forces, which reflects both the academic and cultural climate of the region and time in which the systems evolved (O'Neil, 2023).

There is considerable overlap in diagnostic criteria between the systems, with the *DSM* including corresponding ICD codes alongside each diagnosis. Both systems include classifications for disorders of trauma and dissociation. A comparative overview of current diagnostic categories for disorders associated with complex trauma and dissociation in the ICD-11 and *DSM-5-TR* is provided in Table 14.1.

Complex/Developmental Trauma Disorders

The original concept of "complex trauma," deriving from cases of "prolonged and repeated trauma" (Herman, 1992/2022), was empirically validated with adults within the context of the *DSM-IV* "disorders of extreme stress not otherwise specified" (DESNOS) (van der Kolk et al., 2005), and was proposed as a new childhood diagnosis termed "developmental trauma disorder" (DTD) (van der Kolk, 2005). Neither DESNOS nor DTD was included in the latest ICD or *DSM* nomenclature. Instead, the ICD-11 adopted a diagnosis of complex post-traumatic stress disorder (C-PTSD), which includes a subset of the symptoms of dysregulation described in DESNOS and DTD, and the *DSM-5-TR* incorporated symptoms into the PTSD diagnosis regarding trauma-infused core beliefs (e.g., self-blame), distress-related emotions (e.g., shame), and dysregulation of behaviors (e.g., self-harm). The *DSM-5-TR* also added a dissociative subtype of PTSD, and PTSD criteria specific for children ages six years and younger, that acknowledges that dissociative reactions "may occur on a continuum with the most extreme expression being a complete loss of awareness of present surroundings" (American Psychiatric Association, 2022, p. 303).

Table 14.1 Classifications of Complex Trauma and Dissociation in the ICD-11 (World Health Organization, 2021) and DSM-5-TR (American Psychiatric Association, 2022)

Type of Symptom	Trauma-Related Diagnosis	
	ICD-11 Classifications	DSM-5-TR Classifications
Acute and post-traumatic stress responses[a] (may include peritraumatic dissociation, dissociative amnesia for trauma-related content, and dissociative flashbacks)	Post-traumatic stress disorder (PTSD) Acute stress reaction Adjustment disorder	PTSD (including separate criteria for children six years and younger) Acute stress disorder Adjustment disorders
Attachment concerns related to inadequate caregiving[a,b]	Reactive attachment disorder (RAD) Disinhibited social engagement disorder (DSED)	RAD DSED
Complex post-traumatic stress responses (e.g., alterations in affect regulation, beliefs about oneself, and relationships)	Complex PTSD[c]	None[b,c,d]
Dissociative multiplicity (often occurring alongside dissociative amnesia, which is required for a diagnosis of dissociative identity disorder [DID])	DID Partial DID	DID Other specified dissociative disorder (OSDD) *Chronic and recurrent syndromes of mixed dissociative symptoms*
Dissociation of memory	Dissociative amnesia: specify with/without dissociative fugue	Dissociative amnesia: specify if with dissociative fugue
Depersonalization and derealization (DP/DR)	DP/DR disorder	DP/DR disorder PTSD, with dissociative symptoms
Sensorimotor dissociation	Dissociative neurological symptom disorder	Functional neurological symptoms disorder
Residual kinds of dissociation	Trance disorder Possession trance disorder Other specified dissociative disorders Unspecified dissociative disorder	OSDD *Identity disturbance due to prolonged and intense coercive persuasion Acute dissociative reactions to stressful events Dissociative trance* Unspecified dissociative disorder

[a] Diagnostic criteria specific to infants and toddlers also exist (*DC:0-5*; Zero to Three, 2016).
[b] The proposed developmental trauma disorder (DTD) was not included in the *DSM-5* (Spinazzola et al., 2021).
[c] The *DSM-5-TR* PTSD criteria now include negative alterations in cognitions and mood associated with the traumatic event, but not more globally.
[d] Some clinicians and researchers argue that the *DSM-5-TR*'s borderline personality disorder (which corresponds with the ICD-11's borderline pattern specifier for personality disorders) is itself a stress or trauma response.

Although ICD-11's C-PTSD diagnostic category reflects societal advances in recognizing complex trauma as a disorder with unique symptoms (i.e., emotion and behavioral dysregulation, altered self-perceptions, and altered engagement in relationships), it does not include the disruptions in attachment to the primary caregiver(s), unique aspects of behavioral manifestations of trauma, and somatic dysregulation captured by DTD (Ford, 2023). Further, a diagnosis of C-PTSD requires that a person first meet criteria for PTSD (World Health Organization, 2021). However, children with complex post-traumatic adaptations (i.e., DTD) may not meet criteria for PTSD (D'Andrea et al., 2012; DePierro et al., 2022), tend to have more extensive trauma histories than children with PTSD, and are likely to be more functionally impaired (Ford, 2023). Ongoing research and advocacy for the inclusion of a developmentally appropriate complex trauma diagnosis into the *DSM* has spawned converging evidence from clinician surveys and field trials with children that DTD constitutes a cohesive set of symptoms distinct from but often co-occurring with PTSD (Ford, 2023; Ford et al., 2022; Spinazzola et al., 2021). Although PTSD and DTD share, as antecedents, a history of exposure to traumatic events, DTD differs from PTSD by diagnostically requiring the presence of a combination of interpersonal victimization and disrupted attachment.

The absence of a diagnosis in the DSM capturing the essence of complex trauma means that the sequela of complex/developmental trauma among children are frequently inaccurately attributed to other mental disorders with overlapping symptoms (D'Andrea et al., 2012; Ford et al., 2021). For example, the ICD/*DSM* criteria for reactive attachment disorder (RAD) and disinhibited social engagement disorder (DSED) overlap considerably with DTD. While DTD requires *both* impoverished caregiving that interfered with attachment formation *and* experiencing interpersonal victimization or family/community violence, RAD and DSED require only a historical antecedent of impoverished or unavailable caregiving that limited access to forming selective attachment. Further, while DTD requires three domains of dysregulation (i.e., affective/somatic, cognitive/behavioral, and self/interpersonal), the symptoms of RAD and DSED are narrowly focused on attachment behavior. See Chapters 4 and 5 for information about the role of disorganized attachment in the development of dissociation.

Case Example

"D," age 9, was diagnosed with ODD and encopresis that caused her removal from a second foster home. She had a history of neglect and physical abuse. At risk of being sent to a behavioral residential treatment center, an urgent evaluation revealed that "D" displayed symptoms of dysregulation across all three categories of DTD (i.e., affective/somatic, cognitive/behavioral, relational/identity), as shown in Table 14.2. History was gathered through the lens of DTD. "D" had struggled with toilet training due to a gastrointestinal problem in infancy/toddlerhood that caused intense diarrhea and hospitalizations that separated her from her mother. Additionally, "D" had experienced early sexual abuse and chronic exposure to domestic violence. The symptoms of ODD and encopresis were comorbid with DTD, a condition that, once recognized, shifted the team from an explanatory lens of "willful disobedience" to a lens of empathy.

Dissociative Disorders

Although dissociative symptoms are present in acute stress disorder and PTSD (e.g., amnesia, flashbacks, numbing, depersonalization, and derealization), dissociative symptoms that map onto dissociative disorder diagnoses include dissociative multiplicity (i.e., the presence of more than one center of consciousness), dissociation of memory (i.e., amnesia for personal information beyond what can be attributed to normal forgetting), depersonalization and derealization (i.e., experiencing the world and/or self as unreal), and sensorimotor dissociation (i.e., dissociation of somatic aspects of experience) (American Psychiatric Association, 2022; O'Neil, 2023; World Health Organization, 2021). To qualify as a disorder, the dissociative symptoms must interfere with functioning and/or cause distress; cannot be caused by a medication, substance, or another organic or mental disorder; and must not

Table 14.2 "D"'s Symptoms as Mapped onto the Proposed DTD Criteria

DTD Diagnostic Criteria	Key Features	"D"'s History and Symptoms
A Lifetime contemporaneous exposure to developmental trauma	A1. Primary caregiving system attachment disruptions A2. Interpersonal victimization	A1: Repeated hospitalizations resulting in prolonged separation from caregivers; mother was frequently impaired by substances; multiple foster care placements A2: Early sexual abuse; chronic exposure to domestic violence
B Affective and somatic dysregulation (three key features required for diagnosis)	B1. Emotion dysregulation B2. Somatic dysregulation B3. Impaired awareness or dissociation of emotions or body B4. Impaired capacity to describe emotions or bodily states	B1: Persistent irritability and frequent temper tantrums B2: Gastrointestinal pain and diarrhea without a medical cause; seemingly spontaneous regression in walking (like toddler) B3. Unaware of physical sensations associated with the need to defecate B4. Difficulty identifying and expressing emotional and somatic experiences and needs
C Attentional and behavioral dysregulation (two key features required for diagnosis)	C1. Attention bias toward or away from potential threats C2. Impaired capacity for self-protection C3. Maladaptive self-soothing C4. Habitual or reactive self-harm C5. Inability to initiate or sustain goal-directed behavior	C1. Hypervigilance to foster mom changing sibling's diaper C2. Frequently provokes arguments; aggressive toward siblings/caregivers C3. Smears feces C4. Unpredictably neglects toileting hygiene; does not wash hands after handling feces C5. Unpredictably changes from focused behavior to poor attention and task avoidance
D Self and relational dysregulation (two key features required for diagnosis)	D1. Persistent extreme negative self-perception: self-loathing or view of self as damaged/defective D2. Attachment insecurity and disorganization D3. Extreme persistent distrust, defiance, or lack of reciprocity in close relationships D4. Reactive physical or verbal aggression D5. Psychological boundary deficits D6. Impaired capacity to regulate empathic arousal	D1. Insists she is a "bad" girl D2. Swears and threatens her caregivers upon reunion after separation D3. Often refuses to follow directions; screams and yells when she does not get her way; tells caregivers she hates them D4. Hits and kicks others when upset D5. Sexually reactive behaviors with younger siblings; insists on taking over parental control of baby sibling's care D6. Does not appear to notice or respond to the emotions of others except the baby sibling over whom she is too controlling when the baby is distressed

Table adapted from Ford (2023, p. 405).

be part of an accepted cultural, religious, or spiritual practice. In children, symptoms of dissociative identity disorder (DID) are not better explained by imaginary playmates or other fantasy play (American Psychiatric Association, 2022; World Health Organization, 2021).

The *DSM-5-TR* and ICD-11 diagnoses of depersonalization/derealization (DP/DR) disorder and dissociative amnesia map onto their namesake symptoms. The diagnosis of dissociative amnesia, characterized by an inability to recall autobiographical information, may or may not include a dissociative fugue (i.e., when a person travels or wanders without recall of their identity and/or other important autobiographical memory). A diagnosis of DID may be warranted when someone experiences two or more self-states that recurrently take executive control, as well as (typically) symptoms of amnesia. The ICD-11 and *DSM-5-TR*'s diagnoses of partial DID and other specified dissociative disorder (OSDD) type 1, respectively, may be warranted when someone experiences two or more self-states, but one self-state is dominant and experiences dissociative intrusions from non-dominant self-states; in this case, the non-dominant self-states do not typically recurrently take executive control. Other types of the *DSM*/ICD diagnosis of OSDD may be conferred when the dissociative symptoms do not meet the full criteria for one of the other dissociative disorders but still interfere with functioning and/or cause distress. Finally, the unspecified dissociative disorder diagnosis is reserved for situations in which diagnostic clarification is not feasible at that time.

Although the dissociative disorders criteria are meant for all ages, the *DSM-5-TR* and ICD-11 diagnostic criteria reflect symptoms among adults and may not adequately capture dissociative presentations among children with naturally immature core selves (Silberg & Dallam, 2023). The most recent *DSM* and ICD text revisions attempt to address this gap by providing additional and clarifying information in text about the nature of dissociative symptoms in childhood—stating, for example, that "children usually do not present with identity shifting, instead presenting primarily with independently acting, imaginary companions, or as personified 'mood' states... problems with memory, concentration, and attachment, and may be associated with traumatic play" (American Psychiatric Association, 2022, p. 333). Clinicians should be mindful of how dissociation presents differently in children relative to adults (e.g., children may project dissociated aspects of themselves onto toys or objects) when applying diagnostic criteria (see Silberg, 2022; Waters, 2016; Chapter 12).

Differential and Co-Occurring Diagnoses

Studies of adults find that persons may spend an average of 5–12.4 years engaged in mental health treatment prior to receiving an accurate diagnosis of a dissociative disorder (Boyer et al., 2022). These results highlight the importance of assessing for dissociation and (when appropriate) diagnosing dissociative disorders when they are present in children, as this may expedite access to effective interventions. Dissociation and complex/developmental trauma may be overlooked in large part due to co-occurring and overshadowing symptoms. Children with DTD with or without PTSD may have more co-occurring diagnoses than children with PTSD or other diagnoses (Ford et al., 2021). In the DTD field trial replication study (Ford et al., 2021), children with DTD were nine times more likely to meet criteria for major depressive disorder and ODD, four times more likely to report suicidal ideation, and three to five times more likely to meet criteria for other mental illnesses (e.g., psychosis, anxiety and obsessive compulsive disorders, ADHD, and conduct disorder) relative to children receiving mental health treatment for other disorders; furthermore, DTD was associated with elevated rates of depression, ODD, and separation anxiety disorder beyond what could be attributed to PTSD alone. Thus, complex/developmental trauma presents a challenging mix of internalizing and externalizing problems, including dissociative features.

Delay in accurate diagnosis likely reflects complexities of mental health presentations among this population, as well as the presence of symptoms that overlap diagnostic categories that may fluctuate and change over time (Şar, 2014). Dissociative symptoms may be present in disorders outside of the current *DSM-5-TR* and ICD-11 trauma-related and dissociative disorder categories and may look like non-dissociative symptoms observed across other mental and neurodevelopmental disorders.

Co-occurring diagnoses are conferred when the child's symptoms meet criteria for two or more diagnoses and the symptoms of one disorder are not better explained through another disorder. The identification of co-occurring disorders enriches the case conceptualization and enables clinicians to tailor their interventions to the child's specific presentation and needs. There may be an interaction among co-occurring disorders whereby the symptoms of one disorder escalate the symptoms of the other disorder(s). Similarities and distinguishing features of common differential and co-occurring diagnoses for complex trauma and dissociative disorders among children are outlined in Table 14.3.

Developmental Considerations in Differential Diagnosis

It is not always possible to tease apart precipitating and perpetuating factors of a child's challenges to determine a clear diagnosis. For example, as symptoms of identity alteration are often covert, some clinicians argue that there is a "window of diagnosability" (Kluft, 1991; Loewenstein, 1991) for dissociative multiplicity, where symptoms are only sometimes observable and measurable, and at other times symptoms are unclear. Thus, observation and assessment conducted over time help clarify appropriate case conceptualization and diagnosis in all persons with potential dissociative disorders, but particularly in developing children for whom continuous brain growth is a complicating factor.

Children's vulnerability, due to limited power and undeveloped judgment for self-advocacy, makes it imperative for clinicians to function from the ancient wisdom of Hippocrates (1840) that advises two things when working with disease: (1) be useful; and (2) at least do no harm. Applying stigmatizing labels to a traumatized child (e.g., "oppositional," "defiant," and "explosive") is harmful. Such labeling adds nothing useful to explain perplexing symptoms and inhibits access to more appropriate treatments due to diagnostic overshadowing of the trauma symptoms (Beltrán et al., 2021). It also instills negative expectations in key adults that impact how children are treated, adding to their internal messages of low self-worth, inherent badness, and mistrust of others. The use of stigmatizing diagnostic labels constitutes a nonempathic approach that leaves a child confused and obfuscates symptom etiology. The impact of trauma on a child's behavior must be assessed when considering co-occurring and differential diagnoses, lest the diagnostic process be retraumatizing.

It is imperative to consider the child's developmental age and stage when considering differential diagnoses. Pathological behavior in adults may be developmentally normative among children. For example, while magical thinking may be part of a thought disorder in older adolescents/adults, it is developmentally appropriate in preschool children and may not begin to wane until late childhood. Similarly, imaginary friends and "talking" toys may be developmentally normative, though they may also reflect dissociative multiplicity and represent projected aspects of the self. Further, poor regulation for distress and sudden mood swings are normative in preschoolers but typically begin to even out in school-aged children. These symptom examples could fall into categories of major mental illness; however, both bipolar and primary psychotic disorders have a peak onset at ages 19.5 and 20.5, respectively, with very few persons (only 5.1% and 2%, respectively) showing onset by age 14 (Solmi et al., 2021). Cases of early childhood onset of these disorders are extremely rare because the timing of illness onset reflects brain maturation (Uhlhaas, 2011) that children generally have not yet attained.

Case Example

"S," age 7, was referred by her psychiatrist for a trauma-specific psychological assessment. Referral notes indicated that "S" had symptoms of ADHD (e.g., hyperactivity) and a mood disorder with psychotic features (e.g., mood swings, nonsensical and erratic behavior, and auditory hallucinations). She had a history of severe developmental trauma from birth to age 2, followed by secure kinship placement. Medication trials (e.g., stimulants, antipsychotics, and antidepressants) did not improve

Table 14.3 Symptoms Overlapping with Trauma Responses in Co-Occurring and Differential Diagnoses[a]

Type of Trauma Symptom[b]	DSM-5-TR and ICD-11 Disorders Associated with Trauma	Other Mental Disorders	Neurodevelopmental Disorders
Trauma adaptations (e.g., challenges with mood and cognition, self-regulation, executive functioning, attachment and relationships, dissociative flashbacks)	**PTSD, Acute Stress Reaction/ Disorder, and Adjustment Disorder:** - Associated with post-traumatic re-experiencing, avoidance of trauma-related cues, alterations in mood and cognition, and hyperarousal. - These disorders are distinguished by the onset and duration of symptoms, and the type (i.e., objective severity) of traumatic/stressful event(s). **C-PTSD (ICD-11):** - Criteria met for PTSD. - Includes additional post-traumatic challenges in affect regulation, negative beliefs about oneself, and disturbed relationships. - Attachment disruptions are common. **DTD** (proposed for DSM by van der Kolk, 2005): - Post-traumatic dysregulation in three areas: affective/somatic, attentional/behavioral, and self/ relational. - Does not require a criterion of PTSD to be met.	**Depression:** - Common in people with complex trauma and PTSD (Ford et al., 2021) (note: the *DSM-5-TR* PTSD cluster of negative alterations in cognitions and mood is a direct overlap with depressive symptoms). - Post-traumatic reactivity may manifest as depressive episodes, including despondency and suicidal ideation, in a seasonal pattern coinciding with past trauma occurrences. **Eating Disorders:** - Eating disorder severity is associated with both PTSD and dissociative symptoms in children (Brewerton et al., 2020). - Disordered eating may facilitate avoidance of trauma-related cues (e.g., oral textures), be used to reduce hyperarousal or induce dissociation (e.g., emotional numbing), or reflect identification with the aggressor (Rosenberg et al., 2023). **Obsessive Compulsive Disorder (OCD):** - Compulsions should be distinguished from repetitive behaviors associated with trauma re-experiencing (e.g., flashbacks) and/or attempts to master the trauma (e.g., reenactment or repetition compulsion). **Encopresis/Enuresis:** - Withholding of stool/urine may be a form of avoidance or a response to anxiety and/or pain associated with traumatic experiences.	**Neurodevelopmental Disorders** (see Prock & Fogler, 2018): - The child's timeline of symptom onset alongside adverse childhood experiences (ACEs) may help clarify diagnosis. - Children who are not traumatized rarely display additional trauma symptoms beyond those that overlap with the neurodevelopmental disorder. - Children with true neurodevelopmental disorders are more consistent in their presentations, whereas the neurodivergent symptoms of children with trauma may be more selective and reactive depending on the setting and situation. **ADHD:** - Dissociation (e.g., trance states) may look like inattention, while hyperarousal and hypervigilance may look like hyperactivity. - Shared symptoms with complex trauma include executive functioning difficulties (e.g., inattention, hyperactivity, and impulsivity), irritability and emotional lability, social difficulties, and learning difficulties. - It is common for children to develop symptoms that look like ADHD after experiencing a traumatic event (Endo et al., 2006). These children may also exhibit higher levels of dissociative symptoms, including trance states and intrusions (e.g., from self-states, traumatic content), relative to children with ADHD who had not experienced trauma.

- Must have antecedents of both interpersonal victimization or family/community violence, and disruption in attachment formation.

RAD and DSED:
- Reflect severe attachment disturbances resulting from grossly inadequate caregiving in early childhood.
- Symptom onset is prior to age 5.

Disruptive Disorders (ODD, Intermittent Explosive Disorder, Disruptive Mood Dysregulation Disorder):
- Externalizing responses are associated with a tendency to appraise situations as threatening and react accordingly; this may be a normative adaptation to stressful life events.
- Assess the impact of trauma on a child's behavior. Studies attempting to differentiate between PTSD and the proposed DTD have found that children with high levels of DTD symptoms but low levels of PTSD symptoms were highly likely to meet criteria for ODD (Ford et al., 2021, 2022).
- Disruptive mood dysregulation disorder and intermittent explosive disorder have also both been strongly linked to psychological trauma and abuse (see Bruno et al., 2019).

Emerging Borderline Personality Traits:
- Strong associations with childhood trauma (Winsper et al., 2016) and attachment disruptions (Lyons-Ruth et al., 2013).
- Emotional, behavioral, and relational dysregulation overlap with ICD-11 criteria for C-PTSD, and reflect a trauma/stress response (Ford & Courtois, 2021).

ASD:
- Overlapping features between ASD and complex trauma include a lack of flexibility of thought and behavior, unusual characteristics of play, difficulties in social interactions, less developed theory of mind, lower communication abilities, emotion dysregulation, problems with executive functioning, and sensory integration challenges (Moran, 2010; Prock & Fogler, 2018; Van Scoyoc et al., 2018).
- Early childhood neglect or deprivation can result in ASD-like features (e.g., language delays, difficulties in social reciprocity; restricted, repetitive, and inflexible behaviors and interests) (Van Scoyoc et al., 2018).
- The Coventry Grid (Moran, 2010) can help distinguish between typical presentations of ASD versus those typical of attachment concerns.
- Moving the child to a more nurturing home may lead to symptom improvement for children who are traumatized, but not for children with autism (Van Scoyoc et al., 2018).

Intellectual and Learning Disabilities:
- Neurocognitive deficits may be like those of traumatized children (Kavanaugh et al., 2017).

(Continued)

Table 14.3 (Continued)

Type of Trauma Symptom[b]	DSM-5-TR and ICD-11 Disorders Associated with Trauma	Other Mental Disorders	Neurodevelopmental Disorders
		- Transient forms of dissociation (e.g., amnesia, DP/DR, state dissociation) are common during times of stress or intense emotions. - When a child's history better supports a diagnosis of C-PTSD, an additional borderline personality disorder diagnosis would generally not be considered.	- Children with intellectual and learning disabilities tend to form stable and secure attachments, whereas traumatized children often display insecure or disorganized attachment. **Exposure to Substances In Utero:** - Depending on the substance, the child may have biological (e.g., facial features, growth restrictions, central nervous system abnormalities), cognitive (e.g., intellectual delays; impairments in executive functions, learning, memory, and/or visual-spatial abilities) and behavioral (e.g., mood, behavioral regulation, attention, impulse control) symptoms that overlap with trauma symptoms. - Babies born substance-dependent may experience early attachment disruptions as well as painful withdrawal symptoms and medical procedures, thus adding early adverse experiences to the impact of the substances on brain development (Boris et al., 2018).
Dissociative Multiplicity	**DID:** - Two or more aspects of the child's self recurrently take executive control of the child's consciousness and functioning, with accompanying alterations in subjective experiences (e.g., sensations, perceptions, affect, cognition, behavior) and dissociative amnesia.	**Co-Occurring Diagnoses:** - May be conferred when symptom criteria for both disorders are met, and one is not better explained by the other. **Psychotic Disorders:** - Dissociation may resemble positive symptoms of psychosis (e.g., sensory intrusions such as hallucinations, delusions, disorganized thought process) (Spiegel et al., 2011).	**Neurodevelopmental Disorders:** - Children with neurodevelopmental disorders are more consistent in their presentations, and all aspects of the child's self display the neurodivergence (Reuben, 2023). - Variations in symptoms across different aspects of the child's self is more indicative of a dissociative disorder (Reuben, 2023).

Neurodivergence, Co-Occurring, and Differential Diagnosis

Partial DID (ICD-11) and **OSDD-1** (*DSM-5-TR*):
- One aspect of the child's self is dominant and functions in daily life, with intrusions by other aspects of the child's self. Other aspects of the child's self do not typically take executive control of the child's consciousness and functioning.

PTSD:
- Dissociative symptoms following traumatic events are common (Choi et al., 2017), and include flashbacks, trance-like states, alterations in identity, loss of sense of agency, somatic symptoms, depersonalization, and derealization.
- State changes are limited to episodes of re-experiencing (e.g., flashbacks), and do not take executive control over consciousness and daily functioning.

- Schneiderian first rank symptoms may be as or more prevalent among people with dissociative disorders than among those with psychotic disorders (Dorahy et al., 2009), though people with dissociative disorders rarely report thought broadcasting.
- Negative symptoms of psychosis (e.g., flat affect) are prominent among people with psychosis, but not among those with dissociation (Longden et al., 2020).
- Psychosis does not involve amnesia.
- Voice hearing associated with trauma starts at a younger age (i.e., childhood) than voice hearing associated with psychosis (Dorahy et al., 2009).
- First episode of psychosis typically occurs in late adolescence or adulthood, and very rarely before puberty.
- Symptoms that differentiate dissociation from psychosis include rapid fluctuation in mood and other symptoms, absence of persistent flat affect, unpredictable rapid improvements in symptoms, insight into the illness, and intact reality testing except during dissociative episodes (Şar & Öztürk, 2009).

(*Continued*)

Table 14.3 (Continued)

Type of Trauma Symptom[b]	DSM-5-TR and ICD-11 Disorders Associated with Trauma	Other Mental Disorders	Neurodevelopmental Disorders
	- Both PTSD and a diagnosis of dissociative multiplicity may co-occur when significant dissociative symptoms occur beyond the episodes of re-experiencing.	**Bipolar Disorder:** - The rapid pace of extreme shifts of mood and behavior in dissociative multiplicity (e.g., minutes to hours) is atypical of even rapid-cycling bipolar disorder (where mood episodes last at least several days). - Bipolar disorder is associated with a decreased need for sleep, which is not observed in dissociative multiplicity (though a child with dissociation may have chronic and severe sleep disruptions due to trauma symptoms or self-state activity). - Onset in late adolescence or adulthood, and very rarely before puberty. **Eating Disorders:** - Having an internal eating disorder "voice" has been associated with a history of trauma; this relationship is partly mediated by dissociation (Pugh et al., 2018). - Disordered eating may be driven by self-states (Waters, 2016) or amnesia for eating, especially in children with early neglect who did not develop normal hunger or satiety cues (Silberg, 2022). - Assess functions of behaviors to clarify the role of dissociation.	

OCD:
- Obsessions and compulsions from OCD may appear like intrusions from self-states (e.g., experienced as intrusive and unwanted; child feels driven to perform repetitive compulsive behaviors), but are not experienced as coming from a separate aspect of the self.
- OCD without dissociation does not involve amnesia or discontinuities in the sense of self.
- In dissociative multiplicity, OCD may be carried within self-states (Waters, 2016).

Encopresis/Enuresis:
- Different aspects of the self may hold awareness of the body's needs, while other aspects of the self are unaware of sensations and urges.

Gender Dysphoria:
- In dissociative multiplicity, different aspects of the self may have different gender identities.

Depression:
- A lifelong negative mood state frequently co-occurs with DID, may meet criteria for major depressive disorder, and typically has an onset during childhood.
- Symptoms may fluctuate when they are experienced by some aspects of the self but not others.

(*Continued*)

Table 14.3 (Continued)

Type of Trauma Symptom[b]	DSM-5-TR and ICD-11 Disorders Associated with Trauma	Other Mental Disorders	Neurodevelopmental Disorders
		Emerging Borderline Personality Traits: - Personality styles are pervasive and persistent. There is more variability in personality styles across aspects of the self in dissociative multiplicity. **Factitious Disorder or Malingering:** - Differentiate between intentional deception and amnesia for the activity of different aspects of self.	
Dissociation of Memory	**Dissociative Amnesia** (with/without fugue): - Amnesia for personal information extends beyond the traumatic event. **Acute Stress Reaction/Disorder:** - Transient amnesia for the traumatic event and surrounding period subsides within a few days after the stressor ends. **PTSD:** - Affects only memory for the traumatic event, not memory for personal information beyond the trauma.	**Substance Use:** - Amnesia associated with substance use occurs exclusively during and immediately after substance use (e.g., "alcohol blackouts"). - May co-occur with a dissociative disorder, and the child may rely more heavily on both substances and dissociation during periods of increased stress or exposure to maltreatment; detoxification and detailed history may assist with differential diagnosis. **Functional Neurological Disorder:** - Cognitive symptoms (when present) are not limited to autobiographical information. **Emerging Borderline Personality Traits:** - Transient dissociative amnesia may occur during times of stress or intense emotions.	**Neurodevelopmental Disorders:** - Challenges with memory may occur within the context of executive functioning (i.e., ADHD), cognitive (intellectual disorders), and learning (learning disorders) difficulties. - Memory abilities in neurodevelopmental disorders tend to be consistent between cognitive testing and real-life settings, whereas traumatized children may perform well on cognitive testing (with low emotional demands) but display greater difficulties with memory when in real-life stressful situations (Prock & Fogler, 2018).

Depersonalization and Derealization (DP/DR)	**DP/DR Disorder:** - DP/DR disorder is diagnosed when it precedes the onset and/or continues beyond the cessation of symptoms of other mental disorders. It is not diagnosed when it occurs exclusively within the context of an episode of another mental disorder. - DP/DR disorder is not diagnosed when full criteria is met for another specified dissociative disorder or PTSD with dissociative symptoms. **PTSD, with Dissociative Symptoms:** - When PTSD and DP/DR co-occur, DP/DR are subsumed under the PTSD diagnosis.	**Psychotic Disorders:** - DP/DR are common in primary psychotic disorders (Humpston et al., 2020), but occur in combination with negative symptoms of psychosis (e.g., avolition and flat affect) and a decrease in social and academic functioning. - Non-transient DP/DR may be accompanied by delusional interpretations of this experience during acute psychotic episodes (World Health Organization, 2021). **Depression:** - DP/DR may co-occur with cognitive symptoms of depression but are limited to the depressive episode. **Anxiety Disorders:** - DP/DR as a stress response may occur alongside high levels of anxiety or fear (e.g., panic attacks in anxiety disorders when confronted with feared stimulus), are transient, and subside a short time after arousal decreases. **Substance Use:** - DP/DR associated with substance use occur exclusively during and immediately after substance use. May co-occur with a dissociative disorder (e.g., both are used as means of coping with current stressors). - Distinguished through a period of detoxification and detailed history. **Emerging Borderline Personality Traits:** - Transient DP/DR may occur during times of stress or intense emotions.	**ASD:** - DP/DR may co-occur with anxiety among children with ASD (Storch et al., 2012).

(Continued)

Table 14.3 (Continued)

Type of Trauma Symptom[b]	DSM-5-TR and ICD-11 Disorders Associated with Trauma	Other Mental Disorders	Neurodevelopmental Disorders
Sensorimotor Dissociation[c]	**Dissociative/Functional Neurological Symptom Disorder:** - Involves disruptions in the normal integration of motor, sensory, or cognitive functioning. - Does not occur exclusively during an episode of dissociative multiplicity (e.g., where different aspects of the self may hold different information) or within the context of symptoms of other mental disorders (e.g., PTSD and anxiety). - Symptoms have no identifiable biological etiology. **Complex Trauma and PTSD:** - Greater exposure to ACEs is associated with higher rates of medical concerns (Kerker et al., 2015). - Somatic symptoms (e.g., stomachaches, headaches, dizziness, and heart palpitations) are common symptoms of fear, anxiety, and hyperarousal (Kugler et al., 2012).	**Anxiety Disorders, Depressive Disorders, and Eating Disorders:** - Somatic symptoms are common within these disorders. - Use diagnostic criteria beyond sensorimotor symptoms to clarify differential diagnosis. **Eating Disorders:** - May involve somatic dissociation, (e.g., dissociation of hunger cues), but is fully explained through the eating disorder diagnosis (Waters, 2016). **Encopresis/Enuresis:** - May be associated with decreased sensation associated with abuse or neglect. **Psychotic Disorders:** - May involve somatic delusions or hallucinations. - Somatic symptoms occur only during episodes of acute psychosis.	**Neurodevelopmental Disorders:** - Children may not have language to communicate their experience of somatic concerns.

[a] Information in this table is summarized from the *DSM-5-TR* (American Psychiatric Association, 2022) and/or ICD-11 (World Health Organization, 2021), except and/or in addition to where otherwise indicated.

[b] Rule out medical concerns (e.g., neurocognitive disorders, traumatic brain injuries, epilepsy, other medical conditions) that may cause dissociative symptoms (e.g., amnesia, changes in personality, and DP/DR).

[c] True medical concerns may co-exist with sensorimotor dissociation (e.g., both functional seizures and epilepsy; Zhang et al., 2021). Inability to find a medical cause does not mean that one does not exist or will not be identified with medical advancements (e.g., neurological symptoms of syphilis were originally attributed to mental disorders).

symptoms. (Note that although dissociative hallucinations generally do not respond to antipsychotic medications [Spiegel et al., 2011], the child's response or non-response to psychotropic medications is not an acceptable means of differentiating between diagnoses.) "S" heard internal voices, had highly dysregulated behavior, extreme sleep disturbance, and severe mood swings. She and her caregivers did not report day-to-day memory problems or significant amnesia. Table 14.4 details the symptoms supporting the diagnostic decision of OSDD-1.

Table 14.4 "S"'s Symptoms and History Supporting Differential Diagnosis of OSDD-1

Key Symptoms/ History Domains	"S"'s History and Symptoms	Supports Dissociation Diagnosis?	Supports Psychosis Diagnosis?
Family History of Psychosis	Close family member with a psychotic disorder diagnosis due to the presence of auditory and visual hallucinations	Not specifically: Hallucinations could have been misdiagnosed as psychotic but were dissociative	Yes: Family history of psychosis increases risk for psychosis
Trauma History	History of early and severe developmental trauma	Yes: Early childhood trauma is a known precursor for dissociative disorders	No: Although trauma and psychosis are correlated, this is not a known causal relationship
Thought Process	"S" demonstrated appropriate reality testing and mental organization until presented with ink blots that triggered scary internal "voices," at which point she became disorganized and lost reality testing	Yes: When calm, her thought process was organized and she displayed appropriate reality testing; however, poor reality testing emerged when she experienced a trauma reminder and regressed self-states were activated and may have been illogical	Partially: Disorganized thinking and loss of reality testing was sometimes present, though not consistently
Trauma Responses	"S" showed extreme dysregulation during play and when viewing projective images; her stories contained anxious and catastrophic themes	Not specifically; supports PTSD	Not specifically; may reflect disorganized mental state
Hears Internal Voices (auditory hallucinations)	Terrifying voices of two internal parts that "S" depicted in drawing; described that they fought "on the inside"	Yes: Terrifying statements and yelling attributed to two inside "parts" that the child could describe, name, and produce through drawing	Partially: Psychotic commands and scary statements are not typically attributed to an inside "part" and the voices are not typically described with specific attributes or names
Hears External Voices (auditory hallucinations)	Symptom not present	N/A	N/A
Visual Hallucinations	Symptom not present	N/A	N/A

(Continued)

Table 14.4 (Continued)

Key Symptoms/History Domains	"S"'s History and Symptoms	Supports Dissociation Diagnosis?	Supports Psychosis Diagnosis?
State Dissociation	Zoned out per reports by self and caregiver, and as observed in session	Yes	Sometimes: for example, when attending to auditory hallucinations
Multiplicity	"S" drew a half girl/half boy that she experiences "on the inside"; she drew the terrifying voices; she discussed a baby part; "S" became dysregulated with regressive behaviors several times in session. Caregiver reports of multiplicity detailed specific self-states (e.g., baby and aggressor)	Yes: Experience of internal self-states supports dissociative multiplicity; observed symptoms may indicate switching between self-states	No: Internal voices are not typically conceptualized as imaginary friends
Sleep Disturbance	Caregiver reported "S" had difficulties sleeping (e.g., resisting sleep, frequent waking from nightmares); "S" described that the baby part cries and keeps her awake; the baby part cries due to the scary internal parts that yell	Yes; common	Yes; common

Emerging Personality

Developmental stage is also of utmost importance when considering personality disorders, as these are not typically diagnosed in preadolescent children. Identity formation is a developmental task; children have not had the opportunity to fully integrate their knowledge about themselves and others into a cohesive sense of self and style of relating. Furthermore, the areas in the brain responsible for executive functioning (e.g., impulsivity, self-regulation, emotional control, and inhibition) continue to develop into early adulthood and are considerably underdeveloped in children (Blakemore & Choudhury, 2006), which makes personality disorder criteria associated with self-direction and emotion regulation generally inapplicable to most children. Nonetheless, older children (e.g., ages 11 or 12+ years) may display prominent emerging personality traits that map onto criteria for personality disorders beyond the level that would be expected of typically developing children, and to an extent that causes significant distress and/or impairment. The role of complex/developmental trauma in the formation of the child's personality style should be considered.

Case Example

"V," age 12, was adopted at age 8. His adoptive mother, noting his anger outbursts and lack of empathy, was concerned that "V" might have sociopathic (i.e., antisocial personality) tendencies. "V"'s history revealed that his birth mother suffered from mental illness and substance use disorder; she was neglectful. His maternal aunt (main caregiver) was emotionally and physically abusive. "V" was removed from his birth home at age 3 and placed in orphanages for five years. Evaluation revealed that "V" had an extremely avoidant insecure attachment style. He avoided physical affection, was emotionally flat, and fiercely independent. His aloofness protected him from re-experiencing abandonment, humiliation, and hurt. His perplexing and primitive anger, which felt out of "V"'s control, likely reflected his unprocessed early attachment trauma. Understanding "V" through the complex/developmental trauma lens opened an important opportunity to educate caregivers so that they could increase their empathy, decrease their fear, and obtain effective services.

Factitious Disorders and Malingering

A factitious disorder occurs when a child (or their caregiver) feigns, falsifies, or induces signs or symptoms as a means of eliciting care (i.e., factitious disorder) or to obtain an incentive (e.g., malingering). Although children who feign dissociative symptoms do not meet criteria for a dissociative disorder, their behaviors communicate significant unmet needs that should be taken seriously and require further evaluation. Furthermore, the deception around symptoms does not mean that the child does not genuinely have another true illness or disorder. Particularly relevant to children whose safety and relational needs have not been adequately met, factitious behavior may serve as communication to get their perceived needs met. Furthermore, traumatized children may intentionally deny their behavior not as nefarious deception but as a means of avoiding unwanted consequences (e.g., further abuse and shame).

Caregivers may also deceptively present their children as displaying dissociative symptoms that they do not truly experience (i.e., factitious disorder by proxy). In this case, the child is considered the victim of psychological abuse (World Health Organization, 2021). Observations of the child in the absence of the caregiver may be useful for clarifying symptoms.

Case Example

"L," age 11, was psychiatrically hospitalized when no medical cause could be found for her episodes of syncope and frequent collapsing, during which she could not walk. She often regressed into "baby talk" and wanted stuffed animals for soothing. "L" had been a high-achieving student, successful in a variety of extracurricular activities, and popular among peers. The change in "L" was sudden and perplexing. During the assessment, "L" revealed that she had been visiting an Internet site where people impersonated babies and solicited nurturing infant care from others. Clinicians working with "L" interpreted this online activity as evidence that "L"'s symptoms were possibly learned, factitious, and may be pointing toward unmet dependency needs. She was released without a formal diagnosis, but with the query of a factitious disorder. Following discharge from hospital, "L"'s regressions and episodes during which she was unable to walk increased, and she sometimes required a wheelchair for school. On further evaluation, "L" scored high on screening measures of dissociation, though she denied experiencing any difficulties with her memory. Her only known trauma was that her parents had a rageful marriage when "L" was aged 3–7.

The key to clarifying "L"'s diagnosis as OSDD came when "L"'s mom shared that she suffered the traumatic loss of her own mother when "L" was two years old and she [Mom] became emotionally unavailable for a year, stating, "I lost that entire year." "L" had suffered an attachment insult great enough to cause the symptoms seen in early puberty. Along with this new information came "L"'s growing awareness of a young self-state that needed soothing. "L" successfully learned more effective and healthy ways to both soothe herself and ask for nurturance.

No Diagnosis Warranted

At times, youth may present with dissociative symptoms and believe they have a dissociative disorder, but careful assessment indicates that they do not meet criteria. Their self-diagnosis may have arisen through misinformation; for example, recent concerns have been raised about the potential impact of social media trends on children's mental health symptoms, including symptoms of dissociation (Giedinghagen, 2023). Although the child may not have a diagnosable dissociative disorder, their suffering is real. Their identification with and request for a diagnosis indicates that they have found a model for understanding their suffering from which they may experience validation, acceptance, and belonging. The psychological, social, and cultural factors contributing to their presentations need to be sensitively incorporated into the child's larger case conceptualization and treatment plan.

Neurodivergence

The term neurodivergence refers to having a mind that functions in ways that significantly diverge from prevailing societal standards of "normal" (Legault et al., 2021). A social justice movement (i.e., neurodiversity movement) in relation to ASD and other types of neurodivergence promotes a positive identity for neurodivergents, focusing on their differences or unique talents as strengths rather than deficits, which contrasts with a longer history of demeaning societal attitudes and behaviors toward persons with neurodevelopmental differences. This explosive shift has lessened stigma, especially for those considered higher functioning, and has allowed persons with diagnoses such as ASD, OCD, ADHD, and learning disabilities to celebrate their differences and find belongingness (Baumer & Frueh, 2021). Yet, neurodivergence has a broad spectrum, including those more functionally challenged, such as people with combined ASD and intellectual disabilities. Clinicians are called to create safety and offer effective interventions for traumatized children who may also be challenged by neurodivergence across the spectrum.

Children with ASD and other developmental disabilities are at greater risk of having to endure childhood trauma and adversity (Berg et al., 2016; Kerns et al., 2017), and are predisposed to react with greater sensitivity and reactivity to childhood adversity (Sivaratnam et al., 2015). Also, traumatic experiences may interact with and exacerbate symptoms of neurodivergence as they share underlying neurological mechanisms (Haruvi-Lamdan et al., 2018). In neglected and/or maltreated children, overlapping symptoms of complex trauma and neurodivergence are the norm rather than the exception (Prock & Fogler, 2018). As such, "we can no longer draw arbitrary distinctions between 'mind' (psychiatric)- and 'brain' (neurodevelopmental)-related challenges, because a chronically stressed brain will not only be at risk for a hyperaroused 'fight or flight' system but also impaired learning and executive functioning" (Prock & Fogler, 2018, p. 56). Furthermore, compelling brain research regarding early life adversity (i.e., maltreatment) discusses a "silent epidemic of neurodevelopmental injuries" connected to adult psychiatric illness (Kaffman, 2009, p. 624). (See Chapter 11 in this book.) We have, essentially, a proverbial "chicken and egg" problem. Childhood maltreatment is associated with a variety of neurocognitive deficits, including executive functions, intelligence, language, visual-spatial skills, and memory (Kavanaugh et al., 2017).

Neurodevelopmental Disorders, Trauma, and Differential Diagnoses

Neurodevelopmental disorders (e.g., ADHD, ASD, intellectual and learning disorders, genetic syndromes, neurodevelopmental disorders associated with prenatal exposure to substances) are brain-based disorders with symptoms emerging from birth or in early childhood. A careful review of the child's trajectory across their lifetime (e.g., a timeline of neurodevelopmental symptoms alongside timeline of ACEs) can provide temporal clues to differentiating between complex trauma and neurodevelopmental disorders (Prock & Fogler, 2018). Children who have had safe and secure caregiving throughout their lives and display symptoms of neurodevelopmental disorders throughout the developmental period are more likely to have true neurodevelopmental disorders; these children rarely demonstrate other dissociative symptoms beyond those that overlap with diagnostic criteria. When there is a clear stressor precipitating the onset of neurodevelopmental symptoms, these symptoms may be better assigned to the stress response. It may be more difficult to distinguish between neurodevelopmental disorders and complex/developmental trauma in cases where the child has never received adequate caregiving and/or a historical baseline of their development is not available. Table 14.3 outlines the similarities and distinguishing features between neurodevelopmental disorders and symptoms of complex/developmental trauma and dissociation.

Differentiating between the effects of complex/developmental trauma, the symptoms of neurodevelopmental disorders, and the interactions between these can be particularly challenging because the same regions of the brain may be affected, which results in similar behavioral presentations. Both conditions can cause social challenges, emotional extremes, heightened startle response, repetitive movements, hyperactivity or passivity, and avoidance of eye contact, to name only some overlapping symptoms. Extra care is required to clarify differential diagnoses and case conceptualizations.

Case Examples

"R," age 7, presented for an autism evaluation. Severely neglected, "R" was found in the streets at age 3. His adoptive mother had provided excellent learning opportunities for four years; "R"'s IQ had risen 20 points. "R" had prior diagnoses of ADHD and ODD, and he struggled with relational challenges (peers and family), anger outbursts, and sensory-motor issues (e.g., clumsy and drooling). The evaluation discerned that "R" was not on the autism spectrum and that his neurodiverse symptoms could be explained by neglect that resulted in complex/developmental trauma. Although symptoms on the surface sounded like a fit to ASD, they were qualitatively different, as seen in Table 14.5.

"R"'s adoptive mother died shortly after the initial evaluation and "R" was placed in foster care in another city, where his behaviors worsened and his evaluation results were unknown. Due to "disruptive behaviors," he was shuffled among foster homes and treatment centers. By age 14, "R" had acquired various diagnoses including PTSD, depressive disorder, anxiety disorder, psychotic disorder, and ASD; however, the ASD misdiagnosis had overshadowed consideration of treating complex/developmental trauma. "R" had declined physically, mentally, emotionally, and socially. Once placed in a safe and stable trauma-informed treatment home, "R"'s symptoms stabilized, and he was able to discuss and process the sources of his symptoms.

Consider now the flip side of a differential diagnosis regarding ASD.

"B," age 11, was initially seen by a clinician who specialized in serving youth in foster care. Concerns included a lack of social skills and low adaptive and academic functioning. Although a gold-standard screening measure for autism was administered and many neurodivergent symptoms were flagged, the clinician found no "restricted area of interest." The clinician attributed the social, cognitive, and academic delays to trauma. "B" was diagnosed with PTSD. Indeed, "B" had recently been removed from a physically and emotionally abusive aunt and uncle with whom he'd lived for three years since his former caregiver, his beloved grandmother, had died. "B" had become increasingly withdrawn, and he spoke very little following his grandmother's death. The clinician knew that "B" had been given up at age 3 by his birth mother due to her own mental health concerns and domestic violence; thus, there was early attachment disruption and an unsafe early home. A trauma diagnosis made sense.

Table 14.5 Symptoms of DTD Distinguished from Autism Spectrum Disorders

Key Symptom Domains	"R"'s Symptoms Through a DTD Lens	Similar ASD Symptoms
Attention	"R"'s mom described him zoning out ("brain glitches") and not remembering time passing	Zoning out due to going into an inner world not shared with others
Social and Communication Problems with Peers	"R" desired relationships with peers but felt inferior and feared he could not keep up athletically or academically. His early neglect had left him slow of speech and clumsy. His sense of unworthiness and shame caused him to withdraw	Different or limited understanding of communication/language; awkward or limited social skills; not understanding feelings, another's perspective, or the function or boundaries of relationships; odd mannerisms; restricted interests; difficulty understanding humor/slang; cognitively concrete and literal. (Note: most healthy autistic children desire friends)
Troubled Relationship with Family Members	"R" understood family dynamics and could discuss his part in them (e.g., jealousy toward siblings). "R" was ambivalent about family relationships, easily triggered to fear and anger in the family context, and emotionally and behaviorally dysregulated with parents and siblings	A lack of connecting emotionally and reciprocally with family; more transactional; restricted interests
Emotional Dysregulation and Oppositionality	"R" could label emotions correctly and reflect on his emotions, though he did not have a sense of control over emotions. He could verbalize triggers for his dysregulation, which were relational rather than sensory	Emotional dysregulation for youth with ASD often stems from hypersensitivity or hyposensitivity to sensory experiences (e.g., loud noise and bright lights). Youth have inherent difficulty labeling and processing emotions and reflecting on their internal reactions or emotional cues from others
Sensory-Motor Issues	"R"'s sensory-motor issues (including drooling) stemmed from severe neglect during the formation of his neural-foundational sensorimotor system in the first year of life	Sensory-motor processing issues are often present in children with autism

"B"'s foster mother was concerned when "B" did not respond to standard PTSD interventions and requested a second opinion. The second opinion found clear evidence that "B" met all diagnostic criteria for ASD with Intellectual Impairment; that is, he had historically significant functional impairment due to persistent deficits in social communication, social interaction, and a restricted area of interest (i.e., specific cartoon characters) that greatly narrowed his activities and relationships and caused severe withdrawal into an inner world. Further assessment found that "B" had developed imaginary friends in the form of specific cartoon characters to help him with calming down when angry and to help stave off loneliness, suggesting that his inner world was a combination of both ASD and traumatic dissociation.

The cases of both "R" and "B" remind us that traumatized children with neurodivergence are especially complex. "R"'s neurodivergence was linked to neglect and qualitatively different from ASD. Yet, once he was misdiagnosed with ASD, he was not treated for complex/developmental trauma. In contrast, "B" was seen shortly after removal from an abusive family situation and clearly showed signs of PTSD, which overshadowed his neurodivergence. His ASD plus intellectual disability explained more of his challenges in functioning and needed addressing through direct autism services and resources.

Addressing Complex Trauma and Dissociation among Children with Developmental Disabilities

Children with developmental disabilities are at a substantially increased risk of traumatization, including neglect, overt abuse, and bullying (Jones et al., 2012). This may be particularly salient for children with communication disorders and those children who are unable to verbally report their experiences (Prock & Fogler, 2018). Many children with disabilities are more reliant on adults than their typically developing peers, learning unchecked compliance with authority figures who often handle their bodies as well as their choices. They may be more vulnerable to abuse in the community due to their undeveloped judgment, difficulty understanding what is happening during an abusive situation, and lack of self-protective skills. They are at a higher risk of abuse within their own homes due to a higher level of family strain associated with caring for a child with a disability. Furthermore, children with developmental disabilities often have lower levels of protective factors (National Child Traumatic Stress Network Adapted Trauma Treatment Standards Work Group [NCTSN], 2004). In addition to limited resources (e.g., cognitive and communication abilities, social skills, and mobility) associated with their disability, they may experience increased isolation and a limited social network due to society's stigma associated with their differences.

When children have limited capacity to verbally report their experiences of maltreatment, caregivers and other adults involved with them (e.g., school personnel, therapists, and nurses) rely on behavioral symptoms to identify maltreatment (NCTSN, 2004). Behavioral changes associated with trauma among children with developmental disabilities include an increase in irritability and emotionality, increased anxiety-related behaviors (e.g., objecting to people, places, or activities; perseveration; obsessions and compulsions), reduced responsiveness and interests, changes in sleeping and eating, regression (e.g., toileting accidents among children who were previously toilet-trained), self-harm, aggression, and displaying unusual or age-inappropriate sexual or genitally focused behaviors.

Assessment and interventions among children with developmental disabilities should be modified to account for their disabilities (NCTSN, 2004). This means creating an environment adapted for various sensitivities (e.g., light, sound, and body proximity), slowing down speech and using simple language, presenting one concept or piece of information at a time, being specific and concrete, using visual information in addition to verbal information, and other accommodations as warranted for the child's specific disabilities. Trauma symptom checklists may need to be administered as clinical interviews (Prock & Fogler, 2018), with the inclusion of visual aids or with a translator (e.g., ASL) or caregiver who understands the child's communication. For children whose thought processes are concrete, responses to common assessment questions may sound bizarre due to the child's interpretations of the questions, and projective assessment tools may be ineffective in picking up on the child's difficulties (NCTSN, 2004). Multiple chapters in this volume address sensory-based interventions, systemic approaches, and trauma-sensitive practices with this population.

Conclusion

Accurate identification of complex/developmental trauma and dissociation is a prerequisite for useful case conceptualization and effective interventions. Differential diagnosis of trauma-related disorders is complicated by symptoms that co-occur and overlap with other mental illnesses and neurodevelopmental disorders. Misdiagnoses can cause harm, and diagnostic overshadowing may result in limited intervention effectiveness. Unfortunately, current diagnostic categories in the *DSM* and ICD may not capture the full impact of complex/developmental trauma on children. Clinicians should be mindful of the ways in which trauma symptoms in children may present outside of the typical *DSM* and ICD categories, as well as the ways in which they map onto diagnostic criteria beyond those specifically related to trauma and dissociation. A transdiagnostic approach may be useful in conceptualizing the role of trauma in altered developmental pathways.

Note

1 Case examples have been deidentified and altered to protect client confidentiality.

References

American Psychiatric Association. (2022). *Diagnostic and statistical manual of mental disorders: DSM-5-TR* (5th ed., rev.). American Psychiatric Association.

Baumer, N., & Frueh, J. (Nov. 23, 2021). What is neurodiversity? Harvard Health, Mind and Mood, health.harvard.edu/blog/what-is-neurodiversity-202111232645

Beltrán, S., Sit, L., & Ginsburg, K. R. (2021). A call to revise the diagnosis of oppositional defiant disorder—diagnoses are for helping, not harming. *JAMA Psychiatry, 78*(11), 1181–1182. https://doi.org/10.1001/jamapsychiatry.2021.2127

Berg, K. L., Shiu, C. S., Acharya, K., Stolbach, B. C., & Msall, M. E. (2016). Disparities in adversity among children with autism spectrum disorder: A population-based study. *Developmental Medicine & Child Neurology, 58*(11), 1124–1131. https://doi.org/10.1111/dmcn.13161

Blakemore, S-J., & Choudhury, S. (2006). Development of the adolescent brain: Implications for executive function and social cognition. *Journal of Child Psychology and Psychiatry, 47*(3–4), 296–312. https://doi.org/10.1111/j.1469-7610.2006.01611.x

Boris, N., Renk, K., Lowell, A., & Kolomeyer, E. (2018). Parental substance abuse. In C. H. Zeanah (Ed.), *Handbook of infant mental health* (4th ed., pp. 187–202). Guildford Press.

Boyer, S. M., Caplan, J. E., & Edwards, L. K. (2022). Trauma-related dissociation and the dissociative disorder: Neglected symptoms with severe public health consequences. *Delaware Journal of Public Health, 8*(2), 78–84. https://doi.org/10.32481%2Fdjph.2022.05.010

Brewerton, T. D., Ralston, M. E., Dean, M., Hand, S., & Hand, L. (2020). Disordered eating attitudes and behaviors in maltreated children and adolescents receiving forensic assessment in a child advocacy center. *Journal of Child Sexual Abuse, 29*(7), 769–787. https://doi.org/10.1080/10538712.2020.1809047

Bruno, A., Celebre, L., Torre, G., Pandolfo, G., Mento, C., Cedreo, C., Zoccali, R. A., & Muscatello, M. R. A. (2019). Focus on disruptive mood dysregulation disorder: A review of the literature. *Psychiatry Research, 279*, 323–330. https://doi.org/10.1016/j.psychres.2019.05.043

Choi, K. R., Seng, J. S., Briggs, E. C., Munro-Kramer, M. L., Graham-Bermann, S. A., Lee, R. C., & Ford, J. D. (2017). The dissociative subtype of posttraumatic stress disorder (PTSD) among adolescents: Co-occurring PTSD, depersonalization/derealization, and other dissociation symptoms. *Journal of the American Academy of Child and Adolescent Psychiatry, 56*, 1062–1072. https://doi.org/10.1016/j.jaac.2017.09.425

Cook, A., Spinazzola, J., Ford, J., Lanktree, C., Blaustein, M., Cloitre, M., DeRosa, R., Hubbard, R., Kagan, R., Liautaud, J., Mallah, K., Olafson, E., & van der Kolk, B. (2005). Complex trauma in children and adolescents. *Psychiatric Annals, 35*(5), 390–398. https://doi.org/10.3928/00485713-20050501-05

Costello, E. J., Mustillo, S., Erkanli, A., Keeler, G., & Angold, A. (2003). Prevalence and development of psychiatric disorders in childhood and adolescence. *JAMA Psychiatry, 60*(8), 837–844. https://doi.org/10.1001/archpsyc.60.8.837

D'Andrea, W., Ford, J., Stolbach, B., Spinazzola, J., & van der Kolk, B. A. (2012). Understanding interpersonal trauma in children: Why we need a developmentally appropriate trauma diagnosis. *American Journal of Orthopsychiatry, 82*(2), 187–200. https://doi.org/10.1111/j.1939-0025.2012.01154.x

DePierro, J., D'Andrea, W., Spinazzola, J., Stafford, E., van Der Kolk, B., Saxe, G., Stolbach, B., McKernan, S., & Ford, J. D. (2022). Beyond PTSD: Client presentations of developmental trauma disorder from a national survey of clinicians. *Psychological Trauma: Theory, Research, Practice, and Policy, 14*(7), 1167–1174. https://doi.org/10.1037/tra0000532

Dorahy, M. J., Shannon, C., Seagar, L., Corr, M., Stewart, K., Hanna, D., Mulholland, C., & Middleton, W. (2009). Auditory hallucinations in dissociative identity disorder and schizophrenia with and without a childhood trauma history: Similarities and differences. *Journal of Nervous and Mental Disease, 197*(2), 892–898. https://doi.org/10.1097/NMD.0b013e3181c299ea

Endo, T., Sugiyama, T., & Someya, T. (2006). Attention-deficit/hyperactivity disorder and dissociative disorder among abused children. *Psychiatry and Clinical Neurosciences, 60*(4), 434–438. https://doi.org/10.1111/j.1440-1819.2006.01528.x

Ford, J. D. (2023). Why we need a developmentally appropriate trauma diagnosis for children: A 10-year update on developmental trauma disorder. *Journal of Child & Adolescent Trauma, 16,* 403–418. https://doi.org/10.1007/s40653-021-00415-4

Ford, J. D., Charak, R., Karatzias, T., Shevlin, M., & Spinazzola, J. (2022). Can developmental trauma disorder be distinguished from posttraumatic stress disorder? A symptom-level person-centered empirical approach. *European Journal of Psychotraumatology, 13*(2), Article 2133488. https://doi.org/10.1080/20008066.2022.2133488

Ford, J. D., & Courtois, C. A. (2021). Complex PTSD and borderline personality disorder. *Borderline Personality Disorder and Emotion Dysregulation, 8,* Article 16. https://doi.org/10.1186/s40479-021-00155-9

Ford, J. D., Spinazzola, J., & van der Kolk, B. (2021). Psychiatric comorbidity of developmental trauma disorder and posttraumatic stress disorder: Findings from the DTD field trial replication (DTDFT-R). *European Journal of Psychotraumatology, 12*(1), Article 1929028. https://doi.org/10.1080/20008198.2021.1929028

Giedinghagen, A. (2023). The tic in TikTok and (where) all systems go: Mass social media induced illness and Munchausen's by internet as explanatory models for social media associated abnormal illness behavior. *Clinical Child Psychology and Psychiatry, 28*(1), 270–278. https://doi.org/10.1177/13591045221098522

Haruvi-Lamdan, N., Horesh, D., & Golan, O. (2018). PTSD and autism spectrum disorder: Co-morbidity, gaps in research, and potential shared mechanisms. *Psychological Trauma, 10*(3), 290–299. https://doi.org/10.1037/tra0000298

Herman, J. L. (1992/2022). *Trauma and recovery.* Basic Books.

Hippocrates. (1840). *Oeuvres completes* (Vol. 2) (Littré, Trans.). J.-B Baillière.

Humpston, C., Harrow, M., & Rosen, C. (2020). Behind the opaque curtain: A 20-year longitudinal study of dissociative and first-rank symptoms in schizophrenia-spectrum psychoses, other psychoses and non-psychotic disorders. *Schizophrenia Research, 223,* 319–326. https://doi.org/10.1016/j.schres.2020.07.019

Jones, L., Bellis, M. A., Wood, S., Hughes, K., McCoy, E., Eckley, L., Bates, G., Mikton, C., Shakespear, T., & Officer, A. (2012). Prevalence and risk of violence against children with disabilities: A systematic review and meta-analysis of observational studies. *Lancet, 380*(9845), 899–907. https://doi.org/10.1016/S0140-6736(12)60692-8

Kaffman, A. (2009). The silent epidemic of neurodevelopmental injuries. *Biological Psychiatry, 66*(7), 624–626. https://doi.org/10.1016/j.biopsych.2009.08.002

Kavanaugh, B. C., Dupont-Frechette, J. A., Jersky, B. A., & Holler, K. A. (2017). Neurocognitive deficits in children and adolescents following maltreatment: Neurodevelopmental consequences and neuropsychological implications of traumatic stress. *Applied Neuropsychology: Child, 6*(1), 64–78. https://doi.org/10.1080/21622965.2015.1079712

Kerker, B. D., Zhang, J., Nadeem, E., Stein, R. E. K., Hurlburt, M. S., Heneghan, A., Landsverk, J., & McCue Horwitz, S. (2015). Adverse childhood experiences and mental health, chronic medical conditions, and development in young children. *Academic Pediatrics, 15*(5), 510–517. https://doi.org/10.1016/j.acap.2015.05.005

Kerns, C. M., Newschaffer, C. J., Berkowitz, S., Lee, B. K. (2017). Brief report; examining the association of autism and adverse childhood experiences in the national survey of children's health: The important role of income and co-occurring mental health conditions. *Journal of Autism & Developmental Disorders, 47*(7), 2275–2281. https://doi.org/10.1007/s10803-017-3111-7

Kluft, R. P. (1991). Multiple personality disorder. In A. Tasman & S. M. Goldfinger (Eds.), *American Psychiatric Press review of psychiatry* (Vol. 10, pp. 161–188). American Psychiatric Press.

Kugler, B. B., Bloom, M., Kaercher, L. B., Truax, T. V., & Storch, E. A. (2012). Somatic symptoms in traumatized children and adolescents. *Child Psychiatry & Human Development, 43*, 661–673. https://doi.org/10.1007/s10578-012-0289-y

Legault, M., Bourdon, J. N., & Poirier, P. (2021). From neurodiversity to neurodivergence: The role of epistemic and cognitive marginalization. *Synthese, 199*, 12843–12868. https://doi.org/10.1007/s11229-021-03356-5

Loewenstein, R. J. (1991). An office mental status examination for complex chronic dissociative symptoms and multiple personality disorder. *Psychiatric Clinics of North America, 14*, 567–604.

Longden, E., Branitsky, A., Moskowitz, A., Berry, K., Bucci, S., & Varese, F. (2020). The relationship between dissociation and symptoms of psychosis: A meta-analysis. *Schizophrenia Bulletin, 46*(5), 1104–1113. https://doi.org/10.1093/schbul/sbaa037

Lyons-Ruth, K., Bureau, J. F., Holmes, B., Easterbrooks, A., & Brooks, N. H. (2013). Borderline symptoms and suicidality/self-injury in late adolescence: Prospectively observed relationship correlates in infancy and childhood. *Psychiatry Research, 206*(2–3), 273–281. https://doi.org/10.1016/j.psychres.2012.09.030

Moran, H. (2010). Clinical observations of the differences between children on the autism spectrum and those with attachment problems: The Coventry Grid. *Good Autism Practice, 11*(2), 44–57.

National Child Traumatic Stress Network Adapted Trauma Treatment Standards Work Group (Subgroup on Developmental Disabilities) [NCTN]. (2004). *Facts on traumatic stress and children with developmental disabilities.* nctsn.org/sites/default/files/assets/pdfs/traumatic_stress_developmental_disabilities_final.pdf

O'Neil, J. A. (2023). Dissociation in the ICDs and DSMs. In M. J. Dorahy, S. N. Gold & J. A. O'Neil (Eds.). *Dissociation and the dissociative disorders: Past, present, future* (pp. 355–374). Routledge.

Prock, L., & Fogler, J. M. (2018). Trauma and neurodevelopmental disorder: Assessment, treatment, and triage. In J. M. Fogler & R. A. Phelps (Eds.), *Trauma, autism, and neurodevelopmental disorders: Integrating research, practice, and policy* (pp. 55–71). Springer.

Pugh, M., Waller, G., & Esposito, M. (2018). Childhood trauma, dissociation, and the internal eating disorder "voice." *Child Abuse & Neglect, 86*, 197–205. https://doi.org/10.1016/j.chiabu.2018.10.005

Reuben, K. (2023, April 14). *Treating traumatized and dissociative neurodevelopmentally disabled clients.* Workshop at the International Society for the Study of Trauma and Dissociation 2023 Annual Conference, Louisville, KY, United States.

Rosenberg, T., Lahav, Y., & Ginzburg, K. (2023). Child abuse and eating disorder symptoms: Shedding light on the contribution of identification with the aggressor. *Child Abuse & Neglect, 135*, Article 105988. https://doi.org/10.1016/j.chiabu.2022.105988

Şar, V. (2014). The many faces of dissociation: Opportunities for innovative research in psychiatry. *Clinical Psychopharmacology and Neuroscience, 12*(3), 171–179. https://doi.org/10.9758%2Fcpn.2014.12.3.171

Şar, V. & Öztürk, E. (2009). Psychotic presentations of dissociative identity disorder. In P. F. Dell & J. A. O'Neil, (Eds.), *Dissociation and dissociative disorders: DSM-V and beyond* (pp. 535–545). Routledge.

Silberg, J. L. (2022). *The child survivor: Healing developmental trauma and dissociation* (2nd ed.). Routledge.

Silberg, J., & Dallam, S. (2023). Dissociative disorders in children and adolescents. In M. J. Dorahy, S. N. Gold & J. A. O'Neil (Eds), *Dissociation and the dissociative disorders: Past, present, future* (pp. 433–447). Routledge.

Sivaratnam, C. S., Newman, L. K., Tonge, B. J., & Rinehart, N. J. (2015). Attachment and emotion processing in children with autism spectrum disorders: Neurobiological, neuroendocrine, and neurocognitive considerations. *Review Journal of Autism and Developmental Disorders, 2*(2), 222–242. https://doi.org/10.1007/s40489-015-0048-7

Solmi, M., Radua, J., Olivola, M., Croce, E., Soardo, L., De Pablo, G. S., Shin, J. I., Kirkbride, J. B., Jones, P., Kim, J. H., Kim, J. Y., Carvalho, A. F., Seeman, M. V., Correll, C. U., & Fusar-Poli, P. (2021). Age at onset of mental disorders worldwide: Large-scale meta-analysis of 192 epidemiological studies. *Molecular Psychiatry, 27*, 281–295. https://doi.org/10.1038/s41380-021-01161-7

Spiegel, D., Loewenstein, R. J., Lewis-Fernandez, R., Sar, V., Simeon, D., Vermetten, E., Cardeña, E., & Dell, P. F. (2011). Dissociative disorders in DSM-5. *Depression and Anxiety, 28*, E17–E45. https://doi.org/10.1002/da.20923

Spinazzola, J., van der Kolk, B., & Ford, J. D. (2021). Developmental trauma disorder: A legacy of attachment trauma in victimized children. *Journal of Traumatic Stress, 34*(4), 711–720. https://doi.org/10.1002/jts.22697

Storch, E. A., Wood, J. J., Ehrenreich-May, J., Jones, A. M., Park, J. M., Lewin, A. B., & Murphy, T. L. (2012). Convergent and discriminant validity and reliability of the pediatric anxiety rating scale in youth with autism spectrum disorders. *Journal of Autism and Developmental Disorders, 42*(11), 2374–2382. https://doi.org/10.1007/s10803-012-1489-9

Uhlhaas, P. J. (2011). The adolescent brain: Implications for the understanding, pathophysiology, and treatment of schizophrenia. *Schizophrenia Bulletin, 37*(3), 480–483. https://doi.org/10.1093%2Fschbul%2Fsbr025

van der Kolk, B. A. (2005). Developmental trauma disorder: Toward a rational diagnosis for children with complex trauma histories. *Psychiatric Annals, 35*(5), 401–408. https://doi.org/10.3928/00485713-20050501-06

van der Kolk, B. A., Roth, S., Pelcovitz, D., Sunday, S., & Spinazzola, J. (2005). Disorders of extreme stress: The empirical foundation of complex trauma adaptation to trauma. *Journal of Traumatic Stress Studies, 18*(5), 389–399. https://doi.org/10.1002/jts.20047

Van Scoyoc, A., Marquardt, M. B., & Phelps, R. A. (2018). The challenges and importance of differentiating trauma and stress-related disorders from autism spectrum disorders. In J. M. Fogler & R. A. Phelps (Eds.), *Trauma, autism, and neurodevelopmental disorders: Integrating research, practice, and policy* (pp. 73–91). Springer.

Waters, F. S. (2016). *Healing the fractured child: Diagnosis and treatment of youth with dissociation*. Springer.

Winsper, C., Lereya, S. T., Marwaha, S., Thompson, A., Eyden, J., & Singh, S. P. (2016). The aetiological and psychopathological validity of borderline personality disorder in youth: A systematic review and meta-analysis. *Clinical Psychology Review, 44*, 13–24. https://doi.org/10.1016/j.cpr.2015.12.001

World Health Organization (2021). *International statistical classification of diseases and related health problems* (11th ed.). icd.who.int.

Zero to Three (2016). *DC:0–5: Diagnostic classification of mental health and developmental disorders of infancy and early childhood*. Zero to Three.

Zhang, L. P., Jia, Y., Huang, H., Li, D. W., & Wang, Y. P. (2021). Clinical classifications of children with psychogenic non-epileptic seizure. *Frontiers in Pediatrics, 8,* Article 596781. https://doi.org/10.3389/fped.2020.596781

15
WORKING CONSIDERATIONS IN BUILDING THE ROAD MAP TO TREATMENT

Case Conceptualization, Treatment Guidelines, and Treatment Planning[1]

Jillian Hosey

Introduction

Early and effective childhood treatment of dissociative symptoms and disorders can prevent years of physical, psychological, and economic disruption and challenges (Woolard et al., 2024). Treatment focused on reducing symptoms of dissociation and supporting the development of integrative capacities across all states of being can support the child toward a normative developmental trajectory (International Society for the Study of Trauma and Dissociation [ISSTD], 2004; Silberg, 2021; Waters, 2016; Woolard et al., 2024). Treatment approaches for child dissociation are framed and informed by a child's history and current presentation, as captured through the assessment process (Myrick & Silberg, 2024). The phenomenological data derived from the assessment supports the process of case conceptualization (Henderson & Martin, 2014; Manassis, 2014) and illuminates an initial road map for treatment targets (Silberg, 2021; Steinberg & Hall, 1997) by synthesizing the diverse array of factors contextualizing the child's challenges. This process supplies the clinician with an organizing framework for bridging the process of assessment to treatment.

This chapter outlines the process of case conceptualization and treatment planning for children with complex trauma and dissociation. First, it reviews the child therapy literature on case conceptualization, both generally and specific to children with complex trauma and dissociation. The importance of case conceptualization in elucidating treatment-related tasks and goals follows, exploring important considerations related to proposed treatment guidelines and principles. and factors that affect both the child and their treatment. Lastly, a supplemental sheet is provided alongside a composite case example to demonstrate the initial process of case conceptualization and treatment planning.

Case conceptualization and treatment planning is key in synthesizing all sections of this book into an intentional framework for both understanding the child and guiding treatment. The models of dissociation outlined in the preceding theory section offer readers various theoretical models to conceptualize the child's challenges and inform interventions as they unfold. Readers are encouraged to consider the information from the chapters on symptomatology, screening and assessment, and differential and co-occurring diagnoses to stimulate critical thinking in support of intentional treatment planning attuned to each unique dissociative child. The subsequent sections in this book will introduce a variety of different trauma therapy modalities and essential considerations about how they can be adapted for work with dissociative children and their families. Readers are recommended to keep these modalities and considerations in mind as they continue to read and venture into the case conceptualization and treatment planning process.

Considerations in Case Conceptualization: Pulling It All Together

Following an in-depth screening and assessment process, clinicians face the complex task of pulling together assessment-related data into a case conceptualization and treatment plan. Case conceptualization "involves turning a patient's narrative and all the information derived from examinations, interviews with parents and teachers, and medical and school reports into a coherent and not necessarily lengthy story that will help to develop a treatment plan" (Henderson & Martin, 2014, p. 2). Furthermore, the case formulation

> has to convey relevant signs and symptoms and pertinent negatives (i.e., key absent symptoms); provide meaningful, explanatory contexts for these signs and symptoms, including familial, social, educational, and cultural contexts; justify diagnoses (or no diagnosis, if warranted); and describe treatment options based on the diagnostic considerations.
>
> *(Henderson & Martin, 2014, p. 2)*

In essence, the case conceptualization "synthesiz[es] information into a theory as to how problems developed and how change might unfold" (Winters et al., 2007, p. 114). This process is a strategic one that includes considerations related to what the goals for treatment are, and whether the focus of treatment will be on symptom reduction or comprehensive treatment, where we are working with the systems and environments the child engages with to promote integrative, and systemic change and healing to support the child's development becoming back on track. Approaching conceptualization strategically allows clinicians to start building a picture of how they best understand what is happening for the child, to support the selection of the most relevant, corresponding interventions and modalities that are connected to an overarching treatment plan. As such, case conceptualization is a process rather than a manualized approach or technique.

If careful time and consideration are not taken, clinicians may struggle to organize all the information in a way that supports treatment, and treatment chaos may ensue (Berman, 2018). As such, starting with a theoretical frame or conceptual model is core to the case conceptualization. This process supports clinicians to engage in a mindful formulation that considers the best way to understand the client and develop a trauma- and dissociation-focused treatment plan that honors the unique needs of the child and caregiving system. As wisely stated by Orvaschel et al. (2001), "To intervene without an underlying theoretical framework is akin to building a house without a foundation" (p. 6). This frame informs treatment pacing, targets underlying causes of symptomatology, and ensures goals are oriented toward facilitating developmentally appropriate integrative capacities, all of which support transformation, development, and growth after trauma. The frame organizing a case conceptualization also provides a scaffold for treatment planning as corresponding and complementary treatment models are selected.

In child therapy, case conceptualization is ideally framed through basic neurodevelopmental concepts (Perry, 2009) that acknowledge environmental factors, dependence on caregivers, influences in and outside of the family, developmental norms (Manassis, 2014), and cultural and sociocultural determinants (Bryant & Njenga, 2006; Henderson & Martin, 2014). This process attempts to link the complex and multifaceted components of a child as well as the whole family's past and present experiences to form a synopsis, potentially revealing initially hidden or obscured information. It "assumes that each child has unique reasons for presenting with his or her difficulties...[and] includes examining various contributing factors and possible causes for the child's difficulties" (Manassis, 2014, p. 6). When working with children, this work thus becomes more systemic. Indeed,

> the first difference in the evaluation of children that bears on case formulation is the fact that children, unlike adult patients, are not self-referred but are usually referred by a parent, teacher, or some other agent. The problem is not defined primarily by the patient, and child patients may not even see the behavior expected by the parents or school as desirable.
>
> *(Winters et al., 2007, p. 114)*

As previously stated, the information contained in the case conceptualization assists clinicians in better understanding the child's internal and external experiences and allows them to plan appropriate interventions. It includes a "hypothesis about the intra- and inter-personal dynamics that underlie the client's difficulties" (Havighurst & Downey, 2009, p. 253). To this end, the

> case formulation should include a comprehensive and coherent picture of what the patient is trying to pursue in psychotherapy, the obstruction(s) that prevent him or her from attaining what she or he wants, and how she or he will try to pursue it.
>
> *(Gazzillo et al., 2021, p. 117)*

Such a plan, however, is malleable and may be ever-changing across time as conditions change and additional relevant information emerges in therapy (Manassis, 2014). Thus, case conceptualization is an individualized and nuanced process that generates "a condensation of values, informed by the nature of the encounter between the clinician and the patient; practical goals; training and experience; and implicit and explicit ethics" (p. 8).

Synthesizing and organizing this information requires therapists to ask themselves the following questions: How are a child's symptoms, presenting struggles, and strengths understood across the systems they inhabit? What theory or conceptual model best describes what is happening for a child? What are the goals for treatment and what modality best addresses the child's symptoms, challenges, or needs? What systems and third parties may be involved (Orvaschel et al., 2001), and do they agree on the goals? Furthermore, goal setting is a collaborative effort that also requires careful consideration of the motivation behind the goals, who they are serving (e.g., does the goal serve the clinician, child, parent, or whole system?), and the ways in which the environment and attachment-related dynamics may support or further complicate achieving the established goals. Such questions form the basis of the moment-to-moment clinical decision-making process that clinicians embark on as part of case conceptualization. While we strive for collaboration and congruence, clinicians may discover conflict embedded within this process that highlights the strategies families use to relate and connect. Seeking consultation and peer support in navigating this process is recommended.

Models of Case Conceptualization

Unfortunately, there is no unified approach to case conceptualization, and clinicians may find themselves challenged to reconcile modality-specific models of conceptualization from more general forms. Berman (2018) put forth a four-step structure to support clinicians in developing effective case conceptualization and treatment planning skills. This process involves: selecting the most relevant theoretical perspective; building a premise and conclusion to treatment that is supported by assessment-related material; developing a treatment plan that includes long-term and short-term goals;

and developing a written plan that is described as flexible, comfortable, and motivating for the child client. Henderson and Martin (2014) further share that conceptualization specific to children includes additional considerations such as using precise rather than jargonistic language, detailing the primary complaint and ensuring that both family and school are considered, and relying on a chosen model of child development across the entire formulation rather than as a separate category.

Two fundamental transdiagnostic approaches to organizing assessment information in case conceptualization are the *biopsychosocial formulation* (commonly used by psychologists) and the *Four Ps* (commonly used by psychiatrists; see Henderson and Martin [2014], for an overview of case conceptualization; Macneil et al. [2012]). A biopsychosocial approach (Havighurst & Downey, 2009; Henderson & Martin, 2014) takes a broad rather than reductionist view of the child to understand the biological, psychological, and social factors influencing the child's presentation. The Four Ps approach (Havighurst & Downey, 2009; Henderson & Martin, 2014) organizes the client's presentation according to chronology and etiology by considering the associated predisposing, precipitating, perpetuating, and protective factors (Henderson & Martin, 2014). While not dissociation-specific, the Four Ps approach considers what Braun and Sachs's (1985) outlined in their 3P Factor Theory of Multiple Personality Disorder (now known as Dissociative Identity Disorder), which considers the predisposing, precipitating, and perpetuating factors to developing a dissociative disorder. By synthesizing information across biopsychosocial, developmental, and temporal dimensions, clinicians can identify both strength and resilience factors, as well as areas of growth, to support greater discernment in individualized treatment planning (Nurcombe, 2014).

In addition to the biopsychosocial formulation and Four Ps approaches, the literature offers various other approaches to case conceptualization and treatment planning (see Berman, 2018). These include cognitive, behavioral, cognitive-behavioral, feminist, emotion-focused, dynamic, cultural, structural family treatment, constructivist, and trans-theoretical approaches to case conceptualization and treatment planning. Additional considerations arise in case conceptualization and treatment planning across different

- **Populations**, such as children (Manassis, 2014; Orvaschel et al., 2001), adults (Berman, 2018; Sperry & Sperry, 2020), families (Tamkin et al., 2019), and geriatric (Kendjelic & Eells, 2007);
- **Settings**, such as forensic (Sturmey, 2010), developmental pediatric (Kawamura et al., 2014), agency (Dawson, 2020), and residential (Brown et al., 2013);
- **Professions**, including child and adolescent psychiatry (Winters et al., 2007), psychotherapy (Eells, 2022), and social work (Fung & Ross, 2024; Lee & Toth, 2016);
- **Specific interventions**, including ARC (Arvidson et al., 2011), CBT (Dummett, 2013; Eells, 2022; Zayfert & Becker, 2019), DBT (Eells, 2022), Schema Therapy (Fassbinder et al., 2019), psychoanalytic (Messer & Wolitzky, 2007), brief dynamic psychotherapy (Eells & Lombart, 2003), emotion-focused therapy (Goldman, 2017; Goldman & Goldstein, 2022), creative arts (Karaca & Eren, 2014), cognitive processing therapy (Nixon & Bralo, 2019), EMDR (Gomez, 2012; Shapiro, 2017; Struik, 2014), play therapy (O'Connor & Ammen, 2012); and
- **Treatment approaches/modalities**, including cognitive-evolutionist (Farina, 2021), strength- and hope-based (McCrea et al., 2016), behavioral (Haynes et al., 2011), cognitive (Dudley & Kuyken, 2013), relational/interpersonal (Gazzillo et al., 2021), emotional (Pascual-Leone & Kramer, 2017), person-centered (Simms, 2011), trans-theoretical (Jose & Goldfried, 2008), team-based (Whomsley, 2010), post-structural narrative therapy (Meehan & Guilfoyle, 2015), and systems (Holochwost & Jaffee, 2017; Schiepek, 2003).

While this chapter does not endeavor to advise the right approach to conceptualization, it does provide options and direction to support clinicians in discerning which clinical choices may be in the best interests of each unique child client and their families, as they plan for treatment focused on complex trauma and dissociation.

Case Conceptualization through a Trauma and Dissociation Lens

Clinicians working with child trauma are tasked with an added element of ensuring that they are familiar with the relevant trauma-informed guidelines, treatments, and frameworks (Lucio & Nelson, 2016), including complex trauma–specific care (Cook et al., 2005) and the use of a phase-oriented approach to treatment (ISSTD, 2004). According to Cruz et al. (2022), "as a multifactorial neurobehavioral disturbance, developmental trauma causes significant alterations to children's cognitive, emotional, physiological, and relational capacities, and as a result, they experience widespread disruptions to their academic, social, and occupational functioning" (pp. 4–5). Understanding the impact of trauma on child development is essential to discerning normative as opposed to maladaptive presentations across developmental stages, and recognizing the dynamic manifestations of symptoms across developmental stages and environments (Gregorowski & Seedat, 2013; Orvaschel et al., 2001). Additionally, children's normative dissociative experiences can make it hard to differentiate between a pathological process versus immagination involved in play (Haugaard, 2004).

As such, treatment for child dissociation

> is complex and relies on good clinical assessment of the individual's needs. Efficacious treatment will likely need to be multimodal and focus on different aspects of the child's functioning and involve psychotherapy, psychopharmacology (if needed), and adjunctive therapies such as mindfulness or art therapy to facilitate healing. Although treatment for this population should be developmentally appropriate, methods used with adults who experience dissociation, such as a phasic treatment approach perhaps incorporating developmentally appropriate therapeutic techniques, for instance, play-based tasks.
>
> *(Woolard et al., 2024, p. 8)*

Furthermore,

> recommended treatments for dissociative disorders, particularly DID, have been tied to a very specific theoretical model that posits the onset of these pathogenic processes in early childhood, with the fragmentation of the identity as a coping tool in the face of overwhelming trauma. This theoretical model dictates that treatment should involve the integration of fragmented identity states, and the integration of dissociated traumatic experiences (Kluft, 1999).
>
> *(Silberg, 2001, p. 449)*

Varying definitions of what is meant by identity integration, especially in children, can muddy the process and assume that the automatic desire and outcome of treatment is unity. Orienting oneself in a neurodevelopmental approach allows for deeper consideration around identity development in children, and places the overarching task of treatment as supporting getting development back on track. Assessment-related data can provide information about the degree to which a child's "development and personality ha[s] been structured around cutting off trauma-related memories, thoughts, and feelings and keeping them inaccessible to consciousness and to [their] day-to-day 'apparently normal' self" (Stolbach, 2005, p. 690). Along these lines, Silberg (2001) suggested the use of an "integrated developmental treatment model, in which pathological dissociative processes are viewed as a complex, multi determined outcome for certain children with predisposing capacities and vulnerabilities in an environment which is viewed as threatening" (p. 451).

Clinicians are encouraged to question how they understand the proposed treatment model's "values, assumptions, concepts, principles, and guidelines" (McCrea et al., 2016, p. 12) to discern whether the treatment needs to be adapted to address concurrent symptoms of complex trauma. The selection of a conceptual model to frame treatment is ideally guided by an investigative process that includes critical reflection about the impact of trauma and dissociation. These questions may include: How do I understand my client's manifestation of symptoms across emotional, cognitive, behavioral, somatic, sensorial, and relational domains? What may be maintaining them? Are there themes of loss, shame and guilt, idealization, or concerns about self-harm and suicidality that need to be attended to more acutely? How do I understand my client's self-report capacities, since children and adolescents might not report dissociative symptoms, as they consider them to be normal (Silberg & Dallam, 2009)? How do I understand where the child sits on the continuum of pathology based on outcomes after exposure to traumatic events (Stolbach, 2005)? How do I understand my client's intersectional experiences and identities in the world and how they may or may not contribute to their present symptoms? Are there accessibility and/or cultural considerations (McCrea et al., 2016)? How do I understand the prognostic factors and potential treatment challenges (Putnam, 1997)? How do I understand my client's resources and protective factors? Am I able to conceptualize their symptoms as trauma-related resources that support survival?

Further critical thinking that is systemic in nature is encouraged, as children do not exist outside of the systems that are meant to care for and protect them. These settings may include the immediate and extended family, school and early childcare centers, health care and social services, legal settings (Bellis et al., 2023), and other community locations. A systems perspective also includes becoming curious about how the attachment and caregiving system is understood, and its potential implications for treatment. Understanding the "internalized relationship models, self-esteem, and social and intellectual competencies" (p. 13) of the child may allow the clinician to predict reenactment (McCrea et al., 2016). Family system factors and their interactions (Winters et al., 2007), alongside an understanding of the client's attachment history, may inform considerations for the therapeutic relationship (Farina, 2021) and the role of the child's dissociation within the family system (Putnam, 1997). Furthermore, the spaces and environments the child frequents may support or inhibit their emotion, thought, and behavior regulation. Understanding the systems surrounding and interacting with the child may clarify how their experiences have been assimilated and integrated into their developing view of the world, interpersonal relationships, and self-understandings (Berman, 2018). This knowledge can also help the clinician understand any disclosure responses, triggers, and strategies of avoidance for both the child and part of the larger family system.

The child's and family's mental health and treatment history are essential components of the case conceptualization. Many dissociative children already have a significant treatment history because of misdiagnosis and comorbid symptomatology such as ADHD, conversion, and somatoform disorders; conduct and oppositional defiant disorders; schizophrenia and various forms of epilepsy; and affective disorders (Silberg & Dallam, 2009 Zoroglu et al., 1996). Waters (2016) offered a detailed exploration of these common comorbidities and their presentations in her book, *Healing the Fractured Child: Diagnosis and Treatment of Youth with Dissociation.*

Case conceptualization among children with complex trauma and dissociation should be expected to be rife with uncertainty and confusion, especially "in cases with combinations of complex and severe symptomatic presentations, poor object relations" (Silberg, 1998, n.p.). Clinicians can expect to encounter multiple domains of impairment in children exposed to complex trauma, including in attachment, biology, affect regulation, dissociation, behavioral control, cognition, and self-concept (Cook et al., 2005). These children are often stigmatized and misunderstood. As such, when formalizing a case conceptualization, clinicians are encouraged to carefully consider who this information is for and who else may access it, their rationale for making any specific recommendations, and how their conceptualization may further pathologize the child. As each client's unique symptoms, experiences, and motivations are discovered, needs emerge based on the neurobiopsychosocial, attachment, intersectionality, trauma, and dissociation related facets about the child and family system. It is essential to avoid pathologizing normative behavior and mood shifts in children (ISSTD, 2026). As clinicians begin to identify client and family treatment needs, therapeutic "growth tasks" may emerge as potential treatment goals, which are ideally supported by a complex trauma- and dissociation-specific treatment approach that is informed by principles and guidelines.

Treatment Approach, Principles, and Guidelines

An initial selection of a theoretical viewpoint or perspective helps elucidate what is happening for the client. Clinicians may then begin to identify and highlight the child's and family's strengths and challenges, with supporting material or examples for each (Berman, 2018). (Please note that Berman used the word "weakness" in her text, which has been changed in this chapter to the word "challenge." The rationale behind this is to honor that what may now be perceived as maladaptive was in fact once adaptive, which is not based on weakness.) This chapter does not seek to recommend a specific frame per se, but instead to encourage clinicians to ensure they are grounded in their own theoretical underpinnings and understand how these align (or conflict) with a treatment approach informed by complex trauma and dissociation, as well as with the related principles and established guidelines. Below are key considerations for ensuring that the chosen frame aligns with best practices for treating child dissociation.

The Phased-Oriented Approach to Treatment

The National Child Traumatic Stress Network working group identified six core components required for any intervention in working with children with histories of complex trauma: the establishment of safety; self-regulation; self-reflective information processing; integration of the traumatic experience into a life narrative; re-engagement with relationships; and enhancing positive affect (Cook et al., 2005; Gregorowski & Seedat, 2013). These tasks align with a phase-oriented approach to treatment that matches the most appropriate treatment modality to the corresponding treatment goals to reduce distress and work with the family system (Gregorowski & Seedat, 2013). The use of a phased approach to treatment is associated with a reduction in dissociative symptoms (Gomez, 2012; ISSTD, 2026; Silberg, 2021 Waters, 2016; Wieland, 2015; Woolard et al., 2024). The phase-oriented approach provides a scaffold for treatment and is flexible in allowing for relevant adjunctive modalities and interventions to be integrated within it, including attachment, play-based, and somatic-focused modalities. Woolard et al. (2024) found that most child dissociation-focused "psychotherapy was conducted in a phasic method focusing on safety followed by the treatment of symptoms" (p. 8). Careful discernment is needed to bring together all the data and determine the most appropriate modalities to support the process of therapy, whether it is focused on solely symptom reduction or a comprehensive treatment that brings about full systemic change and healing.

The phases in phase-oriented treatment with children are similar to those in treatment with adults, with a focus on safety and stabilization, remembrance and mourning (trauma processing), and reconnection (Herman, 2015; ISSTD, 2026; Myrick et al., 2015). The final phase focuses on integrating connections to the self and others and moving forward (ISSTD, 2026; Myrick et al., 2015), which may include the use of post-integration therapy (Woolard et al., 2024). According to Waters (2016), a child dissociation–specific, phase-oriented treatment approach allows for the development of integrative functions in children. Inclusive of this approach is that language communicates integration from the outset of treatment, speaking to all aspects of a whole child. Despite being presented as a linear approach, a phase-oriented approach to treatment with dissociative children is progressive and recursive (similar to working with adults; see Steinberg & Hall, 1997), and clinicians may return to the same themes but at deeper integrative layers of experience.

Treatment Principles

Several common treatment principles have been proposed for working with dissociative children and their families regardless of the chosen theoretical frame and corresponding approach. As detailed above, Cook et al. (2005) outlined six core components of complex trauma interventions with children: addressing issues of safety, self-regulation, self-reflective information processing, traumatic experience integration, relational engagement, and positive affect enhancement. Other principles for creating constructive change include establishing safety in the treatment relationship; use of empathic attunement; honoring self-determination as a guide to treatment; acknowledging strengths; building contrastive and effective coping; and building a meaningful trauma narrative (McCrea et al., 2016). Furthermore, Waters (2016) accentuated the importance of focusing on primary trauma-related symptoms rather than secondary ones, as well as developing safety, finding the meaning behind the behavior, educating children and caregivers about trauma and dissociation, integrating developmentally appropriate activities, engaging in all aspects of the child, encouraging responsibility across all states, engaging parents and caregiving systems in treatment, promoting the attachment between caregivers and the whole child (as opposed to with only some aspects of the child), and promoting and building metacognitive skills.

Silberg (2021) put forth the EDUCATE Model to organize treatment with dissociative children. This model includes the following organizing treatment principles: use of the treatment within a phase-oriented approach that expands a child's window of tolerance (Siegel, 2001); building safety and differentiating between "then and now;" the inclusion of all states of being in treatment and encouraging responsibility across all states; the belief in a child's ability to heal; work with caregivers and collaboration across relevant systems; child and caregiver education about trauma and dissociation; the use of relationship as the vehicle to healing; expectation and identification of issues of transference, countertransference, and enactments; intervention of meaningful primary dissociation- and trauma-related symptoms, consideration of symptoms as adaptive under maladaptive circumstances, and that every behavior is meaningful communication; use of both top-down and bottom-up therapeutic approaches and activities that are developmentally appropriate; and promoting metacognitive skills and somatic awareness across all aspects of the self.

Both Waters's (2016) and Silberg's (2021) principles of treatment align with the original philosophy and principles of treatment with dissociative children set forth by Putnam (1997). This included a focus on ensuring safety, meeting the needs of children, understanding the perspectives and binds of children, and supporting the natural resiliency of children. These treatment principles, all specific to complex trauma and dissociation, align with the guidelines for treating dissociative children.

Treatment Guidelines

After the International Society for the Study of Trauma and Dissociation (ISSTD) issued the first edition of *Guidelines for Treating Dissociative Identity Disorder in Adults* in 1994, child therapist Joyanna Silberg led a task force in developing similar guidelines focused on child and adolescent treatment. In 2003, the first edition of *Guidelines for the Evaluation and Treatment of Dissociative Symptoms in Children and Adolescents* was issued (ISSTD, 2004). As of 2024, these guidelines are undergoing their first revision. The purpose of the treatment guidelines is not to create a rigid structure for clinicians to work within, but to provide guidance for clinicians working with traumatized children, as

> [t]reatment strategies aimed at increasing integration and reducing dissociation can be effective in treating some of the most seriously impaired child victims of maltreatment who are engaged in disruptive and self-destructive behavior ... Information on treating dissociation was not available when most clinicians did their training, and it is important to organize clinical information to help familiarize clinicians with current treatment approaches ... [as] without careful consideration of developmental issues, the simplistic application of treatment approaches for adult dissociation to children may be potentially dangerous to children.
>
> *(ISSTD, 2004, p. 121)*

The ISSTD treatment guidelines offer information related to the length and course of treatment; the role of the therapist; special treatment-related cautions; how to build therapeutic goals that support children to develop cohesiveness around their behavior, affect, and cognition; how to build motivation for growth and development, and promote self-acceptance of behavior and knowledge around intolerable and unacceptable affective experiences; trauma memory work to desensitize memories and rework trauma-related beliefs about the world; promoting autonomy and agency in the child toward authentic self-expression and the self-regulation of affective states; and supporting building and/or repair of attachments (ISSTD, 2004). In 2016, the European Society for Trauma and Dissociation (ESTD) issued *Guidelines for the Assessment and Treatment of Children and Adolescents with Dissociative Symptoms and Dissociative Disorders* (revised in 2017). Both the ISSTD and ESTD treatment guidelines illustrate the need for specialized treatment for dissociative children, and offer clinicians and researchers essential information related to the neurobiology of trauma and dissociation; brief theories of dissociation; information related to a trauma- and dissociation-specific assessment framework; guiding treatment principles and a phase-oriented approach; child specific interventions, modalities, and practices; pharmacology; and assessing integration and post-integration work (ISSTD, 2004, 2026).

Treatment Planning

The treatment plan is an evolving document that supports and guides the treatment tasks. Careful attention to flexibility and the recognition that the treatment plan is an ever-evolving document (Henderson & Martin, 2014; Gomez, 2012) allows for constant revisions as clinicians engage in this work. New information about the child and their experiences may arise as the child grows (both internally and externally), and as the relational and environmental dynamics that may perpetuate dissociative symptomatology change (Silberg, 2001, 2021).

Treatment Styles and Goals

The literature describes a variety of different styles of treatment organization, which may be assumption-based, symptom-based, interpersonally based, and historically based, and which shift the focus of how treatment goals are understood (Berman, 2018). For example, Nurcombe (2014) outlined four styles of treatment planning that are either intuitive or deliberate: therapy matching (an intuitive process whereby clinical patterns are matched by therapists to a corresponding diagnostic and treatment plan); problem orientation (a deliberate process whereby treatment is planned around problems that are identified through assessment-related data); focal inpatient treatment planning (a deliberate process, limited to inpatient settings, whereby a problem is identified through diagnosis and explicit objectives are determined to address the problem); and goal direction (a deliberate process whereby problems and potentials are reframed as goals and include considerations related to time, funds, and resources available, and all treatment settings are considered helping clients meet their treatment goals). While they are not specific to complex trauma or dissociation, they complement the principles and guidelines of treatment described above.

Berman (2018) further suggested three key organizational features to a treatment plan, with a selected theory supporting how information is organized: developing a brief treatment plan overview that includes client needs, issues, and goals, and which outlines roles and responsibilities in treatment; developing more comprehensive, long-term goals that speak to what is hoped to be achieved by treatment termination; and the development of brief, specific short-term goals that are measurable via objectives and can be tracked to illustrate change. Although Berman (2018) identified that there is no one standardized format for presenting treatment plan goals, there is a basic understanding that the function of creating treatment goals is rooted in what each unique client will benefit from achieving, learning, and developing.

In alignment with a phenomenological approach to treatment planning, a symptom-based style of treatment planning integrates the subjective information related to child and family personal history across the biopsychosocial, attachment, intersectionality, trauma, and dissociation domains, and the subjective observations of the therapist, while incorporating the objective data derived through testing. This information is then used to develop treatment goals, or growth tasks. According to Nurcombe (2014), developing treatment goals helps identify the "problem," assess its nature, determine a problem-solving goal, design objectives to meet the goal, create an evaluation process, and build a team that collaborates to support the planning and execution of the treatment plan.

It is important to note that assessment-related tools and data (e.g., history, observations, and testing data) are key for both creating, organizing, and monitoring treatment goals. Grasso (2022) encouraged clinicians to use assessment and conceptualization data to create treatment goals that focus on symptom reduction and enhanced functioning; determine how caregivers may be appropriately engaged in the child's treatment; and ensure that goals are "matched to an evidence-based intervention that has been effective with the population they are working with" (p. 9). To ensure this is trauma and dissociation informed, notions of symptom reduction are expanded to consider the (re)development of the self. Ideally, this process is done collaboratively with the child, exploring a shared meaning of "what is wrong" and "what needs to change" as a means of enriching the therapeutic relationship (Myrick & Silberg, 2024). Offering relational approaches to treatment planning, Gazzillo et al. (2021) devised the plan formulation method as a way of evaluating individual needs across domains of impairment and then tailoring specific treatment interventions to the client.

Treatment Planning for Child Dissociation

In dissociation-informed therapy with children, in addition to unique client-focused treatment goals, Silberg (2021) states that the overarching goals for therapy include creating safety in the present, developing the capacity to regulate affect as triggers are encountered, increasing self-awareness, making sense of the traumatic experiences, developing reciprocity in relationships, shifting helplessness into mastery, and developing a more coherent and integrated sense of consciousness. Since children exist within their larger caregiving and family systems, treatment planning for traumatized and dissociative children takes a systemic approach that acknowledges the needs of the specific treatment setting and systems involved. Furthermore, requirements within some treatment settings prescribe specific evidence-based treatments, which may have their own embedded treatment planning guides or tenets.

Silberg (2021) proposed the use of the EDUCATE model to organize dissociation-specific child treatment goals into a three-phase treatment plan. This model follows the treatment principles listed above and guides the process of developing and meeting treatment goals, identifying the method that will achieve the goal, and explaining how the treatment goal and intervention can be linked back to the traumatized child's neurobiology and developing brain. EDUCATE stands for Education; Dissociation motivation (what factors keep dissociation in place as the viable strategy for coping); Understanding what remains hidden inside, which may include hidden affect, identity, or behavioral states; Claiming the hidden aspects as parts of the whole self and helping the child reconnect with what needed to be disconnected for survival; Affect regulation and modulation in attachment/relationship; Trigger identification (precursors to trauma-based responses) and trauma processing work; Ending therapy, planning for developmental changes and challenges, and building flexibility to approach adaptive risk taking and change. Silberg (2021) additionally provides different interventions that readers may consider, and what they target in terms of symptoms and corresponding neurological structure. See Silberg (2021) and Waters (2016) for further detailed essential treatment planning considerations for clinicians working with children with dissociative symptoms.

Integrative Treatment

As you will see highlighted throughout this chapter and comprehensive volume, complex trauma treatment with children is integrative, where multiple approaches and modalities are interwoven (Cook et al., 2005). According to the ISSTD *Guidelines* (2004), "[t]he most successful treatment approach to an individual case is often the most eclectic, with the therapist showing flexibility and creativity in the utilization of a wide variety of available techniques" (p. 122). In a systematic review of the literature on the treatment of dissociation in children, Woolard et al. (2024) found that current dissociation-specific treatment interventions with children are founded in adult dissociation-specific therapies, and the therapies utilized are varied rather than fixed. This lends to the notion of integrative treatment, whereby clinicians create combinations of approaches to best suit a child and their family (Woolard et al., 2024). Since treatment modifications will differ from child to child, research that evaluates the efficacy of therapeutic techniques used in isolation or combination is needed to assess outcomes.

While clinicians are ethically called to use evidence-based treatments, Norcross and Wampold (2018) explored the imperativeness of "adapting psychotherapy to the person of the patient, beyond [their] disorder" (p. 2). Indeed, treatments specifically for children with PTSD may need to be adapted for children with complex trauma and dissociation, shifting away from the notion that there is but one effective treatment or manualized approach (Cloitre, 2015). Of note, however, is that while being integrative allows for a more nuanced treatment, it also means decreased adherence to a model and being able to evaluate its efficacy. Evidence-based treatments may be selected and modified based on a variety of

> child factors, caregiver factors, and environmental factors. Child factors include the child's age, developmental level (particularly regarding speech and language), size, type of symptoms (trauma, behavioral, emotional, relational, etc.), timeline of symptoms, stability of symptoms, and the ability to verbalize aspects of the traumatic event. Caregiver factors include obtaining a supportive caregiver to take part in services, the offending status of the caregiver (i.e., whether the caregiver perpetrated abuse against the child), primary concern of the caregiver, and parent's level of impairment related to traumatic and/or other psychiatric symptoms. Environmental factors include the stability of the child's placement, case plan goal and visitation frequency (for children engaged in the child welfare system), and the use of other trauma treatment modalities within the same family.
>
> *(Vanderzee et al., 2019, p. 518)*

Additional considerations explore bottom-up versus top-down approaches (Gazzillo et al., 2021), implicit versus explicit interventions and how to speak the language of the child (Putnam, 1997), and integration of adjunctive treatments that reflect the needs of the child, which may include family therapy, hypnotherapy, pharmacotherapy, art therapy, group therapy, and psychoeducation (ISSTD, 2004). Many of these treatments are discussed in the section of this volume focused on treatment modalities.

Organizing this information in a mindful, thorough manner includes asking important clinical questions: How do I understand the impact of trauma and the manifestation of dissociation in my client, and how may this fluctuate according to environment? Am I missing any information to develop a nuanced clinical perspective of the child and family system? What template for mapping will organize the information derived through the assessment process? How do I understand the risk and resiliency factors (Compas et al., 2017)? How do I understand the child's stage of development, and how may this stage influence symptomatology and how the tasks of treatment are organized? Have I attended to the biological, psychological, social, and cultural-spiritual domains of the child's life (Manassis, 2014) and how they impact development and the child's unique risk and resilience factors? Have I considered intersectionality, such as faith and spirituality, race, and culture across the entire family system? What do I understand about comorbidity and differential diagnosis considerations (see Chapter 14), as well as about the child's neurotype and learning style? What considerations are necessary regarding use of language and what I want this to convey, as "the language [I] use in writing a treatment plan can increase a client's sense of hope that [I] understand them and what they want" (Berman, 2018, p. 9)? Are there any legal considerations (e.g., court case and custody concerns)? What is my role and responsibility regarding training and consultation (ISSTD, 2026)? How do I understand what the child and caregiving system need from me as a therapist regarding co-regulation as a supportive pathway to developing self-regulation? How do I understand the need for experiences of dependence, interdependence, and independence, a sense of personal value, regulatory capacities, and resources?

Asking these questions requires the therapist to know themselves and remain curious about their own internal reactions and leanings, as these become activated within the therapeutic relationship. It can be helpful for the clinician to develop a strategy for mapping out identified symptomatology and corresponding growth tasks, how they are understood developmentally and supported by an accompanying theoretical model(s), any concurrent risky behaviors that call for careful considerations in pacing, dissociative processes and manifestations and what sustains them, Internal Working Models and attachment-related strategies and dilemmas, comorbidities, environmental factors, and considerations, and matching an intervention to the issue it is targeting. Table 15.1 offers clinicians a way of pulling together the relevant information into a treatment plan.

Treatment Setting

Henderson and Martin (2014) state that

> [t]he shape of a formulation may depend less on the patient's narrative and more on the location of the clinical encounter ... A formulation needs to reflect the imperatives of the system in which the encounter takes place and therefore mirrors clinical priorities.
>
> *(p. 8)*

As such, clinicians are encouraged to consider treatment setting early in the conceptualization process, exploring how it may influence treatment provision and what other adjunct services and supports may be available and/or needed. This includes careful discernment around which setting is best suited for the stabilization of behaviors that bring a great risk of danger to the child—including self-injurious or destructive behavior, or if a child is still residing in an abusive environment (Espenes et al., 2022; ISSTD, 2026; Silberg, 2021)—and how different settings may be helpful or harmful. Questions to consider include: What level of treatment is recommended, where will treatment occur (residential/inpatient and outpatient setting considerations), and how may collaboration be achieved across settings? What are the limitations and boundaries associated with the setting? Will treatment be in person or via telehealth? How will the therapeutic space be created? How may the current environment impact the child and the relationship? How may I promote an environment of physical and psychological safety for the client?

Systemic Approach

Working from a systemic approach acknowledges that working with the child means also collaborating with the persons and environments that interact with the child, which includes building relationship, advocacy, and outreach with schools. This involves identifying where treatment goals across systems and environments may clash, and working to understand the function of conflicting goals, which in turn models collaboration and negotiation in the best interests of the child and their healing. Of note is that schools have been identified as "an under-used resource in treatment planning for traumatized children" (Silberg, 1998, n.p.). Communication across systems involved in treatment is imperative, while also balancing confidentiality. Clinicians would be wise to ask themselves the following questions: What systems and professionals is my client involved with, and how may I interact with them to ensure continuity of care and access to services (Silberg, 2021, p. 285)? How will caregiving systems be involved (Wieland, 2017)? How am I negotiating with families and caregiving systems, and revising plans as needed, concerning the child's level of care (Nurcombe, 2014)? How do I understand the tension between the expectations of others and the awareness of any individual and systemic limitations to treatment (Putnam, 1997)? How can I create checks and balances within myself to ensure I am attending to themes and issues that emerge within the therapeutic alliance and the treatment process (Putnam, 1997)?

Pacing and Treatment Length

Additional considerations around pacing, length, and focus of treatment are important. Treatment ought to be paced and titrated based on the child's regulatory capacities. There may also be restrictions in treatment length (e.g., insurance or setting limitations). While directionality can be outlined in a treatment plan, the length of complex trauma treatment cannot be discerned from the outset. Instead, treatment length can be estimated within the context of the severity and duration of a child's history of trauma, past and present attachment-related dynamics within the caregiving system(s), considerations around present-day internal and external safety, and treatment focus (e.g., solely stabilization-based versus a more comprehensive approach to therapy). Waters and Silberg (1998) found that length of treatment "to achieve full unification will vary depending on the severity of the initial trauma, the consistency and availability of appropriate parenting, and the child's cognitive and emotional strengths" (p. 168). While little information is available regarding generalized length of treatment with dissociative children, Brand et al. (2013) found that 30 months of multi-phasic trauma treatment reduced symptom related challenges and increased functionality (ISSTD, 2026).

Clinical Example

Using the case of Amber put forth in Chapter 13, the processes of conceptualizing and treatment planning will be highlighted using a supplemental planning sheet that takes a mindful stance to formulation, attending to the impact of trauma and dissociation using a combined biopsychosocial and Four Ps approach (Havighurst & Downey, 2009). According to Havighurst and Downey (2009) a "mindful formulation does not advocate any particular theoretical orientation and can be used by clinicians using cognitive-behavioural, psychodynamic, systemic or other frameworks … [and] attends to individual processes within the child and within significant others" (p. 254).

As a reminder, Amber[2] is an eight-year-old girl in foster care who was referred for assessment and treatment to try and prevent a placement breakdown. Amber has a history of neglect, physical abuse, sexual abuse, and drug exposure. She was described by the systems she engages with as "behavioral" and contemptuous toward anyone in a position of authority (please refer to Chapter 13 for further information). Using Table 15.1, Amber's symptoms of trauma and dissociation are mapped and collated into an initial treatment plan (please note, only two symptoms are being mapped as part of this example, and Amber's other symptoms would be mapped using additional sheets to ensure attention is comprehensively paid to all symptom domains). As treatment progresses, goals are met, and/or new information emerges, a new supplemental sheet can be filled out to help organize and track across treatment, honoring the notion of the treatment plan as an ever-evolving document.

Table 15.1 An Example of Case Conceptualization and Treatment Planning

Child Complex Trauma and Dissociation-Specific Conceptualization and Treatment Planner #1
Name: Amber
Age: Eight years old
Presenting problem: Referred by foster care case manager due to being at risk of losing foster placement due to behavioral presentation.
Goals *(across systems):* Stabilize behaviors to prevent placement breakdown.
Diagnostic/Differential Impressions: DSM-5-TR – PTSD (dissociative subtype), DID, Encopresis (without constipation), Other Specified Depressive Disorder.
Clinical Impressions: Disorganized attachment strategies and symptomatology consistent with developmental impact of multiple forms of early abuse and neglect
Family Constellation Map: genogram, timeline, tree, other:
Relevant Third-Party System involvement: Child Welfare/protective services
Organizing Frame/Conceptual model: Dissociation-Focused Therapy informed by the Star Theoretical Model (i.e. Attachment, Discrete Behavioral States, Neurobiology, Erikson's Stages of Development, and Family Systems Theories)
Symptom Domain: Trauma, Dissociation, Attachment/Relational, Somatic/Biological, Emotional/Affect Regulation, Behavioral, Cognition, Self-Concept
(highlight and add into line below)

Symptom Domain: Trauma/Traumatic Experiences	
Predisposing Factors/ Known History	- Neglect, physical abuse, drug exposure (maternal substance misuse), multigenerational domestic violence and exposure to abuse - Loss of primary attachment figure (paternal grandmother) - Sexual abuse - Early medical trauma * These experiences have led to attachment injury, low distress tolerance, social-emotional development concerns, and dissociative symptomology.
Precipitating Factors/ Cues:	*Cues and precipitating factors to be explored and mapped alongside systems involved with the client.*

(Continued)

Table 15.1 (Continued)

Observations (clinician, caregivers, third party, self-reports)	Reported symptoms of: 1 Intrusive thoughts, 2 Hyperstartle response, 3 Restlessness/jumpiness, 4 Nightmares, 5 Poor concentration, 6 Unhappiness, and 7 Headaches/stomach aches.
Testing (screening and assessment outcomes)	Experiences endorsed in testing: 1 Suffering physical abuse by several caregivers that resulted in bruises, 2 Being threatened with physical assault, 3 Witnessing domestic violence toward her mother and grandmother, 4 Being left alone with her younger siblings, 5 Sexual abuse (denied on Northshore, emerged in Systematic Touch Inventory)
Protective/ Resilience Factors and Resources	- Dissociation as protective - Continued connection to siblings - Funny and insightful
Perpetuating Factors (pacing implications)	Nervous system reactivity to traumatic material generates a trauma related response related to state shifting (observed shift into a guarded, "zoned out" state, followed by the emergence of a regressive presentation)

Growth Tasks

Long-term goal: Integration of traumatic memory ("Trauma processing" in the EDUCATE model); new ways of managing trauma-related stimuli.

Goal *Reassess:* *At eight sessions eight ongoing*	Clinical Task	Intervention/ Modality	Client Tasks	Caregiver, Systems Roles/Tasks
Short-term goal 1	Learn more about trauma related precipitating and perpetuating factors (past and present) (**T**rigger Identification, *EDUCATE model*)	Unstructured clinical interviewing with Amber (via play), foster care manager, and foster carers.	Attend sessions	- Bring Amber to sessions - Attend meetings, calls to support information gathering.
Short-term goal 2	Provide trauma informed psychoeducation. (**E**ducation, *EDUCATE model*)	Psychoeducation with child, foster care manager, and involved carers.	Attend sessions	- Carer specific sessions to provide a new frame for understanding behavioral manifestations of trauma symptoms. - Decrease in invalidating responses and approaches from caregivers and systems.

(*Continued*)

Working Considerations in Building the Treatment Road Map

Table 15.1 (Continued)

Short-term goal 3	Affect regulation skills building (co-and self-regulatory capacities) to manage trauma-related cues (**Affect regulation and modulation in relationship, EDUCATE model**)	Synergetic play therapy Theraplay	- Attend sessions - Practice new skills in between session with support	- Receive information about new strategies and engage in planning for in between practice. - Explore additional carer affect regulation skills and resources.

Symptom Domain: *Dissociation*

Predisposing Factors/ Known History	History of early trauma occurring at key developmental periods, lack of attuned caregiving system - Investigate caregiver history of dissociation
Precipitating Factors/ Cues:	- Agitation reported to follow exposure to known trauma related cues (further exploration of agitation is needed) - Additionally clinical interviewing with the carer, Amber, and foster care manager to further discern precipitating factors and trauma-related cues to dissociative symptoms (**Trigger Identification, EDUCATE model**)
Observations (clinician, caregivers, third party, self-reports)	- Dysregulation of body systems such as difficulty walking. - Dysregulation of affect through mood shifts from calm and organized to agitated, zoning out. - Dysregulation in behavior such as changes in speech and eye gaze.
Testing (screening and assessment outcomes)	- **DES/PTSI** measure had a total score of 55; the clinical cut-off score for full PTSD with dissociation is 43. - **CDC** - Goes into a daze or trance-like state; shows rapid personality changes. - Unusually forgetful or confused about things she should have known. - Shows marked day-to-day or even hour-to-hour variations in her skills, knowledge, food preferences, etc. - Shows rapid regressions in age-level behavior. - Difficult time learning from experience. - Continues to deny misbehavior even when the evidence is obvious. - Rapidly changing physical complaints. - Has two or more distinct and separate personalities that take control over the child's behavior. *Items endorsed as "sometimes or somewhat true" included the following:* - Child does not remember or denies traumatic or painful experiences that are known to have occurred. - Child has a very poor sense of time. - Child is unusually sexually precocious. **CDES:** - Derealization - Depersonalization - Disturbances of memory or presence

(Continued)

Table 15.1 (Continued)

	Projective testing: - Inside self-states with distinct names and personalities (Eliza, Kristi) **Clinical interviewing:** Experience of imaginary friends who know things about her past that she does not, are able to help her with body functions (bowel movements), and who are in conflict.
Protective/ Resilience Factors and Resources	The experience of imaginary friends that can help her perform important body tasks (i.e. going to the bathroom) Use of dissociation as a protective mechanism (ongoing access to mother as a perpetuating factor that may be needed to manage access and the affect that ensues as a result)
Perpetuating Factors (pacing implications)	Ongoing caregiver and systems misperception of dissociation as behavioral Ongoing access to mother

Growth Tasks

Long-term goal: Integration of states to support development back on track.

Goal *Reassess:* *At eight sessions and ongoing*	Clinical Task	Intervention/ Modality	Client Tasks	Caregiver, Systems Roles/Tasks
Short-term goal 1	- Support caregivers and systems to better understand and respond to dissociation (**Education**) - Explore and map external responses that may signal danger to Amber and cue dissociative states or responses (**Trigger Identification**)	- Psychoeducation - Sandtray therapies - Dissociation-focused therapies - EMDR therapy	- Attend sessions. - Discuss use of TICES log with Amber, and plan how she may participate in this tracking with her carers, and why.	- Embed dissociation-specific education and trigger identification in carer psychoeducation sessions. - Carer and foster care manager to begin to track triggers and emerging dissociation and symptoms using a TICES log (EMDR therapy)
Short-term goal 2	- Support Amber to better understand her experiences of dissociation - Include **A**ffect regulation and grounding (explore use of scent to manage trance like phenomena) - Discern factors keeping dissociation in place as a strategy for ongoing coping ("**D**issociation motivation," *EDUCATE* model) using the endorsed items on the CDES and CDC.	- Psychoeducation - Sandtray therapies - Dissociation-focused therapies	Attend sessions. - Practice grounding related tools practiced in session to manage trance related symptoms.	- Actively engagement in exploring the environment with carers and foster care manager to build an awareness across systems of perpetuating factors and explore shifts and changes.

(Continued)

Table 15.1 (Continued)

Growth Tasks				
	- Discern what remains hidden (affect, identity, or behavioral states), and currently resides with Amber's imaginary friends that know things that she does not (**U**nderstanding, **EDUCATE** model)			- Provide attuned support to Amber as she begins to better understand the ways in which her mind has helped protect her; learn and support grounding practices.
Short-term goal 3	- Engaging and befriending internal states to build internal system motivation and engage the whole self in therapy. - Explore objections and emerging internal conflict to further understand **d**issociation motivation and engage in building internal problem solving and collaboration across states.	- Psychoeducation - Dissociation-focused therapy - Expressive Arts - Play therapies-type TBD	Attend sessions	Develop new way of engaging Amber's different states of being through participation in caregiver sessions, as well as dyadic sessions where the clinician can model different ways of engagement that facilitate the development of safety.

Table 15.2, found at the end of this chapter, is blank and may be used as a supplemental sheet to aid in the ongoing organization of case conceptualization and treatment planning related information across identified clinically relevant symptom domains. Children with greater traumatic experiences and more severe and complex symptoms will require greater mapping using multiple supplemental sheets that assist in the identification and connection across symptom domains. These sheets become part of supporting the ongoing process of gathering information, as it unfolds across time, supporting clinicians to conceptualize and treatment plan dynamically as more information emerges. Domains and corresponding goals may overlap, detailing the complexity of the ways in which complex trauma and dissociation manifest and are treated. Many areas may be "yet to be determined" and intentionally left blank, revealing where additional exploration is needed. As previously mentioned, the supplemental sheet may be amended many times as clinicians review and update treatment plans and progress, acknowledging that goals, approaches, and pacing may change as more information is revealed, and goals are achieved. It may also be noted that as specific modalities and interventions are identified, mini treatment plans that are modality-specific may be embedded within the overarching conceptualization and treatment plan.

Conclusion

This chapter explored the processes of case conceptualization and treatment with children who have histories of complex trauma and dissociation in an effort to bridge assessment and treatment processes. To achieve this, both dissociation-specific and non-dissociation-specific literatures were reviewed. Principles and considerations in case conceptualization were presented, alongside child dissociation–specific treatment guidelines and approaches, in support of a fluid, flexible, and ever-evolving conceptualization treatment planning process. This chapter closed with an illustration of an example of this process with trauma and dissociation-specific concerns, using the case of Amber (originally presented in Chapter 13). A blanks conceptualization and treatment planning supplemental sheet was provided to support clinicians in the process of synthesis. Due to a lack of literature and research on child dissociation–specific case conceptualization and treatment planning, this author hopes to inspire more writing in this area.

Table 15.2 Child Complex Trauma and Dissociation-Specific Conceptualization and Treatment Planner

Child Complex Trauma and Dissociation-Specific Conceptualization and Treatment Planner #:

Name:
Age:
Presenting problem:

Goals *(across systems):*

Diagnostic/Differential Impressions:

Clinical Impressions:

Family Constellation Map: genogram, timeline, tree, other:

Relevant Third-Party System involvement:

Organizing Frame/Conceptual model:

Symptom Domain: Trauma, Dissociation, Attachment/Relational, Somatic/Biological, Emotional/Affect Regulation, Behavioral, Cognition, Self-Concept
(circle and add into line below)

Symptom Domain:

Predisposing Factors/Known History

Precipitating Factors/Cues:

Observations
(clinician, caregivers, third party, self-reports)

Testing
(screening and assessment outcomes)

Symptom Domain:

Protective/Resilience Factors and Resources

Perpetuating Factors (pacing implications)

Table 15.2 (Continued)

Growth Tasks				
Long-term goal:				
Goal Reassess:	Clinical Task	Intervention/ Modality	Client Tasks	Caregiver, Systems Roles/Tasks
Short-term goal 1				
Short-term goal 2				
Short-term goal 3				

Notes

1 The author would like to thank Alexis Arbuthnott, PhD, for her support in reviewing this chapter, and Ana Gomez, MC, LPC, for her continued wisdom and insight in the complex realm of dissociation-specific case conceptualization and treatment planning.
2 Name and other identifying details are changed in this case compilation.

References

Arvidson, J., Kinniburgh, K., Howard, K., Spinazzola, J., Strothers, H., Evans, M., Andres, B., Cohen, C., & Blaustein, M. E. (2011). Treatment of complex trauma in young children: Developmental and cultural considerations in application of the ARC intervention model. *Journal of Child & Adolescent Trauma, 4*, 34–51. https://doi.org/10.1080/19361521.2011.545046

Bellis, M. A., Wood, S., & Hughes, K. (2023). *Tackling adverse childhood experiences (ACES): State of the art and options for action*. Public Health Wales. Phwwhocc.co.uk/resources/tackling-adverse-childhood-experiences-aces-state-of-the-art-and-options-for-action

Berman, P. S. (2018). *Case conceptualization and treatment planning: Integrating theory with clinical practice*. Sage Publications.

Brand, B. L., McNary, S. W., Myrick, A. C., Classen, C. C., Lanius, R., Loewenstein, R. J., Pain, C., & Putnam, F. W. (2013). A Longitudinal naturalistic study of patients with dissociative disorders treated by community clinicians. Psychological Trauma: Theory, Research, Practice, and Policy, 5(4), 301–308. https://doi.org/10.1037/a0027654

Braun, B., & Sachs, R. (1985). The development of multiple personality disorder: Predisposing, precipitating and perpetuating factors. In R. Kluft (Ed.), *Childhood antecedents of multiple personality* (pp. 38–67). American Psychiatric Press.

Brown, A. D., McCauley, K., Navalta, C. P., & Saxe, G. N. (2013). Trauma systems therapy in residential settings: Improving emotion regulation and the social environment of traumatized children and youth in congregate care. *Journal of Family Violence, 28*(7), 693–703. https://doi.org/10.1007/s10896-013-9542-9

Bryant, R. A., & Njenga, F. G. (2006). Cultural sensitivity: Making trauma assessment and treatment plans culturally relevant. *Journal of Clinical Psychiatry, 67*(2), 74–79.

Cloitre, M. (2015). The "one size fits all" approach to trauma treatment: Should we be satisfied? *European Journal of Psychotraumatology, 6*(1), Article 27344. https://doi.org/10.3402/ejpt.v6.27344

Compas, B. E., Gruhn, M., & Bettis, A. H. (2017). Risk and resilience in child and adolescent psychopathology. In T. P. Beauchaine & S. P. Hinshaw (Eds.), *Child and adolescent psychopathology* (3rd ed., pp. 113–143). John Wiley & Sons.

Cook, A., Spinazzola, J., Ford, J., Lanktree, C., Blaustein, M., Cloitre, M., & van der Kolk, B. (2005). Complex trauma in children and adolescents. *Psychiatric Annals, 35*(5), 390–398. https://doi.org/10.3928/00485713-20050501-05

Cruz, D., Lichten, M., Berg, K., & George, P. (2022). Developmental trauma: Conceptual framework, associated risks and comorbidities, and evaluation and treatment. *Frontiers in Psychiatry, 13*, Article 800687. https://doi.org/10.3389/fpsyt.2022.800687

Dawson, A. (2020). Getting child psychotherapy right for every child: Developing a clinical formulation tool for effective and accountable multi-agency work. *Journal of Child Psychotherapy, 46*(2), 133–151. https://doi.org/10.1080/0075417X.2020.1836502

Dudley, R., & Kuyken, W. (2013). Case formulation in cognitive behavioral therapy: A principle-driven approach. In L. Johnstone & R. Dallos (Eds.), *Formulation in psychology and psychotherapy* (pp. 18–44). Routledge.

Dummett, N. (2013). Formulation: A systemic approach to cognitive behaviour therapy. In P. Graham & S. Reynolds (Eds.), *Cognitive behaviour therapy for children and families* (3rd ed., pp. 69–88). Cambridge University Press.

Eells, T. D. (Ed.). (2022). *Handbook of psychotherapy case formulation*. Guilford Press.

Eells, T. D., & Lombart, K. G. (2003). Case formulation: Determining the focus in brief dynamic psychotherapy. In D. Charman (Ed.), *Core processes in brief psychodynamic psychotherapy* (pp. 135–160). Routledge.

Espenes, K., Kjøbli, J., Rognstad, K., Nilsen, K. H., Tørmoen, A. J., Waaler, P. M., & Wentzel- Larsen, T. (2022). *Effect of emotion regulation interventions across mental health symptoms in children and youth: A meta-analysis*. Manuscript submitted for publication. Centre for Child and Adolescent Health.

Farina, B. (2021). The role of trauma in psychotherapeutic complications and the worth of Giovanni Liotti's cognitive-evolutionist perspective (CEP): Commentary on chapter "Strengths and limitations of case formulation". In R. Dudley & W. Kuyken (Eds.), *Constructivist cognitive behavioral therapies: CBT case formulation as therapeutic process* (pp. 177–189). Springer.

Fassbinder, E., Brand-de Wilde, O., & Arntz, A. (2019). Case formulation in schema therapy: Working with the mode model. In U. Kramer (Ed.), *Case formulation for personality disorders* (pp. 77–94). Academic Press.

Fung, H. W., & Ross, C. A. (2024). Social work service needs of persons with complex dissociative disorders. *European Journal of Trauma & Dissociation, 8*(1), 100379. https://doi.org/10.1016/j.ejtd.2024.100379

Gazzillo, F., Dimaggio, G., & Curtis, J. T. (2021). Case formulation and treatment planning: How to take care of relationship and symptoms together. *Journal of Psychotherapy Integration, 31*(2), 115–128. https://doi.org/10.1037/int0000185

Goldman, R. N. (2017). Case formulation in emotion-focused therapy. *Person-Centered & Experiential Psychotherapies, 16*(2), 88–105. https://doi.org/10.1080/14779757.2017.1330705

Goldman, R., & Goldstein, Z. (2022). Case formulation in emotion-focused therapy. *Journal of Clinical Psychology, 78*(3), 436–453. https://doi.org/10.1002/jclp.23321

Gomez, A. M. (2012). *EMDR therapy and adjunct approaches with children: Complex trauma, attachment, and dissociation*. Springer.

Grasso, D. J. (2022). A trauma-informed approach to assessment, case conceptualization, and treatment planning for youth exposed to intimate partner violence. *Journal of Health Service Psychology, 48*(1), 3–11. https://doi.org/10.1007/s42843-021-00053-2

Gregorowski, C., & Seedat, S. (2013). Addressing childhood trauma in a developmental context. *Journal of Child & Adolescent Mental Health, 25*(2), 105–118. https://doi.org/10.2989/17280583.2013.795154

Haugaard, J. J. (2004). Recognizing and treating uncommon behavioral and emotional disorders in children and adolescent who have been severely maltreated: Dissociative disorders. *Child Maltreatment, 9*(2), 146–153. https://doi.org/10.1177/1077559504264311

Havighurst, S. S., & Downey, L. (2009). Clinical reasoning for child and adolescent mental health practitioners: The mindful formulation. *Clinical Child Psychology and Psychiatry, 14*(2), 251–271. https://doi.org/10.1177/1359104508100888

Haynes, S. N., O'Brien, W., & Kaholokula, J. (2011). *Behavioral assessment and case formulation*. John Wiley & Sons.

Henderson, S. W., & Martin, A. (2014). Case formulation and integration of information in child and adolescent mental health. In J. M. Ray & A. Martin (Eds.), *J. M. Ray's IACAPAP e-textbook of child and adolescent mental health* (pp. 1–20). International Association for Child and Adolescent Psychiatry and Allied Professions.

Herman, J. L. (2015). *Trauma and recovery: The aftermath of violence—From domestic abuse to political terror*. Hachette UK.

Holochwost, S. J., & Jaffee, S. R. (2017). The neurobiological embedding of child maltreatment: A systems perspective. In J. B. Klika & J. R. Conte (Eds.), *The APSAC handbook on child maltreatment* (4th ed., pp. 47–64). Sage.

International Society for the Study of Trauma and Dissociation (ISSTD) (2004). Guidelines for the evaluation and treatment of dissociative symptoms in children and adolescents. *Journal of Trauma & Dissociation, 5*(3), 119–150. https://doi.org/10.1300/J229v05n03_09

International Society for the Study of Trauma and Dissociation (ISSTD) (2026). Guidelines for the evaluation and treatment of dissociative symptoms in children and adolescents. *Journal of Trauma & Dissociation*.

Jose, A., & Goldfried, M. (2008). A transtheoretical approach to case formulation. *Cognitive and Behavioral Practice, 15*(2), 212–222. https://doi.org/10.1016/j.cbpra.2007.02.009

Karaca, S., & Eren, N. (2014). The use of creative art as a strategy for case formulation in psychotherapy: A case study. *Journal of Clinical Art Therapy, 2*(1), 3. digitalcommons.lmu.edu/jcat/vol2/iss1/3

Kawamura, A. A., Orsino, A., & Mylopoulos, M. (2014). Integrating competencies: Exploring complex problem solving through case formulation in developmental pediatrics. *Academic Medicine, 89*(11), 1497–1501. https://doi.org/10.1097/ACM.0000000000000475

Kendjelic, E. M., & Eells, T. D. (2007). Generic psychotherapy case formulation training improves formulation quality. *Psychotherapy: Theory, Research, Practice, Training, 44*(1), 66–77. https://doi.org/10.1037/0033-3204.44.1.66

Kluft, R. P. (1999). Current issues in dissociative identity disorder. *Journal of Psychiatric Practice, 5*(1), 3–19. https://doi.org/10.1097/00131746-199901000-00001

Lee, E., & Toth, H. (2016). An integrated case formulation in social work: Toward developing a theory of a client. *Smith College Studies in Social Work, 86*(3), 184–203. https://doi.org/10.1080/00377317.2016.1191804

Lucio, R., & Nelson, T. L. (2016). Effective practices in the treatment of trauma in children and adolescents: From guidelines to organizational practices. *Journal of Evidence-Informed Social Work, 13*(5), 469–478. https://doi.org/10.1080/23761407.2016.1166839

Macneil, C. A., Hasty, M. K., Conus, P., & Berk, M. (2012). Is diagnosis enough to guide interventions in mental health? Using case formulation in clinical practice. *BMC Medicine, 10*, 1–3. https://doi.org/10.1186/1741-7015-10-111

Manassis, K. (2014). *Case formulation with children and adolescents*. Guilford Press.

McCrea, K. T., Guthrie, D., & Bulanda, J. J. (2016). When traumatic stressors are not past, but now: Psychosocial treatment to develop resilience with children and youth enduring concurrent, complex trauma. *Journal of Child & Adolescent Trauma, 9*, 5–16. https://doi.org/10.1007/s40653-015-0060-1

Meehan, T., & Guilfoyle, M. (2015). Case formulation in poststructural narrative therapy. *Journal of Constructivist Psychology, 28*(1), 24–39. https://doi.org/10.1080/10720537.2014.938848

Messer, S. B., & Wolitzky, D. L. (2007). The psychoanalytic approach to case formulation. In T. Eells (Ed.), *Handbook of psychotherapy case formulation* (pp. 67–104). Guilford Press.

Myrick, A. C., Chasson, G. S., Lanius, R. A., Leventhal, B., & Brand, B. L. (2015). Treatment of complex dissociative disorders: A comparison of interventions reported by community therapists versus those recommended by experts. *Journal of Trauma & Dissociation, 16*(1), 51–67. https://doi.org/10.1080/15299732.2014.949020

Myrick, A., & Silberg, J. (2024). Assessing child and adolescent dissociative disorders and why it matters. In B. Brand (Ed.), *The concise guide to assessment and treatment of trauma-related dissociation* (pp. 189–222). American Psychological Association.

Nixon, R. D., & Bralo, D. (2019). Using explicit case formulation to improve cognitive processing therapy for PTSD. *Behavior Therapy, 50*(1), 155–164. https://doi.org/10.1016/j.beth.2018.04.003

Norcross, J. C., & Wampold, B. E. (2018). A new therapy for each patient: Evidence-based relationships and responsiveness. *Journal of Clinical Psychology, 74*(11), 1889–1906. https://doi.org/10.1002/jclp.22678

Nurcombe, B. (2014). Diagnosis and treatment planning in child and adolescent mental health problems. In J. M. Ray & A. Martin (Eds.), *J. M. Ray's IACAPAP e-textbook of child and adolescent mental health* (pp. 1–21). International Association for Child and Adolescent Psychiatry and Allied Professions.

O'Connor, K. J., & Ammen, S. (2012). *Play therapy treatment planning and interventions: The ecosystemic model and workbook*. Academic Press.

Orvaschel, H., Hersen, M., & Faust, J. (Eds.). (2001). *Handbook of conceptualization and treatment of child psychopathology*. Elsevier.

Pascual-Leone, A., & Kramer, U. (2017). Developing emotion-based case formulations: A research-informed method. *Clinical Psychology & Psychotherapy, 24*(1), 212–225. https://doi.org/10.1002/cpp.1998

Perry, B. D. (2009). Examining child maltreatment through a neurodevelopmental lens: Clinical applications of the neurosequential model of therapeutics. *Journal of Loss and Trauma, 14*(4), 240–255. https://doi.org/10.1080/15325020903004350

Putnam, F. W. (1997). *Dissociation in children and adolescents: A developmental perspective.* Guilford Press.

Schiepek, G. (2003). A dynamic systems approach to clinical case formulation. *European Journal of Psychological Assessment, 19*(3), 175–184. https://doi.org/10.1027/1015-5759.19.3.175

Shapiro, F. (2017). *Eye movement desensitization and reprocessing (EMDR) therapy: Basic principles, protocols, and procedures.* Guilford Publications.

Siegel, D. J. (2001). Toward an interpersonal neurobiology of the developing mind: Attachment relationships, "mindsight," and neural integration. *Infant Mental Health Journal: Official Publication of the World Association for Infant Mental Health, 22*(1–2), 67–94. https://doi.org/10.1002/1097-0355(200101/04)22:1%3C67::AID-IMHJ3%3E3.0.CO;2-G

Silberg, J. L. (Ed.). (1998). *The dissociative child: Diagnosis, treatment and management* (2nd ed.). Sidran Press.

Silberg, J. L. (2001). Dissociative disorders. In H. Orvaschel, J. Faust & M. Hersen (Eds.), *Handbook of conceptualization and treatment of child psychopathology* (pp. 449–474). Pergamon.

Silberg, J. L. (2021). *The child survivor: Healing developmental trauma and dissociation.* Routledge.

Silberg, J. L., & Dallam, S. (2009). Dissociation in children and adolescents: At the crossroads. In P. F. Dell & J. A. O'Neil (Eds.), *Dissociation and the dissociative disorders: DSM-V and beyond* (pp. 67–81). Routledge/Taylor & Francis Group.

Simms, J. (2011). Case formulation within a person-centred framework: An uncomfortable fit. *Counselling Psychology Review, 26*(2), 24–36.

Sperry, L., & Sperry, J. (2020). *Case conceptualization: Mastering this competency with ease and confidence.* Routledge.

Steinberg, M., & Hall, P. (1997). The SCID-D diagnostic interview and treatment planning in dissociative disorders. *Bulletin of the Menninger Clinic, 61*(1), 108.

Stolbach, B. C. (2005). Psychotherapy of a dissociative 8-year-old boy burned at age 3. *Psychiatric Annals, 35*(8), 685–694. https://doi.org/10.3928/00485713-20050801-10

Struik, A. (2014). *Treating chronically traumatized children: Don't let sleeping dogs lie!* Routledge.

Sturmey, P. (2010). Case formulation in forensic psychology. In M. Daffern, L. Jones & J. Shine (Eds.), *Offence paralleling behaviour: A case formulation approach to offender assessment and intervention* (pp. 25–51). Wiley Blackwell.

Tamkin, V. L., Dave, B., Whittaker, A. T. N., & Frankel, K. A. (2019). Constructing a joint clinical case formulation and treatment plan with families. In K. A. Frankel, J. Harrison & W. F. M. Njoroge (Eds.), *Clinical guide to psychiatric assessment of infants and young children* (pp. 327–355). Springer Nature Switzerland.

Vanderzee, K. L., Sigel, B. A., Pemberton, J. R., & John, S. G. (2019). Treatments for early childhood trauma: Decision considerations for clinicians. *Journal of Child & Adolescent Trauma, 12*(4), 515–528. https://doi.org/10.1007/s40653-018-0244-6

Waters, F. S. (2016). *Healing the fractured child: Diagnosis and treatment of youth with dissociation.* Springer.

Waters, F. S., & Silberg, J. L. (1998). Promoting integration in dissociative children. In J. L. Silberg (Ed.), *The dissociative child: Diagnosis, treatment, and management* (2nd ed., pp. 167–190). Sidran Institute Press.

Whomsley, S. (2010). Team case formulation. In C. Cupitt (Ed.), *Reaching out: The psychology of assertive outreach* (pp. 95–118). Routledge/Taylor & Francis Group.

Wieland, S. (2015). Dissociation in children and adolescents: What it is, how it presents, and how we can understand it. In S. Wieland (Ed.), *Dissociation in traumatized children and adolescents* (2nd ed., pp. 23–62). Routledge.

Wieland, S. (2017). *Parents are our other client: Ideas for therapists, social workers, support workers, and teachers.* Routledge.

Winters, N. C., Hanson, G., & Stoyanova, V. (2007). The case formulation in child and adolescent psychiatry. *Child and Adolescent Psychiatric Clinics, 16*(1), 111–132. https://doi.org/10.1016/j.chc.2006.07.010

Woolard, A., Boutrus, M., Bullman, I., Wickens, N., Gouveia Belinelo, P. D., Solomon, T., & Milroy, H. (2024). Treatment for childhood and adolescent dissociation: A systematic review. *Psychological Trauma: Theory, Research, Practice, and Policy.* Advance online publication. https://doi.org/10.1037/tra0001615

Zayfert, C., & Becker, C. B. (2019). *Cognitive-behavioral therapy for PTSD: A case formulation approach.* Guilford Press.

Zoroglu, S., Yargic, L. I., Tutkun, H., Ozturk, M., & Sar, V. (1996). Dissociative identity disorder in childhood: Five Turkish cases. *Dissociation, 9*(4), 253–260.

16
CLINICAL APPLICATIONS OF THE STAR THEORETICAL MODEL[1]

Frances S. Waters

Introduction

Children's stories about their trauma frequently emerge over time in bits and pieces that are clues to understanding the confounding behaviors seen in dissociative children. These children can momentarily lose consciousness, relive their trauma in the moment, behave like an infant or pseudo adult, not recall when or why they slugged their best friend, be unable to dress themselves for school when the previous day they had no trouble, and suddenly attack their caregivers, then run after them for fear of abandonment. These contradictory behaviors and emotions are played out in many scenarios without any apparent rhyme or reason. Yet, they are the vary markers of dissociative states. Therapists and caretakers become frustrated, tired, and at a loss as to what to do next to stabilize the traumatized child.

To make sense of the child's mercurial moods and behaviors, developing a clear conceptualization based on many theoretical models can serve to provide comprehensive analyses and henceforth an effective road map toward recovery. The Star Theoretical Model (STM) provides a road map that examines five theories: attachment, child development, neurobiology, family systems, and dissociation (Waters, 2016). While they have similar overlapping dynamics, each offers a unique understanding of and direction on how to intervene with the dissociative child and their caretakers. When the dissociative child is examined through the five theoretical constructs, the STM helps make sense of what on the surface appears incomprehensible (Figure 16.1).

The STM's star shape itself represents the child exposed to trauma. Attachment theory is intentionally placed at the top of the star to signify both the paramount role that a parent-child relationship plays in contributing to the child's development and ongoing reliance on dissociative coping mechanisms, and the importance of a healthy attachment between the child and caregiver in providing an anchor for the child's ability to heal. When examining each model, it is important to note what age the child was when they experienced trauma and its relevance to each of the theoretical domains. The STM provides a foundation for comprehensive assessment and a multifaceted treatment plan that combines each theory, and can lead to positive outcomes when the child is in a secure and safe environment.

Let's examine the relevant factors of each of these theories and how to apply them clinically.

Star Theoretical Model
Assessing & Treating Children with Dissociation

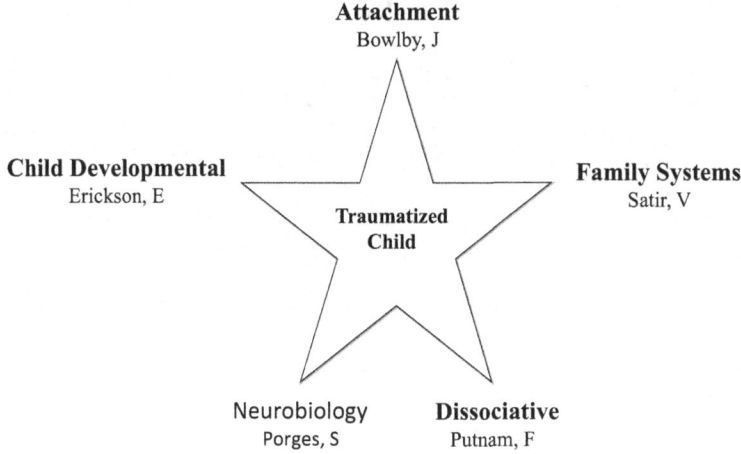

Figure 16.1 Star Theoretical Model Description.

Dissociative Theory of the STM

Putnam's Theoretical Model of Discrete Behavioral States

I have worked with several children who were born drug addicted and, with some embarrassment, described an infant state that suffered the effect of drug exposure. One example is Cindy, a 14-year-old, whose biological mother was a drug addict during her pregnancy. During a session with her foster mother, Cindy's infant state emerged. She was somnolent, which reflected the medication she'd been given at birth to counteract withdrawal symptoms. Cindy's maternal self-state was able to communicate what was transpiring. Her foster mother was able to comfort Cindy's infant state, leading to a healing moment in the teen's recovery.

While we are beginning to better recognize prenatal trauma (Cortizo, 2021; Potgieter Marks, 2022), Putnam's theory of dissociation (1997) describes dissociative defenses and the early formation of discrete behavioral states in maltreated children, adding to our understanding of the impact of early trauma. Putnam examined early infant-mother interactions and how infants learn to modulate their behavioral states based on maternal responses. He describes a mutual sharing of states between mother and child. He notes that a healthy reciprocal pattern develops when the attuned mother reads her infant's cues as the infant experiences the cycle of going from regular sleep to stages of being awake, fussing, crying, feeding, etc. When the mother provides the appropriate response to meet the infant's needs, the infant can smoothly navigate these behavioral shifts. It is through this healthy give-and-take process that children develop the capacity to modulate their own behavioral states. By contrast, Putnam also notes that when a mother is chaotic, frightening, or abusive to her infant, the infant cannot develop the capacity to modulate across these behavioral shifts. Instead, the infant compensates by developing discrete behavioral states that shift and mirror the frightening, chaotic state of the mother. These discrete states become *separate* from one another to manage the mother's unpredictability and avoid the emotionally disturbing feelings that result in the infant. Consequently, the child's capacity to develop self-awareness and self-control is thwarted, and the child often feels confused, helpless, and stressed. This early development of dysregulated patterns sheds light on our understanding of the early root of discrete states and reliance on dissociation.

Regarding clinical application, it is important to explore what the child's prenatal and infancy periods were like. Did the pregnant mother experience domestic violence, medical trauma, loss of a loved one, depression and/or anxiety? What kind of parental care did the child receive? Was the parent able to read the child's cues and respond consistently? Or was the parent unpredictable, frightening, or abusive to the child? Is there an early history in which the child exhibited emotional and behavioral dysregulation that is a result of frightening and abusive parenting? Is the child mimicking the parent's behaviors? Is the child exhibiting discrete behavioral states accompanied by signs of amnesia? What are the triggers that activate extreme shifts in the child, and are these triggers reminders of early child maltreatment? While we may not have a clear history, we can make some educated guesses based on the child's early history and reactivity to stimuli. Our intervention would be to access their behavioral state(s) (self-state), and repair the early trauma to help the child release the painful emotions and develop self-regulation. Children may not have an awareness of what causes them to become highly reactive and/or recall such "regressed" behavior. However, when children behave as a baby or toddler, they are usually willing to reveal when asked if they have a "little me" or "baby me" inside of them.

Case Study of Emily

Seven-year-old Emily came into my office curious and bubbly, with her adoptive mother, Karen. Emily was articulate and enjoyed second grade. Emily's biological mother, Mary, had a significant history of early child abuse and neglect and became a single parent at 20 years old, caring for Emily with little support. Mary felt too overwhelmed to manage Emily and would have bouts of depression, anxiety, and agitation. Mary depended on her live-in boyfriend, who had a temper and problems with alcohol, for financial support. After several child protective investigations of severe neglect and suspected child abuse, through which Emily was deemed a failure-to-thrive baby with significant diaper rashes and bruises on her body, and after several brief placements in foster care, she was permanently placed with her adoptive parents at three years old.

Emily was seen by me after several failed therapeutic interventions to deal with her extreme emotional and behavioral dysregulation, marked by significant temper tantrums during which she would destroy her room. She also exhibited chronic enuresis and encopresis, and "regressed behaviors" of baby talking, sucking her thumb, and walking on her toes.

During my assessment, I noticed Emily had brief moments of staring off into space and dramatic changes in her affect, from high energy to a subdued, shy demeanor. While playing with the dollhouse, Emily gravitated to the baby doll. She began to talk like a baby as she put the doll in the crib. I reflected what she was doing and asked her if she was aware of sometimes talking like a baby. She looked at me and nodded her head. I explained that other kids have told me that they also talk much younger. I asked her if she liked to pretend to be a baby, or if there was a part of her that was like a baby. She told me in a quiet voice that there was a part of her that was a baby—it wasn't a pretend one, "it [was] real." She told me she sees the baby and "she's crying a lot." I told her that it was so good for me to know that, and together we would work to help comfort the baby part of her and let her know that she is safe.

I explained how when little kids get hurt, they can separate out from the scary things and a little part of them can stay stuck at that time, with all of those bad feelings about the things that happened to them. I said we would work together to help her baby part feel better, safe, and comforted. Emily breathed a sigh of relief and smiled. She agreed to call her baby part "Little Emily."

This was the beginning of Emily's healing of her early trauma. I gave her a baby doll that represented Little Emily, and asked Emily to hold the doll and imagine she was holding Little Emily and comforting her, so she could feel loved and safe. Emily agreed to take the doll home, rock her several times a day, feed her a bottle, and keep her in a safe place in her bedroom. I explained that it was through rocking the Little Emily doll and caring for her that Little Emily inside would feel better and grow up to be her age. Emily was excited to do so. She smiled and ran into the waiting room to tell her adoptive mom. Her adoptive mother, Karen, became an active therapeutic partner with me, and during the sessions, she would hold Emily while Emily held her baby doll as they both comforted Little Emily, reassuring her that they loved her and wanted her to know that she was safe. Emily's baby part emerged, and Mary talked to this part about how sorry she felt that Little Emily got hurt and scared.

Over the course of several weekly sessions, Emily reported that Little Emily was growing up from being one year old to being three years old. Emily's baby talk and walking on her toes ceased. I stressed that Little Emily is a part of her body and how important it is for Little Emily to feel Emily's body to experience hugs, hunger, eating food, the need to go to the bathroom, etc. In therapy, Emily practiced with the Little Emily doll, "potty training" her, as Emily became fully aware of her bodily needs. Emily's enuresis and encopresis ceased, as well as her erratic mood and destructive behavior. Emily's adoptive father joined some of the sessions as well, reinforcing how pleased he was to understand Little Emily, and participated in holding her. Over time, Little Emily grew up to be Emily's age and she spontaneously integrated. Emily was well regulated, demonstrated appropriate behavior, and engaged well with her parents and peers. Emily's adoptive parents were able to truly understand their daughter's underlying symptoms and the presence of Little Emily, and effectively engage in healing Emily's early trauma. Let's examine the relationship between trauma and neurobiology and how it furthers our understanding of dissociation and self-states.

Neurobiology in the STM Model[2]

For this chapter, I highlight aspects of polyvagal theory as it relates to clinical application. For a more thorough discussion of polyvagal theory, please refer to George Thompson's chapter in this volume.

Applying the Concept of Neuroception with Dissociative Children

Porges (2004) coined the term *neuroception*, which refers to a physiological response of the nervous system's evaluation of risks in detecting threats and evaluating safety. Porges recognized that certain stimuli, such as low and loud sounds and angry eyes, can activate a defensive reaction—for example, fight, flight, freeze, collapse, or shutdown. He stressed how important it is, then, to modulate our voice and use soft eyes when communicating with others to maintain social engagement. Parents' ability to remain calm and empathize with their child when the child becomes dysregulated can help restore social engagement so that thoughts and feelings are expressed, and conflicts can be resolved.

Understanding that a child's felt sense of safety is paramount to minimize defensive responses is ideal, but it is not easy to provide a safe environment that is devoid of triggers, particularly with traumatized children whose neuroception is "faulty" due to early and repetitive adverse events. Their nervous system is cued to be on alert for danger. They can be triggered and perceive a threat when there is no actual danger and act out in defensive and unpredictable ways. To add to the complexity of faulty neuroception, traumatized children can have hidden self-states stuck in the original trauma and not oriented to time, place, and person. These self-states are highly sensitive to traumatic sensory cues and situations similar to the original trauma, and can spontaneously go into a survival state of fight, flight, or freeze. This self-state-propelled activation of the nervous system is often *beyond* the child's control. The reaction can perplex parents and therapists, as they expect children to know the reality of their current situation, which is non-threatening; to use self-control; and to "learn from their mistakes." Many placements and therapeutic interventions have failed as a result of not identifying and treating self-states who become activated by faulty neuroception and account for persistent behavioral and emotional dysregulation.

It is crucial that therapists working with children with complex trauma evaluate the presence of self-states, carefully pace questions, and modulate their voice as they explore indicators of dissociation. Major tasks with dissociative children are to build internal awareness and cooperation between self-states and orient them to their current environment so that appropriate evaluation of threats can occur. Otherwise, when the child is triggered, they can quickly regress to the shutdown state of complete immobility or switch to a different state that want to fight or flee (Waters, 2016). When the child has returned to homeostasis, it is important to help them track what happened internally and in the environment just before they decompensated and what self-state was activated by the trigger and memory, and create strategies to prevent this from reoccurring. Developing a funny cue word (e.g., goose) or hand signal that both the child and caregiver can use when child shows signs of agitation or shutdown can ward off a defensive reaction or a complete shutdown (Waters, 2016). Also establishing a body movement, such as rubbing hands or shoulders, tapping knees, hopping, stretching, with the adult imitating such movements can bring the child back to bodily awareness and prevent a collapse. Practicing with child's self-states initially with minor stimuli and working toward disturbing triggers, while making it fun and silly, can override the child's urge to go into a defensive state. Also, having a visual and tactile cue, such as a handmade bracelet of beads representing the child's helpers (Adler-Tapia, 2012) or color-coded cards that cue the child regarding the level of dissociating (Ogden & Gomez, 2013) to orient the child to stay present. There are many sensorimotor therapy techniques (Ogden & Fisher, 2015) that are adapted to children (Ogden & Gomez, 2013; Silberg, 2022; Waters, 2016) that can be combined with other techniques, such as EMDR, to help children process their traumatic events.

Case Study of Miranda

Eight-year-old Miranda was accompanied to my office by her adoptive parents for intensive therapy. Miranda's biological parents were drug addicts. They passed out while smoking and the house caught on fire. Miranda was an infant in the crib and survived without any physical injuries. Her biological parents' rights were terminated, and Miranda was placed in foster care and eventually adopted at two years old. While Miranda didn't suffer physical injuries, she suffered emotional scars. As an infant, Miranda encoded into her memory the loud sounds of police sirens and fire alarms. Throughout her childhood, she would become terrified when hearing them. Her entire body would tremble. She would vacillate between running outside, hiding, or collapsing. She was in constant fear of hearing alarm sounds. She generalized her fear to other loud noises. When her parents raised their voices telling her to clean her room or come to dinner, it would set off an internal alarm and she instantly displayed anger and aggression. During these times, she sometimes experienced amnesia. Several years of play therapy and trauma-focused cognitive therapy were ineffective.

As I evaluated her, she disclosed the presence of self-states: a terrified baby, protective maternal figure, and Angry Miranda, who were formed after the original trauma. Miranda stated that her baby state, her original self, would scream and shake in fear. Her maternal state would try to comfort her, and Angry Miranda would become aggressive. When Miranda heard sirens or fire alarms, she would want to run outside or hide. We agreed to work on her original trauma using EMDR Tac scanners, with Miranda's parents by her side. She held a doll representing her baby self-state. We engaged in the flash technique (Manfield et al., 2017) of vacillating between imagining the sound of an alarm and picturing her favorite activity of riding her horse to begin to desensitize and process her fear. Over several sets, her subjective unit of distress (SUDs) decreased from a 10 to a 2. We then added the sound of an alarm on a phone with imagery of her riding her horse. SUDs increased again to 8/10, but went down to a 4/10. Mirada reported feeling tension in her legs and was moving them during the EMDR flash technique. I noted her legs moving and asked her what she wished she could do, and she expressed that she wanted to run. We then agreed to combined EMDR technique with sensorimotor psychotherapy. When she heard the alarm on the phone, with her parents at her side and their arms around her, she ran out my office and down the hall, simulating a safe escape. After three reenactments of a safe escape, Miranda's legs and feet rested when she listened to the sound of the alarm. She rated her fear a 0/10. Her body felt calm, and she and her self-states achieved a sense of empowerment.

Afterward, she was able manage police sirens and school fire drills and felt very proud of herself. She and her self-states were able to master a safe escape and complete what her body wanted to do but was impossible to do when she was an infant. She was on her road to recovery! Combining therapeutic techniques to simulate rescue techniques with dissociative children has helped them feel safe and gain mastery over their trauma.

Attachment Theory of the STM

A healthy attachment with caregivers provides the anchor for children to thrive. Contrarily, when a child is traumatized, particularly by a caregiver, trust and security are abrogated. The child is left without a safety net when they face challenges or adversities. To highlight the critical role of a secure caregiver figure in a child's life, particularly with a child who has been traumatized, attachment theory is at the top of the star of the STM. The STM model is primarily derived from the works of Bowlby, the father of attachment theory, along with the findings of other researchers who have built on his work (e.g. Main & Hesse, 1990).

Bowlby's viewpoint is supported by Schore (2000), who stated, "Attachment theory is essentially a regulatory theory, and attachment can be defined as the interactive regulation of biological synchronicity between organisms" (p. 23). It is through this interplay (whether positive or negative) that the child develops *internal working models* (IWMs) of representation of the self and the attachment figure (Bowlby, 1973), which has relevance to the development of dissociative states when the attachment figure is the abuser.

Bowlby's Internal Working Models and Development of Dissociated Self-States

Bowlby further explains that children can develop different and *incompatible* IWMs based on provocative situations with frightening, neglectful, and/or abusive parents. These internal incompatible models can represent self-states with extreme moods, sensations, behaviors, and roles—for example, the good parent, the abusive parent, the fearful child, the angry child, the student, and so on. The child develops these self-states to segment off what is impossible to manage while portraying a level of functioning. I have treated many children who suddenly display contradictory and incompatible "states of mind." When they feel hurt, they shift into a defensive state in a matter of seconds and attack the parent, who attempts to comfort the child. When the parent retreats because of the attack, the child switches to the state that fears abandonment, panics, and pursues the parent. This cycle repeats. The underlying dynamic is unresolved traumatic grief and mourning held in incompatible states.

Traumatic Grief and Mourning in Children

In his research, Bowlby became acutely aware of loss and mourning in young children who experienced separation from their mothers. He termed this traumatic grief "pathological mourning." According to Bowlby (1961), pathological mourning results from the child's inability to overtly scold the parent for deserting them. The child's urges to recover and reproach the parent become "split off and… continued as active systems within the personality…," influencing the child's feelings and behaviors "in strange and distorted ways" (p. 485) Bowlby aptly describes what appears to be incomprehensible shifts in behaviors that are markers of incongruent self-states that hold traumatic elements.

Robertson and Bowlby (1952) recognized three psychological stages to children's grief and mourning of parental loss—protest, despair, and denial or detachment. Later, Bowlby (1960) noted similarities between children's grief reactions and the reactions of older adults who lost their spouse or another loved one. He revised his and Robertson's model to include five stages of psychological responses to grief and mourning. These stages are: "a) Thought and behavior still directed toward the lost object; b) Hostility, to whomsoever directed; c) Appeals for help; d) Despair, withdrawal, regression, and disorganization; e) Reorganization of behavior directed toward a new object" (p. 17). Bowlby recognized that the child's intense and unresolved grief over the loss of a parent is the underlying dynamic in these stages.

Bowlby's Five Stages of Psychological Responses and Star Theoretical Model

During my numerous years of practice, I recognized that the common denominator in intense and violent hatred in children stems not only from separation from the mother but also from other traumatic events incurred upon children. Subsequently, the universal grief and mourning recognized in Bowlby's research on maternal abandonment is present in children who have suffered various forms of trauma, particularly interpersonal violence. I integrated and compared Bowlby's model of the five stages of psychological responses, including his concepts of IWMs and segregated states, with the understanding of the development of self-states in children in the STM.

Suffice it to say, not all maltreated children experience the five stages of psychological responses of grief and mourning, or experience them sequentially, or display segmented discrete states as outlined. However, the STM recognizes these psychological responses to consider when evaluating and treating traumatized children—to miss such can result in inappropriate intervention. I describe each of the stages to aid the clinician in understanding the underlying dynamics associated with the child who dissociates, across the domains of affect, cognition, behaviors, sensations, and relationships, and the subsequent development of self-states. Self-states can range from fragments of the self with limited roles, behaviors, and affect to more developed states that take executive control over the child's body. Keep in mind that these states are created to manage the traumatic event(s) and associated intense affect, sensations, and behaviors. Often, they are not oriented to time, place, people, or things in the environment. They are reacting from an impulsive need to defend themselves from what is perceived as a threatening environment. They exhibit extreme mood and behavior switches and display what Putnam so aptly called "discrete behavioral states" and Bowlby termed "*incompatible* internal working models." These concepts are incorporated into the comparative stages between Bowlby's five stages and the STM and are intended to help clinicians examine the presence of self-states and understand the confounding shifts that dissociative children display so that appropriate treatment can occur (Waters, 2016) (Table 16.1).

Attachment Theory of the STM: Five Stages

Stage One: Thought and Behavior Still Directed Toward the Lost Object

In Bowlby's (1960) stage one, the child protests loudly in the hopes of being reunited with the parent. All thoughts and behavior are directed toward reunification with the parent, but attempts are futile. The child is at a loss to manage such intense feelings. In my comparison model, traumatized children experience loss and grief over the parent, caregiver, or another who harms them—the loss of the

Table 16.1 Comparison of the Five Stages of Psychological Responses to Grief and Mourning to the Star Theoretical Model of Trauma and Attachment

Comparison of Five Stages of Psychological Responses to Grief and Mourning to STM of Trauma-Attachment-Dissociation

Bowlby's Five stages	Waters STM Five stages
1. Seeking the mother ➔ no mom ➔	Internalized maternal/helper states
2. Hostility ➔ protesting is futile ➔	Internalized anger/rage states, rejects caretaker
3. Appeals for help ➔ unmet ➔	Fearful, dependent, helpless, compliant states
4. Despair, withdrawal, regression & disorganization ➔	Depressed, detached, young states, ADHD type states, states with different skills, etc.
5. Reorganization & directed to a new object ➔	Healing: integration; able to attach/accept parents

Attachment Based Treatment
Processing trauma & mourning, grief and loss leads to integration

idealized caretaker and/or the ability to trust others. These are universal feelings of wanting to be safe, protected, or rescued when threatening events occur. When that doesn't happen and it particularly is incurred by someone the child knows, the child feels vulnerable and loses their sense of self-efficacy, resulting in feeling powerless. The child internalizes the trauma and blames themself, feeling unworthy to be loved and protected. This can lead to despondency and depression.

The unbearable predicament of desiring protection, love, and care and not receiving it can cause the conundrum of wanting to depend on others for protection and care but at the same time feeling distrustful and fear of betrayal. Furthermore, the intense need for immediate comfort propels the traumatized child to compensate by developing internal states—caregivers, hero figures, helpers—to meet those needs. Simultaneously, the child may dissociate from the traumatic events to maintain an attachment to the abusive parent and/or avoid the intolerable feelings of helplessness, rage, grief, and loss. The child may not recall traumatic events and may have protector parts, such as internal idealized caregiver and other helpers to cope with unwanted feelings. Reliance on an internal helper feels safer, particularly when outside help has not been consistently available.

Many of the traumatized dissociative children I worked with over the decades developed helper/protector states to protect, comfort, and keep them from further harm. Children who resided in orphanages during their infancy and toddlerhood described such helpers to cope with their hunger, coldness, isolation, and loneliness. Once these children are adopted, these internalized caretakers can be in intense conflict with the adoptive parents, as described in the case study of Lisa (Waters, 2016).

Stage Two: Hostility, to Whomsoever Directed

Bowlby's (1960) stage two described children in residential care exhibiting hostility toward anyone who tried to nurture them. To deal with overwhelming feelings of loss and despair, the child distrusts others and feels rage, anger, and aggression. They develop such states to express what they are otherwise unable to and to protect themselves from further harm. It is not uncommon that these children vacillate between rejecting care to clinging to their caregivers. They may express rage and betrayal regarding the trauma they have experienced, and the next moment feel fear of abandonment and desperate desire to be loved and comforted. This contradictory behavior is frequently found in dissociative children who shift between states with different roles. Often, because of these children's impulsivity, reactivity, and short attention span, they are often given the diagnosis of attention deficit hyperactivity disorder or disruptive mood regulation disorder. For the traumatized child, the only recourse they know is to dissociate these contradictory emotions into discrete states of fear, angry, aggressive states that act out and protest what happened. Their responses can become generalized toward all caregivers—including foster and adoptive parents who try to nurture the child. The child's states can attack caregivers who are caring for them if they perceive even a minor threat to their survival, such as a raised voice expressing concern for them when they refuse to get ready for school. Traumatized children are highly sensitive to triggers.

For example, very caring parents expressed bafflement over their adopted teenage daughter's overreaction when she came home later than expected, and her mother asked in an elevated, concerned voice, "Where were you?" The daughter repeatedly shouted back, accusing her mom of shouting at her, and saying that she would not take any more shouting—she'd had enough. She had spent the first nine years in an orphanage and was exposed to shouting. So her mother's raised voice brought out her defensive, angry state, and her tirade went on for about an hour, while her mother was baffled and tried to defend her feelings of concern. An empathic approach of resonating with how her daughter must have felt would have defused this angry state until the daughter's brain was back online and was able to process how concerned her mother was.

The hostile or aggressive state may also blame the child for their weakness and thus cause physically self-abusive or harming behavior such as head banging, cutting, burning, purging, or substance abuse. Vogt (2012) stated that these aggressive states "were formed when the child was forced to manage boundary violations by an aggressor… then unconsciously internalized the toxic information contained in the violent scene" (p. 3). They act out on others to release their rage. Much intervention is required to assist the child and caregivers to develop an empathic and appreciative approach toward the hostile state for what this state has taken on for the child. This will build a bridge between them and help the hostile state assume a constructive role and redirect anger toward the child's abuser instead of the child or caregiver. Also, an important task is to reframe the hostile state's role of power to be assertive, instead of aggressive, with others.

Stage Three: Appeals for Help

In Bowlby's (1960) third stage, the child's early appeals for help are unmet and the child becomes painfully resigned to the absence of their mother. This causes the child to feel much fear and vulnerability, which become segmented because containing these feelings is untenable. The child develops internalized self-states that exhibit feelings of fear, helplessness, and dependency. The underlying desire is to please others to avoid further abandonment, rejection, and harm. This child state may seek out comfort and display loyalty to the offending parent or peers who are mean to them. Due to their desire to avoid abandonment, they can put themselves in further harm of being scapegoated and abused.

Because hostile states despise fear and weakness, there can be an internal conflict between hostile and fearful/dependent states within the dissociative child. The hostile state may harm the weak state by hurting the body—for example, by cutting—not recognizing that they share the same body. The child can be amnesic about these times. I once worked with a teenager who would wake up covered in blood because her hostile state saw her as weak, blamed her for the sexual abuse by her dad, and caused self-harm.

The hostile state may also suddenly hurt others. For example, when an argument over fairness occurs with a teen's best friend, the fearful, dependent state wants to please the friend for fear of abandonment, while the other state despises the weakness. That state then becomes aggressive and attacks the friend. The teen's shift from passivity to aggression places stress on their friendship. During these times, the teen may be amnesic about their aggressive acts. If these extreme shifts in relationships between dependency/passivity and aggression continue into adulthood, the individual is often diagnosed with having a borderline personality disorder.

Identifying the presence of self-states that exhibit these contradictory moods and behaviors and their conflicting motivations for survival is the initial step in building internal awareness and cooperation between them. A therapeutic approach that is empathic and collaborative and that understands the hostile state's need to protect through aggression, while also helping that state understand the dependent state's fear of abandonment, is a step toward engaging the aggressive state's cooperation. Orienting the child and self-states to the present reality of threat and safety, recognizing triggers, and practicing using cue words to remind the child of the difference between the past and present can be helpful in stabilization (Waters, 2016). Teaching the dependent state assertiveness and empowerment skills and redefining the aggressive state's role by using their strength to help in this process can facilitate appropriate behavior.

Educating parents who were critical and punitive toward the child about self-states' defensive behaviors can facilitate an approach of compassion and understanding of their child. Caregivers can support these states' new ways of behaving by rewarding them with activities they enjoy.

Stage Four: Despair, Withdrawal, Regression, and Disorganization

In the fourth stage, Bowlby (1960) found that toddlers who were separated from their mothers exhibited rage, despair, withdrawal, regression, and disorganization. Bowlby noted research by Heinicke (1956), who studied children aged between 16 and 26 months who were placed for short periods of time in a residential nursery with a limited number of nurses caring for them. Heinicke observed children seeking their mothers throughout their stay, with most children crying for their lost mothers and displaying autoerotic activity, and intense aggression. In his research, Bowlby observed children swinging between withdrawal, apathy, regression, mourning, and aggression.

In my comparison model, the chaotic, disorganized responses are markers of rapidly dissociative switching, as described above. These children develop self-states with different ages, discrete roles, and varied feelings and needs that attempt to calm, soothe, defend, and protect against perceived threats. The self-states often present with different levels of maturity and preferences regarding food, clothing, activities, and so on. They can quickly shift along those domains, exhibiting extreme dysregulation and chaotic presentation. Ironically, the traumatized child's dysregulation is an attempt to regulate despair, shame, and grief over abandonment and betrayal due to the loss of safety, trust, and care.

There is often a younger self-state who represents the original self, who is frozen in time and displays what appears to be regressive behavior. I recall a ten-year-old girl who had been severely abused from infancy until she was adopted at age 8. She had a complex configuration of self-states that would rapidly switch in response to minor stressors. One moment she would be curled up in a fetal position sucking her thumb and in the next moment she would stand up and shout profanities at her adoptive mother. These mercurial self-states can wreak havoc on the child's ability to form attachments and the caretaker's ability to manage them.

Because these self-states are formed for a particular survival task and not created within a contextual relationship of nurturing care, they haven't learned interpersonal and reciprocity skills. Understanding this can help clinicians and caregivers to not assume that these children are intentionally wanting to disobey or harm others, but rather are operating in a survival task-oriented mode. They misperceive threats. They project onto their current caregiver's what they felt toward their abuser. They will make contradictory remarks that show state shifts. One child said to me about her adoptive mom, "My mom is always mean to me, but she is nice to me." It is challenging for caregivers to be empathic to self-states to decrease their defensiveness and open a door to develop a relationship with caregivers. Appreciating and respecting what each state has taken for the child is critical to helping the defensive states recognize the caretaker isn't a threat but rather wants to understand and collaborate with them.

Stage Five: Reorganization of Behavior Directed Toward a New Object

In the last stage, Bowlby (1960) indicated that reorganization takes place partly in connection with the image of the lost object (mother), and partly in connection with a new object or objects. This is the final phase of mourning, in which the lost object returns or a new object—another person—is found to whom the child can attach. Bowlby observed that if the child could attach to one adult, the mourning ceased; however, if the child were exposed to numerous adults (via placements/numerous caretakers), they could become self-centered and have shallow relationships over their lifetime. This fifth stage corresponds to the later phases of treatment in my model that involve healing and integration (Waters, 2016). Having a supportive, attuned caregiver is the lifeline needed to repair the dissociative child's traumatic past.

All aspects of the STM recognize that the key factor is to build healthy relationships with safe and protective caregivers. The caregivers, along with therapists, educators, coaches, and the like, all play a role in demonstrating the value and worthiness of the fragmented child. The scaffolding of relationships, particularly between caregivers and the therapist working in unison, provides a firm foundation for processing the trauma. Processing the traumatic event(s) and grieving the losses and pain across all parts of the child is essential to the integration of states and the ability to attach to current caregivers. Each of these theories in STM, including that of family systems (described below), focuses on the importance of relationships working in concert to provide a platform for children to process the trauma, face their pain, and mourn their losses.

Case Study of Johnny

I worked with Johnny, who was nine years old and had been physically and verbally abused in infancy until he was placed at 18 months old. He went through a series of foster homes due to his aggression toward and detachment from his caregivers, until he was adopted at four years old. When he came to see me, he exhibited ongoing soiling problems, infantile eating patterns (eating food with his fingers), and sleep disturbances marked by nighttime roaming around the house. He described depersonalization that accounted for his soiling, and amnesia regarding his infantile behavior and aggression toward his adopted parents. He was highly sensitive to even the slightest rise in vocal volume and upon hearing it would zone out and soil himself. His adopted parents were worn out trying to connect with him, as he exhibited extreme and contradictory attachment behavior. He shifted dramatically between fear, hostility, and clinginess toward them in rapid succession.

Johnny's parents and I worked in unison as I provided psychoeducation so they could understand their child's mercurial presentations. They learned strategies for engaging Johnny's self-states in an empathic way to build an attachment with them as he revealed his inner life through an angry voice, a scared voice, a nice voice, and a baby crying. Johnny reported preverbal sensory memories of hearing yelling and his bottom hurting. When the distressed baby state was accessed, represented by a baby doll that Johnny held while he was held by his adoptive mom, dramatic changes began to occur.

In therapy, his mom was directed to talk through Johnny to his baby state about how scary that must have been for him and how hurt he must have felt when he was being hit and yelled at, and how his other voices tried so hard to help him. She thanked them all for helping him and asked if they would accept her and his adoptive dad as their parents, and they could all work together as a team to heal them from the early trauma. Johnny's parents reassured him that they wanted to keep all of him safe and that they loved all of him, even the angry one who must have taken much abuse for Johnny.

Treatment intervention included Johnny and his mom nurturing Little, with the baby doll. Johnny's adoptive mom rocked him as he held the baby doll, who represented his internal baby. His mom talked lovingly to Little through Johnny. I suggested that as Little felt Johnny's and his parents' love and care, he could grow up to be Johnny's age. Johnny's mom and I stressed that it was safe for Little to feel his body, and Johnny reassured him as well. Johnny began to feel his lower body and gain control over his soiling. I suggested that it was through hugging and loving that the little part could grow to be Johnny's age and become one with Johnny. Johnny nurtured his little part through the symbolic baby doll, making sure the baby doll was always kept in a safe place in his room. With a combination of play therapy and EMDR, ongoing interventions focused on building attachment between all of Johnny and his parents. When the other emotional states recognized that the baby and they were safe, they were ready for trauma processing. Johnny was lastly able to grieve what he had been through. His aggression, detachment, and night roaming also disappeared as his parents continued to nurture all of him. Over a month, Little progressed to nine years old and spontaneously integrated, as did the other states. Their survival defenses were no longer needed to protect them, as they felt secure and loved.

Johnny's parents' acceptance, understanding, and care for all of Johnny helped the other states accept Johnny's parents as their parents too. As the states were validated for what they had endured, and with a combination of play therapy, EMDR, and the mom's comfort, they were able to work through their pain, hurt, rage, and depression. Distrust, projection, and opposition toward Johnny's parents subsided. The states were able to co-consciously share together with Johnny in school and other activities with peers and family. After a month, Johnny reported that his parts had spontaneously integrated. The key to Johnny's healing was building an attachment between all of his states and his parents, which provided the anchor for healing to occur.

Building the attachment with his consistent and nurturing adoptive parents provided the anchor for Johnny to grieve his early trauma. He sobbed when he recounted feeling sad and rejected by his birth and foster parents. Being able to grieve is a critical healing step that requires a secure attachment figure to enable the child to release the self-states' defenses for integration to occur. Mourning the relational trauma clears the pathway to being able to trust others and develop healthy attachments. Let's examine the developmental theory of the STM to further understand pathways to forming dissociative states.

Developmental Theory of the STM

For the Developmental Theory of the STM, I chose the work of Erik Erikson, the father of developmental and ego psychology, because his focus is on the development of ego identity—the conscious sense of self—that is formed through social interaction (Erikson, 1968). According to Erikson, ego identity is constantly changing due to interactions between the body (genetics), mind (psychological), and cultural influences. A person's identity is shaped by human experiences and interpersonal interactions, through which new experiences are continually being assimilated, resulting in solidifying, modifying, or disrupting earlier patterns of beliefs, affect, and behavior.

Pittman et al. (2011) provides an extensive comparison between Bowlby's and Erikson's theoretical models. In their seminal article, they noted that the importance of a secure attachment is recognized in Erikson's psychosocial stages. Erikson's theory of ego identity also aligns well with Putnam's (1997) discrete behavioral states theory, which demonstrates the significance of the interplay between the child and the primary caregiver and its influence on the development of self-states. Erikson's (1963) developmental therapy is defined by eight stages of psychosocial development that encompass the lifespan of the individual. New experiences and information are obtained from daily interactions with others and impact competence levels in each stage of psychosocial development. These stages parallel biological maturation and cognitive development. They are mastered within the context of healthy relationships.

Erikson's psychosocial eight stages are (1) basic trust versus basic mistrust in infancy, (2) autonomy versus shame and doubt in toddlerhood, (3) initiative versus guilt in early childhood, (4) industry versus inferiority in preadolescence and late childhood, (5) identity versus role confusion for the adolescent period, (6) intimacy and solidarity versus isolation in young adulthood, (7) generativity versus self-absorption in adulthood, and (8) integrity versus despair in old age. This discussion will only pertain to the first five stages.

Erikson (1968) outlined an order and timing for these psychosocial stages, with the parents playing a major role in the child's early stages of development. Each stage builds on the preceding stage and paves the way for accomplishing subsequent stages. An individual achieves a stage of development after dealing with a biological crisis. To move through each stage, the individual experiences tension and conflicts within the relational context that affect resolution and competency. Ideally, the crisis should be resolved for development in the next stage to proceed. By mastering each stage, a person develops ego strength. However, failure to master a stage can result in less ability to manage the next stage, thereby leading to an unhealthy personality and diminished sense of self. According to Erickson, if an earlier stage's crisis is not fully mastered, it will likely resurface later in life. Healthy attachments provide individuals with the ability to successfully accomplish each phase and prepare them for managing the next phase. Because early and chronic childhood trauma often thwarts the achievement of these stages, it is important to examine the timing of children's trauma at particular stages and how the trauma impacted their ability to master that stage and their subsequent development.

Comparing Erickson's Model with the Star Theoretical Model

Comparing Erickson's model with an understanding of children's traumatic responses and dissociative defenses, the STM analyzes how trauma can impair a child's ability to develop a cohesive identity, resulting in fragmentation. The fragmentation thwarts a child's capacity to master developmental conflicts and stages. The developmental portion of the STM examines Erickson's stages of development in relationship to what occurs with a traumatized child. This model examines when trauma occurs at a developmental stage and the possible development of internal states across multiple domains: behavioral, affective, relational, cognitive, spiritual/beliefs, and neurobiological (see Figure 16.2).

The STM contends that each self-state can have divergent cognitions, affects, behaviors, relational capacity, spiritual/beliefs, and neurobiological differences that can impair the child's ability to effectively achieve developmental stages. To add complexity, certain self-states can be at different levels of psychosocial development, further thwarting the child from performing to age-related expectations. Therefore, when evaluating traumatized children, in addition to recognizing the child's current age according to Erickson's developmental stages, it is important to know child's age(s) when trauma occurred and evaluate how the trauma impaired the child with regard to achieving that developmental milestone. Furthermore, it is critical to evaluate whether a self-state was formed at the time of trauma and what are the characteristics of that state's domains—for example, cognitive,

Developmental Theory of the Star Theoretical Model
Dissociative Child's Domains

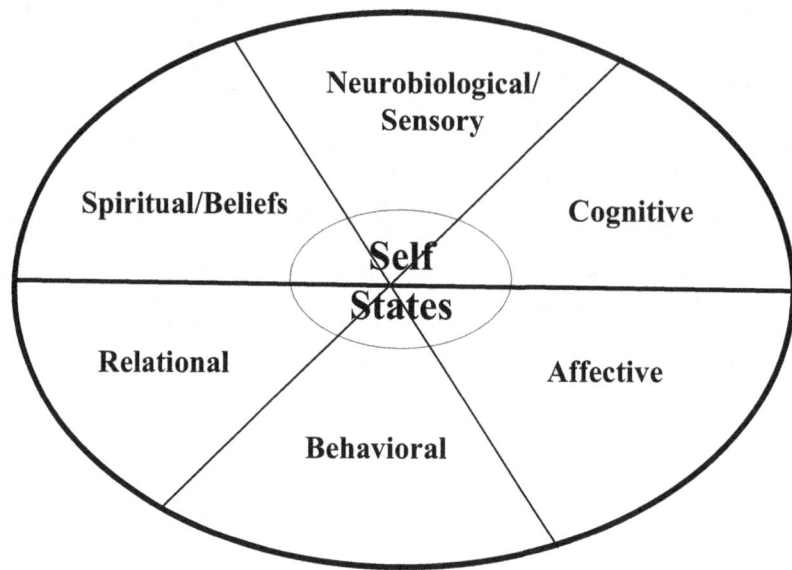

Figure 16.2 Dissociative Domains in the Star Theoretical Model.

behavioral, or relational. With complex trauma, there can be multiple chronological ages at which the child's successful achievement of development was aborted. As well, there can be multiple self-states formed that carry various domains that will disrupt the child's overall functioning. It is helpful to draw, for example, a diagram with the child in the center and their self-states branching out, labeling their ages, characteristics/roles, ages of trauma(s), and their domains of affect, behaviors, and the like. Lines can be drawn between the states that know each other. This developmental map of the child's constellation of states can help the therapist understand the interruption of developmental phases, and the unfavorable outcomes, according to Erickson. This drawing of the child's complex profile can be used to determine parts' developmental ages that may be frozen and how to appropriately intervene.

Case Study of Martha

Martha's biological parents abused her sexually, physically, and emotionally, as well as neglected her, from birth until she was three years old (Waters, 2016). She was placed in foster care and then in an adoptive home for a year, until she was removed and placed in second adoptive home at seven years old, where she remained until adulthood. Fortunately, her second set of adoptive parents were attuned, committed, compassionate, and educated in understanding Martha's trauma.

Martha's life from birth to seven years old was traumatic, compounded by multiple placements, including a severed adoption. According to Erikson's developmental milestones, from birth until seven years old, Martha was unable to achieve a sense of trust, autonomy, initiative, and industry—the basic building blocks of a developing self. She suffered mistrust, shame, doubt, guilt, and inferiority. Martha reported having 19 self-states of different ages, from zero to seven years old. In looking at the developmental domains of dissociation, mostly their affect was of deep sadness, pain, loss, and abandonment. Martha drew a picture of them all crying. Some states' behaviors were sexualized.

Some states were critical of the fearful states and viewed them as weak and would yell at them. Relationally, many of them would blank out when getting close to their adoptive parents. Some states behaved age-appropriately, attended school, and were compliant. Behaviorally, some states, those who suffered the sexual abuse, sexually acted out with peers. Cognitively, they viewed themselves as unworthy and others with distrust and fear. Neurologically, Martha would blank out and lose awareness, but these episodes were due to dissociative amnesia and not a seizure disorder. She would have intense headaches when she switched states, and particularly when the sexualized states would attempt to take over. She had significant developmental gaps in her life, but with intensive therapy and loving, empathic parents as my partners in therapy, she and her self-states were able over time to begin to trust, and then process her significant early traumas.

The last step toward integration was a painful process of mourning all that had occurred to her. An intensive session was arranged with Martha and her mother to help Martha break through her defense of blanking out when she felt painful feelings of loss and abandonment. Her mother held her and reassured all of her that she and her dad loved them, and they were safe. Finally, Martha was able to mourn her early trauma. It was as if the dam had broken, and she sobbed while her mother comforted and rocked all of her. Martha was able to grieve her traumatic past, and that allowed her to move forward.

After Martha had integrated (all of her states united as one with her), years later her mother told me that Martha had made up a song and sung it to her mom in the car on the way home. Martha described some of the things she did to test her adoptive parents to see if they were going to kick her out, as experienced with her previous adoptive parents. Martha repeatedly sang the refrain, "I guess they're going to keep me. I tried everything." Her adoptive mother listened with amusement thinking, "Yes, Martha, you did try everything to make us get rid of you, but we didn't give up!" Most parents who care for children with complex trauma can likely relate to Martha's lyrics, because they are tested repeatedly (Waters, 2016, p. 149).

Family Systems Theory of the STM

Virginia Satir (n.d.) said, "Feelings of worth can flourish only in an atmosphere where individual differences are appreciated, mistakes are tolerated, communication is open, and rules are flexible—the kind of atmosphere that is found in a nurturing family." Satir's profound words recognize the critical role that families and, by extension, children's feelings of self-worth play in children's well-being. In both big and small ways, we must communicate this message to the children and their families. Satir adhered to a growth model that is based on the notion that people change through interactions with other people and through an exploration of their inner life by examining their own thoughts, intentions, and perceptions of others. Her family systems theory coincides with Bowlby's (1960) and Erickson's (1968) models in recognizing that family interactions play a significant role in the pathology of children—often the identified patient.

Satir's therapeutic beliefs about human nature are (1) every individual is geared to survival, growth, and obtaining closeness with others, no matter how distorted it may look; (2) what society calls sick, crazy, stupid, or bad behavior is really the person's signal of distress and call for help; and (3) human beings are limited only by the extent of their knowledge, their ways of understanding themselves, and their ability to relate with others (1983, pp. 124–125). Satir's guiding principles provide a foundation for my work with traumatized children and their families. She postulates that in an open and safe environment, family rules and members' fears are discussed openly, directly, appropriately, and clearly. Conversely, in a closed family system characterized by maltreatment, distortions, and denial, maintaining the status quo is prominent. Such an abusive environment will promote a child's reliance on dissociation to conform to the distortions and denial. When confronted with change, it isn't uncommon that an abusive family system will be resistant to it and attempt to maintain past ineffective ways of interacting, thus resulting in the identified patient—often the child—who suffers. This would require a child protective service report.

Because the identified child's symptoms reflect the distortions, pain, discomfort, and obstruction of growth present within the family system, Satir (1965) contends that the family needs to be treated as a unit, because family members influence each other. While she advises participation of all family members, there are exceptions or important considerations in an abusive environment. Of primary concern is the child's psychological and physical safety. I've worked with abusive parents in therapy who admitted their abuse and were making a successful recovery. Contrarily, I've worked with other families in which the abusive caregiver denied sexual abuse and was a danger to the child, and as such, I recommended in court that they have no contact with the child. Each situation needs to be carefully evaluated with paramount concern for the safety of the child.

A thorough evaluation of the family environment includes the following areas to examine: offender and non-offending caregivers—own histories of abuse and neglect, domestic violence, marital relationship, parenting capabilities, communication concerns, legal issues, employment, mental health, dissociative symptoms, financial health, and education; the offending parent's relationship to the child—the type and length of abuse, harm to the child, future risk to the child, and any suppression/threatening techniques employed to silence the child victim; and the non-offending parent's ability to protect and be attuned to the child, meet the child's emotional and physical needs, and commit to participating in their child's therapy. Regarding siblings, a history of abuse or neglect, their relationship to the child victim, and their emotional status are evaluated. The victim's assessment includes the following history: complete psychosocial and physical health, mental status, abuse and neglect, dissociative symptoms, academic performance, legal concerns, and relationships with parents, siblings, supportive relatives, and peers. It is usually inappropriate to interview the offending parent, particularly if the case is being litigated. Information about the offending parent can be obtained from the non-offending parent or collateral sources.

While caretakers are very involved in their child's treatment, I like to involve other family members who reside with the child to participate periodically to enhance overall communication, understand their needs, and address any conflicts that hamper the child's recovery. It is important to evaluate if the dissociative child is the scapegoat and how the child's dissociation impacts siblings who may be neglected and resentful. A lesson I learned over the years is the importance of involving siblings in the treatment to manage conflicts between them and the dissociative sibling. Because dissociative children can be very time-consuming for the parent(s), siblings may be unwittingly ignored and feel resentful as a result. Having periodic sibling and family sessions can minimize these concerns.

I engage supportive parents in therapy with children, if they are comfortable, to learn from my modeling of how to address their child's symptoms and strengthen the child's attachment to them. Dissociative teens typically like individual sessions, with family sessions only periodically.

With adoptive children, we often don't have details of their traumatic past and must make educated guesses by their interactional patterns and behaviors as to what they bring from their biological families (and other placements) into their adoptive homes. Openly discussing messages, beliefs, and patterns that adoptive children exhibit can help them discard traumatically based distorted beliefs and messages and begin to overcome their fears, distrust, and reliance on dissociative responses and learn healthier communication patterns.

Case Study of Pam

For her first six years, Pam endured much trauma: her mother used drugs and had men cycling through their home. Pam was severely neglected and sexually abused. After several stints in foster care, she was adopted at ten years old. She was the only child. She would roam around at nighttime and raid the refrigerator and pantry. She was amnestic about these forages. When her father came home from work, she exhibited sexually provocative behaviors toward him and would frequently masturbate in a trance state. She had many periods of staring that lasted as long as five minutes. A neurology exam ruled out a seizure disorder. She had periodic rages caused by minor stressors. Pam described internal voices and images that represented a couple of maternal helpers, a perpetrating male, a little scared part, and sad parts. Much psychoeducation occurred to help Pam's adoptive parents understand her significant dissociation and how to manage Pam and her self-states. Both parents became active partners in helping all of Pam learn healthy behavior, and understood her past traumatic reactions being acted out in "real" time.

Based on Bowlby's and Satir's theories, Pam's parents and I agreed to focus on building attachment and trust between Pam and us, and to value and respect Pam for what she had experienced in her young life. We agreed to take a patient and empathetic approach, knowing that her survival behaviors would take time to change, until all of her felt safe, understood, and appreciated, and that her amnestic barriers would eventually erode. We communicated repeatedly the messages that all of her were worthy and respected for what they did to survive. We expressed empathy for how scared Pam and her others must have felt not having their birth mom to care for and protect them, how hungry they must have felt not having enough food to eat, and how terrified and confused they likely felt when they were being sexually abused. We talked about how she and her self-states learned survival skills to get their needs met, how brave and strong they were, and how hard it must be to trust that they could be cared for, and to feel they are worthy of being cared for. We talked about how we wanted to help all of Pam feel safe and have their needs met. We talked about triggers and how that brings all of the states back to everything they experienced. A variety of techniques were implemented to develop internal awareness and cooperation, to connect all states with their body, to expand their window of tolerance in managing triggers (Waters, 2016).

My initial intervention with dissociative children is to connect with the perpetrating parts, who often take the most toxic traumatic events and hold the rage. I did not want Pam's male perpetrator state to be threatened by me. I focused on building a relationship with him and appreciating how strong he was to endure such significant trauma. Because dissociative children have vivid internal worlds, I proposed an internal soundproof (so as not to scare the other states) anger room that was all around safe with padded walls, so he could discharge his rage with a variety of supplies he could choose from (e.g., punching bag, exercise machines, trampoline, art supplies) (Waters, 2016). After he discharged his rage, he was invited to go to an adjoining internal comfort room to watch funny movies, eat snacks, and so on. This strategy blended his anger with enjoyment (an emotion that was foreign to him), and his anger became more nuanced and his destructiveness dissipated.

Other strategies were also implemented. Pam had access to a cabinet with healthy snacks for when she felt hungry. One of her internal moms was able to reinforce that she no longer lived with Pam's birth mom. When the sexualized part wanted to act out, the internal mom built an internal alarm system that would sound, and the other maternal helper would take over and tell Pam's parents, who had art supplies available, so the sexualized part could draw how she was feeling instead. Many of these techniques were installed with EMDR. Over time, Pam and her states developed trust and an attachment with her parents, and she was on her way to integrating.

Parenting a dissociative child is the most challenging role, as the child can switch rapidly from one state to another, displaying different attachment styles, affect, behaviors, and preferences. Suffice it to say, parents must accept all parts of their child, even during these trying times, and recognize that they are coregulators of their child. If parents demonstrate "calm in the midst of the storm," their child will deescalate quicker. Learning how to connect with the child with empathy and reflection before correcting them is a beginning step toward calming them. Because children's acting out behavior can trigger parents' own unresolved traumatic past and attachment disturbances, parents need to be aware of those triggers and ways to manage them effectively to avoid escalation. Recommending therapy for parents can give them the attention and support they need to work on their unresolved issues and learn healthy responses.

Conclusion

In the STM, I integrate dissociative, neurobiology, attachment, developmental, and family systems theories to provide a comprehensive approach to evaluating and treating children with dissociation. These theories interlock, recognizing the impact of interpersonal relationships on the child and the health of these relationships as paramount to providing the anchor for the child's recovery. Each theory highlights specific pathways that contribute to a deeper understanding of the impact trauma has in developing dissociation. Each theory also provides guidance on clinical applications to help traumatized children resolve their traumatic past, grieve their losses, develop healthy attachments, form a cohesive identity, and become productive members of society.

Notes

1 All clinical case studies in this chapter are composites.
2 For a more in-depth view of the neurobiology of trauma in the STM, please refer to Waters (2016, pp. 15–20).

References

Adler-Tapia, R. L. (2012). Integrating theories of developmental psychology into enactments of the child psychotherapy. In *Child psychotherapy: Integrating developmental theory into clinical practice* (pp. 173–204). Springer Publishing Company.

Bowlby, J. (1960). Grief and mourning in infancy and early childhood. *Psychoanalytic Study of the Child, 15*, 9–52. https://clarityrising.wordpress.com/wp-content/uploads/2011/11/bowlby-1960-grief-and-mourning-in-infancy-early-childhood-24-pgs.pdf

Bowlby, J. (1961). The Adolft Meyer lecture: Childhood mourning and its implications for psychiatry. *American Journal of Psychiatry, 118*, 481–497. https://doi.org/10.1176/ajp.118.6.481

Bowlby, J. (1973). *Attachment and loss, Vol. 2:* Separation. Basic Books.

Cortizo, R. (2021): Prenatal broken bonds: Trauma, dissociation and the Calming Womb Model. *Journal of Trauma & Dissociation, 22*(1), 1–10. https://doi.org/10.1080/15299732.2021.1834300

Erikson, E. H. (1963). *Childhood and society* (2nd ed.). W. W. Norton.

Erikson, E. H. (1968). *Identity: Youth and crisis.* W. W. Norton.

Heinicke, C. M. (1956). Some effects of separating two-year-old children from their parents: A comparative study. *Human Relations, 9*, 105–176.

Main, M., & Hesse, E. (1990). Parents' unresolved traumatic experiences are related to infant disorganized attachment status: Is frightened and/or frightening parental behavior the linking mechanism? In M. T. Greenberg, D. Cicchetti & E. M. Cummings (Eds.), *Attachment in the preschool years: Theory, research and intervention* (pp. 161–182). University of Chicago Press.

Manfield, P., Lovett, J., Engel, L., & Manfield, D. (2017). Use of the flash technique in EMDR therapy: Four case examples. *Journal of EMDR Practice and Research, 11*(4) 195–205. https://doi.org/10.1891/1933-3196.11.4.195

Ogden, P., & Fisher, J. (2015). *Sensorimotor psychotherapy: Interventions for trauma and attachment.* W. W. Norton.

Ogden, P., & Gomez, A. M. (2013). EMDR therapy and sensorimotor psychotherapy with children. In A. M. Gomez (Ed.), *EMDR therapy and adjunct approaches with children* (pp. 247–271). Springer.

Pittman, J. F., Keiley, M. K., Kerpelman, J. L., & Vaughn, B. E. (2011). Attachment, identity, and intimacy: Parallels between Bowlby's and Erikson's paradigms. *Journal of Family Theory & Review, 3*(1), 32–46. https://doi.org/10.1111/j.1756-2589.2010.00079.x

Porges, S. W. (2004). Neuroception: A subconscious system for detecting threats and safety. *Zero to Three, 24*(5), 19–24.

Potgieter Marks, R. (2022). "You will not believe me if I tell you!": Prenatal trauma and dissociation. In V. Sinason & R. Potgieter Marks (Eds.), *Treating children with dissociative disorders: Attachment, trauma, theory & practice* (pp. 34–48). Routledge.

Putnam, F. W. (1997). *Dissociation in children and adolescents: A developmental perspective.* Guilford Press.

Robertson, J., & Bowlby, J. (1952). Responses of young children to separation from their mothers II: Observations of the sequences of response of children aged 18 to 24 months during the course of separation. *Courrier du Centre International de l'Enfance, 2,* 131–142.

Satir, V. (1965). The family as a treatment unit. *Confinia Psychiatrica, 8,* 37–42.

Satir, V. (1983). *Conjoint family therapy* (3rd ed.). Science and Behavior Books.

Satir, V. (n.d.). Retrieved from brainyquote.com/quotes/quotes/v/virginiasa175186.html

Schore, A. N. (2000). Attachment and the regulation of the right brain. *Attachment & Human Development, 2*(1), 23–47. https://doi:10.1080/146167300361309

Silberg, J. (2022). *The child survivor: Healing developmental trauma and dissociation* (2nd ed.). Routledge.

Vogt, R. (Ed.). (2012). *Perpetrator introjects: Psychotherapeutic diagnostics and treatment models.* Asanger.

Waters, F. S. (2016). *Healing the fractured child: Diagnosis & treatment of youth with dissociation.* Springer.

PART 3

Treatment Modalities for Children with Complex Trauma and Dissociation

17
TRAUMA-INFORMED CHILD PSYCHOANALYTIC PSYCHOTHERAPY

Valerie Sinason

Introduction

What Is Trauma?

As stated elsewhere in this book, trauma comes from the Greek, meaning "wound," from an earlier derivation meaning "to pierce." It has long been used in medicine and surgery as meaning both an injury where the skin is broken as a result of external violence and as the consequence on the organism as a whole. There is multidisciplinary agreement for the understanding from psychoanalysis that trauma is an external stressor that comes suddenly and cannot be prepared for. The stressor is so strong that it breaks through the protective shield of skin and mind (Freud, 1920); it cannot be adequately mentally processed and affects the whole organism. Finally, and a contribution from psychoanalysis, the stressor interacts with the individual's internal world including unconscious guilt and phantasy (Sinason, 2022a, 2022b).

Psychoanalysis and Its Relationship to Trauma

This chapter is written using a theoretical body of knowledge, Freudian, Independent group, and Kleinian British psychoanalysis, because it has aided me and my patients. However, from my experience of the last 40 years, the model that contains each of us comes as a result of our own personality. It was Dr. Andrew Arthur (2001), a British psychologist and psychotherapist, who decided to research what drew professionals to either cognitive or psychodynamic work. He wondered if it was due to their training or their personality and found it was their personality. Working with extreme trauma requires a range of resources and whilst my resources particularly come from a love of psychoanalytic thinking, I am indebted to music, body, dance, art therapists, and EMDR therapy.

To understand trauma-informed child psychoanalytical psychotherapy with dissociative disorders we need to understand where the child work came from. It did not spring up independently but came from the discovery of adult psychoanalysis. Sigmund Freud (1856–1939) was a doctor who was deeply interested in neurology and later trained in neuropathology at the Vienna General Hospital. He visited the famous neurologist, Professor Jean Charcot (1825–1893) in 1885 in Paris for several months and witnessed Charcot's work with hypnosis and what was called hysteria. It was after this he collaborated with another Viennese physician, Josef Breuer (1842–1925), as a result of which he made a major career change. He formulated his concept of "psychoanalysis" in the 1890s, and he and Breuer co-wrote Studies on Hysteria (1893), which formed the theoretical basis of psychoanalysis. The term "hysteria" came from the Greek word for "womb" and shows how the early Greek misogynist concept of the womb causing florid or volatile emotional states in women has persisted for centuries even when the study of hysteria included male war trauma.

It was the patient Bertha Pappenheim, known under the pseudonym Anna O, who first called her treatment "the talking cure" and "chimney sweeping" (Breuer & Freud, 1893). Freud realised that actions and behaviours could be influenced by unconscious wishes and memories. In particular, aggressive and sexual wishes struggled with the defences against them. He began a self-analysis, noting the unconscious meaning of his dreams. His treatment was revolutionary for the time in offering talking instead of violent physical action that damaged the patient and he built up a group of followers. Indeed, it was in 1910 that the International Psychoanalytic Association was founded with Carl Jung as President although a split developed and Jung developed his own theoretical school of thought.

In 1923, the same year Freud developed cancer of the jaw, he produced a structural model of the mind divided into the id, ego, and superego. In 1933, the Nazis publicly burned a number of his books and in 1938 he left Vienna with his wife and daughter, Anna, for London. Trauma was a subject that concerned Freud throughout his long psychoanalytic career from both a theoretical and applied practical perspective and in the index to his complete works there are an enormous number of theoretical and clinical concepts, much of which is still useful today. Outside the complex controversial area of child abuse, psychoanalysis was concerned with trauma from the start and continuously.

On Jan 11th, 1893, while delivering a lecture on the Psychical Mechanism of Hysterical Phenomena, Freud saw that the trauma must involve the idea of "mortal danger" nearly a century before psychiatry and psychology. In Freud's work with his colleague Breuer (1893 SE2, pp. 3–17) he underlines the impact of fright, anxiety, shame, or physical pain which can cause psychic traumas. It was only in 1980 that the Diagnostic and Statistical Manual of Mental Disorders (DSM III) first included a separate category for psychological trauma in which the person had experienced an event that was outside usual human experience, would be markedly distressing to almost everyone, such as a serious threat to one's life or physical integrity, serious threat or harm to one's children, spouse or other close relatives and friends, sudden destruction of one's home and community; or seeing another person who has recently been or is being injured or killed as a result of an accident or physical violence. Time was able to validate this further. On August 27th, 1998, Hurricane Bonnie swept through North Carolina but did not cause deaths because there had been foreknowledge and careful evacuation. By contrast, at the same time a bombing of Planet Hollywood, an American owned hamburger restaurant in Cape Town in a safe tourist area was profoundly traumatic. It was sudden and there could be no preparation.

In this early stage of his work Freud used hypnotism to lessen the power of these traumas and made the powerful comment that "the psychical trauma, or more precisely the memory of the trauma-acts like a foreign body which long after its entry must continue to be regarded as an agent that is still at work" 1893 (p.6). How this foreign body could be digested and processed was to be the main reason for psychoanalysis following trauma. He concluded "hysterics suffer mainly from reminiscences."

Throughout Freud's life, he drew attention to trauma in prescient ways. Indeed, in his "Thoughts for the times on war and death" (1915, pp. 275–301) he takes us to the core of human inability to confront mortality. Where attachment has been less secure there can be more unconscious ambivalence and therefore a depressive guilt at the triumph of surviving. He followed this in "Mourning and Melancholia" (SE14, pp. 239–58) where he delineates how we can project the best of ourselves into the dead loved one, depleting the survivor and leaving the possibility of pathological mourning. These concepts are crucial in contemporary life and almost all forms of therapy make use of Freud's ideas, even when they do not acknowledge it.

Freud's later rejection of hypnosis for "free association" which he felt did not carry the suggestiveness of the analyst and provided more neutrality caused a rift with the pioneers who used it and meant that the later knowledge that came from clinical hypnosis could not be utilised. That rift has continued. It is Dr. Richard Kluft (2018), a leading psychoanalyst and hypnotist, who currently most voices the damage that came from this split and considers that the rejection of clinical hypnosis by psychoanalysis that continued was not firmly grounded and should be reassessed. That rift also separated Freud's thinking and followers from the groundwork established by Charcot and Janet who rehabilitated the scientific basis for hypnosis. ***This also meant the concepts of dissociation and dissociative disorders had a harder journey*** (emphasis added by this author).

Many of Freud's major discoveries have since been validated by neuropsychology and neuropsychoanalysis (Solms, 1999, 2018a, 2018b). Whilst Freud put on the map the huge areas of controversy that we were not in charge of our mind, that babies were not a blank slate, that there was an unconscious too, perhaps his most complex legacy for our subject of trauma-informed child psychoanalytic therapy and dissociation and dissociative disorders, was to do with child sexual abuse. Initially in the 1890s, he was more focused on external sexual trauma and its consequences but later became more convinced of the internal psychic trauma.

Whilst it has been psychoanalytically important to explore the internal psychic trauma, this change, and the way it happened, was unsurprisingly welcomed by most of his colleagues. It shows the social pressure that this subject evoked. Additionally, we can see how live and modern so many of Freud's ideas are that in the 21st century we still feel let down that Freud could not manage the pressures and traumatic consequences of his own observations. We are expecting Freud to have managed this almost alone. He found himself devastated considering that if everything he heard was as true, as he first thought, then most of his professional neighbours and colleagues who referred their daughters, could be abusers – even his own father. In 1897, he wrote to Fliess (1897) "Surely such widespread perversions against children are not very probable." Middle class abuse in a class-based society can be even harder to accept. This is where he made his major change, added to by the enormous lack of support for these ideas. He decided he had over-valued reality at the expense of phantasy. The Oedipus Complex emerged and his followers (with the notable exception of Ferenczi, 1933) were glad to avoid the controversy caused by sexual abuse, no differently than many contemporary practitioners are. However, Freud himself never reneged on his finding that external child abuse happened and mattered. Indeed, in 1905 he emphasised "I cannot admit that in my paper on the Aetiology of Hysteria (1896) I exaggerated the frequency or importance of that influence" (p. 190).

It is hard enough now in 2024 for professionals to accept the enormity of abuse and trauma, let alone the lack of treatment and care for victims and survivors of sexual abuse even though the National Health Service in the UK accepts that one in four adults experience abuse in a lifetime. It was Sandor Ferenczi, in his seminal paper (1933), who stood alone in his understanding of the traumatic impact of sexual abuse. This paper would eventually be translated into English and republished under the title "Confusion of Tongues between adults and the child-The Language of Tenderness and of Passion." Whilst nearly all the early thinkers tackled the taboo subjects of child sexuality, sexual trauma was still a major problem to write about. Ferenczi's paper is as powerful now as it was then.

Before highlighting the key areas of adult psychoanalysis which child treatments were then able to use, it is helpful to look at the child trainings which, in the UK, were centred at The Tavistock Clinic and the Hampstead Clinic (later known as The Anna Freud Centre.)

Child Analysis and Psychoanalytic Psychotherapy

Historically, treatment for children took a long time to be established, although it is worth noting that the first significant treatment was a largely indirect one of a three-year-old boy known as "Little

Hans" carried out via Freud's communications with the boy's concerned father. The father regularly updated Freud on the boy's development. Little Hans verbalised his worries about his penis, masturbation, castration, and a horse phobia (not helped by the punitive castrating way his mother responded, as was historically acceptable at that time). Through this connection, Freud (1909) developed his ideas on the psychosexual stages of childhood and the father was able to aid the lessening of his child's fears.

The first major figure to formalise analytic treatment with children was Anna Freud, Freud's daughter, who was born in 1895 in Austria, in the same year he discovered psychoanalysis. She was not the first practicing child psychoanalyst, as that accolade goes to her mentor Hermine von Hug-Hellmuth, who published an article on "Play Therapy" in 1913. Carl Jung, Lou Andreas-Salomé, and Sándor Ferenczi had all worked with children as well.

It was Anna Freud (1895–1983) who turned child psychoanalysis into a distinct form of treatment under the encouragement of her father (Malvern & Leff, 2011). In 1927, she published an introduction to the technique of child psychoanalysis, showing (like Maria Montessori) that toys were needed to enable a child to relax and free associate. From 1941 to 1945, on escaping to England, she set up War Nurseries and in 1952 the Hampstead Child Therapy Clinic and a Course began, followed by a preschool nursery to further understand child development. The first trainees were intended to join the newly formed National Health Service.

Melanie Klein (1882–1960), another key pioneer, as a depressed mother of three, sought treatment with Ferenczi after her family moved to Budapest. She was encouraged to observe her children and become a child analyst. She joined the Berlin psychoanalytic society and was invited to give papers on her work in the UK by Ernest Jones. She settled permanently in the UK in 1926 and became a British citizen in 1934.

Freud and Anna Freud came to England as refugees in 1938. Klein met Freud several times, but he was never fully supportive of her ideas, as she was his daughter's most serious critic. The history of psychoanalysis is therefore rooted in the trauma of war, exile, and conflict where the liminal experience of Jewish refugees became relevant. Indeed, Freud had made Carl Jung the first President of his fledgling organisation as an Aryan who might be able to protect the subject better. It was hard for the largely Christian British upper-class psychoanalysts to deal with key disagreements between two Jewish female immigrants and, outside of Ferenczi (1933), and Freud's earliest papers on hysteria, there was almost no concern about sexual abuse and its psychological consequences.

Despite their differences, the two female pioneers believed that training in adult psychoanalysis should come before what they considered was the technically more difficult arena of child psychoanalysis, so that the analyst in training would have had his own analysis and would be familiar with the psychoanalytic theories regarding psychosexual development, the working of the mind, and repression. They agreed that all children needed play materials in order to express the themes that were occupying their inner world. All groups agreed on the importance of psychologically aware teaching. The Hampstead Clinic had their own nursery school, and the Child Guidance Clinic at the Tavistock had a Day Unit where trainees from all theoretical backgrounds were initially welcomed (*The Tavistock Century*, 2021). Children starting treatment were given a box which included small toys, art materials, animals. It was found that exploring family issues was easier to do with animal families. They created a free transitional space.

However, the International Psychoanalytic Association only granted official recognition to training as a Child Analyst in 2000. There were those in the psychoanalytic community, and perhaps still are, who believed that child psychoanalysis was not truly analysis. Truly recognising the need for and relevance of child psychoanalysis to the field of psychoanalysis as a whole took time to accept. It is relevant to this chapter and the subject of trauma and dissociation that treatment and concern for children has always been lower down the hierarchy. It was thanks to the development of the Women's movement that concern for children could be observed more fully.

Key Components of Psychoanalytic Treatment

All clinical examples in this chapter are composite

From psychoanalysis with adults, key theoretical and practical issues emerged that would also be used in child work and psychoanalytic psychotherapy. Central to all ages was the idea that unconscious drives can impact on our behaviour, experience, emotions and cognition. Trying to bring these into conscious awareness to aid emotional development can meet psychological resistance in the form of defence mechanisms. With children, through the medium of play, psychodynamic therapy seeks to address conflicts and developmental obstacles to aid emotional development. The psychotherapist, through their relationship with the child, slowly understands the internal constellations that are disturbing the child and the impact of external factors in their aetiology. Psychoanalytic work does not seek to force the direction of treatment and the Tavistock model underlined both the freedom and rigour of treatment.

Whilst the impact of COVID and the rise of referrals have led to psychoanalytic child psychotherapists taking on short term work and providing formal treatment plans this is not the majority approach. Evaluating intensity of treatment needs and the supportive family work needed is very different to offering fixed term focussed work, however useful that might be. Indeed, children suffering from extreme trauma can require a variety of different approaches. For the psychoanalytic practitioner, there is a dynamic in progress from the moment of referral. Who made it? Why was it made at that moment? What emotional impact does the referral have on the practitioner even before any appointment is offered? There may be many hypotheses. However, it is the actual meetings and assessment period, whether one session or several, that allow the practitioner to consider what might be needed. This includes what is provided in the room. For example, it might be considered helpful to have a room with shared toys as well as a private box to see how the child uses that differentiation. Some children with a history of violence might need objects to illustrate their despair and rage. Others might feel safer with the minimum of objects. Some might like questions or games being initiated. Others might need the practitioner to follow and wait for them. In other words, it is the relationship with the child in the room (or on Zoom) that determines the first stages.

However, two key areas in psychoanalytically informed non-directive work which remain crucial are **the transference** and **countertransference.** Within formal psychoanalytic adult treatment, the patient lay down on a couch or day bed so that their free reverie would not be intruded on by the sight of the therapist. In psychoanalytic therapy treatment with adults now, many prefer to sit on a chair facing the therapist and in trauma work it has been even more important for the patient to see the expression on the face of the therapist. However, in Freud's time, the chaise longue had pride of place in consulting rooms. Freud realised that the patient transferred onto the person of their analyst themes and characteristics that had an earlier role in relationships in their life. Unpicking these transfers could lessen symptomatic pain and discomfort. With child psychoanalytic treatment, there is usually a playroom and drawing equipment and small animals and dolls. Some therapists (Lowenfeld, 1935) use sand and of course there are art, music, and dance psychoanalytic psychotherapists as well as EMDR and other creative models (please see Chapters 20 and 32 in this volume).

Working with the Transference

Sarah sat on the floor in the corner of the therapy room, her hands tightly clasping her arms. She looked terrified.

Therapist (speaking softly and gently) "Hello Sarah, you look ever so frightened sitting there like that,"
She nodded. She reached out hurriedly to pick up a baby doll and hug it.

Therapist: "Is Dolly frightened?"
Patient: "Yes. Me helping Dolly. Dolly very frightened"
Therapist: "That is kind of you to be helping Dolly when you are frightened too"
Patient: "Yes."
Therapist: Do grownups often make you feel scared?"
Patient: "Yes."

She nodded and looked up a little.

Therapist: "Oh dear, then I am sorry if my face looks horrid and scary."
Patient: (laughing) "Not a horrid scary face."

In this excerpt, I used humour to explore and allow the negative transference to me. Humour made it easier for her to accept the interpretation and lessen the negative power of the transference. Understanding the power of transference as a lived experience and not "just" as theory is a major gift of psychoanalysis. Asking about the doll was a transitional way of exploring how Sarah felt without her feeling shamed or exposed. As can be seen, I was free to oscillate between talking about Sarah directly or indirectly according to how I experienced her transferring to me feelings about adults who had frightened her. Her capacity to parent the doll provided a hopeful example of some moments of a good-enough experience of parenting.

Countertransference, by comparison, originally meant the feeling evoked in the analyst by the presence of the patient but more recently has been understood as something primitive that is not bearable which is projected into the other person. This makes it very similar to the Kleinian concept of projective identification. In child psychoanalytic psychotherapy it is important to note the state you are in before seeing the patient so you can see more clearly what emotional luggage has come in that was separate from your own! For example, while sitting in a consulting room waiting to see ten-year-old Maureen, a traumatised young girl with a dissociative disorder (this is a composite case), I was aware I felt calm and thoughtful. I wondered which state of mind would be predominant when she came in and whether any of her "others" would play with the toys in their therapy box. When Maureen came in with her hands clenched in angry fists and a furious look on her face, a feeling of fear entered me. I realised I was in the presence of Max, a furious male teenage alter who took over the ten-year-old body and made it feel dangerous. These feelings had not been in me while waiting for them to arrive – they were an impact of Max in the room and are considered as counter transferential in nature. It is the analytical therapist's own personal intensive therapy or psychoanalysis that aids the therapist's capacity to bear this and recognise it.

Psychoanalytic Disagreements in Child and Adult Work

The disagreements in the adult field were inherited by those working with children. The "Controversial Discussions," refers to the protracted discussions between Anna Freud, Melanie Klein, their followers and members of the indigenous group of British analysts (the Independent Group) who tried to mediate. These took place in the British Psycho-Analytical Society between 1941 and 1946 (King et al., 1991). Anna Freud considered latency was the best time for a child to enter analysis as before that she felt the attachment to the family was too strong and she wanted to help promote the best facilitating environment for the young child and their family. Klein, on the other hand, considered psychoanalysis was relevant at the earliest stage. She interpreted at the deepest level to the youngest children, whilst Anna Freud sought collaboration and gentle exploration first. Anna Freud also considered the role of defences more important than Klein. Klein emphasised the importance of transference in the psychoanalytic treatment for even the youngest children whereas Anna Freud considered that transference did not really exist for young children owing to the parents' powerful place in the child's life. In contrast, Klein used the transference for the "deep" interpretation of hate and envy.

The Anna Freud Clinic did not allow trainees to study with them until their own children were school age whereas the Tavistock Clinic, just a five-minute walk away, did not see age of children or stage of pregnancy as a key issue. However, the different attitude to the age of children of trainees reflected a subtle difference between the weighting of internal or external reality.

Anna Freud clinic practitioners were expected to provide substantial developmental profiles of the child they assessed in addition to clinical details of the assessment meetings. There was a far stronger academic research base historically at the Anna Freud, whilst Tavistock clinic child psychotherapists had a greater freedom to provide a more clinical picture of the child's first sessions. Indeed, in an attempt for the two clinics to liaise more in the 1980s and present shared assessments to each other, I was shocked, as a new Tavistock trainee asked to give the first such presentation to be told by an elderly Anna Freudian, child analyst, "That was very nice dear-a good emotional description of the child-but where is the assessment?"

Kleinian therapists meanwhile looked at the oscillation between different states of mind, seeing the duality of life and death instincts, the fluctuation between the depressive position and the paranoid-schizoid position as well as developmental stages. This controversy left its imprint on the evolution of adult and child psychoanalysis in the UK and led the independent group to uphold the importance of childhood development. In the decades since, whilst there are still theoretical differences between different psychoanalytic groups, they are more nuanced.

I always considered that Anna Freud was planning for families with secure attachments from her own experience, where Melanie Klein was addressing children already traumatised by insecure or disorganised attachments, which mirrored hers. Both women were geniuses and the ideas from both have percolated into almost all fields of child treatment regardless of theoretical background. Whilst having more in common, there have been different historical developments in the two key places. After Anna Freud's death in 1984, the Hampstead Clinic was renamed the Anna Freud Centre. Under the inspired Directorship of Professor Peter Fonagy, the situation at the Anna Freud centre is extremely different now, with trainings in time-limited mentalisation based treatment as well as a 16-week individual therapy protocol for mood disorder, Dynamic Interpersonal Therapy (DIT). Both of these have been the brainchildren of Fonagy, who developed the concepts of mentalisation as a way of highlighting key areas from emotional development and finding a way of aiding the process. These offer brilliantly condensed ideas from psychoanalysis into applicable templates for health service professionals, but they do not take the place of long-term work.

It was in 1948 that John Bowlby, the father of attachment theory, encouraged the start of The Tavistock Clinic Baby Observation course with child and adult psychoanalyst Martha Harris. Up until the 1960s, the Tavistock child training was theoretically independent but from the 1960s it became known as particularly following the theoretical influence of the psychoanalyst Melanie Klein. The Tavistock Clinic remains the largest National Health Service (free to the patient) training and treatment centre for child psychoanalytic psychotherapy in the UK. Although almost all child psychoanalytic psychotherapists then, and now, worked primarily for the National Health Service in child guidance clinics, hospitals, and schools (and rarely in private practice), there are still not enough paid trainee posts and whilst teaching costs are kept extremely low, personal psychoanalysis is required. Training grants have aided the opportunity for more diverse applicants as have attempts to engage black communities.

Other child psychoanalytic trainings in the UK had links with the Anna Freud or Tavistock. Dr. Margaret Lowenfeld (1890–1973) was a paediatrician, with Tavistock links, who became a child psychology and psychotherapy pioneer. She developed sand tray therapy as an approach to dealing with a traumatic event (Lowenfeld, 1935), which is used most for children although suitable for all ages. How children deal with toys in the sand trays aids assessment and treatment of traumatic experiences. Tragically, the Lowenfeld training was not accepted by the newly formed Association of Child Psychotherapists in the UK losing a lot of sandplay knowledge. However, it was further developed by Swiss Jungian psychoanalyst Dora Kalff (1904–1990) who also brought Jungian ideas and Buddhist practices into it. She also had consultations with Lowenfeld and Winnicott. Her seminal book Sandplay, *A Psychotherapeutic Approach to the Psyche* was republished in 2021, 30 years after its original appearance in German in 1966. In 1985, Kalff founded the International Society for Sandplay therapy.

A key concept behind sand tray therapy was that if the therapist provided a safe space the child could use the sand tray to help themselves solve their problems. Whilst other play therapy techniques provided small animals, drawing equipment, dolls and a regular room, sand tray therapy provided a tray or box filled with sand as well as miniature toys to create a world. Children choose toys and place them in the sand wherever they wish. The session follows the child in an unstructured way and when the sandplay picture/scene is complete they discuss it. The child might choose to rearrange its world picture after discussion with the therapist. Sandtray therapy is a combination of art therapy and play therapy and talking therapy. Adlerian play therapy (Kottman, 2011) also uses toys, art, drama, puppets, and roleplay. Adler saw all people as being creative beings who are subjective as well as socially embedded and goal directed.

The small group of pioneers were all interlinked, regardless of their varying theories, just as child trauma and adult trauma therapists are now. Indeed, just as disability psychotherapists from every theoretical model appreciate the intellectual support from each other because our subject is such an unwanted one, we trauma therapists are also grateful for each other's theoretical gifts and edited books (Sinason, 2022a, 2022b) contain a multitude of differing theoreticians. Additionally, as stated, all the major theoretical groupings learn from experience to update themselves. "Contemporary Freudian" is a term which freed up Freudian analysts to state that they were as concerned with the present as the past (Robinson & Schacter, 2020). The book shows how ideas from other theoretical groups were slowly enculturated as well as ideas that remained separate. At the same time, some Tavistock theoreticians called themselves "post-Kleinian" to indicate they incorporated later ideas from Meltzer and Bion (Sanders, 2001).

Relational psychoanalysis began in the USA and focuses on the real as well as imagined relationships in treatment. It began in the 1980s and sought to minimise power differential by accepting the relationship between the therapist and patient was a central real issue as well as a transferential one. Child relational psychoanalysis (Silber, 2015) has also tried to address the power imbalance between child and adult trainings as well as to find ways of aiding the parent-child relationship, working with triads as well as dyads.

A further new trauma-informed child psychodynamic approach and aid to the field of trauma has come from child neuropsychoanalysis. Dr. Allan Schore is known as "The American Bowlby" for the way he has integrated attachment theory with the findings of neuroscience. This fusion of attachment theory and neuroscience also unites many of the previously differing schools. John Bowlby worked at the Tavistock Clinic, where he co-created the child psychotherapy program yet some of the most major attachment research was conducted at the Anna Freud Centre.

Although Bowlby did not work with child abuse explicitly his paper "On knowing what you are not supposed to know and feeling what you are not supposed to feel" (Bowlby, 1979) aids everyone in the field of abuse. When he told Melanie Klein he was worried that a child he was treating and she was supervising would not be able to be helped unless he also saw her mother, Klein refused to allow it and the treatment broke down. He then took a sidestep in researching human attachment patterns and it is thanks to this and the work of those who followed him, such as Mary Main, that there is an exact science of attachment theory in which we now know that children with dissociative disorders have disorganised attachment presentations (Liotti, 2022; Sinason, 2002; Barach, 1991).

Underneath the history of conflicts, we can also see the rapprochements that have been made with the neuroscientific and neuropsychoanalytic work also linking with attachment theory (Panksepp & Solms, 2012). Solms (2012), Damasio (2012), and LeDoux (2012) also show how the mother-infant attachment relationship profoundly impacts on the baby's right brain whether positively or negatively. In the critical period for growth of the right brain relational trauma leads to disorganised attachment that leads to affect regulation problems (please see Chapter 4 for more information).

Infant and Family Psychoanalytic Psychotherapy

Psychoanalytic thinking from all the different theoretical models was struggling with the same issues. How could you best apply psychoanalytic understanding to the youngest? Whilst Klein wanted any work with a parent to be totally separate, John Bowlby wanted it to be combined. Anna Freud wanted to support the mothers of patients with the same therapist. That split had the creative long-term impact of leading to Bowlby's attachment research. It was Selma Fraiberg (1918–1981), Professor of Child Psychoanalysis at the University of California and University of Michigan, who was the American psychoanalyst and pioneer, who focused thinking on the emotional impact of trauma on babies and toddlers. "Ghosts in the Nursery" (Fraiberg et al., 1975) was her evocative way of speaking about "the visitors from the unremembered past of the parents, the uninvited guests at the Christening" (p. 387). Her work was underlined in a seminal 1982 paper that "catalysed a major paradigm shift in the fields of psychoanalysis and child development" (Moore, 2022). As a trained social worker as well as being a psychoanalyst, Fraiberg found a way of using home visits to assess what was needed and consider the way trauma might be passed on. During 1985 in the UK, Dilys Daws and Juliet Hopkins created an infant-parent workshop and in 1990, Stella Aquerone, a Tavistock child psychotherapist began the Parent-Infant private clinic in 1990. This clinic was the first to work psychoanalytically with mothers and babies with pre-autism. It was in the 1980s that I published a paper showing infantile defences (Sinason, 1988).

Composite Case Example

A loved baby was gently washed and wiped except for one shocking microsecond where the mother wiped his mouth roughly. He immediately had a falling reflex and screwed up his eyes and cried. Two weeks later, baby screwed up his eyes moments before his mouth was wiped, showing an awareness of timing and action. His legs became rigid, but he did not cry. At six weeks, the moment the towel touched his mouth he smiled. "It is amazing how he likes that," said mother, as if she recognised the aggression in the movement. By three months he grinned broadly.

This example showed what Selma Fraiberg called "transformation of affect," where the feeling was not bearable for the baby and a brilliant immediate defence transformed it. A shocking part of this, for me, was my inability at first to recognise the impact of one moment of micro-aggression from a loving mother. Becoming aware of this also allowed me to realise a counter transference experience of feeling sick when in the presence of a non-verbal tiny child who had experienced sexual abuse (Sinason, 1988). This was confirmed by the experiences of Caroline Okell Jones in the Tavistock Clinic's first sexual abuse workshop. Baby observation was the highlight for the child training for me. By observing a baby for the first two years of life we felt body-mind transferences that could not be learned theoretically alone.

What Does Trauma-Informed Mean?

In a heartfelt query from Freud in a letter to Fliess, titled "A new motto: What have they done to you, poor child?" (Freud, 1897, in an unpublished letter to Fliess), we see a trauma-informed question at the start of his work, however limited it was by the historical confines of the period. Instead of adding shame and blame by holding the patient guilty for their illness, the trauma-informed therapist is asking "What has happened to you?" or "what has been done to you?" This is not to deny the analytic work needed to disentangle internal destructive processes which have joined in with the traumatic invasion of toxic damage. Trauma-informed analytical work means the therapist cares about authenticity, safety, collaboration, honesty, and competence. There is no painting by numbers in this work. Each treatment is individual. These issues are an Esperanto for all trauma-informed work whatever the theoretical background of the therapist.

Dissociation, Complex PTSD and Dissociative Identity Disorder

Careful reporting of Dissociation in children and adults is not new. It was Professor Jean–Martin Charcot (1825–1893), the 19th century French neurologist, who first brought the concepts of hysteria and its symptoms of neurological damage and amnesia to public attention. He demonstrated that the psychological aetiology of hysteria was linked to trauma, as opposed to an organic aetiology. Although the young Freud came to watch his work at Salpetriere Hospital for four months as a neurologist in 1885, it was Professor Pierre Janet (1859–1947) who isolated and emphasised the process of "dissociation." Before both Freud and Jung, he saw trauma disconnecting the normal functions of memory, affect and knowledge. He showed that the traumatic memory was preserved in its dissociated state, set apart from ordinary consciousness.

With respect to children, in 1840 Antoine Despine, a French physician diagnosed DID in a child, Estelle (Sinason, 2022a, 2022b, p. 3), and expressed concerns that future generations "might not attend to their predecessors' original mistakes" (Fine, 1988, p. 38). It took until 1980 for the introduction of the diagnosis of PTSD in the American psychiatric association (DSM III, 1980), which was influenced by another war, more specifically the impact on veterans of the Vietnam war and the growth of the women's movement. It took a further decade for PTSD to be recognised in the World Health Organization's ICD 10 (International Classification of Diseases 10). In 1988, Dr. Judith Herman suggested a new diagnosis was needed, Complex PTSD, to describe the symptoms of long-term trauma. It has taken time for the utility of the diagnosis of CPTSD to be more accepted (Nestgaard & Schmidt, 2021), and while CPTSD now exists in the ICD, it continues to not be recognised in the DSM.

It was only in 1984 that pioneering child psychiatrist, family therapist, and adult psychoanalyst Arnon Bentovim started a child abuse workshop at the Tavistock Clinic which I joined, having worked with children with intellectual disabilities in the late 1970s who disclosed sexual abuse. Historically, we can see how long it has taken for the safety and dignity of children to be respected. For example, the U.K. signed the UN convention on the Rights of the Child in 1992, corporal punishment was prohibited in all state-supported education in 1986, and the prohibition was only extended to cover private schools in England and Wales in 1998, in Scotland in 2000, and in Northern Ireland in 2003. Looking at signs of trauma and dissociation in children was not helped by the slow progress to reduce "legal" attacks on children. Unfortunately, corporal punishment in the home is still allowed in the UK under the guise of "justifiable chastisement." It was only in 1995 in the UK that psychoanalysts Professors Peter Fonagy and Mary Target (1995) of the Anna Freud researched dissociation in children, Dr. Jo Russell (2015) provided the first Tavistock Professional Doctorate on the subject, Dr. Howard Steele and Professor Mark Solms provided clinical aid and 2002 that my first book on the subject appeared.

However, when we consider the emotional predicament of adults and then children who revealed sexual trauma before society and its representative professionals could hear it, we can start to comprehend the huge backlog of those who developed a dissociative disorder as a defence. The theories we use are the ones we find helped us understand. However, there are child-centred, relational, trauma-aware links between all our works.

Composite Clinical Examples

Peter, Aged 8

Peter was in a new foster home since his father had been imprisoned for physically and sexually abusing him and his mother, who had severe alcohol addiction and disappeared after the father was sentenced. Prior to this he had been regularly in and out of care depending on the stability of his parents. His foster parents knew the biological parents were alcoholics and struggled with severe mental health issues, but they had not been told of his abuse history prior to accepting him, only to realise from his violent masturbation and sexual language that he had far more adverse circumstances than had imagined. They had referred him out of concern for his flashbacks, volatility, heightened responses, or deep withdrawal. There was fear about his violence and sexual acting out. Although the foster-mother realised the violence came from a traumatised child, she felt at times she was in the presence of a dangerous adult and felt frightened. Additionally, it was the foster mother who raised the issue of dissociative identity disorder. She said he had a "boss" who made all kinds of orders and was a slave who obeyed. She felt quite ill when she heard the boss and did not know what to do. It is important to note that when an abusive parent goes to prison and a child feels safer, that symptoms of Complex PTSD or DID emerge. Providing support for the foster parents was crucial.

Having met with the foster parents first, I then had a meeting with Peter. He was a small thin boy with a frightened pale face and clenched fists. As his parents led him to my room he was muttering over and over in a terrified whisper, *"OK Boss, Sorry Boss. Sorry boss."* In my room, I had shared dolls and toys and drawing materials as well as a private box for Peter and his others filled with animal families, wild and tame, plasticine, farm fences, trains, etc. I introduced myself to Peter and asked if he could tell me his name.

Patient (whispering): "Peter." (He slapped himself round the face)
Therapist: "Ouch…Why did that happen and why are you whispering your name?"

My countertransference was shock in identification with Peter as a victim of a part of himself.

Patient (whispering): "Because I don't know if the Boss gives me permission to say my name"

Whilst some groups consider asking questions is intruding on the patient's unconscious, I consider traumatised children can be helped by a question that is on their side.

Therapist: "So you hit yourself before Boss did and were showing you didn't mean to go against him?"

Here I wanted to check out with the child that I had understood his actions properly. Checking that the motive and defence were accurately understood would make the child feel safer he was being actively listened to and thought about.

Patient (whispering): "Yes."
Therapist: "Gosh, that is difficult. That is clever of you to do that just in case. Shall I ask him? Then it won't be you in trouble"

I consider it crucial to accept the world the child inhabits and all his dissociative parts.

Patient: "OK."

He said this, in a normal voice, looking more cheerful. Peter was restored in the room with me because his narrative had been accepted and help was being offered in relating to the intimidating part of him.

Therapist: "He won't be cross with me mentioning you because he says everyone knows him"
Therapist: "Boss! Would you be so kind as to answer a question?"

There was a silence. Then he frowned and his face changed. His face looked a lot older and malevolent. Ignoring dissociative parts in children and adults in the hope they will then disappear leads to negative therapeutic relationships. Welcoming and including whoever appears reveals more about the internal system and the problems.

Therapist: "Don't know if a cunt like you deserves my time. I am very busy; Who the fuck are you anyway?"

He said this in an icy tone. Although only a child, Boss had all the hallmarks of the adult abuser he was modelled on and identified with. Peter looked terrified and held out his hands to me helplessly.

Therapist: "It is alright Peter. It was the boss swearing at me and not you."

I considered it important to treat the Boss with respect and not try to minimise his power.

Patient: *"Pathetic snivelling slave," said Boss to Peter.* Boss turned to face me with a malevolent expression that reminded me of Henry James's haunted little boy in "The Turn of the Screw."
Therapist: "Hello, I am Valerie. You can call me Valerie or Dr. Sinason and my job is to help children who are feeling sad."
Patient: "Sad! Wussy snivelling brats. What I only have to put up with!"
Therapist: "You have lots of angry words...Maybe it is hard to do your job because your job is a very big one." Responding with respect and concern for perpetrator-identified parts allows them to feel heard and start the process of relating and healing.
Patient: "That's right four-eyes," he said, alluding to my glasses but definitely thawed and smiling.

I consider it important to accept all language and insults in a solid way.

Therapist: "We wanted to make your job easier...I asked Peter what his name was and he doesn't know if you give him permission to speak to me."

Patient: "Good slave," said Boss. I considered it important not to be a threat to the hierarchy and be respectful of the internal roles in order to understand better.

Peter appeared for a moment with a wide smile which transformed his face.

Patient: "I give you permission to say anything you want today because you behaved like a proper slave and not a snivelling little wussy and I give you permission to talk to each other because then you might not be such a wuss."

There was a pause.

Therapist: "Thank you…What do I call you?"
Patient: "Boss of course. That is my only name."
Therapist: "And if I need to speak to you, is it alright to call you?"
Patient: *"Call all you like - no one will hear you unless I want to. Bye bitch." He disappeared from the face and body and tiny Peter was there.*
Patient: "Hello. My name is Peter."

This tiny excerpt is illustrative of various theoretical and clinical issues. I took Peter's fear seriously, but I also wanted Boss to feel he could make use of the session and say hello. Implicit in this was my theoretical knowledge that all states needed to be welcomed and had helped to protect Peter. Boss might sound frightening, but he was a child whose identification with an abuser had helped to save them all. I had also accepted initially the internal hierarchy in which Boss existed as part of his defences. The fact that Boss could be easily mollified also offered hope for the future. Just as a child can identify with the aggressor to survive, this is writ large with DID with the abuser internalised. The abuse from an attachment figure, such as the father, is too much to face or digest but can remain internally alive in a dissociated state.

Boss's comment that if I called no one would hear had a chilling impact and I felt it had come from a traumatic threat. Seeing live, on an eight-year-old body, the projected words and personality of an abuser also had an immediate counter transference effect on me as the therapist. The fact that Boss had an idea that therapy might make Peter brave was a systemic positive in which clearly, they both wanted to come and see me. During two years of therapy together, a baby and a little child state appeared, and Boss was able to keep his high place by showing leadership and looking after them as well as Peter.

In working in a trauma-informed way it is understood that everyone has a reason for how they are speaking and behaving. The task is to engage with all states to try and aid the making of meaning and reflection. With multiplicity we are often working, with children or adults, with victims and perpetrators within the same person. When the patient has lived in an environment of extreme violence with attachment figures, a behavioural response is only tackling the surface. Only when Boss could feel sad for himself as a victim of adult violence could he feel empathy for Slave. Additionally, his anger was needed to energise Peter. The fact that he was in a foster home aided the work as if he was still in an allegedly abusive home, a broken defence system could be more dangerous to him and his survival. Unfortunately, DID can be seen as a forensic condition in that whether intentionally or unintentionally, the condition means there has not been a safe attachment system and a child's needs have not been answered. Just as child analysis could only be developed after adult analysis, child work with DID and extreme trauma could only be developed after the specialist adult work on this subject such as Kluft (1984), Putnam (1997), and Ross et al. (1989).

Cathy, Aged 10

Cathy was referred by an educational psychologist. This was an important breakthrough as the school staff mainly belonged to the same unusual ultra-religious Christian group with esoteric rules of its own as her parents. There was concern about abuse and physical punishment as well as her fluctuating grades at school. Cathy was seen as capable of cognitive work to a high level when in the right mood but too often observed to be "in a daydream." She refused to change into her physical education outfit and would not go near the water for swimming lessons. Her parents finally accepted the referral because, "She is just a sinning girl despite all the religion we give her."

Cathy skipped into the assessment room, her blonde plaits bouncing and with a huge, exaggerated smile on her face.

Patient: "Ooops oops,"

she sang as she minced her way inside the room like a cabaret star.

Patient: "What a lovely day," she beamed, "Do you want me on the chair or on your lap." Her voice was full of sexual suggestion and initially shocking to me.

I processed that initial counter transference and transference shock. In the transference, I was being perceived as an adult who wanted her sexual attention. In the countertransference, I felt a sense of shock and disgust at the betrayal of such a young child. In working that through, I felt a deep compassion for her which sounded in my voice.

Therapist: "It sounds like you are good at looking after other people - but where do you want to be?"

She paused for a moment of real contact in which she struggled with her thoughts. She pulled up a chair near mine and looked at me seriously. Her face then changed, and she crossed her legs in a pornographic pose and seriously addressed me.

Patient: "I started my affair with my dad when I was 6. I was asking for it because I liked it."

To hear this young child speaking of an "affair" with her father, as if confiding adult to adult, meant another internal piece of processing to do. It mattered to avoid any shame and to keep her dignity and courage.

Therapist: "Isn't that clever of you to call it an affair, You really are a loyal daughter. You want to protect your daddy. Because an affair is what two grownups have when they have a private sexual relationship. Even if you asked your dad for it every day and even if you liked it, a grownup is not allowed to have sex with a child."

Her face fell. There was a pause. Her face changed into a sad and resigned one. She crossed herself.

Patient: "Hello. I suppose you just saw Cathy. She is going to hell for doing disgusting things. I am praying for her. My name is Mary."

At a moment of connection in which her responsibility for an alleged "affair" was raised, a defence was needed and another state of mind, alter, or part was needed.

Therapist: "Hello Mary- it is very sad what Cathy seems to be doing. It must be worrying for you to see."

Again, in trauma-informed work it is crucial to welcome and accept all parts and realise they are there to help the child survive.

Patient: "Yes. And I tell Jesus she can't help it and I try to stop her, but I seem to disappear."
Therapist: "That is really kind of you to realise she can't help it and to tell Jesus too. And you are doing your best, but you disappear."
Patient: "Yes."

She lowered her head and whispered,

Patient: "I went to Church on Sunday but just as it was my turn to go to confession I disappeared. Does that mean I am a witch, that I am evil?"
Therapist: "How horrid for you to worry that you are a witch, but disappearing is complicated. Do you know, I think it meant you were feeling very loyal to Cathy, and you didn't really want to tell the priest what she had done."

There was a pause. Her face changed.

Patient: "I am the Lord. I am God. I am the Judge. I decide," shouted a furious voice.
Therapist: "Oh,"I was just talking to Mary."
Patient: "And you have no right to talk to Mary without me saying so. Everything comes through me. I am the ruler, the leader." This personality wanted no comment from me and continued shouting its power. Suddenly the face transformed into its beaming smile and Cathy was back. She investigated the therapy box.
Patient: "Oooh- a secret box just for me and you. No handcuffs, no dildo. Do you know what that is? I could make you very happy. And look at the baby dogs - and they wag their tails after they have sex. They are so sweet."

She crossed and uncrossed her legs.

Patient: "I could make you very happy,"

She licked her lips suggestively.

Patient: "What do you really like? I can do it. Are you too shy to say? Don't worry about being old. I can make you feel wonderful."

I said it must be very strange to be with someone who did not need her to look after them or be sexy.

Patient: "Don't you want me? Then I will get into trouble. I have done it wrong."

Her face looked desperate. I took some paper from a shelf and started drawing a pattern.

Therapist: "How would you like to draw a pattern with me. We can colour it in any colours." She started to reach for a felt-tip and then her face changed, and Mary was there.
Patient: "*I like drawing,*" she said approvingly. After she drew a little, she looked up at me.
Patient: "*It isn't really Cathy's fault. You see.*" I leaned forward slightly. Her whole demeanour changed.
Patient: "I Am GOD, the God of your Fathers. I don't give permission."

I felt hopeful for Cathy and her parts after the first meeting despite my concerns that they could be living in an abusive home. If it was her actual father who was abusing her, then social services needing an extra warning. Cathy had found a way of blaming herself that allowed her to feel in control. Fairbairn called this a "moral" defence (1952). She only had to be good and do what the grownups wanted and then the bad thing would not happen again. However, the sexual defence to accommodate the abuse and "like" it was also unbearable to herself and it was Mary who could remind her of a boundary that had been crossed with a harsh God to demand obedience to equal the obedience she had shown her abuser. Again, it mattered to offer space to anyone who wanted to come and to be aware that difficult circumstances had shaped their existence. In all the clinical extracts I have provided all my theoretical understanding from my trainings, Freud, Klein, Anna Freud, Bowlby, Winnicott was there to be drawn from. However, I also had help from more recent wisdom. Judith Herman (1992), as well as van der Hart et al. (2006) are amongst those who added the theoretical trauma-work concept of three stages of recovery, safety, memory, reconnecting, and processing. Most child workers in the field have made use of this theoretically (Sinason & Potgieter Marks, 2021). However, the point of this understanding (as with Klein's paranoid schizoid and depressive condition) is that the three stages do not form a tidy developmental move and oscillations occur between all of them. The longing for rigid applications can intrude on the growth of the therapy relationship. However good a theory is, it is being utilised by fallible humans!

Conclusion

It was an American paediatrician, Professor Henry Kempe, from Denver Children's Hospital, who was the pioneer who named the bruises and damage on children's bodies nearly four decades ago. What was previously seen as clumsiness could now be named and The Battered Child Syndrome (Kempe & Silverman, 1985) transformed awareness. This was not a discovery that came from child psychotherapy, but psychoanalytic child therapy provided some of the tools that could make a difference. In the 1970s, at the largest training and treatment place for child and adult psychoanalytic psychotherapists in the UK, the Tavistock Clinic, there were a few years where only three child psychotherapists were considered to have ever worked with a patient with a definite abuse history. It was considered to be extremely rare. Masson (1988), Alice Miller (1983), and others struggled with their own psychoanalytic allegiance because "…each (therapy) shows a lack of interest in physical and sexual abuse" (Masson, 1988, p. 285) Psychoanalysis can give us the tools to understand our own professional and personal dissociation but cannot ensure we each make use of them. Psychoanalysts Elizabeth Howell and Sheldon Itzkowitz (2022) provide the most substantial understanding of all the contemporary theoretical models that come from psychoanalysis, however, as they state in their introduction, "A most remarkable thing about psychoanalysis is its checkered response to trauma-generated dissociation. Now one "sees" it, and now one doesn't. Why can it not be recognised? Why does it disappear from "sight" or thought?" (p. 7). Unlike war or geographical disasters, sexual abuse is often committed with no-one present except the victim and the perpetrator. Where there are emotional links to the perpetrator through familial abuse it becomes even harder to speak. Abuse plus dissociation brings up legal fears as well. DID is a forensic condition in a child showing that whether intentionally or unintentionally a child has been hurt. Waters's Star Theoretical Model (2022) and Silberg (2021), Young (2022), Silberg and Kluft (1996), and others point to different theoretical models when dealing with extreme organised abuse of children (please see Chapter 45).

Nevertheless, the development of trauma-informed child psychoanalytic psychotherapy for complex PTSD and DID is making its impact. However, much we are each inevitably part of a historical not-knowing or not-wanting-to-know, we realise we are passing on hurt. All professions have let down traumatised children who have suffered from abuse but perhaps because of our wish to face societal and internal truths, we feel more guilt about it. The new look psychoanalysis does not cover all psychoanalysts; however, it gratefully links with the creative arts and energy therapies and its 120 years of history. It is still only in its infancy. As the eminent psycho-historian Lloyd de Mause (1974) commented

The history of childhood is a nightmare from which we have only recently begun to awaken. The further back in history one goes, the lower the level of childcare, and the more likely children are to be killed, abandoned, beaten, terrorized, and sexually abused.

References

Arthur, A. R. (2001). Personality, epistemology and psychotherapists' choice of theoretical model: A review and analysis. *European Journal of Psychotherapy, Counselling and Health, 4*(1), 45–64.

Barach, P. M. (1991). Multiple personality disorder as an attachment disorder. *Dissociation, 4*(3), 117–123.

Bowlby, J. (1979). On knowing what you are not supposed to know and feeling what you are not supposed to feel. *Canadian Journal of Psychiatry, 24*(5), 403–408.

Breuer, J., & Freud, S. (1893). On the psychical mechanism of hysterical phenomena. *The Standard Edition of the Complete Psychological Works of Sigmund Freud, 2*(1893–1895), 1–17.

Damasio, A. R. (2012). Neuroscience and psychoanalysis: A natural alliance. *Psychoanalytic Review, 99*, 591–594.

De Mause, L. (1974). *The history of childhood*. Souvenir Press.

Fairbairn, R. (1952). *Psychoanalytic studies of the personality*. Routledge.

Ferenczi, S. (1933). The passions of adults and their influence on the sexual character development of children. *International Journal of Psychoanalysis, 19*, 5–15.

Fine, C. G. (1988). The work of Antoine Despine. The first scientific reports on the diagnoses and treatment of a child with multiple personality disorder. *American Journal of Clinical Hypnosis, 31*(1), 33–39.

Fonagy, P., & Target, M. (1995). Dissociation and trauma current opinion. *Psychiatry, 8*, 161–166.

Fraiberg, S., Adelson, E., & Shapiro, V. (1975). Ghosts in the nursery: A psychoanalytic approach to the problems of impaired infant-mother relationships. *Journal of American Academy of Child Psychiatry, 14*(3), 387–421.

Freud, S. (1896). The aetiology of hysteria. *The Standard Edition of the Complete Psychological Works of Sigmund Freud, 3*, 187–221.

Freud, S. (1897). *Letter from Freud to Fliess Sept 21, 1897, the complete letters of Sigmund Freud to Wilhelm Fliess, 1887–1904*. Psychoanalytic Electronic Publishing.

Freud, S. (1905). Three Essays on the Theory of Sexuality. The Standard Edition of the Complete Psychological Works of Sigmund Freud, Volume VII (1901–1905): A Case of Hysteria, Three Essays on Sexuality and Other Works, pp. 123–246.

Freud, S. (1909). Analysis of a phobia of a five year old boy. In James Strachey (Ed.), *The Pelican Freud library (1977), Vol 8, case histories 1*, (pp. 169–306). Hogarth Press.

Freud, S. (1915). Thoughts for the times on war and death. *SE, 14*, 275–301.

Freud, S. (1963). Introductory lectures on psycho-analysis (part III). In J. Strachey (Trans.), *The standard edition of the complete psychological works of Sigmund Freud volume XVI (1916–1917): Introductory lectures on psycho-analysis (part III)* (p. 275). The Hogarth Press and the Institute of Psycho-Analysis.

Herman, J. (1992). *Trauma and recovery*. Basic Books.

Howell, E. F., & Itzkowitz, S. (2022). The unconscionable in the unconscious: The evolution of relationality in the conceptualization of the treatment of trauma and dissociation. In Martin J. Dorahy, Steven N. Gold, and John A. O'Neil (Eds.) *Dissociation and the dissociative disorders* (pp. 728–745). Routledge.

Kempe, C. H., & Silverman, F. (1985). The battered child syndrome. *Child Abuse and Neglect, 9*, 143–154.

King, P., Steiner, R., & Tuckett, D., (Eds.). (1991). *The Freud Klein: Controversies: 1941–45*. Routledge.

Kluft, R. P. (1984). Aspects of the treatment of multiple personality disorder. *Psychiatric Annals, 14*, 51–55.

Kluft, R. P. (2018). Freud's rejection of Hypnosis, Part 11: The Perpetuation of a rift. *American Journal of Clinical Hypnosis, 60*(4), 324–347.

Kottman, T. (2011). Adlerian play therapy. In C. E. Schaefer's (Ed.), *Foundations of play therapy* (pp. 87–104). John Wiley & Sons Inc.

LeDoux, J. (2012). Afterword. *Psychoanalytic Review, 99*, 591–594.

Liotti, G. (2022). Infant attachment and dissociative psychopathology, chapter 2. In V. Sinason & R. Potgieter-Marks (Eds.), *Treating children with dissociative disorders* (pp. 10–26). Routledge.

Lowenfeld, M. (1935). *Play in childhood; with a foreword by John Davis*. Cambridge University Press 1991 Originally Published in 1935.

Malvern, N., & Leff, J. R. (2011). *The Anna Freud Tradition: Lines of development-evolution of theory and practice over the decades*. Routledge.

Masson, J. (1988). *Against therapy; emotional tyranny and the myth of psychological healing*. Common Courage Press USA.

Miller, A. (1983). *Thou shalt not be aware: Society's betrayal of the child*. Farrar Straus Giroux.

Moore, M. S. (2022). The importance of attachment in the presence of a perceived threat chapter 3. In V. Sinason & R. Potgieter-Marks (Eds.), *Treating children with dissociative disorders: Attachment, trauma, theory and practice*. Routledge.

Nestgaard Rød, Å., & Schmidt, C. (2021). Complex PTSD: What is the clinical utility of the diagnosis? *European Journal of Psychotraumatology, 12*(1), 2002028.

Panksepp, J., & Solms, M. (2012). What is neuropsychoanalysis? Clinically relevant studies of the minded brain. *Trends in Cognitive Sciences, 16*(1), 6–8.

Putnam, F. W. (1997). *Dissociation in children and adults: A developmental perspective*. Guildford Press.

Robinson, K., & Schacter, J. (2020). *The contemporary Freudian tradition; past and present*. Routledge.

Ross, C. (1989). *Multiple personality disorder*. Wiley.

Russell, J. (May 2015). Dissociative Identities in Children: An exploration of how children with dissociative identities may present in psychotherapy. Are there implications for psychoanalytic technique. Professional Doctorate in Child and Adolescent Psychotherapy, University of East London.

Sanders, K. (2001). *Post-Kleinian psychoanalysis*. The Biella Seminars, Routledge.

Silber, L. (2015) A view from the margins: Children in relational psychoanalysis. *Journal of Infant, Child and Adolescent Psychotherapy, 14*(4), 345–362.

Silberg, J. L. (2021). *The child survivor: Healing developmental trauma and dissociation*. Routledge.

Silberg, J. L., & Kluft, R. P. (1996). *The dissociative child: Diagnosis, treatment, and management*. Sidran Press.

Sinason, V. (1988). Smiling, swallowing, sickening and stupefying: The effect of sexual abuse on the child. *Psychoanalytic Psychotherapy, 3*(2), 97–111.

Sinason, V. (Ed.). (2002). *Attachment, trauma and multiplicity*. Routledge.

Sinason, V. (2022a). Introduction in treating children with dissociative disorders. In V. Sinason & R. Potgieter-Marks (Eds.), *Treating children with dissociative disorders: Attachment, trauma, theory and practice* (pp. 1–6). Routledge.

Sinason, V. (2022b). *The truth about trauma and dissociation; everything you didn't want to know and were afraid to ask*. London: Confer Books.

Sinason, V., & Potgieter Marks, R. (2021). *Treating children with dissociative disorders*. Routledge.

Solms, M. (1999). Dreaming and REM sleep are controlled by different brain mechanisms. Annual Meeting of the American Academy for the Advancement of Science, Anaheim, CA, 25 March 1999.

Solms, M. (2012). Are Freud's 'erogenous zones' sources or objects of libidinal drive? *Neuropsychoanalysis, 14*, 53–56.

Solms, M. (2018a). The neurobiological underpinnings of psychoanalytic theory and therapy. *Behavioral Neuroscience, 12*, 294.

Solms, M. (2018b). The scientific standing of psychoanalysis. *BJPsych International, 15*(1), 5–8.

van der Hart, O., Nijenhuis, R. S., & Steele, K. (2006). *The haunted self: Structural dissociation and the treatment of chronic traumatisation*. W.W. Norton.

Young, E. (2022). I didn't know where you were: In the play space of treatment with a young dissociative boy in treating children with dissociative disorders. In V. Sinason & R. Potgeiter Marks (Eds.), *Treating children with dissociative disorders: Attachment, trauma, theory and practice* (pp. 180–197). Routledge.

Waddell, M., & Kraemar, S. (2021). *The tavistock century*. Phoenix.

Waters, F. (2022). The star theoretical model: An integrative model for assessing and treating childhood dissociation in treating children with dissociative disorders. In V. Sinason & R. Potgeiter Marks (Eds.), *Treating children with dissociative disorders: Attachment, trauma, theory and practice* (pp. 73–97). Routledge.

18
DYADIC DEVELOPMENTAL PSYCHOTHERAPY

Kim S. Golding

Introduction

DDP is a relationship-based model of intervention for children who have experienced trauma and loss (Hughes et al., 2019). These children live in a range of kin or non-kin families or residential homes. This is a population of children who have experienced multiple and chronic exposure to adverse experiences. These experiences largely occurred within their birth families, beginning early in life and impacting their development across seven domains of impairment: attachment, biological, affect regulation, dissociation, behavior control, cognition, and self-concept (Cook et al., 2005). This is trauma where the closest relationships that should offer protection and comfort in traumatic situations are the same relationships from which the trauma originates. This has been described as developmental trauma to distinguish it from other forms of complex trauma (van der Kolk, 2005).

Children who experience developmental trauma typically develop insecure and disorganized patterns of attachment (see the chapter in this volume on traumatic attachment). These are children who have learned to fear being parented. These difficulties move with them into new families where children are offered attuned and nurturing care. Hughes and Baylin (2012) explored how these difficulties lead to blocked trust in the children and blocked care in the adults parenting them.

Blocked trust describes a state in which children react defensively to offers of emotional connection in relationships (Baylin & Hughes, 2016). The children move into defensive nervous system states of sympathetic mobilization or dorsal vagal immobilization rather than social engagement, as described in polyvagal theory (see the chapter in this volume on polyvagal theory). These children cannot enter reciprocal, intersubjective relationships within which they are open both to influencing and being influenced by another (Trevarthen, 2016).

The child's blocked trust can lead to parental blocked care. This is a neuropsychological state in response to the lack of reciprocity from the child, leading to a shutting down of the caregiving systems. Parenting becomes joyless (Hughes & Baylin, 2012).

DDP interventions offer the children and parents new, healthy relational experiences, which help children and parents feel safe enough to move out of defensive states and be comfortable with social engagement. As the children begin to feel safe within relationships, they start to explore the stories of their experience, both current and past. As they process and integrate these experiences, they learn about themselves and others without the shame and terror associated with their past relationship experience. They develop a coherent, autobiographical narrative of themselves and their experience,

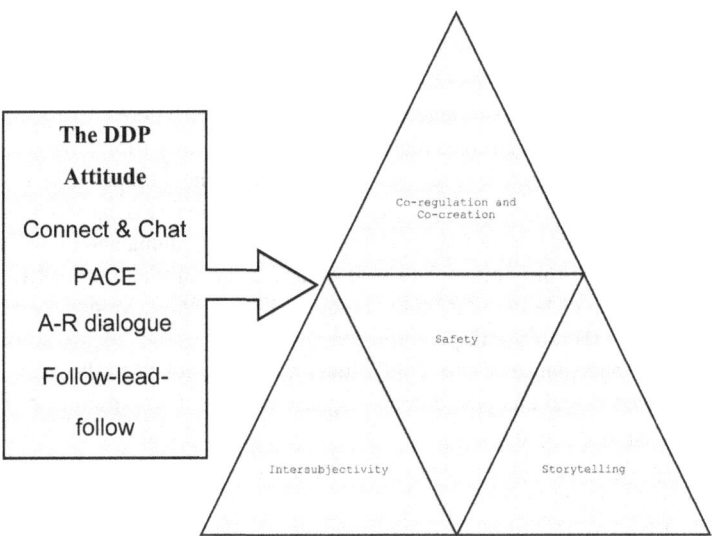

Figure 18.1 DDP Attitude and Principles.

which holds hope for who they are and who they can become. Their development can progress based on this new sense of self and safety with others.

DDP: Principles, Attitude, and Practice

DDP interventions follow a set of principles achieved by the therapist holding a way of being: *the DDP attitude* (see Figure 18.1). These interventions are embedded within a practice model, illustrated in Figure 18.2. These are described more fully in Hughes and colleagues (2019) and Hughes and Golding (2024).

DDP is a relationship-based model of intervention offering a high level of *safety* for children who have experienced developmental trauma, a form of complex trauma. The DDP therapist works closely with the current adoptive, foster, kin, or residential parents to provide the child with dyadic experiences of relationships (therapist to child, parent(s) to child) that are different from their past experience. These relationships are *intersubjective*, helping children overcome their fear of emotional connection.

While the goal of DDP interventions is to achieve therapeutic change, this is held in the background. DDP privileges the importance of safety, unconditionality, and reciprocity in relationships. This provides the child with a high level of *co-regulation* of their emotional experience, allowing them to move deeper into their experience.

The experience of the relationship is carried through the *storytelling* that is a central part of DDP. This is a process of *co-creation*, within which the intersubjective emotional connections between the child, parent(s), and therapist facilitate healing conversations about the child's current and past experiences. This allows the child to experience themselves differently, and with less shame, as they witness themselves safely held in the hearts and minds of the therapist and parent(s).

As the child experiences current relationships as different from past relationships, they form a healthier and more integrated sense of self and a more coherent autobiographical narrative. This leads to increased attachment security. The child's nervous system can adjust to a safer world of social engagement, and new developmental possibilities open up.

The DDP therapist achieves this through holding the DDP attitude or way of being, which consists of these approaches:

- **Connect and chat**: The child experiences the therapist's deep interest in them, not just in the difficulties that have brought them into therapy. This offers an intersubjective relationship within which the child shares stories of their recent experience with the therapist. The rhythm and storytelling tone set during periods of "connect and chat" on light themes is carried over into conversations on more tricky themes related to experiences of complex trauma and dissociation.
- **PACE**: An acronym describing playfulness, acceptance, curiosity and empathy, which together form an attitude or way of being that builds emotional connection. Modeled on healthy parent-infant interactions, the therapist and parent(s) playfully convey their joy and interest in the child with a high level of acceptance of the child's inner world, curiosity to discover and understand this world more deeply, and empathy for this experience. PACE communicates deep interest in the child, their inner world and experiences, and empathy for the struggles that their experience brings. This helps the therapist and parent(s) sit with the child in their experience, even though this can feel deeply uncomfortable for the adults.
- **Affective-Reflective (A-R) dialogue**: The conversations that emerge have both affective and reflective components, as with the telling of any good story. These narratives of experience avoid sole reliance on the catharsis of affect or the intellectualization of cognitive reflection. Instead, affect and reflection are brought together to increase understanding and deepen the emotional experience.
- **Follow-lead-follow:** The dyadic storytelling process involves the therapist following the child's themes, and then leading them into deeper affective understanding of the experience being described. Alongside this, the therapist also leads with themes and connections to the child's life, and then follows the child's response to these. In this way, the therapist finds a balance between being directive and non-directive as a pattern of follow-lead-follow emerges. This sets a rhythm for the telling, which allows the story to emerge.
- **Interactive repair:** Ruptures in the relationship are attended to by the therapist so that the connection between them and the child is maintained.
- **Speaking with, for, and about the child:** The therapist helps the child communicate their experience in a range of ways. When the child struggles to find the words or needs a break from "talking with" the therapist, they can be supported by "talking for" them, based on their previous verbal and non-verbal communications. As the therapist talks in the child's voice, they check in with them to see if they are getting it right or if they are missing anything. The child experiences their story deeply and affectively, aided by the therapist's voice prosody. When the child is moving out of their window of tolerance, either toward dysregulation or dissociation, "talking about" them can assist. This allows them to witness their story being told and helps the child stay emotionally regulated and able to participate in the storytelling again when they are ready.
- Throughout this, the therapist is facilitating communication between the child and their parent(s) in a way that helps the parent(s) respond with PACE. The therapist talks with, for, and about the child in a way that ultimately allows parent(s) and child to talk together.

These same DDP principles and attitude are used when working with the parents. An important part of the DDP model is helping the parents understand their own experience, including any trauma, which can impact their relationship with the child. The therapist explores this before bringing the child into the work. This allows the parent to safely join the child's therapy and also gives them an experience of the model as it will be used with the child.

The parental and dyadic work are embedded in a process of dyadic developmental practice (see Figure 18.2), which also embraces parenting and network support. This helps the parents be

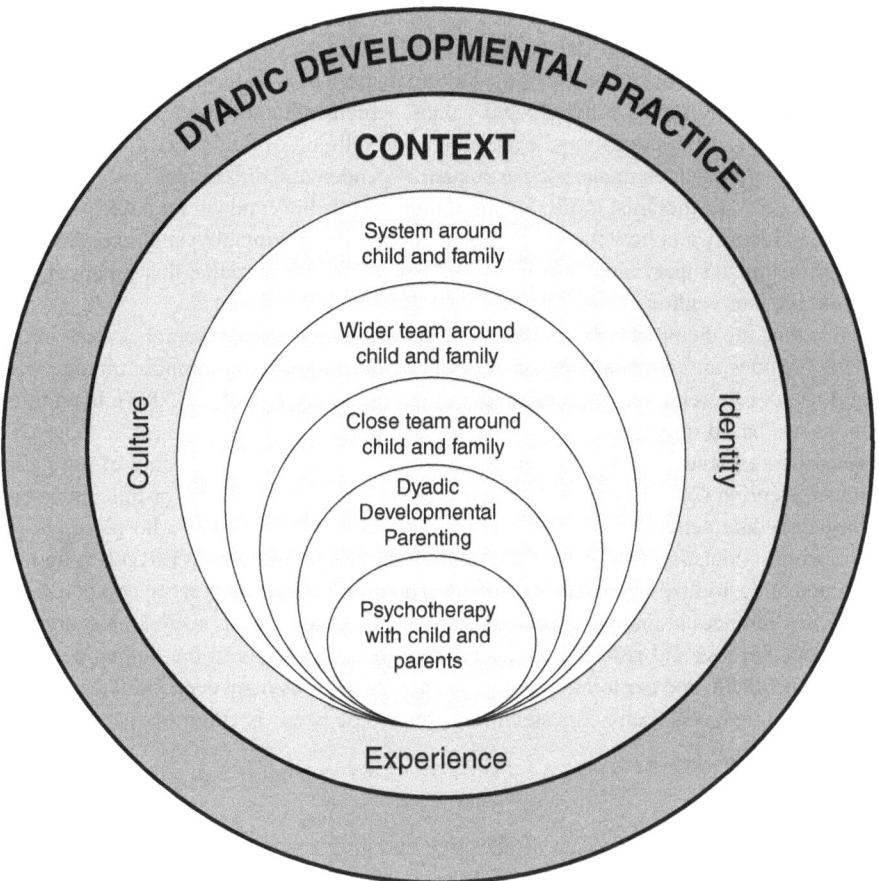

Figure 18.2 DDP Practice Model.

Adapted from Healing Relational Trauma with Attachment-Focused Interventions by Daniel A. Hughes, Kim S. Golding, and Julie Hudson. Copyright 2019 by Daniel A. Hughes, Kim S. Golding, and Julie Hudson. Used by permission of W. W. Norton & Company, Inc.

DDP-informed in their parenting, and their networks to support the family while aligned with the principles of DDP. This is an important part of DDP interventions whether or not psychotherapy with the child is indicated. Hughes and colleagues (2019) and Hughes and Golding (2024) explore parenting and network support in greater detail.

Understanding the context within which DDP interventions are provided is also an important part of the practice model, explored further in the next section.

DDP in the Global World: Working with Culture, Experience, and Identity

As we have been exploring, DDP is a model that aims to help the child heal—supported by their current parent(s)—from developmental trauma through increasingly secure attachment relationships, increasing safety in intersubjective emotional connection, and discovering stories that transform the child's sense of self and open up new developmental possibilities.

The DDP therapist carries out this work adapted to the unique needs of the child and family. In order to do this, they need to understand and work within the context the family brings. As illustrated in the practice model (Figure 18.2), the culture, experience, and identity of the family informs an understanding of the family's beliefs and values, which influence the DDP interventions. This includes the heritage, class, educational experience, and religion of family members, alongside their unique identity-comprising elements such as sexuality, gender, and differences in ability, neurodevelopment, and health. The therapist is also aware of their own beliefs and values based on their culture, experience, and identity and how this might impact the curiosity, empathy, and acceptance they hold for the family. Clinical supervision is an important part of making sure that this enhances rather than detracts from the interventions being offered.

Alongside this, the therapist holds in their awareness the theory and research underlying the DDP model. This includes an understanding of developmental trauma as a complex trauma, which features high levels of dysregulation and dissociation in children (Cook et al., 2005). In addition, DDP interventions are based on psychological theories and models of attachment, intersubjectivity, and interpersonal neuroscience. These have emerged from a Western understanding of psychology and neuroscience. Henrich (2021) reminded us that the research and evidence for this understanding is largely based on data generated from Western middle-class participants—who represent less than 12% of the world population (Arnett, 2008). Henrich described how this WEIRD (Western, middle-class, educated, industrialized, rich, and democratic) population is unusual when compared with other cultures, with differences in many cognitive and social processes such as spatial reasoning, attention, and ideas about fairness and risk-taking. There are universal aspects in the human need for social connection, attachment, and exploration witnessed across cultures. However, DDP therapists need to keep in mind that the social behaviors stemming from these needs is culturally patterned (Harwood et al., 1995).

For example:

- We can understand the importance of sensitive caregiving while also remaining curious about how sensitivity is demonstrated within the cultures of the families we work with. This requires us to move beyond a dyadic perspective of attachment and also consider extended family, kinship network, culture, and community (Fejo-King, 2017).
- Context and culture determine how exploration is encouraged or discouraged. The Aché Indians of Paraguay maintain safety by carrying their infants until they are two years old, avoiding contact with the ground and its inherent dangers of fire and wild animals (Keller, 2022).
- Parenting socializes infants to fit into the cultural societies they are growing up in. For example, from a few weeks of age, Japanese babies show less emotion than European babies (Keller, 2022).

DDP therapists provide interventions in many countries globally, and live and work in multicultural environments. Acceptance and curiosity are essential so that interventions can be adapted to the culture, experience, and identity of the family.

One of the strengths of the DDP model is its emphasis on storytelling within relationships. Storytelling is a human universal. Cultures across the world tell stories to teach, model, share experiences, and heal. For example, the Indigenous peoples of Canada, the United States, Australia, and New Zealand share healing stories together. Atkinson (2002) described a ceremonial process called "Dadirri" within Australian Aboriginal culture, which provides deep listening as part of the healing of loss and trauma.

Following these traditions, DDP is a collaborative model within which the therapist discovers and co-creates with the family the story or narrative of their experience. These stories are witnessed and told within intersubjective relationships, allowing an affective-reflective deepening of experience.

It is not the facts of the story that are important. The family member can tell as much or as little of what happened as is comfortable and known. More important is the experience of what happened and the impact on their sense of self. If the DDP therapist notices there are gaps in the story the child expresses, the therapist accepts these apparent omissions and expresses curiosity about them, safely inviting the child to include them in the expressed story being developed. Trauma stories can be rigid and fragmented, and hold meaning given to the child by those abusing or neglecting them. The intersubjective sharing of these stories leads to a co-creative process of discovery. From this, new narratives of connection, strength, and resilience emerge (Hughes et al., 2019).

Through this intersubjective process of storytelling, the therapist gains a deeper understanding of the experience of the developmental trauma. This understanding is embedded in the context the family brings in terms of their values, identity, and experience, including culture, heritage, sexuality, gender, class, religion, disability, and neurodiversity. DDP's storytelling approach helps the therapist work with the family based on an understanding of the family's experience, values, and hopes for their child.

DDP and Developmental Stages

This section illustrates DDP interventions with children at different developmental stages through fictional and composite examples of families. These examples demonstrate DDP in action via description and dialogue illustrating the work with the parent(s) and psychotherapy with the parent(s) and child. These additionally demonstrate how the DDP therapist explores the context for the work. This includes understanding the values and beliefs of the family and takes these into account when adapting interventions for the unique needs of the family (Figure 18.3).[1]

DDP Intervention with Parents of a Preschool Child

Wren is a developmentally immature 20-month-old toddler who is small for his age. His adoptive parent Jessie has asked DDP therapist Adele to visit because of concerns he and his partner, Kit, have about Wren's development and his lack of connection with them. On her first visit, Wren shows little interest in or wariness of Adele, a stranger in his home. He is holding and mouthing the toys in front of him with apparent disinterest. There is no joy in play. When Jessie moves to pick him up, Wren freezes momentarily but makes no protest. He sits passively on Jessie's lap, neither fussing nor

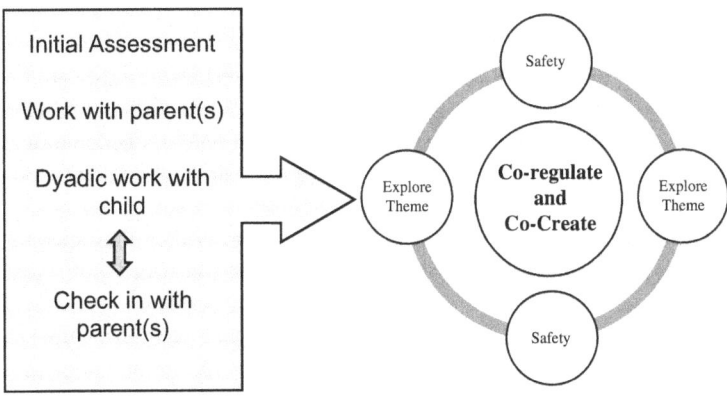

Figure 18.3 DDP Process.

connecting as Adele and Jessie continue to talk together. When Adele offers Wren a toy, he takes it without looking at her.

Jessie talks of how little response they get from Wren. He sleeps for up to four or five hours a day as well as at night. When not asleep, he sometimes curls up in a ball pressed against the wall. They often notice him freeze, appearing "zoned out." A pediatrician has been consulted and has recommended trauma-based intervention to reduce these dissociative behaviors.

Wren was removed from his birth family when he was eight months old. This followed concerns about unexplained injuries and the adequacy of parental care. Wren's parents had received social work interventions to address physical and emotional neglect, but any changes they made were short-lived. Wren was placed in foster care with Jessie and Kit. Following court proceedings, a decision was made to find an adoptive family for Wren. Jessie and Kit applied to adopt him, and after a prolonged period of assessment, this was agreed. Jessie and Kit believe that this assessment was long because of concerns about them being a gay, cisgender couple. They had to strongly advocate for being the best family, with the added advantage of avoiding a further move for Wren.

Jessie is the primary carer, supported by Kit, who has a job requiring long hours out of the home. During Adele's DDP intervention with the family, she mainly works with Jessie, although Kit always joins for reviews and is committed to helping in any way he can.

Adele begins DDP by observing and video recording Jessie and Wren playing together. They sit on the floor, and Jessie tries to engage Wren with some soft toys Adele has supplied. Wren shows interest in the toys, although there is little connection with Jessie. There is no eye contact. When Jessie jumps the tiger toy toward Wren, he briefly giggles and then turns away, burying his head in the cushion behind him. This happens several times, and each time Jessie responds by becoming more animated in an effort to draw Wren into playing with him, but this appears to overwhelm Wren. At the end of the play session, Jessie is despondent and clearly feels a sense of failure.

The following aims for the work are agreed:

1 Build trust and safety. Jessie needs to experience Adele as non-judgmental and interested in working collaboratively with him.
2 Explore Jessie's experience of being a parent to Wren, and the impact of Wren's behaviors and emotional disconnection on him. It is anticipated that this might also involve exploring Jessie's attachment history.
3 Explore and understand the trauma that Wren has experienced and the impact that this has had on him emotionally and behaviorally.
4 Explore different ways of parenting Wren, which will increase his emotional connection and reduce his dissociative behaviors.

Adele spends time getting to know Jessie and developing a therapeutic relationship. This includes talking about being a gay parent in a largely heterosexual world of adoption and what it is like to work with Adele, a heterosexual, cisgender woman. Adele acknowledges heteronormative biases in her view of the world and invites discussion if they notice these arising, while accepting that this is a challenging ask of Jessie.

As Adele and Jessie start to feel safe and comfortable with each other, they spend time watching and discussing the video recording of Jessie and Wren playing, as illustrated in this dialogue:

Adele: Do you see how Wren is responding to the tiger toy? What's your sense of what is happening there?
Jessie: Well, he seems to like the toy, but he's turning away from me. I don't know what I'm doing wrong, but he doesn't want to play with me.

Adele: Oh, Jessie that's hard. You're really noticing Wren turning away and not wanting to play with you. I'd like to think about what is going on for Wren, but first, would it be okay if we spend some time thinking about you and how Wren leaves you feeling?

Jessie: Well, I guess so. I'd like to know what you think is happening for Wren, but you did warn me that you'll be slowing me down. I guess this is one of those moments.

Adele: Yes, in DDP we talk about "slowing down to get there quicker." I do believe that in understanding your responses more deeply it will be easier for us to wonder about Wren. I guess I'm asking you to trust me on this.

Jessie: Okay, in for a penny in for a pound! What would you like to know?

Adele: Thank you, I do appreciate your trust. You noticed Wren turning away from you and you immediately sensed that you were doing something wrong, which meant he didn't want to play with you.

Jessie: Well, yes, I can see it on the recording.

Adele: Tell me more. What were you feeling at the moment you experienced Wren as not wanting to play with you?

Jessie: [after a long pause] Well, I think I felt anxious. I was very aware of you watching. I was wondering what you would think. I guess I was worried that you would see how rubbish I was.

Adele: Oh, Jessie, no wonder you felt anxious if you experienced me as judging you. I'm sorry, parenting while you are being recorded is no easy task. I'm guessing that feeling rubbish is a familiar feeling for you. Would you mind if we focused on that for a bit?

Jessie: Well, Wren certainly makes me feel rubbish. We made a big commitment to him when we adopted him. I'm really worried that we won't get this right for him.

Adele: Okay, such a big commitment, and I know that you felt that the social worker was not fully supportive of your application to adopt.

Jessie: Yes, we worked hard to convince her. She wanted a more "conventional" family for Wren. It did feel quite homophobic at times. We did work through it, and I think she supported us in the end. It is tough, though, like I feel I have to prove something to her.

Adele: Yes, I get that, and when Wren is not responding to you, I imagine you think of her and what she would think if she could see you.

Jessie: You've got it. There is always that nagging worry of not being good enough. You get approved to adopt, but what if they decide they got it wrong?

Adele: Lots of reasons to feel anxious. I'm going to slow us down a bit more. I want to move more deeply into your feelings of being rubbish. What is the hardest thing about parenting Wren, the times when you feel most rubbish?

Jessie: [thinking hard] I think it's when I reach out to him, and he turns away. Just like he did with the tiger toy. I could see he was interested in the toy, but he wasn't interested in playing with me.

Adele: So, you extend an invitation to him: "Come and play with me," and he turns away. He seems to be rejecting the invitation, and it seems like he's rejecting you. I can see how that would feel painful. Can you just hold on to that feeling of being rejected? Notice the feelings that come up, the anxiety. I also sense despondency, maybe a drop in the pit of your stomach. [Jessie nods] Just hold on to that feeling and tell me, is it a feeling you recognize a lot? When else have you felt like this?

Jessie: Oh gosh, you've really taken me back. Yes, I've felt like this many times, the strongest is with my mother. You did warn me we would get to my attachment history. I guess this is it.

Adele: I guess so. Are you up for it? Maybe put the kettle on. We might need another cup of tea while we explore this!

This conversation leads Jessie and Adele into reflecting on his relationship with his mother. Jessie recalls how she brought him and his sister up as a single parent. His mother was hard working and held high standards for her children. He often sensed disapproval from her—in his academic achievements, his choice of friends, even the clothes he liked to wear. Despite this, he did experience her as being there for him and he tried hard to please her. He held back for a long time from telling her he was gay, fearing her disappointment in him. It wasn't until he met Kit and they wanted to build a life together that he told her. This was a hard time, and he isn't sure that she ever fully accepted it. She didn't approve of their adopting Wren and has offered them little support. Adele notices that Jessie's mother is another person in his life whom he might experience as watching and waiting for him to fail. As they talk about this, Jessie begins to notice how other current and past relationships in his life are impacting him as he parents Wren. He understands the anxiety this creates and how this leads him to interpret Wren's behavior in a certain way. Adele and Jessie have co-created a story of Jessie's experiences of rejection and disappointment and linked this to his experience with Wren. Jessie becomes open to the possibility of another narrative about Wren's behavior.

Adele and Jessie return to the video recording and notice the signs of fear and dissociation Wren displays. They consider this in the light of his traumatic background and how this might be triggered when the play becomes emotionally overwhelming. Jessie notices his efforts to engage Wren at these times, which now appear to him as intrusive based on his own anxieties and worries. He needs Wren to show him he is a good parent, and this need and anxiety add further fear for Wren. A trauma dance between them is revealed as each triggers the other into states of anxiety and fear, and subsequent dissociative responses.

Now Adele and Jessie focus on the parent-child relationship. Jessie, supported by Kit, learns to understand the dissociative responses to trauma memories that Wren displays. They learn to recognize Wren's hidden need for and fear of connection. Adele guides Jessie and Kit to talk quietly to Wren about his experiences:

> Oh, did that tiger worry you? I can see you want to play, but he's a bit scary, isn't he? Here we are, let's lie him down. I'm going to stroke him. Do you want to stroke him too? I think he's purring, just like our cat does when we stroke him.

They extend this to many day-to-day experiences developing a prosody in their voices that is melodic and rhythmic. Jessie and Kit notice all the ways they can signal to Wren that he is safe, using their voice and offering as much soothing and comfort as he can manage. They offer many intersubjective experiences, including opportunities and games missed in infancy. They slowly introduce Wren to safe emotional connection, helping him feel comfortable with reciprocal interactions.

Jessie notices those times when he starts to feel anxious again. He now recognizes where this comes from and with self-compassion can soothe himself and stay present for Wren.

Wren's dissociative behaviors reduce, and he becomes more open to emotional connection. He learns to feel safe within the intersubjective relationships offered by Jessie and Kit. Adele makes another recording of Wren and Jessie. They sit facing each other and pulling faces. They are laughing together at the silliness. At one point, Wren hiccups and looks alarmed. Jessie immediately notices. He soothes Wren until he is ready to play again. Wren can now experience comfort and joy with Jessie, and Jessie knows he is a good parent.

DDP Interventions with a Parent and Child at Early School Age

Naomi is a Black British foster carer caring for 8-year-old Mia and her 16-year-old birth son, Zack. Naomi experienced domestic violence by Zack's white father.

Naomi is a strong, resilient, and compassionate woman. After leaving Zack's father, she brought up Zack alone while also qualifying as a doctor. She works three days a week in a clinic in a deprived area of the city. It was here that she first met four-year-old Mia, who came in with a broken arm. No satisfactory explanation was given for this injury. Following investigations, Mia was removed from her birth family, and Naomi applied to foster Mia.

Naomi attended a DDP-informed group aimed at helping parents parenting traumatized children (Golding, 2017). While she attended all sessions, she was skeptical about the parenting approach being introduced and struggled to adopt a PACE attitude. However, following the end of the group, she approached the DDP therapist and group facilitator, Anita, for help with Mia's increasingly oppositional behavior.

As part of an initial assessment, Anita meets with Naomi and Mia. She observes a bright child who opposes all Naomi's requests. Anita and Naomi discuss the impact of loss and abuse on Mia, which has led to a need to be in control, and a sense of not deserving love and care.

Anita notices that in response to Mia's oppositional behavior, Naomi becomes demanding, threatening consequences for non-compliance. In response, Mia becomes angry. As this anger intensifies, Naomi becomes frozen. She sinks to the floor, unable to move, while Mia hits out at her. Anita senses two trauma stories evident in this pattern: Mia's and Naomi's.

Anita decides that a longer period of parent work is needed before beginning therapy with Mia. Naomi reluctantly agrees, although she is frustrated that Mia is not being offered therapy.

This first phase of the work is one of gradually building a therapeutic alliance—helping Naomi develop trust in Anita. Naomi continues to be concerned that Mia is not being helped and expresses regret that there is not a Black therapist available who would understand her better. Anita is empathetic, acknowledging the cultural differences between them and expressing curiosity about the culture Naomi grew up in. She is interested in Naomi's experiences of being parented. She learns of the respect that Naomi has for her parents. She describes them as strict but fair. This is the parenting she wants to provide for Mia. When she met Zack's father, her parents had been disapproving; however, they stood by Naomi and gave her and Zack a home and protection from this violent partner until they could establish their own home.

As Naomi's trust in Anita grows, she talks about her experience of domestic violence, and together they explore the post-traumatic symptoms Naomi displays. Naomi learns to recognize how Mia's anger triggers memories of her previous experience, leading to a dissociative defense. They notice how frightening this is for Mia, triggering her in turn to remember the emotional unavailability of her birth mother when her birth father was abusive. As Naomi understands this pattern, she is able to notice when she is triggered and to recognize the fear behind Mia's behaviors. Anita helps Naomi develop resources to manage her dissociative responses, which then reduce. As a consequence, Mia's anger toward Naomi lessens. Anita wonders if Naomi would benefit from a longer period of trauma therapy but Naomi declines, preferring the focus to be on helping Mia.

Anita agrees to work toward DDP therapy with Mia and Naomi. She asks Naomi to be patient for a little while longer so that she can help her develop a more PACEful approach to her parenting. Naomi remembers this from the group work and expresses distrust and impatience with ideas that do not feel sensitive to her culture. She does not understand how this will help or why the work with Mia cannot begin. Here is some dialogue between them: Anita explains the importance of Naomi and Mia feeling safe together if the therapy is to be successful.

Naomi: So, are you saying that Mia doesn't feel safe with me? I thought this is what we've been working on. I've followed all your suggestions, and you know that Mia's angry behaviors have reduced. Surely, therapy can begin now.

Anita: Of course, you want therapy to begin. I can see how committed you are to helping Mia. It's so frustrating, isn't it? You've worked so hard and made so many changes, and yet I'm asking for more. I'm asking you to trust me that we are working toward therapy for Mia. An important part of DDP therapy is going to be your involvement. I need you to be able to respond to her with PACE when I help her express her emotional world to you.

Naomi: So, that is like the way I notice when she's afraid.

Anita: Yes, that's the curiosity of PACE. Understanding her emotional world can help you connect with acceptance and empathy. I have so appreciated how you've learned to be curious about Mia's fear. I know curiosity is something you didn't experience from your parents when growing up. Do you remember when we explored the cultural differences between us? I think curiosity was something my parents used to help me know my own mind, to encourage me to be independent. In your family, I hear stronger values for children to fit in rather than become independent. You and your siblings were helped to understand the needs of your extended family and social network, and there was less curiosity about your minds and more focus on guiding you to respect your elders. I am now asking you to parent in a way that brings in more curiosity for Mia's emotional experience, to help her overcome trauma, and this is unfamiliar to you.

Naomi: Are you saying my parents were wrong?

Anita: No, not at all. Respect and learning to be part of a group are really important values for children to learn. This is a strength in the values your parents held. I wonder sometimes if we don't focus on this enough when independence is encouraged. Curiosity about the child can detract from helping the child understand the needs of the social group they are living in. I really respect your values, and I see huge benefits for children in developing strong social identities. I guess I'm wondering if there is room for both, a valuing of the child's mind to understand their emotional world, and a valuing of the needs of the social group to help the child fit in. It's complex, isn't it?

Naomi: Well, I can see how understanding Mia's fear has helped, but I'm still uneasy about the whole PACE idea. I just can't see how it will help Mia to learn to fit in.

Anita: Can we explore this a bit more? Help me understand the uneasiness you are feeling.

Naomi: I can't see how empathizing with her will teach her respect. In fact, I think it will be the opposite—that independence you talk about. Won't it just make her more independent and less respectful?

Anita: Naomi, I really appreciate how hard you are thinking about this, and I can see what you mean. Respect is really important, and I want us to hold this in mind as an important parenting goal. As Mia feels understood by you, that you accept her inner world, I do think she will be open to your guidance. She will allow you to influence her, and she will convey respect for your guidance. You can guide her as to what is expected of her, and with your support she will learn to respect both your values and her elders.

Naomi: But will she? Won't she just think she can do what she likes? Where will the boundaries be with all this fluffy stuff?

Anita: [smiling] Yes, PACE alone would feel a bit fluffy, although I prefer to say warm and comforting! I'm not suggesting PACE alone, though. Boundaries are really important. I believe that Mia will accept the boundaries more easily when she starts to believe that she is loved by you.

Naomi: But surely she knows that. I do so much for her. How can she not feel loved?

Anita: You show your love in so many ways. It is your love for her that makes you so committed to helping her grow up equipped for the world. Do you remember the idea of blocked trust

	from the group? I don't think Mia truly believes she is loveable and nor does she trust in your love for her, because of her past experiences. When you provide boundaries and consequences, she sees it as further evidence she is not loveable. Tell me, how did you know you were loved with the parenting you experienced?
Naomi:	Well, I don't know, I just always knew it. My parents were always there for me. No matter how strict they were when I did wrong, I always knew they had my back. I don't know.
Anita:	Yes, from birth you experienced their love and care. It helped you experience yourself as loveable. You never doubted it. When they began to bring in boundaries and discipline, you knew in your very being that they had good intentions toward you.
Naomi:	[with sadness] And Mia didn't have that.
Anita:	No. You're trying to show it, but you also have to provide boundaries. You didn't have the infant stage with her when you could love her without discipline. Learning to trust is hard for Mia. She experiences your discipline as meanness toward her. It confirms her belief that she isn't loveable. She doesn't trust your good intentions toward her—that is the blocked trust. I believe that PACE will help her know that you understand and accept what she's feeling even when you have to correct her. That is how she will know she is loved. When she starts to believe this, she'll become less defensive and less shameful, and she will be open to the boundaries and all the good guidance you want to give her. She will learn to respect you will understand her social responsibility, what is expected of her. It will be a long road. There is a lot of unlearning to do, but I do believe she will grow into the adult you want her to be.
Naomi:	[thoughtfully] While I just pile on the punishments, trying to get her to behave. If she doesn't believe I'm doing this for her, I can see why she gets angry. And my own trauma doesn't help. How can she get that I love her when I freeze in the face of her anger? It's not just her past I am helping her to recover from, is it?
Anita:	It's hard for both of you. When traumas collide, it makes it extra hard for either of you to feel safe. You've worked so hard with this. Mia knows this deep inside. She experiences your commitment and love for her even if she can't yet accept it. We need to help her know she's deserving of this. That's where the therapy comes in. This is why it's important that you can respond PACEfully when Mia allows her fears and doubts to be communicated.
Naomi:	Phew, this is hard work. You want me to be explicit with curiosity and empathy, and that's not something I'm used to.
Anita:	We'll do it together. I'll guide you with PACE and you can help me understand what you want for Mia. We'll make sure that you parent her in a way that helps her overcome her traumatic past and learn the values of respect and social responsibility.

Following this and similar conversations, Naomi begins to parent Mia differently. This is challenging because Mia remains oppositional, causing Naomi to doubt what she is doing. She and Anita hold on to small moments of connection with Mia, noticing and celebrating them.

Within DDP therapy, Mia allows Anita to support her to be vulnerable with Naomi. Mia struggles to talk about her experience. She likes to build dens with cushions and blankets. While she hides in them, Anita can talk for her, expressing Mia's experience based on their understanding of her and what Mia has told them. In the example below, Anita uses Mia's description of a "big fizzing feeling" when she is asked to do something:

> It's so hard, Mia, when you have such big feelings. See if I get this right: 'Mommy, you ask me to do something, and I get such big, scared feelings, like a big fizzing feeling inside me. What if

I can't do it? What if you are cross with me? What if you don't want me to live here anymore? It's such a big muddle in my head. I get so angry. I'm so scared you won't love me anymore.

Mia sticks out her thumb, letting Anita know she has got it right, and Naomi responds beautifully with acceptance and empathy:

So hard, Mia. I see how angry you get, and now I know how scared you're feeling. Such a lot for my girl to cope with. Now I understand why it's hard for you when I ask you to do things. I love my helpful girl, and I love my scared girl, and I love my angry girl.

Sometimes they get out the hand puppets and Mia shows some of her experience with these different states and their triggers. It feels like a special moment for all of them when she demonstrates a puppet getting angry with a mommy puppet who will not get up. Naomi is able to let Mia know of her sorrow that she also frightened Mia, a touching repair of their relationship.

In this way, the three of them explore Mia's experiences of trauma, co-creating her story in a way that helps Mia feel understood in her shame and fear of not deserving love, and start to hold a new narrative of hope and lovability. She experiences the love Naomi has for her, even in the challenging times.

DDP as Parent-Child Psychotherapy with a Preadolescent

Niki is a very chatty 11-year-old who has been living with his paternal aunt and uncle, Monica and Jordan, since he was six years old. Monica is a primary school teacher and Jordan an electrician. Niki's father, Jordan's brother, has a mild learning disability, and his mother struggles with mental health difficulties. They struggled to parent Niki and his two younger sisters. Niki and his sisters were brought into care when Niki was five and his siblings have subsequently been adopted.

Niki is a compliant young man with an avoidant pattern of attachment. Emotions are largely contained and not expressed. This is how Niki survived in a chaotic and neglectful home environment. Niki can be very charming, but Monica and Jordan feel that this is superficial and gets in the way of a real connection with them. They describe Niki's presence in the house like that of a lodger. With the hope that Niki can integrate more successfully into their family, they have turned to DDP therapist Grant for help. The family also includes Monica and Jordan's two birth children, who are 14 and 16 years old. While they don't feature in the dialogue below, other sessions explore Niki's experience of them being favored over him.

We are going to dip into the therapy at around session 10 of parent-child DDP. Niki is always happy to talk to Grant, especially when they can share their love of Marvel comics. He will engage on trickier themes but is reluctant to dip into his emotional experience. Niki talks fast, with lots of stories to keep Grant engaged cognitively. Within these, many themes emerge that could be explored affectively-reflectively, if only Grant could slow him down long enough. It feels like a merry dance, with Niki leading them around the dance floor. However, over the last couple of sessions, Grant has experienced a bit of a breakthrough, with some moments of deeper emotional connection. He hopes in this session to capitalize on this. Niki sits on a sofa between his aunt and uncle while Grant is on a chair near them.

Grant: So, the *Spider-Man* film was cool. I'm glad you got to see it with your friends.
Niki: Yeah, it was good, although I wish Lucas didn't talk so much. I'm sure I missed some of the good bits. I really liked when… [Niki talks quickly describing scene after scene]

Grant:	[holding up his hands] Whoa, it doesn't sound like you missed much there. Take a breath, Niki. I want to ask you something that has just occurred to me. Wow, I have only just noticed. Goodness, why hadn't I noticed this before… [Grant talks with animation, building up some suspense to engage Niki's curiosity]
Niki:	So, tell me. What have you noticed?
Grant:	Spider-Man—Peter Parker, isn't it? [Niki nods] He lives with his aunt, doesn't he? I've just noticed, that's just like you! Do you know why he lives with her?
Niki:	Well, I live with my aunt and uncle, so it's not the same. His parents were killed—a plane crash, I think. There's not much about them in the films. His Uncle Ben was killed by a thief—that's been shown a couple of times.
Grant:	Wow, a lot of loss for a young man. I can see why he wanted superpowers. It was a lot to get over.
Niki:	Yeah, at least my mom and dad are alive, and my uncle. Superpowers would be good, though.
Grant:	[with a smile] Oh, I think you have a few. Those defenses we talked about last time—to avoid emotion—they are pretty super and powerful.
Niki:	Yeah, but you want me to lose them!
Grant:	Oh, have I given you that impression? I'm sorry. Don't lose your superpowers. I just want you to know that you don't need them all the time. It takes super power to feel things, as well. So, tell me, what would it be like if Spider-Man lived with his aunt and his parents were still alive?
Niki:	Confusing, I guess. Like, why is he not living with them? What did he do wrong that means he lives with his aunt?
Grant:	Is that what it's like for you, wondering what you did wrong?
Niki:	No, I'm fine. I didn't do anything wrong.
Grant:	It can be a puzzle, though, can't it. Why am I here and not there. Spider-Man has a clear story about what happened, but he still struggled as a teenager, feeling inadequate and lonely. What's it like when the story is less clear, like when you're left wondering, Is it something I did or didn't do?
Niki:	No, it's fine. It's not something that troubles me.
Grant:	How come? I mean how is it fine? This is what I'm thinking: you were just a little boy, and I know you tried so hard to look after your little sisters, and your mom. And then the social workers decided that you couldn't live there anymore. How does a five-year-old boy make sense of that?
Niki:	[starting to fidget a bit as Grant leads him into affect] He just didn't think about it.
Grant:	How did you do that? I mean, one day you are living with them and trying to make sure they're all okay, and then you're in foster care. You don't know what is going to happen. Everything must have felt so strange.
Niki:	Yeah it did, but I just got on with looking after my sisters. I don't think the foster carers liked that. They kept trying to stop me, like I was doing something naughty.
Grant:	Oh Niki, how hard. You were trying to look after them and it felt like you were doing something wrong. I can't imagine how confused you must have been feeling. [Niki is looking sad and is also tapping his legs with some agitation. Grant talks to his aunt and uncle for a while to help him regulate] It must have been hard, mustn't it, moving so suddenly, not knowing what was going to happen next? I'm thinking how confused Niki must have felt.
Niki:	Well, they found my sisters a new family, so they must have thought I didn't look after them very well.

Aunt Monica:	[taking Niki's hand] Oh Niki, you were so little. No five-year-old should have to look after his baby sisters. You didn't know that, though. I agree with Grant—it must have been so confusing for you. I'm so happy you came to live with us, that we can take care of you.
Grant:	Was that confusing, too, your sisters being adopted and you coming to live with your aunt and uncle?
Niki:	Well, I still get to see mom and dad. I saw them the other week. Mom's put more weight on again. She shouldn't, not with her back problem. Dad's pretty useless, he just keeps getting her more food—they seem to have plenty of food now. Not like when I was there.
Grant:	That sounds hard, too. Yes, you get to see them, but that gives you so many worries. And why do they have food now when they couldn't feed you?
Niki:	Oh, I'm fine. I just told Dad to get her to eat less. [Niki goes into more stories about his mom and dad]
Grant:	Hang on Niki, let's take another breath. Okay, are you with me? [Niki nods] You've been trying so hard to take care of them, and with your aunt and uncle, it's hard to let them take care of you. All these years you've tried to manage not to need them, doing the looking after but not being looked after. And I'm wondering, maybe it never feels like you've done enough?
Niki:	[looking at Grant and replying with a much younger voice] The house was small and dirty, not like here. We never had food in the fridge or sheets on the bed. That's why the social workers moved us. I heard them saying what a state the house was in, and how hungry my sisters were. I tried to tidy up, but there was so much rubbish. I tried to feed my sisters.
Uncle Jordan:	Oh Niki, that was a lot for a little boy to try and do.
Niki:	I didn't, though, did I? They moved me here because I didn't do a good enough job. And this house is so tidy. It felt so big when I came here, and it smelled different. I didn't know what to do. What if I make this house smelly and dirty? [Niki turns to Monica and Jordan] Would you say I can't stay?
Grant:	That's a big worry, isn't it. I think you've been living with that worry for a long time. [Niki leans against his aunt, who gently strokes his hair. He looks young and vulnerable. As they have done before, Grant asks Niki if he can speak for him, to tell his aunt and uncle how hard this has been. Niki nods and snuggles in tighter]
Grant:	Aunt Monica and Uncle Jordan, Niki has said I can talk for him, as he is having some big feelings just now. [Monica and Jordan both look at Niki as Grant begins to talk]
Grant:	[talking as Niki] It has been hard. I lived with Mom and Dad, and it was so difficult. The house was always untidy and dirty. There was never much food. I tried so hard to tidy up, but the social workers were cross. They said we couldn't live there anymore. They said my sisters needed to be cared for better. I felt like I hadn't done a good enough job. And then in foster care, they got cross when I tried to help. They didn't think I could do a good job, either. My sisters went to a new family, and I couldn't look after them anymore. I came here, and it was so clean and tidy. It smelled different. I didn't know what to do. I didn't think I deserved it—after all, I hadn't done well with a small house, how could I be good enough to live here? What if I made this house dirty and smelly? Would you say I couldn't stay?

	[Grant quietly asks Niki if he has got it right, whether there is anything to change or add to the story. Niki nods that it's okay. Grant then asks Monica and Jordan to respond with acceptance and empathy]
Aunt Monica:	You were so little, Niki, when you came to live here. It must have been so confusing. Everything felt so different. No wonder you worried about doing the right thing. When you were at home, you tried so hard to take care of your sisters and your mom and dad, but that is not a child's job. No wonder you didn't feel good enough.
Uncle Jordan:	And you had lost your sisters and worried about your mom and dad. I'm thinking what big worries you had on your shoulders. No wonder you needed a Superman cape.
Niki:	[laughing] It's Spider-Man, Uncle Jordan, and he doesn't wear a cape!
Grant:	[laughing too] You'd better brush up on your superheroes, Uncle Jordan, if you want Niki to stay with you.
Uncle Jordan:	Well, I'm going to study them carefully, because Niki is going to be living with us for a long time. We're going to show him how we can look after him so he doesn't have to worry anymore. I'm looking forward to the day I moan at him to tidy his bedroom—it's way too tidy for an 11-year-old!

Following the therapy, Niki becomes more emotionally connected to Monica and Jordan. If they notice him disconnecting, they all sit down and talk about it. Usually, Niki has a worry he is finding hard to talk about. They all figure it out together. Once a week they visit his mom and dad, helping them with their housework. Oh, and when he is 13 years old, they all laugh when Jordan angrily tells Niki to tidy his room! Niki lives with Monica and Jordan until he leaves home at 19, although he often pops back for Sunday dinner and to get some washing done!

Evidence Base for DDP

Developing an evidence base for DDP is a work in progress, made more complicated because of the complexity of the interventions, range of the work, and the relational focus with interventions tailored to the unique needs of the child and family. There are a range of single case studies and pre- and post-outcome studies, as well as a waiting list comparison study. This is supplemented with qualitative research. Taken together, this research is demonstrating the efficacy of DDP as a psychotherapy, a parenting approach, and for school environments (Hughes et al., 2019; Hughes & Golding, 2024). At the time of writing, a randomized control trial, the Relationships in Good Hands trial (RIGHT), is exploring DDP as psychotherapy for children under 12. The pilot and feasibility work are complete, and the main trial is underway (Turner-Halliday et al., 2014).

Conclusion

Dyadic developmental psychotherapy (DDP) is both a therapy and a practice model that provides a range of interventions to help children who have experienced developmental trauma, many of whom are living away from their birth families. DDP therapists and practitioners provide DDP-informed parenting and network support alongside DDP itself. This is described as dyadic to highlight the importance of working with the child and their current parents or parent figures.

In DDP, the therapist works with the parents first. This focuses on building an alliance and the trust needed to explore the impact of parenting the child. This includes exploring attachment history, any previous traumas, and understanding the context that identity, experience, and culture bring to this. In addition, the therapist prepares the parents for the therapy, guiding them in how to respond to their child within the sessions. As the parent-child psychotherapy progresses, the therapist continues to meet with the parents to review progress and explore issues of concern.

Through this parent and parent-child work, the child is helped to develop trust where they are experiencing mistrust and attachment security instead of insecurity and disorganization. The child develops the safety needed to emotionally connect within intersubjective relationships, safe to influence and to stay open to the influence of the parent(s) without moving into states of dysregulation or dissociation. With these renewed relationships, the child is helped by the therapist to explore their current and past experience. They have conversations together that explore the stories of the child's experience, allowing an integrated sense of self to emerge. The parent(s) join the child in this exploration, providing co-regulation as needed and witnessing and responding to the stories that are co-created. The child can hold a coherent, autobiographical narrative instead of fragmented stories and memories filled with rage, despair, or terror. The child feels a sense of safety and comfort with themselves and others, relaxing the defenses and behaviors they had developed to survive in an unsafe world.

Note

1 The experience, identity, and culture of the characters in the examples are described only when important to the narrative. The reader is invited to add details that help them reflect on these examples from their own experience, identity, and culture.

References

Arnett, J. J. (2008). The neglected 95%: Why American psychology needs to become less American. *American Psychologist, 63*(7), 602–614. https://doi.org/10.1037/0003-066X.63.7.602

Atkinson, J. (2002). *Trauma trails, recreating song lines: The transgenerational effects of trauma in indigenous Australia*. Spinifex Press.

Baylin, J., & Hughes, D. A. (2016). *The neurobiology of attachment-focused therapy: Enhancing connection and trust in the treatment of children and adolescents*. W. W. Norton.

Cook, A., Spinazzola, J., Ford, J., Lanktree, C., Blaustein, M., Cloitre, M., DeRosa, R., Hubbard, R., Kagan, R., Liautaud, J., Mallah, K., Olafson, E., & van der Kolk, B. (2005). Complex trauma in children and adolescents. *Psychiatric Annals, 35*(5), 390–398. https://doi.org/10.3928/00485713-20050501-05

Fejo-King, C. (2017). *Practice live. Attachment and culture. Understanding attachment*. Attachment and Culture, nsw.gov.au

Golding, K. S. (2017). *Foundations for attachment training resource: The six-session programme for parents of traumatized children*. Jessica Kingsley Publishers.

Harwood, R. L., Miller, J. G., & Irizarry, N. L. (1995). *Culture and attachment. Perceptions of the child in context*. Guilford Press.

Henrich, J. (2021). *The weirdest people in the world: How the West became psychologically peculiar and particularly prosperous*. Penguin Random House.

Hughes, D. A., & Baylin, J. (2012). *Brain-based parenting: The neuroscience of caregiving for healthy attachment*. W. W. Norton.

Hughes, D. A., & Golding, K. S. (2024). *Healing relational trauma workbook: Dyadic developmental psychotherapy in practice*. W. W. Norton.

Hughes, D. A, Golding, K. S., & Hudson, J. (2019). *Healing relational trauma with attachment-focused interventions: Dyadic developmental psychotherapy with children and families*. W. W. Norton.

Keller, H. (2022). *The myth of Attachment Theory. A critical understanding for multicultural societies*. Routledge.

Trevarthen, C. (2016). From the intrinsic motive pulse of infant activity to the life time of cultural meanings. In B. Molder, V. Aristila & P. Ohrstrom (Eds.), *Philosophy and psychology of time* (pp. 225–266). Springer.

Turner-Halliday, F., Watson, N., Boyer, N. R. S., Boyd, K. A., & Minnis, H. (2014). The feasibility of a randomised controlled trial of dyadic developmental psychotherapy. *BMC Psychiatry, 14*, Article 347. https://doi.org/10.1186/s12888-014-0347-z

van der Kolk, B. A. (2005). Developmental trauma disorder: Toward a rational diagnosis for children with complex trauma histories. *Psychiatric Annals, 35*(5), 401–408. https://doi.org/10.3928/00485713-20050501-06

19
THE ATTACHMENT VIDEO-FEEDBACK INTERVENTION (AVI)
Reducing Dysregulated Parental Behavior, Attachment Disorganization and Dissociation

Valérie Langlois, Gabrielle Myre and Chantal Cyr

Introduction

Dissociative symptoms are manifested in several forms and may range from benign symptoms (e.g., mind wandering) to more severe clinical diagnosis of dissociative disorders. According to the major classification systems of diseases and disorders, dissociation is seen as a disruption in the normal integration of various mental functions. For example, the International Classification of Diseases (ICD-11), published by the World Health Organization (2018), stipulates that dissociation symptoms "are characterized by involuntary disruptions or discontinuity in the normal integration of one or more of the following: identity, sensations, perceptions, affects, thoughts, memories, control over bodily movements, or behavior" (p. 437).

The pathways to dissociation have been the subject of much theoretical reflection. After many years of research, it is now well recognized that trauma is an etiological and critical factor in the emergence of dissociation, especially trauma related to childhood physical and sexual abuse as well as neglect (Vonderlin et al., 2018). Dissociation is believed to serve as a defense mechanism that may preserve the individual from overwhelming fear and distress associated with the traumatic event. This view of dissociation is consistent with neurobiological theories describing dissociation as a defensive response to threats, such as fight-or-flight behavioral responses. Nevertheless, while maltreatment during early childhood may be an important precursor of dissociation, some individuals without experiences of childhood maltreatment have reported dissociative symptoms (Briere, 2006; Putnam, 1997), implying that broader caregiving experiences, beyond that of abuse and neglect, could explain the phenomenon of dissociation. Based on Bowlby's (1969, 1973) attachment theory and Main et al.'s (1985) subsequent work on attachment disorganization, a contemporary attachment-based model of dissociation now provides a clear parallel between child attachment disorganization and dissociation (Liotti, 2006). It is suggested that a disorganized relationship with the attachment figure in early childhood represents a primary catalyst for dissociation (Liotti, 2006), where dysregulated parental behaviors (frightening/frightened, disrupted, disconnected, or extremely insensitive) may confer early vulnerability to both disorganization and dissociation.

In this chapter, we first review the theoretical and empirical literature on attachment disorganization during infancy. Second, we show how dysregulated parental behaviors, not necessarily involving maltreatment, are a risk factor to the development of attachment disorganization and dissociation in early childhood. Third, we present the Attachment Video-Feedback Intervention (AVI) (Cyr et al., 2020; Moss et al., 2011), an evidence-based parent-child intervention, designed to improve parental sensitivity and attachment security and reduce attachment disorganization. Based on empirical studies and a short case study, we show the extent to which the AVI may diminish dysregulated parental behaviors, child attachment disorganization, and dissociation behaviors in both the parent and child.

Child Attachment Disorganization and Dissociation

According to attachment theory (Cassidy et al., 2017), children are biologically predisposed to seek closeness and physical contact (e.g., crying, approaching, clinging, and reaching) with their caregiver in order to find reassurance and protection in times of stress and danger. These attachment behaviors are thought to be organized within an attachment behavioral system aiming to protect the child, ultimately ensuring its survival. When activated by distress, attachment behaviors signal the caregiver. If the caregiver is available, warm, and responsive, it is likely that the child will cease to exhibit attachment behaviors and return to a calm physiological state, which will deactivate its attachment system, in turn facilitating exploration of the environment in full trust that the caregiver is there if needed. Thus, from the first months of their lives, children learn progressively to regulate dependence (approach behavior) and autonomy (exploratory behavior) needs according to their caregivers' responses.

Since the first seminal study of Ainsworth and colleagues (1978), much work in the field of attachment has shown that sensitive parental responses to child needs promote child attachment security (Sroufe, 2005). Upon reunion, after a brief separation from their parents (the Strange Situation Procedure), secure children show proximity-seeking behaviors and physical contact with their parents, and once reassured, they return to play. Research has shown that a secure attachment is associated with socio-emotional adaptation (Groh et al., 2014) and cognitive skills (Bernier et al., 2012) throughout the preschool and school years. A meta-analysis of the global distribution of attachment recently reported that 52% of children showed a secure attachment relationship with their parents (Madigan et al., 2023). In adulthood, attachment has been described as a set of cognitive representations (attachment state of mind or internal working model of attachment, as stated by Main et al. [1985] and Bowlby [1969]) about the self and others in attachment relationships that organizes expectations and thoughts about the self and others, and ways to behave with others. Parents with an autonomous (secure) attachment state of mind have a coherent narrative about their childhood attachment experiences and make metacognitive (i.e., reflective) judgments to reevaluate the meaning of childhood experiences. As a result of their reflective capacity, these parents show more sensitivity, as they are better able to recognize and respond to child needs without resorting to defensive processes, thereby promoting child attachment security (see Verhage et al., 2016, for a meta-analysis).

However, some parents are more insensitive, failing to recognize child distress, misinterpreting the meaning of child intentions or behaviors, or responding inappropriately or with delay. Such responses limit children's ability to turn to their parents in stressful situations and facilitate child attachment insecurity. Ainsworth and colleagues (1978) described two insecure patterns of attachment: (1) insecure avoidant children who do not reach out to their parents when distressed, express little emotion, and minimize physical closeness, but emphasize exploration and autonomy needs; and (2) insecure resistant/ambivalent children who show dependent and passive behaviors toward their parents when distressed, and exaggerate distress and proximity needs while exhibiting anger and resistance toward their parents' comfort. Although insecure, these children can organize their approach behaviors around the caregiving responses of their parents.

Other insecurely attached children in infancy do not, however, show any coherent attachment strategies, meaning they are not able to organize a secure, avoidant, or resistant/ambivalent strategy to get reassurance from the parent. Either they tentatively exhibit organized strategies and then show a collapse of strategies, or they appear as though they have not developed any of those strategies for reaching out to the parent. In both cases, children fail to regulate behaviors and emotions, and they remain highly distressed. Main and Solomon (1990) have described these children as showing insecure disorganized attachment behaviors. Upon reunion with their parents during the Strange Situation Procedure, these children display contradictory approach/avoidance behaviors (e.g., approaching the parent backward or with head averted) or disrupted or anomalous behaviors that are directly (e.g., fearful facial expression) or indirectly (e.g., disorientation, dazed and trance-like look, freezing, and stilling) indicating fear of their parents (Lyons-Ruth & Jacobvitz, 2016). Liotti (2006) understood disorganized behavior as early behavioral manifestations of dissociation that would predispose the child for later dissociative states and symptoms.

By preschool age, either the disorganized, disoriented, or fearful behaviors are maintained toward the parent or disorganization evolves into a parent-child role reversal relationship (Moss et al., 2005). This evolution is characterized by a dynamic in which the child controls the parent's behaviors by being punitive and hostile or by being emotionally supportive and attentive to the parent's needs (Moss et al., 2004). Disorganized children and disorganized controlling children are known to have a higher risk of externalizing and internalizing problems (Fearon et al., 2010; Groh et al., 2012; Madigan et al., 2013, for meta-analyses; and Moss et al., 2004). They also show more cognitive difficulties and psychopathological symptoms and disorders in middle childhood, adolescence, and adulthood, such as anxiety and conduct problems, borderline personality features, and suicidal ideation (Carlson et al., 2009; Dubois-Comtois et al., 2013; Lyons-Ruth et al., 2013; Moss & St-Laurent, 2001). A few longitudinal studies also show that attachment disorganization in infancy is predictive of later dissociative symptoms in early school age, adolescence, and adulthood (Carlson, 1998; Dozier et al., 2008; Dutra & Lyons-Ruth, 2005; Ogawa et al., 1997).

Pathways to Attachment Disorganization and Dissociation

There are different pathways to attachment disorganization, which may inform the developmental pathways to dissociation. A *first* critical pathway to attachment disorganization is maltreatment directly experienced by the child. Research has shown that children with disorganized attachment are disproportionately represented in samples of abused and neglected children: whereas approximately 22% of children without a history of maltreatment show disorganized attachment, an average of 65% of maltreated children exhibit disorganized attachment (Cyr et al., 2010; Madigan et al., 2023, for meta-analyses). Maltreatment is deleterious in the formation of an attachment relationship. Undoubtedly, it activates the attachment and fear systems of the child. Hesse and Main (2006) suggested that disorganized children appear to be caught in an unsolvable dilemma, a paradox of "fright without solution," (p. 310) in which the parent is both a source of potential comfort and a source of fear. Maltreatment is the perfect example of such a paradox.

Nevertheless, in the meta-analysis that we published in 2010, child maltreatment was not the only predictor of child attachment disorganization. In fact, children without alleged histories of maltreatment presenting five or more family socioeconomic risks (e.g., low income, and no high-school diploma) were as likely as maltreated children to show disorganized attachment behaviors. Research has also shown that risk factors such as parental psychopathology (e.g., borderline personality disorder), poor marital relationship quality, marital conflict, and domestic violence are associated with attachment disorganization in children (Hobson et al., 2005; Myre et al., 2022; O'Connor et al., 2011; van IJzendoorn et al., 1999). Thus, a *second* pathway not involving maltreatment but instead cumulative psychological, social, and economical risks is also at play in the development of attachment disorganization.

A *third* pathway to disorganization, which was also highlighted in studies with non-maltreated children, is that of parents with an unresolved attachment state of mind, who are more likely to have children with a disorganized attachment (Verhage et al., 2016, for a meta-analysis). In response to childhood trauma experiences, such as the loss of an attachment figure or abuse, adults with an unresolved attachment state of mind are unable to integrate thoughts and emotions related to these childhood events into a coherent set of representations. During the discussion of traumatic events, they show lack of resolution through signs of disorientation and disorganization. As explained by Hesse (2016), lack of resolution is observed when temporary lapses in the monitoring of reasoning or discourse are manifested by the adult, who may suddenly experience a shift in conversational style (e.g. talks about a deceased parent in the present tense, gives extreme attention to detail when speaking about a trauma) or express ideas that violate physical causality or time-space relations (e.g., claims to be responsible for the death of a loved one because of something they had said to this person). According to Hesse and Main (2006), such lapses, which indicate the existence of traumatic memories or beliefs that would otherwise be dissociated, have intruded consciousness, suddenly altering the adult's speech. A meta-analysis by Verhage et al. (2016) on the intergenerational transmission of attachment phenomenon has found a significant correspondence between a parent's unresolved attachment state of mind and their child's attachment disorganization (42.4%, although not as compelling as for the transmission of attachment security: 69.1%).

Dysregulated (Frightening, Frightened, Disrupted, Disconnected, or Extremely Insensitive) Parental Behaviors

In our view, there is an underlying common denominator for each of the three pathways mentioned in the previous section—namely, dysregulated parental behavior. Main and Hesse (1990) first described dysregulated parental behaviors as parental frightening or frightened behaviors. According to Hesse and Main (2006), these behaviors would most likely occur when the parent is reminiscent of unresolved traumatic experiences. A wide range of stimuli can trigger traumatic memories and increase the odds of frightening/frightened behaviors. As well, the mere presence of the child, who normally exhibits distress and needs, is sufficient to stress the parent and provoke the reminiscence of painful memories with their own attachment figures, leading to frightened/frightening parental behaviors. These authors argued that when parents are reminded of past traumatic experiences, which they are not able to organize into one coherent set of mental representations, they become overwhelmed by unintegrated material that not only impairs the organization of their mental processes and discourse content, such as during an interview, but also alters their behavior during interaction with the child. Dysregulated parental behaviors have been found to be a key mechanism through which an unresolved attachment state of mind is transmitted to the disorganized attached child (Madigan et al., 2006). According to Main and Hesse (1990), frightening/frightened parental behaviors place the child in a state of "fright without solution" paradox, because the child experiences the parent as both a threat and a rescuer. It is this particular state of confusion that causes attachment disorganization and also seems to be at the root of dissociation. Liotti (2006) suggested that the repeated exposure to such paradoxical experiences is inevitably overwhelming for a young child's limited mentalizing capacity, making these experiences the perfect context for the development of multiple, incompatible models of self and other. The alternation between multiple representations of self further facilitates the onset of disorganization as a predisposing factor to dissociation in early childhood and to dissociative states in later life.

Lyons-Ruth et al. (1999) referred to dysregulated behaviors as disrupted parental behaviors and communication. Extending Main and Hesse's (1990) proposition, they suggested that parental behavior need not be the very source of fear to provoke child disorganization. Other sources of fear related to the incongruence between the child's experience and the parent's response also contributes to disorganization. For example, a parent who engages in contradictory forms of affective communication with the child, such as pulling away from the child when they are in need of comfort, or laughing/smiling when the child is distressed, demonstrates the inability to provide a coherent response to the child's needs under stress. Confronted with such confusing caregiving experiences, the child is left alone to regulate negative sensations and organize attentional processes. These affective communication errors are extreme enough to arouse fear in the child and provoke attachment disorganization if the parent fails to recognize the distress they cause (Lyons-Ruth & Jacobvitz, 2016). Again, this forces the child to create fragmented models of self with the caregiver, giving rise to dissociative behaviors. However, and this could explain why some maltreated children show a secure attachment, if parents recognize child distress (e.g., soothing the child despite distress), they may buffer the effects of sensations that are too intense for the child and help coregulate distress (Schuder & Lyons-Ruth, 2004). This sensitive repair of the relationship by the parent may deactivate the child's attachment system and limit the cascading negative effects of fear on the child's overall organization of behaviors, emotions, and mental processes. In our view, this notion of *repair* is of the utmost importance in attachment intervention.

In the attachment research field, dysregulated parental behaviors have been measured using the Atypical Maternal Behavior Instrument for Assessment and Classification system (AMBIANCE, by Bronfman et al., 1999–2014) and the Frightening/Frightened parental behavior system (FR, by Main & Hesse, 1992–2005). In an attempt to bring together these diverse behaviors, Out et al. (2009a) proposed the Disconnected and Extremely Insensitive Parenting (DIP) behavior coding system, which regroup parental behaviors into two broad categories of dysregulated parental behaviors—namely:

1. The disconnected behaviors category, which includes parents who show an altered state of awareness (e.g. dazed expression), fearful behaviors, or deferential/romantic behaviors toward the child. These behaviors are characterized by sudden changes in normal parenting (e.g., voice alterations and abrupt movements in the child's face) or by role reversal, or are related to dissociation (e.g., stilling and freezing).
2. The extremely insensitive behaviors category includes parents who repeatedly or for a prolonged period of time fail to respond to their child's needs. They are either highly withdrawn from the interaction (e.g., actively creating physical distance from the child, failing to respond to the child's distress, and rarely speaking to the child) or highly negative, such as intrusive, hostile, or aggressive toward the child (e.g., disapproving or blaming them for being in distress and using threatening or stern voice).

Table 19.1 lists the different types of dysregulated parental behaviors according to the three observational coding systems (DIP, FR, and AMBIANCE coding systems).

Overall, dysregulated behaviors are seen as disturbances in the caregiver-child relationship that, although not qualifying as maltreatment, may be as negative as maltreating behavior in the development of attachment disorganization (Schuder & Lyons-Ruth, 2004). Thus, in cases of maltreatment by the parent (pathway 1), we suggest that dysregulated parental behaviors could precede actual parental abuse or neglect. As for the two other pathways, dysregulated parental behaviors could be a relational process through which psychological, social, and socioeconomic risks (pathway 2) and an unresolved attachment state of mind (pathway 3) lead to disorganization and dissociation. Figure 19.1 illustrates our proposition.

Table 19.1 Description of Dysregulated Parental Behaviors According to Three Observational Coding Systems

Frightening/Frightened Parental Behaviors (FR) (Main & Hesse, 1998)	Atypical Maternal Behavior Instrument for Assessment and Classification (AMBIANCE) (Lyons-Ruth et al., 1999)	Disconnected and Extremely Insensitive Parenting behavior (DIP) (Out et al., 2009)
1 Threatening (e.g., aggressive movements, postures, facial expressions) **2 Frightened** (parent indicating fear) **3 Dissociation** (suggesting altered state of consciousness) **4 Deferential** (submission to the child) **5 Spousal or romantic** (excessive intimacy and inappropriate behaviors) **6 Disorganized** (e.g. contradictory behaviors)	**1 Affective communication errors** (contradictory signaling, failure to respond, inappropriate responding) **2 Role boundary confusion** (difficulty in prioritizing child's needs, treats child as a romantic partner) **3 Fearful/Disoriented** (apprehension, dissociation, disorganized behavior, infrequent voice quality) **4 Intrusiveness/Negativity** (physical, verbal) **5 Withdrawal** (physically or verbally maintaining distance from the child)	**1 Disconnected parental behavior** - frightening/threatening the child - frightened behaviors - dissociated behaviors - deferential and romantic/sexualized behaviors - disorganized/disoriented behaviors **2 Extreme insensitivity** **A Withdrawal** - failure to initiate responsive behavior - actively creating physical distance from the child - lack of interaction with the child **B Negative behaviors** - intrusiveness - aggressive behaviors

Note: Names of types (or subscales) of dysregulated parental behaviors are those used by authors in their coding system. References of each coding system appear in the first row of this table. For the listings of types of FR and AMBIANCE parental behaviors, see also Lyons-Ruth, K., & Jacobvitz, D. (2016). Attachment disorganization from infancy to adulthood: Neurobiological correlates, parenting contexts, and pathways to disorder. In J. Cassidy & P.R. Shaver (Eds.), *Handbook of attachment: Theory, research, and clinical applications* (pp. 667–695). Guilford Press.

Numerous studies have shown that parents of children with disorganized attachment exhibit higher levels of dysregulated parental behaviors than parents of children with organized attachment (secure, insecure avoidant, insecure ambivalent/resistant) (see Madigan et al., 2006, for a meta-analysis combining results of both the AMBIANCE and FR measures). In particular, studies indicated that in comparison with parents of organized children, those who displayed more dissociation (Abrams et al., 2006) and withdrawn behaviors (Goldberg et al., 2003) were more likely to have children with disorganized attachment. The work of Out and colleagues (2009b) also found that disconnected parental behaviors were more predictive of child attachment disorganization than extremely insensitive parental behaviors. In a recent study of families referred to child protective services due to maltreatment, we found that parents of children with disorganized attachment showed higher levels of disrupted parental behaviors in comparison with those of children with organized attachment (Langlois et al., 2021). In the same sample, higher levels of disconnected and extremely insensitive parental behaviors were also associated with child attachment disorganization (Zephyr et al., 2021). Dysregulated parental behaviors are also a risk factor for the development of emotion regulation problems and externalizing behavior problems (Green et al., 2007; Guyon-Harris et al., 2022; Jacobvitz et al., 2011;

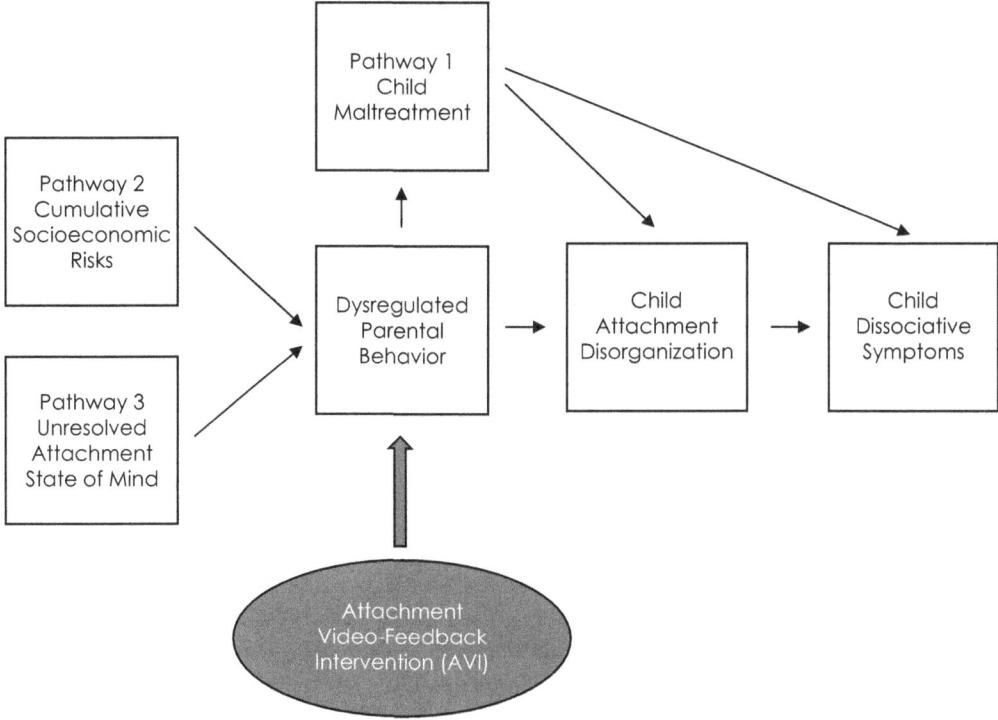

Figure 19.1 Pathways to Child Attachment Disorganization and Dissociation.

Madigan et al., 2007). Other studies with high-risk parents showed that parents who were highly exposed to multiple types of maltreatment during childhood, in comparison with parents with low exposure, were more likely to display disrupted parental behaviors one year postpartum (Guyon-Harris et al., 2021; Khoury et al., 2022). In addition, parental history of physical abuse was also related to more intrusive negative behaviors, while a history of physical neglect was related to more role confusion behaviors (Khoury et al., 2022).

Attachment-Based Intervention with Parents and Young Children

Several attachment-based interventions were designed to increase child attachment security and reduce attachment disorganization (and related dissociation). As parental sensitivity is a core component of attachment security, it has become a key target of attachment interventions. Over the years, the field has sustained two main approaches to attachment intervention (Cyr et al., 2012; Facompré et al., 2018). The first approach is *support-oriented*. It focuses on providing support to caregivers, such as health, social, and educational services and financial and legal resources. It addresses parental sensitivity by guiding parents in reinterpreting the representations of the relationship history with their own attachment figures. For example, the Infant/Child-Parent Psychotherapy (IPP or CPP) (Van Horn & Lieberman, 2008; Cicchetti et al., 2006) is a supportive, non-directive intervention that relies on developmental guidance to promote a trusting relationship with the parent as well as parenting skills and attachment security. This type of intervention is similar to traditional, individual therapy and is usually delivered as part of long-term interventions, generally lasting from a few months to a few years. The second approach is *parent-child-oriented*. It aims to improve the parent's sensitive behavior repertoire while in direct interaction with the child. Here, sessions are structured according to a manualized protocol and practitioners apply specific techniques, for which they have been trained, and engage the parent in the discussion of semi-structured topics. This intervention approach is generally short term, carried out in just a few sessions (e.g., between 6 and 20 weeks), involves weekly home visits, and lasts no longer than just a few weeks or months. In the past years, a growing number of short-term interventions were developed for families with different problems and challenges, such as families referred to child protective services due to maltreatment; adolescent mothers; immigrant families; low-income families; and children with externalizing problems, in foster care, or with an autism spectrum disorder. Many of these short-term interventions were tested using randomized controlled trials (state-of-the-art designs to assess intervention efficacy). The Video-Feedback Intervention to Promote Positive Parenting and Sensitive Discipline (VIPP-SD) (van IJzendoorn et al., 2023) and the AVI (Moss et al., 2018) are examples of short-term interventions. Generally, short-term interventions focus on changing parent-child interactive behaviors, include both the parent and child during the sessions with the practitioner, and offer video feedback or positive comments focused on the parent's strengths. Whether relying on short- or long-term intervention, the practitioner is invited to act as a secure base for the parent, guiding them in the exploration of their and their child's thoughts and emotions as well as their relationship (Berlin et al., 2008).

Taken all together, attachment intervention studies have shown a plethora of positive effects for families exposed to attachment interventions in comparison with families in control groups (either on a waiting list or receiving other types of interventions). In particular, studies have been conducted with families with a history of trauma/adversity or reported for maltreatment and for whom there is a greater risk of child attachment disorganization and dissociation (Cyr et al., 2020; Eguren et al., 2023; Facompré et al., 2018, for a meta-analysis; Steele & Steele, 2017, for a review). Results of these studies have shown that after being exposed to an attachment intervention, parents were generally more sensitive to child needs, showed higher reflective functioning and emotional availability, and reported less family chaos. In addition, parent-child dyads demonstrated more positive shared affect and reciprocity, and children showed more secure attachment, better emotional/physiological regulation and cognitive/motor development, and fewer behavior problems, post-traumatic stress symptoms, and attachment disorganization.

However, only a few studies have tested whether attachment interventions can decrease dysregulated parental behaviors (all studies used the AMBIANCE measure). Tereno et al. (2017) found a decrease in disrupted affective communication for mothers at high psychosocial risk who were exposed to an intensive home-visiting program (44 visits over two years), compared with mothers receiving regular services. This reduction was related to lower child attachment disorganization. In a study of families referred to child protective services due to unsubstantiated and substantiated maltreatment, Yarger et al. (2020) found fewer withdrawal behaviors in mothers after the short-term Attachment Biobehavioral Catch-up (ABC) intervention, in comparison with mothers receiving regular educational services. In a sample of parents with children at high risk for out-of-home placement and receiving attachment intervention using video feedback, Vischer et al. (2020) showed a decrease in affective communication errors, and fearful/disoriented and intrusion/negative parental behaviors. More recently, using the AVI, we have also found a decrease in disrupted parental behaviors (overall score and two dimensions: affective communication errors, withdrawal; Langlois et al., 2022). Furthermore, in another study using the AVI combined with trauma-focused cognitive behavioral therapy (TF-CBT), we found that sexually abused children and their mothers showed decreases in dissociation and post-traumatic stress symptoms, respectively, from the pre-test to post-test evaluations (Caouette et al., 2021).

The Attachment Video-Feedback Intervention (AVI)

The AVI is a short-term attachment intervention for parents and their children and consists of eight-weekly home visits, each lasting approximately 90 minutes. The AVI's overarching goal is to improve parental sensitivity and parent-child interactive quality. It has been tested with parents and children up to seven years of age (Moss et al., 2011) and, although it follows a standardized protocol in which each session is divided in four segments, it can be personalized to meet the families' specific relational challenges and the needs of the various clinical organizations that implement it. Using conceptual and video material, practitioners are trained to observe and distinguish between sensitive, insensitive, and dysregulated parental behaviors, as well as between functional and dysfunctional attachment relationships between parents and children. With the use of the video feedback technique and throughout each session, the practitioner helps the parent read their child's needs and communication strategies by strengthening parental sensitive behavior toward the child—that is, their ability to detect, interpret, and respond to distress signals and needs in the most appropriate way possible and within an acceptable time frame. Figure 19.2 illustrates the different phases of the AVI and usual progression of parents throughout the intervention process.

Each meeting session consists of four segments:

1 **A discussion** (30 minutes) with the parent. In the first session, the practitioner gathers information about the parent and child, describes the intervention process and framework to the parent, and ask the parent about any specific aspects of parenting (e.g., patience and discipline) or child behavior (e.g., emotion regulation, attachment, and compliance) they would like to see improved. The discussion topics of the following sessions focus on attachment and child development and are chosen by the parent and practitioner.
2 **A filmed activity with the parent and child** (10 minutes). Toys are provided to the dyad and simple instruction is formulated for the parent (e.g., describe what your child is doing, mention your child's emotions) by the practitioner in accordance with the behaviors that need to be improved.
3 **Video feedback for the parent** (20–30 minutes), based on the filmed activity at segment 2 and immediately following this activity.

   - During the feedback, the practitioner stops the video at specific moments *to highlight the parent's sensitive behavior and the positive influence on the child* (e.g., "When you touched your child's shoulder, you can see that how your child calmed down and was further able to do the puzzle. What you did is so important for him to learn to regulate his emotions and trust that you are here when he needs it."). The practitioner also asks the parent how they and the child are feeling or what they are thinking during a positive sequence. These questions encourage the parent to take an active part in the intervention process and guide their reflexive process on their own behaviors and mental state, as well as those of the child.
   - To address dysregulated behaviors during video feedback, practitioners are invited to *emphasize the parent's capacity to repair the parent-child relationship*. Once a trusting parent-practitioner relationship has been established and changes in the parent's behaviors begin to emerge, the practitioner, without confronting the parent, asks them to describe more difficult behavioral sequences and think of ways to use their growing repertoire of sensitive behaviors to repair the relationship with their child. In keeping with the strength-based philosophy of the AVI, it is imperative that the practitioner maintain a positive stance at all times, even when addressing dysregulated behaviors.

4 **A wrap-up of the session** (15 minutes). The most important messages are highlighted for the parent, who is encouraged to repeat similar parent-child activities during the coming week. At the

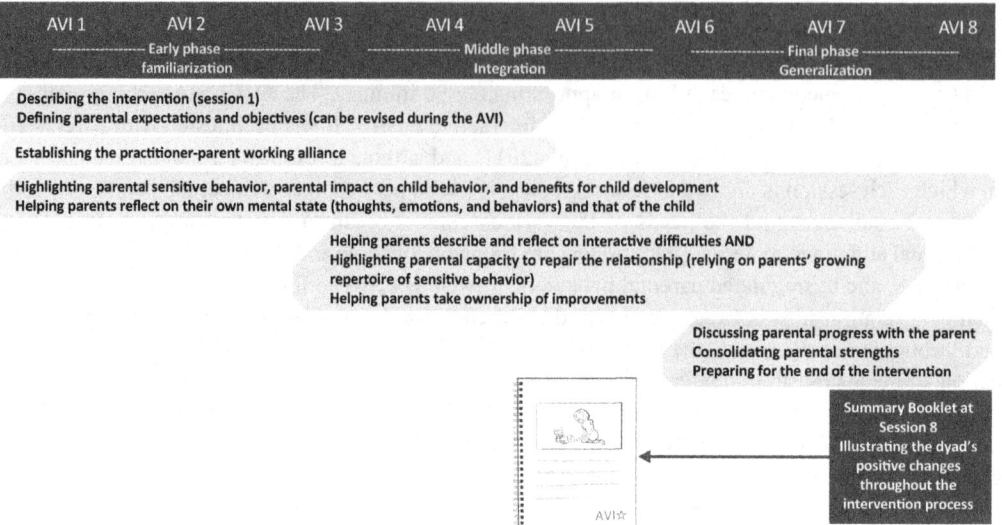

Figure 19.2 Phases of the Attachment Video-Feedback Intervention (AVI) and Parents' Usual Progression Throughout the Intervention Process.

final session, a summary booklet including (screenshot) pictures of the dyad in shared positive moments that were filmed throughout the sessions, each accompanied with a brief description of the parent's positive behavior and its impact on the child, is given to the parent as a visual reminder of their strengths and capacity to generalize and sustain treatment gains.

An AVI Case Study to Reduce Dysregulated Parental Behavior, Child Attachment Disorganization, and Dissociation

In the following case study, we present a fictional mother-daughter dyad for which the background information, data questionnaires, and observations are based on a compilation of actual cases of dyads who have participated in our intervention research projects. For the purpose of this chapter, we focus on changes in child attachment behavior between pre- and post-AVI assessments, as well as changes in dysregulated parental behaviors across these two assessments and throughout all eight AVI sessions. In these projects, practitioners were not involved during the pre- and post-AVI assessments. Figure 19.3 illustrates the parent's changes in disrupted behaviors, assessed from the videos by a research assistant with the AMBIANCE measure. Scores range on a 1 (= no disrupted parental behavior) to 7 (= high disrupted parental behavior) point scale.

Background Information

The mother, in her early 30s, and her two-year-old daughter were referred to the AVI program by a community agency providing resources related to prior domestic violence. On the scale of dissociation symptoms on the Trauma Symptom Checklist (Briere & Runtz, 1989), the mother reported moderate scores for flashbacks, spaced-out experiences, and dizziness. On the Childhood Trauma Questionnaire (Bernstein & Fink, 1998), she reported low to moderate scores for childhood experiences of psychological abuse. On the Child Behavior Checklist questionnaire (Achenbach & Rescorla, 2000), the child

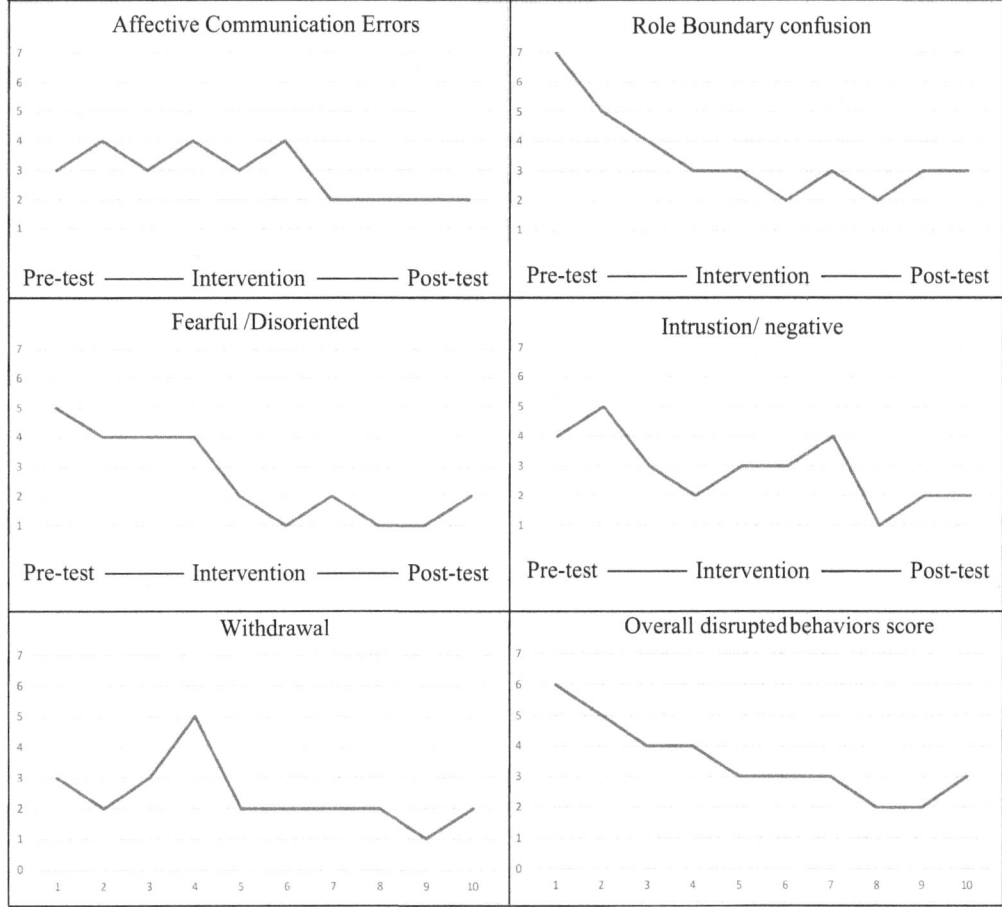

Figure 19.3 Changes in Dysregulated Parental Behaviors across the Assessment (pre-test = session 1; post-test = session 10) and Intervention Process (Sessions 2 to 9).

showed clinical scores of internalizing and externalizing problems. During an interview, the mother also reported dizziness symptoms in her daughter, after which, on a few occasions, the child would shut down and lose consciousness. This was reported to occur more frequently when the child was left alone, such as prior to a nap or in moments when the mother was busy.

Pre-AVI Observation of Behaviors

During the pre-test assessment visit (Strange Situation Procedure), the child was classified as having a disorganized attachment, simultaneously showing avoidance and seeking contact behaviors (with head averted) and freezing behaviors. The child also exhibited some controlling and punitive attachment behaviors.

The mother displayed brief moments of disorientation, combined with other behaviors suggesting fear of her child. While playing with her child, the mother frenetically moved from one toy to another, and when the child attempted to engage her, she remained unavailable, showed flat affect, and avoided eye contact. When approaching her child to play, hesitation movements were observed, culminating in withdrawal behaviors. After backing away from her child, the mother spoke in an unusually high-pitched voice, which was again observed when approaching the child upon reunion. In addition, the mother repeatedly sought comfort from the child, asking for several kisses and insisting when her daughter ignored her requests.

Session 1. *The discussion segment* of the first AVI session focused on the mother's description of her relationship with her daughter, which she considered fusional, friendly, and loving. The mother expressed being preoccupied with her child's dizziness symptoms. She wished to learn to set limits and establish routines with her child, given that the child could sometimes exhibit outbursts of aggressive behavior (e.g., hitting her mother, throwing objects when her mother gives her instructions). *During the parent-child filmed activity segment*, the mother was asked to play with her daughter as she would normally do. She chose sensory motor toys and a soft climbing module. She soon found it difficult to follow her child's initiatives and autonomy needs, physically pulling the child closer to her. When the child managed to move away to explore further, the mother exhibited intrusive behaviors (e.g., holding the child's arm and putting toys on her head). Role reversal was also observed when the mother sought reassurance from her daughter, asking the child to look at her or praise her actions. Following this sequence, the child suddenly threw a toy at the mother's face, and the mother briefly dissociated (blank expression). Then, hesitating movements, a high-pitched voice, and a sudden inexplicable laugh were observed in the mother as her child approached her. *During the video-feedback segment,* the practitioner stopped the video to highlight moments during which the mother let her child explore the toys and the positive impact it had on the child (e.g., the child smiled and looked at her mother after she had finally accepted that her daughter climbed on the sensory module). The mother was asked to reflect on her child's feelings and thoughts at this particular moment. The practitioner highlighted that the mother was available to her child when she showed an interest in her child's verbalizations and maintained eye contact. Toward the end of the feedback segment, the mother commented freely on their dyadic interaction, saying that when the child moved away from her, she noticed that she interrupted her child's exploration. When asked how she felt at this point, the mother spoke of anxiety and rejection associated with the distance her child had taken from her; she believed her daughter was angry and unwilling to make contact with her. This video-feedback experience was the first step in the mother's reinterpretation of her child's rejection behaviors as bids for autonomy and exploration needs.

Based on observations made during this first AVI session, the practitioner formulated a "relationship quality working hypothesis," suggesting that the mother and child were involved in a relationship characterized by avoidance and disorganization: the child showed avoidant and disorganized/controlling behaviors and the mother reported feelings of rejection, combined with the display of negative, intrusive, and dysregulated (seeking the child's affection and dissociation) behaviors. Drawing on this relationship quality hypothesis, the practitioner aimed to improve the mother's availability for her daughter and thought of activities and instructions that would encourage the child's exploration and referencing back to mother. The practitioner provided the dyad with a variety of non-directive yet slightly challenging activities, just enough to trigger the child's need to turn to her mother for support. Such maternal referencing by the child in novel or uncertain situations would likely help the mother see and think of her child's exploration behavior in less threatening ways. The practitioner also aimed to facilitate maternal repair behaviors to decrease the tension generated by her dysregulation (intrusion, dissociation, and role confusion) and the child's associated avoidance and controlling behaviors. To achieve this, chosen activities sought to yield moments of joy and more relaxed parent-child experiences, also conducive to establishing a secure alliance between the parent and the practitioner.

Session 2. *The discussion segment* focused on children's attachment and exploration needs. Using images, the practitioner showed the mother that children normally seek out their parents when they are distressed, and they normally explore their environment when they are comfortable. In both cases, they need their parents either to comfort them or guide them. The mother gradually began to recognize that the more she feels rejected by her child, the more likely she seeks closeness and comfort from her child, when in fact she should be the one assuming a security base role for her child. *During the parent-child filmed activity segment*, the mother was given a set of blocks and was asked to let her daughter decide how she would play, yet at the same time, to participate in the play according to her child's interests. During the play, the child explored the blocks on her own and ignored the mother's invitation to build a tower together. The mother repeatedly asked her daughter's permission to place blocks on the tower, but the child continued ignoring her demands. With a flat affect expression, the mother said, "*I don't exist*," and, with a disengaged gaze, continued to play by herself in a frenetic manner. When the child turned to hand the mother some blocks, the mother responded, "*You don't want Mommy to put blocks on*," attributing a negative motivation to her child. Still, at other moments during the play, the mother encouraged her child, and with a warm voice, she described her daughter's play. *During the video-feedback segment*, the practitioner underlined the mother's ability to praise her child and describe her child's playing. This is important for children, as they can sense their parents' genuine interest in what they are doing, which fosters self-esteem and a positive learning context. The practitioner highlighted that when the mother naturally included herself in her child's play (not asking permission or telling her daughter how to play), the child accepted her presence, and a pleasant and reciprocal play emerged. Noteworthy, the mother kept asking her child for kisses. When the child did not respond to her mother's need for affection, the mother pulled her arm, and gave her a kiss, saying, "*Don't you love me? Don't you want to kiss Mommy?*" The practitioner asked what the mother understood of her daughter's distant behaviors. The mother replied that she believed it was her way of saying no, but that she was not respecting her child's boundaries.

Session 3. *The discussion segment* focused on parental sensitivity to child attachment and distress signals. The practitioner advised that parents who acknowledge their child's distress by showing warmth, comfort, and predictability can help children resolve distress and learn effective emotion regulation strategies when feeling overwhelmed. *During the parent-child filmed activity segment,* the mother was instructed to follow her child's initiatives (as in Session 2), as well as to describe what her daughter was doing. During the craft, the child felt uncomfortable with and stressed by the glue, so she let her mother handle the materials while observing and commenting on what the mother was doing. Although the mother was less intrusive during this session, she minimized the child's distress and physically withdrew herself from the child. In addition, when the child was worried about the glue, the mother switched the topic and said, "*It's over now!*" in a stern voice. After the craft, the child pretended to glue some pieces onto the mother's legs. The mother followed the child's interests and let her explore the material in a context that felt safe for her. *During the video feedback segment,* this last sequence was reviewed with the mother. She observed how her flexibility and ability to follow her child's interests led to a warm moment of proximity. The mother was grateful for this proximity initiated by the child, although she expressed how difficult it was for her to be sensitive to the child's prior distress.

Session 4. *During the discussion segment*, the practitioner initiated a conversation about the child's dizziness symptoms. The mother acknowledged that her child's dizziness leaves her helpless and frightened. She suggested that these symptoms might not have emerged had she been able to spend more quality time with her daughter and not exposed her to domestic violence. The practitioner reminded the mother of the discussion in Session 3, namely, the importance of attending to her child's distress. She suggested that when parents are overwhelmed by their own or child distress, they themselves exacerbate their child's distress. She talked about sensitive repair, where parents, even those who have been a source of stress, can reassert their parental security base role by focusing on repairing the relationship with the child. The practitioner underlined for the mother that parents can do this using what they learn in the AVI—for example, when the mother describes to her child what the child is experiencing in the play. *During the parent-child filmed activity segment*, the mother was instructed, as in Session 4, to follow her child's initiatives and describe what her daughter was doing. In a bowling game with her mother, the child was more interested in exploring the toys than in knocking over the pins. After a few maternal requests ignored by the child, the mother followed the child's interests, began to describe the child's actions more fully, and the dyad played music with the toys, sharing a wonderful moment of physical proximity and pleasure. *During the video-feedback segment*, the practitioner highlighted this last sequence to show how the dyad maintained eye contact and exchanged smiles. She underlined the mother's delight in her child and her ability to describe the child's experience accurately. The mother witnessed her own ability to respect her child's wishes and noted that, rather than imposing her own agenda, she succeeded in following her child's initiatives, leading them to collaborate.

Session 5. *The discussion segment* focused on setting limits and discipline. For example, when setting limits, the mother tended to ask the child what she would like to do (e.g., "*Do you want to get off the table?*") or ask permission (e.g., "*Can I remove the sharp scissors from here?*"). The practitioner advised the mother that questions should rather be used when she wants to offer the child a choice, and that sharing clear and simple instructions makes children feel secure, as parental expectations become more predictable for children. *During the parent-child filmed activity segment*, the mother was asked to play with her child one turn at a time. The child chose to use play dough with her mother. The mother suggested different ways of using the play dough, but did not insist when her child avoided her suggestions. When the child suddenly became irritated and somewhat distressed by the play dough sticking to her fingers, the mother responded sensitively, reflecting the child's emotions. During this sequence, the mother established eye contact and got down to her daughter's level, using a calm, comforting voice to reassure the child. *During the video-feedback segment,* the practitioner highlighted the mother's warmth when her child felt irritated, and praised her for describing her daughter's emotion. This is important because such sensitive behaviors helped the child calm down and learn to develop clear expectations of her mother's ability to meet her needs.

Sessions 6, 7, and 8. During the three last sessions, the discussion segments gradually focused on a synthesis of the strengths consolidated by the mother throughout the intervention process (e.g., increased capacity to respect her child's autonomy needs [less intrusiveness] and increased capacity to respond to her child's distress and repair the relationship [less dissociation]). First, the practitioner asked the mother what she thought of her progress. The mother said she felt less rejected by her child, less overwhelmed by her child's distress, and really enjoyed playing with her child, although she still found it difficult not to solicit her affection (role boundary confusion). *During the parent-child filmed activity segment,* the mother and child were asked to play with figurines and a small bath of water (Session 6), Mr. Potato Head (Session 7), and plastic animals (Session 8). The mother was instructed (as in previous sessions) to follow her child's lead in the play, setting clear limits if necessary (Session 6), and to describe what her child was doing and feeling (Sessions 7 and 8). For example, in Session 6, physically intrusive behaviors were observed when the mother disapproved of her child's behaviors. Another time, when she wanted to stop the child from splashing water, she said in a stern voice, "You're spilling water everywhere!" Nevertheless, at other moments, the mother verbalized clear demands, such as, "*To play with water, you can play with the toy in the bath,*" without having to physically intervene. *During video feedback,* the mother saw that the child reacted positively to the limits she set (Session 6), and also noticed that she was being intrusive when tickling her daughter in the face with a toy, which made her daughter became more aggressive (Session 7). The mother, in a warm yet assertive way, reflected to her daughter how angry she must have been at her invasive tickling and redirected the child to more appropriate behaviors (Session 7). The practitioner highlighted and praised the mother's capacity to see that her child had shown distress, to cease intrusive behavior, and to describe the child's feelings.

Post-AVI Observations of Behavior

In the post-test assessment, the mother showed some disorientation and role-reversal behaviors while playing with her child. However, she also demonstrated the ability to self-monitor and even quickly reorient her mental attention on her child. She was able to respond more frequently and appropriately to her child's signals and exhibiting markedly fewer intrusive and role confusion behaviors. The mother reported that the child was no longer showing dizziness symptoms (since Session 6) and she expressed feeling more available and attentive to her child's needs, especially at critical moments such as during separation (e.g., bedtime routines). She also reported intentionally organizing playtime with her child as part of her daily routine. The mother noticed that her presence had an impact on her child's dizziness symptoms and had decreased her aggressive behaviors. She noted that on days when she spent less quality time with her child, or when she was more intrusive, the child showed more opposition and resistant behaviors.

At the end of the intervention, the practitioner observed an increase in parental sensitivity and a reduction in dysregulated parental behaviors—confirmed by the research assistant's observation of disrupted maternal behavior throughout the AVI (see Figure 19.3) and statistically significant reductions in role boundary confusion (from scores of 7 to 3), disorientation/dissociation (from scores of 5 to 2), and overall disrupted maternal behavior (from scores of 6 to 3). In addition, the child showed fewer externalizing problems and no longer exhibited disorganized attachment behavior (although still showed some avoidant behavior). The progress made by the dyad is consistent with previous findings on the efficacy of the AVI and suggests that the AVI may hold promise for reducing dissociation in mothers and children.

Conclusion

In this chapter, we have argued, on the basis of previous literature linking attachment disorganization and dissociation, that three pathways to attachment disorganization may confer vulnerability to dissociation. Maltreatment, as experienced directly by the child, is the first critical pathway to attachment disorganization. The second and third pathways to disorganization are those taken by children who have not experienced abuse or neglect but are exposed to cumulative socioeconomic risks (second pathway) or to their parents' unresolved (disorganized) attachment state of mind (third pathway). We suggest that dysregulated parental behaviors, such as parental frightening and frightened, disrupted, disconnected, or extremely insensitive behaviors, which have been shown to elicit fear for children, might be a common denominator in each of these three pathways. Several attachment-based interventions have been designed to increase child attachment security and reduce attachment disorganization and related-dissociation behaviors. In this chapter, we focused on the AVI, a program we have refined over the years and that has been shown to improve many aspects of the parent-child relationship and child development, such as parental sensitivity and child attachment security. More recently, we have shown that the AVI is also able to reduce dysregulated parental behavior. In this chapter, illustrated with a fictional case study (based on a compilation of several actual cases), we demonstrated the value of the AVI to diminish parental dysregulation and child attachment disorganization, which are both characterized by dissociation behaviors.

Note

Chantal Cyr, as senior author, and Valérie Langlois have equal contribution to this chapter and thus share equal authorship. During the course of this work, Valérie Langlois and Gabrielle Myre were supported by the Social Sciences and Humanities Research Council of Canada. Chantal Cyr received funding support from the Canada Research Chairs Program. We thank all the families and clinicians who have participated in our intervention projects.

References

Abrams, K. Y., Rifkin, A., & Hesse, E. (2006). Examining the role of parental frightened/frightening subtypes in predicting disorganized attachment within a brief observational procedure. *Development and Psychopathology, 18*(2), 345–361. https://www.cambridge.org/core/journals/development-and-psychopathology/article/abs/examining-the-role-of-parental-frightenedfrightening-subtypes-in-predicting-disorganized-attachment-within-a-brief-observational-procedure/A40D5C5DF14B83CA65F4642B252CB95

Achenbach, T. M., & Rescorla, L. A. (2000). *Manual for the ASEBA preschool-age forms & profiles*. University of Vermont, Research Center for Children, Youth & Families.

Ainsworth, M. D. S., Blehar, M. C., Waters, E., & Wall, S. (1978). *Patterns of attachment: A psychological study of the Strange Situation*. Lawrence Eribaum.

Berlin, L. J., Cassidy, J., & Appleyard, K. (2008). The influence of early attachments on other relationships. In J. Cassidy & P. R. Shaver (Eds.), *Handbook of attachment: Theory, research, and clinical applications* (pp. 333–347). Guilford Press.

Bernier, A., Carlson, S. M., Deschênes, M., & Matte-Gagné, C. (2012). Social factors in the development of early executive functioning: A closer look at the caregiving environment. *Developmental Science, 15*(1), 12–24. https://doi.org/10.1111/j.1467-7687.2011.01093.x

Bernstein, D. P., & Fink, L. (1998). *Childhood trauma questionnaire. A retrospective self-report*. Psychological Corporation.

Bowlby, J. (1969). *Attachment and loss: Vol. 1.* Attachment. Basic Books.

Bowlby, J. (1973). *Attachment and loss: Vol. 2.* Separation. Basic Books.

Briere, J. (2006). Dissociative symptoms and trauma exposure: Specificity, affect dysregulation, and post-traumatic stress. *Journal of Nervous and Mental Disease, 194*(2), 78–82. https://doi.org/10.1097/01.nmd.0000198139.47371.54

Briere, J., & Runtz, M. (1989). The Trauma Symptom Checklist (TSC-33): Early data on a new scale. *Journal of Interpersonal Violence, 4*(2), 151–163. https://doi.org/10.1177/088626089004002002

Bronfman, E., Parsons, E., & Lyons-Ruth, K. (1999–2014). *Atypical Maternal Behavior Instrument for Assessment and Classification (AMBIANCE): Manual for coding disrupted affective communication*. Unpublished manuscript. Harvard Medical School.

Caouette, J., Hébert, M., Cyr, C., & Amédée, L. M. (2021). The attachment video-feedback intervention (AVI) combined to the trauma-focused cognitive behavioral therapy (TF-CBT) for sexually abused preschoolers and their parents: A pilot study examining pre- to post-test changes. *Developmental Child Welfare, 3*(2), 119–134. https://doi.org/10.1177/25161032211013820

Carlson, E. A. (1998). A prospective longitudinal study of attachment disorganization/disorientation. *Child Development, 69*(4), 1107–1128. https://doi.org/10.2307/1132365

Carlson, E. A., Egeland, B., & Sroufe, L. A. (2009). A prospective investigation of the development of borderline personality symptoms. *Development and Psychopathology, 21*(4), 1311–1334. https://doi.org/10.1017/S0954579409990174

Cassidy, J., Brett, B. E., Gross, J. T., Stern, J. A., Martin, D. R., Mohr, J. J., & Woodhouse, S. S. (2017). Circle of security–parenting: A randomized controlled trial in Head Start. *Development and Psychopathology, 29*(2), 651. https://doi.org/10.1017/S0954579417000244

Cicchetti, D., Rogosch, F. A., & Toth, S. L. (2006). Fostering secure attachment in infants in maltreating families through preventive interventions. *Development and Psychopathology, 18*(3), 623–649. https://www.cambridge.org/core/journals/development-and-psychopathology/article/abs/fostering-secure-attachment-in-infants-in-maltreating-families-through-preventive-interventions/1281AD348AD23F959131F575D2D70F85

Cyr, C., Dubois-Comtois, K., Michel, G., Poulin, C., Pascuzzo, K., Losier, V., Dumais, M., St-Laurent, D., & Moss, E. (2012). Attachment theory in the assessment and promotion of parental competency in child protection cases. In A. Muela (Eds.), *Child abuse and neglect: A multidimensional approach* (pp. 63–86). Intech.

Cyr, C., Dubois-Comtois, K., Paquette, D., Lopez, L., & Bigras, M. (2020). An attachment-based parental capacity assessment to orient decision-making in child protection cases: A randomized control trial. *Child Maltreatment, 27*(1), 66–77. https://doi.org/10.1177/1077559520967995

Cyr, C., Euser, E. M., Bakermans-Kranenburg, M. J., & Van IJzendoorn, M. H. (2010). Attachment security and disorganization in maltreating and high-risk families: A series of meta-analyses. *Development and Psychopathology, 22*(1), 87–108. https://doi.org/10.1017/S0954579409990289

Dozier, M., Stovall-McClough, K. C., & Albus, K. E. (2008). Attachment and psychopathology in adulthood. In J. Cassidy & P. R. Shaver (Eds.), *Handbook of attachment: Theory, research, and clinical applications* (pp. 718–744). Guilford Press.

Dubois-Comtois, K., Moss, E., Cyr, C., & Pascuzzo, K. (2013). Behavior problems in middle childhood: The predictive role of maternal distress, child attachment, and mother-child interactions. *Journal of Abnormal Child Psychology, 41*(8), 1311–1324. https://doi.org/10.1007/s10802-013-9764-6

Dutra, L., & Lyons-Ruth, K. (2005, April). Maltreatment, maternal and child psychopathology, and quality of early care as predictors of adolescent dissociation. In J. Borelli (Chair), *Interrelations of attachment and trauma symptoms: A developmental perspective.* Symposium conducted at the biennial meeting of the Society for Research in Child Development, Atlanta, GA.

Eguren, A., Cyr, C., Dubois-Comtois, K., & Muela, A. (2023). Effects of the Attachment Video-Feedback Intervention (AVI) on parents and children at risk of maltreatment during the COVID-19 pandemic. *Child Abuse & Neglect, 139*, Article 106121. https://doi.org/10.1016/j.chiabu.2023.106121

Facompré, C. R., Bernard, K., & Waters, T. E. (2018). Effectiveness of interventions in preventing disorganized attachment: A meta-analysis. *Development and Psychopathology, 30*(1), 1–11. https://doi.org/10.1017/S0954579417000426

Fearon, R. P., Bakermans-Kranenburg, M. J., Van IJzendoorn, M. H., Lapsley, A. M., & Roisman, G. I. (2010). The significance of insecure attachment and disorganization in the development of children's externalizing behavior: A meta-analytic study. *Child Development, 81*(2), 435–456. https://doi.org/10.1111/j.1467-8624.2009.01405.x

Goldberg, S., Benoit, D., Blokland, K., & Madigan, S. (2003). Atypical maternal behavior, maternal representations, and infant disorganized attachment. *Development and Psychopathology, 15*(2), 239–257. https://doi.org/10.1017/s0954579403000130

Green, J., Stanley, C., & Peters, S. (2007). Disorganized attachment representation and atypical parenting in young school age children with externalizing disorder. *Attachment & Human Development, 9*(3), 207–222. https://doi.org/10.1080/14616730701453820

Groh, A. M., Fearon, R. P., Bakermans-Kranenburg, M. J., Van IJzendoorn, M. H., Steele, R. D., & Roisman, G. I. (2014). The significance of attachment security for children's social competence with peers: A meta-analytic study. *Attachment & Human Development, 16*(2), 103–136. https://doi.org/10.1080/14616734.2014.883636

Groh, A. M., Roisman, G. I., van IJzendoorn, M. H., Bakermans-Kranenburg, M. J., & Fearon, R. P. (2012). The significance of insecure and disorganized attachment for children's internalizing symptoms: A meta-analytic study. *Child Development, 83*(2), 591–610. https://doi.org/10.1111/j.1467-8624.2011.01711.x

Guyon-Harris, K. L., Ahlfs-Dunn, S. M., Madigan, S., Bronfman, E., Benoit, D., & Huth-Bocks, A. C. (2022). Disrupted caregiving behavior as a mediator of the relation between disrupted prenatal maternal representations and toddler social-emotional functioning. *Development and Psychopathology, 34*(3), 755–763. https://doi.org/10.1017/S0954579420001674

Guyon-Harris, K. L., Madigan, S., Bronfman, E., Romero, G., & Huth-Bocks, A. C. (2021). Prenatal identification of risk for later disrupted parenting behavior using latent profiles of childhood maltreatment. *Journal of Interpersonal Violence, 36*(23–24), NP13517–NP13540. https://doi.org/10.1177/0886260520906175

Hesse, E. (2016). The Adult Attachment Interview: Protocol, method of analysis, and empirical studies: 1985–2015. In J. Cassidy & P. R. Shaver (Eds.), *Handbook of attachment: Theory, research, and clinical applications* (pp. 553–597). Guilford Press.

Hesse, E., & Main, M. (2006). Frightened, threatening, and dissociative parental behavior in low-risk samples: Description, discussion, and interpretations. *Development and Psychopathology, 18*(2), 309–343. https://doi.org/10.1017/S0954579406060172

Hobson, R. P., Patrick, M., Crandell, L., Garcia-Pérez, R., & Lee, A. (2005). Personal relatedness and attachment in infants of mothers with borderline personality disorder. *Development and Psychopathology, 17*(2), 329–347. https://www.cambridge.org/core/journals/development-and-psychopathology/article/abs/personal-relatedness-and-attachment-in-infants-of-mothers-with-borderline-personality-disorder/464B7B008F64BD-A7973B02DAE5B3C21B

Jacobvitz, D., Hazen, N., Zaccagnino, M., Messina, S., & Beverung, L. (2011). Frightening maternal behavior, infant disorganization, and risks for psychopathology. The origins and organization of adaptation and maladaptation. In D. Cicchetti & G. I. Roisman (Eds.), *The origins and organization of adaptation and maladaptation* (pp. 283–322). John Wiley & Sons, Inc.

Khoury, J. E., Dimitrov, L., Enlow, M. B., Haltigan, J. D., Bronfman, E., & Lyons-Ruth, K. (2022). Patterns of maternal childhood maltreatment and disrupted interaction between mothers and their 4-month-old infants. *Child Maltreatment, 27*(3), 366–377. https://doi.org/10.1177/10775595211007567

Langlois, V., Cyr-Desautels, L., Bronfman, E., Dubois-Comtois, K., & Cyr, C. (2022, June). The efficacy of the attachment ideo-feedback intervention: Decreases in atypical parental behavior in families reported for maltreatment and neglect. In Audrey-Ann Deneault (Chair), *Assessing foundational claims of attachment theory*. Paper symposium –Canadian Psychological Association, Calgary.

Langlois, V., Cyr-Desautels, L., Cognard-Bessette, S., & Cyr, C., (2021, March). *Disrupted parental behavior, child attachment disorganization and child psychopathology in families reported for child maltreatment*. Poster Presentation – Society for Research in Child Development Virtual Biennial Meeting.

Liotti, G. (2006). A model of dissociation based on attachment theory and research. *Journal of Trauma & Dissociation, 7*(4), 55–73. https://doi.org/10.1300/J229v07n04_04

Lyons-Ruth, K., Bronfman, E., & Parsons, E. (1999). Maternal frightened, frightening, or atypical behavior and disorganized infant attachment patterns. *Monographs of the Society for Research in Child Development, 64*(3), 67–96.

Lyons-Ruth, K., Bureau, J. F., Holmes, B., Easterbrooks, A., & Brooks, N. H. (2013). Borderline symptoms and suicidality/self-injury in late adolescence: Prospectively observed relationship correlates in infancy and childhood. *Psychiatry Research, 206*(2–3), 273–281. https://doi.org/10.1016/j.psychres.2012.09.030

Lyons-Ruth, K., & Jacobvitz, D. (2016). Attachment disorganization from infancy to adulthood: Neurobiological correlates, parenting contexts, and pathways to disorder. In J. Cassidy & P. R. Shaver (Eds.), *Handbook of attachment: Theory, research, and clinical applications* (pp. 667–695). Guilford Press.

Madigan, S., Atkinson, L., Laurin, K., & Benoit, D. (2013). Attachment and internalizing behavior in early childhood: A meta-analysis. *Developmental Psychology, 49*(4), 672–689. https://doi.org/10.1037/a0028793

Madigan, S., Bakermans-Kranenburg, M. J., Van IJzendoorn, M. H., Moran, G., Pederson, D. R., & Benoit, D. (2006). Unresolved states of mind, anomalous parental behavior, and disorganized attachment: A review and meta-analysis of a transmission gap. *Attachment & Human Development, 8*(2), 89–111. https://doi.org/10.1080/14616730600774458

Madigan, S., Fearon, R. M., van IJzendoorn, M. H., Duschinsky, R., Schuengel, C., Bakermans-Kranenburg, M. J., Ly, A., Cooke, J., Deneault, A-A., Oosterman, M., & Verhage, M. L. (2023). The first 20,000 strange situation procedures: A meta-analytic review. *Psychological Bulletin, 149*(1–2), 99–132. https://doi.org/10.1037/bul0000388

Madigan, S., Moran, G., Schuengel, C., Pederson, D. R., & Otten, R. (2007). Unresolved maternal attachment representations, disrupted maternal behavior and disorganized attachment in infancy: Links to toddler behavior problems. *Journal of Child Psychology and Psychiatry, 48*(10), 1042–1050. https://doi.org/10.1111/j.1469-7610.2007.01805.x

Main, M., & Hesse, E. (1990). Parents' unresolved traumatic experiences are related to infant disorganized attachment status: Is frightened and/or frightening parental behavior the linking mechanism? In M. T. Greenberg, D. Cicchetti & E. M. Cummings (Eds.), *Attachment in the preschool years: Theory, research, and intervention* (pp. 121–160). University of Chicago Press.

Main, M., Kaplan, N., & Cassidy, J. (1985). Security in infancy, childhood, and adulthood: A move to the level of representation. *Monographs of the Society for Research in Child Development, 50*(1–2), 66–104. https://doi.org/10.2307/3333827

Main, M., & Solomon, J. (1990). Procedures for identifying infants as disorganized/disoriented during the Ainsworth Strange Situation. In M. T. Greenberg, D. Cicchetti & E. M. Cummings (Eds.), *Attachment in the preschool years: Theory, research, and intervention* (pp. 121–160). University of Chicago Press.

Moss, E., Cyr, C., Bureau, J. F., Tarabulsy, G. M., & Dubois-Comtois, K. (2005). Stability of attachment during the preschool period. *Developmental Psychology, 41*, 773.

Moss, E., Cyr, C., & Dubois-Comtois, K. (2004). Attachment at early school age and developmental risk: Examining family contexts and behavior problems of controlling-caregiving, controlling-punitive, and behaviorally disorganized children. *Developmental Psychology, 40*, 519–532.

Moss, E., Dubois-Comtois, K., Cyr, C., Tarabulsy, G. M., St-Laurent, D., & Bernier, A. (2011). Efficacy of a home-visiting intervention aimed at improving maternal sensitivity, child attachment, and behavioral outcomes for maltreated children: A randomized control trial. *Development and Psychopathology, 23*(1), 195–210. https://doi.org/10.1017/S0954579410000738

Moss, E., & St-Laurent, D. (2001). Attachment at school age and academic performance. *Developmental Psychology, 37*(6), 863–874. https://doi.org/10.1037//0012-1649.37.6.863

Moss, E., Tarabulsy, G. M., Dubois-Comtois, K., Cyr, C., Bernier, A., & St-Laurent, D. (2018). The attachment video-feedback intervention program: Development and validation. In H. Steele & M. Steele (Eds.), *Handbook of attachment-based interventions* (pp. 318–338). Guilford Press.

Myre, G., Cognard-Bessette, C., Dubois-Comtois, K., St-Laurent, D., Tarabulsy, G., Bernier, A. Moss, E., & Cyr, C. (2022, June). Domestic violence, atypical parental behaviours and child attachment disorganization in families receiving child protective services. In Audrey-Ann Denault (Chair), *Expanding Attachment Research to Fathers, Different Risk, Contexts, and Family Systems.* Paper symposium, Development 2022: Canadian Psychological Association, Calgary, Alberta, Canada.

O'connor, E., Bureau, J. F., Mccartney, K., & Lyons-Ruth, K. (2011). Risks and outcomes associated with disorganized/controlling patterns of attachment at age three years in the National Institute of Child Health & Human Development study of early child care and youth development. *Infant Mental Health Journal, 32*(4), 450–472. https://doi.org/10.1002/imhj.20305

Ogawa, J. R., Sroufe, L. A., Weinfield, N. S., Carlson, E. A., & Egeland, B. (1997). Development and the fragmented self: Longitudinal study of dissociative symptomatology in a nonclinical sample. *Development and Psychopathology, 9*(4), 855–879. https://doi.org/10.1017/s0954579497001478

Out, D., Cyr, C., Pijlman, F. T. A., Beijersbergen, M. D., Bakermans-Kranenburg, M. J., & Van IJzendoorn, M. H. (2009a). *Disconnected and extremely insensitive parenting (DIP).* Center for Child and Family Studies, Leiden University.

Out, D., Bakermans-Kranenburg, M. J., & Van IJzendoorn, M. H. (2009b). The role of disconnected and extremely insensitive parenting in the development of disorganized attachment: Validation of a new measure. *Attachment & Human Development, 11*(5), 419–443. https://doi.org/10.1080/14616730903132289

Putnam, F. W. (1997). *Dissociation in children and adolescents.* Guildford Press.

Schuder, M. R., & Lyons-Ruth, K. (2004). "Hidden trauma" in infancy: Attachment, fearful arousal, and early dysfunction of the stress response system. In J. D. Osofsky (Ed.), *Young children and trauma: Intervention and treatment* (pp. 69–104). Guilford Press.

Sroufe, L. A. (2005). Attachment and development: A prospective, longitudinal study from birth to adulthood. *Attachment & Human Development, 7*(4), 349–367. https://doi.org/10.1080/14616730500365928

Steele, H., & Steele, M. (Eds.). (2017). *Handbook of attachment-based interventions.* Guilford Press.

Tereno, S., Madigan, S., Lyons-Ruth, K., Plamondon, A., Atkinson, L., Guedeney, N., Greacen, T., Dugravier, R., Saias, T., & Guedeney, A. (2017). Assessing a change mechanism in a randomized home-visiting trial: Reducing disrupted maternal communication decreases infant disorganization. *Development and Psychopathology, 29*(2), 637–649. https://doi.org/10.1017/S0954579417000232

Van Horn, P., & Lieberman, A. F. (2008). Using dyadic therapies to treat traumatized young children. In D. Brom, R. Pat-Horenczyk & J. D. Ford (Eds.), *Treating traumatized children* (pp. 228–242). Routledge.

Van IJzendoorn, M. H., Schuengel, C., & Bakermans–Kranenburg, M. J. (1999). Disorganized attachment in early childhood: Meta-analysis of precursors, concomitants, and sequelae. *Development and Psychopathology, 11*(2), 225–250. https://www.cambridge.org/core/journals/development-and-psychopathology/article/abs/disorganized-attachment-in-early-childhood-metaanalysis-of-precursors-concomitants-and-sequelae/87A710EAEC0C4167E02811B62CB284CF

Van IJzendoorn, M. H., Schuengel, C., Wang, Q., & Bakermans-Kranenburg, M. J. (2023). Improving parenting, child attachment, and externalizing behaviors: Meta-analysis of the first 25 randomized controlled trials on the effects of video-feedback intervention to promote positive parenting and sensitive discipline. *Development and Psychopathology, 35*(1), 241–256. https://doi.org/10.1017/S0954579421001462

Verhage, M. L., Schuengel, C., Madigan, S., Fearon, R. M., Oosterman, M., Cassibba, R., Bakermans-Kranenburg, M. J., & van IJzendoorn, M. H. (2016). Narrowing the transmission gap: A synthesis of three decades of research on intergenerational transmission of attachment. *Psychological Bulletin, 142*(4), 337–366. https://doi.org/10.1037/bul0000038

Vischer, A. F. W., Post, W. J., Grietens, H., Knorth, E. J., & Bronfman, E. (2020). Development of atypical parental behavior during an inpatient family preservation intervention program. *Infant Mental Health Journal, 41*(1), 5–23. https://doi.org/10.1002/imhj.21823

Vonderlin, R., Kleindienst, N., Alpers, G. W., Bohus, M., Lyssenko, L., & Schmahl, C. (2018). Dissociation in victims of childhood abuse or neglect: A meta-analytic review. *Psychological Medicine, 48*(15), 2467–2476. https://doi.org/10.1017/S0033291718000740

World Health Organization. (2018). *The ICD-11 classification of mental and behavioural disorders: Clinical descriptions and diagnostic guidelines.* World Health Organization.

Yarger, H. A., Bronfman, E., Carlson, E., & Dozier, M. (2020). Intervening with attachment and biobehavioral catch-up to decrease disrupted parenting behavior and attachment disorganization: The role of parental withdrawal. *Development and Psychopathology, 32*(3), 1139–1148. https://doi.org/10.1017/S0954579419000786

Zephyr, L., Cyr, C., Monette, S., Langlois, V., Cyr-Desautels, L., & Archambault, M. (2021). Disinhibited social engagement behaviors in young maltreated children: Dysfunctional behavior of biological parents and child attachment. *Child Abuse & Neglect, 111*, Article 104791. https://doi.org/10.1016/j.chiabu.2020.104791

20
A MULTIMODAL-INTEGRATIVE APPROACH TO EMDR THERAPY

Ana M. Gómez

Introduction

This chapter presents a multimodal approach to EMDR therapy with complexly traumatized children, where clinicians navigate through the eight phases of treatment and procedural steps of EMDR while supported by the latest understandings in neuroscience. EMDR therapy now has extensive possibilities to access traumatogenic networks while preserving the stability and homeostasis of the child's system. The utilization of EMDR therapy is reaching new heights of understanding and complexity, which is resulting in new prospects in healing for children exposed to chronic and repetitive trauma during critical periods of development. EMDR therapy uses a three-pronged approach, working systematically with the past, present, and future that coexist in the biology of the child (F. Shapiro, 2001, 2018). EMDR therapy accesses top-down and bottom-up processes to promote the assimilation of memory and the integration of identity and, ultimately, the self. The multimodal approach to EMDR therapy for children with complex trauma and dissociation is enriched with developmentally sound practices emerging from play, expressive arts, gestalt, and somatic therapies.

EMDR Therapy History and Research

EMDR therapy was developed by Francine Shapiro in the 1980s to treat the symptoms generated by trauma. EMDR therapy is an integrative and client-centered psychotherapy that brings together new therapeutic possibilities while utilizing key treatment elements from other psychological modalities (F. Shapiro, 2001, 2007, 2018). It has robust empirical support for the treatment of complex trauma as well as recognition as an evidence-based approach for children (World Health Organization, 2013; California Evidence-Based Clearinghouse for Child Welfare, 2010).

Meta-analyses, systematic reviews, and randomized control trials have found EMDR therapy to be an effective approach with children and adolescents who have suffered trauma (Karadag et al., 2019; Manzoni et al., 2021; Rodenburg et al., 2009; Teke & Avşaroğlu, 2021). A systematic review of randomized controlled trials in children and adults with complex trauma suggested that EMDR therapy is also a promising treatment for older children impacted by chronic and repetitive trauma (Chen et al., 2018). Rolling et al. (2024) found EMDR treatment to be highly effective with adolescents with complex PTSD secondary to childhood abuse in a case series study. Several research findings have also shown effectiveness with complexly traumatized children. For instance, Lichtenstein and Brager (2017) found that the combination of EMDR and relationship therapy in children with complex trauma resulted in symptom reduction and an increase in general global functioning. Olivier et al. (2022) found an 85.7% diagnostic remission in young children (ages 4–8) with post-traumatic stress disorder (PTSD). Karadag et al. (2019) reported anxiety reduction in children with PTSD. Moreover, an integrative approach that united EMDR and family therapy showed that children's trauma symptoms decreased and they demonstrated improvement in their overall global functioning (Silvestre, 2022; Wesselmann et al., 2018).

An important and distinctive component of EMDR treatment is the utilization of bilateral dual attention stimulus (BLS/DAS). There is still debate regarding the underlying mechanisms of action that according to Landin-Romero et al. (2018) fall under psychological, psychophysiological, and neurobiological models. There is evidence, however, that eye movements are the most effective form of BLS/DAS (de Jongh et al., 2013). In general, dual-attention stimulation (DAS) appears to be one of the most critical mechanisms influencing treatment outcomes in EMDR therapy (Shapiro & Laliotis, 2015). Some researchers suggest that engaging in demanding tasks while recalling traumatic memories taxes working memory, leading to a sense of emotional and cognitive distancing from the memory, as well as a reduction in its vividness and associated arousal (de Jongh et al., 2013). This perspective raises the possibility that DAS may not necessarily need to be bilateral to achieve therapeutic effects. However, further research is required to deepen our understanding of how the brain and nervous system respond to EMDR therapy and to explore the efficacy of various forms of DAS.

In EMDR therapy, children are not asked to provide descriptions of their traumatic stories, form verbal narratives of it, or solely focus on their traumatic events. Instead, free association and mindfulness are invited as the child "notices" and "lets whatever happens happen" during trauma processing. The integration of memories in EMDR treatment often leads to the development of a coherent and cohesive cognitive, emotional, and somatic autobiographical narrative, even though creating a verbal story is not the primary focus.

The Adaptive Information Processing Model and Complex Trauma and Dissociation

EMDR therapy is a comprehensive reprocessing psychotherapeutic approach founded on the adaptive information processing (AIP) model and procedural steps, which include the use of BLS/DAS, and the eight phases of treatment (F. Shapiro, 2018). Although EMDR therapy is mainly organized around accessing, processing, and integrating memory, there are also components that lead to interpersonal, state, and identity integration. When children heal from the imprints left by trauma, a transformed sense of identity emerges, as well as a renewed connection to self and their life stories.

Trauma and its concomitants inhibit the human apparatus biologically organized to assimilate and integrate the various elements of a wounding event held in the child's biology. The AIP model posits that clinical symptoms manifest from unintegrated and unassimilated memories (F. Shapiro, 2018) that produce the fragmentation of neural coherence (Cozolino, 2014). These trauma-formed neural systems remain isolated and frozen in "trauma time," becoming reactivated by present stimuli and perpetuating trauma-induced states. (F. Shapiro, 2018). The memory of trauma in EMDR therapy is not just a narrative from a past event; it is the neurobiological imprint containing cognitive, affective, and sensorimotor information that becomes the lens through which the child sees, feels, and experiences the present (F. Shapiro, 2001, 2018).

The neural network becomes the crux and center of the clinical landscape, and the integration and assimilation of memory are the focus of treatment. The memory systems are represented as fragmented recollections of images, body sensations, emotions, and embodied cognitions seeking integration.

A Circular Phase Approach to EMDR Therapy for Complex Trauma

EMDR therapy follows a unique and extended phase approach where stabilization, trauma processing, and integration are embedded within eight phases of treatment. This phase-oriented approach to treatment was originated by psychologist Pierre Janet and is considered by the International Society for the Study of Trauma and Dissociation (ISSTD) to be the gold standard for the treatment of complex traumatization and dissociation (2004). Even though the eight phases of treatment may be used linearly, especially with children with single trauma experiences, complex trauma cases often call for a spiral (Courtois, 2004) and circular approach in EMDR treatment (Gomez, 2023a). This orbitual movement honors the child's often dysregulated states and disjointed and fragmented stories and identities. As such, clinicians may find themselves circling and coming back to previous phases. We may go back to history-taking over and over again as the child, parents, or case managers deliver new historical data. Clinicians may also have to pendulate between the trauma processing phases and the preparation and stabilization phases, as the lives of these children are full of crises and instability. Clinicians navigate through the eight phases depending on the child's moment-to-moment emerging data while utilizing case conceptualization in intentional decision making. Even in one session, shifts from one phase to another may occur as the moment demands it. The EMDR clinician becomes the artist and alchemist accompanying the child each moment in presence and synchrony. The clinicians delivering EMDR therapy awaken the child's innate healing capacities that, once stimulated, move information to an adaptive resolution and health (F. Shapiro, 2001, 2018).

A Multimodal-Integrative Approach

The multimodal approach to EMDR therapy includes other supporting theories besides the AIP model, including the neurosequential model, interpersonal neurobiology (IPNB) and attachment, dissociation, affect regulation, and polyvagal theories. This approach to EMDR treatment also integrates strategies from other approaches such as somatic, play, sandtray, expressive arts, systemic, and gestalt therapies. The masterful blending of these approaches into EMDR treatment enriches and honors the unique journey of each child affected by chronic traumatization while preserving the essence and heart of EMDR therapy.

The Eight Phases of Treatment for Children Affected by Complex Trauma and Dissociation

Phase One: Client History and Treatment Planning

Considering the complex histories of children affected by developmental trauma, it requires great effort to gather a comprehensive psychosocial history. Many of these children come from foster care, child protective systems and orphanages, so they have multiple historians and there may be no coherent accounts. Often, these children are part of a family equally impacted by trauma, which makes a systemic approach to EMDR therapy imperative and the collection of information about the functioning of the caregiving system equally relevant (Gomez, 2013; F. Shapiro, 2007; Silvestre, 2022; Wesselmann et al., 2018). EMDR clinicians need to move beyond the view of history-taking as a linear process with a beginning, middle, and end to practice comprehensive, nonlinear information gathering. Often, children will expose their assets, resources, and wounds through play-based stories and themes, body-based and somatic holding patterns, and behavioral and relational displays. The therapeutic space and relationship become a fertile ground for reenactments and the play-based portal with tools such as the sand tray, the doll house, a puppet show, and free play. Each tool offers avatars (sand characters, puppets, etc.) through which the child's embodied mind can tell their stories, capitalizing on the distance they offer (Gomez, 2021a, in press). Non-directive and directive play gives the child a space for their story to emerge while they remain in the place of non-ownership.

An example is a child with a history of abuse who creates a play story in which a mighty and violent lion overtakes a vulnerable llama who is powerless and unable to escape. The child does not consciously acknowledge that the fear of the vulnerable animal in the hands of a powerful perpetrator is a representation of their own fear. These portals offered by play reenactments provide refuge for the child's mind, and as such, these themes become part of history-gathering and later serve as processing targets.

Often, the most profound parts of the wounding story emerge through the right-brain-generated experience, which may be implicit and non-conscious (Schore, 2012). Another example is a child who moves incessantly, exhausting their caregivers and therapist, or, on the contrary, a child who moves slowly and seldomly plays and participates in their therapy sessions. Both children tell a story, and the clinician's exhaustion in response to their autonomic states becomes part of a storytelling process (Dion, 2018). These nervous system interactions show the child's depleted homeostatic repertoire and the biological imprints left by their stories of trauma. The hypo-aroused and sympathetically mobilized child gives the clinician an entrance into their life accounts. Embodied holding patterns and autonomic neural pathways of defense are linked to internal working models and neural networks holding experiences of trauma that also emerge in play and relational enactments.

The EMDR clinician pays close attention to the various shades of the story while staying connected to themselves, listening to the unique and often subtle portals the child's mind uses to tell their stories. The use of play, body-based, and expressive arts therapies within an integrative approach to EMDR treatment provides diverse pathways to explore the history of the child and their relational and internal milieu. Direct inquiries about traumatic events early in treatment are highly discouraged when working with severe traumatization (Courtois, 2004). Instead, utilize the natural and developmental pathways the child offers, which will not come in well-organized and coherent verbal narratives but rather in embodied and play-based reenactments. With this population, the exploration of trauma is reserved for when the child has developed enough safety, affect regulation, affect tolerance capacities, and homeostatic resources. Instead, actively utilize other sources such as caregivers, case managers, teachers, or any other story holder. The exploration and assessment of dissociation is paramount, and is initiated during the intake and continues throughout the eight phases. The level at which dissociation exists will impact the organization of each treatment phase.

The EMDR clinician should also carefully and thoroughly study the caregiving system, creating a baseline of its functioning and the strategies used to deliver care. Deficits and a lack of co-regulatory and co-homeostatic capacities in the caregiver could lead to wounding patterns in interacting, relating, and differentiating with the child. If they perseverate, they will continue to strengthen memory networks holding trauma-based meta-perceptions; affective, sensorimotor, and behavioral concomitants; patterns of autonomic activation; and modes of relating to self and others.

Clinicians should also investigate all the complex forms of oppression, marginalization, and discrimination that have surrounded the child and their family. Cultivating culturally responsive and affirming practices that recognize and honor the child's cultural experiences and heritage throughout the eight phases of treatment, as well as the intersectionality of multiple identities connected to gender, culture, race, religion, ethnicity, and immigration, foster a more supportive and inclusive experience for clients. Equally essential is the exploration of experiences with child welfare, foster care, and legal systems, which often lead to traumas of separation, abandonment, severance of parental rights, and utter powerlessness. The very experience of living in a group home, having to move from foster home to foster home, and an absolute lack of control expose children to further traumatization. Despite their short lives, these children possess long and convoluted life histories that may involve trafficking, ritualistic abuse, and despicable acts that should be handled with much care to avoid re-traumatization and dysregulation.

Clinicians are encouraged to explore and identify defensive patterns created to support survival, as these patterns become burdens to the child's healing and therapeutic process, such as avoidance (in all its multiple forms), perfectionism, control, manipulation, pleasing, competitiveness, the frantic pursue of acceptance, and idealization of wounding attachment figures or the self (see Chapter 40 for more information). In phase one, the clinician also initiates the exploration of inner dynamics and polarizations existing within the dissociative milieu. Furthermore, the clinician recognizes the body as a valuable source of insight, information and as an essential historian by carefully observing and noticing attentively how the body carries tension, executes repetitive movements and actions, and changes and responds from moment to moment. For instance, the child may show different movement patterns, tension, etc., in the mother's presence compared to the father or any other important attachment figure.

Phase Two: Preparation

The ultimate goal of this phase is to increase the child's integrative capacities and accessibility to their homeostatic repertoire. There is still discussion about how much preparation and stabilization are needed before proceeding to trauma processing in complex trauma and dissociation. Adult studies delivering intensive EMDR treatment interspersed with psychoeducation and rigorous physical activity to C-PTSD and high comorbidity clients showed high remission after two weeks of treatment in a highly contained environment (Bongaerts et al., 2017). The preparation phase in its standard format was not provided, although it may be argued that the highly contained environment and exercise are considered preparation and stabilization tools. Some studies suggest that direct trauma processing without the preparation phase results in the most rapid reduction in symptomatology in children with single-incident trauma (de Roos et al., 2017). These findings, however, have not been established in children with C-PTSD and other comorbidities. My clinical practice with hundreds of children with complex trauma and dissociation has consistently shown that the majority of children affected by chronic traumatization need a stabilization and capacity building period that may be circularly interspersed with trauma processing sessions. Indeed, we need research in this area across multiple clinical orientations that work with severe traumatization.

Throughout the eight phases of EMDR treatment, clinical strategies are organized to support regulation, homeostasis, and social engagement, helping the child achieve greater balance and stability while down-regulating defenses. Due to the intricacies of dissociation and complex traumatization, preparation often has multiple components and layers, as listed below. However, the length, the number of these areas addressed, and the extent to which they are utilized will depend on the unique characteristics and qualities of each child.

Creating Safety

Safety is a multidimensional concept and experience that extends beyond the creation of a real or imagined safe place. It is the visceral and embodied felt sense of safety, connectedness, and belonging across multiple domains in the child's life that more rapidly begins to reset the child's biology and create sufficient balance and homeostasis to support the processing of trauma. Physical safety, relational safety, and internal safety (inner cues of safety or danger connected to trauma and the dissociative milieu's inner dynamics and internal conflicts) all contribute to restoring the child's bodily rhythms associated with safety.

The clinician works actively to remove or decrease sources of threat and dysregulation starting in the initial phases of treatment, which may be a challenging task considering the often unstable lives of these children. The clinician also co-creates a safe and growth-promoting relational space and makes moment-to-moment micro and macro adaptations to meet the child's demands for safety. The clinician utilizes active and passive pathways organized to activate mechanisms that down-regulate defenses, supporting social engagement and connection. The passive pathways work with the social engagement system by providing cues of safety, such as a compassionate environment and kindhearted facial expressions and voice intonation (Porges & Dana, 2018). The clinician's genuine presence, self-connection, and capacity to recruit their social engagement system to provide cues of safety to the child all begin to supply corrective and reparative experiences.

With this foundation, the clinician moves gradually into active pathways, where invitations to the child to engage in play, intentional breathing, movements, reciprocal dialogues, and vocalizations are delivered (Porges & Dana, 2018) and then enhanced with BLS/DAS. These active pathways need to rest in the foundation of safety created by the passive pathways. The clinician may invite the child to find even small memories of shared love, nurturance, connectedness, and belonging (if present in the child's life), representing active ways to enter safe embodied states that can be enhanced with BLS/DAS. Grounding exercises also build the child's embodied sense of self and their connection to a felt sense of their physical body. This preparatory work supports the child in renegotiating their relationship with their bodies and eventually restoring their embodied sense of safety. When the child experiences these moments of homeostasis and safety in the body, BLS/DAS (if appropriate) can enhance the connection to these physiological and affective states. Initially, the child may not be able to assess or welcome safe states considering the severe violations and assaults inflicted on their sense of safety. Nevertheless, persistent, compassionate, and growth-promoting relational experiences of safety and belonging will begin to interrupt trauma-formed autonomic reactions, recruiting the social engagement system and strengthening the vagal break.

However, inner system conflicts and polarizations resulting from trauma can develop into a neuroception of danger. Despite the physical and relational safety that may surround the child, polarized dissociative self-states can activate sympathetic or dorsal vagal–mediated states. Reducing the inner conflict among parts and increasing collaboration also contributes to an increased sense of internal and external safety. For children with mild to moderate dissociation, an integrated sense of identity, greater access to homeostatic resources, and the early processing of triggers and even trauma using a titrated approach can also begin to change internal conflicted ego state dynamics. The early and titrated processing of trauma and triggers may constitute another loop and a portal into reestablishing the neuroception of safety.

Systemic and dyadic therapeutic engagement with parents is often necessary to establish or restore their role as *external psychobiological regulators* (Schore, 2003) and co-organizers of experience (Gomez, 2021b). For the traumatized parent, the child's behavior, emotions, and needs and their attempts to elicit care may awaken the parent's traumatogenic networks and patterns of nervous system activation. The cognitive, emotional, somatic, and behavioral representations left by trauma become the lens through which the parent sees, experiences, and makes meaning of the child's requests for care. This phenomenon organizes parental behavior and moves the parent out of connection and co-regulation into survival, self-preservation, and defense (Porges, 2021). Often, children are the generational storytellers; they are the ones brought to therapy when the wound is generationally shared. The EMDR clinician has many offerings, including EMDR group or individual work and protocols, to support the caregiver. The parenting wheel (Gomez, 2021b) uses principles of regulation, attachment, and Polyvagal Theory utilizing images and metaphors. The EMDR Group Parent

Empowerment Protocol (GPEP) (Gomez, 2022) supports caregivers in increasing relational and parenting capacities and was inspired by and founded on the Group-Traumatic Episode Protocol (E. Shapiro, 2018) and the Resource Development and Installation Protocol (RDI) (Korn & Leeds, 2002). The parenting wheel and the GPEP can be combined with the G-TEP for low-intensity processing to reduce disturbance associated with parenting triggers that move the caregiver out of connection and co-regulation. For the parents who need comprehensive and individualized treatment, EMDR therapy has a gamut of processing possibilities, from child- and parenting-specific targets (child's daily needs, emotions, or challenging behaviors) to peripheral memories of recent traumatic experiences and core attachment wounds. These all influence parental behaviors, and their integration can highly support the reorganization of parenting states, internal representations, working models, and behavior.

Active pathways also include invitations to both the child and parent to play, intentionally breathe, and connect (Porges & Dana, 2018). These encounters recruit the child's and parent's social engagement systems to create a secure base. While the parent-child dyad is regulated, the EMDR clinician joins in synchrony, curiosity, and emotional reflectivity with invitations to engage in bilateral movement or touch:

> I see a smile showing up, and big and shiny eyes as you play with Dad. I wonder what is happening for you now. Are there feelings visiting you now? Where are they landing or hanging out in your body?

When the child can tolerate the positive affect resulting from interpersonal experiences, BLS/DAS strengthens such states using tactile stimulation, eye movement, or embodiments—for example,

> Let's paint in [brushing the child's hands or feet bilaterally] or march in [marching bilaterally] as you continue to play with Dad, holding happy feelings in your tummy. This experience offers the child an opportunity to have a positive and safe shared experience.

The Therapeutic Relationship

Relational safety is continuously co-created in each moment throughout the EMDR therapeutic process. The clinician or caregiver provides a safe relational holding space while utilizing EMDR procedural steps, creating fertile ground to awaken the child's innate healing capacities. The therapeutic relationship is an extensive and complex topic with profound ramifications, covered throughout this volume.

Psychoeducation

Psychoeducation is an essential component of the preparation phase. However, psychoeducation should be tailored to the short attention span and dissociative characteristics of most children with complex trauma. In "segmented and embodied psychoeducation" (Gomez, 2021a, in press), information is delivered in small amounts, supported by embodiments, play, and expressive arts therapies. Clinicians may also provide short and easy-to-understand pieces of information such as: "I know something we can try to help your mind, heart, and body sort out painful or scary things that happen. When we are in 'sort out mode,' we might move our eyes back and forth; we can march, drum, or brush back and forth while we think about these hurtful stories. We can also play out or tell life stories in the sand tray, doll house, puppet theater, or playroom. We paint in or march in slowly when we connect to 'goodies' and safe, happy, or special moments, and we go fast when we sort out hurtful stuff." The clinician may read books that explain EMDR therapy (Flynn, 2023; Gomez, 2010, 2018), at a pace appropriate for the child, so they become acquainted with EMDR processes and procedures and gain a greater sense of predictability, safety, and control.

Dual Attention Stimulus (DAS)

A myriad of possibilities for engaging the child in BLS/DAS exist; the following are some of them:

- **Tactile stimulation:** BLS/DAS may be provided by using brushes to "paint in" resources and "sort out" memories (Gomez, 2013), or by squeezing Play-Doh back and forth, drumming, doing the butterfly hug (Artigas & Jarero, 2014), the gorilla dance (chest taps simulating a gorilla), kitty kneading (metaphorically describing the rhythmic, alternating movements reminiscent of a cat's kneading), and pat-a-cake.
- **Eye movement:** light wands projected onto a drawing, paint or sand tray worlds (Gomez, in press), finger or hand puppets the child follows with their eyes. Using a wand with a picture of a resource (Monaco, 2021) or a superhero figure.
- **Movement and embodiments:** BLS/DAS such as pool noodles (Dion, 2018) to tap back and forth. Clinicians also utilize movement-based BLS/DAS such as bilateral dance, rhythmic movements with arms, marching, running, or just using EMDR on the floor (Gomez, 2013, 2023b; Monaco, 2021; Stricklin, 2021).
- **Auditory stimulation:** Clinicians use music, rattles, and maracas.
- **Apps and technological devices:** Various BLS/DAS devices that facilitate bilateral stimulation, such as through sound or eye movement, are readily available online.

The type and form of BLS/DAS for children with complex traumatization, in addition to being a procedure for memory processing (F. Shapiro, 2001, 2018), is a tool for co-regulation (Gomez, in press) that the clinician changes based on the data emerging in the moment and how it is unfolding for the child. For example, let's say the child starts processing while sitting on the floor, and the clinician begins to use brushes to "sort out" traumatic memories. Suddenly, the child stands up, pretends to run away from a monster, and begins to rush about. Brushing is no longer the most suitable form of BLS/DAS for the child, given how processing is evolving in real time. The clinician instead follows the child, inviting them to stomp their feet while running.

Each BLS/DAS method makes contact with the child's nervous system and biology in diverse ways. For instance, BLS/DAS that involves movement invites the forces of the vagus nerve and the sympathetic system to join in a hybrid physiological and playful state transforming it into a neural excercise. This experience supports presence and engagement, especially for a child with dissociative tendencies and a short attention span. The BLS/DAS is used synchronically moment to moment while the memory is metabolized and transformed. When the child's information processing stalls, a shift to another form of BLS/DAS or the increase and decrease in the number of sets not only stimulates information processing (F. Shapiro, 2018) but also up-regulates or down-regulates the child's physiology through embodiments, movement, rhythm, tactile stimulation, and sounds. The use of BLS/DAS with dissociative children, even when utilized to install a resource, may have the potential to promote the linkage into traumatic networks. Caution should be exercised, especially when working with children with a history of self-harm, aggression, suicidality, or a highly contended and compartmentalized inner structure with intense polarization and conflict. Keep in mind that eye movements are the most potent form of BLS/DAS (de Jongh et al. , 2013) and the fastest in activating traumatogenic memory systems.

Increasing State-Change and Self-Regulatory Capacities

In order to develop the capacity to self-regulate, the child must have experiences of co-regulation with a safe external psychobiological regulator (Schore, 2012). As the child grows and expands their sense of agency, they begin to intentionally influence and modulate their arousal. The EMDR clinician utilizes active and directive pathways that promote self-regulation while continuing to engage in passive pathways of regulation. EMDR-based protocols such as the safe place, the team of companions, the container exercise, and a myriad of playful breathing exercises scaffold the child's emerging self-regulatory capacities. Many of these resources can be created in the playroom or the clinician's office. The child needing containment may choose a tent, while the child seeking physical activity might prefer a balancing board or a ball. The child can create a unique space in the office with all the elements that convey and promote safety. Once it is created and completed, the child is invited to connect with their feelings and bodily states associated with safety.

Children on the severe side of the trauma and dissociation spectrum may present with dissociative parts that coexist within a conflicted milieu—for example, what one part finds safe and calming, another may find terrifying. A part may need a specific object or stuffie for safety, while another may find that shameful. The clinician supports inner negotiations so the child can realign the fractionated identities that may pull them into different directions, making the inner world chaotic. These frequent internal battles disrupt internal safety, so repatterning these inner relational choreographies can support the neuroception of safety.

Neurodevelopment and vertical integration (Siegel, 2010) are impacted by early and chronic experiences of trauma. Children who experienced trauma when the lower brain—highly devoted to regulation—was in development have severe deficits in affect regulation. As a result, sensory modulation strategies coming from the field of occupational therapy represent one of the first lines of intervention that actively tap into the child's somatic intelligence. An embodied approach to EMDR therapy that engages the five senses with sound, movement, breathing, and rhythm, to mention a few, will begin to increase interoceptive and exteroceptive consciousness and intelligence, as well as help reclaim the body as a safe place. These sensory-based resources invite a bottom-up approach to resource building. The child is invited to engage in BLS/DAS in a regulated and homeostatic state while actively utilizing rhythm and connection to the body's wisdom and intelligence. Once the child begins to have access to higher cognitive capacities, we incorporate resources that capitalize on top-down resources.

Skill Building

Children with complex trauma often lack access to somatic, affective, and cognitive awareness; the capacity to identify feelings; and, in general, interoceptive awareness. These children are disengaged from their inner world or live in hypervigilance, distorting interoceptive and exteroceptive cues. Mindfulness, identification of feelings, mentalization, and the expansion of cognitive, affective, and somatic literacy support the child's connection and dialogue with their inner world. However, this level of work often follows the bottom-up resourcing of lower brain structures and autonomic states.

Affect Tolerance

Children with complex trauma often present with a narrow window of tolerance (Siegel, 2010) as well as trauma-related phobias (Steele et al., 2017)—for example, phobia of traumatic memories, affect, dissociative parts, and, in general, their inner world. In order to access and tolerate a broader range of emotions and physiological states, the young human mind needs a safe adult who can first hold them, contain them, and regulate them for the child. However, the life of children exposed to severe trauma is colored by acts of omission and the absence of a safe, regulating adult. These children often grow up in relational environments with very narrow "emotional bandwidths," where expressing feelings results in punishment, rejection, abandonment, or in emotionally chaotic systems without any sense of containment.

Throughout the eight phases of treatment, EMDR clinicians support children in overcoming such phobias by using an approach that expands their access to a broader range of affective states. Most of this work falls within a titration continuum where the entrance into the embodied mind of the child and their stories (affective, somatic, behavioral, and cognitive) of adversity is gradual and tailored to the child's capacities and window of tolerance. For example, suppose a child finds an emotion overwhelming. In that case, the clinician makes moment-to-moment adjustments in the treatment method and supports the child in making contact with a much more tolerable volume of this emotion. The clinician becomes a bridge that connects the child to themselves so a relationship is possible with their inner realities while in the containment offered by the child's relational milieu. The child taking a "drop" of sadness (Gomez, 2013, in press) or a much smaller "spoon" of frustration while in the companionship of the clinician and the parent (when present in the session) begins to soften their rigid defenses and build affect tolerance. Invitations to feel a broader range of emotions will challenge the child's sense of safety. This experience, however, opens up possibilities and opportunities for the child to contain previously disrupted autonomic states and receive corrective and reparative experiences from the clinician and the parent. The EMDR clinician utilizes the play system actively to give the child the experience of containment. For instance, the clinician or parent might hold the represented feeling, providing the child with scaffolding and a corrective experience of support and companionship. Alternatively, the therapist invites the parent to hold the child and the embodied and physicalized sadness while providing companionship and co-regulation: "I am right here with you"; "I am here with you and all the sides of you and your little drop of sadness." This level of work begins to build a connective tissue among states that exist in separateness and fragmentation as they join to receive validation, containment, and connection. Some parts may not tolerate connection, which can also be honored and titrated.

Working with Dissociation

Dissociative states exist within a continuum from mild to moderate to severe (Putnam, 1997), in which divisions and structural dissociation exist (Steele et al., 2017; van der Hart et al., 2006, chapter 6). Whether we conceptualize a shift in attention, mental absorption, or hypo-arousal as dissociative or as a shift in consciousness, the EMDR clinician utilizes this information as essential data about the self and inner organization of the child. This data informs therapeutic decisions and actions. The severity and dissociative patterns the child exhibits highly influence the organization of the preparation phase. When dissociation or alterations in consciousness are present, the EMDR clinician works on supporting the child's nervous system in receiving the corrections and contingency. The child borrows from the clinician's presence, co-regulation, and homeostatic repertoire.

If severe dissociation is present, establish playful routines by inviting the child to have "moments of curiosity" to contact their inner system. "Can we be curious together? Let us do an inside visit and see if all the sides of you are okay with this or in agreement." In general, it is not necessary to assign names to each part (unless requested by the child), as doing so may be counterproductive (Steele et al., 2017). Instead, the focus should be on increasing interoceptive intelligence, fostering curiosity about inner relational dynamics, and creating pathways into the inner world, which may present with discrepancies and polarities. This process must be gradual and carefully paced, as initial encounters with the inner system may be laden with remnants of trauma.

The clinician invites the child to make contact with their inner world, utilizing language that acknowledges inner divisions and, at the same time, guides the child through the spectrum of realization. For example, "It seems like there is a side of you that wants to be here while another side does not want any help or support." Physicalizations may start in phase one, inviting these inner polarities and self-states to unblend into figures, puppets, and posters. Pacing is important, as promoting communication too fast and too soon among parts may potentially unleash memories of trauma prematurely that the system is not yet equipped to deal with or address (Steele et al., 2017). Initially, the communication happens around the present moment, resources and the titrated exploration of the child's internal organization. With the data emerging, the clinician is often working on realigning the inner and outer world by using mirroring and reflective communication so the child can find the self in the reflections of the clinician's mind.

Often, dissociative parts or ego states in children emerge in the metaphor of play (Gomez & Lyles, 2025). They arise unacknowledged and unnamed, protected in the sacred and safe space offered by play. For instance, a sandtray world may become a vessel and a refuge where parts unblend without being owned or named. The characters may fall into the perpetrator, rescuer, and victim trauma triangle (Danylchuk & Connors, 2024). A puppet show, sand tray world, or free play where, for example, a dog is imprisoned and abused by evil aliens may play out the victim-perpetrator dynamic, and the characters may represent the physicalization of a part that imitates the perpetrator and a part that holds the experiences and powerlessness of a young victim. Often, for children, this is the portal the inner system of parts utilizes to enter the outer world (Chapter 31). Clinicians may use sequencing protocols (Gomez, in press) in the sand tray, doll house, or through expressive arts therapies. The child creates sequences of inner decision-making leading to dysfunctional behaviors such as aggression and self-harm. The clinician explores parts' dialogues, voices, input, and contributions to the ultimate harming behaviors alongside their internal conflict. The clinician supports and invites negotiations, agreements, and alternative ways to dialogue with the inner system of parts. When working with older children, clinicians may invite a connection to the "wiser or guiding self" to mediate or develop new ways of interacting with the inner and outer world. New realizations and mentalizing capacities may be enhanced with BLS/DAS as the clinician invites the child to be with and embrace new knowing.

Dual Attention

F. Shapiro (2018) emphasized the importance of supporting the client's dual attention. As soon as the traumatized mind touches traumatic layers, its defenses, adaptations, and internal organization made in the service of survival often become activated. Accessing traumatic networks may result in the activation of dissociative processes and states. Inexorably, EMDR clinicians will be working with some level of dissociation. However, we seek enough presence to access the child's inner experience without recreating or promoting the same states that occurred during the traumatic event. The child must be grounded in the safety of the present before venturing into traumatic states.

During the preparation phase, the clinician uses playful tools to assess presence. For instance, "the Fanometer" or the "presence string puppet" (Gomez, 2013) are playful instruments that support the child in assessing and communicating to the clinician how present they are in the moment. When the string puppet is upright or the fanometer is fully open, it signifies a strong connection to the present moment, while their complete collapse or closure depict the severance of connection to the present. When the child reports a felt sense of drifting away into dissociative states or shifts in consciousness states of disengagement and detachment, the clinician utilizes movement and rhythm among other tactics to up-regulate, reengage, and restore presence and the child's connection to the present safety.

Defenses

In order to coexist with the remnants and biological imprints left by trauma, children develop rigid forms of defense and self-protection. These defenders prevent intrusions from post-traumatic material (Knipe, 2018) and, if not addressed early in EMDR treatment, have the potential to block the integration of traumagenic memories. During the initial phases of treatment, the clinician needs to dim defenses first by using passive and active pathways to promote safety and regulation. However, additional work with these defenders is often necessary, to befriend them and renegotiate their trauma-based relationship before accessing or processing traumatic memories. In this volume, A. M. Gomez's chapter on defenses provides multiple hands-on strategies that are paramount within EMDR treatment. Defenders may exist within a dissociative inner matrix or as states of consciousness that are part of a unified self. Trauma-based defenses and forms of self-protection, as well as trauma-related phobias, may keep EMDR therapy stagnant and circling the defense system. Clinicians often need to work actively with these defenders throughout the eight phases of treatment, especially during the transition into trauma processing.

Phase Three: Assessment

Establishing the Readiness for the Exploration and Processing of Trauma

The assessment phase is the access point to the targeted information (F. Shapiro, 2018), identifying the most salient manifestations of the trauma. During the assessment phase, the memory network's cognitive, emotional, behavioral and somatic elements are accessed and stimulated (F. Shapiro, 2001, 2018) so dysfunctional trauma-based manifestations can be rapidly metabolized, assimilated, reconsolidated, and integrated.

Shifting from resource building to memory exploration and processing requires a conscious and intentional decision with clear markers. The clinician carefully mentalizes the child's assets, capacities, and challenges before entering into memory networks that hold trauma. Only after the child shows signs of increased capacity to engage in co-regulation, tolerate emotional and somatic disturbance, and have greater co-consciousness and communication among parts (when presenting with a dissociative structure), and when there is a relational milieu that can support the child, do we take steps toward direct trauma exploration or processing. Readiness is ever-changing and shifts between and within sessions, so it is not dichotomous or static but a highly dynamic process. It is about how we dance therapeutically while honoring the child's inner system's capacities and resources. Readiness to access trauma involves a continuum and a field of exploration and processing possibilities that go from complete and direct access to a fractionated and titrated approach to entering the traumatized mind.

The following are markers and guidelines that support the clinician in their decision-making to move forward into processing phases as well as how to enter traumatogenic networks best:

- Indicators of capacities such as self-regulation and the ability to engage in co-regulation with others. The lack of state-change and self- and co-regulatory capacities will be evident when suicidal ideations and gestures, self-mutilation and self-harm, or prolonged and extreme behaviors and emotion dysregulation persist.

- Increase in the capacity of the child's inner system of parts to communicate and resolve conflict. Strong internal polarizations and conflict may make the processing of trauma highly contended, potentially resulting in increased and severe dysregulation (Gonzalez & Mosquera, 2012).
- Despite exhibiting dissociative symptoms, the child responds to the clinician's efforts to foster presence and keep them grounded in the safety of the present moment. The relational and caregiving systems exhibit signs of stability, even subtle ones, and responsiveness to the child. Polarized and chaotic or disengaged and disconnected caregivers may keep the child at a significantly heightened baseline of nervous system activation or shutdown, which will narrow the child's integrative capacities and window of tolerance.
- For the child with ongoing trauma, processing is still possible and, for some, a way to stabilize. However, titration and the use of advanced approaches to avoid re-traumatization are paramount.
- Increased emotion and somatic tolerance. The child can explore and "be with" disturbing as well as comfortable and positive sensations and affect without becoming highly dysregulated or dissociated. Even though we will be working with some level of dissociation, we want to ensure the child has enough connection to the present safety when accessing any disturbing material.
- Adaptive information is available. F. Shapiro (2001, 2018) emphasized the importance of having access to corrective information within comprehensive, and adaptive networks. Hence, there is an associative process as the traumatogenic networks link up with the adaptive systems during processing phases. This represents the reconsolidation and rearrangement of memory systems that appear to occur during EMDR processing.
- The clinician has established their own level of readiness to accompany these children through their often turbulent journeys. Does the clinician possess the therapeutic capacities and an appropriate understanding of complex trauma and dissociation? Has the clinician been trained and received advanced consultation on treating severe traumatization and dissociation? In addition, is the clinician emotionally ready to accompany children with tumultuous stories of trauma? And aware that the children's behavior may trigger their own traumatic memories?
- There is consensus among the child's parts and inner system in general to move forward into processing trauma memories.

Creating the Platform for Processing

As we move into the assessment and later processing phases, we set up the session to optimize the child's integrative capacities and widen their window of tolerance. We should arrive at such sacred moments of transformation only with appropriate planning. Clinicians should not move into processing by opportunity but by intention. The following variables will support clinicians in setting up the foundation for the assessment phase:

- Who will accompany the child? Will a parent/caregiver, pet/animal, or extended family member be present during processing? If so, have they been prepared? Parents are often invited, with the child's consent, to provide a greater sense of safety and actively accompany the child in such vulnerable moments. Caregiver-delivered interweaves can be incredibly powerful when planned well (Gomez, 2013). If the parent provides interweaves under the clinician's guidance, has this been clearly and carefully planned to repair and promote attachment completions?
- The clinician sets up the assessment session to bring the nervous system within tolerable windows with enough safety and ventral vagal energy for engagement to optimize integrative capacities. For the child with a tendency toward hyper-arousal, setting up the session to contain and down-regulate may include the use of physical spaces that promote containment (tents, umbrellas,

hiding places), as well as having playful resources available and accessible to the child, such as their team of helpers, their animal companion, their "safety chair" or "safety fairy," and more. For the child who moves quickly into hypo-arousal, up-regulating the system through movement and strategies borrowed from play and expressive arts therapies will optimize their engagement and integrative capacities.

- If the clinician is working with divided identities, a lot of care should be dedicated to ensuring the stability of the inner system of parts during processing phases. The child can decide how their inside world will participate in the process and what resources they will bring to accommodate the demands for safety of each part and the system as a whole.

Processing Phases with Complex Trauma and Dissociation: Desensitization, Installation and Body Scan

EMDR therapy has expanded and grown to offer a myriad of portals into the unintegrated memories of trauma. These entry roads actively consider and honor the child's unique capacities and characteristics. In this field of possibilities, the clinician holds the strategies, protocols, and procedural steps while at the same time relying on curiosity, co-regulation, and mentalizing capacities. Standard EMDR therapy offers a complete and direct entrance into the memory that may be tolerable for many children, especially the ones with single-incident trauma. However, as we move into complex trauma and dissociation, the child's reduced integrative capacities and window of affect tolerance make the entrance into traumatogenic material intricate, requiring both greater dexterity on the part of the clinician and the use of advanced strategies and protocols. We do not access traumatogenic data just as a verbal narrative of an event but as a biological imprint carrying cognitive, emotional, somatic, and behavioral elements. The clinician invites the child's embodied mind to visit what can be witnessed and realized. The clinician remains supportive as a safe anchor while allowing the child's inner healing capacities to awaken at the pace and rhythm tolerable to the child. Nevertheless, the clinician remains active as a companion, supporting the child's mind movement toward assimilation and integration. Bottom-up and top-down processing takes place, and when information processing stalls, the EMDR clinician utilizes interventions/interweaves that support the restoration of the movement toward integration.

The clinician makes active and intentional choices about the portal and access route to better suit the child's organism and system's capacities. For a child with reduced affect tolerance and lack of self- and co-regulatory capacities, the EMDR clinician will utilize titration strategies and protocols that support a gradual entrance into the pain, fear, shame, and the biological imprint holding the trauma.

The following are portals and titrated entry strategies into the child's inner world and their traumagenic stories.

The Titration Continuum

EMDR clinicians have multiple tools for co-regulation, modulation of arousal, restoration of presence, and information processing at their disposal. While employing strategies and protocols, the EMDR clinician stays attuned to their own nervous system signals and inner experience, emphasizing that even within a structured approach, the work remains rooted in the intersubjective field, fostering intentional, moment-to-moment responses. The clinician remains a companion, witness, and bio-emotional regulator of the child, especially as they access deeper layers of the self and their wounds. Each titration level creates distance and borders around traumatic material, or fractionates it into digestible data. The following are access routes organized around a titration continuum to enter memory systems and their accompanying physiological states.

- Standard and complete processing with open access to multiple layers and channels of association: In this type of access, the child has met markers for readiness to own, represent, and tolerate the accessing of multiple channels. In this standard EMDR processing, there is full activation of the cognitive, emotional, behavioral and somatic aspects of the memory.
- The access to associative channels (information linked associatively with the initial targeted event) may be limited and restricted. F. Shapiro (2001, 2018) initially used what is known as EMD, which focuses on desensitizing and reducing the level of disturbance while restricting access to other associative channels. When using EMD, the clinician returns to the target memory after every set of BLS/DAS, refocusing the child on the specific memory or aspect of the memory, ultimately preventing the mind with a narrow window of affect tolerance from becoming flooded with other memories and accompanying affect. Several delivery formats of restrictive protocols have been proposed to avoid overwhelming the traumatized mind: EMD, EMDr, and EMDR (F. Shapiro, 2001, 2018; Shapiro & Laub, 2014). They represent a continuum that goes from high restriction to lesser limitations created around how much of the trauma memory is accessed, as well as other channels of association.
- Clinicians may also utilize *EMDR recent event protocols* to break down the memory into smaller fragments, such as the Recent Traumatic Episode Protocol (RTEP) (Shapiro & Laub, 2014). The "Google search" used in RTEP invites the client to examine the traumatic episode and find a "point of disturbance," which becomes the focus of processing, instead of the larger episode. The clinician invites the child to do "detective work" and find "a nugget" that is bothersome or hurtful. The focus becomes this kernel of the episode, which places restrictions on the amount of information the child is accessing. Clinicians may impose more significant restrictions by working with a memory instead of an episode.
- *Pendulation/oscillation* is also a strategy imported into the work of EMDR from somatic therapies (Levine, 2015; Ogden et al., 2006). For instance, the Constant Installation of Present Orientation and Safety (CIPOS) (Knipe, 2018)—a pendulation EMDR protocol—enhances the dissociative client's connection to the present safety. For children, multiple protocols that pendulate the entrance into traumatogenic states and memory systems include: "This was me then, and this is me now" or the pendulation from a resource into small segments of the traumatic memory (Gomez, 2013, in press). These protocols support the child's embodied mind in entering the cognitive, emotional, and somatic stories while grounding the client in the safety of the present and their resources.
- *Frequent time orientation* has been shown to be very effective in clinical practice (Knipe, 2018). Clinicians can use the "safety chair" or "safety fairy," or "safety checks" (Gomez, in press) that orient the child to the present safety. For example, "Let's look around and check where you are. Let's find or touch something in this place that reminds you that the experience/story we are visiting is over, and it is not happening now," (Shapiro & Laub, 2014) or "Let's sit in the safety chair and turn around [360 degrees] to check where you are and how safe you are, and to see that the story we are visiting today is over." The clinician may also have a transitional object reminding the child that they are safe now. During processing, the clinician often pendulates directing the child to connect to the safety in the present.
- *Segmentation of the memory*: Clinicians may intentionally fractionate memories (Kluft, 1999) into smaller fragments that the child visits. The child may divide the experience and draw a picture of just one portion, which becomes the focus of the processing. The "green, yellow, and red" protocol (Gomez, 2013) uses paper in these colors so the child can draw the accessible parts of the memory on the green paper and the ones with a much greater disturbance, yellow or red. The colors can

be adjusted based on the child's preferences. The clinician creates borders by inviting the child to focus on this little "nugget" of the memory while engaging in BLS/DAS. Once the level of disturbance is low or zero, the next green nugget is uncovered and drawn until all the green parts are processed. Then, the clinician invites the child to access the yellow parts and, finally, the red parts, with much greater disturbance. In this titrated approach, the child's mind dialogues with tiny kernels of their story at a time.

- *Time titration:* Children's nervous systems often need breaks from processing, especially when working on highly charged memories. Having a resting place in the office is paramount. The child knows in advance that resting, stopping, or shifting into another activity is always an important option. The child has signals to indicate they want to stop, rest, or take a break. Ideally, clinicians will have a chair or small bed where the child can rest and reset their nervous system. Healing should not be another task or accomplishment to achieve. Instead, we hold the space for the needs of the child's nervous system, providing opportunities for correction, repair, and attachment completions. The child may process for ten minutes and rest or distance by playing with different toys or directing their attention to another part of the room. The space of "sorting" out and dancing with our memories and feelings remains open for the child's return when they are ready, so processing does not become an obligation.
- *Distance*: With children, this is one of the most essential ways to titrate the entrance into the memory network holding the trauma. The clinician actively utilizes play, embodiments, and expressive arts so the child can reenact their painful stories through play. The sand tray, for instance, provides a safe refuge to the traumatized mind, and the miniature collection becomes avatars so the child can represent the inner world's happenings in the outer world.
- *Gradual entrance into the memory*: The tip of the finger strategy (Gonzalez & Mosquera, 2012) proposes that rather than targeting the traumatic memory, the client process its outer layers first. Honoring the client's capacities, the clinician gently guides the client to work with small segments of trauma-related peripheral material such as an emotion, sensation, or irrational belief while preventing the direct accessing of the trauma memory. Along the same lines, Knipe (2018) offered strategies and protocols that work on targeting defenses and trauma-related phobias first to lower affective arousal before accessing trauma memories. With children, the clinician can target small fragments of peripheral emotions, sensations, or beliefs emerging in play states—for example, during free play or while creating puppet stories or sandtray worlds (Gomez, in press).
- *Micro-processing*: Clinicians may reprocess negative but isolated and low-arousing experiences so the child gets acquainted with the process. When the child and their inner system of parts are familiar with and get to test what EMDR processing is like, they feel safe with the process. The clinician may process something distant, such a very small and low-disturbing trigger in the child's play theme. It may be a subtle nuance of the play character. The processing of such small kernels also gives the clinician a view of the child's integrative capacities and processing style. The micro-processing of low-disturbing kernels of experience may be, for example, the little llama who is upset because she could not play with her favorite toy. This experience may be fractionated further into the llama's emotions, behaviors, thoughts, behaviors or bodily reactions. The clinician can invite awareness to the smallest fraction of information equivalent to the child's integrative capacities and window of tolerance.
- *Manipulation of the speed and length of the BLS/DAS*: The clinician can move to slower and shorter sets of BLS/DAS in order to slow down the accessing of traumatogenic material (F. Shapiro, 2001, 2018).

Despite the technicalities and myriad options, the clinician, just like a dancer, moves masterfully with the highly technical steps and transforms them fluidly for the audience into an experience of art.

The EMDR Interweave

During trauma processing, rapid BLS/DAS triggers a physiological state that facilitates information processing (E. Shapiro, 2018). The child is simultaneously attending to trauma-related and safety cues. The relational ecosystem accompanying the child in their processing experience utilizes active and passive pathways (Porges & Dana, 2018) to deliver safety signals. Often, the processing and integration of previously ruptured elements of memory occur spontaneously. However, when working with children with complex trauma and dissociation, information processing becomes stuck more often. The EMDR interweave is a strategy clinicians deliver to restore information processing when it stalls (E. Shapiro, 2018). The interweave either promotes the linkages between traumatic and adaptive memory systems or bridges the missing information and experiences. The EMDR interweave is also a co-regulatory and co-homeostatic strategy that modulates the affect-regulating system of the individual (Gomez, 2023a, in press). Bottom-up and top-down processes are actively attended to in EMDR therapy when information processing is stuck. The EMDR interweave may work with body-base, affective, or cognitive data, embracing lower-, mid-, and higher-brain-generated data. Trauma processing intrinsically challenges the child's sense of safety. However, it also opens up the opportunity to repair trauma-based and previously disrupted autonomic states, supporting the return to safety and social engagement as well as the rewiring of synaptic structures holding traumatogenic information. At times, the sympathetic or dorsal system may dominate the processing experience. In response, the EMDR clinician delivers interweaves combined with BLS/DAS that contain, modulate, correct, and support the completion of unfinished actions that move the child's organism to safety, homeostasis, and wholeness.

The following are some child-friendly interweaves:

- *Interweaves that work with the sensory-motor system* address the body, awakening possibilities for completing truncated defensive responses. When a fight or flight defense or a dissociative part that holds the trauma becomes active during processing, the clinician can utilize strategies from somatic therapies as interweaves (Ogden & Gomez, 2013). The clinician invites the child to track bodily sensations and execute new empowering actions that could not be performed during the traumatic event. The clinician invites therapeutic embodiments such as running, pushing, breaking free, breathing or spitting while keeping the child in a safe, playful, and mindful state. The clinician delivers invitations to the child to mindfully observe their body-based states using binoculars, magnifying glasses, or "the watching hat," actively bringing in the play system while engaging in rapid and longer sets of BLS/DAS.
- *Interweaves that work with emotions and the affective system*: emotions may show up in a state of dysregulation or constriction during processing. The clinician utilizes interweaves that expand the child's window of tolerance while titrating the access to disturbing emotions. Up- or down-regulating interweaves give the child access to their inner world while they remain connected enough to the ventral vagal system and the present safety. The clinician awakens possibilities for emotional expression through embodiments and movement. Emotions may travel into the outer world in the way the child can tolerate witnessing them. The representation of an emotion through a puppet, figure, or drawing may show up completely covered or fully exposed. An interweave may invite just a kernel of an emotion into the child's field of consciousness. As an external bio-emotional regulator, the clinician awakens and opens the possibilities that have remained invisible and inaccessible to the child's embodied mind through interweaves. Nevertheless, the clinician intervenes only when the child's integrative capacities stall. In EMDR therapy, clinicians join in while honoring the innate healing capacities of the child with intention, compassion, and respect for the child's journey.

- *Interweaves that work with the attachment system* actively utilize the caregiver's presence or are directed toward fulfilling the child's missing experiences and needs. When information processing stalls, signaling the presence of an unmet developmental need, the clinician invites the parent to offer interweaves that repair, provide missing information or experiences (feed, hold, or rock the child), validate, mirror, give the child's body corrective completions, or fulfill an unmet need.
- *Interweaves that restore dual awareness* are often directed to up- or down-regulate the child's system and awaken presence. The clinician uses child-friendly scales to invite interoceptive awareness. If the child is signaling the loss of connection to the present safety, the clinician utilizes interweaves to restore dual attention and the reconnection to states of safety, presence, and social engagement. The child may engage in movement, jump on the "safety chair," and do a "safety check," or connect to the figure, puppet, or stuffie previously installed in the preparation phase to remind themself that this experience is in the past and now they are safe. The clinician can also utilize their interoceptive signals and ventral vagal energy to support the child's connection to the safety of the present moment. The clinician's voice intonation, prosody, breathing patterns, posture, proximity, and facial expressions of safety, compassion, and validation maintain or restore the connection to safety when lost.

Once the level of disturbance decreases to zero, the EMDR clinician will work on strengthening the adaptive information and positive meta-perceptions, felt beliefs, and embodied cognition. For highly dissociative children, the clinician consults the inner system and delivers invitations to interocept and look within to find the embodied cognition and "good thought" that they now want in association with the imprint of the traumatic experience that by now is on its way to being reprocessed, reconsolidated, and rewired. The child creates songs and dances with an embodied belief while holding the memory in mind and engaging in BLS/DAS (Gomez, 2013). For instance, if the good thought is "I am strong," the clinician and the child may create a song and dance using the belief "I am strong."

The body scan is the last step in processing a memory. In this phase, the child connects very closely to their body, so residual somatic elements of the memory are integrated. The child directs their awareness within, listening closely to their body as an essential storyteller and historian.

Children often report a greater connection to the present sense of safety as the memory is appropriately located in time and space. The child arrives at a state of temporal organization and integration that allows them to experience the present free of the remnants of past traumas. They also report a sense of empowerment, freedom, agency, hope, and connection to themselves.

Reevaluation and Closure

EMDR therapy has built-in mechanisms and strategies for frequently checking the child's progress or the challenges the child may be experiencing that could result in treatment stagnation or negative outcomes. Every session of EMDR ends with closure, ensuring sufficient time to support safety and stabilization at the end of the session. Adequate closure and the return to homeostasis are paramount, especially when trauma has been explored or processed with a dissociative child. If parts were active, the clinician must utilize closure strategies to bring the parts back to containment, safety, and homeostasis. The clinician invites the inner world to connect with the "inside safe place" or "the inner okay place."

The reevaluation phase is utilized at the beginning of every session to keep track of changes, progress, or the need to modify and adjust treatment delivery. If the caregivers report an increase in the child's challenging issues, the clinician frequently explores the underlying issues responsible for the exacerbation of symptoms. The clinician reevaluates at the end of treatment to ensure all targets, symptoms, and triggers have been addressed.

Case Study: Ruby

Ruby was a seven-year-old girl who spent her first five years in an orphanage. She also experienced physical, emotional, and sexual abuse in her adoptive family, and as such, child protective services (CPS) had to take custody of her. Ruby spent one year in foster care, and then a new family adopted her. She presented with severe dysregulation in sleep patterns, food intake, and emotions. Temper tantrums usually lasted for over two hours, and she did not accept or seek regulation from her adoptive parent. Ruby was aggressive with her classmates and extremely controlling, so no one from her school wanted to foster relationships with her, which created social isolation. Ruby also presented with sexualized behaviors with children. However, she reported no memory of such events. Ruby was diagnosed by her psychiatrist with reactive attachment disorder and PTSD. Her mother reported that Ruby sometimes talked to herself and had three imaginary friends who visited her. One was an older adult who usually came to provide companionship and protection, a very young child who did not communicate verbally, and a voice that often told her to hurt or act out sexually on other children.

EMDR Treatment

Phase 1

The EMDR clinician initially met with the caregiver to gather information about Ruby's life, current symptoms, triggers, known traumatic events, and resources, as well as relational dynamics and strategies Ruby used to defend and to elicit care. The clinician thoroughly explored when, how, and what Ruby did when her symptoms were activated, as well as how the caregiver, teachers, and other adults in a caregiving role responded. The clinician invited verbal narratives and, at the same time, worked on exploring right-brain-generated data and patterns of autonomic activation. The clinician invited Ruby and her mother to engage in directive and non-directive play, using such tools as puppets and the sand tray, to observe their relational choreographies and nervous system tendencies.

From the first meeting with Ruby, the clinician remained connected, aware of herself and her internal rhythms and how they interacted with Ruby's biological sequences. Ruby received signs of safety through the clinician's intentional use of her voice, body posture, movement, and every interaction that conveyed presence and congruency. Ruby created worlds in the sand tray where children and animals were victims of horrific acts. She created a puppet show with her mother where a dragon bullied vulnerable others. At times, Ruby very quickly moved into hyper-arousal and high sympathetic activation. Sometimes, she became hypo-aroused and depressed. The clinician provided active and passive pathways for Ruby to reengage and recruit her social engagement system, which allowed her to collect data about Ruby's capacities for regulation and engagement.

Ruby would become angry and agitated if the clinician or parent did not do what she wanted, and would employ control, manipulation, lying, and avoidance of any conversation about or reference to her inner world of feelings. The clinician carefully observed how the caregiver responded and her co-regulatory and relational capacities. The clinician remained curious and present. When Ruby became verbally aggressive toward her, the clinician self-regulated so as to remain safe for the child and herself. Ruby refused to answer any tests to assess for dissociation, so the clinician gave the parent and teacher dissociation checklists and instruments to explore dissociative tendencies in Ruby. The clinician received Ruby's requests and denials with acceptance, compassion, and reflective listening and communication.

A clinical landscape emerged, showing highly dysregulated ANS and defensive regulatory strategies such as control, manipulation, and avoidance. The inner system of parts began to surface in the stories and through the avatars offered by the sandtray worlds, puppet play, non-directive play, and embodiments. The clinician paid attention to Ruby's body—where and when her body would become agitated, and the movements, as well as holding patterns of tension and collapse, that were present. The history-taking phase was circular as the clinician received new information and data about Ruby's story throughout treatment.

Preparation Phase

With the information gathered from Phase 1, the clinician continued working with Ruby and her mother to co-construct safety, regulation, and homeostasis to reset her nervous system and support the mother and Ruby in developing co-regulatory capacities. The clinician also used psychoeducation and showed Ruby how to engage in BLS/DAS using developmentally appropriate language (see earlier sections of this chapter). The co-construction of safety and regulation from moment to moment took great effort and presence, as Ruby found it unfamiliar. When her mother attempted to connect, Ruby would push her away, and the trauma-related phobias of her inner world, affect, and connection blocked her caregiver from providing the nurturance Ruby longed to receive. Ruby could not find a place where she felt safe, so the clinician invited her to construct one in her playroom. The clinician chose to use distance and titration to support Ruby in overcoming her phobia of positive affect. She invited Ruby to create a happy or relaxed place for a character of her choice. Ruby brought a bear she called Molly.

Once Ruby had built the place, the clinician invited her to bring her "wonder mind," to wonder how Molly felt in this place. The clinician also addressed Ruby's internal system and the potential conflicts, saying: "Sometimes one side of us feels happy and safe while another may not. Let's ask Molly if all the sides of her inside feel happy in this place." Ruby reported that Molly felt happy and identified where these feelings were "hanging out" in Molly's body. The clinician invited Ruby to use movement and marching as a form of BLS/DAS while holding Molly in her safe place. The choice of marching was intentional, as eye movement had previously moved Ruby quickly into traumatic material, while marching was welcomed and regulating.

Eventually, Molly invited her mother to join her in her happy place, and Ruby invited her mother to represent and impersonate Molly's mom. Ruby became curious about how she would feel inside Molly's happy place, so she practiced being in the same place with Molly. However, this time, the clinician invited Ruby's "wondering and curious mind" to see how she was feeling. The clinician's frequent mentalization and intentional decision-making created greater synchronicity, synergy, and contingency in her responses, which allowed Ruby to experience repair and corrections that, in turn, created new synaptic connections and a more robust adaptive network. These experiences of safety also began to challenge Ruby's internal working models created from trauma and disrupted autonomic states.

The clinician continued to use distance and titration through the worlds Ruby created in the sand tray, and invited Ruby to identify feelings in the animals and characters of her stories, often a kangaroo, not yet her own. The clinician reflected aloud that sometimes feelings may feel too big, so they invited the kangaroo to decide how much anger she was ready to see and feel, and she chose only a tiny spoon. The mother and clinician actively accompanied the kangaroo and her tiny spoon of anger. The clinician wondered out loud,

How does the kangaroo feel knowing that she has companions and is not alone with her anger? How is it for her to know that it is okay to feel anger? Feelings are messengers even when they feel uncomfortable. I wonder if the kangaroo knows this?

This work began to enhance Ruby's affect tolerance and connection to her emotions.

Parallel to Ruby's work, the clinician met with the mother to work more actively in supporting the mother's capacities for co-regulation, reflective communication, and mentalization.

The clinician also enhanced playful experiences with Ruby using BLS/DAS, in which she expressed joy and calmness, and triumphant moments when she could "dance" with her uncomfortable emotions while co-regulating with her mother during therapeutic sessions. Throughout the preparation phase, the clinician continued to invite and direct Ruby to check her inner world to increase interoceptive awareness and connection. Ruby started to speak about her other "Me's" and what they did for her. While honoring their presence, the clinician continued to support Ruby's relationship with her inner storytellers. Ruby began to show a greater capacity for tolerating positive and negative affect, allowing her mother to have physical and emotional closeness with her.

Traumatic memories began to emerge through play themes, where malevolent people were hurting babies living in an orphanage. However, there was no ownership or recognition on Ruby's part of this trauma as her own. This level of distance gave Ruby refuge from her stories while they were acted out by her characters/avatars. The clinician maintained close communication with Ruby's mother, who was actively working with a therapist to address her own experiences of trauma. This work aimed to ensure that Ruby's actions would not trigger these memory systems, causing her mother to shift from co-regulation to a state of defense and self-preservation. The clinician also worked with Ruby and her defenses, utilizing segmented embodied psychoeducation (Gomez, 2025), where Ruby realized her protectors while in the compassionate companionship of the clinician and the mother.

Assessment Phase

Ruby had made significant improvements in her sleep and food intake patterns, but she still presented with aggressiveness and dissociative symptomatology. However, she had greater affect tolerance and participated more often when her mother or the therapist made invitations to co-regulate. Ruby's mother reported that when Ruby challenged her, she used her parenting wheel to stay grounded in her guiding self and her capacity to up- or down-regulate, mirror and use reflective function, support Ruby in co-organizing her experience and co-create meaning, and actively give her signals of safety. Ruby's inner voices were no longer active, and she stated that her imaginary friend did not visit her as much but stayed in the background.

The clinician continued to invite somatic awareness and connection to her inner world whenever they needed to make decisions. Ruby did not necessarily name her inner voices, but her inner world was embraced and honored at all times. Organically, Ruby began to create stories through the sand tray or with puppets representing babies living in an orphanage who were hurt. The clinician and the parent, utilizing readiness decision-making markers, agreed that Ruby could benefit from moving into the trauma processing phases of EMDR therapy while preserving the distance she had chosen so organically through the sand tray and doll house. Ruby had multiple resources that accompanied her through her processing sessions: her safe place in the office where she could take a "resting time" and the companionship of her helpers. Ruby could go to her "safety chair," where she could do safety checks at any point to connect to the felt sense of safety in the present.

In one session, Ruby created a story in the tray depicting hurt babies. One of the babies (main character and voice of the tray) tried to fight, but was unsuccessful. The clinician asked Ruby's inner system if they could "sort out" what was happening in the story, and Ruby and her inner storytellers accepted the invitation to do so. They also identified what they needed to have nearby for safety. The clinician created a platform for Ruby's inner system to optimize her integrative capacities, incorporating resources, special powers, and helpers previously identified during the preparation phase. The clinician intentionally reduced the assessment phase, considering that Ruby tended to shut down when asked too many questions, but did ask questions such as: What part of this world stands out for the bigger baby? What feelings does the baby have? How hurtful, painful, or bothersome is this for the baby? (the clinician used ten measuring spoons to identify the level of disturbance associated with this story), and where is this "hanging out" in the baby's body? Within a titration continuum, the clinician utilized distance and an implicit portal into the memory that honored Ruby's capacities.

Processing Phases

The clinician initiated rapid sets of BLS/DAS while Ruby was moving the figures in the sand tray and telling her story, at times without words. The clinician paused, inviting moments of breathing and "dancing with air" and wondering aloud what was happening in the tray. When information processing stalled, the clinician utilized interweaves that supported integration at cognitive, emotional, and sensorimotor levels. These interweaves supported attachment and defensive completions. The babies of Ruby's story were nurtured, defended, protected, and loved. In addition, the babies were able to escape and fight, giving Ruby the opportunity to experience these completions of truncated responses and savor the acts of triumph through the characters and avatars of the story.

Ruby came to each session eager to tell and "sort out" a new story. Her mother reported more rapid changes in her affect, aggression, and also the acknowledgment and expression of her emotions. There were some ups and downs when Ruby had to be moved to a new school due to changes in her mother's job. At this point, Ruby did not want to "sort out" stories, and the clinician used a circular approach to the eight phases and went back to preparation phase–based strategies to stabilize her. This time, Ruby went back to balance quicker and was able to return to processing.

Ruby began to talk about her memories of abuse at the hands of her prior adoptive parents. Ownership and greater temporal awareness emerged as Ruby spoke about these occurrences as having happened in the past to her. Ruby brought her team of companions, her personal treasure, and special powers to her processing session. The clinician created a platform with resources, companionship, and connection to the present safety to bring Ruby to an optimal connection to her social engagement system, safety, and to herself. Her mother and the clinician emphasized that Ruby was not alone and that they both were there to hold a safe space for Ruby. Ruby knew she could take breaks and go to her resting and safe place anytime. When she was hungry, she would become easily dysregulated, so her mother gave additional attention to Ruby's basic biological needs before the session to expand her window of tolerance and increase her integrative capacities.

While processing a memory of abuse, Ruby expressed fear. The clinician delivered invitations to visit this fear mindfully and engage in rapid BLS/DAS while at the same time ensuring that Ruby had enough connection to the present safety. Signals of safety were conveyed through voice intonation, facial expressions, and physical proximity of the caregiver and the clinician, plus verbal reminders to Ruby such as "This is over, and you are safe now; we are right here with you, by your side. Your storytellers are just sorting this out." During processing, Ruby went into other parts of the memory as well as into other experiences of abuse. Considering Ruby's capacities for affect tolerance, the clinician let Ruby's mind go where it needed to go without any restrictions. Throughout multiple processing sessions, Ruby traveled through memories and moments of attachment completions when her mother repaired and fulfilled Ruby's longings for love, belonging, validation, and protection. When information processing was blocked, the clinician utilized interweaves that supported Ruby in completing truncated and unfinished actions. She ran with her mother and the clinician sometimes, pushing and moving as her body longed to move while engaging in BLS/DAS. Throughout the processing sessions, Ruby not only traveled through memories, but her therapeutic work represented a journey into herself.

A three-pronged approach to EMDR treatment supported Ruby and her mother in accessing the biological imprints from the past, the turbulent present, and their visions for the future. Ruby processed present triggers and created stories in the sand tray and the doll house about her future with a new sense of self, agency, empowerment, and freedom to be who she was meant to be. The clinician did not push Ruby to abandon the self-states and story keepers that had held her life's stories; instead, Ruby organically attained the level of integration in her sense of self that made sense and honored her. Ruby rearranged the relationship she had with her inner world and herself. She organized a party of gratitude and compassion for her inner storytellers.

Despite the positive outcome, the treatment of Ruby had a lot of ups, downs, and challenges. However, the clinician remained consistent, present, and compassionate for Ruby and her mother.

Conclusion

EMDR therapy has proved to be an effective treatment for children affected by trauma. Having been on both ends, as a recipient and a practitioner delivering EMDR therapy to children affected by chronic traumatization, I have been a witness to its transformative power. EMDR treatment has many technicalities, and its combination with the most recent findings in neuroscience makes it powerful and its practice intricate. Just like the artist who unites complex techniques with presence, passion, and a deep connection to themselves so fluidly, the EMDR clinician delivers an approach with such intricate choreographies in a way that the child experiences it as a work of art that takes them into a much greater connection to themselves. This approach, as any other, requires mastery, presence, and dedication, especially when provided to the children most affected by chronic traumatization.

References

Artigas, L., & Jarero, I. (2014). The butterfly hug method for bilateral stimulation. emdrfoundation.org/toolkit/butterfly-hug.pdf.

Bongaerts, H., Van Minnen, A., & de Jongh, A. (2017). Intensive EMDR to treat patients with complex posttraumatic stress disorder: A case series. *Journal of EMDR Practice and Research, 11*(2), 84–95. https://doi.org/10.1891/1933-3196.11.2.84

California Evidence-Based Clearinghouse for Child Welfare. (2010). cebc4cw.org/program/eye-movement-desensitization-and-reprocessing

Chen, R., Gillespie, A., Zhao, Y., Xi, Y., Ren, Y., & McLean, L. (2018). The efficacy of eye movement desensitization and reprocessing in children and adults who have experienced complex childhood trauma: A systematic review of randomized controlled trials. *Frontiers in Psychology, 9*, 534. https://doi.org/10.3389/fpsyg.2018.00534

Courtois, C. A. (2004). Complex trauma, complex reactions: Assessment and treatment. *Psychotherapy: Theory, Research, Practice, Training, 41*(4), 412–425. https://doi.org/10.1037/0033-3204.41.4.412

Cozolino, L. J. (2014). *The neuroscience of human relationships: Attachment and the developing social brain.* W. W. Norton.

Danylchuk, L. S., & Connors, K. J. (2024). *Treating complex trauma and dissociation: A practical guide to navigating therapeutic challenges* (2nd ed.). Taylor & Francis.

de Jongh, A., Ernst, R., Marques, L., & Hornsveld, H. (2013). The impact of eye movements and tones on disturbing memories involving PTSD and other mental disorders. *Journal of Behavior Therapy and Experimental Psychiatry, 44*(4), 477–483. https://doi.org/10.1016/j.jbtep.2013.07.002

de Roos, C., van der Oord, S., Zijlstra, B., Lucassen, S., Perrin, S., Emmelkamp, P., & de Jongh, A. (2017). Comparison of eye movement desensitization and reprocessing therapy, cognitive behavioral writing therapy, and wait-list in pediatric posttraumatic stress disorder following single-incident trauma: A multicenter randomized clinical trial. *Journal of Child Psychology and Psychiatry, 58*(11), 1219–1228. https://doi.org/10.1111/jcpp.12768

Dion, L. (2018). *Aggression in play therapy: A neurobiological approach for integrating intensity.* W. W. Norton.

Flynn, J. (2023). *Little gecko's broken tail: A book to introduce EMDR therapy to children.* Self-published.

Gomez, A. M. (2010). *Dark, bad day... go away: A book for children about trauma and EMDR therapy* (2nd ed.). Self-published.

Gomez, A. M. (2013). *EMDR therapy and adjunct approaches with children: Complex trauma, attachment, and dissociation.* Springer.
Gomez, A. M. (2018). *Stories and storytellers: The thinking mind, the heart and the body: A book for children about healing and EMDR therapy.* Self-published.
Gomez, A. M. (2021a). Dissociation in children: A multimodal approach to EMDR therapy. *Go With That* magazine, *26*(4), 17–25. emdria.org/magazine/emdr-therapy-and-dissociation
Gomez, A. M. (2021b). *The parenting wheel training manual.* Unpublished manuscript.
Gomez, A. M. (2022). *The EMDR group parent empowerment protocol (GPEP) training manual.* Unpublished manuscript.
Gomez, A. M. (2023a). *EMDR therapy basic training manual.* Unpublished manuscript.
Gomez, A. M. (2023b). The journey of the butterfly: G-TEP with children. In R. Morrow Robinson & S. Kemal Kaptan (Eds.), *EMDR group therapy: Emerging principles and protocols to treat trauma and beyond* (pp.139–148). Springer.
Gomez, A. M. (In press). *EMDR-sandtray-based therapy: Healing Complex Trauma and Dissociation across the lifespan.* W. W. Norton.
Gomez, A. M. (2025). The trauma-formed defense and self-protective system. In A. Gomez & J. Hosey (Eds.), *The handbook of complex trauma and dissociation in children: Theory, research, and clinical applications* (pp. 752–773). Routledge.
Gomez, A. M., & Lyles, M. (2025). An integrative and phase-oriented approach to sandtray therapy. In A. Gomez & J. Hosey (Eds.), *The handbook of child complex trauma and dissociation* (pp. 590–611). Routledge.
Gonzalez, A., & Mosquera, D. (2012). *EMDR and dissociation: The progressive approach* (English ed). Amazon Publishing.
International Society for the Study of Dissociation, Task Force on Children and Adolescents. (2004). Guidelines for the evaluation and treatment of dissociative symptoms in children and adolescents. *Journal of Trauma & Dissociation, 5*(3), 119–150. https://doi.org/10.1300/J229v05n03_09
Karadag, M., Gokcen, C., & Sarp, A. S. (2019). EMDR therapy in children and adolescents who have post-traumatic stress disorder: A six-week follow-up study. *International Journal of Psychiatry in Clinical Practice, 24*(1), 77–82. https://doi.org/10.1080/13651501.2019.1682171
Kluft, R. P. (1999). An overview of the psychotherapy of dissociative identity disorder. *American Journal of Psychotherapy, 53*(3), 289–319. https://doi.org/10.1176/appi.psychotherapy.1999.53.3.289
Knipe, J. (2018). *EMDR toolbox: Theory and treatment of complex PTSD and dissociation.* Springer.
Korn, D. L., & Leeds, A. M. (2002). Preliminary evidence of efficacy for EMDR resource development and installation in the stabilization phase of treatment of complex posttraumatic stress disorder. *Journal of Clinical Psychology, 58*(12), 1465–1487. https://doi.org/10.1002/jclp.10099
Landin-Romero, R., Moreno-Alcazar, A., Pagani, M., & Amann, B. L. (2018). How does eye movement desensitization and reprocessing therapy work? A systematic review on suggested mechanisms of action. *Frontiers in Psychology, 9.* https://doi.org/10.3389/fpsyg.2018.01395
Levine, P. A. (2015). *Trauma and memory: Brain and body in a search for the living past.* North Atlantic Books.
Lichtenstein, A., & Brager, S. (2017). EMDR integrated with relationship therapies for complex traumatized children: An evaluation and two case studies. *Journal of EMDR Practice and Research, 11*(2), 74–83. https://doi-org.libproxy.nau.edu/10.1891/1933-3196.11.2.74
Manzoni, M., Fernandez, I., Bertella, S., Tizzoni, F., Gazzola, E., Molteni, M., & Nobile, M. (2021). Eye movement desensitization and reprocessing: The art of efficacy in children and adolescent with post-traumatic disorder. *Journal of Affective Disorders, 282,* 340–347. https://doi.org/10.1016/j.jad.2020.12.088
Monaco, A. (2021). Understanding and responding to dissociation. In A. Beckley-Forest & A. Monaco (Eds.), *EMDR with children in the play therapy room: An integrated approach* (pp. 251–290). Springer.
Ogden, P. K., & Gomez, A. M. (2013). Using EMDR therapy and sensorimotor psychotherapy with children. In A. Gomez (Ed.), *EMDR therapy and adjunct approaches with children: Complex trauma, attachment and dissociation* (pp. 247–271). Springer.
Ogden, P., Minton, K., & Pain, C. (2006). *Trauma and the body: A sensorimotor approach to psychotherapy.* W. W. Norton.
Olivier, E., de Roos, C., & Bexkens, A. (2022). Eye movement desensitization and reprocessing in young children (ages 4–8) with posttraumatic stress disorder: A multiple-baseline evaluation. *Child Psychiatry and Human Development, 53*(6), 1391–1404. https://doi.org/10.1007/s10578-021-01237-z
Porges, S. W. (2021). *Polyvagal safety: Attachment, communication, self-regulation.* W. W. Norton.
Porges, S. W., & Dana, D. (2018). *Clinical applications of the polyvagal theory: The emergence of polyvagal-informed therapies.* W. W. Norton.

Putnam, F. W. (1997). *Dissociation in children and adolescents: A developmental perspective*. Guilford Press.

Rodenburg, R., Benjamin, A., de Roos, C., Meijer, A. M., & Stams, G. J. (2009). Efficacy of EMDR in children: A meta-analysis. *Clinical Psychology Review, 29*(7), 599–606. https://doi.org/10.1016/j.cpr.2009.06.008

Rolling, J., Fath, M., Zanfonato, T., Durpoix, A., Mengin, A. C., & Schröder, C. M. (2024). EMDR–Teens–cPTSD: Efficacy of eye movement desensitization and reprocessing in adolescents with complex PTSD secondary to childhood abuse: A case series. *Healthcare, 12*(19), 1993. https://doi.org/10.3390/healthcare12191993

Schore, A. N. (2003). *Affect dysregulation and disorders of the self*. W. W. Norton.

Schore, A. N. (2012). *The science of the art of psychotherapy*. W. W. Norton.

Shapiro, E. (2018, April 19–22). *The EMDR group-traumatic episode protocol (G-TEP)*. EMDR Early Intervention World Summit, Natick, MA.

Shapiro, E., & Laub, B. (2014). The recent traumatic episode protocol (R-TEP): An integrative protocol for early EMDR intervention (EEI). In M. Luber (Ed.), *Implementing EMDR early mental health interventions for man-made and natural disasters: Models, scripted protocols, and summary sheets* (pp. 193–207). Springer.

Shapiro, F. (2001). *Eye movement desensitization and reprocessing: Basic principles, protocols and procedures* (2nd ed.). Guilford Press.

Shapiro, F. (2007). EMDR, adaptive information processing, and case conceptualization. *Journal of EMDR Practice and Research, 1*, 68–87. https://doi.org/10.1891/1933-3196.1.2.68

Shapiro, F. (2018). *Eye movement desensitization and reprocessing: Basic principles, protocols, and procedures* (3rd ed.). Guilford Press.

Shapiro, F., & Laliotis, D. (2015). EMDR therapy for trauma-related disorders. In U. Schnyder & M. Cloitre (Eds.), *Evidence based treatments for trauma-related psychological disorders: A practical guide for clinicians* (pp. 205–228). Springer International Publishing/Springer Nature. https://doi.org/10.1007/978-3-319-07109-1_1

Siegel, D. (2010). *Mindsight: The new science of personal transformation*. W. W. Norton.

Silvestre, M. (2022). Systemic family therapy and EMDR therapy: An integrative approach. *European Journal of Trauma & Dissociation, 6*(4), Article 100291. https://doi.org/10.1016/j.ejtd.2022.100291

Steele, K., Boon, S., & van der Hart, O. (2017). *Treating trauma-related dissociation: A practical integrative approach*. W. W. Norton.

Stricklin, A. (2021). "Splatting" out the trauma with movement in EMDR processing. In A. Beckley-Forest & A. Monaco (Eds.), *EMDR with children in the play therapy room: An integrated approach* (pp. 378–438). Springer.

Teke, E., & Avşaroğlu, S. (2021). Efficacy of eye movement desensitization and reprocessing (EMDR) therapy for children and adolescents with post-traumatic stress disorder. *Journal of School and Educational Psychology, 2*(1), 1–12. https://doi.org/10.47602/josep.v2i1.1

van der Hart, O., Nijenhuis, E. R. S., & Steele, K. (2006). *The haunted self: Structural dissociation of the personality and treatment of chronic traumatization*. W. W. Norton.

Wesselmann, D., Armstrong, S., Schweitzer, C., Davidson, M., & Potter, A. (2018). An integrative EMDR and family therapy model for treating attachment trauma in children: A case series. *Journal of EMDR Practice and Research, 12*(4), 196–207. https://doi.org/10.1891/1933-3196.12.4.196

World Health Organization. (2013). Guidelines for the management of conditions that are specifically related to stress. who.int/publications/i/item/9789241505406

21
PSYCHO-SENSORY INTERVENTION®

An Occupational Therapy Approach

Kim Barthel

Introduction: Occupational Therapy Practice in Mental Health and Childhood Trauma

Occupational Therapy (OT) enables people to participate in the things they want to do in life. As a relatively new health care profession (early 1900s), the mission of OT is to help people become their best selves. With intentional therapeutic use of self, occupational therapists (OTs) enter into a therapeutic relationship with their clients, becoming potential facilitators of change. Clinical reasoning that is holistic and evidence-informed in both physical medicine and mental health (mind-body) provides OTs with an arsenal of resources for the creation of individualized intervention plans. Through a systems approach lens, OT considers the person, environment, culture, and context as interacting pieces of influence in a person's overall well-being. OTs weave together clinical evidence and art, seeking tools and models of intervention that will guide their therapeutic process.

Pediatric OTs specialize in evaluating a child's developmental strengths and difficulties and design interventions that promote the skills needed for success in daily activities (occupations). Complex childhood trauma and dissociation have a profound and devastating impact on a child's occupational performance and engagement in daily living. Areas such as self-regulation, social engagement, learning, playing, motor skills, and daily living activities are often impacted by complex trauma and thus benefit from the clinical reasoning and interventions of OT. One approach designed by an OT to specifically meet the individualized needs of people with complex trauma and dissociation is Psycho-Sensory Intervention (PSI).

The Story of Daniel[1]

Almost 35 years ago, Daniel was referred to me for OT by his teacher to help him manage his behavior. He was born to a mom who was crystal meth-addicted, and she overdosed when he was three months old. After the loss of his mom, his primary caregivers became three other children: an 8-year-old, an 11-year-old, and a 13-year-old. They often lived homeless in conditions of poverty and hunger, and danger and uncertainty were a part of their daily lives. This predominant state of homelessness happened for the first eight years of Daniel's life, until he was suddenly brought into residential care. When I met him, Daniel had just started to attend school and found himself in a classroom environment for the first time. His teacher described him as a "feral animal" who destroyed the classroom and was "incapable of interaction" with his peers. She said, "He must be undiagnosed ADHD and needs medication for his behavior." Knowing a little about the work of OTs in Sensory Integration, the teacher asked me to "take him into the magic lab [sensory gym] and do something with him." She wasn't convinced it would change anything, but she'd heard enough about my beliefs in SI's ability to help some kids learn to stay focused and to manage their behavior, that she was willing for me to try.

Eager to prove the value of Sensory Integration therapy, I invited Daniel into the sensory gym for our first meeting. I had learned in my Sensory Integration certification training that the child guides the treatment by engaging with sensory equipment in a "self-organizing way." Daniel impulsively ran toward the six-foot climbing wall that had a big foam pit below. This equipment was designed to provide experiences of safe climbing and crashing, offering opportunities for intense proprioception and vestibular integration. Daniel was certainly intense. He wanted as much height, danger, and frequency as he could get. He climbed to the very top and would turn around and free fall into space without even extending his arms forward for protection. This experience went on repeatedly, uninterrupted, for 45 minutes. Thinking the activity was doing all the work to reorganize Daniel's nervous system, I sat passively nearby on a mat, ensuring safety, but had minimal interaction with him. He became slower in speed and more fatigued as the session progressed, and eventually, he lay still on the mat near me. His eyes were present, and he seemed contemplative in his state of being. Observing this change in state left me thinking that the session was successful in its objective.

What happened next changed the course of my career. Daniel left the therapy room and went upstairs to his residence and attempted to hang himself. He did not succeed, thankfully. And later, when we'd established a therapeutic relationship, he was able to share with me that from crashing into the foam pit so much, he had started to remember so many horrible things that had happened in his past that he hadn't recalled or focused on before. In my many conversations with multidisciplinary colleagues that followed (a clinical counselor and psychologist in particular), the idea that sensory intervention could support children who experience complex trauma and dissociative states was explored. The key would be to have it be carefully guided in the context of relationship combined with psychotherapy, and at a pace that allowed for greater ease of processing. This case started me on my journey in this direction.

The focus of this chapter is to:

- Introduce the Psycho-Sensory Intervention (PSI) approach
- Describe the key components of PSI
- Summarize the frames of reference supporting PSI
- Explain sensory, postural, and movement challenges related to complex childhood trauma and dissociation
- Highlight PSI assessment and intervention in practice

What Is Psycho-Sensory Intervention?

Psycho-Sensory Intervention® (PSI) is a holistic approach designed to support trauma survivors across the lifespan. For this chapter, the focus of discussion will be on PSI specifically for children. Developed by this author (an OT from Canada) beginning in the mid-1990s, PSI integrates the author's knowledge from (and experience with) several interdisciplinary frames of reference. Foundationally, PSI is informed by neurobiology. Philosophically, PSI is inherently trauma-sensitive. The PSI approach needs to be practiced by clinicians with good self-awareness who include elements of co-regulation through relationship blended with play-based, sensory-motor interventions and psychotherapy. Treatment is custom-made for each child within their zone of proximal development, based on assessment and clinical reasoning. PSI focuses on a child's strengths and challenges in participation, as opposed to childhood developmental diagnoses and conditions. A clinician's own self-awareness and emotional intelligence in understanding their role as an attuned therapeutic agent of change is critical.

Psycho-Sensory Intervention Is Neurobiologically Informed

Client assessments and interventions that are neurobiologically informed support clinicians and caregivers in developing evidence-informed clinical reasoning. Technological advances over the past 20 years have validated many psychological, sociobiological, and therapeutic theories that were previously based in hypothesis. Professions identified as social sciences such as OT are now able to derive evidence for their existence and therapeutic offerings. The neurobiological study of trauma, attachment, and mental health has exploded with research and is foundational to the ongoing development of the PSI approach.

Two particular neurobiological frames of reference that have been a constant backdrop to PSI are interpersonal neurobiology and polyvagal theory. The work of Drs. Daniel Siegel and Allan Schore in the 1990s introduced the scientific concepts supporting the interactions between mind, brain, and relationships (Siegel et al., 2021). This specific field of neurobiology revolutionized the concept that relationship is in and of itself a healing force. Simultaneously, Dr. Stephen Porges began writing about polyvagal theory identifying the role of "felt safety" (neuroception) (Porges, 2011) within relationships as the foundation of regulation and social engagement. Both theories are fully conceptualized in other chapters in this book.

Psycho-Sensory Intervention Is Trauma-Sensitive in Its Practice

Trauma-Sensitive Practice® (TSP) is a set of guiding principles developed by this author and her Relationship Matters Team in the early 2020s. TSP began as information about supporting people who have experienced trauma, and evolved during the COVID-19 pandemic to take the ideas from its principles and encourage practitioners to live them consciously. TSP has at its foundations the following principles.

1 **Be curious** about what underlying variables contribute to observable behavior.
2 Create a **culture of comfort** and safety embedded in the relationship, communication style, environment, and context.
3 Attempt to avoid instigating **retraumatizing** memories or triggers.
4 Appreciate the need for attention to the **language** used in describing behavior.
5 Adopt a **strengths-based** view of the people around you, no matter their apparent capacity.
6 Recognize secure **relationship**s as a healing force for change.
7 Implement a consistent philosophy that seeks to apply these principles with **consistency**.

TSP is the guiding philosophy of PSI.

A note about the "Spokes on the Wheel" model below (Figure 21.1). It was designed by this author to illustrate various elements that contribute to any given therapeutic goal. It may be used by anyone seeking a holistic visual representation of both assessment and treatment ideas. A practitioner may put any goal in the center of the wheel, and then insert their own 360-degree lens of what "spokes" may be impacting that goal being reached or not. With all spokes being strong, wheels go around with relative ease. For the purposes of describing PSI, this model has been revised to illustrate the key elements that make an intervention "psycho-sensory".

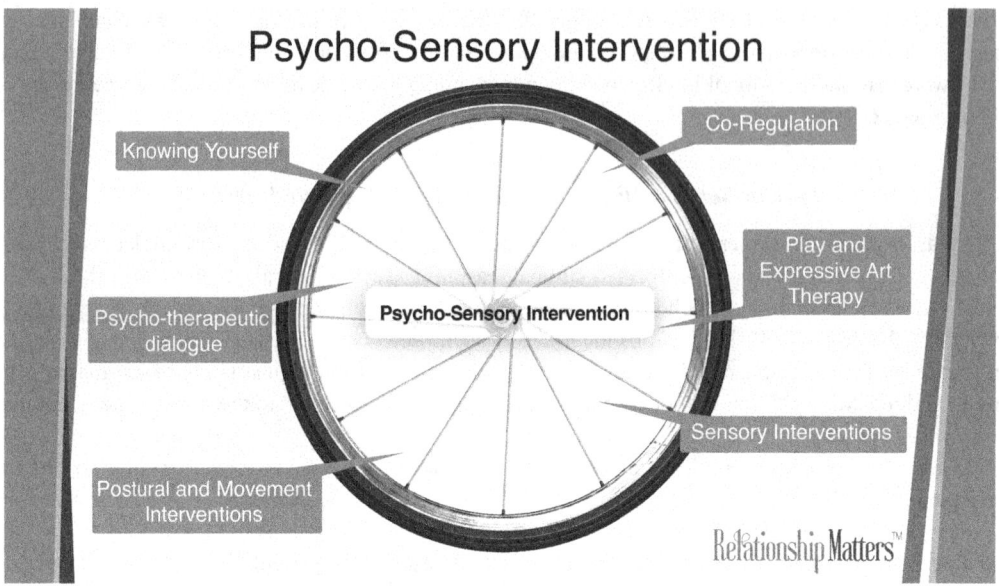

Figure 21.1 "Spokes on the Wheel": Elements of Psycho-Sensory Intervention.

Elements of Psycho-Sensory Intervention

Clinician's Self-Awareness

At the core of PSI are the co-regulating, attuning, and self-regulating skills of the clinician. Through developing increased capacity for self-awareness and social and emotional intelligence, the psychotherapeutic capacity to hold space and co-regulate the child expands. Making sense of one's own life allows clinicians to have the mentalizing skills to see, attune with, and empathize with others, qualities of a sensitive caregiver that are associated with secure attachment. As a clinician evolves in self-awareness, their own window of tolerance expands, and their self-regulatory skills become accessible with increasing ease. A clinician's effective therapeutic use of self is of paramount importance in the practice of PSI.

Regulation Through Relationship

Dr. Daniel Siegel's game-changing book *The Developing Mind: Toward a Neurobiology of Interpersonal Experience* (1999) catapulted the evolution of PSI, emphasizing the critical variable of attuned attachment as foundational in the development of regulation. In PSI, establishing a healthy and safe therapeutic relationship is the first task when working with a client. A consciously present and available clinician has a focused mind that facilitates the process of mentalization. This capacity allows the clinician to track their own thoughts and feelings while simultaneously putting their mind in the mind of the child. This shared space is like a resonant experience that flows between the two brains and allows each person to feel "felt" by the other (Siegel, 2010).

When emotions build in the child, moving them outside of their window of tolerance, the clinician discerns the activation within themselves and regulates the energy using their own inner resources. The child's brain observes how the clinician's nervous system manages these psychobiological shifts and follows suit. Through the clinician holding space for the child's emotions, the child learns to hold space for themselves, feeling the interoceptive experience of their feelings and tolerating them. As the state of arousal moves, the clinician moves the child forward into re-engagement in social connection or activity. Careful tracking of nonverbal affective cues enables the clinician to respond with subtle adjustments in their own nonverbal cues while staying authentic in their being. The clinician can match the energy of the child's varying affective states and shift the dial within themselves to return to connection and collaboration.

Play-Based Activities

Since the early days of the OT profession, creativity has been intrinsic to the beliefs and practice of OTs. Creativity is defined as "the use of expressive arts in therapy" (Schmid, 2004, p. 85). Dr. Bruce Perry's neuroscientific findings (2009) suggested that traumatic memories are predominantly stored in the right hemisphere, making verbal declarative memory of trauma difficult to access. Expressive therapies (such as play, visual art, dance, and music) are pathways into the right brain. Hence, when an attuned clinician engages in expressive activities with a client, unconscious material that is coded and potentially dysregulating can be accessed (Perry, 2009).

Dr. Cathy Malchiodi describes expressive therapies and creative therapies as action-oriented methods through which individuals can explore issues and communicate thoughts and feelings (Malchiodi, 2015). Highly charged emotional experiences such as trauma are encoded by the limbic system as a form of sensory reality. This would then suggest that successful intervention and resolution would benefit from expression and processing of sensory memories of the traumatic events through action-oriented methods (Malchiodi, 2015; Rothschild, 2000).

Most sensory motor based, psychotherapeutic interventions are embedded in play schemes, especially when supporting young children. Some of these concepts related specially to play are well described in Chapters 27–30, so please refer to them for more fulsome descriptions. Although play-based interventions may continue to be accessed in older children, this selection may be a less prioritized spoke on the wheel within PSI as the child begins to adopt the use of sensory-motor supports with greater independence across contexts.

Sensory-Based Interventions

A primary spoke on the wheel of the PSI approach is the provision of sensations with a therapeutic intent of supporting safety, regulation, learning, and social connection. Sensory input is incorporated in a play activity, offered as stand-alone exercises or available in particular environments (ex. home, school) dependent on the chronological age of the child. Parents are educated and instructed in the use and understanding of why sensory strategies can support regulation and function. OT and author Tina Champagne described sensory-based interventions as sensory strategies that address an individual's sensory systems in a therapeutic manner to create change and enable adaptation to one's physical environment (Champagne, 2011). Paired together with regulation through relationship and posture and movement strategies, sensory interventions work together to assist the child in connecting to their body sensorily (felt sense), experiencing themselves separate from others, and exploring and expanding connection with the world.

The Sensory Systems

Important to the understanding of sensory-based interventions is the appreciation of the various sensory systems and their functions (Table 21.1).

Table 21.1 Sensory Systems

Sensory System	Function

Vestibular system	• Lies in the inner ear
	• Provides awareness of:
	  ○ Position in space
	  ○ Direction of movement
	  ○ Speed of movement
	• Detects influence of gravity and body weight
	• Influences ocular motor function for stable horizon
	• Influences postural control, readiness to move, balance and coordination
	• Contributes to interoception, sense of self, and consciousness (Riva & Dakanalis, 2018)
	• Can be soothing or alerting depending on speed, direction, or rhythmicity
	• Influences emotions and cognition
	• Anchors all other sensory systems

Proprioceptive system	• Information arising from the body, especially the muscles, joints, ligaments, and fascia in the body • Perceived when we stretch, push and pull, move our bodies against resistance, and engage in heavy work • Tells us how our joints and muscles are moving and how heavy or light objects are • Reinforces a person's sense of self and the feeling of "being" in a body • Proprioceptive activities that also incorporate deep touch have the potential to calm the fight-or-flight response.
Tactile system	• Skin covering the entire body • Affective touch contributes to felt safety • Light touch can activate the defense system, indicating threat • Deep pressure touch can be soothing and grounding • Discriminative touch allows the subject to sense and localize touch, and identify what is being touched
The auditory system	• Located within the inner ear • Converts sound waves to electrical impulses processed in the brain • Locating potential threat • High and low frequency sounds elicit an instant orienting response and self-protection • Mid-range frequencies of sound relate to human voice and are received by the brain as language
The visual system	• Processes light waves that enter the eye, converting them to electrical impulses that are transmitted to the brain for interpretation • Visual perception is the ability of the brain to process and interpret these impulses • Occurs with increasing complexity and interpretation as it proceeds through the lower levels of the brain up toward the cortex • Requires smooth integration of two distinct pathways of vision: ambient (peripheral) and focal (central detail vision) needed to orient to a stimulus and make meaning out of what is being seen • Interaction between the visual and vestibular systems supports the coordination of smooth eye movements, facilitating fixation and following of moving images with the eyes
The olfactory system	• Detects the presence of odor molecules in the air • Enhances awareness of the environment and alerts to potential danger such as fire, a gas leak, or rancid food • Directly connects into the limbic brain, involved in emotions and memory

(*Continued*)

Table 21.2 (Continued)

Sensory System	Function
The gustatory system	• Interprets taste and texture within the mouth • Taste buds on the tongue act as receptors to sweet, salty, sour, bitter, and umami (savory/meat) • Interpretation of the chemical reactions of taste feedforward to the oral motor system, supporting the function of eating and feeding
The interoceptive system	• The process of receiving, accessing, and appraising sensory signals that come from inside the body • Makes sense of internal state • Plays a role in influencing our mood, emotions, and sense of well-being (Cameron & Minoshima, 2002) • "May precede the ability to know what we are feeling, to become aware of shifts in internal bodily states that influence our affective arousal" (Siegel, 2012) • Involves activation of the right anterior insula in the prefrontal cortex • "Correlated with the capacity for empathy for the feelings of others" (Siegel, 2012)

Postural and Movement Interventions

OTs receive a significant amount of training in musculoskeletal anatomy, kinesiology, biomechanics, motor control, and motor learning. Since trauma lives in the body as well as the brain, OTs are poised to evaluate the kinesiological adaptations that arise from self-protective affective states. When intentional sensory experiences are offered in treatment for the purpose of trauma reorganization, the body must have access to the necessary musculature in order to ground and contain the sensations experienced. Knowing that the trunk of the body is the foundation for the function of our head and limb movements, careful evaluation of postural alignment and access to trunk musculature is a critical component of PSI for the regulation of affective arousal states. Being up against gravity requires sound sensory processing and motor activation to "hold on and stay put" and move through the world. Clinicians provide hands-on facilitation to enhance perceived movements, when necessary, incorporate equipment to support postural alignment, and give home-program exercises to sustain newly acquired postural and movement capacities.

Psychotherapy

OTs are trained mental health practitioners and often practice psychotherapy as an aspect of their holistic intervention. Psychotherapy, within the Occupational Therapy Act, is defined as

> planned and structured interventions aimed at influencing behavior and function, by **psychotherapeutic** means. Psychotherapy is delivered through a **therapeutic relationship** to change an individual's disorder of thought, cognition, mood, emotional patterns, perception, or memory that may impair the individual's judgment, insight, behavior, communication, or social functioning as it relates to the performance of daily activities
>
> *(College of Occupational Therapists of Ontario [COTO], n.d., original emphasis)*

Additionally, effective communication and collaboration with other members of a multidisciplinary team (psychologists, psychotherapists, play therapists, counselors, social workers, educators, etc.)

are valuable for integrated interventions that best serve the needs of children with complex trauma and dissociation. Professional roles and boundaries are commonly communicated between professional's dependent upon the context, experience of the clinicians, engagement with the family, and the system within which teams are employed. Typically, therapeutic approaches to the treatment of trauma have been identified as either top-down or bottom-up inventions. Top-down integration of the brain requires cortical structures to process, inhibit, and organize reflexes, impulses and emotions generated by the brainstem and limbic system (Cozolino, 2002). Approaches of psychotherapy that are language reliant (cognitive) are often referred to as top-down. Bottom-up integration refers to approaches that specifically address sensory and emotional information processing at the level of the brainstem and limbic system, where safety and danger are perceived. In the PSI approach, which serves to inform clinicians from a range of disciplines, the intention is to support the child in feeling safe in their body with the help of sensations and movements (bottom-up) that we can perceive. At the same time, meaning-making, reframing, and co-regulating are constantly incorporated throughout the sensory-motor play-based experiences (top-down). By joining the child in their play, combined with sensorimotor interventions, the therapist makes meaning out of what is happening in the body and in the play through narration and co-regulation. PSI is a whole-brain and body approach to the treatment of complex trauma and dissociation.

Contributing Frames of Reference to Psycho-Sensory Intervention

In appreciating the holism of PSI, the foundational bodies of knowledge that inform and guide PSI will now be highlighted to provide a sense of how intervention is designed and delivered for each individual child who comes into our practice. The frames of reference are presented in alignment with Table 21.2, in the approximate order that this author brought them into her own multifaceted practice when supporting children who experienced complex trauma.

Table 21.2 Contributing Frames of Reference

Contributing Frame of Reference	Originator	Time Frame Developed
Sensory Integration (SI)	Dr. A. Jean Ayres	First developed in 1972; trademarked as Ayres Sensory Integration in 2005
Dynamic Maturational Model of Attachment and Adaptation (DMM) ("FRI," 2019)	Dr. Patricia M. Crittenden	2005
Neuro-Developmental Treatment (NDT) (Neuro-Developmental Treatment Association, 2023)	Mrs. Berta Bobath and Dr. Karel Bobath	1940s
Dynamic Core for Kids (Mannell & Wiebe, 2010)	Shelley Mannell, PT, and Julie Wiebe, PT	2009
Bodynamic Somatic Developmental Psychology (Bodynamic International, 2023)	Lisbeth Marcher	1968
Polyvagal Theory (Polyvagal Institute, 2023)	Stephen W. Porges, PhD	1994

Sensory Integration

PSI was foundationally influenced by the OT Sensory Integration frame of reference. Sensory Integration therapy was developed by Dr. Anna Jean Ayres, an OT with postdoctoral training in educational psychology and neuroscience. From the 1950s through the 1980s, Dr. Ayres published numerous articles, standardized assessments, chapters, and books related to the neurological relationships between sensation, movement, learning, and behavior (Smith-Roley et al., 2020). All human experiences rely on the processing of sensory information by the brain. All of these "bites" of sensory data must come together in the brain in an integrated manner for humans to make sense of and engage with the world. Dr. Ayres defined Sensory Integration as "the neurological process that organizes sensations from one's body and from the environment and makes it possible to use the body effectively in the environment" (Smith-Roley et al., 2020). When the senses are well integrated neurobiologically, adaptive responses to the environment arise naturally, contributing to new learning and progressive functional capacity. Over the decades, since the origination of Ayres Sensory Integration (ASI), there has been a growing body of evidence documenting the efficacy of the approach. Recently, Sensory Integration has been qualified as a new evidence-based practice for autism (Hume et al., 2021; Steinbrenner et al., 2020). The Ayres Sensory Integration Fidelity measure guides research effectiveness, ensuring the integrity of the frame of reference (Parham et al., 2007). Therapists educated in ASI are required to be certified in its theory, assessment, and treatment.

Key features of ASI Intervention (adapted from Parham et al., 2007):

- Treatment is provided in a "sensory gym" environment that is matted, ensuring safety for the child to explore sensation and movement with varying levels of intensity and risk. Suspended equipment that moves in three dimensions combined with opportunities to climb, crash one's body, and move through space are integral to the treatment experience.
- Therapy is attuned to the child's arousal and behavioral states throughout the session, presenting opportunities for child-guided exploration.
- Therapy must incorporate tactile, vestibular, and proprioceptive inputs that are embedded in developmentally appropriate motivational play activities.
- Play schemes are created to include more than one sensory modality at a time.
- Sensory, play-based experiences are tailored-made to be "just-right challenges," ensuring each child has an experience of "felt" success.
- Therapeutic alliance with the clinician is integral to the experience of safety, exploration, and playfulness.

Through interaction with the equipment and environment, the therapist tracks the child's changing states of alertness, regulation, and affect. Treatment is also designed to support changes in postural, ocular, coordination, and motor planning skills through scaffolded activity choices and environmental demands. Many aspects of the key features of the Sensory Integration frame of reference are also a part observed in the treatment sessions of the PSI approach.

PSI for complex childhood trauma and dissociation is classified as a sensory-based intervention but is different from ASI. Ayres Sensory Integrative theory and practice requires stringent adherence to the core process elements of the frame of reference. While some or many of these Sensory Integration core elements may be present within a PSI session, other frames of reference are holistically incorporated within a PSI experience as well, dependent on the holistic needs of the individual child.

How Does Sensory Processing Relate to Complex Childhood Trauma and Dissociation?

Drs. Ogden, Pain, and Fisher describe developmental trauma as being processed at a somatosensory level, potentially contributing to increased aggressive behavior, decreased ability to regulate and decreased ability to tolerate sensory input (Ogden et al., 2006).

Children with complex trauma and dissociation are often referred to OTs to support them with their self-regulation. This term "self-regulation," however, is used in many different contexts without a consensus of the definition. In the PSI approach, self-regulation requires the physiological management of arousal states.

Arousal is the energy in the brain and body that allows a person to match the demands of the environment and context they are in. Functionally, humans must adjust these states rapidly, flexibly, and comfortably to participate in life. Throughout the field of trauma therapy, the terms "arousal" and "arousal regulation" are typically identified and understood as energy in the brain and body related to "affective states" that are predominantly modulated by the autonomic nervous system and impacted by the stress continuum. Neurobiology emphasizes the massive impact that sensory input, through neural pathways separate from the autonomic nervous system, have upon states of being. Beginning at the brainstem, some sensations have the potential to wake up and excite the brain, while others have a role in inhibiting and quieting the activity of the brain. Excitation messages are needed for survival, motivation, focus, attention, and connection. Inhibition is also sometimes needed for relaxation, focus, attention, and connection. The reticular activating system (RAS) in the brainstem is a cluster of neural networks designed for survival and organized to modulate attention and wakefulness (Pfaff, 2009). The design of the brain inherently seeks to balance interacting chemicals and neural networks in an attempt to create arousal state homeostasis (just-right state). Sensory processing plays a distinct role in achieving this arousal balance. Dr. Smith-Roley indicates that there are four sensory systems feeding the alerting (up-regulating), ascending arousal pathways in the brainstem. These sensory systems are the vestibular, somatosensory, auditory, and gustatory systems, all of which have distinct regulating and novelty detection orienting survival functions (Smith-Roley et al., 2001).

Alternately, the brainstem also has a role as a sensory filter, inhibiting irrelevant stimuli so that only the most important sensory information is brought to consciousness. In the case of children with developmental differences or children exposed to early adversity, the RAS in the brainstem may not be so competent in this filtration or modulation process, potentially heightening awareness of unnecessary sensory input (Perry, 2001; Thome et al., 2019). This potential modulation limitation can keep the child suspended in vigilance and activated in their arousal state. Challenges with appropriate neurobiological inhibition of sensory stimuli can result in exaggerated fight-or-flight responses when a sensory stimulus is presented (Garcia-Rill, 2019). "Chronic overactivity in the RAS can also produce 'hypofrontality' decreased blood flow to the frontal lobes" (Garcia-Rill, 2019, p. 74). Heightened activity in the survival brainstem RAS can short-circuit the capacity for reasoning, decision making, impulse control, and connection. When prefrontal cortical circuits are impaired through exposure to childhood trauma, this disruption to top-down cognitive neural networks may cause bottom-up subcortical neural processes to predominate, where sensory stimuli from the external physical world and affective sensations from the internal world are paramount for driving these processes (Harricharan et al., 2021).

Panksepp and Biven (2012) state, "All sensory information is first processed subcortically." Given the design of the nervous system, sensations meet emotions and become affective states. Jaak Panksepp's historical work proposes the existence of primitive affective circuits that generate raw sensory experiences and relay them higher in the brain for conscious perception (Panksepp, 2004). Further, Harricharan and colleagues describe how emotionally salient stimuli activate the primitive affective circuits in the subcortical brainstem structures, including the periaqueductal gray of the brainstem

(Harricharan, et al., 2021). Arousal is generated and impacted by various stimuli, making it difficult to discern whether any dysregulating stimulus is sensory or emotional in origin. Inefficient sensory processing at the level of the brainstem, no matter the cause, can take a child outside of their "window of tolerance," where the brainstem influence will dominate the processing (Siegel, 2012). Appropriate sensory processing is a critical component of arousal regulation. PSI addresses this challenge by always providing sensory input in the context of an attuned therapeutic relationship.

In addition to the understanding of sensory influences on arousal states, extensive brain research has identified the impact of complex childhood trauma on the specific sensory regions of the brain. If trauma occurred during critical periods of brain development, the child's developing functions of language, self-regulation, and social engagement may be impaired (Perry, 2009; Teicher & Samson, 2016). Many researchers and authors have emphasized the relevance of sensory processing adaptations and the need for sensory intervention as a component of the treatment of childhood trauma and dissociation. Examples of sensory emphasis within treatment approaches are the Neurosequential Model (Perry, 2009), Sensorimotor Psychotherapy (Ogden & Fisher, 2015), Trust-Based Relational Intervention (Purvis et al., 2011), the Sensory Motor Arousal Regulation Therapy SMART Approach (Warner et al., 2013) and Somatic Experiencing (Levine, 2010), among others. Additionally, Dr. Bessel van der Kolk, MD, Ruth Lanius, MD, and Martin Teicher, MD, are examples of authors who have written, spoken, and researched the impacts of childhood trauma and dissociation, specifically on the sensory systems and their respective neurobiological underpinnings. More information on these neurobiological underpinings can be found below (Table 21.3).

These neurobiological sensory differences cited in the literature help explain how modifications to sensory systems and pathways convey aversive experience to consciousness and collectively offer a theoretical rationale for the use of PSI sensory-based interventions (Teicher & Samson, 2016).

Table 21.3 Neurobiological Research Highlighting Impact of Complex Childhood Trauma and Dissociation Upon the Sensory Systems

Author	Sensory-Related Brain Structures That Adapt in Response to Trauma	Functional Implications of Interrupted Neural Functions
McLaughlin et al. (2019) Note: These findings are observed in relationship to varying forms of abuse not observed in children exposed to deprivation and neglect	Reduced amygdala volume Reduced medial prefrontal cortex (mPFC) volume Increased hippocampal volume	The amygdala tags sensory input as threatening or safe, resulting in poor discernment of safety and danger The mPFC modulates, organizes, and inhibits multisensory input, leaving the survival aspect of the brain in hyper-alert states Potential altered memory encoding and retrieval
Teicher et al. (2022) Neurobiology of childhood trauma	Decreased volume of corpus callosum Attenuated development of the circuitry between the anterior cingulate, orbitofrontal cortex, dorsolateral prefrontal cortex, and the amygdala	Poor right-left hemisphere integration of information flow May result in hyper-vigilance and blunted responses to reward anticipation

(*Continued*)

Table 21.3 (Continued)

Author	Sensory-Related Brain Structures That Adapt in Response to Trauma	Functional Implications of Interrupted Neural Functions
Choi et al. (2009) Exposure to parental verbal abuse	Alterations in gray matter volume in left auditory cortex Reduced left arcuate fasciculus that interconnects Broca's and Wernicke's areas	Altered language processing Hyper-focus on vocal tone instead of language context Diminished lAF integrity is associated with lower verbal IQ and comprehension
Teicher et al. (2022) Children who witness domestic violence Sensitive period analysis found that observing interparental violence between ages 7 and 13, a peak period of active myelination, had the greatest impact (Teicher & Samson, 2016)	Reduced gray matter in the primary visual cortex Reduced integrity of the inferior longitudinal fasciculus that interconnects the limbic and visual pathways	Potential reduction in capacity for memory coding of emotional things that are "seen"
Teicher and Khan (2019) Sexual abuse before age 12	Reduced bilateral gray matter volume in the primary visual cortex and visual association cortex Specific gray matter loss is also observed in the left fusiform and middle occipital gyri	Deficits in visual memory and capacity for visualization Altered capacity for face recognition and processing of facial expressions
Teicher and Samson (2016) Exposure to emotional abuse	Thinning in the left anterior and posterior cingulate cortex and bilateral precuneus	Diminished processing in these brain regions involved in self-awareness and self-evaluation
Kearney and Lanius (2022) Drawing from research in the field of adult PTSD, subjects exhibiting the dissociative subtype demonstrate vestibular processing challenges	Limited vestibular nuclei connectivity with the temporoparietal junction within the parieto-insular vestibular cortex Limited vestibular nuclei connectivity with dorsolateral prefrontal cortex	May negatively impact the ability to understand one's own self-orientation in space and can lead to feelings of disembodiment Reduces an individual's capacity for multisensory integration and navigation through their external environments

Dynamic Maturational Model of Attachment and Adaptation

The field of OT places therapeutic use of self at the core of the profession. The unfolding science of Interpersonal Neurobiology has solidly validated the importance of therapeutic relationship as a credible tenant of OT practice. An understanding of attachment theory and its contribution to child development and behavior naturally became another layer of knowledge influencing the development of PSI.

The Dynamic Maturational Model of Attachment and Adaptation (DMM), developed by Dr. Patricia Crittenden, offers an integrated perspective of attachment adaptations in response to a child's perception of danger relative to what they experience with their caregivers. The DMM hypothesizes that as individuals mature across their lifespan, new and more complex mental and behavioral processes evolve in response to each person's context. According to this theory, attachment adaptations change and reorganize in relationship to the neurological, cognitive, and emotional maturation relative to a person's contextual factors and exposure to trauma, requiring an increasing need for the adoption of self-protective strategies. Exposure to danger differs by age as well as person, family, and cultural experience with persistent local dangers (Crittenden, 2005).

The following DMM concepts inform the PSI approach (adapted from Crittenden, 2005):

- The attachment system motivates an infant to seek proximity to parents (and other primary caregivers) to be soothed and protected from harm.
- Early interactions, especially with the mother, directly shape the architecture of the growing brain and have lasting effects across the lifespan (Rass, 2017).
- Contingent interactions between a sensitive attachment figure and the child allow the child to feel seen, soothed, and valued.
- Early experiences children have with their caregivers shape the long-term development of several mental processes across the lifespan. The DMM emphasizes the capacity for attachment adaptations to change as a person matures.
- Secure attachment is associated with the following: the ability to balance one's emotions, reduce fear, be attuned to others, have insight and self-understanding, have empathic understanding of others, and have well-developed moral reasoning.
- Insecure attachment can arise when caregiving behaviors are not attuned, are inconsistent, or are a source of terror for the child.
- Self-protective strategies will evolve as adaptations in response to the mindset and actions of the caregiver.
- Unreliable responses to a child create a sense of anxious attachment, filling the child with uncertainty and an underlying fear of loss of connection with their caregiver.
- In response to unpredictable caregiving, a child may adapt and display connection-seeking behaviors to solicit a reliable contingent response from their caregiver. Miscues of threat and aggression from the child are often pleas for comfort and connection.
- Unattuned or threatening caregiving may stimulate an avoidant adaptive response from the child.
- To preserve the relationship with the caregiver, the child may diminish the display of their feelings as an adaptation of avoidance or withdrawal.
- Experiences of chaos and complex relational trauma may require complex adaptations, such as alternating between anxious (connection-seeking) and avoidant self-protections.
- All forms of insecure attachment impact the development of arousal regulation.

The DMM model informs PSI to best support the clinician in appreciating how each child they treat adapts to their attachment experiences. These self-protective attachment strategies are displayed within the relational, sensory, and movement systems influencing daily function. It is fundamental that the PSI clinician understand the influence of attachment in the treatment of childhood complex trauma and dissociation as a part of assessment and treatment, and as part of their own self-awareness of the adaptive strategies they most currently employ.

Postural and Movement Frames of References That Inform the Psycho-Sensory Intervention Approach

Four distinct posture and movement frames of reference support the PSI approach: neurodevelopmental treatment, Dynamic Core for Kids, Bodynamic Somatic Psychotherapy, and polyvagal theory.

Neuro-Developmental Treatment

As a frame of reference, neuro-developmental treatment (NDT) is also fundamental to PSI. NDT is described as a dynamic, hands-on treatment approach guiding OTs globally in their assessment and intervention of children with neurological deficits who experience posture and movement impairments (Barthel, 2020). Through an understanding of typical posture and movement development, NDT focuses on helping a child shift their compensatory movement strategies to achieve the most energy-efficient motor performance within functional occupations that are meaningful to them. These functional occupations include attachment, social engagement, play, and all other daily tasks that children like and need to do.

NDT draws on kinesiological and biomechanical concepts as a theoretical foundation for analysis and treatment. Important concepts are planes of movement, alignment of the body, range of movement, base of support, muscle strength, postural control, weight shifts, and mobility. The NDT frame of reference is based on "systems theory" (Barthel, 2020)—knowing and appreciating that the movement system is influenced by self-regulation and emotional arousal, and compromised by experiences of complex trauma. Readiness to move (postural activation) is highly influenced by the autonomic nervous system. The sympathetic nervous system (fight/flight) readies the muscles to move while the freeze system deactivates the motor system toward collapse. Felt safety, comfort, and a "just-right challenge" (Ayres, 1972) are needed to support the learning of new posture and movement strategies, and the learning of new posture and movement strategies supports the feelings of safety, comfort, and functional participation.

A key kinesiological concept of NDT to the PSI approach is the importance of postural alignment. When the joints of the body are aligned, muscles have greater biomechanical capacity to work. Postural alignment in the trunk is especially critical, as all limb movements rely on stable trunk control. The rib cage is stacked on top of the pelvis and the head is aligned on top of the trunk. These observable markers not only create the potential for active motor systems but also support regulatory functions within the body. Within the PSI approach, clinicians utilize kinesiological and biomechanical knowledge from NDT to track the postural alignment of their clients and offer individualized interventions of support. A photo example of an adult seated in postural alignment with a roll for pelvic support can be observed in Figure 21.2.

Dynamic Core for Kids

Dynamic Core for Kids (developed by Mannell & Wiebe, 2010) has contributed significantly to the understanding of core muscle activation for postural control and regulation. Their work describes how the inner-core muscles are a group of neurobiologically linked synergies, where when one muscle fires, the others are pulled into play. These inner-core muscles include the respiratory diaphragm, pelvic floor musculature, transverse abdominis, and multifidus (Hodges & Gandevia, 2000). The diaphragm initiates the coactivation of this sequence. The diaphragm must be aligned on top of the pelvis for optimum access to this inner-core synergy of centered postural stability. With every draw of inward breath, the diaphragm flattens and lowers, expanding the rib cage. The descent of the diaphragm creates pressure on the organs below the diaphragm, which are rich in interoceptive feedback, relaying information of internal affective states to the brain. With a prolonged exhale, the diaphragm returns to neutral and allows the vagal brake to ease any sympathetic arousal in the system.

The diaphragm, having both a breathing and a postural function, places breath and autonomic regulation at risk when posture is not aligned and balanced. When the diaphragm remains high in the chest with the rib cage tipped up and the spine extended, a sympathetic arousal bias within the autonomic nervous system is created. When the position of the rib cage is tipped downward over the

Psycho-Sensory Intervention®: An Occupational Therapy Approach

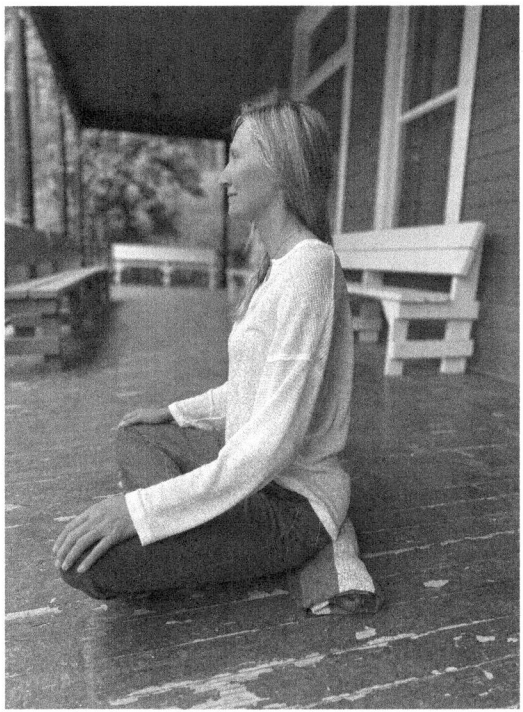

Figure 21.2 Postural Alignment.

pelvis with the diaphragm compressed and collapsed, autonomic functions related to breath are also compromised. Stacking the rib cage over the pelvis is key to optimum arousal capacity. The body must have a postural container in which to support and manage our varying affective states. Ultimately, Dynamic Core for Kids is a frame of reference informing PSI and practitioners of many other approaches that posture and alignment matter a great deal for regulation as well as function.

Bodynamic Somatic Psychotherapy

Bodynamic Somatic Psychotherapy is a developmental theory that brings together motor development with social-emotional development. Developed toward the end of the 1960s by Lisbeth Marcher in Denmark (bodynamic.com), this frame of reference was created to understand psychological defense mechanisms and their attachment to specific muscles. Through muscle testing that evaluated the response of muscles through a manual pull in the direction of the muscle's fibers, Marcher was able to determine the degree of tenseness and elasticity of a muscle response paired with the timing and sequencing of the development of these muscles during early childhood. Through extensive case study research, Marcher created a graphic chart called the Bodymap to determine a person's somatic resources and weaknesses. Through years of data gathering, Marcher and her team observed the elicitation of psychological themes that were activated in a client each time a specific muscle was physically stimulated during treatment. These themes are entitled Ego Functions. As with NDT, the understanding of typical motor development was foundational to the creation of the Bodymap. Certain muscles were ascribed to particular developmental stages (rolling over, sitting, crawling, pulling to stand, standing, walking, etc.) and helped clinicians to determine when ruptures in attachment may have occurred in each client. This understanding of muscles related to social-emotional development was found to align with the close analysis of typical development essential to NDT theory. Although not formally researched in Barthel's clients, Bodynamic teachings shed light on what was clinically observable to Barthel in her clients with complex childhood trauma and dissociation. Bodynamic training contributed to Barthel's fine tuning of movement observations in relation to attachment patterns and developmental trauma and serves to inform practitioners of how trauma can live in the body, from the earliest of ages.

Polyvagal Theory

Nonverbal communication is deeply connected to states of mind and embodied emotions. Dr. Stephen Porges's Polyvagal Theory illuminates the impact of safety on the social engagement system for connection (please see Chapter 10). The expression of emotions through the eyes and upper face, the ability for the middle ear to attune to the human voice, the vocal folds to produce melodic sound in speech, and the muscles of the head and neck that contribute to social gesturing are tied to an evolved branch of the parasympathetic system (ventral vagal branch), indicating that muscles are aligned with states of arousal. When a sense of safety is felt, these social motor systems are unveiled and enlivened to enhance the quality of attunement and relationship (Porges, 2011). Ultimately, the polyvagal theory describes and reinforces the physiological need for safety and regulation through relationship, which is an embodied experience and a key tenet of PSI.

Complex Childhood Trauma Shows Up in the Posture and Movement Systems

Posture has a powerful influence on emotions and well-being. The sensory systems interface closely with the posture and movement systems. Challenges arising within the sensory systems from childhood trauma will have "fall-out" in the movement system. As previously stated, activation of the motor system and muscle tone relies on the accurate processing of vestibular input (Mori et al., 2001). In childhood complex trauma and dissociation, it is possible that "alterations in vestibular processing, dissociation and disembodiment will be observable within the body and how it moves" (Kearney & Lanius, 2022).

The sympathetic nervous system has direct connectivity with musculature that increases muscle tension necessary for fight and flight. When survival-oriented actions are completed, vestibular and somatosensory systems send sensory feedback to the brain signaling the completion of the fight or flight response from the body as being successful and finished. When a sympathetically activated state in response to a threat is thwarted or incomplete, the body in response to trauma may reflexively enter into an exaggerated reactive motor pattern or defensive state such as tonic immobility or collapse. These exaggerated responses may reoccur in the presence of everyday stressors or trauma triggers (Kearney & Lanius, 2022). Dr. Wilfred Barlow, M.D., an Alexander bodywork practitioner, described fixed postures, such as a chronically slumped spines or a stiff and extended spines as positions that restrict emotions and behavioral adaptive responses, limiting the access to flexible emotional adaptations (Barlow, 1973). Tonic immobility is observed in adults with PTSD in studies evaluating memory recall, suggesting that traumatic memories remain connected to subconscious postural response (de Kleine et al., 2018). As one example of trauma living in the body, hypo-arousal or collapsed muscle tone can occur during emotional shutdown, as "drastically reduced arousal and tonicity diminish the conscious experience of physical injury and psychic distress during inevitable or prolonged attack, sometimes to the point of an out-of-body experience or complete loss of consciousness" (Kearney & Lanius, 2022, p. 13).

When a child has adopted a taut, immobilized posture of self-protection through continuous sympathetic nervous system activation, the extensor muscles of the trunk can become biased in their capacity for recruitment, overriding the possibility of balanced coactivation in the trunk's antigravity flexors. This happens when a child unconsciously taps into their primitive motor withdrawal patterns. This preprogrammed reflex arises early in fetal development, seen as the fetus arching (extending) their spine away from perceived threat. This primitive movement pattern, known as the Moro reflex, is accessible across the lifespan and will continue to rapidly engage in times of threat. During the first phase of the Moro reflex (avoidant withdrawal phase), the baby's spine extends, arms and legs move away from the body (abduction), respiration rate is fast and shallow, diaphragm is elevated, and eyes are wide and open; this is a state of immobilization. Hands are open wide as if to say, "Go away." The withdrawal phase is for avoidance of a stimulus. In a newborn, the stimuli that activate the Moro reflex are typically sensory in nature, such as sounds, movement through space, bright lights, or anything that is startling to any aspect of their sensory system (Figure 21.3).

Although this movement pattern is part of typical development in a newborn without the presence of more evolved movements for protection, the Moro reflex can become dominant within a person's motor system when chronic, repetitive, and pervasive threat is experienced. In an older child, the first phase of the Moro reflex can also emerge in response to emotional experiences and is no longer strictly sensory stimulus bound. Aspects of the first phase of the moro reflex can be observed in the postural system when the autonomic state is predominantly in a freeze response. When a child presents with a remnant postural presentation of the Moro's first phase, PSI interventions may support the child in shifting toward a more regulated state by altering the tonic activation of the motor system (into flexion).

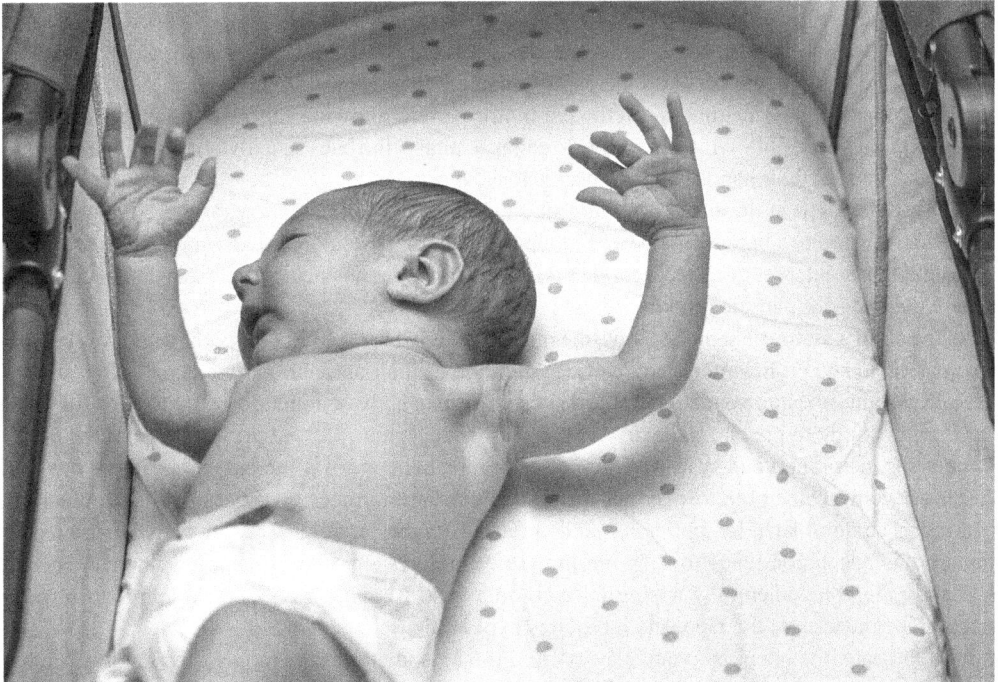

Figure 21.3 The First (Avoidant Withdrawal) Phase of the Moro Reflex.

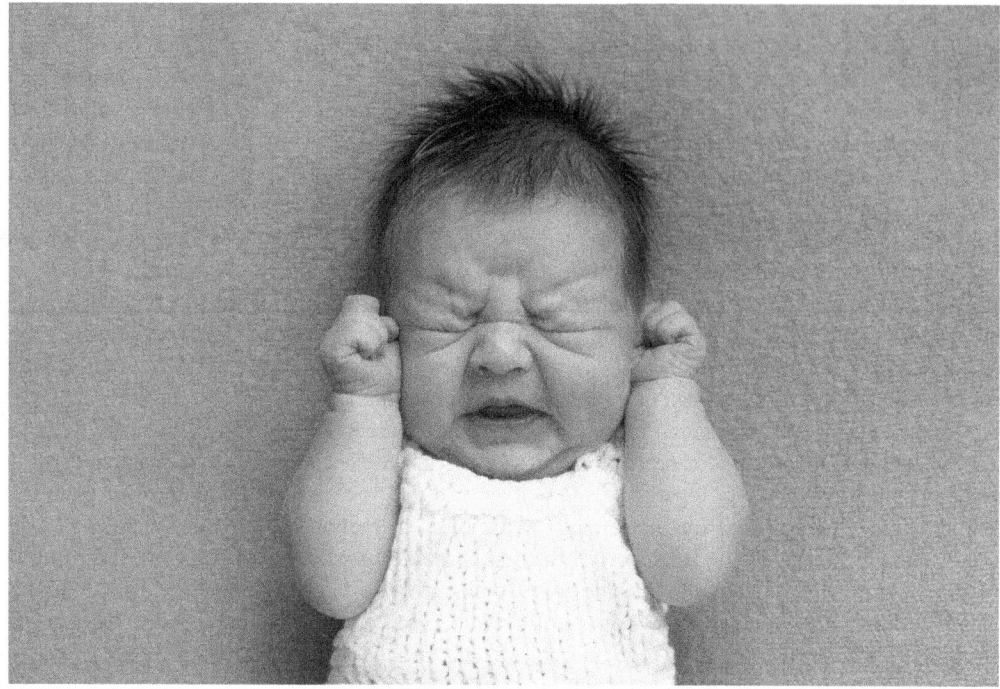

Figure 21.4 Recovery Collapse Phase of Moro Reflex in Infancy.

The second phase of the Moro reflex is called the recovery collapse phase, when the spine and limbs are pulled into a protective, curled-up position of flexion. Flexion through activation of the proprioceptive system connects into the parasympathetic pathways of recovery and restoration. The recovery collapse phase begins as a reflexive motor pattern allowing the infant to cling to the caregiver for protection. Following the recovery collapse phase, the baby usually cries in distress, closes their eyes, and fists their hands (Masgutova, 2016) (Figure 21.4).

The muscles used in these early movement patterns form the foundation for more mature movements that develop in a baby's first year. To help the postural system mobilize from collapse to active engagement, PSI interventions incorporate upright and movements that recruit extension patterns that prepare the body for participation in life.

As the child's motor system develops, the muscles needed for the fight-or-flight responses become more available and proficient, reflecting the maturation of their autonomic states.

Fight responses require a stable postural system with an activated inner core for the arms to separate from the body to punch. The extensor muscles of the spine receive innervation from the nerves of the sympathetic nervous system. Thus, when sympathetic arousal increases repeatedly the back muscles become vulnerable to over-activation and over-recruitment (Mori et al., 2001). When the fight response dominated by aggression and defense becomes a child's predominant self-protective strategy this adaptation tends to show up in the postural system. Over time, the spine can become rigid and inflexible, potentially arising from chronic mistrust and hypervigilance. Threat is also detected in the muscles of the face, and it requires hypertonicity to generate this signal.

In flight state, the intent is to move away from threat; sometimes the movements involve running away while being chased, and sometimes the movements are observed in the trunk and neck alone as the body leans away from a stimulus it perceives as threatening.

Collapsed posture can readily be observed in the bodies of children who have experienced complex trauma. Deactivation of the postural system can occur when conditions of prolonged disembodiment occur. The dorsal vagal branch of the parasympathetic vagus nerve is a pathway of "shutdown." A dorsal vagal state may be accessed for survival under the conditions of life and death or become a force of protective influence during childhood maltreatment, hopelessness, or shame (Porges, 2011). The inner-core musculature, specifically the diaphragm, which is innervated by the vagus nerve, may drop in tone, resulting in a slumped posture and curved spine (Bordoni & Zanier, 2013). Collapse in sitting involves a deactivated pelvic floor, downward-tipped diaphragm, posterior pelvic tilt, and a forward head position. In standing, the child places their weight on their heels, the knees are hyperextended, hanging on the front of the hip joints with the belly protruding, the spine has a marked curve starting from the shoulder blades, and the thorax collapses near the upper part of the breastbone. The heaviness of the muscles in collapse makes it difficult to reach out in approach toward another person or to participate in an activity. Dorsal vagal dominance can also overshadow access to the muscles of the face necessary for social connection, giving the face a flat affective appearance, as is frequently observed in depression and that of a trance-like state, often perceived as zoned out or spaced out. This low-arousal, immobilized movement system offers progressively less and less somatosensory input to the brain across time, further disconnecting the child from the interoceptive experiences necessary for a healthy sense of self.

Psycho-Sensory Intervention Assessment and Treatment in Practice

From the very first moment of contact with a child, each interaction is a moment of both assessment and treatment. Co-regulatory experiences occur in the first seconds of connection between a therapist and child. A present, attuned, and connected clinician can create the potential for felt safety, setting the stage for therapeutic work. Relationship is the powerhouse of complex trauma and dissociation work and is the place upon which all other "Spokes on the Wheel" of PSI scaffold. The clinician continuously tracks the nonverbal cues in the body, breath, posture, and movement system as it relates to the developmental age and stage of the child. As different sensory-motor interventions are introduced, the clinician also continuously monitors the child's arousal and regulation and shifting states.

The clinician also notices self-protective attachment adaptations that begin to emerge within the therapeutic relationship as themes. This gathered information guides the clinician in their selection of the most appropriate style of attuned, authentic connection that optimally aligns with the child's attachment style. Sensory-motor-relational strategies are embedded within play or expressive art activity, further increasing the child's experience of safety while inviting potential access to previously unconscious, implicit memories, states of being, and influences of their trauma history. Psychotherapeutic dialoguing, narrating, and meaning making within the child's appropriate zone of proximal development are integrated with the clinician's authentic self as they help the child increasingly connect and tolerate uncomfortable states. In the words of this author's NDT mentor, Regi Boehme, OTR: "When it works, it's treatment, and when it doesn't, it's assessment." When what we do as intervention helps achieve a goal, it is treatment, and when it does not achieve a projected outcome, the intervention becomes further assessment. Clinical reasoning informs the basis for selection of all intervention.

Psycho-Sensory Intervention: Putting Theory into Practice

Helping is to get to the symptoms, not the story.

—*Ditte Marcher (2020)*

Integrating the varying components of PSI weaves the fabric of the individualized treatment for children with histories of complex trauma and dissociation. Within the frame of reference, there is a relative hierarchy of priorities that support the movement of the child's nervous system through safety toward regulation, from regulation toward boundaries, and from self-identity toward agency through exploration and expansion of the self within relationships and the world.

Creating Safety in the First Session

Felt safety begins with relationships. Revisiting the Spokes on the Wheel model, attunement and co-regulation with a mindful clinician are the points of entry to every interaction between therapist and child. By tapping into their own body senses, the clinician interoceptively perceives the child's state of arousal as a form of resonance (Dion, 2017). Hopenwasser describes these connected experiences with our clients as "dissociative attunement." These profound rhythmic encounters that occur within therapy are described as "systematically self-emergent moments in which multiple self-states are shared by means other than projection." (Hopenwasser, 2008 p. 349). Through this attunement with the clinician, the child feels "felt" by the clinician, setting the stage for further connection. Many children who have experienced complex trauma and exhibit dissociation may not experience safety as "safe." Through attunement, the clinician may notice cues from the child that relational connection is uncomfortable. Tracking this observation, the clinician has an opportunity to adjust their style of engagement, changing the amount of observable animation in their affect, offering more distance in their physical proximity, speaking less, or lowering their tone of voice and shifting into activity more quickly. Within PSI, this is called the "sideways approach," where the clinician comes alongside the child and decreases the intensity of relational cues to provide more space for trust to develop.

The chronological age and developmental capacity of the child will also factor into the way the clinician creates felt safety. When working with a baby, relationship safety is directed predominantly toward the caregiver, as dyadic work will become the focus of PSI for infants with developmental trauma. As the child ages, the play and language alter to fit the child's zone of proximal development. With older children, psychoeducation expands to support the child's understanding of how therapeutic interventions can be supportive. When working with children who have multiple self-states, attention to differing ages and stages of development held by different states of being is crucial.

Upon meeting for the first time, an explanation of what will happen when the child, clinician, and likely parent are together is a critical aspect of establishing felt safety. If treating the child in a clinical space, a tour of the therapy facility, toys, and equipment is a part of setting the stage for familiarity.

The clinician observes the child's posture and movement system to notice indications of tension or deactivation. Is the child holding their breath? Are their shoulders elevated? Are their eyes wide with vigilance, and/or rapidly scanning the environment? Do they orient to every stimulus in the environment with an energy of startle in their body? What do you notice happen just before shifts and changes in tension, activation, and deactivation? These cues are perceived by the clinician as arousal dysregulation. By tracking a client's changing non-verbal cues, the clinician is able to determine whether the client is moving toward further dysregulation or toward a more integrated state.

The clinical reasoning of the clinician shifts in priority throughout the session as the child's presentation changes. The clinician notices and narrates their impressions of the changes in sensory processing and motor control within the activities to bring the child's conscious awareness in alignment with the functional changes. When appropriate, the clinician may emphasize the psychotherapeutic aspect of the content of the play or interaction while simultaneously adding or removing sensory-motor supports. If the child happens to express feelings verbally or nonverbally, the toys or sensory play equipment may serve as symbols that portray a different meaning within the psyche of the child. Displays of anxiety, aggression, or dissociation are closely monitored with immediate support to acquire self-soothing, conflict resolution, visualization, and self-understanding. Interventions are provided at the developmental level of the individual child and the different states within, and as therapy proceeds, the child's story often emerges and is met with attuned co-regulation and sensory-motor resourcing.

Sensory-Based Interventions

When noticing hyper-aroused states within the therapeutic process, the clinician may begin to highlight sensory-based interventions. The choice of intervention depends on the degree to which a child displays dysregulation.

Selection of Sensory-Based Options and Clinical Reasoning for Usage

Various sensory-based options, how to use them, and their application to varying chronological ages will be presented in the following tables.

The first priority within the therapeutic sequence is to support the child in experiencing felt safety in their body. The sensory-motor strategies most likely to offer felt safety emulate the sensory womb-like experience. Developmental trauma can occur at multiple times (complex trauma) throughout a child's developing life, and traumas at different stages will present differently. For some children, sensory experiences perceived while in utero will be their only coded implicit memory of safety. For other children, felt safety was never experienced, even before birth. When a sensory-motor intervention elicits perturbations in regulation or exacerbates dysregulation, this is not necessarily a signal to discontinue the intervention. This may signify that the sensory stimulus has tapped into an implicit memory activation connected to developmental trauma and attachment. With discernment, the clinician who knows they are able to regulate their own fear in the face of the child's dysregulation will be able to meet this shift in state with energetic and relational containment, thereby allowing the child to feel the increasing intensity and discomfort relatively safely.

All these sensory-based experiences are carefully titrated in their delivery and co-regulated within the therapeutic relationship. Any access to memory may prematurely break down dissociative barriers and result in flooding of the nervous system and an overwhelmed state. When clients are exposed to memory prematurely, dysregulation, attempts to avoid memory, dissociative switching, or shutdown are often triggered. Titration of sensory stimulation may be required to allow the child to learn tolerance of overwhelming sensations.

Examples of sensory-based interventions for felt-safety and regulation include, but are not limited to: rhythmic sounds, rhythmic movements, enclosed spaces, beanbag chairs, motherese, Safe and Sound Protocol™, vestibular movement experiences in different directions and speeds, moving through space independently, rolling inside a therapy barrel, hanging upside down, deep pressure touch, oral motor supports of sucking, swallowing, and breathing. Refer to Table 21.4 for more contextual information.

PSI directed toward felt safety contributes to the learning of self-regulation. Self-regulation, however, requires the experience of dysregulation in order to return to a restored place of physiological balance. Sensations support regulation, but the motor system further contributes to the capacity to regulate actively. When attending to posture and movement patterns with the intention to support regulation within the body, it is important to remember that the child's postural adaptations are self-protective in nature. Altering a postural adaptation can be frightening to parts of the self that developed that adaptation in protection. The following table provides posture and movement-based interventions in support of regulation. Activities are hierarchically provided in the order of typical motor development in early childhood. It is not necessary to offer these activities in progressive order.

Table 21.4 Sensory-Based Interventions for Felt Safety and Regulation

Sensory-Based Interventions For Felt Safety and Regulation	Rationale for the Intervention	Situations When the Intervention May be Useful	Intervention Variations Dependent Upon Age
Rhythmical Sound: • Clapping rhythms • Metronome • Drumming • Humming	The first sensation to be perceived by a developing fetus is the mother's heart rate. As the fetus is situated in an aqueous environment (the embryonic fluid), the sounds of mother's heart rate is physically perceived as waves against their body as muted sound.	When movements or states of arousal appear disorganized or out of sync When breathing is shallow, held, and/or dysrhythmic To increase the rhythm of serve and return in dyadic interactions to create increased security in attachment When the child's eyes appear hyper-vigilant, lost, and/or empty When the child presents as shut down and tuned out (collapse body posture image) Difficulties with oral motor rhythms in chewing Difficulties with falling asleep and staying asleep (circadian rhythms)	*Babies:* Rhythmical sounds provided in the ambient space while feeding, being held, during periods of dysregulation, or during dyadic interaction with caregivers *Toddlers and Preschoolers:* Rhythmical sounds provided in the ambient space during play, movement through space, periods of dysregulation or dyadic interaction with caregiver. Child is invited to move in rhythm to sound (e.g., clap-along songs) *School-Aged:* Rhythmic sounds may be provided in either the ambient space or through headphones (e.g., metronome) Offered proactively to support regulation, while attempting to focus on learning, to increase motor coordination and to enhance rhythmical interactions in relationships
Rhythmical Movements: • Rocking side to side • Rocking back and forth • Bouncing up and down on trampoline or therapy ball • Tapping on the body rhythmically	In the first trimester, fetuses are observed to move their bodies in rhythmical patterns of flexion and extension These are the most primitive movement patterns to access Rhythm is calibrated predominantly by the cerebellum and creates temporal and spatial order to a stimulus. This aids in creating felt safety and predictability	When the child initiates rhythmical movements for self-soothing (e.g., rocking body, shaking leg up and down, flapping hands, etc.). When the child displays erratic breathing When the child is moving rapidly through space without purpose (e.g., pacing the room) When the child is displaying emotional dysregulation (i.e., crying, shouting, punching, biting, hitting, kicking, anxiety)	*Babies:* Bouncing and rocking movements while held in arms *Toddlers and Preschoolers:* Movements can be offered during moments of observed dysregulation and/or proactively to prolong regulated states of arousal across time. Therapists typically support the child on the equipment physically Rhythmical rolling of a ball back and forth between the child and the caregiver can support the establishment of rhythms seen in secure attachment *School-Aged:* Rhythmical movements may be embedded into activities for learning or during play. At this age, the child may be taught how to use rhythmical movements as self-soothing adaptations independently

Enclosed Spaces: • Lycra swing • Peapod • Beanbag cushion • Hooded swivel chair with cover for hiding	The intrauterine space is an enclosed space providing full body proprioceptive input As the fetus stretches and moves within the uterus, they are pushing their muscles and joints against resistance, which is called "heavy work." This level of sensory processing contributes to the development of a sense of self distinct from others	When the child presents with an over-activation of extension within their spine (e.g., rib cage tipped upward). When the child has trouble being "still" in their body and emotions When the child is shut down and tuned out When the child is displaying emotional dysregulation (e.g., crying, shouting, punching, biting, hitting, kicking, anxiety)	*Babies:* Held in arms in flexion *Toddlers and Preschoolers:* Invite the child to climb into an enclosed space to either experience stillness or move their body against the boundaries of the equipment. The clinician supports the child's body with their hands and/or verbal cues This equipment is blended with a play scheme that is typically imaginative or goal directed The clinician may not be able to see the face and body of the child while they are enclosed and as such may need to attune to any sounds, dialogue, or movements requiring co-regulation, narration, or meaning making *School-Aged:* Enclosed spaces can be used for self-regulatory needs, times for learning, and focused attention or play Psychotherapeutic dialogue happens frequently while children are in enclosed spaces
Mother's Voice: • Safe and Sound Protocol (SSP) • Singing • Motherese	Mother's voice is the first sound perceived by the developing baby Taps into the ventral vagal system of regulation through processing in the middle ear	When a child appears anxious, dissociated, and/or aggressive	*Babies:* Prosodic singing SSP is not typically provided to babies. However, the use of SSP for the caregiver may be used in dyadic work with the mother listening while co-regulating the baby *Toddlers and Preschoolers:* Might begin with SSP's "Connect" (unfiltered music) SSP and singing are embedded within other activities that are in the context of a co-regulated relationship *School-Aged:* May need to begin with SSP's "Connect" to develop comfort, and then move to the use of SSP's "Core" (filtered music) to support the child's nervous system in attenuating to mother's voice to access felt safety

(Continued)

Table 21.4 (Continued)

Sensory-Based Interventions For Felt Safety and Regulation	Rationale for the Intervention	Situations When the Intervention May be Useful	Intervention Variations Dependent Upon Age
Vestibular Experiences in Variable Directions and Speeds: • Self-rocking • Rocking chair • Office chair (for rotation) • Swings (i.e., platform, tire, bolster, hammock, Lycra, etc.) • Rolling (on the ground, in a sheet, in a barrel, etc.) • Dancing and twirling • Roughhousing • Hanging upside down • Scooter boards	The intrauterine space is aqueous and offers movement experiences in 360 degrees, thus stimulating all aspects of the vestibular apparatus Developmental trauma has been demonstrated to interrupt vestibular processing, thus diminishing the intrinsic use of movement as an accessible resource for regulation When rhythm is added to a movement experience, the stimulus becomes grounded in time and space Important Note: The use of vestibular input requires careful monitoring, as it can easily become over-arousing or move a child toward shutdown	When the child is repeatedly drawn toward a particular position (e.g., hanging upside down or twirling) and demonstrates a sense of increased presence during or following engagement in sensory experience When the child is unable to find rhythm within the body (e.g., cannot coordinate rhythmic movements) Has difficulty with interpersonal rhythms (e.g., challenges with serve and return) Difficulties holding their body up against gravity Body parts are constantly in motion (e.g., shaking leg up and down) Difficulties with eating and sleeping	*Babies:* Rocking, rolling on the floor, crawling *Toddlers and Preschoolers:* Vestibular experiences are always provided within a play scheme and a psychotherapeutic relationship Movements may elicit emotions that will need to be met and held within a co-regulated relationship The speed, direction, and intensity of the vestibular input may need parameters and modification based on the attuned tracking of the child's shifts in arousal state The use of therapeutic sensory equipment may enhance the experience for the child toward increased integration *School-Aged Child:* Same parameters as above Important Note: As the child increases in their capacity for self-reflection, movement may elicit implicit memory and require coherent meaning making and psycho-education from the clinician

Deep-Pressure Touch • Hug-like feeling • Wrapped in Lycra • Weighted blanket	The compression sense of the uterine space provides deep pressure to the mechanoreceptors of the skin, which contribute to felt safety Deep-pressure touch is known to increase serotonin and oxytocin production (Field, 2014).	When dysregulation in arousal state is observed When the child is observed to lean on people and objects constantly When the child repeatedly curls their body into a flexed position Seeks physical contact frequently Difficulties with sleep	*Babies:* Swaddling and held in flexion *Toddlers and Preschoolers:* Supervised use of deep-pressure tools such as weighted blankets or sheets of Lycra. Use of these tools may be preventative of dysregulated states or incorporated during a state of dysregulation. *School-Aged:* Same protocol as above. Weighted supports may be used during activities or interactions that are emotionally evocative to support felt safety in the body Use of weighted blankets: "Recommended weights for a weighted blanket can vary between 5% and 12% of their body weight, with most people preferring a weighted blanket that weighs approximately 10% of their body weight. Regardless of its weight, a proper blanket should allow for comfort and movement" (Noyed, 2023)
Oral Motor Soothing: • Sucking and chewing • Chewelry • Gum • Twisted straws • Popsicles • Lollipops • Fruit leather	From nine weeks onward, fetuses suck their thumb and move their jaw (Nowlan, 2015)	Difficulties with eating and feeding Dysregulated states of anxiety, depression, aggression and/or dissociation. The child engages in frequent mouthing Uses food for self-regulation	*Babies:* Feeding and pacifier *Toddlers and Preschoolers:* Oral motor supports or nutritious food. Can be introduced preemptively or made available in response to a moment of dysregulation *School-Aged:* Sucking a candy, or a liquid that provides resistance when sucking through a twisted straw during stressful activities or conversations

The Handbook of Complex Trauma and Dissociation in Children

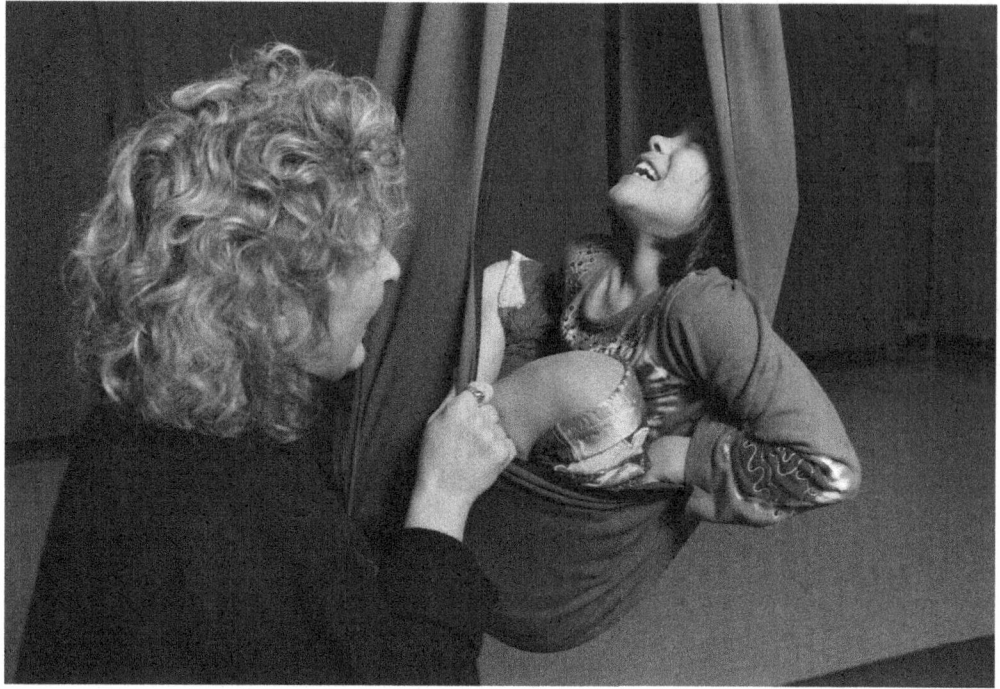

Figure 21.5 Child in Supine Position Pushing Feet into Lycra Swing to Activate the Deep Inner-Core Muscles.

Observations of the child's postural adaptations will offer theoretical hypotheses about the possible developmental timeline on which traumas may have occurred within the child's life.

Using the Posture and Movement System as Intervention

Based on the research relating to posture, movement, and felt safety, the clinician is provided with yet another "spoke on the wheel" to support trauma and dissociation.

Examples of posture and movement interventions for felt safety and regulation include, but are not limited to: positioning the body in a flexed position (Figure 21.5), practicing umbrella breathing (Figure 21.6), activating the pelvic floor muscles, sitting with the rib cage aligned over the pelvis, blowing bubbles through a straw, standing tall with arms raised overhead, and lying in a prone position on a scooter-board or therapy ball while lifting the upper body and limbs against gravity. Refer to Table 21.5 for more contextual information.

Boundaries

Many children with complex trauma and dissociation feel disembodied and require titrated sensory motor supports to feel connected to themselves safely. As body boundaries are developed, therapy expands into spatial boundaries and boundaries between self and others.

Examples of sensory, motor and activity-based interventions that support the development of boundaries include, but are not limited to: deep pressure touch, bone conduction headphones, "Launch and Land" activities (Sheila Frick, 2021), spatial boundaries with hoola-hoops, moving

Psycho-Sensory Intervention®: An Occupational Therapy Approach

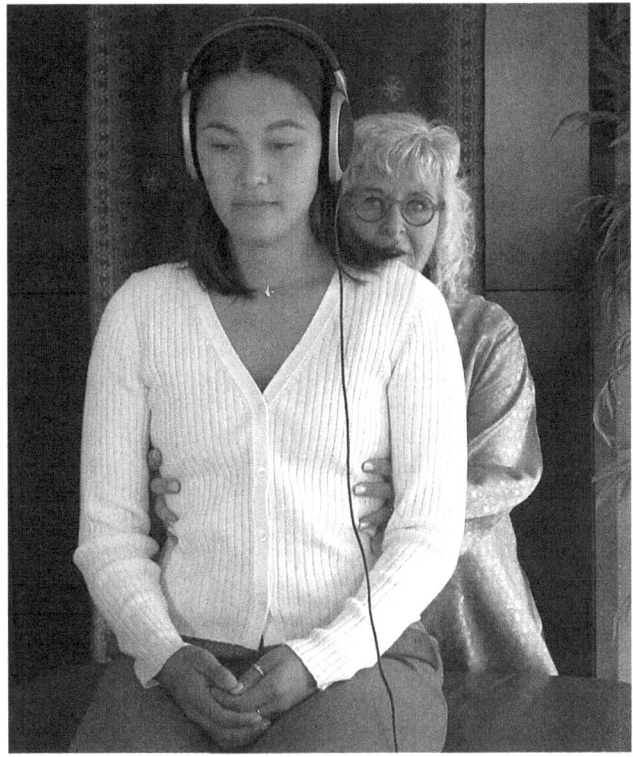

Figure 21.6 Clinician Guiding Client in Umbrella Breathing.

Table 21.5 Posture and Movement Interventions for Felt Safety and Regulation

Posture and Movement Interventions for Felt Safety and Regulation	Description of the Intervention	When Intervention May be Useful	Intervention Variations Dependent on Age
Support into Flexed Posture for Interoception and Proprioception: • Lycra swing • Beanbag chair	Wrapped tightly into a Lycra swing in a flexed position This position emulates physiological flexion, which is the postural control that develops in utero The flexor muscles provide the majority of the body's proprioception The curled position increases interoception due to intra-abdominal pressure	When the child's spine presents as stiff and rigid When they have trouble turning their head separately from their body When they behaviorally demonstrate persistent states of fight/flight	*Babies*: Positioned in caregiver's lap on their back, curled, facing caregiver for engagement *Toddlers and Preschoolers*: Equipment is provided to place the child's body into flexion within a play scheme *School-Aged*: The child may use equipment in the clinic, at home, or at school to support their body in a secure feeling of flexion when required to perform different tasks or engage in emotionally evocative conversations

(*Continued*)

415

Table 21.5 (Continued)

Posture and Movement Interventions for Felt Safety and Regulation	Description of the Intervention	When Intervention May be Useful	Intervention Variations Dependent on Age
Inner Core Activation: • Sitting in alignment • Umbrella breathing • Ball between knees • Yoga wedge • (Mannell & Wiebe, 2009) • Facilitation with handling • Blast Off activity (Frick, 2022)	Sitting in alignment requires that the pelvis be aligned underneath the rib cage. Sitting on a yoga wedge (as an example) will tip the pelvis forward toward neutral for optimum muscle recruitment. When appropriate, placing a small ball to hold between the knees can assist in the activation of the pelvic floor muscles. This aspect of motor intervention is the cornerstone of alignment for arousal management Umbrella breathing is a technique coined by Julie Wiebe, PT, to describe the expansion of the rib cage laterally as the child takes and in breath. The therapist places their hands on the side of the ribs. When the child breathes in, the therapist expands their hands like a balloon, inviting the child the find the therapist's hands with their ribs. During the exhale, the clinician provides compression inward and downward toward the base of support to help create the feeling of a connected inner core Blast Off activity has the child wrapped within a Lycra swing for compression in a flexed position. The child pushes into the Lycra with their toes, activating the deep inner core muscles	When the child's body is either collapsed in posture or hyper-extended	*Babies*: Alignment is just beginning to develop in babies; thus, exposure to overall movement development is necessary (sitting, crawling) *Toddlers and Preschoolers*: Introduce equipment during play activities. Umbrella breathing is typically introduced at this time to support with the access to inner core stability *School-Aged*: The child may begin to use these movement supports independently when they perceive dysregulation within themselves
Blowing with Prolonged Exhale: • Blowing bubbles	Have the child engage in blowing activities positioned in aligned sitting	When the child presents as dysregulated in their state of arousal	*Babies*: N/A *Toddlers, Preschoolers, and School-Aged*: Introduce blowing games in the context of co-regulated play

(*Continued*)

Table 21.5 (Continued)

Posture and Movement Interventions for Felt Safety and Regulation	Description of the Intervention	When Intervention May be Useful	Intervention Variations Dependent on Age
• Blowing against resistance • Blowing games		When they present as collapsed or hyper-extended in their postural systems	
Activation of Upright Posture and Extension Through the Spine: • Standing tall • Sitting on a yoga wedge • Prone on scooter board • Prone on platform swing • Prone on therapy ball • Yoga	Play activities such as "superheroes," standing tall Ride the scooter board while lying on the tummy to promote the extended position. Can ride the scooter board down a ramp to increase the impetus to lift the body into extension against gravity Lie on the tummy on a platform swing that moves in 360 degrees and swings through space. This activity offers intentional vestibular input to support activation of the extensor muscles of the back. This activity can be replicated on a therapy ball	When the child presents as collapsed in their body	*Babies*: Introduce tummy time to support in the development of the extensor postural muscles. Educate caregivers in this activity if appropriate *Toddlers and Preschoolers*: Introduce the equipment and activities in play schemes that are within the child's zone of proximal development *School-Aged*: Introduce activities and equipment in the clinic, home, and school environments as appropriate

the body against resistance in lycra (Figure 21.7), and wall push-ups. Refer to Table 21.6 for more contextual information.

Examples of activities that support the expansion of regulation, exploration and interpersonal collaboration include, but are not limited to: climbing on a climbing wall, pillow fights, tug-of-war, rock-climbing with a belayer, and team sports. Refer to Table 21.7 for more contextual information.

The Story of Trevor[2]

Trevor was a bright-eyed four-year-old living in foster care following the loss of his biological mom and the incarceration of his biological dad. Prior to apprehension, Trevor witnessed his dad murder his mom with a knife during a domestic violence incident. Trevor came to live with his current foster family immediately following the violent incident in his home.

At the time of the referral, Trevor was sleeping only about three to four hours a night. He made constant pleas to sleep with his foster parents. Night terrors were frequent. He was described as a picky eater and toileting was challenging for him. Small things seemed to bother Trevor, and he would have meltdowns with intense screaming for up to an hour. He had a strong dislike of the family cat and would frequently attempt to hurt the cat by pulling its tail.

The Handbook of Complex Trauma and Dissociation in Children

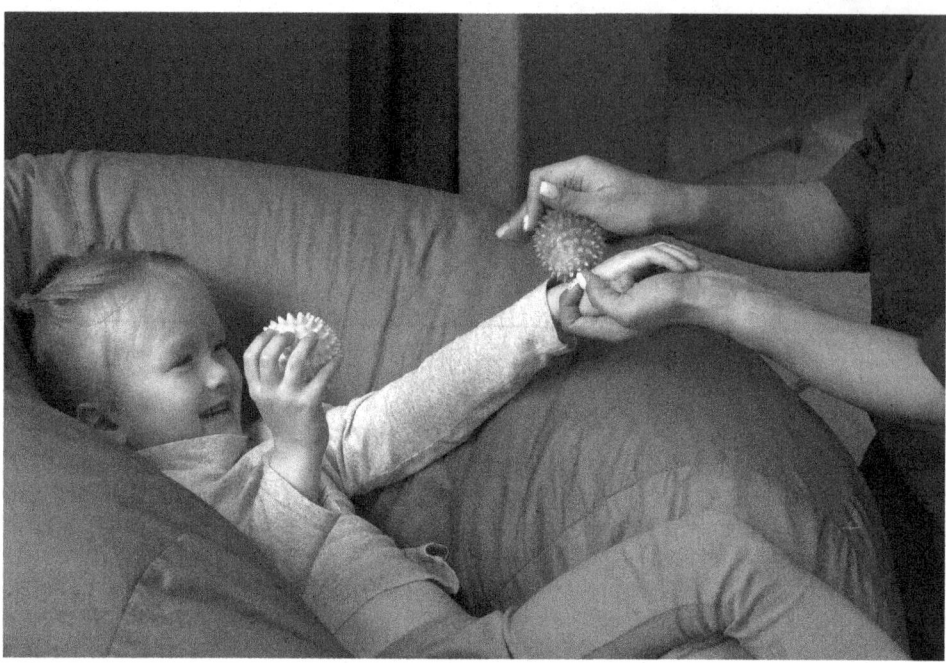

Figure 21.7 Developing Body Boundaries Through Deep-Pressure Touch.

Table 21.6 Developing Boundaries with Sensory-, Motor-, and Activity-Based Interventions

Developing Boundaries with Sensory-, Motor- and Activity-Based Interventions	Sensory Contributions to the Development of Boundaries	Motor Contributions to the Development of Boundaries	How These Activities Assist in the Development of Boundaries
Developing Body Boundaries and Sense of Self	Deep-pressure touch to the body: "This is me, this is not me" Sound through bone conduction provides vibration into the head and body. (Used with Therapeutic Listening vitallinks. net; Focus Integrated Listening Systems integratedlistening.com; Forbrain forbrain.com.) Develops a sense of self Gravity: Lying on the floor with a weighted blanket Lying over a therapy ball	Pushing the body against resistance: Lycra swing Body Sock Pushing the body against a support surface: Push-ups Climbing Stairs Pushing feet against the wall	Deep pressure to the skin increases the awareness of the skin boundary Heavy work increases interoceptive awareness of self Gravity with weight connects the body to ground and allows the child to feel their full body weight

(Continued)

Table 21.6 (Continued)

Developing Boundaries with Sensory-, Motor- and Activity-Based Interventions	Sensory Contributions to the Development of Boundaries	Motor Contributions to the Development of Boundaries	How These Activities Assist in the Development of Boundaries
Developing Spatial Boundaries between Self and Other	Hula-Hoop spatial boundaries Launch and Land (Sheila Frick, 2022) Listening to ambient sounds Visually tracking moving images (Therapeutic Listening vitallinks.net)	Pushing away with hands and feet against resistance develops the needed muscles for physical boundaries to "push away"	Having a Hula-Hoop around the body provides a concrete representation of personal space Launching through space provides as sense of moving the body through space Visual and auditory localization support the mapping of space

Table 21.7 Expansion of the Window of Tolerance, Exploration, and Interpersonal Collaboration

Expansion of Window of Tolerance, Exploration, and Interpersonal Collaboration	Sensory-Based Activities	Posture and Movement Activities	Psychotherapeutic Activities
Preschooler and School-Aged Child	Climbing wall: Heavy work: vestibular, proprioceptive, interoceptive, visual, tactile	Climbing wall: • Inner-core stability • Integration of eye muscles • Bilateral integration • Balance • Strength	As the child struggles with competency in this task, there are opportunities to experience regulated struggle and persistence, failure and success, metaphorical strength and weakness as it relates to self-awareness and development of self-regard
Preschooler and School-Aged Child	Pillow fight: Heavy work: proprioceptive, vestibular, and tactile	Pillow fight: Inner-core stability Push and pull Bilateral coordination Strength	Development of collaborative arousal management through co-regulation at higher arousal states
Preschooler and School-Aged Child	Tug-of-war: Heavy work: proprioceptive, vestibular	Tug-of-war: Inner core stability Pull Bilateral Coordination Strength	Development of containing shared tension between two people
School-Aged Child	Making Contact: visual and tactile	Making Contact: Inner-core stability Shoulder girdle stability	Development of staying stable within oneself while making contact with another

Trevor was referred for OT to assist him with the regulatory functions of sleeping, eating, and toileting. Upon presentation, Trevor had dark circles under his eyes and his eyes appeared empty. His eyebrows were held in an elevated position with a vigilant gaze. His shoulders were elevated toward his ears, and he rarely turned his head to look around. His spine was stiff, his arms were held close to his body, and his fingers were splayed in a widely open defensive posture. His rib cage was tipped upward, and his breathing was shallow and placed high in his chest. His pelvis was positioned in posterior pelvic tilt in both sitting and standing, suggestive of inner-core weakness. He maintained an open mouth posture.

Trevor was guarded in his interaction with me; however, he loved the sensory gym. He would run freely and enjoyed crashing and falling on the therapy mats in the room. In the sensory gym was a sand tray. During the first session, he chose three human-like figures and placed them in the sand. Although not verbally identified, the female figure appeared to represent "Mom." He buried her in the sand. The adult male figure was presumed to be "Dad," whom he immediately threw out of the sand tray onto the floor. The little boy figure (whom I presumed to be Trevor) sat alone in the corner of the sand tray.

This play scheme repeated itself over several sessions and appeared to me to become a "stuck" trauma reenactment. During this play reenactment, my role was primarily that of observer, holding space for this expression. During the fourth session, after once again repeating this reenactment, Trevor climbed into the Lycra swing, which was positioned nearby. I moved slowly toward him and cinched up the Lycra, pulling him into a tightly flexed position. I positioned myself underneath him, placing my hands in a cradling position, rocking gently. Within a couple minutes, Trevor began to sob, then wail, then rage. I shifted the movements of the swing to allow for physical support for each emotion. Rocking when sobbing, bouncing when wailing, and vigorous swinging while raging. After several minutes, Trevor rolled out of the swing and headed back toward the sand tray. He promptly picked up the "Dad" figure and placed it beside the little boy. Then Trevor spoke out loud. Pretending he was the dad, he looked at the figure of the boy and said, "Sorry." That was it. Witnessing this scene was profound and demonstrated the impact of play-based, sensory-motor supports in a psychotherapeutic context.

During follow-up sessions, Trevor no longer displayed interest in the sand tray at all, moving his play to activities involving more expansive sensory exploration. Our sessions discontinued when the foster family moved to a different community, but I did have the opportunity for warm closure, and no further contact was made. Thank you to Trevor for allowing me to be a part in his healing journey.

Conclusion

PSI has evolved over the past 35 years, ever expanding in its trans-disciplinary knowledge base. It is hoped that the PSI approach enables clinicians from diverse professions to feel validated in their treatment of the body as a valued component of their trauma work. As trauma does live in the body, a holistic mind-body approach is needed for the treatment of complex childhood trauma and dissociation.

Notes

1 The child's name is an alias to maintain confidentiality.
2 The child's name is an alias to maintain confidentiality.

References

Ayres, A. J. (1972). *Sensory integration and learning disorders*. Western Psychological Services.

Barlow, W. (1973). *The Alexander principle*. Victor Gollancz.

Barthel, K. (2020). A frame of reference for neuro-developmental treatment. In P. Kramer, J. Hinojosa & T. Howe (Eds.), *Frames of reference for pediatric occupational therapy* (4th ed., pp. 205–245). Wolters Kluwer.

Bodynamic International. (2023). https://www.bodynamic.com

Bordoni, B., & Zanier, E. (2013). Anatomic connections of the diaphragm: Influence of respiration on the body system. *Journal of Multidisciplinary Healthcare, 6*, 281–291. https://doi.org/10.2147/JMDH.S45443

Cameron, O. G., & Minoshima, S. (2002). Regional brain activation due to pharmacologically induced adrenergic interoceptive stimulation in humans. *Psychosomatic Medicine, 64*(6), 851–861.

Champagne, T. (2011). The influence of posttraumatic stress disorder, depression, and sensory processing patterns on occupational engagement: A case study. *Work, 38*(1), 67–75. https://doi.org/10.3233/WOR-2011-110

Choi, J., Jeong, B., Rohan, M. L., Polcari, A. M., & Teicher, M. H. (2009). Preliminary evidence for white matter tract abnormalities in young adults exposed to parental verbal abuse. *Biological Psychiatry, 65*(3), 227–234. https://doi.org/10.1016/j.biopsych.2008.06.022

COTO (College of Occupational Therapists of Ontario) (n.d.). Psychotherapy within occupational therapy practice. coto.org/standards-and-resources/webinars-and-podcasts/psychotherapy-within-occupational-therapy-practice

Cozolino, L. (2002). *The neuroscience of psychotherapy: Building and rebuilding the human brain*. W. W. Norton.

Crittenden, P. M. (2005). Attachment theory, psychopathology, and psychotherapy: the dynamic-maturational approach. International Association for the Study of Attachment. PDF. iasa-dmm.org/images/uploads/Attachment-theory-psychopaathology%20andpsychotherapyThedmm-approach.pdf

De Kleine, R. A., Hagenaars, M. A., & van Minnen, A. (2018). Tonic Immobility during re-experiencing the traumatic event in posttraumatic stress disorder. *Psychiatry Research, 270*, 1105–1109.

Dion, L. (2017). Be yourself – Therapist authenticity in the playroom. Synergetic Play Therapy Institute. synergeticplaytherapy.com/be-yourself

Field, T. (2014). *Touch*. The MIT Press.

FRI. (2019). https://familyrelationsinstitute.org

Garcia-Rill, E. (2019). *Arousal in neurological and psychiatric diseases* (Kindle ed., p. 74). Elsevier Science.

Harricharan, S., McKinnon, M. C., & Lanius, R. A. (2021). How processing of sensory information from the internal and external worlds shape the perception and engagement with the world in the aftermath of trauma: Implications for PTSD. *Frontiers in Neuroscience, 15*, Article 625490. https://doi.org/10.3389/fnins.2021.625490

Hodges, P. W., & Gandevia, S. C. (2000). Changes in intra-abdominal pressure during postural and respiratory activation of the human diaphragm. *Journal of Applied Physiology, 89*(3), 967–976. https://doi.org/10.1152/jappl.2000.89.3.967

Hopenwasser, K. (2008). Being in rhythm: Dissociative attunement in therapeutic process. *Journal of Trauma & Dissociation, 9*(3), 349–367. https://doi.org/10.1080/15299730802139212

Hume, K., Steinbrenner, J. R., Odom, S. L., Morin, K. L., Nowell, S. W., Tomaszewski, B., Szendrey, S., McIntyre, N. S., Yücesoy-Özkan, S., & Savage, M. N. (2021). Evidence-based practices for children, youth, and young adults with autism: Third generation review. *Journal of Autism and Developmental Disorders, 51*(11), 4013–4032. https://doi.org/10.1007/s10803-020-04844-2

Kearney, B. E., & Lanius, R. A. (2022). The brain-body disconnect: A somatic sensory basis for trauma-related disorders. *Frontiers in Neuroscience, 16*, 1–34. Article 1015749. https://doi.org/10.3389/fnins.2022.1015749

Levine, P. A. (2010). *In an unspoken voice: How the body releases trauma and restores goodness*. North Atlantic Books.

Malchiodi, C. (2015). *Creative interventions with traumatized children*. Guilford Publications.

Mannell, S., & Wiebe, J. (2010, December 10). Dynamic Core for kids. HeartSpace Physical Therapy. Retrieved from heartspacept.com/dynamic-core-for-kids

Masgutova, S. (2016). Post-trauma recovery in children of Newtown, CT, using MNRI Reflex Integration. *Journal of Traumatic Stress Disorders & Treatment, 6*(1), 1–12. https://doi.org/10.4172/2324-8947.1000163

McLaughlin, K. A., Weissman, D., & Bitrán, D. (2019). Childhood adversity and neural development: A systematic review. *Annual Review of Developmental Psychology, 1*, 277–312.

Mori, R., Bergsman, A., Holmes, M., & Yates, B. (2001). Role of the medial medullary reticular formation in relaying vestibular signals to the diaphragm and abdominal muscles. *Brain Research, 902*(1), 82–91. https://doi.org/10.1016/s0006-8993(01)02370-8

Neuro-Developmental Treatment Association. (2023). https://ndta.org

Nowlan, N. (2015). Biomechanics of foetal movement. *European Cells and Materials, 29*, 1–21. https://doi.org/10.22203/ecm.v029a01

Noyed, D. (2023, January 31). How heavy should a weighted blanket be? Sleep Foundation. Retrieved from sleepfoundation.org/bedding-information/weighted-blanket-weight-chart

Ogden, P., & Fisher, J. (2015). *Sensorimotor psychotherapy: Interventions for trauma and attachment* (Norton series on interpersonal neurobiology). WW Norton & Company.

Ogden, P., Minton, K., & Pain, C. (2006). *Trauma and the body: A sensorimotor approach to psychotherapy*. W. W. Norton.

Panksepp, J. (2004). *Affective neuroscience: The foundations of human and animal emotions*. Oxford University Press.

Panksepp, J., & Biven, L. (2012). *The archaeology of mind: Neuroevolutionary origins of human emotions*. W. W. Norton.

Parham, L. D., Cohn, E. S., Spitzer, S., Koomar, J. A., Miller, L. J., Burke, J. P., Brett-Green, B., Mailloux, Z., May-Benson, T. A., Smith Roley, S., Schaaf, R. C., Schoen, S. A., & Summers, C. A. (2007). Fidelity in sensory integration intervention research. *American Journal of Occupational Therapy, 61*(2), 216–227. https://doi.org/10.5014/ajot.61.2.216

Perry, B. D. (2001). The neurodevelopmental impact of violence in childhood. In D. Schetky & E. P. Benedek (Eds.), *Textbook of child and adolescent forensic psychiatry* (pp. 221–238). American Psychiatric Press.

Perry, B. D. (2009). Examining child maltreatment through a neurodevelopmental lens: Clinical applications of the neurosequential models of therapeutics. *Journal of Loss and Trauma, 14*, 240–255. https://doi.org/10.1080/15325020903004350

Pfaff, D. W. (2009). *Brain arousal and information theory: Neural and genetic mechanisms*. Harvard University Press.

Porges, S. W. (2011). *The polyvagal theory: Neurophysiological foundations of emotions, attachment, communication, and self-regulation*. W. W. Norton.

Purvis, K. B., Parris, S. R., & Cross, D. R. (2011). Trust-based relational intervention: Principles and practices. In E. A. Rosman, C. E. Johnson & N. M. Callahan (Eds.), *Adoption factbook V* (pp. 485–489). National Council for Adoption.

Rass, E. (Ed.). (2017). *The Allan Schore reader: Setting the course of development*. Routledge.

Riva, G., & Dakanalis, A. (2018). Altered processing and integration of multisensory bodily representations and signals in eating disorders: A possible path toward the understanding of their underlying causes. *Frontiers in Human Neuroscience, 12*. https://doi.org/10.3389/fnhum.2018.00049

Rothschild, B. (2000). *The body remembers the psychophysiology of trauma & trauma treatment*. W. W. Norton.

Schmid, T. (2004). Meanings of creativity within occupational therapy practice. *Australian Occupational Therapy Journal, 51*(2), 80–88. https://doi.org/10.1111/j.1440-1630.2004.00434.x

Siegel, D. J. (1999). *The developing mind: Toward a neurobiology of interpersonal experience*. Guilford Press.

Siegel, D. J. (2010). *Mindsight: The new science of personal transformation*. Bantam.

Siegel, D. J. (2012). *The developing mind: How relationships and the brain interact to shape who we are*. Guilford Press.

Siegel, D. J., Schore, A. N., & Cozolino, L. (2021). *Interpersonal neurobiology and clinical practice*. W. W. Norton.

Smith-Roley, S., Blanche, E. I., & Schaaf, R. C. (2001). *Understanding the nature of sensory integration with diverse populations*. Therapy Skill Builders.

Smith-Roley, S., Schaaf, R., & Baltazar-Mori, A. (2020). Ayres sensory integration frame of reference. In P. Kramer, J. Hinojosa & T. Howe (Eds.), *Frames of reference for pediatric occupational therapy* (4th ed., pp. 87–153). Wolters Kluwer.

Steinbrenner, J. R., Hume, K., Odom, S. L., Morin, K. L., Nowell, S. W., Tomaszewski, B., Szendrey, S., McIntyre, N. S., Yücesoy-Özkan, S., & Savage, M. N. (2020). Evidence-based practices for children, youth, and young adults with autism. University of North Carolina, Frank Porter Graham Child Development Institute, and National Clearinghouse on Autism Evidence and Practice Review Team.

Teicher, M. H., & Khan, A. (2019). Childhood maltreatment, cortical and amygdala morphometry, functional connectivity, laterality, and psychopathology. *Child Maltreatment, 24*(4), 458–465.

Teicher, M. H., Gordon, J. B., & Nemeroff, C. B. (2022). Recognizing the importance of childhood maltreatment as a critical factor in psychiatric diagnoses, treatment, research, prevention, and education. *Molecular Psychiatry, 27*(3), 1331–1338.

Teicher, M. H., & Samson, J. A. (2016). Annual research review: Enduring neurobiological effects of childhood abuse and neglect. *Journal of Child Psychology and Psychiatry, 57*(3), 241–266. https://doi.org/10.1111/jcpp.12507

Thome, J., Densmore, M., Koppe, G., Terpou, B., Théberge, J., McKinnon, M. C., & Lanius, R. A. (2019). Back to the basics: Resting state functional connectivity of the reticular activation system in PTSD and its dissociative subtype. *Chronic Stress, 3*, https://doi.org/10.1177/2470547019873663

Warner, E., Koomar, J., Lary, B., & Cook, A. (2013). Can the body change the score? Application of sensory modulation principles in the treatment of traumatized adolescents in residential settings. *Journal of Family Violence, 28*, 729–738.

22
A SENSORIMOTOR PSYCHOTHERAPY PERSPECTIVE ON FAMILY INTERVENTIONS

Bonnie Goldstein

Introduction

Our younger clients affected by complex trauma and dissociation are highly dependent on their families. Therefore, sensorimotor family therapy aims to address the family system (Ogden & Goldstein, 2017; Goldstein & Ogden, 2016; Ogden & Fisher, 2015; Ogden et al., 2012). Because trauma and early attachment challenges can leave their mark on family members and shape interactions, treatment aims to enhance communication, work with self-regulation strategies, address difficulties in boundary setting, and foster resilience in all family members. This chapter will focus on the use of Sensorimotor Psychotherapy within the family context, seeking corrective experiences to override some of the troubling experiences of the past and to offer fresh hope and renewed connection and closeness. Jon Kabat-Zinn (1990/2013), trailblazer in the science of mindfulness, wrote, "As long as you are breathing, there is more right with you than wrong with you, no matter how ill or how despairing you may be feeling" (p. xlix). This is a message that Sensorimotor Psychotherapy family therapists can aim to offer to family members—a sense that no matter how hopeless they may feel, there is more right with their family than there is wrong. You can invite them to work together with you so they can discover what feels right. Making the decision to enter family therapy is a huge step in this process of discovery.

Sensorimotor family therapy prizes a body-oriented approach that is less reliant on language than many therapies, instead exploring the nonverbal role of trauma on interactions (e.g., emotions and affect regulation, procedural learning, sensations, and sensory processing), in addition to the verbal narrative when available. The cases described in this chapter will address the nonverbal "somatic narrative" family members have a difficult time identifying or articulating, yet which continuously anticipates the future and powerfully impacts behavior.

Sensorimotor Psychotherapy recognizes that family therapy does not occur in a social or cultural vacuum and that any treatment must be dedicated to promoting diversity, inclusion, equity, cultural sensitivity, and a therapeutic environment that aims to be free of bias. In their seminal article, Laszloffy and Hardy (2000) discussed the critical need for family therapist training to include the development of racial awareness and racial sensitivity; the failure to include it will result in the replication of systemic racism within the therapeutic setting. The demographic makeup of the profession itself illustrates the importance of diversity training. While much of the US population is projected to be non-white by 2044, only 14% of psychologists were people of color in 2017, although that percentage was higher (37%) for marriage and family therapists (Erolin & Wieling, 2021). Recognizing the need for attention to this issue, Kelly et al. (2020) described the skills essential for all family therapists, including sensitivity to privilege, critical consciousness, a humble stance, recognition of the strengths of multigenerational caregiving and kin networks in Black families, and helping parents actively cultivate a positive Black identity in their children (pp. 1379–1381). These authors (themselves Black therapists) recommended that therapists enhance traditional therapeutic interventions by incorporating racial socialization, as follows:

> Therapists need to assume that it is always a background factor in Black lives. First, clinicians should continually educate themselves on the issues that Black families face as a part of their formal and informal continuing education to enhance their capacity to serve Black families effectively. Next, the topic of race needs to be addressed directly at the beginning of treatment, granting permission for families to talk about these issues should they become central to the discourse in the therapy process.
>
> *(p. 1382)*

Diversity is of course not limited to differences in race; differences due to ethnicity (Raffaelli et al., 2005), gender identity (Mills-Koonce et al., 2018), and other sources of bias are equally important for therapists to address (McDowell et al., 2017; McGoldrick & Hardy, 2019; Stratton & Low, 2020).

This chapter will begin with an overview of ways to work with families of children affected by complex trauma and dissociation through a Sensorimotor Psychotherapy approach, emphasizing the primary skills Sensorimotor Psychotherapy family therapists use to make progress in issues related to communication, boundary setting, self-regulation, dissociation, and resilience. Brief case examples of family sessions in Sensorimotor Psychotherapy will be offered to elucidate the principles of Sensorimotor Psychotherapy with our younger clients. Various points in this chapter will introduce ways to motivate family members to engage in therapy (long-distance treatment, animal assisted treatment, etc.) while cultivating a comfortable, collaborative, and safe environment for all family members.

Overview

This chapter's focus on family therapy aims to address a wide range of challenges the clinician faces, including working with family members who have experienced complex or severe trauma, while subscribing to the overarching philosophy that the family is the "client." This is an idea best served by the understanding (often through a prearranged agreement) that the focus of our work through the lens of Sensorimotor Psychotherapy will be on the family's present-moment interactions rather than on their historic material. We share this expectation with clients at the outset and clarify that the role of the therapist will be to interact by scanning for verbal or nonverbal threats, looking to see if a family member is trying to enlist the therapist to side against another member, and so on. We collaborate with the families by asking, "How much do you want me to intervene?" or "Would you prefer that I sit back and observe or that I jump in?" A partnership is established from the onset, with fluidity and give-and-take modeled by these questions. Our initial goal is to build a therapeutic alliance as we help family members work toward their vision, goals, and established ideals for the family. We work collaboratively, tracking and looking for signs (from words to somatic indicators) of threats, both implicit and explicit. We use somatic cues and other evidence to guide our treatment directions. For example, I often encourage family members to face one another so they can see each other; then, after a problematic interaction, I might turn to a family member and say, "What you said seemed to get a negative reaction. Did you notice that in his posture or in the way he moved when you made your comment?" Sometimes family members look at the therapist rather than at one another, which can be perceived as betrayal, a sign they are not tuning into one another, anxiety, or possible avoidance behaviors. Any of these are possibilities, and we want to evoke family members' curiosity about how they are affecting one another, particularly during very rapid interactions and escalations of emotion, anxiety, upset, and the like. By employing the principles of neuroplasticity, which capitalizes on our capacity to experience something new in the present moment (Siegel, 2020), we are shifting both the child's and caregiver's experiences with one another and within themselves.

Sensorimotor Psychotherapy family work explores how therapy can help a family by looking for ways to motivate each member to engage in therapy. Our work starts the moment we come into the therapy room, as we offer family members a choice of where to sit while observing where each family member chooses to sit; from the outset, we aim to create a safe environment to calm the nervous system of even the most hesitant family members. Also from the outset, we are aware and sensitive to the cultural, gender, and power dynamics in the room, including whatever background and bias we bring to this new relationship, and aim to address it in the present moment. Authenticity and presence, foundational principles in Sensorimotor Psychotherapy, foster working toward reciprocally embodied consciousness, which is conveyed to each family member through body-to-body affective communication (Ogden & Goldstein, 2020). We offer a therapeutic demeanor of equanimity (open, accepting, curious, fluid, collaborative) and a playful environment (e.g., spacious and colorful, and with child- and family-friendly props, pillows, blankets), thereby establishing a welcoming visual picture. These elements of therapy build on the work of leading family therapists such as Virginia Satir (1964) Murray Bowen (1993), and Salvador Minuchin (Minuchin & Fishman, 1981).

As huge amounts of information are communicated during the session through body language, family members often interpret information incorrectly and miss and/or ignore each other's cues. When families come to therapy, they often want to get right to the story and hope the therapist can "fix" whatever feels broken, while not necessarily eager to attend to the body's role. For example, family members can start conflicts without saying a word to each other or realizing they are doing it. Their nonconscious, procedurally learned habits of body-to-body communication formed during childhood (in ways that vary from family to family, as well as culture to culture) dictate their behavior, often beneath conscious awareness. Similarly, family members may feel anxiety stemming from early-life experiences during which they felt threatened and learned to avoid, suppress, or mask their feelings. When they become parents, they fall into patterns, knowingly or unknowingly, that recreate some version of their earlier experiences. Sensorimotor Psychotherapy brings to awareness these unconscious procedural tendencies and body-to-body communications, elucidating how they fuel conflict and adversely affect the family system. Sensorimotor Psychotherapy aims to explore what happens in each member of the family, tracking individual family members' nervous systems and working with each individual (child, teen, or caregiver) to understand variations in responses. It involves working with the body through physical sensation, muscle tonicity, information from the five senses, gestures, and movement, which all vary from individual to individual and may be more or less evident. However, this is not to say that feelings, thoughts, and words are absent from this approach. Rather, therapists are encouraged to look beneath a client's story to the somatic level of experience and then seek insight based on those discoveries. Clients learn ways to self-regulate, set boundaries, and overcome the inevitable ruptures that arise in family system dynamics.

As mentioned, pioneering family therapists and family systems theorists (e.g., Satir, Bowen, Minuchin, and others) paved the way for us to address the family hierarchy, the need for parents to take charge, the challenges within a family system in which a child becomes parentified, and family sculpting. Over the past two decades, Sensorimotor Psychotherapy family therapists have integrated the work of these pioneers, offering a lens through which family members can recognize, identify, feel, and deal with emotions (e.g., anxiety, fears, depression, and anger). These emotions and feelings are often the first signposts of deeper feelings. For example, adult family members may feel anxiety around emotions that stems from earlier times in life, when feelings were perceived as threatening and they learned to avoid, suppress, dissociate from, or mask them. These early experiences and responses lead to adverse associations (e.g., the belief that being with one's feelings is dangerous), which are then perpetuated in subsequent relationships with friends, mates, children, and so on. Sensorimotor Psychotherapy posits that it is through the body that we can enhance understanding and emotional awareness. By dropping into or staying with the emotions, sensations, feelings, and perceptions that arise within the body, clients can learn to allow and move through them. Psychoeducation can enable this way of working, especially when family members want to go right to the "story," rather than to understand the body's role.

Addressing Difficulties with Communication

Escalating stress and a lack of felt security can compromise our ability to communicate and hijack our sense of empathy or caring for another. For example, family members who have been diagnosed with autism spectrum, pervasive developmental disorder, dissociation, and similar disorders, can experience a range of difficulties using language to communicate. Therefore, fostering nonverbal communication offers new pathways toward building relationships. The aim of the Sensorimotor Psychotherapy family therapist is to help grow each family member's ability to be emotionally present, mindful, and available, even when triggered by overwhelming feelings. Since the body's answers do not come through a verbal narrative, attending to the moment-to-moment interactions between family members helps them develop a broader range of communication skills, as elucidated in the following case composite.

When initially coming to therapy, Bill, parent to Lizzy, age 11, recognized that his parenting skills and his ability to communicate with his children were compromised by rigidity. His lack of flexibility resulted in difficulty being present with his children. Prior to the first family session, he shared with the therapist that his ex-wife had suggested he resented that his children had been born because being their parent seemed to make him feel inadequate. In the midst of family conflict, which often occurred at family dinners, he described himself as "floating—not in a good way" and feeling discomfort or "on the outside, looking in." When conflict arose, he would first feel tense and then become silent and immobile. To address these issues, I introduced an exercise in grounding (encouraging Bill to notice where his rear touched his chair and to sit with his spine in an aligned posture, put his hands on his knees, and push his knees toward the floor, thus further shifting his alignment towards sitting straighter), all of which brought Bill back into the present moment. As Bill did this grounding exercise, remembering the dynamics in his family led to a memory from early childhood. As a child, he learned that neither fighting back nor running away were acceptable responses and only made the trauma and chaos in the family worse. As he described the rage and abuse in his childhood, his body became visibly rigid and he had a recollection of his mother becoming numb, collapsing, and becoming immobilized. This was her best means of assuring her survival in the face of her husband's (Bill's father's) alcoholic rages. At the time of therapy, Bill was sheltering at home due to the COVID-19 pandemic. His irritation and inflexibility had grown even more pronounced and problematic because he had lost his outlet (surfing at the beach, which is available all year long in Los Angeles) due to the beaches being closed to the public. He felt trapped, claustrophobic, and suffocated. Through our work, he began to see how his childhood informed his current communications and behaviors. He recognized the impact of his rigidity on communication within his family, causing him to hold back, especially during times of conflict, because he feared the ensuing chaos would feel too overwhelming.

I used Bill's memories, brought up by his body-based experience, to address his communication behaviors. Together, we worked toward increasing his capacity to be present during sessions. As his memories of anger, grief, and blame arose, he learned to identify where these feelings started in his body. In addition, he learned to express his thoughts and to share with less censoring and greater acceptance. He came to understand that even if someone else in his family felt something, that did not delegitimize his own feelings. Using qualifiers when discussing his implicit experience during our sessions made the process collaborative in nature and also suggested that I, the therapist, might not have the answers or might be wrong—I made statements such as "I'm making a guess," "I'm possibly wrong," "I'm interested in your feedback." This invited the dialogue and let Bill know that he had the option to correct or select a better word or meaning.

Bill's daughter Lizzy communicated very differently from her father. She was often in high arousal, enthusiastic, and emotional. Sensorimotor Psychotherapy helped her become more aware of the impact of her emotions on her body (e.g., her breathing quickened, muscles tightened, and shoulders hunched up). In the family system, Lizzy's high-arousal defenses sprang into action when Bill's body shut down as his way protecting himself or, through the lens of depersonalization, provided a layer of self-protection. Their respective responses to communication mirrored each other in opposing ways. This happened so quickly that it was difficult for them to assess the situation accurately, yet I was continually tracking, watching, noticing, and evaluating. Through psychoeducation, I shared information judiciously to ensure the family members were able to assimilate information. This family came to see that they had developed a pattern or habit of rapid-fire, non-thinking responses to perceived threats. Their styles of communication had become a liability within their family dynamics, especially with respect to navigating emotional experiences. In therapy, as Bill and his daughter reevaluated their habitual thoughts (e.g., "anger is bad," "emotions are dangerous," and "expressed feelings bring disdain or loss of approval"), they began to shift their perceptions and reassess their interactions with greater accuracy. Our work strengthened their capacity for self-observation as a launching point for an enhanced awareness of how they experienced family dynamics. Treatment goals included helping Lizzy develop her capacity, in the midst of family communications, to observe instead of reacting; to notice what was transpiring inside her body; and to identify her thoughts, sensations, and emotions. Over time, Lizzy reported that "instead of being completely absorbed in stress and distress," she was able to sense these feelings in her body, and to identify and name the experience.

Therapy helped Lizzy and Bill step out of their experience just enough to create some space to drop beneath their words (i.e., not thinking, assessing, or judging) and look at their reactions more objectivity. They learned to recognize the way feelings of overwhelm and helplessness showed up in the body, and they were able to increase their awareness of their feelings without being unduly affected by them. By changing their relationship with their feelings, their experience itself changed as well, as did their ability to communicate with each other and with other members of their family, friends, and colleagues.

When working with family members of all ages (e.g., parents/caregivers, children, and teens and young adults), the Sensorimotor Psychotherapy family therapist can introduce props to enhance communication, concentration, and listening skills—for example, using musical instruments such as drums of varying shapes and sizes (which are strategically placed throughout the office) and encouraging family members to use them for fun/joy, stress release, and collaborative communication. An example of enhancing communication between family members is making a beat using the drum and then seeing if another family member can copy it. This form of "communication" also fosters emotional co-regulation and interactive concentration skills, and can help elucidate the family process. Some family members may withdraw or submissively comply, while others may respond aggressively or critically. For example, numerous younger children have used the drums in my office to begin to "thaw" traumatic memories and communicate thoughts and feelings. Other families use the exercise of drumming for communication—for example, the caregivers lie on the carpet and spontaneously begin tapping a drum beat on the carpet using their hands and/or feet. Following this lead, other family members lie on the carpet alongside them, collaboratively co-creating the beat, while being encouraged by the therapist to notice the emerging thoughts and feelings, sensations, and emotions that arise. Often, teens in parent-caregiver sessions can create a drumbeat by tapping on their phones, thereby drumming out their emotions. For example, one teen, after about ten minutes of drumming while expressing her anger about her father, exclaimed "That's it... that's why I'm so upset at what Dad does... I feel so much better now... I can catch my breath now... maybe I should become a drummer." For her, this seemed to be a pivotal session; she felt that the somatic release of her feelings opened new pathways for self-understanding, parent-child communication, and well-being.

Myriad props can be used therapeutically in Sensorimotor Psychotherapy to address conflict, enhance communication, foster understanding, and impact behavior (Goldstein & Ogden, 2016; Ogden & Fisher, 2015; Ogden & Goldstein, 2017). For example, to highlight the importance of flexibility in family relationships, the egg toss game can be used; The idea is for family members to move farther and farther from one another while tossing an egg so that another family member can catch it, keeping it whole and not allowing the shell to break. Insights are derived throughout this exercise, and gently helping parents and children to recognize the trick of moving their hands with the egg as it arrives allows for success, because capitalizing on the movement offers better chance of keeping it intact—if you caught it with your hands fixed, the egg would almost certainly break. This exercise is illustrative for parents and children to understand their relational dynamics experientially, as inflexibility breaks the relationship, whereas movement protects. Similarly, using a dowel, or a peg of wood or metal, can be used for relational balance, family teamwork, and collaborative communication as family members navigate moving the object in synchronicity.

When therapy is conducted online, the therapist can still readily see how the dynamics of a family system, including family communications, play out, even in the first moments of the session. For example, squabbles between a parent and child can quickly escalate while another parent or caregiver looks at their phone rather than taking seriously the nature of the conflict. We can observe this, not realizing the impact on family dynamics; in fact, as it turns out, some conflict may revolve around the other family members' attempts to pull them into the fray. All these dynamics can be observed and addressed by the therapist in person or online effectively.

Virginia Satir's work elucidating ways to physicalize family dynamics by sculpting the family system blends well with Sensorimotor Psychotherapy; I am always watching to see where family members sit and how their bodies interact with one another as indicators of the patterns and habits of the family. Noting the seating arrangement of family members (in live or long-distance sessions) and then collaboratively rearranging the positions of the parents or children can offer insight to family dynamics. I encourage family members to notice what different thoughts, feelings, and sensations arise in these new positions. For example, when we are working online, perhaps the mother appears bigger on the screen than other family members (e.g., based on seating and proximity to the screen). In that case, I might suggest rearranging the seating to move the children closer to the screen and have the mother sit farther back in the room. If multiple screens are available, I might encourage using the gallery view to equalize their viewing size, position on the screen, and so on.

Similarly, to illuminate triangulation as family members communicate, Sensorimotor Psychotherapy interventions can include encouraging family members to move around the room in ways that emphasize their family structure. This can help clarify family members' roles and perhaps identify (i.e., based on physical positioning) a child who is perceived as "the problem" or identified patient. The therapist can ask a parent and child to swap seats, or have one family member stand on a chair while another family member crouches on the floor, thereby enabling a shift in their relational dynamic.

Working with Difficulties with Setting and/or Respecting Boundaries

A universal challenge for families is setting and respecting boundaries, and working with navigating personal space is foundational in Sensorimotor Psychotherapy. Ogden and Fisher's 2015 book, *Sensorimotor Psychotherapy: Interventions for Trauma and Attachment*, has myriad exercises on boundary setting which can be applied to family work. For example, we can see the struggles family members experience. when children's boundaries are not respected (e.g., they may learn either to stop asserting themselves or assert themselves antagonistically or aggressively and destructively, or they may dissociate needs or affect when not respected or attuned to). As we approach family treatment through Sensorimotor Psychotherapy, we work to drop beneath the words to the somatic narrative, aspiring to foster a somatic sense of boundaries (e.g., setting boundaries, understanding and respecting boundaries that are set by others).

A case example, of a boy I will call Josh, age 11, illustrates this. Josh started family therapy because he was having difficulty coming to terms with the trauma of losing his father, who died when Josh was 8. He presented as a disheveled youth with long, uncombed hair (which his mother attributed to a prolonged shiva, the Jewish mourning period). I sensed his wildness represented a bodily manifestation of his internal trauma. However, he stated that he just didn't care, and his mother's concerns were unwarranted., Josh's hopelessness intensified whenever he turned on the news, as well as when he saw an uptick in hateful or anti-Semitic comments on social media, and his disheveled appearance further devolved. In fact, he agreed to come to family therapy because it was online, which he felt required less effort on his part.

Josh had difficulty making eye contact and complained that his previous therapist had "constantly interpreted—or misinterpreted" his lack of eye contact, furthering his discomfort. He recalled feeling that the therapist's eyes were probing him too intensely, as were his mother's, and he objected to feeling "badgered." In fact, at the onset of our first family Zoom session, his mother exclaimed, "Josh, stop looking away!" As she said this, his head dropped and his shoulders curved in, making his long hair cascade over his left eye, further distancing him by covering his gaze. I used this as the entry point for therapy with Josh and his mother; he and I identified his resistance to his mother's attempts to shape his behavior both in and out of the sessions. Collaboratively, we agreed to look at his experience of his mother, which he described as feeling poked and prodded, as he felt his mother pushed his boundaries daily. Conversely, we looked at his mother's worry that Josh's life was stalled, manifesting in a sensed pressure that she must cajole, push, and mobilize him.

From the outset of our sessions, I established ways of working that fostered a sense of safety. For example, I helped Josh see how averting his eyes served to make him feel safer and less vulnerable. He acknowledged this, and we were able to explore how that affected his way of being in the world. I encouraged him to notice what happened in his body when he looked away from his mother. Offering permission for him to continue his gaze aversion for the time being, led to his reflecting that it was one of the things he did to feel safe, as well as to set boundaries so he could feel more empowered and in control. Questions and directions such as "What's happening now?" and "Notice what happens when you avert your eyes in my presence" led to Josh identifying two feelings. On the one hand, he felt safer, calmer, and less "probed." On the other hand, as I slowly invited his curiosity, he was able to experience his anger at the loss of his father, and the ensuing changes in his mother, along with concomitant feelings of upset and guilt.

As we worked together, it became clear that he felt he had no outlet through which to deal with his feelings of anger, upset, and loss, because he believed his mother was "all he had" and he did not want to risk alienating her. He felt responsible for being "the man of the house," which felt overwhelming. His avoidant behaviors enabled Josh to set boundaries and shield himself and his mother from the feelings that were simmering right below the surface. When I asked Josh and his mother if they would be willing to try an experiment (in Sensorimotor Psychotherapy, experiments are fundamental to treatment) in which she handed him a pillow, at first Josh was reluctant to participate, exclaiming that this was a silly exercise. Slowly, however, he started to explore his feelings when his mother handed him the pillow. His predominant feeling was "Why should I take it? You'll just take it away from me again." It became clear that this exercise echoed his experience of loss wherein he did not have the chance to say goodbye to his father when he was younger. Something was taken away from him that he could not get back. As a result, the boundaries that he set, consciously and unconsciously, were an attempt to against future painful losses.

Josh attempted to be the strong warrior, with Samson-like long hair, yet he had no ability to conquer the torment of his emotions. He had waded into fantasies of death and contemplated suicide, at times surrendering to the feelings of hopelessness that immobilized him. In therapy, we explored Josh's fear of being smothered by the upsetting feelings that engulfed him, while also addressing his mother's issues. As her son's feelings came to the surface, she grew agitated and said that she was physically uncomfortable. It appeared she wanted to bolt from the session. It became clear that she was mired in the haze of her own feelings and had brought Josh to family therapy to be "healed" or "fixed." For example, she would exclaim, "I lost your father and now I feel like I'm losing you" whenever he began to open up about his feelings.

As she struggled with her own stability, Josh's mother began to smoke more marijuana, which was readily available and legal in California, however, marijuana provided an illusory escape that only exacerbated her anxiety, frustration, and parental concern. She seemed to be overwhelmed often by feelings she could not control or understand, and Josh was the one thing she felt she had control over... until she didn't. He pointed out the irony that his mother was smoking daily yet he was expected to be responsible, proactive, and sober.

Working with this parent-child dynamic proved challenging because their emotional turbulence disrupted all aspects of their relationship. Josh would disappear for hours on end into his room, where he engaged with an online gaming community. This heightened his mother's anxiety because she could see that freezing off his painful emotions was his only mechanism for dealing with his pain. Psychoeducation helped Josh see that this freezing had an adverse side effect, as he subsequently lost access to any pleasurable feelings because all feelings were numbed. As we worked through these issues, he came to perceive his "freeze" as all encompassing, necessitating an ice pick in order to chip away at the frozen traces of his past experiences that had been so immobilizing. Concomitantly, his mother's role in this freeze was palpable: the more she encouraged, pushed, and cajoled, the more he dug his heels in.

Our sessions served as a thawing process as Josh gained access to the range of his emotional reality that had been "frozen solid" so he could avoid his overwhelming feelings, and as he learned to set realistic and healthy boundaries.

Working with Difficulties with Self-Regulation

Relationships in which one person overreacts and the other underreacts, and neither is able to self-regulate, can be increasingly problematic, as these patterns become automatic over time. These difficulties present in level of arousal, affect, and energy, and can vary from moment to moment throughout a family therapy session. Therefore, helping family members identify arousal states and increase their capacity to regulate their arousal is an essential treatment goal. Some family members have a *sensory processing sensitivity*, which can contribute to their feeling more overwhelmed and sensitive to their surroundings while also increasing the likelihood of high anxiety and stress levels. Such an individual is frequently called a *highly sensitive person*, and therapists can help one or more family members who are struggling during the session to modulate their arousal using a variety of bottom-up exercises (Aron & Hewitt, 2023).

For example, a girl I will call Brenda was a sixth grader who had no brake on her yelling, screaming, and crying behavior. Her parents described her lack of self-regulation as "When she's good, things are very, very good; when she's upset/triggered/dysregulated, her rageful behavior overwhelms the family." Brenda was always remorseful after an incident, and her parents capitalized on her regret. Her mother tended to focus on how she got caught in the rising hysteria (e.g., "I was having a great day until you went crazy"), or contributed to the escalation (e.g., by saying to Brenda, "You need to go to a mental institution" or "You are nuts"). Moreover, her mother continued to overreact even though she realized her words further exacerbated the situation and, in fact, were words her own mother had said to her. Brenda's father's reaction was the opposite: he would underreact, get quiet, withdraw, and refuse to be drawn into the conflict.

Working collaboratively, our initial goal was to help Brenda find more balance in her nervous system. Sometimes she would jump up and leave our session tearfully, angrily shouting at her mother, "I hate you!" Her mother would shout, "Get back here, right now!" Sometimes that resulted in an agitated, overwhelmed girl returning to the session, at other times, not. I asked the parents to imagine what would happen if they didn't demand Brenda return but instead gently encouraged her to return when she was ready. Her mother expressed fear that her daughter would not return, which led me to propose we try it as an experiment. She agreed, and Brenda did return (both out of curiosity and out of fear of punishment, I suspect).

I was then able to help Brenda understand that leaving was her body's way of expressing her degree of upset. I asked her to track her body during the session, using a scale of 0 to 60 to measure how upset she was. We agreed to try to notice together what was happening in her body in the moments right before she felt she had to jump up and get out. I encouraged her to check inside, evoking her curiosity about what happened in her body as her upset rapidly increased. She said she had difficulty breathing and could feel her face becoming hot. Indeed, when she dropped into these feelings within her body as she reflected on her upset, she began gasping for breath. Her breath then became the access route on which we focused for her therapy. Brenda and her mother each agreed to work on recognizing their own anxiety and anger as it arose during their interactions. They each reported a range of feelings and sensations they were not previously in touch with. Mom recognized getting still and quiet, yet feeling like exploding. She seemed surprised when I commented that her fists were balled up. Brenda identified starting to shake, feeling breathless, her face feeling hot, having tears, and wanting to hit or kick. I was then able to introduce the concept of the window of tolerance/window of optimal arousal, in child-friendly language (Ogden et al., 2006; Ogden & Fisher, 2015; Siegel, 2020), which helped Brenda begin to self-regulate. When she noticed the signs of initial upset within her body, she grew curious about different ways to shift toward self-regulation.

Anxiety's debilitating effects can interfere with family members' day-to-day functioning. Younger family members who are experiencing difficulties caused by heightened anxiety can benefit from the self-regulation tools that Sensorimotor Psychotherapy family sessions can offer. I like to use an exercise incorporated in Sensorimotor Psychotherapy as "orienting" (Ogden et al., 2006; Ogden & Fisher, 2015), which can foster a "state shift" in order to address the escalation of upset, anger, anxiety, and so forth. In essence, using this exercise in family sessions helps foster family members' heightened awareness of their senses. I suggest that they drop into their senses and name three things they notice—that is, three things that they are seeing, feeling, hearing, smelling, or tasting. Alternatively, I suggest that they look around the room and find three things to orient toward. This practice can help interrupt the automatic catastrophic thinking that fuels anxiety and can enable better self-regulation. For example, encouraging Brenda to take a sip of water and notice how the coolness affected her "hot" anger helped her interrupt the automatic escalation of anger that had become a relational habit. We worked toward titrating between states, noticing what was happening in her body and finding ways for her to manage her anxiety and anger—tools that may be helpful in working with children experiencing dissociative symptoms, or who may be depersonalized from their body.

At the end of family sessions, I offer suggestions for follow-up with at-home opportunities to revisit and practice some of the work we have done together. One exercise that seems universally beneficial involves asking each family member to come up with activities they can do to alleviate stress, reduce anxiety, and practice self-regulation strategies. Such activities include baking or cooking together, watch a captivating show together, and doing something physical, such as taking a walk, engaging with nature, or shooting hoops. Naming these aloud then propels families to come up with ways to proceed, co-creating schedules that are mutually agreeable.

In addition to exploring the ways that orienting can be woven into family therapy, we can also address the ways that the body participates in suppressing primary emotions through *dissociation* and *splitting*, responses often associated with complications of complex trauma (also often used to describe clients who are difficult to treat). Recognizing and assessing dissociative symptoms and diagnosing dissociative disorders becomes essential when treating family members who have experienced complex trauma and the aftermath because, through the lens of Sensorimotor Psychotherapy, dissociation can also be reframed as a coping mechanism or an adaptive strategy or response to get through intolerable moments (e.g., the numbing that occurs). Recognizing and assessing dissociative moments or diagnosing dissociative disorders when treating family members who have experienced trauma and the aftermath is essential; Bessel van der Kolk (2014) stated, "As long as the trauma is not resolved, the stress hormones the body secretes to protect itself keep circulating, and the defensive moments and emotional responses keep getting played out" (p. 66). Dissociation is the essence of trauma and can be seen as a resource, helping family members tolerate unbearable moments (e.g., when emotions grow too upsetting, or when traumas of the past interfere with the here-and-now, in the session). When the therapist suspects that it is too difficult for family members to stay present, making meaning of the moment-to-moment experiences as they transpire offers the therapist opportunities to be curious and concerned about family members' dissociative symptoms, as they compromise the ability to manage basic activities (e.g., a caregiver's self-care or taking care of children, food, and grooming).

Our treatment goals include helping every member in the family session find ways to self-regulate, moment to moment, allowing for continuous consciousness and fewer instances of dissociative moments. This can be fostered through the repetition of new practices that facilitate awareness of being in the present moment, allowing for new habits to be formed (Fisher, 2017; Ogden & Fisher, 2015). When other adaptive strategies or resources (e.g., nature, relationships with friends and family, connection to a higher power, movement, and prayer) or somatic mechanisms (holding in, compressing, collapsing or inflating posture, kinetic movement, etc.) are unavailable, dissociation can take the form of numbing or spacing out; this can also be correlated to the numbing that transpires through addiction (e.g., to drugs or alcohol, technology or the Internet, watching sports hour after hour). All the above may be consciously or unconsciously utilized by family members when primary emotions are too painful to experience, cause loss of control, stimulate unbearable needs, and/or lead to dysregulation.

Addressing the neurobiological legacy of trauma, Fisher (2017) stated that "without a clear chronological record of what happened but vulnerable to the uninvited activation of trauma-related feeling and body memories, individuals are left with a legacy of symptoms and reactions with no context that identifies them as memory" (p. 20) and concluded that "trauma treatment must address the effects of the traumatic past, not its events" (p. 21).

Over the course of treatment, which focuses on the effects of their traumatic past, our clients can begin to soften. For example, one very angry, upset client who refused to come to therapy found that when she did finally come, swinging on our indoor office swing offered both a fun and soothing movement. Swinging is often a natural regulator that calms most people, providing a suspended state of yielding or relaxation. This was evidenced in this client by her yielding into the swing, her head back, wearing a huge smile, and unclenching her tight fists. While she had a hard time letting down her guard, the swing provided her an opportunity that allowed for a new experience to emerge.

Fostering Resilience

Listening to our clients' concerns while also noting our own needs as therapists starts with developing somatic resonance (i.e., using our body to attune to the state of another person). Although we can never fully know another person's experience, we can help validate their anxiety and fears while concomitantly accompanying them on their unfolding path, helping them discover their own path toward resilience. This foundational principle in Sensorimotor Psychotherapy helps family members expand their resources for self-care to foster resilience and propel state-shifts toward greater empowerment. We have a hand in helping clients process implicit memories (e.g., memories that are not in awareness or are just below awareness), because those are what influence and affect their conscious explicit behaviors and experiences. Resilience has been defined as "an effective adaption to, or a navigation (or management) of, significant sources of traumatic stress or adversity and the capacity to absorb disturbance to harness resources effectively" (Denckla et al., 2020). While this definition arose out of the 2019 annual meeting of the International Society for Traumatic Stress Studies (ISTSS), the panel acknowledged the need to better determine the cross-cultural validity of the concept of resilience. Nevertheless, much has been written about resilience with respect to BIPOC as well as those in the LGBTQ2+ community, and family support clearly can play a significant role in the development of resilience in the face of racism, discrimination, and oppression. Burt et al. (2017) reported that racial socialization practices within families fostered resilience among youth, especially when the focus was on building positive racial identities and spirituality/religiosity. Discussing youth dealing with discrimination and economic hardship, Hostinar and Miller (2019) cited the importance of retaining their culture (cultural resilience) within their families as a means of counteracting stress. Zeeman et al. (2017) discussed the importance of systemic support (e.g., teachers, nurses, community organizations) for trans youth, especially including those who do not receive support from within their families. Perhaps no single circumstance has called for resilience more than the unprecedented worldwide disruptions to family systems because of mandates for social distancing, extended forced isolation, and compromised social interactions during the COVID-19 pandemic. Many community members view the pandemic as a defining moment in their lives affecting how they view family and other relationships, how they define security, how they deal with anxiety, and more. Wade et al. (2020) cited not only the negative effects of the pandemic on the mental health of children and youth but also the cumulative risk and "sleeper effects" that can be expected to cause long-term consequences for families. Moreover, recognizing the likelihood that families will need to deal with an increasing number of sociopolitical and environmental crises, all of which will demand resilience in the coming years, family therapists are tasked with addressing these escalating global concerns.

Although negative experiences may have been at the forefront of many family members' minds during crisis, they may have also found moments of light—even small moments—such as the relief experienced during the pandemic from no more clothing conflicts while getting ready for school or such as those helpless moments when a teen shouted, "I have nothing to wear." Moreover, the chance to sleep later, more family meals together, and opportunities for family members to take walks or spend time together offered some positive light to these disruptive years. Through Sensorimotor Psychotherapy we can help families increase their resilience and pivot toward equanimity so they can hold both the negative and positive aspects of their experiences. Sensorimotor Psychotherapy can move family members toward solidarity through their collective loss, grief, uncertainty, anxiety, sense of claustrophobia, and so on, as they each breakthrough an existential sense of aloneness. As therapists, we are the bridge that can help, even in the most unimaginable times, by lighting a pathway to hope as we remain open to our clients and their family members, meeting them in whatever state they currently find themselves.

As an example, I'll describe the case of a child I'll call Terry, age 7, who like most young children looked for other people to regulate their emotions, yet their drug-addicted mother was unavailable, and over time, Terry's method for regulating their own emotions became dissociation. Additionally, Terry's grandmother stepped in to raise them when their mother was serving a jail sentence for her part in a domestic squabble that involved hitting Terry's father with a bat. The grandmother adhered to their family creed of "letting the infant cry," which was inspired by the well-known recommendations of Richard Ferber and Benjamin Spock and passed down through generations in their family. Hence, as their attachment cries went unmet, there was no secure base Terry could come home to. Terry had little awareness of their own emotions and struggled with a range of issues including those of identity and gender fluidity, and relational challenges. Terry became so accustomed to holding things in and being tightly wound and rigid that they were unable to ever feel comfortable or at ease or draw on resilience in the face of crisis.

After traditional "talk" therapy had proved unhelpful, Terry came to individual Sensorimotor Psychotherapy with the presenting issue of anxiety which escalated during the forced isolation during the COVID-19 pandemic. Terry's somatic responses during our online sessions opened a door, ever so slightly, allowing them to see how their "shutdown," or dissociation, served as an adaptive strategy. Contact statements such as "Sounds like you don't want to open any door that you don't feel you can walk through" slowly forged a relationship on which Terry could widen their window of tolerance/ window of optimum arousal. Terry was able to recall the adaptive style of surviving horrific early experiences—"checking out," a sensation they described as an overarching feeling of "just not being there" for their life. It was a different sensation than trying to be small, which they also experienced. Checking out morphed into disappearing and being invisible, a shift that happened beneath their awareness much of the time. This had become Terry's patterned response and served as their defense against rejection and criticism.

The overarching beneficial effects of encountering novel, new experiences (which often eluded our clients through month after month of social distancing) are linked to satisfaction and a sense of aliveness, passion, and joy (Goldstein & Siegel, 2017). Changes in our environment were harder to make when family members were required to stay at home; however, even small changes (e.g., taking a walk, shifts occurring in their home) that introduced variability were linked to positive emotional states and are correlated with enhanced well-being: "While increased physical activity and social interaction afforded by enriched environments facilitate positive behavioral outcomes, environmental activity alone is sufficient to produce many benefits of enrichment" (Heller et al., 2020, p. 800).

With this in mind, I worked with Terry to introduce novel experiences, starting with something as simple as coming out of their room and spending more time in other parts of the house or garden each day. In addition to encouraging novel experiences, Sensorimotor Psychotherapists can identify somatic mechanisms to modulate arousal in order to build resilience. The ability to self-regulate is widely recognized as an important strategy for treating traumatic stress in children and adolescents (Blaustein & Kinniburgh, 2018). Somatic strategies, including grounding exercises, can be introduced to enhance self-regulation and calming (Ogden & Fisher, 2015). Together, Terry and I shifted our body posture, each of us placing our feet firmly on the ground beneath us. Tensing and releasing the muscles in our arms, legs, and torso, we then brought our attention to these shifts in posture and to the somatic effects (e.g., the parts of our body where we held stress and tension). Through further collaboration, aimed at stress reduction, we found ways to experience calm and center ourselves through these body-based exercises, and then worked together as new insights, memories, and thoughts came forth.

Globally, our awareness of the fragility of the Earth has grown in recent years, and grounding exercises can serve as a reminder to all of us to connect with our immediate environment on a regular basis. Because many clients of all ages find being outdoors somewhat grounding, therapists can develop this as a resource for families. For example, noticing the seasons as they shift (e.g., appreciation for the autumn leaves, the first rain or snow, the phases of the moon, the physical contact of our body with the earth) invites the possibility of spiritual resources (e.g., nature, taking part in the seasonal shifts) for families as they reconnect with the universality of being connected to something larger than themselves.

In the therapeutic milieu, co-creating with family members an environment of experimentation and concomitantly fostering an openness to the experience can lead to an emergent experience through which family members feel more deeply connected. For a grounding exercise that included focusing on a tree, Terry mentally conjured up an image of themself as a tree, planted solidly in the earth, with legs like roots. This image offered strength and resilience whenever the winds of adversity arose (e.g., family conflict, peer challenges, and self-doubt). Terry reported feeling a surge of energy while doing this grounding exercise, so we extended the concept, encouraging them to take walks in their neighborhood. They mentioned a eucalyptus tree outside their apartment. We came to refer to it as their grounding tree, which they returned to often (in their mind and in person). Terry would touch the trunk, notice myriad variations in the bark and how the color changed at different times of day, and embrace the natural desire to physically connect with the earth's healing energy. Most importantly, I followed Terry's lead when we were working together, using qualifiers while contacting their implicit experience during our sessions in order to propel curiosity and invite collaboration (e.g., statements such as "I'm making a guess," "I'm possibly wrong," "I'm wanting your feedback," etc.). This lets our clients know that they have the option to fine-tune or select a better word or meaning.

Revisiting Boundaries

Helping co-create consistency at home, knowing that children thrive on regularity especially in distressing or irregular circumstances, family therapy can explore ways to enforce schedules while still establishing boundaries. Of course, there is a wide range of responses to boundaries (e.g., some family members feel protected and safer while others may feel trapped or constricted by boundaries). Sensorimotor Psychotherapy family therapy aims to illustrate the understanding of how each member somatically responds to situations, and can guide families through the exercise of physicalizing (e.g., by using scarves, jump ropes, pillows, space in the room and between family members) so that each person can establish individual, separate circles that represent boundaries. Looking for the somatic markers of tension or stress in the body (shoulders tight, head down, eye gaze toward ground, etc.), we can elucidate that tension is often a precursor to movement that wants to happen. Aiming to evoke curiosity, the therapist can say, "I notice your body shifted when we discussed some of the boundaries in your home… let's see if something wants to happen right now," while watching with curiosity what transpires in the moment, we're bringing attention to the body. This curiosity is an invitation both for the therapist and also the client and family members to slowly observe, together creating an opening for possible thoughts and feelings along with ensuing movements, which can be further explored in the session. The words "Let's see if something wants to happen right now" bring our attention to the present moment in the session.

Here we will consider a case illustrating how to pull together various Sensorimotor Psychotherapy skills available in family treatment and underscoring ways to address boundary setting and respecting of set boundaries. In one session, I worked with a single mother of three children through an exercise of physicalizing aimed to establish individual, separate circles that represented boundaries and that would help her family address the chaos and conflict in their home. I offered the family a box of long yoga straps, inviting everyone to select their own straps and extend the lengths by tying the ends of several together. All were encouraged to create circles around themselves that represented boundaries. The mother created a very small circle while her teens each made large circles, leaving very little space in the room.

When I pointed out that the mother had the tiniest circle, she said, "Yup, this is how I feel. There is a mess everywhere, and I feel suffocated in this circle and in this family." She became more aware of her emotions through this somatic experience, starting to tear up, and dropped her head, saying, "No, I'm not going to let it get to me!" Encouraging her to stay with the emotion that was emerging while also gently guiding her to notice what was transpiring in her body, we created a space where tears could flow; as she identified tightness in her chest and an overall sense of heaviness, she started to recognize how much of her energy had been spent "doing, creating, cooking, and serving others." Her sense of depletion was palpable. She was able to identify the message she gave herself: "I must be everything to everyone." This exercise propelled small shifts, for the caregiver's sake and for the sake of her family members, and she realized that she was complicit in the chaos at home. For example, she had dropped all expectations of her teens because she was overwhelmed by all their complaints and the overarching anxiety in the house. Throughout this session, as we physicalized her felt experience (the day-to-day sense of dread and chaos in the household), she began to shift, identifying for herself that maintaining family expectations (e.g., chores, homework) was not only important but also conveyed the message that their family was resilient and had continuity.

We worked to help her find equanimity, which she defined as an ability to maintain mental and emotional calm and balance—especially under stress—and an openness to experiences without being lost in reaction. She realized that she was demanding that the family remain "just fine" even as the aftermath of the pandemic's many months of homestay had an adverse impact on her teens' well-being (e.g., behind in school academically, social awkwardness returning to campus, resistance to engage in school activities, generalized anxiety).

As this mother expressed to her children the hopes that they could stay connected with one another, a range of responses ensued as the teens sat in their very large, disparate circles formulated with the yoga ropes. There was a discussion on the way the family used the space in the large room, with each child in their own very large, albeit separate circle, while the mother sat in her tiny circle. She stated, "This way, there's less likeliness that conflict will erupt." A very telling comment, as the mother was then able to express her response to conflict (e.g., when conflict started, she would feel light-headed, as though she were spacing out or dissociating). Linking this to her childhood experiences, the mother was better able to understand how this well-worn pattern from her childhood in her volatile household now accompanied her as an adult in her family, work, and relational experiences. We worked together to identify the many "parts" of her experience (i.e., one part felt she needed to flee; another started to shut down or freeze; yet another felt she "should" stand up and fight).

Through this boundary exercise and many others described in Ogden and Fisher's handbook on Sensorimotor Psychotherapy (2015), the mother came to understand how her responses, including the features of disassociation, served her safety and survival needs, as these patterned responses helped her survive the most intolerable situations. She came to see the adverse impact on her teens and her family's well-being. As the mother started to differentiate between the current negative encounters with her family members and her adverse childhood experience, I offered her tools and resources to combat her propensity to, in her words, "check out." Initially, as we worked together on themes of family conflict and dissociative moments manifested during our sessions, we worked in the present moment, using short breath exercises (i.e., noticing as her breath came in and out, gently exhaling longer than the inhale so that her sympathetic nervous system had a chance to regain calm (Porges & Porges, 2023). In the situation described above, the mother was able to stay present in the family discussion as she sat in her circle, following her breathing as it brought her back to the present moment.

Concomitant to describing both her adverse early childhood experiences and her current feelings of overwhelm the mother started to feel more grounded and more resilient. I added grounding exercises similar to the ones discussed earlier in this chapter, in order to deepen her experience of returning to the present (i.e., pushing her bare feet into the floor and noticing her toes as they pushed into the fuzz of the carpet, the solidness of her heels grounding into the floor, and the impact of this grounding on her spinal alignment). For example, during these grounding exercises, she exclaimed in a playful voice, "I'm a tree, grounded into the earth, held by nature's past and carried into the future." As she said this, her face broke into a huge smile, and she sat tall and appeared powerful and balanced. We came to call these experiences her "equanimity moments." She and her three children—also the focus of attention at varying times throughout our session—played with the emerging family dynamics; the mother grew more comfortable recognizing and holding true to what was happening within herself amid the family discussion, and grew more able to remain calm and, in her own words, "firm like the image of the tree, grounded in the earth."

Exploring the aftermath of this successful exercise, homework exercises were co-created (e.g., she started by embodying this "tree" stance during quiet, uneventful moments a few times a day). Eventually, she found ways to remind herself to recreate the embodied strength and solidarity of the tree even during especially trying moments in her household. On some days when it felt difficult to remember to use these homework exercises, she proposed placing notes judiciously throughout her house to serve as reminders without sharing the purpose of the notes with her children because she felt that keeping their purpose secret served to empower her. However, in moments of family conflict, she would gaze at or orient toward the notes. This proved so successful that we added another element: the placement of the notes. Since it was noted that the mother's posture was often somewhat hunched over and her eyes gazed downward, we discussed relocating the notes higher on her walls. This way, she would raise her gaze and her body would follow, causing her stance to straighten and making her appear to others as more empowered. She reported, "My eyes led my whole body." She used the word "pride" on more than one occasion to express how she felt as she shifted her posture to a more elongated stance. Over time, we coupled the "tree of equanimity and balance" with her "pride tree," words and images that served as a foundation that allowed her to remain in conflict-laden encounters with family members and feel resilient during trying moments in her household. We continued to co-create small homework assignments she could do, such as embodying an empowering stance in uneventful moments a few times a day; reminding herself to use this exercise as an aid to stay present despite the inevitable conflicts and troubles of the times; and writing the notes she wrote herself on colorful Post-its instead to add a small element of novelty and variety to the exercise.

Conclusion

A Sensorimotor Psychotherapy lens can propel the reformation of goals and objectives with family members, including co-creating and expanding on experiences which foster hope. Of course, despite our best intentions, as old wounds come to light in the therapeutic milieu, one or more family members may become upset or feel triggered by the interactions transpiring during the family session. Ruptures will arise, and may be more likely to happen in times of worldwide trauma (e.g., feelings of uncertainty, worries about the economy, and illness) or human trauma (e.g., racial conflict and protests). Therapeutic challenges and enactments may occur especially with clients who have had early trauma (e.g., dissociative disorders and other co-morbidities). Along with addressing the presenting issues that brought the family members to therapy, Sensorimotor Psychotherapy family work aims to help family members learn to communicate and foster greater resilience during uncomfortable moments. Concomitantly, we aim to move families toward solidarity with a greater understanding of collective loss, grief, and the aftermath of sorrow (e.g., elucidating the wide range of different responses to the same situations, encouraging understanding, and through psychoeducation give permission for these differences). Overarching objectives of effecting positive change include inviting family members to notice their internal experience; to develop awareness of their bodily sensations, movements, perceptions, and cognitions; to learn new ways to communicate while fostering understanding; and to share insights that emerge throughout the session. Through self-reflection (often by identifying repetitive and unhelpful ways of perceiving experiences and behaviors), family members can revisit old behaviors and beliefs with new emotional responses, with a reframe aimed at developing expanded ways of being with one another. By helping family members become connected to the wisdom of the body and to appreciate the body's innate intelligence, we shift the verbal narrative during family therapy from primarily dialogue and cognitive tasks toward an exploration of present-moment awareness and increased understanding of rapid body-to-body nonverbal communication. As family members engage with one another in new ways, new possibilities emerge for expanded awareness of the body as a source of important insight and information. Family therapy co-creates with families the opportunities for shifts through a treatment paradigm that maximizes the possibility of members collaboratively taking their next steps toward self-regulation, enhanced communication, mutual understanding, and healing.

References

Aron, E., & Hewitt, C. (2023). *The highly sensitive child: Helping our children thrive when the world overwhelms them.* Harmony Books.

Blaustein, M. E., & Kinniburgh, K. M. (2018). *Treating traumatic stress in children and adolescents: How to foster resilience through attachment, self-regulation, and competency.* Guilford Press.

Bowen, M. (1993). *Family therapy in clinical practice.* Jason Aronson.

Burt, C., Lei, M. K., & Simons, R. (2017). Racial discrimination, racial socialization, and crime: Understanding mechanisms of resilience. *Social Problems, 64*(3), 414–438. https://doi.org/10.1093/socpro/spw036

Denckla, C. A., Cicchetti, D., Kubzansky, L. D., Seedat, S., Teicher, M. H., Williams, D. R., & Koenen, K. C. (2020). Psychological resilience: An update on definitions, a critical appraisal, and research recommendations. *European Journal of Psychotraumatology, 11*(1), Article 1822064. https://doi.org/10.1080/20008198.2020.1822064

Erolin, K. S., & Wieling, E. (2021, January). The experiences of couple/marriage and family therapists of color: A survey analysis. *Journal of Marital and Family Therapy, 47*(1), 3–20. https://doi.org/10.1111/jmft.12456

Fisher, J. (2017) *Healing the fragmented selves of trauma survivors; overcoming internal self-alienation.* Routledge.

Goldstein, B., & Ogden, P. (2016). Playing with possibilities: Sensorimotor Psychotherapy with younger clients in individual, family and group psychotherapy. In S. Hart (Ed.), *Inclusion, play and empathy neuroaffective development in children's groups* (pp. 228–249). Jessica Kingsley.

Goldstein, B., & Siegel, D. J. (2017). Feeling felt: Cocreating an emergent experience of connection, safety, and awareness in individual and group psychotherapy. In M. Solomon & D. J. Siegel (Eds.), *How people change: Relationships and neuroplasticity in psychotherapy* (pp. 275–289). W. W. Norton.

Heller, A. S., Shi, T. C., Ezie, C. E. C., Baez, L. M., Gibbons, C. J., & Hartley, C. A. (2020). Association between real-world experiential diversity and positive affect relates to hippocampal–striatal functional connectivity. *Nature Neuroscience, 23*, 800–804. https://doi.org/10.1038/s41593-020-0636-4

Hostinar, C. E., & Miller, G. E. (2019). Protective factors for youth confronting economic hardship: Current challenges and future avenues in resilience research. *American Psychologist, 74*(6), 641–652. https://doi.org/10.1037/amp0000520

Kabat-Zinn, J. (1990/2013). *Full catastrophe living: Using the wisdom of your body and mind to face stress, pain and illness* (Revised ed.). Random House.

Kelly, S., Jérémie-Brink, G., Chambers, A. L., & Smith-Bynum, M. A. (2020). The Black Lives Matter movement: A call to action for couple and family therapists. *Family Process, 59*, 1374–1388. https://doi.org/10.1111/famp.12614

Laszloffy, T. A., & Hardy, K. V. (2000). Uncommon strategies for a common problem: Addressing racism in family therapy. *Family Process, 39*(1), 35–50. https://doi.org/10.1111/J.1545-5300.2000.39106.X

McDowell, T., Knudson-Martin, C., & Bermudez, J. M. (2017). *Socioculturally attuned family therapy: Guidelines for equitable theory and practice*. Routledge.

McGoldrick, M., & Hardy, K. V. (Eds.). (2019). *Re-visioning family therapy*. Guilford Press.

Mills-Koonce, W. R., Rehder, P. D., & McCurdy, A. L. (2018). The significance of parenting and parent-child relationships for sexual and gender minority adolescents. *Journal of Research on Adolescence, 28*(3), 637–649. https://doi.org/10.1111/jora.12404

Minuchin, S., & Fishman, C. H. (1981). *Family therapy techniques*. Harvard University Press.

Ogden, P. Goldstein. B. Fisher, J. (2012) Brain-to-Brain, Body-to-Body: A Sensorimotor Psychotherapy Perspective on the Treatment of Children and Adolescents. In Longo, Bergman, Creeden and Prescott (Eds.), *Current Perspectives and Applications in Neurobiology; Working with Young Persons who are Victims and Perpetrators of Sexual Abuse*.

Ogden, P., & Fisher, J. (2015). *Sensorimotor Psychotherapy: Interventions for trauma and attachment*. W. W. Norton.

Ogden, P., & Goldstein, B. (2017). Embedded Relational Mindfulness (ERM)© in child and adolescent treatment: A sensorimotor psychotherapy perspective. In K. Buckwalter & D. Reed (Eds.), *Attachment theory in action, building connections between children and parents* (pp. 65–79). Lanham: Roman and Littlefield.

Ogden, P., & Goldstein, B. (2020). Being present: Philosophical and spiritual principles to guide practice. In D. Siegel & M. Solomon (Eds.), *Mind, consciousness and well-being* (186–232). W. W. Norton.

Ogden, P., Minton, K., & Pain, C. (2006). *Trauma and the body: A sensorimotor approach to psychotherapy*. W. W. Norton.

Porges, S., & Porges, S. (2023). *Our polyvagal world: How safety and trauma change us*. W. W. Norton.

Raffaelli, M., Carlo, G., Carranza, M. A., & Gonzalez-Kruger, G. E. (2005). Understanding Latino children and adolescents in the mainstream: Placing culture at the center of developmental models. *New Directions in Child and Adolescent Development, Fall*(109), 23–32. https://doi.org/10.1002/cd.134

Satir, V. (1964). *Conjoint family therapy*. Science and Behavior Books.

Siegel, D. J. (2020). *The developing mind: How relationships and the brain interact to shape who we are* (3rd ed.). Guilford Press.

Stratton, P., & Low, D. C. (2020). Culturally sensitive measures of family therapy. In K. S. Wampler, M. Rastogi & R. Singh (Eds.). *The handbook of systemic family therapy* (pp. 77–101). https://doi.org/10.1002/9781119788409.ch4

van der Kolk, B. A. (2014). *The body keeps the score: Brain, mind, and body in the healing of trauma*. Viking Press.

Wade, M., Prime, H., & Browne, D. T. (2020). Why we need longitudinal mental health research with children and youth during (and after) the COVID-19 pandemic. *Psychiatry Research, 290*, Article 113143. https://doi.org/10.1016/j.psychres.2020.113143

Zeeman, L., Aranda, K., Sherriff, N., & Cocking, C. (2017). Promoting resilience and emotional well-being of transgender young people: Research at the intersections of gender and sexuality. *Journal of Youth Studies, 20*(3), 382–397. https://doi.org/10.1080/13676261.2016.1232481

23
SOMATIC EXPERIENCING®

Maggie Kline

Introduction

This chapter offers a view of complex trauma and dissociation through the synergistic lens of Somatic Experiencing (SE) and the Resilience Roadmap Model (Kline, 2020). SE untangles conditioned (overcoupled) channels of perception—namely, Sensations, Images, Body Behaviors, Affects, and Meanings (SIBAM®)—and recovers dissociated/frozen (undercoupled) elements that consolidate around traumatic experiences. The acronym SIBAM, used for this prototype, was developed by Dr. Peter A. Levine. The basics of SE safely and gently guide children back into their sensing, feeling bodies that hold both the symptoms and the key to their release. SE integrates whole-brain function by utilizing interoceptive, proprioceptive, and kinesthetic sensations. Attachment-focused SE during the early years includes dyadic completion of interruptions in the bonding process.

Four vignettes detail the SIBAM model with step-by-step illustrations. The first shows how Carlos's maternal abandonment manifests when he is a fifth grader whose freeze/dissociation and shame are misdiagnosed as oppositional defiant disorder. Another vignette illustrates how terror from an accident when he was three years old is so deeply embedded within an 11-year-old's psyche that it causes a split between his daytime and nighttime reality. Next, a summary of post-surgical toddler trauma treatment illustrates how SE, "Rescue Role Play," and dyadic completion hold promise for complex trauma and dissociation prevention by working with the shock *and* the reunification of mother and child. The final vignette demonstrates how the combination of SE with the Gingerbread Body Map (Levine & Kline, 2007) resolves school phobia and somatization of a sexually molested nine-year-old girl.

The Resilience Roadmap features tools for co-regulation and self-regulation. The first supports a secure attachment using the "Eight Essentials"; the second builds interoceptive intelligence, a self-regulation skill in SE built through play and drawing. Autonomic nervous system (ANS), sensory-motor, and relational completions are at the heart of addressing dissociation from episodic trauma and the integration of a shattered sense of self. A brief explanation of the polyvagal theory is given, with examples of research suggesting that childhood maltreatment dampens ventral vagal efficiency, highlighting the importance of early relational safety. A collection of child-friendly emBODY research studies from Finland, referenced later in this chapter, provides evidence that as interoceptive awareness increases, it significantly shapes the way children label, perceive, and interpret their emotions *and* their environment. Impairments in emotional awareness are associated with serious internalizing problems, such as depression, anxiety, alexithymia, and somatization. Games and activities that promote sensation awareness provide access to a core sense of self.

What Is Somatic Experiencing?

SE is an innovative, biopsychophysiological method of resolving and preventing symptoms of trauma and relieving stress. It was developed by Dr. Peter A. Levine from his studies of ethology, stress physiology, psychology, biology, neuroscience, medical biophysics, and indigenous healing practices. Levine teaches that while the magnitude of an event is an important factor, *it does not define trauma;* rather, trauma occurs and exists in its effect on the nervous system (Levine, 2015). He observed that animals in the wild have a natural ability to "shake off" the effects of a traumatic experience, whereas humans often get stuck in a state of hyper-arousal or dissociation. However, through clinical practice, Levine learned that we have this same innate ability to discharge high levels of arousal by evoking fight/flight mechanisms that had been overwhelmed, frozen, and/or dissociated. SE accesses these natural healing abilities through interoceptive awareness of implicit bodily defenses. It tracks polyvagal nervous system states and gently guides the completion of thwarted movements, resetting the ANS.

In attachment-focused SE, "trauma is not so much what happened to us but, rather, what we hold inside in the absence of an empathic, mutually connected witness" (Riordan et al., 2019, p. 59). When frightened, the child's nervous system is wired to first seek safety from a caregiver. If that approach is ineffective, the child might kick, scream, or bite in protest. If no one comforts the child, he shuts down. SE is a lens to assess where the physiology got stuck in the "orienting, readiness, flight, fight, freeze/dissociation, discharge, integration, social engagement" cycle. Without a release from heightened activation, fear can result in collapsed immobility. "When the dorsal (or 'reptilian') vagus is activated, dissociation follows. The metabolism is speedily shut down, heart rate drops rapidly, hiding behavior and passive withdrawal are initiated, and a hypo-aroused physical collapse may be triggered" (Schore, 2019b, p. 237). Because the degree of traumatization is directly related to the capacity and maturation of the nervous system, the youngest are the most vulnerable.

To avoid being stuck in the threat response cycle, the mobilized energy must be discharged, resetting the physiology and reestablishing homeostasis. If this energy is not fully released, the hippocampus imprints an easily triggered implicit procedural memory of the failed strategy. The lingering effects of an overwhelmed nervous system create the symptoms. Levine often says in his presentations and writing, "Trauma is a fact of life—but so is resilience." Resilience increases when challenges are met with courage and children can safely open to their sensations and emotions with adult support rather than remain shut down, depressed, hopeless, and/or dissociated.

Whether one witnesses a terrifying event such as an assault or a catastrophe, *or* directly experiences a medical procedure, playground bully, nearby explosion, or the urgency to evacuate a place, the shock is primarily *physiological* rather than psychological (Levine, 1997). With SE trauma first aid, long-term symptoms are preventable. This is in contrast to domestic violence, familial emotional abuse, neglect or assault, and/or intergenerational societal trauma. Abuse or scapegoating at home, school, or in society deeply affects children psychologically, as well as physiologically. When the threat comes from those who are supposed to love and nurture, there is a real dilemma causing disorganized attachment. This adds to the complexity because establishing safety and trust in relationships may be challenging. Safety is *not* a thought! It is an interoceptive, or sensory-based, experience of the body signaling that all is well. It represents much more than the absence of threat.

The Resilience Roadmap combines SE skills with the "Eight Essentials of Healthy Attachment" (Kline, 2020) to create a dyadic ventral state in which children can trust enough to gingerly explore their internal world. Using SIBAM, the SE therapist slowly assists in teasing apart the conditioned responses coupling immobility with fear. When trauma occurs preverbally, the default may be an implicit stimulus/response pattern of shutdown and freeze. The older child can be left with a pattern of braced hypervigilance alternating with shutdown and/or dissociation, accompanied by feelings of helplessness and hopelessness. If the primitive vagus nerve is repeatedly activated as the dominant protection for blocking out overwhelming stimuli and pain, then freeze/immobilization and dissociation become habituated. These are not coping skills that children learn. They are automatic survival mechanisms meant to be time-limited. But due to the evolution of our neocortex, our judging, shaming "higher" brain impedes the release of the survival energy crystallized around the traumatic past.

Complex Trauma and Dissociation through the Lens of Somatic Experiencing

Trauma leaves its mark on everyone, but infants, toddlers, and young children are the most vulnerable. Their growing brains and bodies are like sponges, absorbing implicit and explicit imprints through their senses. These imprints shape the anatomy and physiology of brain and body, beginning in utero. It is generally believed that complex trauma occurs in the years before the age of 5 (Perry, 2013). Terrifying early experiences are a blueprint for lifelong symptoms and dissociation because they disrupt the process of forming a secure attachment—the most critical protective factor for resiliency.

Stephen Porges developed the polyvagal theory, leading to our burgeoning understanding of the nervous system's evolutionary role in our survival (Porges, 2016, 2011). The brief description below will help readers navigate this chapter, as polyvagal concepts are woven into the warp and woof of SE practice. Polyvagal theory reveals that the ANS developed over millions of years in a hierarchical order. In recent mammalian history, we have *three*, not two, neural platforms that developed for evolutionary adaptation. Historically, the ANS has been described as having two branches: (1) *sympathetic*, responsible for a chain reaction of hormonal and chemical secretions to mobilize energy for movement, acting as the accelerator in fight/flight for emergencies; and (2) *parasympathetic*, responsible for inhibiting the activity of the sympathetic branch—that is, "the vagal brake"—and returning it to a resting state. The *parasympathetic* vagus, over time, divided into two branches, *dorsal* and *ventral,* with distinctly different functions. The primitive dorsal vagus induces a state of energy conservation, withdrawal, shutdown, freeze, and immobilization. The "smarter" component of the parasympathetic, cardioinhibitory ANS is the newest, myelinated vagal system. This system, as predicted by the polyvagal theory, develops last in the fetus, and continues functional development well into the first postnatal year (Porges & Furman, 2011). The ventral branch induces a state of safety and social engagement associated with a calm, relaxed body. The social engagement system (SES) is made up of the ventral vagal pathways together with four cranial nerves involved in facial expression, vocalization, and listening. When stimulated, the SES returns the ANS to a state of equilibrium for resting, socializing, cooperating, digesting food, learning, and loving.

According to the neuroaffective model, the infant's nervous system develops in three maturational phases that correspond to Paul MacLean's triune brain (1990). The reptilian brain is the first to develop; the second is the mammalian mid-brain circuitry; and the last to mature is the neocortex for thinking, reasoning, and socially connecting. Marianne Bentzen emphasizes that in understanding the sequential order of the maturation process, "there are steps in emotional development that we cannot skip or leave out." The brain's ability to *feel* precedes its capacity to *think,* and this order cannot be reversed (2019, p. 14). During the first stage of child development (trust vs. mistrust), it is imperative that the nervous system become tuned to safety—not danger and distrust. When frightened, the child's system sets off an autonomic response to seek safety by reaching toward, crawling, or running to their primary caregiver for comfort-seeking. This is a neuro-motor, survival imperative. The primary caregivers act as the ventral vagal soothing system for the unmyelinated infant's nervous system. Children must engage with a face–heart connection to allow for neuronal integration of the ANS until it is myelinated and can regulate itself.

Without a calming adult, the primitive dorsal vagus serves to reduce the pain with numbing endorphins instead of oxytocin, the neuropeptide that is the emotional adhesive for bonding. If the rupture in attachment continues, shutdown may become the default mode, replacing interpersonal neurobiological connectedness. Consistent co-regulation within a trusting, pleasurable dyadic relationship precedes self-regulation. Being soothed, cradled, and rocked within the safety and surrender of a secure attachment may be the most protective factor in the development of resilience.

The Relationship between Dissociation and Freeze/Immobility

A wide continuum of dissociative behaviors ranges from denial, spaciness, and attention deficit to more severe symptoms such as amnesia, psychosis, and identity confusion. Everyone can relate to scattered attention and diminished concentration on stressful days. Dissociation becomes a problem when it prevents access to our sentient feelings and emotions. Freeze (or tonic immobility) and dissociation are adaptive survival responses meant to be time-limited. They are related but different. While dissociation is commonly agreed among professionals to be a psychological process, the freeze/immobility response is physiological and is described as tonic immobility by ethologists. The latter is an unconscious automatic process deeply rooted in the brain stem.

With infants and young children, freeze is akin to a shutdown of the viscera to conserve energy and prepare for the eventuality of death. In an article on attachment-focused SE, Riordan et al. (2019) reported that

> more than any other traumatic state, the freeze response in all its forms—avoidance, passive aggression, depression, and disassociation—promotes relational disconnect and dyadic trauma. Freeze kindles significant neurochemical changes in the brain and shifts hedonic valences from attraction to repulsion. This leads to the loss of attachment bonds and social isolation.
>
> *(p. 83)*

When a young child lives in fear, the freeze response and dorsal activation become the default state. Later in life, with minimal stress or a minor trigger, the mind can go blank and cloud with shame.

There are many different forms of dissociation. The out-of-body, third-person perception (like the child as onlooker) is a common example of depersonalization. In the case of a high-velocity vehicular accident, dissociation can present as a perceptual distortion of time, as if everything is happening in slow motion, accompanied by emotional confusion and numbness. Not all children who freeze will dissociate, but it is quite common that freeze and dissociation go hand-in-hand. Robert Scaer (2001), a neurologist who specialized in the rehabilitative treatment of accident victims, wrote that "the freeze or immobility response itself very likely represents a type, or perhaps a part, of dissociation." (p. 98).

Two lists below show how SE distinguishes the characteristics of each state (Levine & Kline, 2007):
When dissociation/shutdown predominate:
While some kids live in an agitated, restless state, others may live in a fog after an extreme event. When *dissociation* predominates, some or all of these symptoms may emerge:

- Distractibility and inattentiveness
- Amnesia and forgetfulness
- Reduced ability to organize and plan
- Depersonalization: feeling detached and not real, as if watching yourself from outside your body
- Derealization: feeling like the world around you is not real or that it is distorted

- Muted or diminished emotional responses, making relationships difficult
- Easily and frequently stressed out/low frustration tolerance
- Frequent daydreaming and/or fears of going crazy
- Low energy, easily fatigued/unmotivated
- Night terrors, with or without sleepwalking
- Excessive shyness with time spent in a fantasy world or with imaginary friends
- Identity confusion
- Disembodied, impotent rage

Constriction, freeze, and immobility are closely related and grouped for simplicity. The listed symptoms may emerge over time. These may be in addition to or alternating with dissociation and hyper-arousal.

When constriction, freeze, and/or immobility predominate:

- Altered sense of time and space like in a dream
- Feeling numb or detached from the body
- Headaches and stomachaches
- Spastic colon, asthma, digestive problems, or diminished appetite
- Feelings and behaviors of helplessness and hopelessness
- Feelings of shame and guilt
- Feeling like you can't move, speak; sense of annihilation
- Avoidance behavior/withdrawal and depression
- Diminished curiosity and capacity for pleasure
- Postural and coordination problems
- Low energy/fatigue/unmotivated/failure to complete schoolwork
- Clinginess/regression to younger behaviors
- Repetitive play
- Bed-wetting and soiling

Trauma and Memory: Explicit and Implicit Systems

There are basically two main memory systems: *explicit* and *implicit*. Declarative is an explicit subcategory referring to data recall such as birthdays, the soccer practice schedule, and math facts. Another subcategory, episodic memory, is colored by emotional feelings and tends toward storytelling—for example, feeling excitement decades later when recalling the first fish caught, or perhaps remembering the pride of feeling grown up but nervous when Mom let you walk to school alone. Although details of these memories may morph like shifting sands, words can describe them. Levine notes that despite exceptions, it is generally believed that episodic memories extend back to the age of 3½, when the hippocampus becomes functional for storing narratives (Levine, 2015).

Implicit memories, unlike explicit memories, are usually outside conscious awareness. The two broad subcategories are emotional and procedural. Rather than arising at will from the neocortex, they are organized around emotions or skills (procedures) like riding a bike. Together, these two types have a powerful, often automatic influence on the psyche and behavior of children. Levine stated, "Like bookmarks, emotions are charged signals that select a particular procedural memory out of a book of possible motor memories. They prompt organizing themes for action" (2015, p. 22). These emotional survival memories are experienced in the body as physical sensations.

Traumatic memories consist of dissociated fragments stored physiologically as body memories—they are implicit. In SE, we guide clients to access, track, and befriend interoceptive sensations.

These primarily arise from the smooth muscles or viscera (ANS) and the striated skeletal muscles, joints, and impulses for movement (sensory-motor system). Body awareness is key to releasing the energy bound in the traumatic memory. When overwhelming experiences occur, the imprints (called *engrams*) are emblazoned in a frozen state. They are made up of a myriad of images, physical sensations, emotions, impulses, and thoughts that crystalize into chronic patterns outside awareness. The SIBAM model facilitates retrieving the shattered self through the integrity of the body's wisdom. The elements of SIBAM that are beyond conscious experience are referred to as "undercoupled" or dissociated; and those elements that habitually arouse a threat response under non-threatening circumstances are referred to as "overcoupled."

These conditioned reflexes can be sympathetically driven impulses and muscular pre-movements that were impossible to execute due to age, strength, dependency, or limited motor skills. Earlier implicit memories may have "bookmarked" that shutdown is safer. In other words,

> these emotions had, in the past, evoked procedural memories, i.e., survival-based fixed action patterns. While some may signal successful strategies, in the case of trauma, they were tragically unsuccessful and often default to freeze. Such maladaptive, habitual reactions leave the individual entangled in unresolved emotional angst, disembodiment, and confusion.
>
> *(Levine, 2015, p. 23)*

Trauma leaves implicit body memories without an explicit narrative. Because SE works directly with implicit memories, it's effective for episodic *and* complex trauma.

Using the SIBAM Model to Access Dissociated Implicit Memory

In SE, awareness of the various nervous system states helps clients renegotiate the fragmented elements that make up the gestalt of an experience. Levine coined this process SIBAM. *S* represents Sensations. *I* represents Images—visual, auditory, tactile, gustatory, or olfactory, and also metaphorical. *B* is for Body Behaviors, *A* for Affect, and *M* for Meaning. Briefly, behaviors include gestures, movements, facial expressions, and the like. Affect includes emotions, moods, and the "felt sense," an expression coined by Eugene Gendlin in his book detailing the Focusing process (1982). Meaning can be thoughts, beliefs, or judgments that are consolidated in traumatic memory.

Sensations and images are used to safely guide a dissociated child back into their body by *following* the child's body language. Triggering associations—like those experienced by Carlos, whose story is below—don't go away by *talking*. Once it's understood that the traumatized brain has a *distinctly different* physiology from a non-traumatized brain, it becomes clear why cognitive-behavior therapy (top down) is inadequate for a child driven by the "survival alarm" (bottom up) of trauma. When fear activation is not fully released, it imprints a highly charged amygdala; while, *implicit procedural memory* is primarily stored in the cerebellum and basal ganglia. The trick is to work with both the conscious triggers and the unconscious/dissociated associations that are bound up in strong, instinctual, defensive behaviors, such as going blank, postural collapse from shame, refusal to work, withdrawal, and hiding, like Carlos.

Carlos's Story: An "Oppositional Defiant" Ten-Year-Old Fifth Grader

Carlos was failing math and in trouble at school three out of five days for disruptive behavior. His refusal to work was punctuated by angry outbursts. With the slightest pressure, he became defiant. His teacher suggested that Carlos had ADHD because he would "get up and bolt out of class and hide."

He alternated between a blank spaciness (dorsal vagal) and angry flight behavior (sympathetic fight/flight), displaying oppositionality to escape the helpless feelings of shutting down.

Carlos was abandoned by his mother, whose whereabouts were unknown. His abusive teenaged brother, a gang member, was in charge of Carlos after kindergarten. His father worked long hours and was unavailable to meet. The extent of therapy possible in a school setting is restricted. However, the principles of SE were used successfully: safety, containment, titration, pendulation between trauma vortex (traumatic activation) and counter-vortex (pleasurable activation), and SIBAM. To build trust, many of the "Eight Essentials of Healthy Attachment" (such as safety, soothing voice, laughter, and warm authentic smiles) were consciously used to engage one's SES for co-regulation. Also, consistent phone connection with a caring uncle was arranged.

Meeting Carlos

Carlos had bolted out of class. After searching, I found him hiding in a remote area of the playground. His head hung down as he told me that he hated math. Instead of asking, "What is it about math you hate?" I began a sensation-based process with him. His mood was cast in despair because "nothing ever changes." The mood-shifting process below helped Carlos discover his internal resources.

1. **Building safety:** Attuning to Carlos with empathy, rather than trying to talk him out of his feelings or extol the benefits of math, built trust. Listening and offering to explore his struggle helped relax him. Given paper to show his sensations, he drew as many butterflies as he could fit that were "flying around in his belly." After sharing, he said his belly had calmed down and he agreed to accept help.
2. **Working with Sensations, Images, and Affect from SIBAM:** Carlos imagined, upon invitation, that there was a math paper on his desk, and he was asked to describe what he noticed. He said his mind "just goes blank; there's a wall that comes up." Asked to describe the sensations of the wall, he said, "Like a paper shredder in my head above my left temple."
3. **Pendulation, Titration, and Developing Resources in the Counter-Vortex:** Carlos said he couldn't remember ever liking math. When I challenged him to take time, no matter how far back he had to stretch, he finally looked up, made eye contact, and said he remembered when his first-grade teacher was teaching regrouping in addition; the class didn't understand. Carlos didn't either, until the second demonstration. When his best friend, Oscar, didn't get it, Carlos's teacher asked Carlos to show him. As he shared the good feelings of teaching his friend, he lit up with a grin from ear to ear.
4. **Reinforcing Positive Shifts in Body Behavior from SIBAM:** Carlos's shift in posture from shame to pride was quite remarkable. His spine elongated and his chest expanded. His smile was radiant. When asked what he felt, he replied, "Warm, with only one or two butterflies left in my belly." What a dramatic difference from his slumped position. (*Note:* Levine calls this organismic shift from contraction [freeze] to expansion [opposite] "pendulation." Slowing down allows time for integration of the new experience of expansion [counter-vortex].)

After a gentle invitation, Carlos revisited the image and sensation of the "paper shredder" (trauma vortex), which now looked like a square. As he focused on its size and shape, a long-forgotten "bad experience" surfaced (undercoupled or dissociated). He recalled his brother, who was supposed to help him with kindergarten math, becoming abusive. Carlos described him as mean and violent. He blasted Carlos verbally (and possibly physically) for needing help, calling him stupid, and became enraged that he had to babysit.

Tears streamed down Carlos's face, his head slumped over, and his torso collapsed in shame. As we sat together through this painful experience, he released more tears (discharge). He slowly sat up, made eye contact, and took my outstretched hands for comfort. (*Note:* kind eyes, nurturing touch, attunement, rhythm, and synchronicity are five of the "Eight Essentials.") Carlos remembered hating math after that. But he had an "aha" moment that shifted the "M" in the SIBAM from "I'm stupid in math; my mind goes blank" to a new meaning: "I can do math; my brother was stupid for hurting me."

Carlos again focused on the square blank in his head. With his tears released, and a co-regulating, empathetic adult reassuring his safety now (brother left home), the painful image shrank to a tiny grain of sand. Next, he imagined working a hard math problem. Again, the wall came up. This time, when he looked at the wall, he saw black. When asked for an opposite image, Carlos saw himself punching (a defense against meanness) through the wall to get to the other side—the opposite of feeling humiliation. He was given a little resistance so he could feel his muscles pushing his brother away. Within 30 seconds, he saw himself on the other side of the wall.

Carlos had felt shame since kindergarten. Until released, the repressed implicit memory of humiliation had remained locked in his posture and psyche, shaping his beliefs and eroding his confidence. Carlos's painful dissociated memories lost their grip once all the elements of his experience became conscious and released. Giving Carlos a pleasant experience provided him with new resources. Elaborating on helping Oscar increased his budding confidence, and he pronounced, "I feel happy and proud." As he located the physical sensations, he pointed to his chest, exclaiming, "It's warm around my heart. It feels like I just fell into a little hole of happiness!" Carlos's facial expression grew into a broad glowing smile as he said, "I'm ready to go back and do my math paper now!"

New neuronal pathways and synaptic connections are strengthened through *experiential* processes. New beliefs arise organically. Strong positive emotional experiences become imprinted. Witnessing and reflecting these moments profoundly change children's sense of self. The trick is to make sure that the *bodily sensations* (warmth around the heart and "falling into a little hole of happiness") underlying *emotions* (happiness and pride) are given time to be felt deeply and expressed.

Collaboration with Carlos's teacher regarding the "Eight Essentials" helped support healthy social engagement. With her support to take "time-in" for "mood shifting," Carlos began asking for help (ventral vagal) rather than going blank and bolting out the door (sympathetic) to hide in shame (dorsal vagal). With empathy from his teacher and uncle, Carlos experienced adult co-regulation. The shame and "defiance" ceased as his window of tolerance and confidence grew.

Part I of the Resilience Roadmap: Co-Regulation with the "Eight Essentials of Healthy Attachment"

When the child's environment fails to provide the safe and nurturing ingredients for a secure attachment, a major protective factor for resiliency is missing. This gap is physiological as well as emotional, heightening susceptibility to future traumatization. The need for safety, affection, and playfulness remains throughout life. If missed during the early years, social-emotional growth requires age-appropriate supplementation. For activities to accompany each of the following "Eight Essentials," please refer to *Brain-Changing Strategies to Trauma-Proof Our Schools: A Heart-Centered Movement to Wire Well-Being* (Kline, 2020).

1. **Safety, containment, and warmth.** Transmitted nonverbally through an adult's co-regulating presence, a calm nervous system with relaxed muscles helps children settle and feel safe. Wrapping a blanket around the back and upper arms for containment; holding; rocking; using weighted blankets; bilateral tapping of upper arms as a butterfly self-hug; etc., are nonverbal ways to help calm a child.

2. **Soft mutual eye-gazing for infants; soft kind eyes for children**. Words are powerful, but nonverbal cues "speak" louder. Adults can calm children and shape a relaxed nervous system through the quality of their presence. A kind face, warm smile, and a ventral state relaxes a tense, frightened child. Via consistent repetition within the adult's heart field, the child's nervous system "learns" self-soothing.
3. **Shared intention, attention, and focus**. Awareness of body language is key. This intimate attunement is a process experienced as a desire to learn the wishes, intentions, and energetic rhythms in dyadic synchrony or somatic resonance. When misattunement happens, it should be quickly repaired to restore safety and trust.
4. **Skin-to-skin molding for infants; safe nurturing touch for children**. Nurturing touch can transmit a sense of safety via the face–heart electromagnetic field. An adult can soothe a child through holding, rocking, hugging, cuddling; hair brushing, stroking, or braiding; gentle massage, supportive touch of the head, back, shoulders, or feet; and high-fives and contact games such as hand-clapping and piggyback rides. If touch is inappropriate, plush toys, furry pets, comfy cushions, and beanbag chairs help.
5. **Sweet, soothing sounds and rhythmic movement for all ages**. Rocking; using a soft, soothing voice; music; chanting; drumming; rattles and other percussive instruments; hammocks; dancing; and swings all help calm the nervous system. The tone, pace, and rhythm are key. Singing and humming to or with children while moving, dancing, or resting can be a mighty healing force for experiencing the joy of connection.
6. **Synchronized movement and facial gestures for all ages**. Spontaneous silly games and mirroring activities such as funny expressions or introducing the element of surprise, such as following a child's drumming pattern with a simple beat and then suddenly changing the speed or rhythm can trigger synchronization at first. However, the unexpected turn of events may cause mild, but pleasant, astonishment eliciting simultaneous bursting out with laughter and an increasingly enjoyable connection.
7. **Pleasure**. Smiles + Play + Laughter = fun for all ages. Play may be structured or spontaneous as long as it's fun; any variety of active and passive games from patty-cake to puppy piles; silliness for no reason. When sympathetic activation is pleasant, it uncouples the association that a rapid heartbeat always means danger. Dyadic play supports social engagement.
8. **Alternating between stimulating (sympathetic) and quiet activities (ventral vagal)**. For the little ones, "Itsy Bitsy Spider" or "Fox in a Box" can be stimulating; for school-age: chase and hide-and-seek games such as "The Wolf Comes at Midnight," and athletics and team sports such as ball play, relay races, rough-and-tumble, jump rope, juggling sticks, are arousing activities. Quiet debriefing and sharing afterward solidify body/mind integration. Ideas for quiet activities are coloring, story time, drawing the body map, meditation, yoga, and calming music.

In summary, the ventral pathways and cranial nerves for facial expression, vocalizing, and enervating the heart and lungs for down-regulating fear arousal make up the SES. Creating play activities using the Eight Essentials as ingredients stimulates the ventral pathways. These are the connections setting the stage for the relational field of "we" to develop.

> Transformation occurs when both parties reach a moment of joint attention where the child becomes aware that another person is aware of what the child is aware of within him/herself. This is 'the sacred moment,' a moment of meeting that involves a new degree of coherence in the child's experience of his or her attention to inner states as well as the external world.
>
> *(Winnicott, 1971)*

Night Terrors: Repercussions from Unrepaired Toddler Trauma

Repetitive night terrors are a symptom of complex trauma. There is debate on whether they are a dissociative process. In a study of 22 patients with night terrors, only six reported a trauma history (Hartman et al., 2001). In this author's opinion, this number is a gross underestimate due to common misconceptions regarding trauma's scope. Birth complications, early accidents, falls, and medical/surgical procedures are often overlooked as the source of symptoms. Though young children cannot narrate their terror, their bodies do, as Jason's story illustrates. His daytime and nighttime selves were diametrical opposites. During treatment, it became clear that his night terrors were dissociated fragments from a terrifying event at three years of age.

Jason's Story: 11-Year-Old with Mysterious Night Terrors and Sleepwalking

Jason was referred due to eight years of persistent night terrors. He was mystified about his family's concerns. He had total waking amnesia after every episode. Jason had no inkling of his aggressive verbal threats and thrashing movements that took two adults to contain. His parents were equally mystified by the origins of his adrenalized sleepwalking. Jason was popular, academically and athletically talented, and loved by his family and friends. This strong, handsome boy appeared to be and reported he was happy. Yet, at night he metamorphosed from a pre-pubescent Dr. Jekyll into a monster-like Mr. Hyde.

The suggestion of trauma was denied until Jason's medical history was queried. With probing and given a menu of possibilities including stitches, accidents, or emergency room trips, his mother recalled a horrific backyard accident involving jagged glass. The nighttime terrors began shortly afterward, but the link had not been made. Jason's nocturnal episodes became more frequent and terrifying as he got older and stronger. His sleepwalking personality was aggressive with threatening language—even expressing wanting to kill someone. Jason denied any need for help. He acted as if his family were making it all up as a joke. He had no awareness of his terrified crying, screams, or sleepwalking.

At his first session, Jason sketched his most recent nightmare (which, unlike the night terrors, he remembered vividly). His drawing of two ninja warriors chasing him around jagged rocks became the Image for SIBAM. Next, using Gestalt techniques with SE, Jason role-played the postural Behavior of the warrior's tall stance rather than being chased. When asked to describe his Sensations, he reported that his legs felt strong and he was ready for action. His neck turned as his eyes looked in anticipation of danger from something "coming around the corner." Jason was willing to return for another session despite being confused about why, because he felt "good," which is an Affect. The belief or Meaning was that his family had the problem, not him.

At the next session, Jason's mother reported another night terror that was qualitatively different. He cried out as usual, but when his mom shook his shoulders, "he came out of it." For the previous eight years, his eyes would open but he would be totally unresponsive. It had been impossible to wake him, making it "the scariest part." When Jason's father and brother described his sleepwalking behavior, he showed surprise (*A*) by his facial expression (*B*) that he was causing distress. After each of the other family members were guided to deactivate their stress, Jason was invited to share more about his drawing. He described the actions (*B*) of the ninja warriors from the previous session's drawing (*I*), which stimulated a titrated, manageable level of activation. Jason said one warrior "saw something coming from here" (*I*), pointing (*B*) to the jagged stone (*I*). Then Jason's father described his son's running into a horizontally placed broken mirror, his deep cut, and subsequent emergency room trip requiring stitches across his jugular vein so many years ago as a three-year old!

Cognitively, Jason couldn't relate (*M*–nothing happened), but his body did! He shuddered (*B*) and reported an "icky" (*S*) feeling. He was able to track his bodily sensations. This led to heavy (*S*) and numb (*S*) odd, hypoesthesia sensations that he described as a "3 inches tall and 3 fingers wide" area covering the faint scar on the skin over his jugular vein. (*B*) As he gently stroked his neck, he also noticed his breath getting quicker and shorter. The numb feeling (*S*) changed to throbbing (*S*) and then cooling (*S*) as sensations spread upward into his jaw. As Jason continued to notice changes, the throbbing (*S*) spread and became weaker. Returning to the ninja warriors in his dream (*I*) (who looked like doctors in blue scrubs), he described one coming around the corner as he rotated his neck (*B*) to look. He felt the impulse (*S*) to jump up and run (*B*), which he demonstrated. Jason detailed heavy, uncomfortable feelings (*S*) in his forearm. As he concentrated on these "weird" sensations, his wrists began spontaneously twitching (*B*). His fingers also flicked as if pushing something away (*B*). Suddenly, his shoulder and arm involuntarily lurched backward (*B*). (Perhaps this was a retraction (*B*) from the glass, or a reaction to immobilization from an IV or stitches.) The releases (*B*) continued in his hands and fingers for several minutes. When the spontaneous movements and twitching ceased, Jason began voluntarily opening and closing his hands because "they wanted to do something," so we did a bit of playful back-and-forth catch.

The numbness (*S*) in his neck and forearm transformed to watery sensations of fluidity (*S*), and the weird weak (*S*) feelings were replaced by sensations of strength (*S*), indicating dissolution of a partial freeze. Jason's drawing had a tiny yellow dot in the midst of a dark sky (*I*). While looking at the image, Jason gestured toward his whole body (*B*). He described the dot as a yellow light that felt like a golden shield (*S*) protecting him (*A*), and said "it felt like the light disintegrated the warriors." With a bright smile (*B*), he proudly exclaimed, "It felt cool!" (*A*). With the numbness and weakness (*S*) changing to fluidity and strength (*S*) and the light becoming a golden shield (*S* & *I*) of safety (*A*), the dissociated (undercoupled) nighttime terror coupled with impotent rage shifted from the old *Meaning* of being chased by "warriors" (*M*) to a triumphant *Meaning* of disintegrating the warriors (new *M*) with the light. Jason's eight years of persistent night terrors ceased.

Dissociation/Freeze Can Be Global or Partial

Tracking bodily sensations uncovers unresolved experiences. With few or no words to create a narrative, the terror is buried deep within the psyche. When stiches come out or the surgery is life-saving, everyone celebrates. They are unaware of the fragmentation in the child's psyche. Dissociation can occur in any nervous system state. It can be whole or partial, chronic or triggered by a specific implicit memory. For example, breaking an ankle can cause shock from the fall, affecting the vestibular system and causing partial dissociation. Trauma first aid can release the activation, restore equilibrium, and catalyze frozen reflexes. Without it, the child may be "braced" or "clumsy" due to lack of proprioceptive awareness and frozen reflexes. When children shut down globally, it's because the ANS has sensed a mortal life threat. The psychic response is to avoid the terror of annihilation. In either case, when dissociation/freeze occurs, there is a flooding of hormones in the brain, creating natural analgesics with varying degrees of altered states.

Using SE with Play Therapy to Prevent Post-Surgical Toddler Trauma

A basic premise of SE is that being in a state of terror *and* simultaneously immobilized is a recipe for trauma. A child who is maltreated cannot escape. Neither can a child restrained for a life-saving procedure. Because it is common practice to use restraints during medical treatment, universal use of trauma first aid could significantly reduce these repercussions. Separation from the primary attachment figure during such a frightening time can rupture the relationship. Attachment breach of the dyad disrupts secure connectedness, attunement, reciprocity, synchronicity, and love (Porges, 2016). If the traumatic attachment continues, the networks responsible for interpersonal neurobiological growth are compromised because the trauma is held in the interpersonal neurobiology *between* the pair rather than only in their individual nervous systems. Attunement stimulates the neural activity, providing the linkage to promote neurogenesis, synaptogenesis, and myelinogenesis with neural integration for both (Siegel, 2010). Without repair, the emergence of oppositional behaviors in either one of the pair has been postulated (Tronic, 2007).

According to the National Center for Health Statistics (2022), an estimated 10.5 million children aged zero to five years visited the emergency department in 2020, making hospital trauma ubiquitous—such as in the example of "Little Bill," who at 23 months was in a high state of chronic fear during medical procedures. After the procedures, his mother was unable to soothe him. Deactivating the threat response and re-establishing a secure heart–face connection (*dyadic completion*) are both vital (Riordan et al., 2017) to connect the lower brain circuitry with the prefrontal SES (Siegel, 2012). Attachment breach is a homeostatic disruption that may involve disintegration of neurological communication, leaving the primitive subcortical brain structures to hijack the interpersonal biological process of neurogenesis (Levine, 1997; Porges, 2011; Riordan, 2017; Siegel, 2012). Unfortunately, this steers a toddler's development to be dominated by the survival circuitry, rather than the SES.

In "Toddler Trauma: Somatic Experiencing, Attachment and the Neurophysiology of Dyadic Completion," Dr. Riordan illustrates step-by-step post-surgical trauma treatment using Rescue Role Play (Riordan et al., 2017). SE play therapy is fundamentally different from traumatic play or re-enactment. Modeling his work after Peter Levine's demonstration with Baby Jack and the dyadic completion with his mother (Levine, 2015), Dr. Riordan renegotiated 30-month-old Little Bill's *incomplete* autonomic survival "action plans" in a guided, titrated way following the toddler's pace and rhythms. Beginning with an unprepped doll, the progression slowly introduced more activating props such as Band-Aids and surgical instruments, which previously caused panic. In this way, Little Bill was able to "live his feelings through" by gradually and sequentially mastering his fear (Levine, 2015, p. 37).

Little Bill's sleep returned to normal, his biting ceased, his meltdown tantrums disappeared, and his oppositional behaviors normalized. After the fifth session, office sessions could be terminated and Rescue Role Play continued at home until Little Bill allowed his mother to apply Band-Aids. His trust in his mom as safe and their mother–child reconnection constituted a milestone representing dyadic completion. At three years old, Little Bill was admitted again to the hospital for surgery. His mother reported no overreaction, no overwhelm, and his willingness to have her remain with him. Completing an incomplete response with young children is as much about *running toward safety* (completing the neurobiological imperative of surrendering a relaxed body into warm, loving arms) as it is about *running away from danger*.

Part II of the Resilience Roadmap: Self-Regulation through Interoceptive Awareness

Interoceptive awareness may be foreign to children who dissociate; they may not even notice tense muscles, hunger, fullness, or thirst. Traumatized children may lack the biochemical mechanisms to develop enriching, emotionally meaningful relationships. Dr. Ruth Lanius and her colleagues (Bluhm et al., 2009) used fMRI scans to investigate differences in the "default networks" of people with histories of complex trauma from childhood abuse compared with those who had none. Their discoveries are illuminating. While at rest, the brain structures that cooperate to create a sense of self were active only in the trauma-free group. The scans of those with severe early childhood trauma showed almost no activity in the self-sensing brain areas. The insula, a brain structure that facilitates access to

Somatic Experiencing

sensations and emotions (Craig, 2009; Lamm & Singer, 2010), did not activate in *any* of the trauma survivors. According to Dan Siegel (2023), "our early relationships impact our emotional lives, our bodily experiences of regulating those emotions, our capacity for insight and empathy, and even our ability to reflect on the mind itself." A wholesome relationship with oneself is free of distortions and fragmentation. It is a body/mind integrated experience. The next section gives tools to help children develop interoceptive and emotional intelligence.

Safe Ways to Build Interoceptive Awareness and Empowerment

Grounding

Trauma uproots grounding. Children with complex trauma often live with their "head in the clouds," disconnected from their body. With sexual or physical assault, it is common for them to view themselves from outside themselves. Inhabiting the body can feel scary, especially if it was violated. Simple, fun grounding exercises can be used for safely exploring sensations. Please refer to *Trauma through a Child's Eyes* (Levine & Kline, 2007) or *Brain-Changing Strategies* (Kline, 2020) for activities such as "The Magic in Me—Become a Tree" through which children can imagine and feel their branches high and their feet low with roots reaching to the center of the earth. A simple way to assess embodiment is to ask: "Where are your feet?" If children glance down at their feet rather than sensing them, it's an indication that mind and body are separate; feet become an abstraction instead of a felt experience. To help children feel a sense of gravity, bring awareness slowly to ankles, toes, heels, and balls of the feet. This prompts a feeling of balance, well-being, and connection to the ground. It's a safe readiness step for exploration.

Sensation-Tracking Activities

Below are three ways to explore the brain/body connection. I teach kids to "be the boss of their own brains and bodies."

1 Drawing and coloring sensation/emotion body maps to track the body's reactions
2 Inviting exploration through mutual tracking in SE sessions using art and/or movement
3 Teaching ANS tracking of activation/deactivation cycles using physical games.

DRAWING AND COLORING SENSATION/EMOTION BODY MAPS TO TRACK BODY REACTIONS

Drawing is an easy and fruitful way for kids to express what words cannot. "The Gingerbread Person Body Map" is a specific, efficient, non-threatening strategy to access the body's story, befriend sensations and emotions, and evoke movement. Discovering physical sensations underlies emotional regulation. Damasio (1999) conceived "core consciousness" as the unadorned feeling of self. He theorized that the brain can't be conscious unless it represents not just objects, but also a primitive self. This primal self is pivotal. The skill of safely sensing, *in present consciousness*, the *past* survival impulses lying beneath freeze/dissociation is key to a self-observing consciousness.

Materials are simple: paper and a set of colored markers or crayons. A plain outline of a gingerbread person is ideal for locating where emotions *and* sensations are held. The body in the shape of a cookie encourages a wide spatial distribution of sensations especially to the viscera, limbs, neck, and face, where traumatic activation is held. Coloring bypasses thoughts and interpretations, freeing up safe access to the deep psyche. This sensory-motor act creates immediate contact with sensations, bringing conscious awareness of the body as the container for feelings. And it gives a quick assessment of the depth and location of the child's pain. If the drawing shows mostly unpleasant feelings, the child can be guided to notice, explore, and expand their undiscovered internal resources.

Using colors, size, shapes, or sketches, children exhibit their experience. Nervous kids typically draw squiggly lines, zigzags, or tiny butterflies. Coloring and sharing with a caring adult can quiet down the fear response. Held-back aggression often shows up as tension in the shoulders, arms, fists (for fighting or pushing), legs (for kicking), or jaw (for biting). By coloring and naming, for example, tightness in the shoulders, or drawing red and orange flames coming out of their sketch's mouth in the shape of a fire-breathing dragon's hot breath, the pent-up feelings can begin to dissolve—and so does the trauma, because trauma is held in the organs (ANS) and muscles (sensory-motor system) for fight and flight.

A matching color-coded key to label the newly discovered feelings is an integrating whole-brain experience. Finding words connects the upper and lower brain circuitry. If a child names only emotions, guide her to find sensations. For example, ask how she knows she feels scared or sad. It might be jitteriness in the stomach, a racing heart, or "like butterflies." If the fear became a stomachache, it might be "hard like a rock." Sadness might be described as heaviness, teary eyes, a lump in the throat, or a hurting heart.

Guidelines for body map drawings using colors, shapes, or pictures:

1 Include physical sensations and emotional feelings.
2 Include comfortable and uncomfortable feelings.
3 Include strengths and resources.
4 Make a color-coded key in the margin to match nonverbal sensations and emotions with labels. Example: blue = sadness/heavy heart.

The body map is a self-portrait of the ANS. Sometimes it shows the sensory-motor impulses to complete incomplete defensive responses. These can lead to empowering movements, such as pushing away and setting boundaries.

INVITING EXPLORATION THROUGH MUTUAL TRACKING IN SE SESSIONS WITH ART AND MOVEMENT

The body tells the story; just remember the ABCs—that is, **A**ll **B**ehavior = **C**ommunication. The body's narrative unfolds in an organized sequence of sensory-motor impulses. As children gain access to sensations from their own ANS and sensory-motor system, magic happens, as Krista's story illustrates. Her drawing facilitated organic movements, boundary-setting, release, and completion.

"Gingerbread Girl Body Map": Krista's Story

*Note: This is a composite case example of my typical school-age assault clients.

Krista was a nine-year-old fourth-grader who didn't want to attend school because she was "very scared all the time." When the teacher called on her to answer questions, she froze and went blank. Her nervousness was so unbearable that she feared vomiting in front of classmates. During her session, Krista pushed down hard on her marker as she intensely drew her tummy filled with swirly black squiggles. Her gingerbread cookie body map tells the story of her symptoms *and* her resources. It also illustrates her dissociation as mental fog and confusion impairing her concentration. The layered colors in Krista's abdomen (orange, red, and yellow underneath the black) are a telling example of how thwarted defensive actions contain the sympathetic fight/flight energy (anxious, jumpy, and angry) that had been repressed, causing bellyaches (Figure 23.1).

Somatic Experiencing

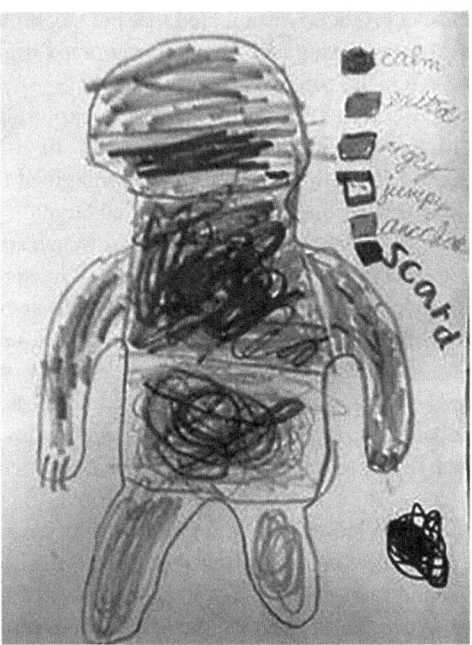

Figure 23.1 Nine-Year-Old Sexually Molested Girl.

Krista's Body Map Color Key
  Turquoise = Excited (to finally get help)
  Red = Angry (although red is colored in the square, only the tiniest bit shows in her belly)
  Yellow with **Orange** squiggles on top in belly and legs = Jumpy and Anxious
  Blue = Calm
  Black on shoulders and arms and layered on belly above yellow and orange = Scared and Tight
  Black Dot = Bellyache
  Gray upper head and face = Foggy and Confused
  (Krista forgot to draw gray in the color key but described herself as foggy, scared, and confused.)
  Examining Krista's drawing through an SE lens, it appears that she held a variety of states simultaneously. Her freeze showed up as her mind going blank and her head gray like the fog, with the scary, chaotic, frozen black tummy accompanying this sensation. Yet, underneath the black are the yellow and orange colors of her jumpy sensations and anxious emotions, showing sympathetic charge mobilizing for movement. The turquoise in her arms, hands, the lower half of her face, and the edges of her torso represented excitement. The substantial portion of darker blue represents calm. Krista reported being excited to meet. This provided a nice counter-balance to her discomfort. In SE, tracking sensations brings awareness to impulses, activated by the ANS, bringing energy to the limbs in preparation for self-defense. The orange and yellow in Krista's legs, labeled as jumpy and anxious, indicate the activation in her gut sending impulses into her legs for fight or flight. Krista drew a red box representing angry feelings, but colored a barely visible dot. She drew claws for hands. With sexual trauma, it is not unusual to have impulses to claw, scratch, and bite the offender because attacks elicit primal self-protective reflexes.
  Krista's drawing brought implicit memories of molestations by her teenaged stepbrother. Coloring and sharing with a safe witness appeared to relieve some distress. But her restless legs wanted to

"do something." Following the sympathetic energy with curiosity, it became clear they wanted to run away rather than face her abusive brother. Krista feared that her stepbrother might be released from jail. She wanted her stomach to stop hurting and the nervousness to disappear, giving her courage to stand tall and look him in the eye in the courtroom.

Beginning with grounding exercises, Krista was guided to explore the sensations in her ankle and toe joints and heels. With her feet firmly planted like roots, she became aware of her body in gravity. This gave a felt sense of strength in her legs as she imagined the anxious energy moving from her abdomen into her legs. The roiling in her belly settled but didn't stop. When Krista looked at the colors representing her jumpy legs, she felt immobilized. When sensations are frozen, images are invited. Krista was able to imagine kicking her stepbrother's hands until he stopped. A Pilates ball was held on the floor to give resistance. Krista was guided to sense her strength as she consciously organized movements from hip joints, flexed knees, ankles, and feet to slowly "kick" by pressing her feet hard to move the ball with fully extended legs. Slow, steady, firm, and purposeful pushing, alternating with pauses to sense the proprioceptive and kinesthetic feedback, gave Krista a new sense of self. Four repetitions, with resting between each, allowed the shaking and vibrations from the adrenalized activation to release, along with heat and deeper spontaneous breathing as her ANS reset.

Feeling empowered after these releases, Krista wanted help to prepare to be "strong in court." With her new courage, she was able to stand upright and rehearse what she wanted to voice. Her stomachaches, school phobia, and scary feelings dissolved. As energy from the frozen physiology is released, it doesn't disappear. When the ANS resets, the amygdala quiets, freeing the brain's electrochemical energy to support clear thinking. Krista was no longer confused or fearful that she would go blank or vomit at school.

Body Map Research of Emotion-Related Sensations

Finnish investigators studied the development of bodily sensations associated with happiness, anger, sadness, fear, disgust, and surprise in 6–17-year-olds. Data were acquired using a child-friendly paper-and-pencil version of the emBODY tool, showing that preschool and young school-aged children associate discrete patterns of bodily sensations with specific basic emotions (Nummenmaa et al., 2014). These interoceptive representations show rudimentary differentiation in preschool with increasing differentiation during development. Emotions are based on sensory, visceral, and kinesthetic sensations before children can verbally label them (Bucci, 1997). These investigators suggested that as interoceptive awareness increases, it significantly shapes the way children label, perceive, and interpret their emotions and environment. Impairments in emotional awareness were associated with more serious internalizing problems, such as depression, anxiety, and somatic complaints (Rieffe & De Rooij, 2012; Rieffe et al., 2010; van der Veek et al., 2012). The emBODY tool is seen to have significant potential in supporting and advancing the positive development of children's self-concept (Hietanen et al., 2016). This research supports principles of SE with its emphasis on interoceptive awareness and tracking sensations. It also affirms the successful empirical results using the "Gingerbread Body Map," which appeals to all ages and is an effective tool to access ANS states.

Teaching ANS Tracking of Activation/Deactivation Cycles Using Physical Games

Children stuck in freeze or who report feeling "nothing" need extra support to notice and locate sensations. Using active play and movement eases them into their bodies. When children are numb, fatigued, or depressed in a dorsal vagal state, movement is their medicine. Games such as tag, beanbag toss, relay races, ball play, parachute games, juggling sticks, jump rope, or even jumping jacks can shift a dorsal state to a pleasurable sympathetic state. Movement gets the heart pumping, lungs expanding, blood circulating, and is fun. It's a great way to teach kids to track activation/deactivation cycles and train the nervous system to settle.

To be effective in creating shifts, pause frequently so the kids can feel their heartbeat and breath, and their temperature as it changes. Tracking aerobic activity can rewire perceptions of terror due to faulty neuroception, a term coined by Stephen Porges to describe perceptual distortions (Porges, 2004). For example, traumatized children may implicitly associate their elevated heartbeat with danger. During the pause, they can experience this same sensation of their pumped heart but, instead, associate it with fun. Invite them to place a hand on their fast-beating heart to feel the sympathetic activation from playing. They continue tracking until heart and breath settle into a calm, ventral state. While resting, sensations of release may arise. Prepare children by teaching that shakiness, trembling, and other "nervous" sensations are extra energy to move limbs quickly to run, hide, or fight. They can show how and where the energy wants to move, like Krista did.

Remember to incorporate the "Eight Essentials." Using soft, kind eyes, a warm smile, and playfulness at the child's pace will help create safety and containment. In the rest phase, as the adult–child dyad calms down, feelings such as aliveness, tingling energy, warmth around the heart, stamina, strength, or stability in the limbs are likely to arise as a treasure chest of body-based resources become internalized. New sensations can be colored on a gingerbread-shaped "selfie" to reinforce them. If the child has difficulty locating positive sensations, offer extra support or nurturing touch (if appropriate) to locate feelings of safety, strength, comfort, warmth, openness, or calm relaxation. Gently orient the child to discover internal *and* external resources. This can include the face of the co-regulating adult, a pet, or something fascinating, beautiful, or calming nearby that shifts the focus from past to present.

Conclusion

Events that interrupt a child's early development, whether egregious or incidental, are a recipe for complex trauma, shutdown/freeze, and dissociation. In addition to using the principles of SE to release activation of the fight/flight/freeze trajectory, repair of attachment rupture between a child and the primary attachment figure (dyadic completion) is critical during the early years. This can prevent the long-term repercussions of limbic and ANS maturation that might otherwise produce "enduring neurobiological alterations that underlie right brain affective stability, inefficient stress tolerance, memory impairment, and dissociative disturbances" (Schore, 2019a, p. 51).

Levine, Porges, and others emphasize the importance of treating trauma from a biopsychosocial perspective (Dale et al., 2022). SE and the Resilience Roadmap, which includes the "Eight Essentials of Healthy Attachment," fit this specification. This synergistic combination also utilizes the Gingerbread Body Map to foster interoceptive intelligence through building sensation awareness. Impairments in emotional and interoceptive awareness have been associated with serious internalizing problems, such as depression, anxiety, alexithymia, and somatic complaints (Rieffe & De Rooij, 2012; Rieffe et al., 2010; van der Veek et al., 2012).

Investigative studies are recommended employing the emBODY tool as a pre- and post-assessment with children receiving trauma treatment using SE's biopsychophysiological approach with the Resilience Roadmap (combining co-regulation and self-regulation strategies). And, finally, SE first aid for infants, toddlers, and preschoolers that ensures dyadic completion holds promise for mitigating episodic trauma to prevent it from becoming complex with long-term symptoms.

References

Bentzen, M. (2019). *The neuroaffective picture book*. Jessica Kingsley Publishers.

Bluhm, R. L., Williamson, P. C., Osuch, E. A., Frewen, P. A., Stevens, T. K., Boksman, K., Neufeld, R.W. J., Théberge, J., & Lanius, R. A. (2009). Alterations in default network connectivity in posttraumatic stress disorder related to early-live trauma. *Journal of Psychiatry & Neuroscience, 34*(3), 187–194.

Bucci, W. (1997). Symptoms and symbols: A multiple code theory of somatization. *Psychoanalytic Inquiry, 17*(2), 151–172. https://doi.org/10.1080/07351699709534117

Craig, A. D. (Bud). (2009). How do you feel—now? The anterior insula and human awareness. *Nature Reviews Neuroscience, 10*(1), 59–70. https://doi.org/10.1038/nrn2555

Dale, L. P., Kolacz, J., Mazmanyan, J., Leon, K. G., Johonnot, K., Bossemeyer, B. N., & Porges, S. W. (2022). Childhood maltreatment influences autonomic regulation and mental health in college students. *Frontiers in Psychiatry, 13*, Article 841749. https://doi.org/10.3389/fpsyt.2022.841749

Damasio, A. (1999). *The feeling of what happens: Body and emotion in the making of consciousness*. Harcourt.

Gendlin, E. T. (1982). *Focusing*. Bantam Books.

Hartman, D., Crisp, A. H., Sedgwick, P., & Borrow, S. (2001). Is there a dissociative process in sleepwalking and night terrors? *Postgraduate Medical Journal, 77*(906), 244–249. https://doi.org/10.1136/pmj.77.906.244

Hietanen, J. K., Glerean, E., Hari, R., & Nummenmaa, L. (2016). Bodily maps of emotions across child development. *Developmental Science, 19*(6), 1111–1118. https://doi.org/10.1111/desc.12389

Kline, M. (2020). *Brain-changing strategies to trauma-proof our schools: A heart-centered movement for wiring well-being*. North Atlantic Books.

Lamm, C., & Singer, T. (2010). The role of anterior insular cortex in social emotions. *Brain Structure and Function, 214*(5–6), 579–591. https://doi.org/10.1007/s00429-010-0251-3

Levine, P. A. (1997). *Waking the tiger, healing trauma: The innate capacity to transform overwhelming experiences*. North Atlantic Books.

Levine, P. A. (2015). *Trauma and memory: Brain and body in a search for the living past*. North Atlantic Books.

Levine, P. A., & Kline, M. (2007). *Trauma through a child's eyes: Awakening the ordinary miracle of healing; Infancy through adolescence*. North Atlantic Books.

MacLean, P. D. (1990). *The triune brain in evolution*. Plenum Press.

National Center for Health Statistics. (2022). Emergency department visit rates by selected characteristics: United States, 2020. cdc.gov/nchs/products/databriefs/db452.htm

Nummenmaa L., Glerean, E., Hari, R., & Hietanen, J. K. (2014). Bodily maps of emotions. *Proceedings of the National Academy of Sciences of the United States of America, 111*, 646–651. https://doi.org/10.1073/pnas.1321664111

Perry, B. (2013). Bonding and attachment in maltreated children: Consequences of emotional neglect. Adapted in part from *Maltreated children: Experience, brain development and the next generation*. W. W. Norton. fosteringandadoption.rip.org.uk/wp-content/uploads/2016/01/bonding-and-attachment-in-maltreated-children.pdf

Porges, S. (May 2004). Neuroception: A subconscious system for detecting threats and safety. *Zero to Three, 24*(5), 19–23.

Porges, S. (2011). *The polyvagal theory: Neurophysiological foundations of emotions, attachment, communication, self-regulation*. W. W. Norton.

Porges, S. (2016). *The neurobiology of trauma, attachment, self-regulation & emotion*. RNV042910, DVD, recorded April 8, 2016, PESI Publishing & Media. pesi.com

Porges, S., & Furman, S. (2011). The early development of the autonomic nervous system provides a neural platform for social behavior: A polyvagal perspective. *Infant and Child Development, 20*(1), 106–118. https://doi.org/10.1002/icd.688

Rieffe, C., & De Rooij, M. (2012). The longitudinal relationship between emotion awareness and internalizing symptoms during late childhood. *European Child and Adolescent Psychiatry, 21*(6), 349–356. https://doi.org/10.1007/s00787-012-0267-8

Rieffe, C., Oosterveld, P., Meerum Terwogt, M., Novin, S., Nasiri, H., & Latifian, M. (2010). Relationship between alexithymia, mood and internalizing symptoms in children and young adolescents: Evidence from an Iranian sample. *Personality and Individual Differences, 48*(4), 425–430. https://doi.org/10.1016/j.paid.2009.11.010

Riordan, J. P., Blakeslee, A., & Levine, P.A. (2017). Toddler trauma: Somatic experiencing, attachment and the neurophysiology of dyadic completion. *International Journal of Neuropsychotherapy, 5*(1), 41–70. https://doi.org/10.12744/ijnpt.2017.0041-0069

Riordan, J. P., Blakeslee, A., & Levine, P.A. (2019). Attachment focused-somatic experiencing: Secure phylogenetic attachment, dyadic trauma, and completion across the life-cycle. *International Journal of Neuropsychotherapy, 7*(3), 57–90. https://doi.org/10.12744/ijnpt.2019.057-090

Scaer, R. (2001). *The body bears the burden: Trauma, dissociation, and disease* (p. 98). The Hawthorne Medical Press.

Schore, A. N. (2019a). *The development of the unconscious mind.* W.W. Norton.

Schore, A. N. (2019b). *Right brain psychotherapy.* W.W. Norton.

Siegel, D. J. (2010). *The mindful therapist: The clinician's guide to mindsight and neural integration.* W.W. Norton.

Siegel, D. J. (2012). *The developing mind: How relationships and the brain interact to shape who we are.* W.W. Norton.

Siegel, D. J. (2023). Online description of IPNB neuroaffective attachment course. https://www.mindsightinstitute.com

Tronic, E. (2007). *The neurobehavioral and social-emotional development of infants and children.* W. W. Norton.

van der Veek, S. M. C., Derkx, H. H. F., de Haan, E., Benninga, M. A., & Boer, F. (2012). Emotion awareness and coping in children with functional abdominal pain: A controlled study. *Social Science and Medicine, 74*(2), 112–119. https://doi.org/10.1016/j.socscimed.2011.10.023

Winnicott, D. W. (1971). *Therapeutic consultations in child psychiatry.* Basic Books.

24
CLINICAL NEUROFEEDBACK

Anna K. Morrell

> If you want to find the secrets of the universe, think in terms of energy, frequency and vibration.
> — *Nikola Tesla*

Introduction

Imagine a six-year-old child just placed in a residential treatment program after demonstrating violent, dysregulated behaviors in the face of trauma. In the program, the behaviors continue, with the child threatening self-harm and destroying keepsakes from their adoptive family. The child has difficulty sleeping, fearful of the recurring nightmares and shadows as they move across the walls. The child is angry that they are not living at home and terrified that they might not return. They are terrified of family visits. The child's fear and reactivity are all-consuming, making learning to read and write impossible. Developing meaningful relationships is off the table at the start of treatment. The child desires nothing more than to be cared for and attended to; however, they approach others as if they are walking away. Traditional play therapy sessions seem to wind up the child's energy levels. They are resistant to grounding and relaxation techniques. Medicating has been complicated because of the complexity of symptoms and their age. They have difficulty focusing but become fixated, and are hyper-motoric but with apraxia, hypervigilant but dissociative. The list of DSM diagnoses is long and not an accurate description of the child's daily functioning or quality of life.

This child uses incredible resources at their program and school, needing one-to-one support to maintain safety and provide opportunities for co-regulation and success. This is a child with an ACE score of 4 or more by age 6, and a trajectory of high-risk adolescent behaviors so they can feel something other than the rage or absence of themselves. The experience of trauma can alter the very structures of the brain and develop neural pathways of the fear circuitry that are more like superhighways, ultimately rerouting neuronal communications away from a healthy growing sense of self. When we address the dysregulation at its origin with neurofeedback, we offer the opportunity for this child to experience safety and regulation within themselves, rerouting the fear circuits to fire only when necessary.

"In the field of trauma, especially developmental trauma, we are coming to recognize that the problem is in the brain, not in the mind," psychotherapist and neurofeedback practitioner Sebern Fisher told me in March 2023.

The primary issue of people with developmental trauma is fear. It is also pain, and rage, and shame, but fear is at the core. We cannot quiet that fear with our therapeutic presence alone as we have relied on in decades of talk psychotherapy. Neurofeedback addresses fear at the level of the brain.

To understand how neurofeedback can quiet fear and improve affect regulation for children who have experienced complex trauma, we must first understand basic biofeedback and neurofeedback principles. Biofeedback is commonly defined as using a monitoring device to give immediate information to a subject about their bodily functions. These physical functions are often outside of the individual's conscious awareness. However, the information given via feedback can then be used to manipulate or learn how to alter these processes, such as heart rate, muscle tension, or temperature regulation. Neurofeedback is a form of biofeedback that uses the electroencephalogram (EEG) to record and reflect real-time brain wave activity to the person. The International Society for Neuroregulation and Research (ISNR) describes neurofeedback training (NFT) as using "monitoring devices to provide moment-to-moment information to an individual on the state of their physiological functioning" (ISNR, n.d.). The distinguishing feature of NFT compared to other forms of biofeedback is that the information monitored is focused on the central nervous system and the brain's electrical activity. Clinical neurofeedback is a neuroscience-driven and technology-delivered modality relying on clinical skills and therapeutic relationships. NFT is often performed with a brain-computer interface system, in which the computer displays brain activity using visual and auditory cues, often via video games. The games range from simplistic to more visually appealing, but they all have the same basic premise: to reflect the brain's activity meaningfully so that the brain can learn from its awareness. Neurofeedback has an inherent "cool" factor for many children because they get to play a video game with their brains during sessions. Because of this, it is often a modality that even the most treatment-avoidant children will engage with.

Neuroplasticity is crucial to why neurofeedback can effectively improve regulation and treatment outcomes with complex trauma. The brain creates electrical activity whenever a neuron or brain cell communicates with another cell. Suppose these communications are helpful for the brain or body, such as cells communicating with each other to initiate a fight, flight, tonic, or collapsed immobility response to a threat. In that case, these cells will continue to speak to each other, creating greater connectivity (Roelofs, 2017). This is neuroplasticity in action. By operant and classical conditioning techniques, the NFT process helps the brain learn or try on new cell communications at an unconscious level. As neurofeedback providers, we support the child in making these new communications in areas of their developing brain impacted by the assault of trauma.

All neurofeedback systems include monitoring devices to access the brain's electrical activity. Silver or gold electrodes or sensors, combined with a conductive paste or gel, are typically applied to the patient's scalp. These sensors are then plugged into an amplifier, which conveys the signal to a computer with software that translates the frequencies of the brain waves into a visual representation for both the clinician and the patient. The visual representations on the clinician's computer can be monitored, interpreted, and recorded. For the patient, these representations are the moment-to-moment information of their physiological state that they can learn volitional control over. During NFT sessions, the brain is rewarded through auditory and visual feedback when it makes desired adjustments to amplitude and is given error feedback (or lack of reward) when it is not making the desired changes. This is the neurofeedback process. The brain learns to make changes in how it operates, and if those changes serve the patient, as seen in symptom reduction or increased affect regulation, the brain will want to remember those changes. However, the brain is also highly efficient, meaning that the changes it makes during training might take more effort to operate as it is learning the new physiological state. Because of this, NFT is often recommended two or more times a week, to offer the brain more practice in making the desired changes. Repetition is the essence of learning—just as professional athletes are not at the apex of their game if they attended practice only once. They achieve their peak performance because they continue to practice.

Many neurofeedback systems are available for clinical use, which may reflect different underlying theoretical approaches. The varying systems often have introductory courses to teach their underlying assumptions and the operation of their specific software. They focus on a distinctive lens or theory to view the brain and its functioning. In essence, the field of neurofeedback is heterogenous, with dynamic clinicians, researchers, and applied neuroscientists seeking efficient ways to address several issues in a variety of populations. However diverse the field may be and regardless of the neurofeedback system one chooses, to be a clinical neurofeedback provider, per the Biofeedback Certification International Alliance (BCIA), one needs to complete a 36-hour training course, which includes history, basic principles, neuroanatomy, sensor placement, measurement, assessment, and more. BCIA is an organization that sets education and training standards in the field of biofeedback. For many clinical systems, independent licensure in health care is also required. Learning clinical neurofeedback can have a steep curve and even more so when working with a complex-trauma population, due to the extent of trauma's impact on brain development and function. However, adding neurofeedback into a clinical practice focusing on childhood trauma is achievable. Considering the modality's implications for regulation at the brain level, it becomes an exquisite complement to other trauma therapies, especially those focused on co-regulation and relational attunement.

History and Research of Neurofeedback

The electroencephalogram (EEG) allows us to access, record, and observe electrical activity in the brain. Hans Berger, a German psychiatrist, developed the electroencephalogram in 1924. He invented a recording device where sensors were placed on the scalp, and the electrical activity was amplified and traced onto a sheet of scrolling paper. In the 1960s, investigations and applications of the EEG for neurofeedback began. Joe Kamiya (1971) explored mindfulness and teaching people to increase their alpha state, producing a relaxed and pleasant physiological state by bringing the alpha activity into the person's awareness. Barry Sterman (2000) investigated EEG activity related to sleep onset, identifying the sensorimotor rhythm (SMR). Sterman designed an experiment to determine whether cats could learn to control EEG activity through operant conditioning. The cats naturally learned to increase SMR activity when rewarded with food after being cued by a red light. Wyrwicka and Sterman (1968) published a paper adding brain functioning to the growing list of pliable physiological functions through feedback and volitional control. Sterman charged forward with his SMR investigations, demonstrating that the brain can learn to control seizure activity (Sterman, 2000).

In 2005, Hirshberg, Chiu, and Frazier published a meta-analysis of emerging interventions in the *Journal of Child and Adolescent Psychiatric Clinics of North America,* using the American Academy of Child and Adolescent Psychiatry (AACAP) clinical guidelines to establish evidence-based treatments. It concluded that neurofeedback meets the criteria based on those guidelines for treating various DSM diagnoses (Hirshberg et al., 2005). Research on the application of neurofeedback with children has focused primarily on ADHD, with approximately 80% of published randomized controlled studies since 1995 investigating the effects of neurofeedback on attention and executive functioning. Neurofeedback as an intervention for ADHD/ADD is considered a top-tier intervention by the American Academy of Pediatrics (2014), partly because of the depth of research in the field. Monastra et al. (2006) published a review of the evidence for using neurofeedback with the ADHD population. More recently, a large National Institute of Health grant was awarded to the Neurofeedback Collaborative Group to study the effectiveness of neurofeedback on attention, called the ICAN study. While this double-blinded study found the NFT did not have statistically significant outcomes over traditional interventions for ADHD (medication, behavior training), at the 13-month follow-up, those in the neurofeedback group took less medication to manage attentional issues (Neurofeedback Collaborative Group, 2021) indicating improvement in the brain's ability to regulate the attentional systems.

The history of neurofeedback in trauma treatment has primarily been focused on the adult population. In 1991, Peniston and Kulkosky published a landmark study of the effectiveness of alpha-theta training, a specific form of neurofeedback, with Vietnam veterans with PTSD and substance abuse. The outcomes included statistically significant improvements across numerous measurements, including the Minnesota Multiphasic Personality Inventory, where participants in the neurofeedback group reduced scores in suicidality, pathology, and depression and showed reductions in medication usage and substance relapse. These improvements were measured 30 months post-NFT. In 2009, neuroscientists at the University of Western Ontario identified brain network differences between PTSD and non-PTSD groups using fMRI imaging (Bluhm et al., 2009). The images of the average fMRI data demonstrated that in the non-PTSD group, the Default Mode Network (DMN) had blood flow activation across the posterior cingulate cortex (PCC), precuneus, medial prefrontal, and inferior parietal cortices. The PSTD group showed minimal or no blood flow activation to the medial prefrontal cortex and limited connectivity between the PCC and the right amygdala, hippocampus, and insula. Bluhm et al. (2009) hypothesized that the "involvement of the right hemisphere may be important given the suggestion that the early-life trauma experienced by the patients with PTSD may have interfered primarily with the development of the right hemisphere" (p. 192). The right hemisphere is believed to be the center of emotion regulation. According to Allan Schore (2018), a leading researcher in the field of interpersonal neurobiology, "the early developing right brain generates the implicit self" (p. 178), or one could argue, the origin of the self.

This group of researchers has taken the current neuroscience about brain connectivity and functioning within the trauma and dissociative population and developed training protocols through fMRI and EEG neurofeedback studies to determine how to activate greater connectivity in the DMN (Harricharan et al., 2016). A recent randomized control trial of one EEG biofeedback protocol, commonly known as Alpha-Down training, demonstrated improved connectivity in the PTSD group to the frontal nodes of the DMN (Shaw et al., 2023). Most importantly, it diminished PTSD symptoms and enhanced quality of life. While this research has been focused on an adult trauma population, one can hypothesize that applying NFT with the child population can support the development of the connectivity needed for a healthy DMN in adulthood. In an interview with Dr. Ruth Lanius, she reflected that "the DMN in children looks like a traumatized adult" (personal communication, June 9, 2023), as our prefrontal cortexes are not fully connected until we are in our early 20s—meaning, the hub of activity is located at the back of the brain. This means the child lacks the ability to create a context of time, space, and another, especially when exposed to trauma. There is no autobiographical self yet, but it is being written. It can be written by continuing to myelinate neurons in the fear circuitry, reinforcing the connectivity at the back of the brain, or it can be written in regulation, awareness of the self and another, and social connection.

Research on the efficacy of neurofeedback with trauma treatment in a child population is sparse but growing at the time of publication; however, clinical observations and case studies offer reported improvements across multiple domains. Research with a child population has hurdles, including consent, consistency, attrition, community, familial influence, and financial backing. In a recent pilot study of NFT, children aged 6–13 diagnosed with PTSD were randomly assigned to the NFT group or treatment as usual (Rogel et al., 2020)—the NFT group trained at T4-P4, rewarding their peak alpha plus and minus 1 Hz. The training time of participants ranged from 6 to 18 minutes. All included in the experimental group received NFT twice a week, totaling 24 sessions in combination with ongoing weekly psychotherapy, while the control group was Treatment as Usual (TAU). At the study's conclusion, for those in the NFT group, PTSD criteria were met for only 25% of participants, and they demonstrated improved executive functioning, improved social interactions, and emotional regulation in various measurements. These improvements did not last; however, it was hypothesized that more training sessions could be more effective for longer-term benefits. In the case examples throughout this chapter, it is essential to note the number of training sessions. Research studies have specific designs that often limit the number of training sessions, typically 20–40. For the brain to rewire functioning cemented for survival in the most horrific circumstances will require significantly more sessions than 40. However, arousal improvements may be observed as early as the first training session. In a systematic review of neurofeedback research with children and trauma, as of 2022, only seven peer-reviewed articles met search criteria, which included a minimum of pre-post research design, participant criteria of at least one traumatic event, a population of 18 or younger, and original research for the efficacy of NFT (Schutz & Herbert, 2022). Rogel et al. (2020) and Schutz and Herbert (2022) concluded that further research is needed to determine better protocols and the average length of treatment for optimal and lasting outcomes.

Frequency and Amplitude

As Nikola Tesla stated, the secrets of the universe lie in frequency. Moreover, in neurofeedback, the secrets of regulation lie in frequency, amplitude, and connectivity. Frequency is a measure of the speed of the electrical output. An electrical charge is created when brain cells send information to other cells. Frequency is measured in hertz, or cycles per second, of how quickly brain cells under the sensor are firing. In Hans Berger's (1929) initial investigations, he applied sensors to patients under anesthesia and later to family members, recording their brain waves. He observed a dominant, rhythmic waveform, or frequency, which he named the "waves of the first order," or alpha waves, which became more prevalent when the eyes were closed. This frequency was recorded at 8–12 hertz (Hz), meaning 8–12 peaks and valleys were traced per second. Subsequent early EEG researchers began to name other waveforms and frequencies: delta, theta, alpha, beta, and gamma.

Amplitude is the measure of power or strength in electrical output. Brain waves are measured in microvolts (μm). All brain wave frequencies exist in the brain at all times. However, they can vary in amplitude, giving rise to the brain's arousal level. For example, delta's frequency range (1–4 Hz) has the largest brain wave amplitude during deep sleep. Like radio stations whose sound travels by frequency, one can tune their radio dial to a specific station, say 88.7 MHz, and if they like the song playing, one might turn up the volume, or the amplitude, of that frequency.

The frequencies, in combination with the amplitude levels, translate to various arousal states in the brain. As mentioned above, the slow-wave delta (1–4 Hz) is often seen in the highest amplitudes in deep and dreamless sleep and is associated with unconsciousness (or unawareness). Theta (4–8 Hz) is most associated with inattention, internalized focus, and daydreaming, but also with creativity, and is beneficial in complex problem-solving (Sammer et al., 2007). Alpha (8–12 Hz) is most associated with a sense of well-being, internal safety, and security, not actively engaged in an external task but being present with the self. Alpha is also vital in the brain's ability to shift between arousal states. Alpha frequencies have become a focus of neurofeedback and neuroscience research in complex trauma and altered states of consciousness (Gapen et al., 2016; Hargraves, 2017; Nicholson et al., 2016). SMR (12–15 Hz at the sensorimotor strip) is closely associated with actively engaging in tasks but with calm and clear focus. Hamlin (2018) wrote that 12–15 Hz is often experienced as a rhythmic quiescence for the brain. In other brain areas, 12–15 Hz is also associated with a calm, clear focus. However, when the waves are not recorded at the sensorimotor strip, they are referred to as beta or low beta; 15–18 Hz is often called beta or mid-beta, associated with an active wakeful state engaged in tasks; and 22–36 Hz is called high beta and is often used in training to help the body learn to manage muscle tension. This frequency is a fast waveform closely associated with increased levels of alertness accompanied by physical strain or stress.

These various electrical frequencies can be seen throughout the brain, over all brain regions and locations. In EEG, an international system of 10–20 or 10–10 is used to maintain consistent sensor placement sites. In essence, the 10–20 system is based on measurements of the skull from key points: front to back—the nasion (bridge of nose/forehead) to the inion (base of the skull resting on the neck in the center); side to side—left preauricular point over the center of the head to right preauricular point; and from front to back around the sides—frontal pole to inion (left and right side). Each site is labeled by its location over the brain (F = frontal, T = temporal, C = central, FP = frontal pole/prefrontal, P = parietal, O = occipital). Left-side placements are designated by odd numbers (e.g., left temporal = T3), and right-side placements are designated by even numbers (e.g., right temporal = T4). The center line of placements is referred to as Zero or Z (central parietal = PZ). Each site is measured in intervals beginning at 10% of the key point to start the measurement, followed by 20% of the total distance. In the case of measuring from front to back down the midline, 10% from the nasion is the central frontal pole (FPZ), 20% from FPZ is frontal (FZ), 20% from FZ is central (CZ), 20% from CZ is parietal (PZ), 20% from PZ is occipital (OZ), and 10% from OZ reaches the base of the skull at the inion (IZ).

NFT sessions have protocols comprising the site placement, targeted frequencies, type of process (sum training, differential, synchrony, inhibition, etc.), and length of time. For example, the protocol "T4-P4 inhibit 1–4 Hz, 4–7 Hz, and 22–36 Hz, rewarding 7–10 Hz for a total of 12 minutes" means that the child had electrodes placed at the right temporal (T4) and the right parietal (P4) and they were getting feedback to reduce slow wave (1–4 Hz and 4–7 Hz) and high beta (22–36 Hz) while learning to increase 7–10 Hz for 12 minutes. T4-P4 also indicates that T4 is the primary sensor with P4 as a reference, and A1 (the left ear) would be the ground. At a minimum, all protocols must have three points of contact. The primary signal is where most of the electrical activity is picked up. The reference in a bipolar montage (two head placements, not necessarily interhemispheric) is subtracted (−) from the primary signal total amplitude. In monopolar montages, or a single head sensor placement and reference on an earlobe, the reference helps localize where the electrical activity originates. The ground is often applied to an earlobe, which helps reduce atmospheric electrical activity.

During a NFT session, the client controls the modulation of the amplitudes of different brain waves through the inhibition (reduction of) or reward (increasing of) based on parameters set by the neurofeedback provider or the neurofeedback system itself. The inhibits and rewards mentioned are essential for symptom reduction and arousal state changes the client is seeking. The child patient, especially the child who often feels they have no voice or choice, must understand that they control their brain wave activity.

Approaches and Theories

Our understanding of the brain and interest in developing brain/computer interfaces grows as technology advances. As stated previously, there are a growing number of neurofeedback systems and approaches to brain regulation within neurofeedback. No outcome studies indicate that one system or approach is better; however, the largest body of peer-reviewed research has utilized the arousal model. New neurofeedback trainees must consider a system and approach most aligned with their clinical orientation and population. Here, we explore the arousal model approach and summarize several other approaches.

In 1908, psychologists Robert M. Yerkes and John Dillingham Dodson investigated the impact stress or pressure had on performance. They were initially investigating the impact of punishment on learning using non-harmful shocks with mice. They hypothesized that the ability to perform a task or engage in habit formation would also increase as the stressors increased. They found a distinct and consistent curve that, over time and as stress is applied, initially, performance improves, but only to a point. This curve is known as the Yerkes-Dodson law. After surpassing the optimal performance zone and as stress continues to be applied, the person's performance begins declining.

While not a scientific law, the theory of the Yerkes-Dodson law continues to have relevance over a century later. In the 1950s, psychologist Donald Hebb (1955) applied this research to the concept of arousal. The Yerkes-Dodson law has since evolved to be strongly associated with arousal. In application to human performance, as the stress level escalates, motivation and activation increase from inaction and low arousal levels. Arousal continues to increase into the peak or optimal zone where mental and physical capabilities are most efficient.

When stress continues to be applied, arousal decreases into fatigue, anxiety, sickness, and burnout. Research indicates that medial tasks require the brain to shift into the higher end of the optimal zone, while complex tasks require the brain to shift into the lower end (Gardner, 1986; Yu, 2015). To keep one's attention and focus during repetitive or tedious tasks—for example, a child completing multiplication tables—one's arousal needs to be in the higher end of the optimal zone, holding a narrower point of focus to keep attention from drifting or wandering. To keep one's attention and focus during complex, higher processes, such as a child engaging in reciprocal and relational interactions, one's arousal needs to be in the lower end of the optimal zone to keep focus without increasing anxiety or stress. From the lens of the arousal model on childhood trauma, understanding the exposure and impact chronic stressors have on brain functioning is paramount. Most children with complex trauma demonstrate symptoms of high arousal, often combined with instabilities or a disordered profile.

The nervous system needs to be flexible to adapt to the levels of stress it is experiencing, meaning arousal needs to shift from higher to lower states depending on the person's everyday experience and situation. When a child has been exposed to complex trauma and neglect, those experiences create a template for developing brain structures. This allows the child to determine what is safe and not, thus preserving their survival. With the application of arousal model neurofeedback with a child with complex trauma, the child's brain can learn new oscillations and neuronal firing patterns. This is the premise of the arousal model of NFT. While this chapter is focused on arousal model neurofeedback, it is not the only approach. As stated previously, the field of neurofeedback is diverse and complicated. A more in-depth description of the arousal model neurofeedback approach follows a summary of other neurofeedback approaches.

Amplitude training is where the patient focuses on learning to control the amplitude of various brain waves. For example, a patient might learn to increase SMR (12–15 Hz) amplitude to strengthen calm and clear focus while learning to decrease slow waves (2–6 Hz) and high beta (22–36 Hz) to reduce inattention and muscle tension while engaging in tasks. This is the most common type of neurofeedback in a clinical setting, with the largest body of empirical data.

FMRI neurofeedback uses a functional magnetic resonance imaging machine and is often used in research to demonstrate blood flow and various brain structure excitation or inhibition.

ILF (infra-low frequency) is a newer approach focused on training the brain at frequencies below 1 Hz utilizing specifically engineered amplifiers. This model is symptom-based and results-driven, with flexibility in the systems to adjust training parameters toward the patient's "optimal reward frequency" for regulation. The late Sue Othmer and her husband, Siegfried, developed this approach (2017). The Othmers are pioneers in the application of neurofeedback, investigating the theoretical approach of the arousal model and turning investigations toward the lowest measurable frequencies in support of regulation.

The LENS (Low Energy Neurofeedback System), created by Len Ochs in 1990 (2019), incorporates a brain map; various 10–20 sites of the brain are determined to need a low-energy stimulus to help shift the frequency or amplitudes in that location and its relation to other areas of the brain.

LORETA (low-resolution electromagnetic tomographic analysis) uses information from a qEEG and mathematical analysis to determine the source location within the brain of various amplitude or communication deficiencies or overloads. Training then focuses on bringing the brain's electrical activity toward the normative amplitudes, phase, or coherence. Non-linear dynamic approaches theorize that the brain is a self-organizing organism. When given guidance or reflective information, the brain will adjust its functioning toward more efficiency and regulation.

Slow cortical potential (SCP) neurofeedback monitors event-related, direct-current shifts of the EEG, and this type of training aims to support the regulation of cortical excitation. SCP training has the largest body of evidence with ADHD as the brain learns to inhibit or regulate direct-current shifts (Mayer et al., 2013).

QEEG (quantitative) guided neurofeedback is where a patient wears a cap of 19, 32, or 64 site locations, measuring brain activity simultaneously. The data recorded from the brain is then interpreted via various software and normative databases. The information is then further analyzed by someone specializing in qEEG interpretation, and protocols are provided based on how different brain areas perform, communicating with one another. QEEG is sometimes referred to as brain mapping. The data is often recorded for research, measuring electrical activity pre- and post-experimental intervention to determine if and where amplitude or coherence changes were created. Several training approaches and systems require measuring qEEG data, including Coherence, LORETA, and Z-Score.

Z-Score training often involves two- or four-channel training. The computer system continuously calculates different variables (amplitude, phase, coherence, asymmetries) by comparing the patient's brain activity to a normative database. The system then provides feedback to the patient to help them adjust their EEG toward the norm.

Arousal Model

The arousal model training approach, whose origins are found in the research and clinical applications from Yerkes and Dodson (1908), Joe Kamiya (1971), and Barry Sterman (2000), can incorporate qEEG and other measurements and is framed around an in-depth clinical assessment to determine the general tone of the patient's nervous system. The arousal model is often considered the most transferable approach to a classically trained psychotherapist. It does not utilize the DSM to inform treatment, but rather, it requires the clinician to use therapeutic listening and observation, tuning into the story of the patient's nervous system. This model allows for the whole person to be seen. There are four known categories of arousal: under-arousal, over-arousal, unstable arousal, and disordered arousal. These categories have been defined through decades of research and symptom cluster analysis. Arousal symptoms include physiological, emotional, cognitive, and psychological symptoms. The arousal model approach is symptom-based and results-driven, meaning that the experience of the child patient is continually being assessed through symptom tracking and measurements from the child's perspective and the child's caregivers (parents, foster parents, adoptive parents, teachers or coaches, clinicians). In complex trauma, leaders in neurofeedback, such as Sebern Fisher, Bessel van der Kolk, and Ruth Lanius, have championed the arousal model.

Under-arousal can be defined as someone whose brain tends to have higher amplitudes of slower frequencies (delta, theta) for their age range. These are often children who have symptoms of difficulty staying asleep, are easily distracted, have low mood or energy levels, are daydreamy, and have difficulty sequencing and following through with tasks. Because children naturally have higher levels of delta and theta, amplitudes are age-normed when using amplitude in comparison. When working with children with trauma or attachment wounded histories, they might present with any of the typical under-arousal characteristics. Dissociative children will also often present with higher levels of slow-wave activity. However, it is essential to recall the Yerkes-Dodson arousal curve in that most traumatized children will be on the far-right side of the curve, in the burnout, fatigue, and illness range. Due to chronic stress and pressure, the brain has had to adapt for survival. The presence of high amplitude slow-wave activity can be misleading with dissociative and complexly traumatized children. Emerging research on ADHD and trauma has indicated that ADHD is often over-diagnosed in children with complex trauma (Boodoo et al., 2022; Miodus et al., 2021). Under-arousal is commonly addressed by training on the left side (or center) of the brain and helping the brain learn to make less slow-wave amplitude while increasing mid-beta amplitude.

Over-arousal can be defined as someone whose brain tends to have higher amplitudes of faster frequencies (high beta) for their age range. These children often have difficulty falling asleep, demonstrate aggression, and are seasonally sensitive, hypervigilant, agitated, and tense. Over-arousal is a common arousal category for the population when working with children with complex trauma. This is a nervous system that works very hard to stay activated, stay aware, and stay alive. Over-arousal is commonly addressed by training on the right side (or center) of the brain and helping the brain learn to make less fast-wave amplitude while increasing SMR, alpha, or lower.

Unstable arousal can be defined as someone whose brain has a narrower arousal curve, in that it tends to take a fair amount of stress or pressure to activate into performance, followed by a narrow window of optimal performance and then a sudden decrease in performance. This brain can flip from under-aroused to over-aroused quickly. Unstable arousal is also a common category for the complex trauma and dissociative child population. These children often have a history of seizures, migraines, TBI or concussions, early medical needs requiring oxygen, and attachment or interpersonal difficulties. For this category, training is typically conducted using an interhemispheric or stabilizing placement (left and right hemispheres), focusing on decreasing slow- and fast-wave amplitude while increasing SMR, alpha, or lower.

Disordered arousal is a newer category identified by Dr. Ed Hamlin after he analyzed hundreds of brain maps of traumatized children. It can be described as a nervous system displaying symptoms of over-, under-, and unstable arousal simultaneously in different brain regions—for example, a child with high vocal irritability and agitation but who is also unable to move or has collapsed immobility. This is also a nervous system that commonly has paradoxical effects on training. Like over-arousal and unstable, disordered arousal is frequently seen in the complex trauma patient, including the dissociative child. Often this arousal profile is not determined until after training, unless using a qEEG assessment, when the clinician monitors the impacts of the brain learning new neuronal firing patterns. Training is typically focused on calming (right side) or stabilizing (interhemispheric) to address the various symptoms, carefully tracking the training impacts.

The patient learns to make less and more of various frequencies in the arousal model or amplitude training. They are making less of the frequencies that impact their day-to-day functioning (e.g., too much fast-wave or high beta at night can impair sleep onset). The child is also learning to make more amplitude of the frequencies that help bring them into a present state of awareness (often SMR, alpha, or lower, especially for those impacted by complex or developmental trauma). In a dissociative child, the brain is learning to be more present in the face of perceived danger by reducing the amplitude of slow-wave activity.

In the arousal model, assessing how the patient responds to NFT is ongoing and imperative for progress. Initial protocols (the site location, the frequency bands to reward and inhibit, and the amount of time training) are often determined by a combination of the clinical assessment, categorizing arousal symptoms, and valid measurement tools. While there is a place for qEEG measurements, I conduct informal mini maps to access the electrical activity of two or more brain sites to get a snapshot of the amplitudes of different frequencies sequentially over different brain regions. The data gathered from a mini map can be beneficial in determining the patient's posterior dominant rhythm (PDR) or peak alpha. The PDR is the brain's idling speed when it is at rest. The PDR can be found by measuring at

PZ with eyes closed and observing the highest amplitude level in a single frequency band. The PDR is important to distinguish when working with children because the PDR speed increases through early brain development. Researchers have found that children aged 1 have a PDR range of 5–6 Hz, and it slowly increases with healthy development up to age 10–12, when the PDR speed solidifies around 10–12 Hz (Britton et al., 2016). However, if a child is exposed to abuse, neglect, or attachment wounding, the PDR speed might not increase as the brain develops around this idling rhythm (Bazanova, 2012).

This chapter previously defined various waveforms by specific frequencies (e.g., alpha 8–12 Hz). However, those are merely labels to help categorize. In the case of child brain development, if the patient's PDR is measured to be 7 Hz, this frequency becomes their alpha. Suppose the NFT aims to help increase calm focus by increasing low beta. In that case, this patient's low beta can be considered to begin at 8 or 9 Hz, typically one or two frequencies above their peak alpha. This approach allows for neurofeedback to be used as a modality across the lifespan.

Ongoing assessment and awareness of the impact of the training protocol with the child patient is an essential element of the training process. Learning to listen simultaneously to the child's nervous system and their story about their training experience is crucial while attuning the therapeutic relationship toward a language of regulation and awareness. Providers often have symptom tracking sheets developed for the caregiver/parent/teacher and child to complete after two hours and two nights of sleep. The information noted in the symptom trackers monitors physiological, emotional, behavioral, and cognitive responses. Patients and caregivers are often asked to record sleep onset, quality, and waking compared to before the last NFT session, using an SUD rating or Likert scale. Mood, impulse control, mental clarity, and mental flexibility are frequently tracked in addition to any specific symptoms the patient seeks to change. Suppose a patient or caregiver notes that there has been an increase in under-arousal symptoms. In that case, the reward frequency can be adjusted by increasing the reward band from 0.125 to 1 Hz, depending on the nervous system's sensitivity. If a patient or caregiver notes an increase in over-arousal symptoms (or no reduction), the reward frequency should be reduced from 0.125 to 1 Hz, depending again on nervous system sensitivity.

The following case vignette of Caroline demonstrates the importance of tracking training impacts and making adjustments, especially with a susceptible nervous system. All named case vignettes are real-case examples, with pseudonyms for privacy.

Case Study: Caroline

Caroline is an 11-year-old internationally adopted female with a history of significant preverbal trauma and attachment wounding. She is a highly creative and imaginative preteen who enjoys fantasy novels involving animals, and classic literature. She is also a talented artist who has perfected evoking a sense of animals' personalities in their facial expressions and caring eyes. She has an extremely sensitive nervous system, emotionally impacted by the external energy of her classmates and family and internally by subtle shifts of arousal state. We proceeded slowly and carefully when training, observing minute changes in her arousal after every training session. Caroline adapted a rating scale to describe a combination of her energy level, sensory experience, and hypervigilance/response, ranging from a 5, meaning a "swarm of bees stinging under my skin," to a 1, meaning calm, peaceful, happy, and content.

Her training protocols began at C4-A2 based on the clinical assessment indicators of over-arousal. A disordered arousal profile became known after the first session of one minute of training. Caroline's energy and mood flipped from an over-aroused state to an under-aroused state. Her training was adjusted to C3-C4 and T4-P4 to address her heightened sensory experience and responsivity to others. While this protocol combination had some benefits (no longer having recurring nightmares and fewer over-arousal symptoms), the impact of her early and deep attachment wounds continued to play out in interactions within the family, especially with her adoptive mother. After adding IZ-A2 training in addition to C3-C4, there was an immediate and significant shifting of arousal, even after 30 seconds of training. Caroline continued to train at IZ-A2 and C3-C4 for several sessions, slowly and methodically increasing the time training at IZ from 30 seconds up to three minutes. She could now train at C3-C4 for six minutes. The reward at IZ-A2 was 2–5 Hz. After 12 sessions, she became calm and regulated, almost slipping into under-arousal, as observed by increased sleep, difficulty waking and with focus, increased irritability, and tearfulness. Based on her sensitivity, the reward band was increased by 1/8 Hz. After 30 seconds of the 1/8 Hz higher frequency, Caroline became increasingly agitated, hyper-motoric, and panic-stricken. She shrieked that she needed to tear her skin off to release the swarm of bees. She was beyond a 5 on her scale after 30 seconds and such a slight change in frequency. Luckily, my system allows for adjustments during training, and I reduced the reward band back to 2–5 Hz. After 30 more seconds of training, Caroline collapsed onto her Squishmallow pillow; her breathing rate returned to normal, and her voice softened. When she could lift her head, she reached for her mother's hand to hold and squeeze. She was seeking and aware of her need for connection and was accepting of co-regulation offered by her caregiver.

We will take another look at Caroline's story and outcomes when discussing brain training regions.

Training Considerations

Neurofeedback is a process of exploration and learning; two vital components of a child's development made more impactful in a relationship with another. How wonderful it is to explore and experience affect regulation—a sense of calm, peace, and ease. After a training session, children will often release a content sigh of relief. It is important to know there can be dysregulation after training, as seen in Caroline's session above. For a child to experience a sudden change in their arousal level can be dysregulating in and of itself. There can also be dysregulation after a training session if the protocol (site, reward, amount of time training) is not in service of the child's nervous system. As with the disordered arousal category, different brain regions can be operating with both under- and over-aroused symptoms simultaneously. As we set the stage for adding NFT to a treatment plan for a child with complex trauma or dissociative symptoms, integrating NFT into psychotherapy and various modalities (play, creative arts, SMART, TF-CBT, etc.) is essential. While NFT can be a stand-alone treatment, when working with this population, it is recommended that other therapeutic modalities be used in conjunction. When the child patient is learning to regulate their brain's patterns, modulate arousal levels, and increase their awareness of themselves and others, a trusted, secure "other" is vital to support this experience. There can be fear in the changing nervous system; experiencing a new physiological state and having a safe therapeutic other through this emergence is fundamental. When the brain is regulated, the mind can more readily access trauma processing safely and securely. These pseudonymed case vignettes will highlight the value of engaging in neurofeedback within the framework of psychotherapy and the therapeutic relationship.

Neurofeedback is always performed with the consent of both the parent or caregiver and the child. Legally, consent is needed only from the parent or guardian, yet the child patient is worthy of understanding the process within their capacity. Explaining or demonstrating the sensor hookup and how to play the game needs to be done with age-appropriate language and can most certainly be done with a playful curiosity. To apply the sensors, neurofeedback requires a consenting therapeutic touch. A gentle, purposeful touch of the head to find site locations to prepare the sites is needed to receive the EEG signal without impedance. Moreover, helping return the patient's hairstyle, especially for those preteens, is a necessary promise.

Neurofeedback is never done "to" or "on" someone. It is a discovery and learning process that can be done only "with" or "for" a patient. We must be cautious with our wording and explanations for children with abhorrent histories of actions done to them. Their brain unconsciously takes on the learning challenge, and we work together "with" or "for" greater rhythmicity and modulation. As the provider, I can only help guide the child's brain toward regulation by setting specific parameters.

Our child patients do not live in a vacuum. Children need and have all different types of caregivers, whether their birth, adoptive, foster, or program parents. Even teachers, coaches, mentors, and neighbors should be considered caregivers if they are giving care. Neurofeedback can and should be offered for caregivers to support the caregiver's regulation and attunement needs. Just as with other modalities when working with children who have experienced complex trauma and perhaps demonstrate dissociative symptoms, addressing the caregiver's regulation needs is just as prudent in supporting the child's healing and regulation needs. Caregiver regulation needs can be addressed simultaneously or even primarily to support a more regulated, predictable, responsive, and attuned child-caregiver relationship. We will see a case example of NFT with caregivers later in the chapter. In a conversation with Dr. Lanius (2023), I asked her how she wished the therapies had gone for her adult clients with complex trauma. She responded that she would have wanted the parents to engage in neurofeedback, even pre-pregnancy, as an early intervention. Suppose her adult clients had had a present, attuned, and regulated caregiver. In that case, the traumatized adult might not have experienced the attachment wounding that is all too common in complex trauma. The regulated caregiver is a good enough caregiver because they can be present and attuned to their needs as well as to the needs of their child. Ortiz (2019) noted that regardless of the number of ACEs a person might experience, if that person also has the experience of a present, attuned, and regulated caregiver, the negative impact on their physical and mental health will be greatly diminished.

Age Ranges

I work with children as young as age 2 and know colleagues who have used neurofeedback with infants, especially those with a disordered sleep/wake cycle. When working with infants, a parent or caregiver holds the child, and the gaze is directed toward the feedback monitor. Customizing and simplifying an infant's visual and auditory feedback is also essential in engaging the young brain in learning. The physiological responses are often felt during the training, with a rigid body softening into the arms of the attuned parent.

Children ages 2–4 are best engaged through spirited curiosity. I will explain the process using words and examples to employ interest. Instead of calling the electrodes sensors, I call them "Brain Buttons" and explain that the buttons must stay on to make the game work. The PDR in this age range is often around 6 or 7 Hz, so adjusting the reward frequencies according to the desired outcome is paramount. The games are engaging, but additional rewards are sometimes needed to keep a young child's interest. The most challenging part of training with this age range is helping the child sit relatively still. When there is movement, the brain produces large amounts of high beta, and the electrodes can quickly lose their connections or "pop off." However, motoric inhibition becomes easier for the young child as the brain becomes more regulated. One measure of progress can often be how quickly the child can settle into the session.

For all children, using the feedback of different arousal states can be explored through playful experiments. Showing the child what the brain waves look like when they move their bodies at different intensities is an interactive way to provide feedback and a way for them to see what they have control over. I will often supplement these explorations with sensory modulation, trying different skills or tools to achieve a calm and still body. Placing the sensors on younger children requires some finesse, especially for those children with sensory sensitivities. I permit my young patients to play with small quantities of the conductive paste to feel more at ease when the sensors are applied to their heads.

School-aged children begin to develop an awareness of how their behavior impacts what other people think of them, or at the very least, what their behavior might be preventing them from having, inciting a feeling of unjustness. I have found that using this developmental awareness to find intrinsic motivation for engaging in neurofeedback sessions is beneficial. When the child gets into trouble at school for being unable to transition from play to classwork or becoming overstimulated in play situations, the child often feels shame or embarrassment. I explain that neurofeedback can help them learn to be more flexible so they can enjoy recess and settle into reading time when the situation presents itself.

Many older latency and preteen patients have the experience of playing video games, and neurofeedback has easy buy-in. There is a specific "cool" factor to learning how to control a video game with your brain. With all ages, motivation becomes intrinsic once the nervous system experiences a shift in arousal state and a reduction in fear, rage, and pain. To be in a state of calm and peace can be reinforcing and, coupled with the knowledge that they have learned control over these states, empowering. Most of the published research in the field has been conducted with school-aged children, focusing on ADHD. Only a few case studies or clinical presentations of neurofeedback with younger children and infants exist.

Brain Regions for Training

The brain is one of the most complex organisms on the planet and in the known universe. Science has been studying the brain for decades; however, it is thought that we still know very little about the brain. As discussed in other chapters in this book, brain development is impacted by genetic and environmental factors. As a fetus develops in utero, they begin their attachment and co-regulation process with the mother and the mother's environment. After birth, it is the exposure and exploration of the world that helps to shape various brain structures through synaptic growth, pruning, and myelination of beneficial neuronal connections. Brains exposed to attachment wounds, neglect, and physical, sexual, and emotional abuse find ways to survive. The brain develops strong connections within the fear circuitry of the brain, namely, the locus coeruleus, superior colliculus, periaqueductal gray, and amygdala (Corrigan & Christie-Sands, 2020; Frewen & Lanius, 2015; Harricharan et al., 2016; Teicher et al., 2016), often at the detriment to other areas of the brain, including areas involved with emotion regulation, the sense of self, and executive functioning. While these brain structures are deeper limbic systems and brain stem regions, their activation sends electrical signals to the outermost part of the brain, the cortex.

When working with complexly traumatized children, neurofeedback clinicians need to think about brain training in correlation with the development of the brain. The brain develops communication from the bottom up, back to front, and right to left (Schore, 2005). Moreover, when presented with an arousal profile as over-aroused, unstable, or disordered, as most children with complex trauma and dissociation do, it is imperative to hold the developmental age in mind and the impact the traumas have had on brain development. As a fellow child and developmental trauma neurofeedback provider, Leanne Gregory, DClinPsych, of Ireland, stated in consultation and collaboration, "With this panoramic presentation, this brain seems to need training everywhere, so I can only start at the beginning" (personal communication, April 14, 2023) when thinking about which areas of the brain to be targeting in NFT.

During the clinical assessment, if possible, gaining information about when trauma experiences occurred in the developmental history is essential to correlate to what is happening in the brain at that time of development. We are also thinking about in utero exposures, trauma, attachment disruptions, or wounding that can be exchanged through the amniotic fluid (Brand et al., 2006). One can hypothesize that the very rhythm of the mother and infant can become desynchronized when such trauma occurs. In her book, Sebern Fisher (2014) wrote about training a pregnant mother patient with a highly active, "aggressive" fetus. When the mother's fear and nervous system quieted during an NFT session, it was observed that the fetus's activity also quieted. It was later reported that this fetus developed into a well-regulated infant and toddler with the capacity to self-regulate and co-regulate with the mother and others.

Clinical neurofeedback often focuses on training (listed anatomically back to front) at the inion ridge, occipital, parietal, temporal, central strip, and frontal pole orbital (FPO1 or 2) for regulating arousal and the development of connections between brain areas. Recent research of simultaneous fMRI and EEG recordings found that the amygdala sends signals throughout the cortex, but most concentrated at P1 and PZ locations in the 10–10 system (Meir-Hasson et al., 2016). Furthermore, while researchers continue to discover the cortical relationships between deeper brain structures, especially those associated with trauma, neurofeedback providers look to brain areas that might contribute to the areas of arousal related to complex trauma and dissociation.

There is a hierarchy to protocol choice and development, especially when working with a vulnerable child's traumatized brain. Knowing how the individual nervous system will respond to learning a new firing rate is essential. While research and patterns exist for how a nervous system metabolizes its new functioning, every brain is unique. For this reason, clinicians will often begin NFT centrally or at T4-P4, carefully listening to how the nervous system responds to the changes. For example, if a child is assessed to have an over-aroused profile, the provider would begin training at C4-A2 or C3-C4 if instabilities are noted, as the previous case example demonstrated. If the child continues to be over-aroused after the first training, the provider can adjust. Once the tone of the nervous system is established, different protocols can be explored. Here, we look at various brain regions on which to focus training, organized from the back of the brain toward the front. However, a neurofeedback treatment plan would not necessarily follow this order.

Inion ridge training is a newer region of the brain being explored for child trauma and developmental trauma throughout the lifespan. The inion ridge is the thicker piece of the skull at the base of the head and top of the neck, protecting the brain's early developed areas, the brain stem, and the cerebellum. The cerebellum appears to be significant in the coding of memory early in the development process, in addition to regulating motor control and balance (Ohashi et al., 2019). When we train at IZ, we are typically rewarding low frequencies, thought to be supporting the rhythmicity of early brain development as the neonate PDR's average has been measured in the 2 Hz range (Britton et al., 2016). Research is needed in this area; however, case study reports indicate significant improvement in regulation and quieting fear responses.

The story of Caroline is one such example, especially when we can observe profound changes in her fear response. NFT at IZ and interhemispheric has continued, never increasing the reward band but adjusting the amount of time training to address any under-arousal symptoms that occasionally appear in her tracking. Her overall arousal has continued to lower. She no longer has nightmares. She can access learned sensory modulation and regulation skills, sometimes needing prompting and engaging independently when she notices her arousal state shifting. Her benchmark testing in school showed marked improvement in grade level performance from the beginning of the year (pre-neurofeedback) to mid-year (during neurofeedback). This case example highlights the disordered arousal and the sensitivities of a nervous system that has been exposed to horrific traumas in utero and before the age of 1, and beautifully exemplifies the organizing and regulating quality of the back of the brain (bottom up, back to front) that training can have on executive functioning.

Current research in complex trauma with the adult population has concentrated on established oscillations at PZ to help increase extended range connectivity within the default mode network (DMN) (Shaw et al., 2023), increasing the sense of self and agency, and reducing C-PTSD symptoms. It is noted that the DMN can be connected (back to front) only once the prefrontal cortex is fully developed, around the early to mid-20s (Kolk & Rakic, 2022). Clinically, there are hypotheses about how NFT during brain development can support increasing connectivity in the proto-DMN, especially if the fear circuitry can be quieted. We might train at the parietal lobes when there are concerns about sensory processing, both external and internal sensory systems, supporting the development of interoception and awareness of our body on this earth and in relation to another.

We train at the temporal lobe when emotional regulation and communication concerns occur. Temporal training is often focused interhemispherically (T3-T4) for emotional stability and on the temporoparietal junction (TPJ) (Gapen et al., 2016; Rogel et al., 2020; van der Kolk et al., 2016). The right TPJ is associated with social cognition, awareness, and a sense of another. In our children with complex trauma, especially those of interpersonal or attachment wounding, research has demonstrated that with training at the right TPJ, participants displayed decreased internalizing and externalizing symptoms, increased positive interpersonal relationships, and effective communication. The following case example incorporates TPJ training and its impact on improved emotion regulation and communication.

Case Study: "Fimbo"

"Fimbo" was a young boy, age 8, when his parents sought NFT. He came complete with a history of a difficult birth resulting in separation from his mother and prenatal exposure to domestic violence, which continued until his parents separated. Initially, the mom and Fimbo's concerns were related to attention, regulation, sleep onset and nightmares, and negative interpersonal interactions. These interactions could be either verbally aggressive or dismissive, especially toward the mom. They did not want to place this young child on medication. Because he struggled with verbal expression, Fimbo described many of his nightmares through visual art therapy directives. His pictures had themes of being kidnapped or taken at night, and much of his fear began before he closed his eyes. He would describe the tree outside his window as leaving "arm and finger shadows" and being increasingly aware of the slightest noise from outside of the house.

Fimbo was a bright and curious child. He loved moving his body, doing everything from rock climbing and biking to playing in the woods and building forts, all the while gaining mastery over how he moved and regulated himself when there was an opportunity. Fimbo wanted to be a Formula 1 driver and learn to play the guitar better than Jimmy Page. He was a sensation seeker but could quickly become overwhelmed.

After the assessment, baseline measurements from a mini map were used to help determine starting protocols. It was noted that the slow-wave amplitudes frontally and centrally were significantly elevated for a child his age. This arousal state of the brain activity matches some of his difficulties with attention, especially with the "boring" tasks he had to complete in school. He also had significantly higher levels of high beta centrally and parietally, which also correlates with his concerned symptoms of hypervigilance, being quick to rage, and difficulty with sleep. The clinician determined his PDR to set the initial reward frequency for training.

Starting with C4-A2, the focus became reducing his over-arousal symptoms and helping coach him through lowering his high-beta amplitudes. Fimbo learned quickly to reduce the slow- and fast-wave activity while experiencing and practicing calm, relaxed focus during training. Immediately after training, Fimbo said he felt calm. I noted that while he still enjoyed moving his body around in session, the movement felt less pressured and more purposeful. Fimbo and his mom reported that his sleep was improving every week. After a few sessions, we lowered the reward band to help further address issues of nightmares and regulation, reactions, and reenactments. Once the reward band was more congruent with what supported greater rhythmicity for his nervous system, sleep onset became easier, nightmares became rare, and Fimbo reported feeling rested. His focus and attention were also improving. However, lurking in the shadows, his amygdala, PAG, and superior colliculus were still seeking and reacting to situations of threat.

Just as Fimbo had active fear responses and a hypervigilant threat detection system, so did his mother. As Fimbo's arousal began to improve and he was sleeping through the night, his mom's arousal was stuck in the hypervigilant state, and often, a cascade of fear and anxiety would take over her ability to be as present as she desired in her life and as a mother to her children. Mom began to engage in NFT after completing an arousal assessment and giving consent. Within five training sessions at C4-A2, she was reporting feeling better able to calm herself if an anxious thought took hold in her mind. This afforded her to be better attuned to not only her needs but also the needs of Fimbo and his siblings.

Fimbo often had difficulty communicating his fears and feelings to his mom but would call out at night for comfort, signifying his distress. When he felt threatened, his sleep regulation would regress, and the nightmares would return, creating a vicious cycle of needing sleep and being too fearful of sleeping or being alone at night. I changed the protocol to T4-P4, based on the TPJ research, straddling his PDR for the reward while giving feedback to the developing brain to make less slow- and fast-wave amplitude.

After the first training at T4-P4, Fimbo's mom reported that his mood had improved; he was brighter and more engaged and making eye contact instead of looking down. The night after training, he noted improved sleep, no nightmares, and was "not even afraid of the rain on the windowpanes that sound like someone trying to break in and take me away." The training was quieting the fear circuitry, providing rest his brain and body deserved. Mom also began to train at T4-P4 and began to find sleep onset easier. Staying organized as a mom of three became easier, too, and she found herself better able to be in the present moment without anxious thoughts taking over.

Fimbo continued training at T4-P4 for about 40 sessions, scheduled weekly due to time conflicts, slowly increasing training time as he tolerated, up to 15 minutes a session. Throughout the 40 sessions, his mood steadily improved, and the nightmares and difficulty falling asleep all but disappeared. Fimbo was also able to advocate for himself differently. His mom and teachers reported that instead of yelling or becoming verbally aggressive if he felt unfairness, he would often take a deep breath and then say what he wanted to say without pressure or a change in his tone. This improved his relationships with his family and peers. He could access other learned regulation skills when exposed to a perceived threat. In contrast, before neurofeedback, he reacted with his threat detection systems. When asked how he felt after NFT compared with before, he reported that he knows he has more control and choice, which makes him feel more confident and secure. He is now a high school student, active in athletics, enrolled in honors classes supported by his family, and has meaningful friendships.

For decades in the field of neurofeedback, training was conducted almost exclusively on the central strip, based on the initial investigations of this approach. Sterman's investigations into regulating seizure activity were all conducted centrally (2000). The central strip is located over the fold between the frontal and parietal lobe, making it ideal for training motor control or regulation. Because the field of neurofeedback began at central placements, there is more documentation of arousal level response to training, making it easier to monitor training impacts and to adjust the targeted frequencies. Central placements are often the first protocols taught in introductory classes and the first treatment protocols before transitioning or adding other sites.

The occipital lobe is home to reward and visual processing, and social interactions, and is an integral part of the sensory experience of children's development. One might choose to train the brain in the occipital region if there is a history of witnessing violence, domestic or community, or other traumatic experiences, to support greater rhythmicity and regulation of brain waves. There are also reports of training interhemispherically at the occipital lobe to improve spatial awareness and motor stability.

With dissociation, imaging has also allowed the invisible to become visible. As discussed in other chapters in this book, dissociation is the state of not being present, often in response to overwhelming fear and shock or a flooding memory. There is a continuum of dissociation, from a structural state of preservation, as often seen in high amplitude slow-wave activity, to a more organized state shift, where a child might shift into a different ego state or identity formed in the presence of threat. Frank Putnam (1997) has eloquently described dissociation in children as a discernible failure in the integration of memory, information, perception, and experience, which, while a brain is in its vulnerable development, can have a longitudinal impact on the functioning of the brain's ability to maintain a presence as an older child, adolescent, or adult. It has been documented that the electrical firing patterns of a brain during a dissociative event frequently have a significant drop in overall amplitude of alpha and the lower beta range and can have either a sudden and simultaneous increase in fast wave (more often seen in rigid tonic immobility) or a sudden and simultaneous increase in delta/theta amplitude (more often seen in collapsed immobility). Often, it is both. Neurofeedback, by its very nature, assists the brain in learning to be more present. When working with children with dissociation, it is essential to know what the patterns of dissociation can look like in the EEG and various techniques to bring consciousness back into the body. If dissociative patterns are identified early in an episode, using the feedback to help bring the child into the moment can be enough. I will often direct the child to focus on an additional visual in the game or another external sensation (proprioception, sound of the birds outside, smell of hand lotion or scented markers) while holding the thresholds of the slow- and fast-wave activity to engage the brain in its feedback. If this is not enough to pull the child into the current moment, I will often pause the training and engage in sensorily grounding activities to bring them back into the therapy office and into their body and present moment. The case of "Drake" highlights the impact of neurofeedback on increasing awareness of dissociation, affect regulation, and the development of a sense of self.

Case Study: Drake

Drake was adopted at around 18 months old and came for neurofeedback at age 9 after significant increases in affect regulation issues in the home environment, including aggression toward his mom and younger brothers and placing himself in high-risk, life-threatening positions. He had an insecure, disordered attachment style, and when under perceived relational stress, he would shift into an ego state of a much younger self. This younger self communicated with "baby talk" and limited comprehension compared to his other ego states. He could be indifferent at times but also needed the containment of another adult. There were questions and concerns regarding dissociative symptoms during times of threat. He was constantly scanning and alert but never present. He struggled with executive functioning, reading, math, processing speed, and the social prosody needed to develop peer relationships. In play therapy, themes of kidnapping and violent storms included frenetic activity revolving around villains and kidnappers and freeze-state activity from the "children" in the stories.

Once he understood that I could not read his thoughts and that he got to play a video game using his brain as the controller, he was excited, albeit nervous, to begin neurofeedback. At the initial intake session, Drake was cautious about the prospect of someone applying sensors to his head, so I connected them to mine, demonstrating what some of the games looked like and what I would be looking at on the therapist's "wave screen." I gathered a sequential baseline measurement of amplitude at CZ and PZ (eyes open, eyes closed) to help determine his PDR, which measured at 8 Hz. Because of his over-aroused and unstable arousal assessment, the initial training site was C3-C4 9–12 Hz reward with 1–6 Hz and 22–36 Hz inhibits.

After training, I observed a brief calm in the room and a quieter body. His mom's report indicated that on the day of training, he was calmer on the car ride home and during the evening routine, had difficulty sleeping, and the next day returned to baseline. It was beautiful that he was responding well to training. However, his anxiety and fear needed more quieting.

We gradually reduced the reward by 0.25 Hz to start, then 0.125 due to nervous system sensitivities, and eventually landed on a 7.125–10.125 Hz reward, increasing the time to nine minutes total.

Drake appeared more regulated between and coming into sessions. Play therapy and art therapy directives were less frenetic. However, themes of fear, loss, and kidnapping continued in sessions and were communicated between sessions between parents and school personnel. At Session 10, we added a T4-P4 7–10 Hz reward and 1–6 Hz, 22–36 Hz inhibit, three minutes to start, building to six minutes, and concluding with C3-C4 training based on his sensory and emotional responsivity. The parents reported some reduced fear and reactive behaviors and increased communication of feelings. However, Drake's arousal state continued to be elevated, often dropping into freeze and dissociation. As at C3-C4, his reward frequency needed to be lowered to better regulate and calm his nervous system.

My office was arranged with the client chair facing a long wall, with the neurofeedback monitor a few feet from a window overlooking large sugar maple and Norway spruce trees. For one training session, there was a forecast of high winds and severe thunderstorms throughout the day. The gusts of wind must have been up to 65 mph, with the trees bending to the velocity. Drake was settled into his chair, sensors applied, and ready to begin training when he asked me to close the blinds because he was distracted and thinking about the wind. One of his significant traumas was a car accident during severe weather and high winds. In his play therapy sessions, he developed a story of his biological mother being crushed by a falling tree from hurricane winds in the country of his birth.

Drake took a few grounding, slow out-breaths and was able to begin his training. He selected a game called 4Mation, which has a hidden photograph, pieces of which are unveiled when the brain meets the conditions of less low/fast-wave and enough thalpha (theta-alpha combined). After a few minutes, a roar of wind could be felt without seeing it through the window. Almost immediately, his EEG changed. His raw EEG began to wander, and the slow-wave amplitude suddenly increased. Following this was a sudden increase in Drake's fast-wave frequency. It all happened within a two-second window of time. I attuned myself to Drake. He was staring in the direction of the window, vacant, with shallow breathing and tightened neck and shoulders. His hands were gripping the arms of the supportive lounge chair. He was experiencing a dissociative episode.

I paused the game and worked with Drake through grounding and sensory modulation techniques to help him return to his body. Once present, he quickly expressed that the wind and weather were too scary for him. After a few months away from neurofeedback due to the COVID-19 pandemic, training resumed, and we added IZ-A2. Immediately, there was renewed increased interest in social connections, reduced agitation, and, most importantly, reduced fear and fewer observed dissociative episodes. Drake's play and art continued to have themes of kidnapping. However, every chapter or drawing now had a "hero" and helpful characters to return the kidnapped to a place of safety and security. The younger self ego state showed up less and less, even as he was engaging in more interpersonal relationships.

Neurofeedback is a versatile modality used in different settings such as residential programs, acute hospitals, community mental health centers, in-home therapy, outpatient offices, and, increasingly, schools. There have been a few research studies in which neurofeedback was offered explicitly within the school setting, with results such as improved executive functioning measurements, reduced time away from learning, and improved social interactions (Steiner et al., 2014). The public school district in Moab, Utah, has a neurofeedback program within the school counseling department. Students can engage in neurofeedback during school hours and often as a part of their IEP social or emotional goal. While working within the school environment, students are pulled from electives such as music, art, or gym. Symptom tracking and support are coordinated with the classroom teachers. In this setting, the provider also has the unique opportunity to observe how the child engages in the classrooms with academic tasks, peer and adult interactions, and if they can utilize various coping skills for regulation. Program director and certified neurofeedback provider Kelly Vagts describes the neurofeedback process in her elementary school through a case example; names were not provided.

> Case Study: Eight-Year-Old Boy
>
> An eight-year-old boy with little motor coordination, high levels of dissociation, self-injurious behaviors, significant early trauma history, and exposure to substances in utero and postnatally needed more therapeutic intervention. He was quick to rage over events and could not control his body when walking down the hallway; he would throw himself on the floor or against walls. School personnel would engage in make-believe, pretending to be cats, playfully crawling on all fours and meowing, to get him safely around the school building. The boy had such a vacancy in his presentation that he was not benefiting from traditional trauma therapy approaches. He was certainly struggling to access academic learning. Kelly began his training at T4-P4, slowly adding time to the training sessions, and pausing between game rounds to help ground and keep him present with supportive touch or proprioceptive input. NFT was completed twice weekly for about two years, with breaks over school vacations. The reward band was set around his PDR based on age and developmental stage, although it varied at different placements.
>
> Over the next two years, the protocol placements varied to address different symptoms that were appearing as he came more into the present moment in his body and mind, including C4-P4 (trauma memory in the body), T3-T4 (emotional expression), back to T4-P4, F4-T4 (executive functioning and reading), CZ-A2 (limbic regulation), and lastly IZ-A2, rewarding at 2.5–5.5 Hz. With each protocol change and training session, there was incremental progress toward presence and regulation. With IZ training, he ended psychiatric medications and has since been medication free.
>
> NFT with the boy concluded when the COVID-19 pandemic shuttered the school buildings for months. Nonetheless, his regulation gains carry on. Three years after his last training session, Kelly describes him as insightful, aware of himself and others, and empathetic. He is curious about the world and allows his village of secure relationships to cheer him on. He is described as knowing joy, love, and safety. Behaviors such as head-banging, nail scratching, and rage are part of his history, but they are no longer his present.

Conclusion

NFT in the treatment of complex trauma and dissociation with children is in its infancy in terms of empirical research; nonetheless, the clinical evidence is mounting. While the modality itself can feel cumbersome and it can feel overwhelming to learn such a technology-driven intervention, the outcomes are often unparalleled for this traditionally difficult-to-treat population. Because we can lead the brain toward regulation with neurofeedback and therapeutic relationships, we can increase resiliency, awareness, and the sense of self and another. The last case of the young boy receiving neurofeedback in his school demonstrates the impact and experience of regulation three years after his last session. Imagine the impact ten years after his last session, when his prefrontal cortex is fully connected. Imagine the hypothetical case of the six-year-old boy entering a residential program, fearful, and feral. Suppose this boy received neurofeedback in his residential program. He is getting restful sleep for the first time in his life. He can transition from play to classwork. He can form meaningful relationships with his peers and caregivers. He practices and uses relaxation strategies to manage his reactivity. Suppose his adoptive parents received neurofeedback as well. Family visits become an opportunity to play and be present with each other, rewriting their relationships from a place of fear and reactivity toward a place of safety, security, and attunement. Imagine a world where children are given the opportunity to shape their future by managing their present. We have that opportunity when we introduce neurofeedback into our practices.

References

American Academy of Pediatrics. (2014). Evidence-based child and adolescent psychosocial interventions. bio-medical.com/media/blog/evidence-based-child-and-adolescent-psychosocial-interventions.pdf

Bazanova, O. M. (2012). Alpha EEG activity depends on the individual dominant rhythm frequency. *Journal of Neurotherapy, 16*(4), 270–284. https://doi.org/10.1080/10874208.2012.730786

Berger, H. (1929). On the EEG in humans. *Archiv fur Psychiatrie und Nervenkrankheiten, 87*, 527–570.

Bluhm, R. L., Williamson, P. C., Osuch, E. A., Frewen, P. A., Stevens, T. K., Boksman, K., Neufeld, R. W. J., Théberge, J., & Lanius, R. A. (2009). Alterations in default network connectivity in posttraumatic stress disorder related to early-life trauma. *Journal of Psychiatry & Neuroscience, 34*(3), 187.

Boodoo, R., Lagman, J. G., Jairath, B., & Baweja, R. (2022). A review of ADHD and childhood trauma: Treatment challenges and clinical guidance. *Current Developmental Disorders Reports, 9*(4), 137–145. https://doi.org/10.1007/s40474-022-00256-2

Brand, S. R., Engel, S. M., Canfield, R. L., & Yehuda, R. (2006). The effect of maternal PTSD following in utero trauma exposure on behavior and temperament in the 9-month-old infant. *Annals of the New York Academy of Sciences, 1071*(1), 454–458. https://doi.org/10.1196/annals.1364.041

Britton, J. W., Frey, L. C., Hopp, J. L., Korb, P., Koubeissi, M. Z., Lievens, W. E., Pestana-Knight, E. M., & St. Louis, E. K. (2016). *Electroencephalography (EEG): An introductory text and atlas of normal and abnormal findings in adults, children, and infants.* American Epilepsy Society.

Corrigan, F. M., & Christie-Sands, J. (2020). An innate brainstem self-other system involving orienting, affective responding, and polyvalent relational seeking: Some clinical implications for a "deep brain reorienting" trauma psychotherapy approach. *Medical Hypotheses, 136*, Article 109502. https://doi.org/10.1016/j.mehy.2019.109502

Fisher, S. F. (2014). *Neurofeedback in the treatment of developmental trauma: Calming the fear-driven brain.* W. W. Norton.

Frewen, P., & Lanius, R. (2015). *Healing the traumatized self: Consciousness, neuroscience, treatment.* W. W. Norton.

Gapen, M., van der Kolk, B. A., Hamlin, E., Hirshberg, L., Suvak, M., & Spinazzola, J. (2016). A pilot study of neurofeedback for chronic PTSD. *Applied Psychophysiology and Biofeedback, 41*, 251–261. https://doi.org/10.1007/s10484-015-9326-5

Gardner, D. G. (1986). Activation theory and task design: An empirical test of several new predictions. *Journal of Applied Psychology, 71*(3), 411. https://doi.org/10.1037/0021-9010.71.3.411

Hamlin, E. (2018). Growing the evidence base for neurofeedback in clinical practice. In J. J. Magnavita (Ed.), *Using technology in mental health practice* (pp. 101–122). American Psychological Association. https://doi.org/10.1037/0000085-007

Hargraves, H. K. (2017). *Therapeutic induction of altered states of consciousness: Investigation of 1–20Hz neurofeedback* [Doctoral dissertation, University of Western Ontario]. Scholarship@Western, Electronic Thesis and Dissertation Repository. 4517. ir.lib.uwo.ca/etd/4517

Harricharan, S., Rabellino, D., Frewen, P. A., Densmore, M., Théberge, J., McKinnon, M. C., Schore, A., & Lanius, R. A. (2016). fMRI functional connectivity of the periaqueductal gray in PTSD and its dissociative subtype. *Brain and Behavior, 6*(12). Article e00579. https://doi.org/10.1002/brb3.579

Hebb, D. O. (1955). Drives and the CNS (conceptual nervous system). *Psychological Review, 62*(4), 243–254. https://doi.org/10.1037/h0041823

Hirshberg, L. M., Chiu, S., & Frazier, J. A. (2005). Emerging brain-based interventions for children and adolescents: Overview and clinical perspective. *Child and Adolescent Psychiatric Clinics, 14*(1), 1–19. https://doi.org/10.1016/j.chc.2004.07.011

ISNR (International Society for Neuroregulation and Research) (n.d.). What is neurofeedback? Retrieved April 2023 from isnr.org/what-is-neurofeedback

Kamiya, J. (1971). Biofeedback training in voluntary control of EEG alpha rhythms. *California Medicine, 115*(3), 44.

Kolk, S. M., & Rakic, P. (2022). Development of prefrontal cortex. *Neuropsychopharmacology, 47*(1), 41–57. https://doi.org/10.1038/s41386-021-01137-9

Mayer, K., Wyckoff, S. N., & Strehl, U. (2013). One size fits all? Slow cortical potentials neurofeedback: A review. *Journal of Attention Disorders, 17*(5), 393–409. https://doi.org/10.1177/1087054712468053

Meir-Hasson, Y., Keynan, J. N., Kinreich, S., Jackont, G., Cohen, A., Podlipsky-Klovatch, I., Hendler, T., & Intrator, N. (2016). One-class FMRI-inspired EEG model for self-regulation training. *PLoS One, 11*(5), e0154968. https://doi.org/10.1371/journal.pone.0154968

Miodus, S., Allwood, M. A., & Amoh, N. (2021). Childhood ADHD symptoms in relation to trauma exposure and PTSD symptoms among college students: Attending to and accommodating trauma. *Journal of Emotional and Behavioral Disorders, 29*(3), 187–196. https://doi.org/10.1177/1063426620982624

Monastra, V. J., Lynn, S., Linden, M., Lubar, J. F., Gruzelier, J., & La Vaque, T. J. (2006). Electroencephalographic biofeedback in the treatment of attention-deficit/hyperactivity disorder. *Journal of Neurotherapy, 9*(4), 5–34. https://doi.org/10.1007/s10484-005-4305-x

Neurofeedback Collaborative Group. (2021). Double-blind placebo-controlled randomized clinical trial of neurofeedback for attention-deficit/hyperactivity disorder with 13-month follow-up. *Journal of the American Academy of Child and Adolescent Psychiatry, 60*(7), 841–855. https://doi.org/10.1016/j.jaac.2020.07.906

Nicholson, A. A., Ros, T., Frewen, P. A., Densmore, M., Théberge, J., Kluetsch, R. C., Jetly, R., & Lanius, R. A. (2016). Alpha oscillation neurofeedback modulates amygdala complex connectivity and arousal in posttraumatic stress disorder. *NeuroImage: Clinical, 12*, 506–516. https://doi.org/10.1016/j.nicl.2016.07.006

Ochs, L. (2019). My 50 years of history in the field. *Neurofeedback: The First Fifty Years* (pp. 307–316). Academic Press. https://doi.org/10.1016/b978-0-12-817659-7.00041-5

Ohashi, K., Anderson, C. M., Bolger, E. A., Khan, A., McGreenery, C. E., & Teicher, M. H. (2019). Susceptibility or resilience to maltreatment can be explained by specific differences in brain network architecture. *Biological Psychiatry, 85*(8), 690–702. https://doi.org/10.1016/j.biopsych.2018.10.016

Ortiz, R. (2019). Building resilience against the sequelae of adverse childhood experiences: Rise up, change your life, and reform health care. *American Journal of Lifestyle Medicine, 13*(5), 470–479. https://doi.org/10.1177/1559827619839997

Othmer, S., & Othmer, S. (2017). Development of the Othmer method of neurofeedback. https://doi.org/10.13140/RG.2.2.31226.90562

Peniston, E. G., & Kulkosky, P. J. (1991). Alpha-theta brainwave neurofeedback for Vietnam veterans with combat-related post-traumatic stress disorder. *Medical Psychotherapy, 4*(1), 47–60.

Putnam, F. W. (1997). *Dissociation in children and adolescents: A developmental perspective.* Guilford Press.

Roelofs, K. (2017). Freeze for action: Neurobiological mechanisms in animal and human freezing. *Philosophical Transactions of the Royal Society of London. Series B, Biological Sciences, 372*(1718). https://doi.org/10.1098/rstb.2016.0206

Rogel, A., Loomis, A. M., Hamlin, E., Hodgdon, H., Spinazzola, J., & van der Kolk, B. (2020). The impact of neurofeedback training on children with developmental trauma: A randomized controlled study. *Psychological Trauma: Theory, Research, Practice, and Policy, 12*(8), 918–929. https://doi.org/10.1037/tra0000648

Sammer, G., Blecker, C., Gebhardt, H., Bischoff, M., Stark, R., Morgen, K., & Vaitl, D. (2007). Relationship between regional hemodynamic activity and simultaneously recorded EEG-theta associated with mental arithmetic-induced workload. *Human Brain Mapping, 28*(8), 793–803. https://doi.org/10.1002/hbm.20309

Schore, A. N. (2005). Attachment, affect regulation, and the developing right brain: Linking developmental neuroscience to pediatrics. *Pediatrics in Review, 26*(6), 204–217. https://doi.org/10.1542/pir.26-6-204

Schore, A. N. (2018). The right brain implicit self: A central mechanism of the psychotherapy change process. In J. Petrucelli (Ed.), *Knowing, not-knowing and sort-of-knowing* (pp. 177–202). Routledge.

Schutz, C. A., & Herbert, J. (2022). Review of the evidence for neurofeedback training for children and adolescents who have experienced traumatic events. *Trauma, Violence, & Abuse, 24*(5), 3564–3578. https://doi.org/10.1177/15248380221134295

Shaw, S. B., Nicholson, A. A., Ros, T., Harricharan, S., Terpou, B., Densmore, M., Theberge, J., Frewen, P., & Lanius, R. A. (2023). Increased top-down control of emotions during symptom provocation working memory tasks following a RCT of alpha-down neurofeedback in PTSD. *NeuroImage: Clinical, 37*, Article 103313. https://doi.org/10.1016/j.nicl.2023.103313

Steiner, N. J., Frenette, E. C., Rene, K. M., Brennan, R. T., & Perrin, E. C. (2014). In-school neurofeedback training for ADHD: Sustained improvements from a randomized control trial. *Pediatrics, 133*(3), 483–492. https://doi.org/10.1542/peds.2013-2059

Sterman, M. B. (2000). Basic concepts and clinical findings in the treatment of seizure disorders with EEG operant conditioning. *Clinical Electroencephalography, 33*, 45–55. https://doi.org/10.1177/155005940003100111

Teicher, M. H., Samson, J. A., Anderson, C. M., & Ohashi, K. (2016). The effects of childhood maltreatment on brain structure, function and connectivity. *Nature Reviews Neuroscience, 17*(10), 652–666. https://doi.org/10.1038/nrn.2016.111

van der Kolk, B. (2014). *The body keeps the score: Brain, mind, and body in the healing of trauma.* Viking Press.

van der Kolk, B. A., Hodgdon, H., Gapen, M., Musicaro, R., Suvak, M. K., Hamlin, E., & Spinazzola, J. (2016). A randomized controlled study of neurofeedback for chronic PTSD. *PLoS One, 11*(12), e0166752. https://doi.org/10.1371/journal.pone.0166752

Wyrwicka, W., & Sterman, M. B. (1968). Instrumental conditioning of sensorimotor cortex EEG spindles in the waking cat. *Physiology & Behavior, 3*, 703–707. https://doi.org/10.1002/cne.920180503

Yerkes, R. M., & Dodson, J. D. (1908). The relation of strength of stimulus to rapidity of habit formation. *Journal of Comparative Neurology & Psychology, 18*, 459–482. https://doi.org/10.1002/cne.920180503

Yu, R. (2015). Choking under pressure: The neuropsychological mechanisms of incentive-induced performance decrements. *Frontiers in Behavioral Neuroscience, 9*, 19. https://doi.org/10.3389/fnbeh.2015.00019

25
TRAUMA-FOCUSED COGNITIVE-BEHAVIORAL THERAPY
Not Just for Acute Trauma Anymore!

Matthew D. Kliethermes

Introduction

Trauma-focused cognitive-behavioral therapy (TF-CBT) is the most well-supported, evidence-based treatment for trauma reactions in children (de Arellano et al., 2014; Thielemann et al., 2022). However, due to common misconceptions about TF-CBT, many mental health professionals wrongly assume that the treatment is not appropriate for children experiencing outcomes associated with complex trauma exposure. This chapter will begin with a basic overview of TF-CBT and then explore various application strategies for TF-CBT with children experiencing complex trauma outcomes, including dissociation.

Core Principles of TF-CBT

TF-CBT (Cohen et al., 2017) is the most widely disseminated and implemented intervention for childhood trauma exposure (Cohen et al., 2010). TF-CBT is appropriate for children aged 3–18 who have experienced trauma, including complex trauma, and are exhibiting significant trauma-related difficulties such as post-traumatic stress disorder (PTSD), depression, and behavior problems. TF-CBT has recently been piloted with transitional-aged youth (aged 15–25), with initial results suggesting TF-CBT is feasible, acceptable, and potentially clinically effective for this demographic (Peters et al., 2021).

TF-CBT is a "hybrid" cognitive-behavioral intervention, combining trauma-sensitive treatments with cognitive-behavioral theory, but also including elements of attachment, developmental neurobiology, family, empowerment, and humanistic theory to best meet the needs of traumatized children and families (Cohen et al., 2017).

There are several core principles inherent to TF-CBT (Cohen & Mannarino, 2022). These principles are (1) phase- and components-based treatment, (2) component order and proportionality of phases, (3) the use of gradual exposure, and (4) the importance of caregiver involvement in treatment.

TF-CBT is a phase- and components-based treatment. The three phases of TF-CBT are Stabilization, Trauma Narration, and Integration. These three phases are made up of the TF-CBT PRACTICE components: psychoeducation, parenting skills, relaxation skills, affect modulation skills, cognitive coping skills, trauma narration and processing, in vivo mastery of trauma reminders, conjoint child-parent sessions, and enhancing safety and future development (see Table 25.1).

Table 25.1 TF-CBT Components and Phases

Stabilization Phase	Psychoeducation
	Parenting skills
	Relaxation
	Affect modulation skills
	Cognitive coping skills
Trauma Narration Phase	Trauma narration and processing
Integration Phase	In vivo mastery
	Conjoint child-parent sessions
	Enhancing safety and future development

Fidelity to the model is believed necessary to achieve positive treatment outcomes and includes the following: (1) PRACTICE components are provided in sequential order, barring circumstances that indicate the need to prioritize stabilization skills and safety; (2) all PRACTICE components are implemented (other than in vivo mastery, which is not always clinically indicated); and (3) the Stabilization, Trauma Narration, and Integration phases are implemented in appropriate proportion and duration. Typical TF-CBT duration is 12–15 sessions for trauma treatment cases, and each treatment phase receives a roughly equal number of sessions (typically four to five sessions per phase).

The core principles of TF-CBT remain in effect when working with children exhibiting complex trauma outcomes, but specific interventions within the TF-CBT components are tailored to address their specific symptom presentation (Cohen et al., 2012). These applications for complex trauma and dissociation will be discussed in more detail throughout the remainder of this chapter.

Gradual Exposure to Traumatic Content

A fundamental principle of TF-CBT is gradual exposure (Cohen et al., 2017). Gradual exposure involves progressively exposing the child to trauma cues and memories of increasing intensity. Trauma is discussed in every TF-CBT session. During the skill-building components of treatment, the child identifies their trauma cues and develops skills for coping with them. In the trauma narration component, the child gradually progresses from processing minimally distressing memories to the most distressing. Over time, the child experiences decreasing distress in response to trauma processing. Learning to tolerate this distress results in the child developing improved mastery over traumatic memories, weakening the association between traumatic memories/reminders and strong emotional or physiological reactions. Through gradual exposure, the child learns that trauma content can be approached in a safe, controlled manner.

It is critical to highlight the gradual aspect of this process as opposed to "flooding" the child with trauma content. Gradual exposure is intended to prevent the child's coping resources from being overwhelmed by trauma content, causing them to decompensate in session and/or fall back on maladaptive coping strategies (e.g., dissociation and self-injury). Neither outcome accomplishes the goal of weakening the child's mental associations between traumatic memories and current distress.

This gradual approach is crucial when working with dysregulation associated with complex trauma and dissociation. The early components of TF-CBT are focused on skill-building and increasing tolerance of trauma content through indirect exposure (e.g., talking about trauma in general). Aspects of dissociation-focused therapy (Wieland & Silberg, 2013) can be easily integrated into gradual exposure. It is critical that the TF-CBT therapist attend to the child's emotional, behavioral, and physiological presentation during the gradual exposure process, looking for indicators of dysregulation or dissociation. When indicators are identified, the TF-CBT therapist can utilize grounding activities to help the child remain regulated and present during gradual exposure. Gradual exposure can also include the identification and discussion of environmental cues that trigger dissociative responses both inside and outside of therapy. TF-CBT therapists can also help children attend to moments of dissociation during gradual exposure including dissociated feelings, sensations, cognitions, and memories.

Of note, the presence of dissociation does not dramatically change the gradual exposure process. Dissociation in the context of gradual exposure would be approached much like any other maladaptive coping strategy (e.g., avoidance, aggression). Namely, it would be identified as a coping strategy that previously made sense but may no longer be of benefit to the child, and then adaptive coping strategies would be developed to be used in its stead.

Caregiver Involvement

Although TF-CBT is child-focused, it values caregivers' roles with their children, particularly as models for coping with trauma. Following a traumatic occurrence, children look to caregivers to know how to respond. Lessons learned by observing their caregivers can be potentially helpful or problematic (Deblinger & Heflin, 1996). Caregiver involvement in TF-CBT is intended to increase their ability to model positive coping strategies and limit reliance on maladaptive responses. There are clear indications that positive caregiver functioning has a strong ameliorative influence on children's trauma-related symptoms (Cohen & Mannarino, 2000). The inclusion of caregivers in TF-CBT is a key mechanism for recovery (Cohen et al., 2017).

The main goals of caregiver involvement are to promote the ability to engage in trauma-informed parenting, help the caregiver understand the need for gradual exposure, and promote the ability to regulate their thoughts and emotions regarding the child's trauma. Ideally, the caregiver becomes a more helpful model for trauma-related coping and support for the child. These goals are accomplished in parallel with work done with the child. Caregivers develop positive parenting skills and stress management, experience their own gradual exposure, and identify and correct trauma-related cognitive errors. With therapist support, the caregiver then applies these skills in conjoint sessions with the child and ideally will continue after treatment has ended.

These aspects of caregiver involvement in TF-CBT are perhaps even more relevant for children with complex trauma outcomes and dissociation. Strengthening attachment bonds between children and their caregivers can increase the child's sense of safety and lower their need for problematic coping strategies like dissociation (Wieland & Silberg, 2013). The caregivers can also model adaptive forms of coping by promoting open discussion of feelings and sensations and active problem-solving. A primary aspect of caregiver work within TF-CBT is making sure that the caregiver is able to conceptualize their child's difficulties in the context of post-traumatic stress and respond in a trauma-informed manner. Helping caregivers understand and respond to dissociation would be no different from helping the caregiver understand other common trauma reactions, including nightmares, hypervigilance, and irritability.

TF-CBT PRACTICE Components

The three phases of TF-CBT comprise the PRACTICE components: psychoeducation, parenting skills, relaxation, affect modulation skills, cognitive coping skills, trauma narration and processing, in vivo mastery, conjoint child-parent sessions, and enhancing safety and future development (Kliethermes & Wamser, 2012). These components will be discussed in greater detail during discussion of TF-CBT implementation with children experiencing complex trauma outcomes and dissociation.

During psychoeducation, the child and caregiver receive information about trauma, common trauma reactions, and trauma reminders. The therapist then works with the family to connect this information with the child's own trauma experiences and reactions, including an understanding of trauma reminders in the child's daily life. This information is tailored to the needs of the child and caregiver and is designed to normalize trauma exposure and responses and instill hope for recovery and improved functioning.

In the parenting skills component, caregivers learn effective strategies for responding to trauma-related behavioral and emotional dysregulation evidenced by the child. This work is typically conducted in the context of instruction, practice, and role-play. Typical parenting skills addressed include the use of time out, praise, positive attention, selective attention, and behavioral contingencies.

Relaxation addresses physiological hyper-arousal associated with trauma exposure, possibly experienced by the child and caregiver. The therapist works with the child to develop personalized relaxation strategies in session and then encourages regular practice at home. Common relaxation strategies include focused breathing, progressive muscle relaxation, and visualization, but a variety of skills can be included based on child development and interest. Caregivers are taught the child's preferred relaxation exercises, to learn to recognize when the child would benefit from these exercises, and how to coach the child in using these skills. Caregivers may also find these exercises valuable for their own anxiety or hyper-arousal.

During the affect modulation skills, the therapist helps the child identify and express emotions and develop skills for managing uncomfortable mood states. Affect modulation skills include problem-solving, seeking social support, healthy distraction techniques, mindfulness, and general anger management, with a focus on using these skills in response to trauma reminders. The therapist educates and practices with the caregiver how to encourage and support the child in using these skills. Therapists often work with caregivers on developing their capacity to tolerate emotional expression by the child and to respond to these expressions empathetically rather than punitively.

In cognitive processing skills, the focus is on developing the child's ability to recognize connections between thoughts, feelings, and behaviors (the cognitive triangle) and to replace inaccurate or unhelpful thoughts with more adaptive replacements. Trauma-related beliefs are not the focus during this component, as it is more effective to process these beliefs during trauma narration. Common techniques include progressive logical questioning, responsibility pie, best-friend role-play, and balanced thinking. The therapist also meets with the caregiver to introduce the cognitive triangle and begin processing the caregiver's maladaptive beliefs. Initially, this work addresses everyday beliefs but may progress to trauma-related beliefs (e.g., I failed as a parent because my child was abused).

Trauma narration and processing involves the therapist and child interactively processing the child's traumatic experience(s), emphasizing thoughts, feelings, and physical sensations that occurred during the trauma(s). This is done by gradually increasing intensity with less distressing memories first followed by more distressing memories. This leads to the child processing the most distressing traumatic memories and the development of mastery rather than avoidance. During this process (or in prior components), the child and therapist identify unhelpful beliefs about the trauma (e.g., the abuse was my fault because I am a bad kid). Previously learned cognitive skills are used to help the child process unhelpful beliefs and identify more helpful, balanced beliefs about their traumatic experiences. This often includes the development of a tangible summary of the process, typically in the form of a story, poem, song, or artwork. However, it is important to recognize that this tangible product is less critical than the interactive process between the child and therapist.

In each session, as the child develops the narration, the therapist meets with the caregiver to review the content. This familiarizes the caregiver with the child's trauma experiences, helps them develop mastery of their own distress and avoidance related to the information, identifies and addresses the caregiver's unhelpful beliefs about the trauma, and prepares the caregiver for conjoint child-parent sessions.

In vivo mastery is the sole optional component of TF-CBT. Following trauma, some children develop fear and avoidance related to innocuous situations or cues. If this impacts functioning, it may be addressed in TF-CBT. For example, a child who was involved in a car accident may avoid getting into a car. This could have a significant impact on functioning, making in vivo mastery appropriate. Rather than imaginal exposure, in vivo mastery involves direct exposure to the innocuous situation (e.g., getting into a car) that the child fears and avoids. Gradually facing the situation and realizing the feared outcome does not occur results in reduced avoidance. Borrowing from systematic desensitization, in vivo mastery involves the therapist, child, and caregiver developing a fear hierarchy, from the least feared to the most feared scenario, typically using a scale from 1 to 10. With the support of the caregiver, the child gradually works through the hierarchy until they master the final spot.

Conjoint child-parent sessions occur multiple times during the integration phase of TF-CBT. The component focuses on enhancing communication between the child and caregiver about trauma. Conjoint sessions typically involve meeting individually with both the child and caregiver (five to ten minutes each) to prepare for the rest of the session, which involves 40–50 minutes of conjoint work. The initial conjoint session typically involves the child sharing their trauma narrative with the caregiver. The goal of this session is to encourage deeper discussion about trauma, which is often identified by families as the most beneficial aspect of TF-CBT. Subsequent conjoint child-parent sessions may address healthy sexuality, family communication, or enhancing safety. These topics are determined by the therapist based on what would be beneficial for the child/family.

Enhancing safety and future development focuses on enhancing the child's physical and emotional safety and providing the necessary skills to promote adaptive future functioning. This component often includes traditional safety skills such as assertive communication, seeking support from safe adults, and the development of family safety plans.

Effectiveness Research: General TF-CBT

TF-CBT is the most extensively studied intervention for childhood post-traumatic stress. As of 2023, TF-CBT has been evaluated in approximately 23 randomized controlled trials comparing it to other active treatments or wait-list control conditions. TF-CBT has been evaluated across the entire childhood developmental range (3–18 years), for multiple types of trauma, in a variety of settings, and in multiple countries and cultures (Cohen & Mannarino, 2022). In all studies conducted, TF-CBT was found more effective than comparison conditions for addressing symptoms of PTSD and other trauma-related difficulties, including depression, anxiety, and behavioral, cognitive, and relationship problems. A recent meta-analysis (Thielemann et al., 2022) was conducted based on a selection of 61 studies that met inclusion criteria. Results for the meta-analysis indicated strong support for TF-CBT, suggesting that it is an efficacious treatment for childhood post-traumatic stress with promising results for depression, anxiety, and grief.

TF-CBT Applications for Complex Trauma and Dissociation

A common misconception regarding TF-CBT is that it cannot be used with children exposed to complex trauma. Instead, it is assumed that TF-CBT is effective only with acute trauma (e.g., a car accident). However, complex trauma applications for TF-CBT have been developed, and the effectiveness of TF-CBT with complex trauma has been evaluated. These applications and evaluation outcomes will be the focus of the remainder of this chapter.

Complex Trauma and TF-CBT Implementation

The National Child Traumatic Stress Network defines complex trauma as "exposure to multiple traumatic events, often of an invasive, interpersonal nature, and the wide-ranging, long-term impact of this exposure" (National Child Traumatic Stress Network [NCTSN], n.d.). While the number of traumas experienced by a child does impact the implementation of TF-CBT, implementation is most impacted by the wide-ranging impact of this exposure. Specifically, in addition to traditional PTSD symptoms, complex trauma outcomes often include dysregulation in multiple areas of function, including emotions, physiological arousal, attention, behavior, self-concept, and relationships (DePierro et al., 2022). Dysregulation does not refer to just emotional outbursts, hyperactivity, or other examples of hyper-arousal, but also includes hypo-arousal including emotional constriction, withdrawal, and other forms of dissociation.

Dysregulation can be impactful in all therapy. Given the dysregulating nature of trauma processing itself, dysregulation in the context of a trauma-focused intervention such as TF-CBT often carries increased weight. The dysregulation associated with complex trauma outcomes can be conceptualized as a survival adaptation that has become habitual and chronic (Courtois & Ford, 2013). Neutral environmental cues, such as redirection by a therapist, can be perceived as threats, leading to maladaptive survival responses (e.g., running out of the therapist's office). For dysregulated children, day-to-day stress levels tend to remain high. The developing therapeutic alliance may trigger concerns about trust and safety. Therapist attempts to structure sessions may be perceived as threatening. Dissociation may result in the child not being "present" enough in sessions to benefit from trauma processing. Subsequently, the application of TF-CBT components may need to be altered, and the emphasis on phase-based implementation becomes even more critical (Kliethermes & Wamser, 2012).

Dysregulation can be a therapy-interfering behavior or create an increased risk of harm to the child. Dysregulation may result in a child client who is unable to remain in the therapist's office without emotional and behavioral outbursts, or a child who is completely shut down and unable to engage with the therapist in therapeutic activities. Dysregulation is also associated with behaviors that can substantially increase the risk of harm. Distress reduction behaviors (Briere, 2019), including aggression, risky sexual behavior, binging and purging, self-injury, and substance use, may occur and are often the best efforts of youth to self-regulate. While these behaviors may alleviate immediate distress, they often increase stress in the long term (e.g., school suspensions, relational conflict) and can also increase the risk of harm to self or others (e.g., drug overdose, violence perpetrated on others). These behaviors often become a necessary clinical focus, particularly early in treatment (Kinnish et al., 2021).

For these reasons, dysregulation must be considered when implementing TF-CBT for complex trauma and dissociation. The remainder of this chapter will focus on how the TF-CBT model in general, and the PRACTICE components specifically, can be best applied to address complex trauma and dissociation outcomes.

Overview of PRACTICE Component Applications for Complex Trauma and Dissociation

The phase-based approach is believed to be important when implementing TF-CBT with complex trauma. Expert consensus recommends phase-based interventions for complex trauma survivors (Cloitre et al., 2012) and in the context of dissociation-focused treatment (Wieland & Silberg, 2013). Research indicates that phase-based approaches are effective in treating complex trauma outcomes in adults (Cloitre et al., 2010), but are not clearly more effective than "stand-alone" therapies such as eye movement desensitization and reprocessing (EMDR) (van Vliet et al., 2021) and prolonged exposure (Oprel et al., 2021).Phase-based approaches appear to be effective for youth exposed to trauma (Dauber et al., 2015; Fischer et al., 2022). However, no research appears to exist comparing the efficacy of phase-based interventions to "stand-alone" therapies for children.

Not all complex trauma survivors present with severe dysregulation. While most children exposed to complex trauma will exhibit some signs of dysregulation, both hyper- and/or hypo-arousal, it may not reach the level of creating significant therapy-interfering behaviors, or risk of harm to the child (e.g., occasional "zoning out" during sessions). In practice, the decision to use phase-based treatment should be based on the presentation of the child. A child with severe dysregulation would likely benefit from a phase-based approach, while it may not be necessary for a child with better self-regulation. However, given that TF-CBT is a phase-based treatment, that framework will be used to discuss TF-CBT applications for complex trauma and dissociation.

Stabilization Phase

The Stabilization phase of TF-CBT includes psychoeducation, parenting skills, relaxation, affect modulation skills, and cognitive coping skills. In traditional TF-CBT, each treatment phase is approximately one-third of the total number of sessions (Cohen et al., 2017). Therefore, in TF-CBT completed in 12 sessions, roughly four sessions would be spent in the Stabilization phase.

When treating complex trauma and dissociation, particularly with dysregulation, the proportion of time spent in this phase is often extended to one-half of the total sessions. The remaining sessions are divided equally across the trauma narration and integration phases. In addition, the overall length of TF-CBT may be extended to 25 sessions with approximately 12 sessions spent in Stabilization, six sessions in Trauma Narration, and six sessions in Integration (Cohen et al., 2012). These additional sessions address eminent safety risks, enhance the therapeutic alliance, and provide extensive skill-building before the initiation of the Trauma Narration phase.

Within the Stabilization phase, the PRACTICE components can be applied in a manner consistent with the needs of complex trauma survivors. At times, this requires that the enhancing-safety component be moved to the beginning of treatment. This is necessary when children present with environmental (e.g., severe bullying) or individual conditions (e.g., severe substance abuse, suicidal ideation) that raise concern for immediate safety. The following paragraphs discuss addressing initial safety concerns and applications recommended for psychoeducation, relaxation, affect modulation skills, and cognitive coping skills.

Enhancing Safety (Stabilization Phase)

Child complex trauma survivors often present with a variety of safety concerns, including poor self-care, high-risk behaviors (e.g., risky sexual behavior, substance abuse, self-injury, suicidality, running away), revictimization, and dissociation (Myrick & Green, 2014). The presence of these concerns can increase the immediate risk of significant harm or destabilization including such outcomes as injury, illness and disease, loss of placement, academic expulsion, juvenile detention, and even death. Given the severity of these consequences, it is essential to address these issues immediately and revisit them throughout treatment.

Some safety concerns may be due to unsafe situations, which are often caused by external forces that the child has limited control over. These can include bullying at school, domestic violence, or community violence. Addressing these concerns involves traditional safety planning to remove, prepare for, or otherwise respond to the dangerous situation. For example, if domestic violence is occurring, a plan may be developed to help the child keep themselves safe as it is occurring (e.g., identifying a safe place in the home, having a place to go if it becomes unsafe to stay in the home, ensuring access to a phone if it becomes necessary to call for help).

However, some youth may engage in unsafe behavior in response to situations that are not inherently dangerous but are perceived as threatening. Many safety concerns are tied to dysregulation and may represent the child's best efforts to regulate their emotional and physiological responses to stressors or trauma cues (Kinnish et al., 2021). For example, strategies such as running away may have been the best available way to deal with past circumstances but are not adaptive to their current situation. These behaviors should not be conceptualized as "bad" behavior, but as strategies that briefly protected them or helped the youth cope but increased their risk in the long term. Before working to develop more adaptive strategies, it is important to validate these efforts, recognizing that the child was doing the best they could in the moment. The therapist should also work with the caregiver to increase their understanding of the function of these behaviors, as caregivers often misinterpret them as willful misbehavior.

To address unsafe behavior triggered by environmental situations, it is critical to work with the youth, caregiver, and other relevant individuals (e.g., teacher) to fully understand the context of the behavior, including antecedents and consequences. An example of this would be the use of functional behavior analysis (Cohen et al., 2010). For example, if the concerning behavior is aggression toward a younger sibling, the therapist would work with the child and caregiver(s) to identify precursors to that behavior (e.g., the caregiver ignoring the child in favor of the younger sibling). Once the relationship between the situation and the unsafe behavior is recognized, the therapist works to reduce the occurrence of unsafe behavior in three ways. First, they can identify strategies to reduce the occurrence of situations that precipitate unsafe behavior (e.g., increase opportunities for positive attachment between the caregiver and child). Second, they can enhance the child's ability to cope with the precipitating situation when it does occur (e.g., encourage the child to use focused breathing when they feel frustrated about being ignored). Finally, if all else fails, they can work with the child and caregiver to implement harm reduction strategies when unsafe behavior occurs (e.g., remove the child from the vicinity of the younger sibling when the child is becoming agitated).

Given the longstanding nature of these behaviors, therapists should not be surprised or disheartened if it takes time to replace dangerous behaviors with more positive coping (Kinnish et al., 2021). These behaviors will likely need to be addressed at multiple points throughout treatment. It is important to balance the need for enhancing safety and stability with continuing to move through the TF-CBT components. Once "good enough" stability has been accomplished, the therapist needs to remain vigilant regarding safety concerns, while also proceeding through the remainder of the model. This requires considerable clinical skill and judgment but is necessary, as aspects of the youth's dysregulation are often best addressed through later TF-CBT components (e.g., trauma narration and processing).

One way to accomplish the goal of balancing stability and moving through the model is the use of what the author lovingly refers to as "TF-CBT Judo." Judo is a martial art based on the philosophy of using your opponent's energy against them (e.g., using their momentum to make it easier to throw them to the ground). While we are not going to be using any martial arts on our clients, the philosophy can be relevant to therapy. Dysregulated children (and their caregivers) often come to sessions with situations that they are highly distressed about. Sometimes referred to as COWs (Crises of the Week), these are situations that the child or caregiver is motivated to talk about and thus may eat up large amounts of a session. Further, for dysregulated children, these events are often important (e.g., school suspension, pending placement change), but may not be immediately relevant to the TF-CBT component that is being worked on. However, with flexibility, a TF-CBT therapist can take most events and shift them into the component that they are currently working on (this is the judo part!).

For example, imagine that a child comes in furious about an encounter they had with a peer. If they are in the relaxation component, the therapist can process the situation with them and discuss relaxation strategies the child could use the next time they encounter the peer. If they are in the affect modulation skills component, the therapist can help the child identify and rate different emotions they experienced during the encounter.

Psychoeducation

The goals of TF-CBT psychoeducation are to provide basic information about trauma and trauma reactions, normalize and validate child and caregiver reactions to the trauma, provide information about TF-CBT, and instill hope for recovery. The therapist works with the family to connect the information that is given with the child's own trauma experiences and reactions, including an understanding of trauma reminders in the child's daily life. This information is tailored to the needs of the child and caregiver and is designed to normalize trauma exposure and responses and instill hope for recovery and improved functioning. With complex trauma, these basic goals remain the same, but the content and process of the component may be shifted.

As in all components of TF-CBT, psychoeducation involves gradual exposure to trauma content. However, a dysregulated child may have difficulty tolerating the gradual exposure typically implemented in this component. Rather than discussing information about specific types of trauma (e.g., sexual abuse), it may be easier to focus on general education about stress and trauma (Kliethermes & Wamser, 2012). Helpful topics include an overview of complex trauma, the human stress response (e.g., fight, flight, freeze), distress reduction behaviors, and trauma "leftovers" such as trauma reminders, core beliefs, self-fulfilling prophecies, and habitual emotional and behavioral responses.

Obviously, concepts like these can be difficult for younger children to grasp. However, it is important to cover these concepts in detail with caregivers, as they are likely to see these concepts in action in their child's behavior. Further, critical concepts can be simplified to help younger children better grasp them. This is often done by creating simple dichotomies (e.g., Lizard Brain and Wizard Brain) or metaphors building on concrete experiences from the child's life. For example, the author once worked with a five-year-old who didn't like spaghetti and hated it when his mom made it because they had to eat leftover spaghetti for the rest of the week. The experience of having to eat leftover spaghetti was used to explain the idea of trauma reminders. Even though the night his mom made spaghetti was several days before, the leftovers were still on the table every day. Similarly, even though his sexual abuse happened in the past, "leftovers" were still present in his day-to-day life (e.g., cars like the one driven by the perpetrator). Subsequently, "leftover spaghetti" became a phrase used to describe any situation that served as a trauma reminder and helped the child and caregiver better communicate about and plan for those situations.

Traditional psychoeducation often focuses on providing information about the trauma experienced by the child (e.g., sexual abuse prevalence data). However, by definition, children exposed to complex trauma have experienced multiple types of trauma. Therefore, even if a child is not excessively dysregulated, it may not be beneficial or even possible to provide information about every type of trauma experienced. Instead, it tends to be most helpful to identify the trauma types most critical to the child's symptom presentation and limit education to those. Critical trauma types are typically those that appear to be most connected to the child's trauma reactions (e.g., they have nightmares about sexual abuse, but not other traumas).

It is important to keep in mind that the child or caregiver doesn't need to be an expert on trauma. With complex trauma, it can be very easy to get lost in the available information that could be presented. Instead, it is best to view this component as "setting the stage" for discussions about trauma that will continue throughout treatment. The therapist should focus on the information they deem critical to helping the child move through the remaining components. For example, if the therapist suspects that the child will be resistant to engaging in the Relaxation component, it would be helpful to stress the impact of trauma exposure on physiological arousal.

Relaxation, Affect Modulation Skills, and Cognitive Coping Skills

The last three components of the Stabilization phase focus on skill-building, and the considerations for applying these components for complex trauma are similar. All three components focus on the development of self-regulation, albeit in different domains (e.g., physiological, emotional, cognitive). As mentioned previously, dysregulation is a common outcome of complex trauma exposure. Subsequently, these three components can be challenging, but are also very important.

Why do dysregulation and dissociation make these components challenging? Both dysregulated and dissociative children often have limited awareness of internal processes (e.g., physical sensations, emotions, thoughts) (Kliethermes et al., 2014; Wieland & Silberg, 2013), resulting in a variety of associated skills being underdeveloped. For example, using relaxation skills requires recognizing a tension state in your body that would benefit from relaxation. Therefore, across these three components, it is often necessary to work on skills at a younger developmental level than the child's chronological age. For example, in affect modulation, it may be necessary for the therapist to focus on mirroring and labeling emotions, which would typically be done only with very young children.

Youth with complex trauma outcomes and dissociation also often have extensive prior experience in therapy and may already have a negative mindset about the use of therapeutic skills in these components. With their additional tendency to be triggered by authority figures and being controlled, clients may behave in opposition to the therapist's efforts to promote the use of adaptive coping skills. Engaging in power struggles is not conducive to promoting self-regulation. Subsequently, it is critical to approach these components from a collaborative perspective (Kliethermes & Wamser, 2012). The therapist must consider the child's strengths and interests and devise strategies appealing to the child. Creativity and willingness to incorporate media that is familiar to the child (e.g., movies, music, technology) are invaluable.

Relaxation addresses physiological hyper-arousal associated with trauma exposure, possibly experienced by the child and caregiver. The therapist works with the child to develop personalized relaxation strategies in session and then encourages regular practice at home. Common relaxation strategies include focused breathing, progressive muscle relaxation, and visualization, but a variety of skills can be included based on child development and interest. Caregivers are taught the child's preferred relaxation exercises, learn to recognize when the child would benefit from these exercises, and coach the child in using these skills. Caregivers may also find these exercises valuable for their own anxiety or hyper-arousal.

Dysregulated children often have difficulty differentiating between tense and relaxed states. A relaxed state may be unfamiliar to them and potentially cause them to feel vulnerable, prompting increased dysregulation. Further, many of these children are already utilizing distress reduction behaviors to regulate distress. These are often more appealing to the child despite the possible consequences of their use. It is often necessary to go beyond "traditional" relaxation skills (e.g., focused breathing, progressive muscle relaxation). Possible "non-traditional" skills include mindfulness, grounding, distraction, self-soothing, and kinesthetic and sensory exercises (Kliethermes & Wamser, 2012). It is also important to consider helpful strategies that the child already uses. Many children already use adaptive strategies, such as listening to music or exercising, in addition to maladaptive strategies. If they are already using these skills, it would be foolish not to capitalize on that.

Grounding strategies are particularly relevant for children exhibiting dissociation (Wieland & Silberg, 2013). For example, the author worked with a seven-year-old client who frequently "shut down" and became non-responsive when the topic of sexual abuse was raised. Working with the child's caregiver, it was realized that the client was very tactile in nature; they liked to touch a variety of different textures. Subsequently, a grounding activity was introduced into session that involved creating a "touch box" that held objects of different textures (e.g., pine cone, sandpaper, silk).

When the child noticed themselves becoming distressed, they would take one or more objects out of the box and hold them, successfully staying grounded, while engaging in therapeutic activities.

When addressing maladaptive distress reduction behaviors, even if they are not inherently dangerous (e.g., excessive video game playing), the approach discussed to address unsafe behaviors is also appropriate. First, it is important to validate the behavior as a best effort to cope (Kliethermes et al., 2013). The next step is to establish the long-term detrimental impact of the behavior (e.g., failing school due to ignoring schoolwork in favor of video games). Next, it is important to identify situations (e.g., feeling depressed) that promote the use of maladaptive behavior. Then the child should practice delaying the behavior, ideally engaging in adaptive behaviors instead. A helpful concept is "urge surfing" (Bowen et al., 2011), which focuses on developing the ability to delay acting on an urge, creating awareness that urges decrease naturally when not acted on.

During the affect modulation skills, the therapist helps the child with identifying and expressing emotions and developing skills for managing uncomfortable mood states. Affect modulation skills include problem-solving, seeking social support, healthy distraction techniques, mindfulness, and general anger management, with a focus on using these skills in response to trauma reminders. The therapist educates the caregiver on encouraging and supporting the child in using these skills and practices this with them. Therapists often work with caregivers on developing their capacity to tolerate emotional expression by the child and to respond to these expressions empathetically rather than punitively.

Emotional dysregulation makes it challenging for children exposed to complex trauma to access, regulate, and communicate emotions (NCTSN, n.d.). Subsequently, attunement between the therapist and youth, and ultimately between the caregiver and youth, is critical. Frequent mirroring and labeling emotions helps children become more aware of their internal emotional states. Therapists and caregivers need to demonstrate a strong capacity to regulate their own emotions to promote co-regulation and eventually help the child develop the ability to self-regulate emotions (Kliethermes & Wamser, 2012).

Important concepts to address in this component include the function of emotions, that emotions are temporary and tolerable, and that expressing emotions can reduce the intensity and help secure support from others. Important skills include recognizing physiological sensations associated with emotions, labeling emotional states, recognizing intensities of emotions, and frameworks for expressing emotions (e.g., "I feel _____ because _____"). Emotional mindfulness skills may help children observe emotions in a non-judgmental fashion as they occur.

It is not unusual for caregivers to need special attention in developing their own emotional skills. They may have their own difficulties with emotion regulation due to past trauma, or simply struggle with managing their emotions in response to the child. Emotional attunement skills including active listening, acceptance, reflection, and empathy can be developed in caregivers through didactics, role-plays, and live practice in conjoint TF-CBT sessions (Kliethermes et al., 2013).

In cognitive processing skills, the focus is on developing the child's ability to recognize connections between thoughts, feelings, and behaviors (the cognitive triangle) and to replace inaccurate or unhelpful thoughts with more adaptive replacements. Trauma-related beliefs are not the focus during this component, as it is more effective to process these beliefs during trauma narration. Common techniques include progressive logical questioning, responsibility pie, best friend role-plays, and balanced thinking. The therapist also meets with the caregiver to introduce the cognitive triangle and begin processing the caregiver's maladaptive beliefs. Initially, this work addresses everyday beliefs but may progress to trauma-related beliefs (e.g., I failed as a parent because my child was abused).

Working with cognitive skills is often challenging for dysregulated children due to underdeveloped metacognition. Specifically, awareness of thoughts, particularly in the moment, can be limited. Subsequently, helping the child apply the cognitive triangle in the moment is an important skill.

Dysregulated children often present to sessions with recent events that prompted distress or are distressed by events in session. Therapists should take these opportunities to help the child process the situation using the cognitive triangle. For children struggling with this process, supplementing the cognitive triangle with a more detailed, step-by-step analysis of the situation can be helpful. Utilizing "chaining" from dialectical behavior therapy could be one way to accomplish this.

This component can be particularly challenging for young children. Specifically, they are unlikely to grasp the cognitive triangle in its entirety and can struggle with determining if thoughts are accurate or inaccurate. However, even relatively young children are able to understand the concept of thinking (e.g., "what I say to myself") and the idea that certain thoughts can be helpful or unhelpful. A common approach with young children is to use a dichotomy that is meaningful to the child to illustrate helpful ("hero" thoughts) and unhelpful thoughts ("Bad Guy" thoughts). For example, this author once worked with a developmentally disabled ten-year-old, who loved food and developed his own dichotomy of "Twinkie" thoughts and "broccoli" thoughts. Not surprisingly, "Twinkie" thoughts were those that made him feel happy or relaxed, and "broccoli" thoughts were those that made him feel sad or angry. This became useful shorthand for the remainder of treatment (e.g., "Did you have any broccoli thoughts when your foster mom told you to go to bed?").

Trauma Narration Phase

Trauma narration and processing involves the therapist and child interactively processing the child's traumatic experience(s), emphasizing thoughts, feelings, and physical sensations that occurred during the trauma(s). This is done in gradually increasing intensity with less distressing memories first, followed by more distressing memories. This leads to the child processing the most distressing traumatic memories and the development of mastery rather than avoidance. During this process (or in prior components) the child and therapist identify unhelpful beliefs about the trauma (e.g., the abuse was my fault because I am a bad kid). Previously learned cognitive skills are used to help the child process unhelpful beliefs and identify more helpful, balanced beliefs about their traumatic experiences. This often includes the development of a tangible summary of the process, typically in the form of a story, poem, song, or artwork. However, it is important to recognize that this tangible product is less critical than the interactive process between the child and therapist.

In each session, as the child develops the narration, the therapist meets with the caregiver to review the content. This familiarizes the caregiver with the child's trauma experiences, helps them develop mastery of their own distress and avoidance related to the information, identifies and addresses the caregiver's unhelpful beliefs about the trauma, and prepares the caregiver for conjoint child-parent sessions.

With dysregulated children, the transition from the Stabilization phase to the Trauma Narration phase can be difficult to gauge. It is important to keep in mind that the goal of the Stabilization phase is not perfect stabilization (the author has yet to accomplish that himself!). Instead, we are working toward "good enough" stability to allow for safe trauma processing (Kliethermes & Wamser, 2012). Good enough stability means that the child may be experiencing some minor dysregulation "hiccups" in their daily life, but no significant stressors (e.g., placement disruption) are eminent. Further, the child should feel safe enough in therapy to allow the therapist to help them regulate when needed.

A common concern of therapists when working with traumatized children is that the child is not ready for trauma processing (Patel et al., 2022). However, therapists often tend to underestimate the capacity of children to tolerate trauma processing. Therefore, the default assumption is that children can be ready to initiate trauma processing with support from the therapist. Therapists can recognize readiness for trauma processing in a variety of ways. Basic signs of readiness include the following:

1. The child is consistently able to remain in the therapist's office and engage in therapeutic activities.
2. If the child engages in therapy-interfering behavior, they can be successfully redirected to therapeutic activity.
3. If the child becomes distressed during a session, the therapist can help the child regain their composure through relaxation or other co-regulation activities.
4. If the child exhibits signs of dissociation, the therapist can engage the child in grounding activities so they are able to remain present and engaged in session.
5. The child has demonstrated the ability to successfully tolerate gradual exposure throughout the earlier components of TF-CBT.

Even with "good enough" stability, the trauma narration component will result in the child experiencing some distress. Desensitization to trauma memories requires the child to experience some discomfort that alleviates as exposure work progresses. In truth, successful trauma narration is another means of developing self-regulation. However, dysregulated children may be more sensitive and reactive to this process. Subsequently, the therapist needs to attend to the therapeutic window (Briere & Scott, 2015), which suggests that exposure work needs to fall into a "window" that is tolerable for the child. It must be deep enough to create distress, but not enough to cause the child to completely dysregulate. For dysregulated children, this window can be excruciatingly small. Subsequently, therapists need to make the process as predictable as possible, allow the child to have appropriate control over the process, process the trauma in gradually increasing "waves," and practice skillful co-regulation.

Even when taking the best of precautions, "broken windows" may occur. The child may have a negative reaction and become more dysregulated than anticipated. While unfortunate, this is not the end of the world. Instead, this becomes a fantastic opportunity for the therapist to create a corrective emotional experience by taking responsibility for the "broken window" and collaborating with the child to prevent it from recurring. This is often a novel experience for the child and tends to enhance the therapeutic alliance rather than weaken it.

Trauma narration is essentially the process of the child telling the story about their traumatic experiences. However, if telling the story was all that was involved, children wouldn't need to go to therapy to do so. Instead, it is important to recognize that telling the story in the context of the therapeutic alliance contributes to the healing process (Cohen & Mannarino, 2022). Ideally, the child's relationship with the therapist should be the opposite of the traumatic relationships described in their narration. Rather than becoming reactive and lashing out at the child, the therapist provides "safe containment" for the child's emotions. This experience promotes the child's ability to remain regulated and develop mastery over trauma content.

Even without dissociation, processing complex trauma can be challenging. It involves multiple, chronic events that often occur early in the child's life and overlap with each other. Subsequently, challenges include establishing the chronological order of events, gaps in memory, and "interaction effects" between traumas (e.g., being removed from their biological home because of physical abuse and then being sexually abused by the new foster parent). It may not be feasible or advisable to process every trauma in a detailed account (Kliethermes & Wamser, 2012). The primary purposes of trauma narration are desensitization and healthy meaning-making (Cohen et al., 2017). However, both may not be necessary for every trauma experienced by a child. With complex trauma, this author's clinical experience has suggested that while some desensitization work may be necessary, a larger focus on meaning-making is often warranted.

A helpful analogy to consider is the idea of not "missing the forest for the trees." Desensitization is needed for specific "trees" in the forest. These would be traumatic events that are particularly tied to avoidance, intrusive symptoms, or event-specific problematic thoughts (e.g., It's my fault I was sexually abused). For these events, a more detailed account of the trauma may help alleviate these symptoms by allowing the child to develop a sense of mastery over the memories and engage in cognitive processing of the event-specific problematic thoughts. This would be "traditional" TF-CBT trauma narration, revolving around the thoughts, feelings, and sensations that the child experienced during the trauma. Not every traumatic event needs to be processed in this way, just the ones most clearly tied to trauma reactions.

Meaning-making involves considering the entire "forest." Traumatic events are often interrelated, and humans strive to make sense of experiences and "connect the dots" between events. As children experience traumatic events, their core beliefs about the world, themselves, and others begin to conform to those experiences. This tends to result in "themes" that incorporate these experiences and continue to influence the child's daily functioning long after the trauma has ended. While these themes can cover a broad range of concepts, constructivist self-development theory (McCann & Pearlman, 1992) offers five helpful schema categories—Safety, Trust, Intimacy, Power/Control, Identity/Esteem—that can be used to help children understand how their beliefs have been impacted by traumatic experiences. In this scenario, trauma narration could be organized around a theme (e.g., power/control) rather than a traumatic event. For example, while considering the traumas they have experienced, the therapist may help the child recognize a theme related to power and control that developed due to experiences with trauma (e.g., due to abuse by caregivers, the client believes it is not safe to allow anyone to have control over you). Ideally, the therapist can help the child recognize that while this theme was helpful in the past, it may no longer be functional. At that time, cognitive processing would be used to help the child develop a more balanced belief that integrates the past and the present (i.e., Some people with power have hurt me in the past, and there have also been people who did not abuse their power).

An extremely helpful format for "tree" and "forest"–level trauma processing is a timeline. Early in trauma narration, the therapist and child can develop a timeline of important events in the child's life, including traumatic experiences. Timelines easily allow both "tree"- (i.e., processing a specific event on the timeline in greater detail) and "forest"-level processing (e.g., discussing what themes appear to be present across all events on the timeline).

When dissociation is added to this scenario, an additional layer of challenge is present during trauma narration. Dissociation prohibits a child from being able to benefit from desensitization and meaning-making, as being engaged in the present moment is necessary for both. If a child is prone to dissociation during sessions, it is anticipated that this tendency would have been identified during the assessment or early components of TF-CBT. Subsequently, the child would have practiced grounding exercises until identifying one or more that they could reliably use to help them remain engaged and present in sessions. These skills would then be utilized to help the child remain grounded during work on trauma narration, allowing the benefit of gradual exposure and meaning-making.

If the child experienced dissociation during the traumatic event(s), they may have difficulty assessing traumatic memories during trauma narration. This can be frustrating for both the child and the therapist. It is important to revisit psychoeducation about the purpose and function of dissociation, noting that it was the best response the child had at the time of the trauma. Rather than attempting to process memories they are unable to access, it is appropriate to process what it is like for the child to have those gaps in their memory.

Dissociation may also relate to the themes processed during trauma narration. For example, a child may have decided that they are weak because they dissociated or froze during a traumatic event and have habitually engaged in this response when confronted by subsequent stressors. Cognitive processing can then be done with the child to help them recognize that they have no control over their body's decision to engage in a survival response like dissociation. Alternately, it may be helpful for the child to recognize that dissociation may have been their best survival option rather than a fight-or-flight response at that time (e.g., as with a five-year-old being physically abused by an adult male). Ideally, the child recognizes dissociation as an understandable response at the time of the trauma, but that they are now able to replace it with more adaptive responses to a more stable environment.

Integration Phase

The Integration phase of TF-CBT consists of in vivo mastery, conjoint child-parent sessions, and enhancing safety and future development. This phase is of considerable importance for complex trauma, which can be thought of as a range of environmentally caused developmental delays. Subsequently, relationships with caregivers, personal safety skills, and other important skills (e.g., problem-solving, effective communication) may remain impaired after completion of trauma narration. Subsequently, this phase is designed to address some of those shortcomings, hopefully moving the child closer to an appropriate developmental trajectory. This section will focus on conjoint child-parent sessions and enhancing safety and future development, as the application of in vivo mastery does not change significantly in the context of complex trauma.

Conjoint Child-Parent Sessions

As mentioned previously, caregivers of dysregulated children with a history of complex trauma often struggle in their parenting interactions. Many have their own trauma histories or are buckling under the challenge of parenting a dysregulated child. Either can result in caregivers who are also dysregulated, often in the context of parenting (e.g., angrily lashing out at the child). Unfortunately, this response typically triggers the child even further, resulting in back-and-forth escalation.

Working with these caregivers often mirrors the work the therapist is doing with the child. Namely, it is important to focus on developing a trusting, collaborative relationship with the caregiver. Dysregulated parenting behaviors should be viewed in the same light as the child's problematic behaviors (i.e., understandable responses to stress, current best efforts to cope, due to lack of skill rather than ill intent). The caregiver often needs support in developing their own self-regulation skills, particularly in conjunction with parenting. A primary focus of work with caregivers should be to enhance their ability to engage in effective co-regulation. This skill can be practiced in role-play between the therapist and caregiver and then in conjoint sessions with the child. Caregivers may also benefit from processing their experiences with being parented as a child. These experiences may have been problematic and resulted in themes that impact their current caregiving. Developing more adaptive beliefs about parenting (e.g., I didn't deserve to be yelled at and neither does my child) helps the caregiver change current parenting behavior.

Enhancing Safety and Future Development

This component is of substantial importance for complex trauma. These children often have an impaired ability to recognize danger, may continue to live in high-risk families or communities, and may have limited access to supportive caregivers and systems. Further, there is always the potential that they could return to the use of maladaptive distress reduction behaviors (Kinnish et al., 2021). Due to these concerns, complex trauma survivors tend to be at high risk for re-victimization. Subsequently, it is critical to focus on skills and knowledge to alleviate these concerns. Common topics addressed include personal safety skills, healthy relationships and sexual decision-making, Internet safety, and alcohol and substance use.

It is important to help the child identify, normalize, and prepare for future life challenges associated with complex trauma (e.g., managing dysregulation in dating or work relationships). After trauma narration, the child is in a position to consider future situations that may be triggering for them, such as a micromanaging boss. It is often helpful to consider life-skill training opportunities that may be beneficial for the child following the completion of TF-CBT. This could include training in job or life skills or a course on healthy sexuality. Children need to be consistently reminded that the skills they developed in TF-CBT can be applied to future challenges as well. It is also helpful to normalize the need for a later return to therapy or ongoing supportive counseling while highlighting their increased mastery over their traumatic experiences.

This component is also important for the caregivers of child survivors of complex trauma. Caregivers should be guided to consider future parenting challenges that they may face, including dating, possible contact with the family of origin (in the case of foster care/adoption), and child relapses into maladaptive coping. Once these future challenges have been identified, the therapist and caregiver can work together to discuss possible strategies and plans that could be implemented at that time.

Effectiveness Research: TF-CBT for Complex Trauma

Research regarding TF-CBT for complex trauma is in the early stages, but multiple effectiveness studies have been conducted. For example, Hébert and Amédée (2020) found that TF-CBT was associated with improvements in children with complex trauma who experienced PTSD symptoms, dissociation, and behavior problems, but also in children with domains related to complex trauma, including affect regulation, negative self-concept, and interpersonal relationships. Bartlett and colleagues (2018) found that TF-CBT resulted in significant reductions in child behavior problems across all domains, and in PTSD symptoms for youth exposed to complex trauma. Another study compared the effects of TF-CBT for youth with PTSD and complex PTSD (Sachser et al., 2017). Results indicated that youth with PTSD and complex PTSD benefited equally from TF-CBT, but youth with complex PTSD ended treatment with clinically and statistically greater symptoms than those with PTSD. Similarly, Ross and colleagues (2021) evaluated the effectiveness of TF-CBT on simple and complex PTSD with a diverse, treatment-seeking sample of youth who experienced interpersonal trauma. Results indicated that post-treatment outcomes were equivalent for youth with simple and complex PTSD, suggesting that TF-CBT is an appropriate intervention for youth with complex trauma histories and reactions. Finally, a recent study (Jensen et al., 2022) found that youth with complex PTSD who had completed TF-CBT experienced a significant decline in PTSD symptoms, affect dysregulation, negative self-concept, and relationship disturbances, and did not drop out more than youth with PTSD. Overall, these findings suggest that TF-CBT is indeed effective for complex trauma.

Conclusion

TF-CBT is an extremely well-established intervention for trauma-exposed youth. Decades of research have demonstrated that it is effective in reducing common symptoms associated with trauma, including PTSD, depression, behavioral difficulties, and many more. Despite the challenges associated with children exposed to complex trauma, the evidence currently suggests that TF-CBT can still be used effectively to address trauma-related difficulties. This is not to suggest that implementing TF-CBT for complex trauma is easy. Dysregulation and dissociation do present many challenges to a TF-CBT therapist, but those challenges are present regardless of the treatment model being used. TF-CBT therapists who are skillful, creative, and patient can have great success with this population.

References

Bartlett, J. D., Griffin, J. L., Spinazzola, J., Fraser, J. G., Noroña, C. R., Bodian, R., Todd, M., Montagna, C., & Barto, B. (2018). The impact of a statewide trauma-informed care initiative in child welfare on the well-being of children and youth with complex trauma. *Children and Youth Services Review, 84*, 110–117. https://doi.org/10.1016/j.childyouth.2017.11.015

Bowen, S., Chawla, N., & Marlatt, G. A. (2011). *Mindfulness-based relapse prevention for addictive behaviors: A clinician's guide*. Guilford Press.

Briere, J. (2019). *Treating risky and compulsive behavior in trauma survivors*. Guilford Press.

Briere, J. N., & Scott, C. (2015). *Principles of trauma therapy: A guide to symptoms, evaluation, and treatment* (2nd ed.) Sage Publications.

Cloitre, M., Courtois, C. A., Ford, J. D., Green, B. L., Alexander, P., Briere, J., Herman, J. L., Lanius, R., Pearlman, L. A., Stolbach, B., Spinazzola, J., van der Kolk, B., & van der Hart, O. (2012). *The ISTSS expert consensus treatment guidelines for complex PTSD in adults*. ISTSS.

Cloitre, M., Stovall-McClough, K. C., Nooner, K., Zorbas, P., Cherry, S., Jackson, C. L., Gan, W., & Petkova, E. (2010). Treatment for PTSD related to childhood abuse: A randomized controlled trial. *American Journal of Psychiatry, 167*(8), 915–924. https://doi.org/10.1176/appi.ajp.2010.09081247

Cohen, J. A., Berliner, L., & Mannarino, A. (2010). Trauma focused CBT for children with co-occurring trauma and behavior problems. *Child Abuse & Neglect, 34*(4), 215–224. https://doi.org/10.1016/j.chiabu.2009.12.003

Cohen, J. A., & Mannarino, A. P. (2000). Predictors of treatment outcome in sexually abused children. *Child Abuse & Neglect, 24*(7), 983–994. https://doi-org.ezproxy.umsl.edu/10.1016/S0145-2134(00)00153-8

Cohen, J. A., & Mannarino, A. P. (2022). Trauma-focused cognitive behavioral therapy for children and families. *Child and Adolescent Psychiatric Clinics of North America, 31*(1), 133–147. https://doi-org.ezproxy.umsl.edu/10.1016/j.chc.2021.05.001

Cohen, J. A., Mannarino, A. P., & Deblinger, E. (2017). *Treating trauma and traumatic grief in children and adolescents* (2nd ed.). Guilford Press.

Cohen, J. A., Mannarino, A. P., Kliethermes, M., & Murray, L. A. (2012). Trauma-focused CBT for youth with complex trauma. *Child Abuse & Neglect, 36*(6), 528–541. https://doi.org/10.1016/j.chiabu.2012.03.007

Courtois, C. A., & Ford, J. D. (2013). *Treatment of complex trauma: A sequenced, relationship-based approach*. Guilford Press.

Dauber, S., Lotsos, K., & Pulido, M. L. (2015). Treatment of complex trauma on the front lines: A preliminary look at child outcomes in an agency sample. *Child & Adolescent Social Work Journal, 32*(6), 529–543. https://doi.org/10.1007/s10560-015-0393-5

de Arellano, M. A. R., Lyman, D. R., Jobe-Shields, L., George, P., Dougherty, R. H., Daniels, A. S., Ghose, S. S., Huang, L., & Delphin-Rittmon, M. E. (2014). Trauma-focused cognitive-behavioral therapy for children and adolescents: Assessing the evidence. *Psychiatric Services, 65*(5), 591–602. https://doi.org/10.1176/appi.ps.201300255

Deblinger, E., & Heflin, A. H. (1996). *Treating sexually abused children and their nonoffending parents: A cognitive behavioral approach*. Sage Publications, Inc.

DePierro, J., D'Andrea, W., Spinazzola, J., Stafford, E., van Der Kolk, B., Saxe, G., Stolbach, B., McKernan, S., & Ford, J. D. (2022). Beyond PTSD: Client presentations of developmental trauma disorder from a national survey of clinicians. *Psychological Trauma: Theory, Research, Practice, and Policy, 14*(7), 1167–1174. https://doi-org.ezproxy.umsl.edu/10.1037/tra0000532.supp (Supplemental).

Fischer, A., Rosner, R., Renneberg, B., & Steil, R. (2022). Suicidal ideation, self-injury, aggressive behavior and substance use during intensive trauma-focused treatment with exposure-based components in adolescent and young adult PTSD patients. *Borderline Personality Disorder and Emotion Dysregulation, 9*(1), Article 1. https://doi.org/10.1186/s40479-021-00172-8

Hébert, M., & Amédée, L. M. (2020). Latent class analysis of post-traumatic stress symptoms and complex PTSD in child victims of sexual abuse and their response to trauma-focused cognitive behavioural therapy. *European Journal of Psychotraumatology, 11*(1). Article 1807171. https://doi.org/10.1080/20008198.2020.1807171

Jensen, T. K., Braathu, N., Birkeland, M. S., Ormhaug, S. M., & Skar, A.-M. S. (2022). Complex PTSD and treatment outcomes in TF-CBT for youth: A naturalistic study. *European Journal of Psychotraumatology, 13*(2). Article 2114630. https://doi.org/10.1080/20008066.2022.2114630

Kinnish, K., Cohen, J. A., Mannarino, A., & Kliethermes, M. (2021). *TF-CBT for the commercial sexual exploitation of children: An implementation manual*. Allegheny General Hospital.

Kliethermes, M., Nanney, R. W., Cohen, J. A., & Mannarino, A. P. (2013). Trauma-focused cognitive-behavioral therapy. In J. D. Ford & C. A. Courtois (Eds.), *Treating complex traumatic stress disorders in children and adolescents: Scientific foundations and therapeutic models*. (pp. 184–202). Guilford Press.

Kliethermes, M., Schacht, M., & Drewry, K. (2014). Complex trauma. *Child and Adolescent Psychiatric Clinics of North America, 23*(2), 339–361. https://doi.org/10.1016/j.chc.2013.12.009

Kliethermes, M., & Wamser, R. (2012). Adolescents with complex trauma. In J. A. Cohen, A. P. Mannarino & E. Deblinger (Eds.), *Trauma-focused CBT for children and adolescents: Treatment applications* (pp. 175–196). Guilford Press.

McCann, L., & Pearlman, L. A. (1992). Constructivist self-development theory: A theoretical model of psychological adaptation to severe trauma. In D. K. Sakheim & S. E. Devine (Eds.), *Out of darkness: Exploring satanism and ritual abuse.* (pp. 185–206). Lexington Books/Macmillan.

Myrick, A. C., & Green, E. J. (2014). Establishing safety and stabilization in traumatized youth: Clinical implications for play therapists. *International Journal of Play Therapy, 23*(2), 100–113. https://doi.org/10.1037/a0036397

National Child Traumatic Stress Network (n.d.). Complex trauma. NCTSN.org. Retrieved April 28, 2023, from nctsn.org/what-is-child-trauma/trauma-types/complex-trauma.

Oprel, D. A. C., Hoeboer, C. M., Schoorl, M., Kleine, R. A. de, Cloitre, M., Wigard, I. G., van Minnen, A., & van der Does, W. (2021). Effect of prolonged exposure, intensified prolonged exposure and STAIR+prolonged exposure in patients with PTSD related to childhood abuse: A randomized controlled trial. *European Journal of Psychotraumatology, 12*(1). Article 1851511. https://doi.org/10.1080/20008198.2020.1851511

Patel, Z. S., Casline, E., Shaw, A. M., Jensen, D. A., & Ramirez, V. (2022). Measuring clinician stuck points about trauma-focused cognitive behavior therapy: The TF-CBT stuck points questionnaire. *Journal of Traumatic Stress, 35*(5), 1357–1367. https://doi.org/10.1002/jts.22835

Peters, W., Rice, S., Cohen, J., Murray, L., Schley, C., Alvarez-Jimenez, M., & Bendall, S. (2021). Trauma-focused cognitive–behavioral therapy (TF-CBT) for interpersonal trauma in transitional-aged youth. *Psychological Trauma: Theory, Research, Practice, and Policy, 13*(3), 313–321. https://doi-org.ezproxy.umsl.edu/10.1037/tra0001016.supp (Supplemental).

Ross, S. L., Sharma-Patel, K., Brown, E. J., Huntt, J. S., & Chaplin, W. F. (2021). Complex trauma and trauma-focused cognitive-behavioral therapy: How do trauma chronicity and PTSD presentation affect treatment outcome? *Child Abuse & Neglect, 111.* Article 104734. https://doi.org/10.1016/j.chiabu.2020.104734

Sachser, C., Keller, F., & Goldbeck, L. (2017). Complex PTSD as proposed for ICD-11: Validation of a new disorder in children and adolescents and their response to trauma-focused cognitive behavioral therapy. *Journal of Child Psychology and Psychiatry, 58*(2), 160–168. https://doi.org/10.1111/jcpp.12640

Thielemann, J. F. B., Kasparik, B., König, J., Unterhitzenberger, J., & Rosner, R. (2022). A systematic review and meta-analysis of trauma-focused cognitive behavioral therapy for children and adolescents. *Child Abuse & Neglect, 134,* 1–13. Article 105899. https://doi.org/10.1016/j.chiabu.2022.105899

van Vliet, N. I., Huntjens, R. J. C., van Dijk, M. K., Bachrach, N., Meewisse, M.-L., & de Jongh, A. (2021). Phase-based treatment versus immediate trauma-focused treatment for post-traumatic stress disorder due to childhood abuse: Randomised clinical trial. *BJPsych Open, 7*(6). Article e211. https://doi.org/10.1192/bjo.2021.1057

Wieland, S., & Silberg, J. (2013). Dissociation-focused therapy. In J. D. Ford & C. A. Courtois (Eds.), *Treating complex traumatic stress disorders in children and adolescents: Scientific foundations and therapeutic models* (pp. 162–183). Guilford Press.

26
ANIMAL-ASSISTED THERAPY

Michael Remole

Introduction[1]

On a hot summer afternoon, Thomas, a young child, arrived at our farm. He was wearing a hoodie and had a stoic expression. His slumped shoulders and distant, disinterested eyes painted a somber picture—he appeared devoid of any signs of joy.

During the intake session, I asked Thomas's adoptive dad to accompany him for a walk around the pasture, allowing his mother to more freely answer some questions I had. Through these inquiries, it was revealed that Thomas had endured abuse within his biological family and had multiple failed placements, and now, his adoptive family was contemplating making significant changes in their relationship. My heart ached hearing the extensive list of traumatic events Thomas had experienced in his young life, which shed light on the reasons behind his struggles. The weight of relational trauma had rendered human connections as unpredictable, unsafe, and overwhelming for him.

From a distance, I observed Thomas and his father walking outside of the pasture. One of the horses trotted toward the fence and began walking parallel to them.

When Thomas returned to the office, he was smiling. Excitedly, he asked if I had noticed what had transpired. "That horse liked me!" he said. Seizing the opportunity, I asked him if he wanted to learn more about the horse, Ranger.

Ranger, a large gelding, had his own challenging journey of relational trauma. Rescued from an abusive situation as a yearling, he went through a series of failed adoptions due to his frequent unpredictable and unsafe behaviors. Eventually, Ranger found his way to our program. As I shared Ranger's story with Thomas and his parents, we realized the striking similarities between Thomas and Ranger. Both were in dire need of genuine connection and relational healing. That is when Thomas said, "I want to work with Ranger."

As the relationship between Thomas and Ranger progressed and therapy sessions continued, Thomas experienced significant changes in his home life. He changed living arrangements to assist him with addressing some of his tricky behaviors and struggles in building healthy relationships. Through that transition, Thomas was able to maintain services at the farm. One morning, Thomas arrived visibly frustrated and annoyed. As I greeted him, he unleashed a torrent of anger, proclaiming therapy to be "boring" and me to be "stupid," and declaring his refusal to engage in any session activities. Thomas was clearly in pain, grieving the disruption of his family life. He seemed conflicted, yearning for meaningful relationships while also resisting most attempts of connection from others.

Standing with his gaze fixed on the tree line, Thomas crossed his arms tightly over his chest. I was positioned at a slight distance and had a view of the horses in the pasture behind him.

Ranger, who had been eating with his herd in the pasture, went from walking to trotting toward Thomas. Thomas noticed Ranger, and with each step Ranger took, Thomas's posture and expression softened. Thomas started walking toward the fence and found himself face to face with Ranger. Ranger rested his head on Thomas's cheek, appearing to convey a message of understanding. The two embraced for several minutes, a powerful moment of genuine connection and relation for both horse and human.

Theory and Tenets of Animal-Assisted Therapy (ATT)

> In fact, the research on the most effective treatments to help child trauma victims might be accurately summed up this way: what works best is anything that increases the quality and number of relationships in the child's life.
>
> *(Perry & Szalavitz, 2007, p. 85)*

Children navigating complex trauma and dissociation often find themselves in a paradoxical situation: while they desperately require relationships for healing, these connections can act as powerful triggers, overwhelming their systems and leading to negative reactions. Children with traumatic relational experiences such as abuse or neglect often associate relational interactions as a threat. Consequently, many children receive life-altering labels such as "antisocial," "criminally minded," or having "avoidant attachment." The founder of Trust-Based Relational Intervention (TBRI), Karen Purvis, and colleagues emphasized that healing from relational trauma involves fostering loving, stable relationships (2013). The pivotal role of professionals working with children who have experienced significant trauma lies in striking a balance between the need for relational connection and implementing a therapeutic dosage of connection as the child navigates their intimacy barrier.

Animal-Assisted Interventions (AAI) offer a unique approach to activating the brain's relational networks without triggering negative associations with intimacy, thus providing an opportunity for individuals to manage intimacy more effectively in a supportive environment. This enables children to reconstruct neural networks, fostering trust and a sense of safety and security without succumbing to emotional overwhelm or retraumatization. Engagement with animals activates various brain regions within the neurosequential process, starting from somatosensory and movement-related areas, navigating through emotional centers, and extending into reasoning and problem-solving faculties. Thoughtfully integrating animals into therapeutic settings opens pathways to healing for children contending with complex trauma and dissociation by providing abundant relational opportunities that harmonize biologically for both human and animal.

Animals and humans have a long history of relational connection with one another. Although AAT has become increasingly popular in the last few decades, there is evidence that animals have been vital co-regulatory partners for hundreds of years (Perry, as cited in Tedeschi and Jenkins, 2019). Understanding the complexities, neuroscience, and healing power of these co-regulatory relationships is vital as more professionals begin to integrate animals into their therapeutic practice.

In the book *Transforming Trauma: Resilience and Healing Through Our Connections With Animals*, Tedeschi and Jenkins (2019) wrote:

> The inclusion of animals in therapeutic applications is known as animal-assisted intervention or AAI (Kruger & Serpell, 2010 as cited in Tedeshi and Jenkins, 2019). AAI ranges from informal activities with animals to provide enrichment (animal-assisted activities or AAA); to individualized and structured sessions with animals, targeted at meeting the client's therapeutic

goals (animal-assisted therapy or AAT); to the incorporation of animals in educational settings to achieve academic objectives (animal-assisted education or AAE). The premise of AAI is that the animal's presence is expected to provide a unique and therapeutic benefit, above and beyond other complementary approaches (Chandler, 2012 as cited in Tedeschi and Jenkins, 2019). For people who have experienced trauma, these benefits may include a source of nonjudgmental support, stress-reducing companionship, positive outlets for joy and laughter, a safe haven for physical touch and emotional vulnerability, and "bio-affiliative safety."

(p. 15)

According to the American Veterinary Medical Association (AVMA) (n.d.), "animal-assisted interventions (AAI) is a broad term that is now commonly used to describe the utilization of various species of animals in diverse manners beneficial to humans. Animal-assisted therapy, education, and activities are examples of types of animal-assisted intervention" (para. 5). In the APA Dictionary of Psychology (n.d.), the American Psychological Association's definition of animal-assisted therapy is:

The therapeutic use of pets to enhance individuals' physical, social, emotional, or cognitive functioning. Animal-assisted therapy may be used, for example, to help people receive and give affection, especially in developing communication and social skills. It may be most effective for people who have suffered losses or separation from loved ones. Also called pet-assisted therapy; pet therapy.

(para. 1)

This author advocates for the critical rephrasing of the definition in substituting the term "use of" with "partnership with," resulting in "the therapeutic partnership with pets." AAT is dedicated to cultivating a profound therapeutic bond between the person and the animal. The word "use" implies a unidirectional relationship, potentially overlooking the balanced and reciprocal nature inherent in the human-animal bond. It is crucial for the language employed in integrating animals into therapeutic settings to align with the ethos of relationships in contexts beyond therapy. The fact that animals are sentient beings challenges us to reevaluate how the APA definition endorses an individual to leverage a relationship solely for their benefit. We must acknowledge the animal as an equitable partner in the therapeutic alliance. Neglecting the animal's equal footing might potentially lead to compromises and exploitation, undermining their well-being.

In AAI, the APA definition and the word "use" within sparks a crucial discussion on animal welfare. According to AVMA (n.d.), animal welfare reflects an animal's ability to cope with its living conditions. An animal is considered to have good welfare if scientifically evidenced: it is healthy, comfortable, well-nourished, safe, able to express innate behaviors, and free from unpleasant states like pain, fear, or distress. For professionals engaging in AAT, it is essential to prioritize the animal's welfare. This should encompass more than just physical comfort, extending also to consider their emotional well-being.

While the concept of vicarious trauma—commonly discussed regarding its impact on clinicians—is well-known, it is equally pivotal to recognize the emotional impact on animals in therapeutic environments. Mental health professionals understand the mental, physical, and emotional toll of clinical sessions. When integrating AAT into practice, acknowledging the stress experienced by partnering with animals becomes imperative. As sentient beings, animals possess the ability to sense, perceive, experience, and respond to various emotional states present in a session. Their capacity to provide feedback about the session's emotional atmosphere constitutes an invaluable aspect of AAT. Thus, neglecting the physical, emotional, and mental impact of AAT on animals is unjust and can promote an unhealthy relationship model.

Carl Rogers a prominent figure in humanistic psychology, advocated the principle that "in any relationship, if it is not good for both, it is not good for one," emphasizing the importance of mutual well-being and establishing healthy, interconnected relationships. In the context of AAI, this concept translates into recognizing and ensuring mutual benefit and equality in relationships involving animals. Rogers emphasized that for any relationship to flourish, the needs of all involved parties must be acknowledged and given precedence. Professionals engaged in animal-related work must vigilantly monitor the animals' well-being and permit the expression of their innate behaviors, ensuring a balanced and respectful therapeutic relationship. During AAT, the professional assumes the role of the "voice of the animal," articulating without labeling what the animal might be communicating. (The concept of labeling will be further explored later in this chapter.) The objective is that as the child's relationship with the animal strengthens, the child will progressively observe and appropriately respond to the cues and signs from their animal partner.

Here are several essential questions to contemplate while engaging in AAI:

- Am I allowing the animal to seek relief from the stress of the session?
- Is the animal free to naturally exhibit their innate behaviors?
- Does the session or intervention respect the animal's autonomy by giving them the space to decline participation?
- Does this principle of relationship positively influence other relationships?
- Am I creating room within the session to explore the animal's communication?
- Am I disregarding any cues from the animal for the sole benefit of the client?

Active engagement in monitoring the signs and cues of the animal partner provides children with natural opportunities to practice empathy, meet the needs of others, enhance awareness of and accurately interpret social cues, and demonstrate problem-solving skills within the human-animal connection. Discussions around the signs and cues should be framed in relational terms, necessitating careful consideration of language used when identifying contentment or dissatisfaction in animals. The words used during these discussions can unintentionally reinforce negative beliefs, paralleling patterns seen in human relationships tied to core beliefs such as "I am not good enough," "I'm unlovable," "I'm too much," or "I can never do anything right." Sigmund Freud (Levy, 1998) shed light on the unconscious repetition of relational patterns to master, resolve relational conflicts, or heal from past traumas. Similarly, children often repeat these relational patterns with animals. Enabling a child to forge a genuine relationship with a sentient being offers them an opportunity to modify, break, or heal negative relational patterns. These multifaceted experiences provide holistic development and relational scaffolding that extends beyond comprehending the animal's welfare, significantly benefiting the child's social and emotional growth. Additionally, the animal experiences growth as well in their relationships with other animals.

Navigating Relational Patterns

Kylan, a timid eight-year-old boy, arrived for his first session at the ranch. His slumped posture and poor eye contact demonstrated his hesitance around the therapy team. During the intake, a history of abuse and multiple out-of-home placements emerged, providing the heartbreaking story of this young boy.

After a few weeks, Kylan appeared to be ready to select his relationship horse. He quickly picked the smallest horse—Winnie. We discussed what a friendship with Winnie might look like, and the young, timid kid gave awkward glances between the therapist and the ground, then stated he wanted to just try the friendship out.

Kylan walked hesitantly out into the middle of the horse arena and approached his new friend, Winnie. He petted her for a moment and then lay himself completely flat on the ground right beside her. The clinical team asked Kylan what was happening, and he said, "She needs to feel that I am safe. If I do this, I am not a threat to her."

While Kylan lay on the ground, Winnie began to smell and walk all around his head. The clinical team closely monitored Kylan's safety in his vulnerable position. Soon, it became clear to them that this was a typical pattern for Kylan in his relationships. Due to his early developmental trauma, he had learned that to keep the peace, he had to compromise what he needed. Throughout his life, from home to foster care and at school, he operated in a state of "robotic compliance," and was doing what it took to avoid disrupting the system.

The clinical team was able to engage Kylan in creating a secure, calm place for *both* him and Winnie. Over months of therapy, the secure, calm space was created. Through the process, Kylan began to recognize what he needed to feel safe and how to balance the safety and needs of others as well.

After nearly three years of working with Kylan, he was doing well. One day, he arrived to his session and asked if he could spend time with Winnie. Kylan walked into the arena, now with confidence. As he walked in, he asked if the clinical team remembered him lying down during his first encounter with Winnie. "Now I don't need to do that," he said. "I know that Winnie and I can work together to keep each other safe."

AAT sessions provide a unique setting for the child's relational patterns to emerge. Whether your clinical practice has one or multiple animals with whom to partner, there are some steps that can be taken to protect the therapeutic relationship in the AAT setting.

Plan for relationship patterns and disruptions to emerge in the sessions. Invite the child into the process of planning for those moments when they get frustrated, disappointed, sad, etc., with their animal friend. It can be helpful to explore their ideas and hopes for the relationship, as well as their fears or worries. This will provide an opportunity for anticipatory guidance and normalizing those challenging moments in the relationship, as well as help identify any unrealistic expectations of their animal partner. It can also provide a space for identifying what the child may need in those moments of intense emotion, and for inviting them to help their animal partner in those moments as well—for example, How can I help you and your friend when you get frustrated, sad, or angry? Proactive work provides predictability in those unpredictable, highly emotional moments for the child and their animal partner. It may be helpful to create an Exit and Wait to Connect plan to identify the steps, strategies, and interventions needed in those moments.

The Exit and Wait to Connect Plan

When I get frustrated or upset, I can call a "time out" to help myself and my animal friend.

Develop a code word or phrase for you to know when you need a time out:

What are the signs my body gives me to help me know I should take a time out?

What are the signs my animal partner gives me to help me know that we should take a time out?

How long do we need to regulate? *(Decide as a clinical team what is appropriate)*

Where will I go when I am Exiting & Waiting to Connect:

The plan:

When I feel _____, *(the anticipated emotion)*
I will say _____ *(code word)*
I will go to _____ *(approved spot in the clinical space)*
and I will do _____ *(strategies to help regulate)*
When I feel _____ *(emotion)*

I would like _____ *(professional's name)*
and my animal partner _____ *(animal partner's name)*
to help me co-regulate by
(using a few words, taking belly breaths, setting a timer, turning on music, walking with my animal partner, etc.).

The child can be invited to write a letter to themself and/or their animal partner listing things they want to remember when they become frustrated, overwhelmed, or upset during therapy. Alternatively, they could draw a picture of these things. The letter or picture can be incorporated into future sessions to help the child recall the information they have learned. Empowering the child to create the plan for their animal partner can make them more receptive to feedback from their animal companion, rather than attributing negative relationship dynamics to the professional facilitating the process.

Communicate clearly about the interactions between the animal and child. If or when negative relationship patterns emerge, it can help the child to know that the animal is responding to what is happening in the moment and they are not trained to respond in a specific way. This can help protect the therapeutic relationship between the child and professional, as, again, it can often feel to the child as if the professional caused this negative thing to happen. While educating the child about the animal's behavior does not eliminate this risk, it can help avoid significant disruption between the child and the professional.

If your therapeutic setting has multiple animals available, involve the child in selecting their animal partner when possible. This fosters a sense of autonomy and control in the relationship, offering valuable insights into the child's relationship patterns. Allowing the child to choose their animal partner enables them to observe, experience, and repair any negative relationship patterns within their interactions with the animal.

Addressing the Signs and Cues of the Animal

Maintain Present Focus

It is crucial to maintain focus on the present relationship between the child and the animal. When things go well in the relationship, allow the child and the animal to revel in the experience of dopamine release (the "feel-good" chemicals) generated from positive relational connections. The child is creating new and healthier neural networks that can impact not only this present relationship but also all relationships in their life. Within the session, it is vital to celebrate or address the current relationship—a genuine bond in which the child can presently alter their behavior, fostering healthy relational connection, repair, and healing. AAT not only offers the child a relationship in the present moment but also can help create a relational template transferable outside of the session. Even though the child may not discuss their outside relationships, the work is still being done, as the relational networks are being activated, allowing the child to experience alternative, more appropriate responses to take place within the relational context.

Avoid the temptation to compare the relationship between the child and the animal to other of the child's relationships with similar patterns. Shifting attention to external relationships during powerful moments of connection in sessions can abruptly disrupt and potentially damage the profound present relational connections being established. The thought of other relationships will likely trigger the child's stress response, activating cortisol, the stress hormone, instead of the desired dopamine release. This stress response could then disturb the present relationship with their animal partner, causing distress for both the client and the animal. Consequently, this may reinforce a negative association with relationships—that they are unsafe and stressful.

Avoid Labeling Behaviors

The role of the professional is to assist the child in identifying the nonverbal communication of the animal without specifically assigning meaning to the animal's behavior. An important aspect of this is the professional's own emotional response to what is taking place with the animal partner, which will be discussed later in the chapter. Statements about the animal such as "he is scared" or "he seems mad" or even "he seems to really like you!" can halt the therapeutic process and eliminate the space for the child to interpret what is taking place. When developmentally appropriate, invite the child into the problem-solving process by asking questions like "What do you think might be happening with our friend?" "Have you noticed this behavior? What do you think might be going on?" It can also be helpful to compare current behavior to previous behavior. This process will provide powerful insight into the lens through which the child views relationships, and awareness of their own behaviors and the impact of their behavior on others.

When the professional labels the behaviors of the animal, they are applying their own lens with which to view that behavior and potentially robbing the child of the valuable opportunity to practice reading and responding to social cues. The professional must practice restraint in this area, allowing the space for the child to experience the relational connection and identify what is taking place with their animal partner. There will be times when the child's interpretation is accurate. Celebrate these moments, then engage the child in creative problem-solving to see what needs to be done next in the relationship with their friend. There will also be opportunities when the child misreads the animal partner's cues. When the interpretation is inaccurate, it can be helpful for the professional to simply point out the nonverbal communication of the animal—for example, "Here is what I noticed. Stella put their tail down quickly, showed her teeth, and backed away. I wonder what those signs might say about how she is feeling about what is taking place?" Children who have a limited emotional vocabulary may benefit from the professional translating the behaviors of the animal with their own body. If an animal expresses frustration or annoyance, the professional may furrow their brow and make an exaggerated angry face. This can become a fun game: inviting the child to join the professional in making the face of what they believe the animal is communicating. The professional can then exaggerate the nonverbal communication of the animal to assist the child in learning the cues and signs.

It is important to create a space where the child feels comfortable expressing their own experience within their relational context. While an experience might appear positive from the professional's standpoint, the child's interpretation might be entirely different; they may perceive the experience as scary or uncomfortable. If the professional narrates the moment in a way that does not resonate with the child's feelings, it can place the child in the very tough position of either correcting the professional or disregarding their own internal response, assuming it to be incorrect. For instance, consider a child meeting a large dog for the first time. While the professional might view this as a powerful, fun, and positive experience, the child might be overwhelmed with terror. Thus, it becomes crucial for the professional to ask, "What was that experience like for you? What do you think it was like for your animal partner?" These instances provide opportunities to address emotional discrepancies, such as the child appearing to be laughing and smiling while internally finding the experience dreadful or scary.

Providing impartial feedback based on simple nonjudgmental observations during these moments can help enhance the child's awareness of their nonverbal communication. For example, saying, "It's interesting to hear you describe that as terrifying and awful. Can I share what I noticed? I observed you were smiling and laughing. How do you think I might interpret those signs?" In other cases, a child might describe the experience as amazing while showing signs of inner turmoil, like fighting back tears and holding their breath. During this process, it is common for cognitive distortions and core beliefs to begin to emerge, providing rich opportunity for the child to explore refuting those distortions and to experience relational connections where those cognitions are not true. The child's previous relational experiences and developmental insults have created templates that can make challenging those negative core beliefs difficult. Through a partnership with an animal, the child can begin to explore new ways to view relationships and social cues.

Navigating the Relationships When Things Do Not Go as Planned

In this work, honesty and transparency about the animal's experience are essential for fostering balanced, healthy relationships. Even when it is challenging, it is crucial to be truthful in addressing what is happening. Communicating with the child might involve statements like, "I am not quite sure what might be going on for our friend, but something seems different from our previous times with them. I'm wondering if we could figure out a way to help them?" or "I'm noticing some things from our friend that make me wonder about how they might feel. I'm wondering what might happen if we tried something different."

It is important to emphasize that animals, especially prey animals like equines, do not lie or have ulterior motives. When professionals are not truthful, they become incongruent, and from the perspective of prey animals, they may be perceived as predators. This incongruence can create an unsafe environment for all involved parties, highlighting the importance of honesty in the therapeutic process.

When it is determined that a different animal should be involved in the sessions, it is important to include the child in this process and explore opportunities for the relationship, to make the adjustments. Many times, children are not given the opportunity for healthy goodbyes or "see ya laters." If it is clinically appropriate to change animals in the therapeutic setting, helping the client and previous animal partner work on the relationship in a different manner is important. It can also be helpful if while this relationship is changing, it is still one the child can continue to build, just with distance. This still holds clinical significance. Detachment is a core concept of Natural Lifemanship (Jobe et al., 2021), a comprehensive, Trauma Focused-Equine Assisted Psychotherapy model that discusses the importance of attachment (working on the relationship in close proximity) and detachment (working on the relationship with distance). When the relationship with the animal partner moves from attachment to detachment, it can be helpful for the child to write cards or give pictures or drawings to their animal friend and schedule visits or other things that one might do when a friend has moved away.

A young child, Josiah, had been working with one of our older horses, Bogie, for over a year. During the time together, the youngster grew and pushed beyond the weight tolerance of an older horse. To protect the child and the horse in this delicate situation, the team decided that addressing this like a graduation would be the best for the relationship. Bogie could pass the child to a "new friend" to continue the work. As the graduation took place, the therapy team allowed Bogie to participate in the transition through simple strategies such as session "check-ins," when Josiah would say hi to both horses and share about his week, as well as allowing Bogie to stay in the barn and watch Josiah ride his new equine partner. This allowed Josiah to maintain the relational connection with Bogie while also building a new relationship.

Navigating Sickness and Death of the Animal Partners

AAT provides real-life situations in which sickness, grief, and loss will take place. Navigating these situations can provide rich growth opportunities and therapeutic healing. There are times when an animal partner becomes sick and adjustments must be made in the therapeutic relationship. It is in these moments that a child can practice the skills of empathy, compassion, and concern toward their friend when they are not feeling well. It is important to keep in mind the child's window of tolerance. Some children may be able to participate in the care by actively assisting, but for some this may be overwhelming and it may become necessary for them to explore the relationship through detachment.

A young boy, Tyler, had been removed from his biological family around the age of 5. It was discovered he had countless broken bones as a result of physical abuse from his stepfather. His presentation at the age of 8 was classic conduct disorder. While Tyler was involved in our services, a miniature horse, Mr. Buttons, broke his leg and required over a year of vet care, which included going on short walks and needing cold compresses and frequent bandage changes. This disconnected, struggling boy began asking how he could help Mr. Buttons with his vet care, and that became part of his own treatment. Tyler would take care of Mr. Buttons's injury, closely monitoring for signs of comfort and discomfort. Tyler's often cold and detached presentation began to soften, and he began to share about his days at school and even stories of his earlier childhood. Tyler began to become more present as he responded to the needs of Mr. Buttons during the walks and application of cold compresses. Throughout this process with Mr. Buttons, Tyler also began to build relationships outside of the sessions. It became evident in the way he interacted with the clinical staff and his teachers at school. Tyler began to make eye contact, communicate more freely, and demonstrate care and concern for others.

There may also be situations when it is determined that an animal is too sick and can no longer actively participate in sessions. And of course an animal may pass away. This can be devastating on multiple levels, but it is a powerful opportunity to model grieving, to allow the client to express their grief, and to provide closure. In my practice, there have been a number of losses around the farm and each loss has led to some powerful healing.

Content warning: What follows in this next case story may be upsetting for some. Please proceed with care.

A young child, Lizette, had been referred to services due to anxiety following the unexpected loss of a grandparent. When Lizette began with us, she was given an opportunity to pick a friendship horse. As she began exploring the herd, it was quite clear that she was being picked by one of the horses, Kitty. Miss Kitty, as she was often called, was a 32-year-old Appaloosa with a bit of an unknown history. She came to the herd through a donation from a therapeutic riding program and seemed to have a heart for those grieving. As Lizette explored the herd, Kitty would not leave her side. It was evident to Lizette, her parents, and the clinical team that this was the friendship horse for her.

The two worked together throughout therapy. After much success in treatment, it was decided that it was time for Lizette to graduate from services. Plans were made for her graduation (her closing session), but no one was quite prepared for what would take place that day.

Twenty minutes before the graduation session was to start, a staff member came running into the office and said, "Kitty is down. She's not okay!" The team rushed out to Kitty and found her lying on her side. They hustled to get Kitty medicine to help get her comfortable. Through tears, the staff told Kitty, "Your friend is going to be here soon. She needs to be able to say goodbye."

After a few moments, Kitty stood up on her own. Lizette arrived for her graduation celebration. The clinical staff discussed the situation with Lizette's family. The vet was on his way to help Kitty cross over the rainbow bridge. Lizette's family agreed: she needed to be with Kitty. They shared the news with the child, and with tears they all made their way over to Kitty, who was waiting for her friend in the arena.

Lizette went over to Kitty and took the lead rope. The two walked together as the child thanked the horse for their time together. There were tears; there was laughter remembering funny times together; and there were goodbyes—there was closure. In the last few hours of Kitty's life, she was able to do something that words cannot fully express. Lizette, who had not gotten an opportunity to say goodbye to her grandpa, was given an opportunity to say goodbye to her friend Kitty, and in that moment, there was both loss and healing. It was gut-wrenching and beautiful at the same time.

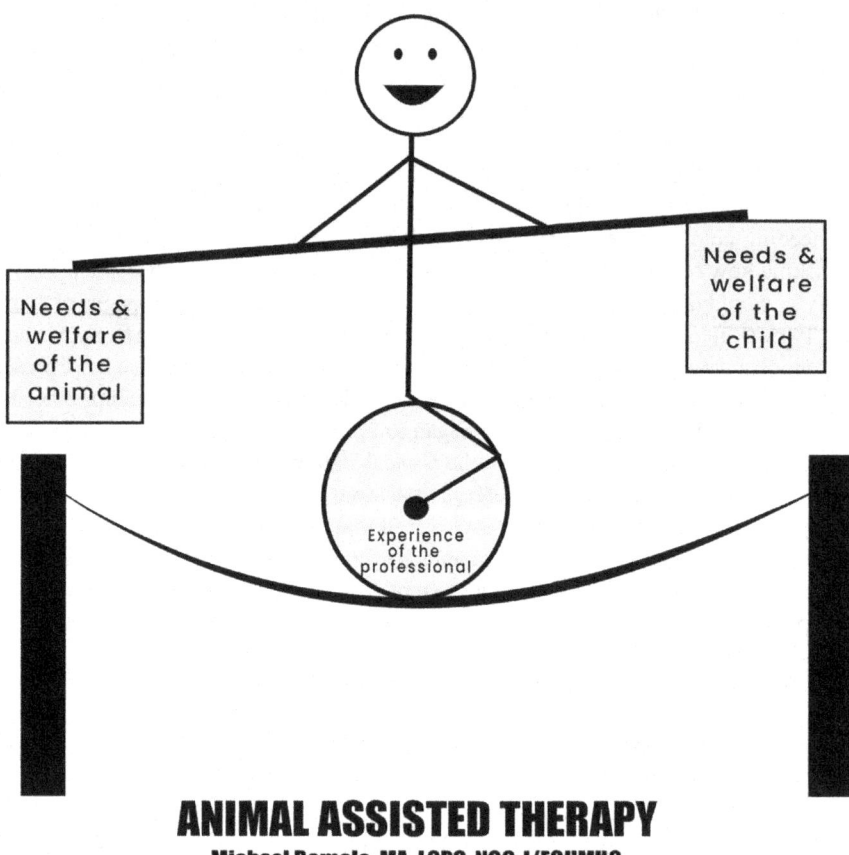

ANIMAL ASSISTED THERAPY
Michael Remole, MA, LCPC, NCC, I/ECHMHC

Figure 26.1 Stick Figure Riding a Unicycle on a Tightrope Holding a Pole.

Doing Your Own Work

A crucial aspect of AAT involves the professional's adeptness in navigating the complexities involving their own animal. Professionals engaged in AAT must deftly balance the needs of both the client and the animal partner, all while being cognizant that their emotional responses toward both parties can significantly impact the clinical work (see Figure 26.1). The professional's internal state during sessions affects not only the child but also the animal partner. It is imperative for the professional to closely monitor and effectively manage their emotional and physiological responses to what transpires in the sessions. When appropriate, this can model healthy behavior for the child.

For the professional, AAT can feel as if they are riding a unicycle on a tightrope while carefully balancing the needs of the animal partner and child and also managing their own physical and emotional response to what is taking place in the therapy session.

When engaging in AAT, it is essential for the professional to identify signs that they may be influenced by the work and impacting the session. While it is easy to appreciate the positive aspects of AAT, there are times when sessions do not go as planned, and children may become frustrated and act out. Balancing these factors is complex, and one must consider potential triggers and stressors that may influence the session. Introducing an animal into the therapeutic setting may result in sessions deviating from plans, leading children to express discomfort toward the animal. In such moments, it is crucial for the professional to address and repair any challenges arising from their own "stuff" in relationships. AAT should provide opportunities for genuine connection. Genuine connection is not a goal to be accomplished. Rather, it is the continual work of both beings to carefully balance one's own needs while holding in mind the needs of the other.

It is important to note that animals cannot differentiate the "identified client" in the session and will respond to the emotional environment as a whole. Animals can detect emotions, potentially interpreting them as predatory. Thus, authenticity in the moment becomes crucial in AAT, and professionals need to acknowledge their emotions appropriately during sessions—for instance, stating, "I'm feeling a bit frustrated right now" or "I am a bit concerned about what this might be like for our friend." However, caution is necessary when discussing these situations. Sticking to factual observations rather than labeling behavior is vital in these instances.

The Neurosequential Model

Perry and colleagues (1995) stated, "Understanding the organization, function, and development of the human brain, and brain-mediated responses to threat, provides the keys to understanding the traumatized child." The Neurosequential Model © (NM), developed by Bruce D. Perry, is a developmentally informed approach and respects the biology of individuals navigating complex trauma. The neurosequential part refers to core concepts of the sequential development and hierarchical organization of the functional capacities of the brain. This sequential process begins in the lowest region of the brain, responsible for basic survival (brainstem) and motor skills (diencephalon), advancing to the middle regions (limbic system), managing relationships and attachment, and culminating in the upper regions (neocortex), responsible for problem-solving, reasoning, and reflection. The sequential development and organization commence in utero, with critical development and construction of neural networks continuing throughout childhood and into adolescence. While the majority of growth occurs early in development, the brain continues to evolve and adapt throughout the lifespan.

The mature brain comprises over 86 billion neurons and ten times the number of glial cells; these units collaborate to orchestrate brain-mediated functions (Perry et al., 1995). Neurons create networks through associations and experiences, responsive to signals from other neurons, establishing systems to govern function. The more these associations occur, the more dominant and habitual they become, forming the templates for development, memory, and learning. Perry et al. (1995) stated, "Depending on the severity, frequency, nature, and pattern of traumatic events, at least half of all children exposed [to traumatic experiences] may be expected to develop significant neuropsychiatric symptomatology" (p. 271). Individuals experiencing severe, prolonged, and unpredictable stress may develop a hypersensitive stress response, leading to disorganized brain function. Consequently, the cortical regions' capacity to override the brainstem's reactive responses diminishes. The body's threat response mechanisms aim to maintain safety and homeostasis.

State-Dependent Functioning

Perry et al. (1995) delineated stress responses along a spectrum, ranging from a state of calmness to heightened alertness, alarm, fear, and, in extreme cases, terror. This continuum is governed by the rapid and unconscious interpretation of stress signals by the ever-evolving brain and body, arising from internal and external information. Subsequently, the brain rapidly interprets this data and signals through the core regulatory systems—including dopaminergic, noradrenergic, and serotonergic—guiding responses to novelty, challenge, and threat (Perry, 2017a). These core regulatory systems, located in the brain's lower regions, modulate and regulate the various brain functions essential for addressing or adapting to stressors to ensure the individual's safety. The level of activation is influenced by one's developmental history and exposure to specific threats. This state of activation dictates the individual's functioning, transitioning from internal calmness to alertness, alarm, fear, and ultimately, terror. As the stress response activates, the core regulatory systems shut down the "smarter" portions of the brain, concurrently activating more primitive brain regions. Perry encapsulates this phenomenon as "state-dependent functioning," illustrating how an individual's cognitive and emotional functionality adapt based on their current physiological and emotional state. Perry (2017b) stated,

> When exposed to extreme or prolonged distress (e.g., physical or sexual abuse), or unpredictable and uncontrollable stress (e.g., with poverty, community violence), these stress response systems can become 'sensitized.' This means they become overactive at baseline and overly (and inappropriately) reactive. The sensitized response to stress triggers rapid movement along the hyperarousal or dissociative continuums.

Perry et al. (1995) discussed the two universal adaptive stress response continuums: hyperarousal and dissociation. The hyperarousal response, commonly known as fight or flight, is more prominently recognized and taught. In contrast, the dissociative response is activated when an individual perceives a stressor as an inescapable, unavoidable, and painful situation (Perry, 2017c). These response patterns—dissociation and hyperarousal—operate in tandem to help an individual maintain equilibrium amid everyday stressors and survive traumatic experiences (Perry, 1999). Perry also noted that many individuals faced with stress may employ a combination of both hyperarousal and dissociative responses, despite these being two distinct reactions.

After the threat has been eliminated, the core regulatory networks play a crucial role in determining the pace of returning along the continuum toward the baseline state. The individual's brain and body, influenced by factors such as the timing, intensity, and duration of exposure, dictate the rate at which they move toward a state of calm. Repeated exposure to evocative cues compromises the ability to return to a state of calm, leading to an alteration in baseline functioning.

Clinical Applications of the Neurosequential Model

Throughout clinical sessions, the team, consisting of the child, clinical staff, and the animal partner, navigates the continuum of state-dependent functioning. Each individual responds to internal and external stressors with the goal of co-regulating and supporting one another in the face of various stressors. An integral part of the work of AAT is facilitating therapeutic experiences that are sensitive and respective to the animal partner, the child's developmental status in various domains and to state regulation capacity of both the animal and child.

In the context of AAT, it is critical to monitor the therapeutic dose for not only the client, but also the animal. Throughout the relationship, small, predictable amounts of stress will need to be applied, along with the scaffolding support to navigate the stressor. The professional must closely monitor the situation to balance the appropriate dose of relational connection with returning to more regulating activities such as walking, grooming, or petting. As the beings in the relationship demonstrate the ability to effectively manage the current stress, then additional stress can be introduced to the relationship.

Practical Strategies and Interventions

It is important that AAT be incorporated into sessions through the relational framework: Is this good for both beings in this relationship? Are we compromising the well-being of the animal to accomplish something for the child? If day-to-day activities in session are introduced as "tasks" to be completed, then the relational connection between child and animal can become compromised. One of the focuses of AAT is to explore how the day-to-day activities can be completed in relational manner, rather than as a "task." A part of the therapeutic process is to help the child be attuned to the needs of their animal partner while putting the collar and leash on their dog, brushing their animal partner, going for a walk with their animal friend, or putting on the saddle to ride their equine partner. Relationally engaging in these small day-to-day "tasks" can provide powerful moments of relational connection and intimacy.

It is also imperative for the therapist to note that the items that are discussed are not prescriptive. The interventions listed below assist with bottom-up regulation for the child, to help them develop a more fully integrated brain, and have been compiled in collaboration with Marti Smith, OTR/L and Natural Lifemanship Institute. The clinician's particular theoretical orientation will influence the ways in which these interventions are introduced and implemented. All these strategies should be done with the focus on the relationship with and well-being of the animal partner. Many of the examples provided are discussed in the context of working with equines or canines but can be modified to fit the needs of a variety of animal partners. If you work with dogs and they are not off leash, you may explore various ways to engage in the activities by utilizing leashes that secure to a belt that the child can wear, or the therapist can hold onto the leash at times to allow the child to have their hands free.

The role of the therapist is to consistently monitor the various states of the child and the animal partner and then provide appropriate therapeutic interventions to engage and regulate the child's brain in the sequential order. A simple exercise that can be incorporated in session is to have the child list five things they can see, four things they can hear, three things they can feel or touch, two things they can smell, and one thing they can taste.

This is a quick way to help the clinician assess the client's current state of functioning and provide the framework for the session. Does the child mention things that are close to them or things that are a significant distance away from them? Do they include their animal partner in the things they can see? This exercise can also provide rich information for the professional regarding the client's felt safety, as well as how they are interpreting the world around them. Are they aware of their surroundings? Sometimes, it can be valuable to ask the child which of those sounds they identify is the loudest or most distracting. What are they noticing for touch? Is it their animal partner or something else? This can provide immediate feedback to the professional about what the child is experiencing in the here and now. It can be fun to determine if the smells they are identifying are positive or even gross. When working around the farm with animals, there are a plethora of smells that to some are pleasant, while repulsive to others. This exercise can create a fun, relational connection by inviting the child to guess what their animal partner might see, hear, touch, smell, and taste.

What follows is an extensive list of AAT strategies and interventions categorized by brain area.

Brainstem: Rhythmic, Patterned, Repetitive Sensory Input

- When a child is highly dysregulated and operating from the brainstem, keep in mind that the rhythmic, predictable, patterned sensory input may need to be provided without the child's active involvement—the clinician may help with rhythmic breathing, swaying, and the cadence of the professional's voice. Rhythmic, patterned, repetitive sensory input can also be provided through the heart rates of the professional and animal. If comfortable, the child can place their hands on the animal to feel their heart beat and breathing. As the child moves toward a more regulated state, they can begin to gently tap to the beat of the animal's heart.
- Provide physical movement through walks with the animal partner, or if working with horses and the child is comfortable, through mounted work.

- The clinician can also assist the client in brainstem regulation through various visual exercises such as looking from side to side or looking up and down. When they are walking their horse or dog, invite the child look to the left, then move their head and look to the right. This can also form a relational connection for client and their horse: if the child is riding, the more attuned the horse is to the rider, the more they will adjust based on the direction the child is looking. For canine-assisted therapy, the animal partner may notice the change in where the child is looking and look as well.
- Crossing the body's midline in a predictable manner can be regulating, as it engages both sides of the brain. There are a variety of ways to incorporate this rhythmic input into your session. It can be done through rhythmic petting or brushing of the animal partners. A bear or butterfly hug (Jarero et al., 2006) can be done while sitting with the animal or riding a horse. The child can place their hands on both sides of the animal's shoulders to feel the different steps taken.
- Weighted products can be used during sessions. When working with children and animals, wearable weighted products are helpful to allow for free movement. The use of CapeAble Weighted products allows the client to wear the products while engaging in the activities with the animals. When incorporating weighted products, please seek guidance from an occupational therapist.
- As they show signs of improved regulation, the child may massage their animal partner. This activity is also relational, so it is activating the limbic system as well.
- Activities may also include belly breathing, rhythmic breathing, or taking "horse breaths, lowering your head" (Jobe et al., 2021).
- Identifying the various sensations of the animal's coat. Is it fluffy, rough, scratchy? Is it long or short? The same can be done with the various items for the animals. Is this brush soft, scratchy, or hard? Are the reins (or is the leash) smooth or bumpy?
- Incorporating the sense of smell into the session. The clinician can work with the child to identify scents that the child finds pleasant and can be used in a diffuser during an indoor session to enhance the therapeutic work. When a session is taking place outdoors, smell can be introduced through essential oils on a paper towel and placed inside the helmet of the child, in a pocket, or clipped on the shirt of the child.
- Tactile sensations also activate and engage the brainstem. This can be done by utilizing a more textured leash, lead rope, reins, or harness for the animal with which you are partnering. These can be made simply by using a hot glue gun and gluing dots on a lead rope, reins, or leash.

Diencephalon: Rhythmic, Patterned, Repetitive Movement

- Activities can include interventions during which the child crosses their body's midline. This can be done organically through grooming their animal partner or reaching for various tack, and it can also be done through a game. When the child is riding their horse partner, the clinician can call out directions: "Take your right hand and touch your left knee," going back and forth as the child demonstrates they are maintaining a more regulated state. The professional and client can mirror one another throughout this process.
- The animal's coat can be very helpful in providing opportunities for regulation for the child. For animals with longer hair, the child could try braiding and combing. Done within the context of the relationship between the child and the animal, the professional can help the child assess how the animal is responding to the grooming. This can provide insight into what may be happening in the session.
- Riding a horse is regulating for the diencephalon. An important thing to consider when working with children with complex trauma is to take note of their balance prior to engaging in riding. Gateway Family Services of Illinois utilizes bareback riding pads to allow for close contact for

children with their equine partner. While this provides for greater sensory input, it is critical to note that for those with vestibular and proprioception challenges, it may be more dysregulating, as the bareback pads do not have stirrups to assist with balance. The Cowboy Compression Cape, developed by this author and Marti Smith, OTR/L, was created to provide appropriate support and sensory input to assist in regulating the vestibular and proprioceptive systems. Lycra or CapeAble Weighted products can be incorporated here as well.
- Incorporating music with a strong heart rate rhythm, such as Native American drumming. Younger children have a higher resting heart rate, and as they move toward adolescence, their numbers lower (Rao & Zahka, 2023). When working with an animal partner, can the two beings walk or move to the beat, essentially dancing with one another. The application Tempo Magic can be downloaded on most devices and can integrate songs selected by the child and provide an opportunity to change the rhythm of the music to better meet the needs of the child.
- Incorporating drums, a metronome, tapping, or clapping into the activities. As a child improves their state of regulation, they will be able to provide the rhythm. During times of more extreme dysregulation, the professional will need to provide the external rhythm until the child is able to join in. When the child is in a more regulated state, they can also determine how their animal partner feels about that rhythmic activity to increase opportunities for attunement, empathy, and reading social cues. This activity can easily become a full-brain activity: the professional provides the rhythm (brainstem), the child joins in, also providing the rhythm (diencephalon), the child checks in with their animal partner on how they feel about what is taking place (limbic system), and then together the child and professional can problem solve and reflect on how to support the animal friend (neocortex).
- Using grab bins while mounted on horseback or walking with their animal partner. The client can grab various identified items specifically focused on the tactical sensations. Examples of items can be stress balls, shaker bottles, rice, sand, or slime. Involve the child in the selection process of the items in the bin, and if appropriate, invite them to introduce the items to their animal partner. A variation of this activity would include asking the child to use their opposite hand to cross over their body and reach into the bin.
- Farm activities—raking the stall, carrying buckets, moving feed, etc. Engaging in the heavy work on the farm is helpful for providing physical activity, as well as involving the child in the relational connection of how the activities are helping their animal partner.
- Giving the animal a bath. This intervention will need to be planned to ensure a positive experience for the animal receiving the bath. This form of care and nurturing can be fun and healing.

Limbic System: Rhythmic, Patterned, Repetitive Relationships

- Spending time grooming the animal partner may appear to be a simple strategy; however, it is engaging in emotional intimacy and seeking to meet the needs of others. Invite the child to find the places the animal enjoys being groomed.
- Tending to the needs of the animal, through simple daily care or even vet care if the animal is sick. This can help cultivate empathy and nurturing.
- Identifying the various emotions of the animal partner—this can be done with the animal present or through pictures of them. Variations of this activity would include creating storyboards of what is taking place for the animal. In the situation where there appears to be a negative emotion, how can the child help the animal?
- Creating the story of the animal using various pictures of the animal's emotions. Using storyboards can provide opportunities to identify the various feelings that their animal partner may experience in various situations. This can be done as future planning—for example, "If _____

happened, what might come next in this story? How might your friend feel after _____?" It can also be done by reflecting backward: "How did your friend feel when _____ happened?" If developmentally appropriate, invite the child to create their own emotional sequence as the animal's timeline is being created. This can help the child see their role in co-regulation.
- Bringing a camera to session and inviting the child to capture the various expressions of their animal partner. A variety of clinical interventions can be done with those images, including printing them and creating stories based on what is taking place for their animal partner, or having the child mimic the emotion or expression they perceive in the pictures. If the professional has permission, capturing pictures of the child expressing various emotions and printing them for a matching game can assist the child in their accuracy of interpreting social cues. This can lend itself to a variety of strategies for the professional to engage the client in identifying the emotions.
- Identifying and discussing the feelings of the animal and the child. This may be done in a small dose of relational connection, such as, "How is your animal friend doing?" or "What do you think is going on for your friend?" The child can be invited to help their friend with the various emotions that are being discussed: "What do you think your friend needs from us today?" It may also move to more child-centered questions about the way the child feels around their animal partner. What can the animal partner do to help them?
- Sometimes, the child may want to share their story with their animal friend. They may want their friend to know about the trauma they have experienced. The child can share while they are riding or moving in session, or grooming their animal partner. Some may become dysregulated, while others may experience relief to be able to share their story with their friend. For those who can engage in mounted work with horses, being carried by the horse during these moments is very helpful in maintaining a more regulated state because of the passive rhythm being provided by their animal partner.
- Inviting the child to create a playlist of music to listen to during the session. See if they can identify if the animal likes or dislikes the music selected. This playlist can be incorporated into Rhythmic Riding sessions (Jobe et al., 2021) or on the ground while the partners walk together. Can the animal and child move to the rhythm of the music together?
- Drawing pictures or writing letters to the animal when the child and animal are not sharing the same space or can be helpful to foster the relationship and its benefits.
- As the child and animal begin to experience moments of emotional connection and intimacy, the child may be able to share where they feel that in their body. Explore what that particular feeling is like in their body or in their animal's. Where in their body do they feel their connection to their friend? Does that feeling have a color? Does that feeling need to say anything to the child or to their animal partner? Does the emotion the animal is experiencing need to tell the child something? This can create an opportunity to allow the child to express in words, art, or other creative outlets what message they are receiving from their animal partner.

Neocortex

- A child may choose to invite their animal partner into their places of trauma. What might the support of their animal partner be like for them in those places of hurt? How might their friend support them or carry that hurt, sadness, grief, anger? If appropriate, the child may choose to create a visual representation of their various emotions (using paper or pieces of material) and allow their animal partner to help carry those heavy things. The child can then reflect on what that feels like to know their animal partner can help carry those big feelings or situations.
- Creating a secure, calm place that includes their animal partner. What do both beings need in this space to feel safe, connected, and protected? On the farm, it is possible for the client to create a

physical space and invite their partner into that space. However, the strategy can also translate into a sandtray or art activity in which the child invites their animal partner into the safe space they've created.
- Partnering with the therapy animal provides an opportunity for the child to be a part of the life story of the animal. How does the child feel about their relationship with the animal helping improve the animal's life? Invite the child into a future template of what life is like for the animal because of the connection with the child. What does the child's life look like in the future because of the relational connection with the animal?
- Asking the child to put on the animal's training vest, leash, collar, halter, saddle pad, etc. This can be an excellent way for the child to problem solve.
- Walking with the animal and playing a game of Simon Says to see if the child and animal can help one another through the game. The child is also following directions, attending to multiple cues at the same time.
- Creating and completing patterns or obstacle courses with the animal. *This will need to be monitored closely for what obstacles are available and what is realistic for the animal. This can also provide a great opportunity to see if the animal's needs are also considered in this process.*
- Offering choices to the client and simple problems for them to solve. "Where should we go for a walk? Where can we put these items now that we are finished brushing?"
- Having the child place their hands together and out in front of their chest while walking, standing, or (if with a horse) riding. Ask the child to spell the animal's name in the air with their hands.
- Ask the child to count their animal partner's steps while walking with or riding the animal. Can they ask their partner to walk eight steps? Can they ask their partner to go faster, slow down, stop, etc.? Various amounts of healthy stress can be added to this simply by inviting the child to silently count the steps or asking their animal partner to walk, if they are comfortable, with their eyes closed to allow for greater input.
- Inviting the client to share with their animal partner what they are learning at school and practice while walking or riding. This is especially helpful for kids who might be having some school anxiety or struggles in school.
- Moments of reflection. As the child can access their neocortex, they are able to be reflective about their experience and the experience for their animal partner. For some, this may be done through verbal processing and reflection. This can also be where other means of expression are brought into the session, such as drawing or painting a picture or creating sandtray worlds to reflect and express what took place in that moment with their partner. If surrounded by nature, children can also incorporate sticks, rocks, and leaves into their art or sandtray stories.

Animal Partner Selection to Address Dissociation and Hyperarousal

Both humans and animals may respond to stress through hyperarousal or dissociation. Some may display a combination of these responses. The professional's role is to remain attuned to both the animal and the child, monitoring for signs of dysregulation. The professional will then work to engage both beings in the co-regulation process.

Is the child prone to hyperarousal or dissociation? When working with individuals who exhibit a predominant tendency toward dissociation, the appropriate animal paired with them might also lean toward dissociation. While this may seem counterintuitive, within this relational context, it can benefit both beings. The child is encouraged to assist their animal partner in staying more present, necessitating their own heightened attentiveness to their animal friend's cues and needs. An animal prone to dissociation will face the challenge of remaining present through the connection with their human friend. If the child dissociates, the animal's response system is challenged to stay more present as well—in the animal world, more than one animal dissociating signals a significant threat to their safety. This dynamic offers numerous opportunities for both human and animal to develop the skill of staying in or coming back to the present, and will need to be closely monitored by the professional—horses have nudged, nibbled, or even bucked to bring their dissociative partner back. Cats or dogs have used their paws, claws, or teeth to regain their friend's attention. The animal's innate ability to detect dissociation becomes valuable when working with children exhibiting a complex presentation of dissociation.

It is equally important to monitor whether the animal can navigate the child's stress response without joining in their dysregulation. Considerations for monitoring:

- Is the client more predisposed to dissociation, or do they display signs of hyperarousal?
- Assess the animal partners to determine their response to an individual exhibiting dissociation or heightened activation. Can safety be maintained?
- Can the professional maintain a connection and safety with the animal amid stress to be a source of co-regulation?
- How does the animal manage multiple children exhibiting similar stress responses?

It is imperative for any professional working with animals in the clinical setting to be extremely familiar with each animal partner. When choosing animals to invite into the therapeutic setting, it is critical to recognize and embrace their natural instincts. This chapter has primarily discussed partnering with canines and equines. Both animals have different ways of being—dogs are a predatory animal, while equines are a prey animal. Being cognizant of these differences is critical, since that impacts the animals' responses and cues.

Conclusion

Animal-assisted therapy (AAT) stands as a powerful and nuanced strategy in the realm of therapeutic interventions, particularly for children navigating the complexities of relational trauma. AAT can be the primary mode of treatment or it can be done in combination with other therapies such as art, play, sandtray, EMDR, TF-CBT, or Motivational Interviewing. This chapter has delved into the intricate layers of AAT, emphasizing the necessity for clinicians to possess a profound understanding of the neurosequential process and a robust clinical foundation. We explored the art of seamlessly integrating various interventions and strategies throughout clinical sessions, with a meticulous balancing act catering to the unique needs of the child, animal, and professional. Central to this process is a keen awareness of the state-dependent functioning within the session, harmonizing the relational dance between child, animal, and professional. The hope is that this chapter serves as a guiding beacon for AAT clinicians dedicated to fostering healing, connection, and growth in the lives of those grappling with relational trauma.

Note

1 Case stories in this chapter are used with permission of the clients. They have been adjusted or modified to protect the clients' identities while maintaining the core concepts for the chapter.

References

American Psychological Association. (n.d.). Animal-assisted therapy. In *APA dictionary of psychology*. Retrieved October 28, 2023, from dictionary.apa.org/animal-assisted-therapy

American Veterinary Medical Association (AVMA). (n.d.). Animal-assisted interventions: Definitions. avma.org/resources-tools/avma-policies/animal-assisted-interventions-definitions

Jarero, I., Artigas, L., & Hartung, J. (2006). EMDR integrative group treatment protocol: A postdisaster trauma intervention for children and adults. *Traumatology, 12*(2), 121–129. https://doi.org/10.1177/1534765606294561

Jobe, T., Shultz-Jobe, B., McFarland, L., & Naylor K. (2021). *Natural lifemanship's Trauma Focused-Equine Assisted Psychotherapy (TF-EAP) and Trauma Informed Equine Assisted Learning (TI-EAL).*

Levy, M. S. (1998). A helpful way to conceptualize and understand reenactments. *The Journal of Psychotherapy Practice and Research, 7*(3), 227–235.

Perry, B. D. (1999). Memories of fear: How the brain stores and retrieves physiologic states, feelings, behaviors and thoughts from traumatic events. In J. M. Goodwin & R. Attias (Eds.), *Images of the body in trauma* (pp. 26–47). Basic Books.

Perry, B. D. (2017a). Trauma- and stress-related disorders. In T. P. Beauchaine & S. P. Hinshaw (Eds.), *Textbook of child and adolescent psychopathology* (3rd ed., pp. 683–705). Wiley.

Perry, B. D. (2017b). *Understanding dissociation: The NMC Ten Tip Series.* CTA Press.

Perry, B. D. (2017c). *Understanding hyperarousal: The "Flock, Freeze, Flight and Fight" continuum. The NMC Ten Tip Series.* CTA Press.

Perry, B. D. (2019). Foreword. In P. Tedeschi & M. A. Jenkins (Eds.), *Transforming trauma: Resilience and healing through our connections with animals* (pp. x–xi). Purdue University Press.

Perry, B. D., Pollard, R. A., Blakley, T. L., Baker, W. L., & Vigilante, D. (1995). Childhood trauma, the neurobiology of adaptation, and "use-dependent" development of the brain: How "states" becomes "traits." *Infant Mental Health Journal, 16*, 271–191. https://doi.org/10.1002/1097-0355(199524)16:4<271::AID-IMHJ2280160404>3.0.CO;2-B

Perry, B. D., & Szalavitz, M. (2007). *The boy who was raised as a dog.* Basic Books.

Purvis, K. B., Cross, D. R., Dansereau, D. F., & Parris, S. R. (2013). Trust-Based Relational Intervention (TBRI): A systemic approach to complex developmental trauma. *Child & Youth Services, 34*(4), 360–386. https://doi.org/10.1080/0145935X.2013.859906

Rao, R., & Zahka, K. (March 13, 2023). Heart rate and kids: How high is too high? Cleveland Clinic. health.clevelandclinic.org/pushing-childs-heart-rate-high

Tedeschi, P., & Jenkins, M. A. (2019). *Transforming trauma: Resilience and healing through our connections with animals.* Purdue University Press.

27
CHILD-CENTERED PLAY THERAPY

Kristi L. Perryman

Introduction: Play Therapy

The Association for Play Therapy (2023) defines play therapy as "the systematic use of a theoretical model to establish an interpersonal process wherein trained play therapists use the therapeutic powers of play to help clients prevent or resolve psychosocial difficulties and achieve optimal growth and development" (para. 2). Play has been credited with therapeutic powers that include facilitating communication, fostering emotional wellness, enhancing relationships, and increasing personal strengths (Schaefer & Drewes, 2014). It has long been a part of the therapeutic process, first documented by Sigmund Freud in 1909 through his work with Little Hans, a five-year-old boy with phobias. Melanie Klein (1932), a student of Freud, incorporated play with children as a mode of free association. Anna Freud, daughter of Sigmund Freud, utilized play to build a relationship with children prior to transitioning to interpretation (1946).

Others focused specifically on the role of play as therapy, furthering the knowledge in the crucial role of play in the lives of children through relationship therapy, release therapy, and structured play therapy (Allen, 1942; Hambridge, 1955; Levy, 1938; Taft, 1933). Piaget's work contributed greatly to the growth of play therapy, as his work was the first to refute the belief that representational thought derived from a child's verbal ability, stating, "Thought is both prior to language and broader than language" (1972, p. 47). Teaching infants sign language is an example of this. Children can cognitively understand signs and their meaning and utilize them to express their needs for food, drink, and so on prior to their ability to verbalize. Erikson's work also contributed to the understanding of play in a child's life, specifically their natural inclination to make sense of their world through their natural language of play: "play may well facilitate in a child an impulse to recapitulate and, as it were, to reinvent his own experience in order to learn where it might lead" (1972, p. 132). Similarly, Landreth (2012) described play as a child's language with toys as their words. Play therapy has continued to evolve and develop with the establishment of the APT; an international peer reviewed journal; an annual international conference; numerous research articles, books, presentations; and, most recently, the movement toward neurobiology and biomarkers as a measure of change in traumatized children.

based registered play therapist (SB-RPT). The APT also now designates approved university centers of play therapy education and approved providers of continuing education to ensure quality education for those specializing in play therapy. The APT has over 7,000 members. These include those from 42 US branches in addition to numerous international members. The APT has rigorous standards for approved university and continuing education courses, ensuring therapists obtain quality education to establish their scope of practice in working with children.

Seminal Theories and Evidenced-Based Approaches

It is crucial that therapists have a strong base and functional understanding in their theoretical perspective, as it is the road map used to determine their role in the therapeutic process. Theory serves to answer what an individual believes about human nature, where adaptive behaviors come from, where maladaptive behaviors come from, and finally, the healing factor that allows change to occur. Theory provides meaning, purpose, and goals for the therapeutic work, promoting advanced thoughts, questions, and ultimately research to validate and/or update our theoretical vision and models of child development, trauma, and play therapy interventions. Without a grounding in theory understanding and application, therapists have no direction for their work with clients.

The APT (n.d.) recognizes seven seminal play therapy theories that include Adlerian, child-centered, cognitive-behavioral, exosystemic, gestalt, Jungian, and psychoanalytic play therapies. Three play therapy approaches are also listed that include attachment theory and Theraplay, as well as filial therapy, which is based on CCPT theory. These theories and approaches are foundational elements for all training and credentialing to ensure best practice. Of these seminal theories and approaches, the Substance Abuse and Mental Health Services Administration (SAMHSA) recognizes Adlerian and CCPT theories as evidenced-based. They also recognize child-parent relationship therapy and filial family therapy-based approaches, as well as Theraplay, an attachment-based approach. Play therapy is established as an evidence-based approach for working with children aged 3–12 with trauma-related behaviors, social emotional issues, developmental delays, and relational issues (Ray et al., 2015).

What does evidence-based mean and why does it matter in play therapy? An effective intervention is well defined and theoretically grounded with a clear model, has comparison groups with different interventions, uses randomly assigned participants, and has reliable and valid measurements, and favorable statistical outcomes (Ray, 2018). In determining the effectiveness of a therapeutic intervention, at least one randomized controlled trial is required, testing play therapy by randomly assigning participants to comparison groups, and analyzed statistically to evaluate change (Ray, 2018). The California Evidenced-Based Clearinghouse (CEBC) lists evidenced-based therapies for working with children. In 2017 the Substance Abuse and Mental Health Services Administration (SAMSHA) did as well and both have served as resources for therapists to evaluate their practices.

Evidence-based interventions indicate the gold standard for best practice. There are numerous marketed approaches to play therapy that have not had studies conducted, and while some have been researched, many have not had randomly controlled trials to evaluate their effectiveness. The increase in the need for mental health services has created more consumer awareness and more need to be able to explain our theoretical approach and the neuroscience supporting it, which includes sharing research regarding both the effectiveness and the approximate number of sessions needed for change. In the 21st century, play therapists may be considered illiterate or ineffective without this knowledge and the ability to articulate it to the adults in a child's life such as parents, teachers, pediatricians, and judges. This is especially crucial for working with children who have experienced trauma, as they are more vulnerable and in need of scientifically based effective therapies.

Children Who Have Experienced Complex Trauma

According to Substance Abuse and Mental Health Services Administration [SAMSHA] (2023), a minimum of one out of seven children experienced abuse within the last year in the United States. Among children, more than two-thirds reported having had at least one traumatic experience by the time they were 16 years of age. Such events include:

1. Psychological, physical, or sexual abuse
2. Community or school violence
3. Witnessing or experiencing domestic violence
4. National disasters or terrorism
5. Commercial sexual exploitation
6. Sudden or violent loss of a loved one
7. Refugee or war experiences
8. Military family-related stressors (e.g., deployment, parental loss, and injury)
9. Physical or sexual assault
10. Neglect
11. Serious accidents or life-threatening illness (Substance Abuser and Mental Health Services Administration, 2023).

The physical, emotional, social, and financial impact of childhood trauma is enormous and often results in long-term health problems, more involvement with juvenile justice and child welfare systems, an increase in the utilization of both health and mental health services, and educational problems such as low academic achievement and expulsions (Substance Abuse and Mental Health Services Administration, 2023). It is estimated that the financial cost to North America alone is $758 billion annually (Bellis et al., 2019).

Adverse childhood experiences (ACEs) are traumatic exposures prior to the age of 18 that result in lifelong negative social, emotional, and health outcomes for those who experience them. ACEs include exposure to physical neglect, emotional neglect, emotional abuse, physical abuse, sexual abuse, domestic violence, loss of a parent, a family member with addiction, depression or mental illness, or a family member incarcerated prior to one turning 18 (Centers for Disease Control and Prevention, 2021; Felitti et al., 1998). The more ACEs experienced by an individual, the higher the incidence of poor health outcomes such as depression, anxiety, suicide, post-traumatic stress disorder, infectious disease, chronic disease, and risky behaviors such as drug and alcohol use, which also impact future victimization and perpetration (Centers for Disease Control and Prevention, 2023). ACEs are also experienced by some populations more than others. There is a higher incidence of exposure to ACEs for minoritized children. Black children have an average of 1.69 ACEs, with white children having an average ACE score of 1.52 (Merrick et al., 2018). Minoritized children suffer from systemic racism and are more likely to live in poverty, which increases the likelihood of family stress and dysfunction leading to more neglect, violence, and abuse (Merrick et al., 2018; Patterson et al., 2018; Post et al., 2019).

When a traumatic event occurs, there are three ways a person may respond. A fight response may occur: the person fights back against others (Levine, 2015; Porges, 2009). They may appear overly reactive or volatile (Perryman et al., 2019). A second possibility is a flight response (Levine, 2015; Porges, 2009): they attempt to flee from the situation to feel safe. They may be perceived as being distant, distracted, or unreliable (Perryman et al., 2019). Finally, a person may have an immobilization or freeze response (Porges, 2009), storing trauma in their body in the form of sensations and repressing all feelings as though the event is not happening. Van der Kolk and Fisler (1994) explained that when people experience trauma, it creates a "speechless terror," leaving one unable to describe the experience in words. He also stated that the primary indicator of how one responds to trauma is whether they were alone when it occurred or had someone there to help. For a child, having a caring adult to help them is crucial to how they are impacted by the event. If there is no one available, the child is likely to be perpetually stuck with their trauma response, even in non-threatening situations, as though the event is still happening. Ordinary occurrences that once would not have bothered them may now leave them with the fight, flight, or freeze response (Perryman et al., 2019). These responses are helpful in the moment the trauma occurs as their brain attempts to cope, but left unresolved, the ability to function is impaired, causing both interpersonal and intrapersonal problems (Badenoch, 2018; Siegel, 2010).

Children who experience ongoing trauma are likely to present with mistimed, maladjusted behaviors related to truncated fight, flight, or freeze responses, leading to issues in the classroom and all other relationships. Clinicians may notice that once in the playroom, the children are more likely to play with only a few toys, or not play at all, as they are often cautious and do not trust adults to do what they say or keep them safe. They lack spontaneity in their play and may want to be told what to do (Landreth, 2023). They may even associate intimacy with threat if the adults in their lives have been the source of their trauma (Perry et al., 2016). Their experience of adults has often not been that they are there to keep them safe, so, understandably, they are not naturally trusting of the therapist.

There are observable themes to the play of children who have experienced trauma. According to D'Elia et al. (2022), "post-traumatic play is characterized by repetition, containing aspects, scenes, or sequence of the traumatic event, expressed explicitly or symbolically" (n.p.). They also describe play as repetitive, ritualistic, and frequently with an iniquitous ending. Others have described post-traumatic play similarly—as factual, organized, repetitive, and without joy (Baggerly & Exum, 2007; Gil, 2006). Additionally, Perry (1988) found that children expressing maladaptive behaviors demonstrated more themes of conflict, negative views of themselves, dysphoric feelings, and play disruptions, and they spent much of their time in play therapy feeling anxious, unhappy, scared, angry, or sad. This could be compared to an adult verbally articulating their feelings in therapy in an attempt to reach resolution, with their expressed feelings mirroring their ongoing or past experiences.

The children's play may also be aggressive and violent, either with the toys or directly toward the therapist or themselves. In this way, children use play to problem solve and attempt to make sense of their world, and thus may reenact the abuse they have experienced or witnessed within the safe confines of the playroom. This play is typically repetitive for several sessions, as the child attempts to resolve the past trauma. If the trauma is ongoing, this will be reflected in their play with no resolution. Children also may share their feelings indirectly, through symbolism with water, clay, sand, or paint (Landreth, 2023). Complex trauma often appears messy and with intensity with these mediums rather than organized and free, representing how their experience feels in their body.

Children who have experienced chronic trauma are likely to encounter emotional blocks as they process their memories and feelings through play therapy (Landreth, 2023). This is similar to the way in which adults in therapy may distance themselves from an experience to protect themselves when the work becomes too threatening or uncomfortable. Developmentally, young children are naturally prone to fantasy and imagination in their play to make sense of their world, and thus are more likely to dissociate (Cudzik et al., 2019). This can result in feeling detached from their body, feeling as though they are watching what is happening from afar or dreaming they are watching the experience happening to someone else, or even losing pieces of the memory or event altogether (Cudzik et al., 2019; National Child Traumatic Stress Network, 2023).

Dissociation can initially be seen as an adaptive way to respond to experiences that are unbearable, but when it goes beyond normal, in terms of frequency and intensity and with no dividing line between fantasy and reality, it becomes harmful (Cudzik et al., 2019; Shusta-Hochberg, 2003). In extreme cases, a child may lose touch with aspects of their self, which can become a way to cope and can happen when they are reminded of the trauma or are encountered with other stressors (National Child Traumatic Stress Network, 2023; Shusta-Hochberg, 2003). While dissociation can be an effective way to cope in the face of overwhelming pain and anxiety, it can also be counterproductive to school environments, impacting social relationships as well as learning. All the examples mentioned describe a child's attempt to make sense of what has happened to them, and it is crucial that play therapists understand complex trauma and its impact in working with children to understand the child's physical, emotional, and developmental needs as they attempt to heal.

Needs of Children Experiencing Complex Trauma and Dissociation

Van der Kolk (2014) explained that the primary predictor of how someone is impacted by trauma is whether they had someone there to comfort and help them after the event occurred, emphasizing the human need for connection. Gaskill (2022) emphasized the relationship as "the most powerful therapeutic impact play therapists can create" (p. 5). He also recognized this in his emphasis on understanding what rewards the child in therapy, with a reminder that the human brain naturally gravitates toward feeling safe, nurtured, and supported (Gaskill, 2022). The lack of a safe adult to protect is instrumental to the impact of the trauma, and so it only makes sense that the presence of the relationship with a safe adult is required for healing.

When a safe, consistent, warm adult is not available to co-regulate with the child, there is a likelihood that more severe issues will occur as the child seeks ways to cope and heal. Panksepp and Bevin (2012) asserted the importance of the attuned relationship, which creates synchrony of bodily functions such as heart rates, brain waves, and hormones, in turn creating the ability to understand and learn from one another, experiencing and enhancing empathy through mirror neurons. Children can heal their wounds through the co-regulatory relationship with a skilled therapist who has created the safe space to heal and grow. Through this process, children develop skills to self-regulate and new pathways for building and maintaining trusting relationships beyond the playroom.

In addition to the relational qualities needed by a play therapist, knowledge of child development in terms of physical, social, and identity development are also needed. These understandings offer insight into how children are impacted by complex trauma and serve as a guide for choosing developmentally appropriate treatments for them. For example, a treatment that is focused on verbal communication will not be beneficial for a child under the age of approximately 10, as it is only around this age that a child's left hemisphere is developed enough that they can really express themselves through talking.

Ray (2016) developed *A Therapist's Guide to Child Development: The Extraordinary Years*, which provides clinicians with an extensive overview of physical, social, and identity development for children between the ages of 3 and 12 and aligns with suitable evidence-based play therapy interventions. Gaskill (2022) also asserted the importance of recognizing development at a functional age, rather than solely chronological age, because traumatic experiences interfere with typical and expected development processes. Because the brain develops from the bottom up, play therapy treatment must also be hierarchical, with interventions working from the bottom up as they address the areas of the brain impacted by the trauma (Gaskill & Perry, 2017). Perry (2001) described this as crucial because the areas of the brain must interpret and consolidate information successively. Taking into consideration the child's chronological age from when the trauma occurred along with the onset of symptoms, the functional age can be determined and offer an understanding of the child's behaviors and needs. This is important for understanding therapeutic needs but also for working with parents and teachers, equipping them with appropriate expectations for the child.

In early years, the lower brain region primarily forms connections, and when traumatic events occur during this period, the lower brain areas are compromised, resulting in a disorganized or dysregulated brain (Gaskill & Brown, 2016; Perry & Winfrey, 2021). In these situations, therapy requires a great deal of repetition in the form of recurring somatosensory stimulation for change rather than focusing on verbal modalities (Gaskill, 2022). Because the lower brain region does not learn through verbal language and trauma is stored implicitly, as senses rather than words, this is a slow process. Landreth (2023) pointed out the child's natural inclination to repeat play until they reach resolution. Returning to the play and exploring and creating new endings offers the opportunity for the child to feel in control and to make an unbearable story into one that is manageable as they work toward emotional resolution.

In severe cases where a child felt alone in dealing with their trauma or an inability to escape, dissociation can occur (Choi et al., 2017). In such cases, Waiess (2006) posited, "the process of remembering is as important as the memories themselves and is the key to healing," adding that the relationship with a caring and patient therapist remains key to the emergence of unconscious memories to the conscious. Waiess cautioned against abreactive models for retrieving memories, as more harm could be incurred, asserting that, "within a valuable relationship the patient's life in its entirety becomes valuable to him or her" (p. 499) and traumatic events are reconsolidated in a way that can be felt and acknowledged as past rather than present. "Remembering is the first part, but it's not enough," Waiess maintained. "Moving beyond the memories into their meaning and into relationship with others is the second and by far the more important part" (p. 500). Regardless of the severity of the trauma reaction, having a play therapist who is relationally focused, knowledgeable regarding child development and the impact of trauma, and skilled at setting limits is necessary for healing to occur.

CCPT is a relationally focused and developmentally appropriate approach with the child, rather than problems or issues they may have, at the center. The relationship with the therapist offers a safe environment in which to resolve and reconsolidate trauma through repetition as the child expresses their feelings and experiences. The therapist's unyielding belief in the child is empowering and teaches them self-control. As the most widely researched form of play therapy, CCPT is therefore the seminal theory of focus in this chapter for working with children who have experienced trauma.

Child-Centered Play Therapy

Carl Rogers's (1961) person-centered or humanistic theory is based on the premise that the counselor-client relationship is the impetus for change, with the core belief that humans are born with an innate tendency to grow emotionally, just as they do physically. The neuroplasticity of the brain to change has been well documented through recent neuroscience (van der Kolk, 2014), as has the importance of the relationship (Cozolino, 2002; Schore, 2003). The core conditions are the foundation of the therapeutic relationship and include the ability of the therapist to demonstrate empathy, genuineness, and unconditional positive regard toward their client. It is a non-directive approach, with the focus on the relationship, creating safety for the client to take risks, change, and grow. Virginia Axline, a student of Rogers, adapted the person-centered theory for work with children, now known as child-centered play therapy (CCPT), which shifted the focus to being with the child rather than trying to change them. Axline (1947) was a pioneer in the field of play therapy, and in CCPT specifically. She described play therapy as "the child's natural medium of self-expression" (p. 16), offering an outlet for self-expression through play equivalent to an adult verbalizing their feelings in talk therapy. As such, CCPT focuses on the child rather than the behavior. Verbal language is not needed for CCPT, as the child uses toys to create their internal world (Schoonover & Perryman, 2022). The CCPT therapist is trained to understand play themes and use them to help the adults in the child's life better nurture the needs of the child within the safety of the playroom.

Guerney (1983) further developed the work of Axline (1947) as did Landreth (1991), serving as one of the founders of the Association for Play Therapy as well as the Center for Play Therapy at the University of North Texas, where he currently serves as director emeritus. Landreth's extensive work in the form of textbooks, research, and as a training play therapist has been instrumental in the field of play therapy, emphasizing the importance of CCPT skills needed for the "complete therapeutic system" (p. 53), rather than viewing them as only preparatory or for building a rapport with the child. The CCPT therapist has deep faith in the child and their resilience, and their ability to be self-directing in a positive way (Landreth, 2023). This faith is true for all children regardless of what they have endured. In the case of complex trauma, this abiding belief is most crucial—a great deal of patience and faith are required of the therapist, as they are a guest on a very painful journey with a child who has been repeatedly traumatized.

Toys

Specific toys are needed in the CCPT process and should be carefully selected to ensure therapeutic value. Landreth (2012) identified the types of toys needed as real-life toys, acting out aggressive-release toys, and toys for creative expression and emotional release. These toys are organized on shelves according to theme or, in the case of a tote bag playroom, placed in plastic bags and containers. Landreth suggested the following list of toys and materials (pp. 167–169).

Balls
Band-Aids
Barbie doll
Bendable doll family
Blunt scissors
Bop Bag
Broom, dustpan
Building blocks (various shapes and sizes)
Cereal boxes
Chalkboard, chalk
Colored chalk, eraser
Construction paper (several colors)
Crayons, pencils, paper
Cymbals
Dart guns
Dinosaurs, shark
Dishes
Dishpan
Doll bed, clothes blanket
Doll furniture (sturdy wood)
Dollhouse (open-on-floor type that child can lean into)
Dress-up clothes
Drum
Egg cartons
Empty fruit and vegetable cans
Erasable nontoxic markers
Flashlight
Gumby (bendable nondescript figure)

Hand puppets (doctor, nurse, police officer, mother, father, sister, brother, baby, alligator, wolf)
Handcuffs
Hats: fireman, policeman, tiara, crown
Lone Ranger-type mask and other masks
Medical kit
Medical mask
Nursing bottle (plastic)
Pacifier
Paints, easel, newsprint, brushes
Pitcher
Plastic knives
Play camera
Play money and cash register
Pots, pans, silverware
Pounding bench and hammer
Puppet theater
Purse and jewelry
Rags or old towels
Refrigerator (wood)
Rope
Rubber snake, alligator
Sandbox, large spoon
School bus
Soap, brush, comb
Spider and other insects
Sponge, towel
Stove
Stuffed animals (two or three)
Telephone (two)
Tinker toys
Tissues
Tongue depressors, popsicle sticks
Toy soldiers and army equipment
Toy watch
Transparent tape, nontoxic glue
Truck, car, airplane, tractor, boat, ambulance
Watercolor paints
Xylophone
Zoo animal and farm animal families

In cases where the counselor is providing counseling at home or a location without a playroom, a tote bag playroom may be utilized, with the toys organized on a tablecloth on the floor by theme. The suggested toys are listed below by Landreth (2012, pp. 166–167):

Aggressive hand puppet (alligator, wolf, or dragon)
Band-Aids
Bendable doll family
Bendable Gumby (nondescript figure)

Blunt scissors
Costume jewelry
Cotton rope
Crayons (eight-count box)
Dart guns
Doll
Dollhouse (use box that holds reams of paper, box lid serves as dollhouse, draw lines on inside of lid to mark rooms; box doubles as storage container for toys)
Dollhouse furniture (at least bedroom, kitchen, and bathroom)
Handcuffs
Lone Ranger-type mask
Medical mask
Nerf ball
Newsprint
Nursing bottle (plastic)
Pipe cleaners
Plastic knife
Play dough
Popsicle sticks
Small airplane
Small car
Spoons
Telephone (two)
Toy soldiers (20-count is sufficient)
Transparent tape
Two play dishes and cups

When working with children who have experienced complex trauma, a therapist may consider adding a few other toys to this list. A yoga ball offers opportunities for sensory integration as well as rhythmic movement, as it is large and strong enough for child to lie on it and rock, roll it back and forth to the therapist, and so on. The Bop Bag, on the first list, is also frequently used to lie on, as well as punch or kick, but the yoga ball offers a different sensory experience because it is a sphere and easy for a child to maneuver. A weighted blanket can be added for a child to soothe and nurture themselves, providing sensory stimulation. A beach blanket is also a valuable addition, as the child can use it for a blanket but also parents can be taught to use it as a rhythmic soothing tool as they rock the child in it, offering opportunities for attunement and connection.

Basic Principles

Using therapeutic toys, the CCPT therapist abides by basic constructs, which include the person, the phenomenal field, and the self (Rogers, 1961). The person encompasses the behaviors, feelings, thoughts, and physical being of the child, with them as the center. The phenomenal field includes all things experienced by the child, both internally and externally, offering a paradigm for viewing their world. According to this paradigm, the self evolves from interaction with the phenomenal field as the child encounters the reactions of others, such as parents, teachers, and so on in an evaluative way and comes to see themselves as either good or bad based on these experiences (Landreth, 2023). Therefore, it is imperative that the therapist hold attitudes toward the child that are congruent with a deep belief in their ability to self-actualize. Axline (1947) posited the *Eight Basic Principles* to serve as a foundation for therapy with all children. Landreth (2012, p. 80) revised these principles:

1 The therapist is genuinely interested in the child and develops a warm, caring relationship.
2 The therapist experiences unqualified acceptance of the child and does not wish that the child was different in some way.
3 The therapist creates a feeling of safety and permissiveness in the relationship, so the child feels free to explore and express himself completely.
4 The therapist is always sensitive to the child's feelings and gently reflects those feelings in such a manner that the child develops self-understanding.
5 The therapist believes deeply in the child's capacity to act responsibly, unwaveringly respects the child's ability to solve personal problems, and allows the child to do so.
6 The therapist trusts the child's inner direction, allows the child to lead in all areas of the relationship, and resists any urge to direct the child's play or conversation.
7 The therapist appreciates the gradual nature of the therapeutic process and does not attempt to hurry the process.
8 The therapist establishes only those therapeutic limits necessary to anchor the session to reality and which help the child accept personal and appropriate relationship responsibility.

Objectives and Skills

The CCPT therapist embraces these principles with a focus on the child, rather than on the problem(s), utilizing both verbal and nonverbal skills in a playroom intentionally created and organized with therapeutic toys. The following objectives offer a foundation for comprehending the characteristics and process of CCPT, and its benefits for children:

1 Develop a more positive self-concept.
2 Assume greater self-responsibility.
3 Become more self-directing.
4 Become more self-accepting.
5 Become more self-reliant.
6 Engage in self-determined decision making.
7 Experience a feeling of control.
8 Become sensitive to the process of coping.
9 Develop an internal source of evaluation.
10 Become more trusting of himself. (Landreth, 2012, pp. 84–85)

These principles are conveyed through facilitative responses provided by the therapist, which tracks the child's play, reflects feelings and content, facilitates decision making, returns responsibility, and sets needed limits (Landreth, 2012). Through the relationship with the CCPT therapist, a child learns to respect themselves, that their feelings are acceptable, to responsibly explore feelings, to assume self-responsibility, to be problem solving, to be responsible for the choices they make, and to build self-control skills (Landreth, 2012). The CCPT therapist responds to the child in ways that are esteem building—for example, "You worked really hard to get that just the way you wanted it," which praises the effort rather than the child.

Limits

In this process, the therapist accepts the child but does not show acceptance of all exhibited behaviors, setting limits as needed. These limits are crucial to the therapeutic relationship, as they allow the child to learn self-control and feel safe. The ability of the therapist to set and enforce firm and consistent limits is crucial. To establish and maintain trust, these limits should be "minimal and enforceable" (Landreth, 2023, p. 304).

Limits are consistently used to protect the safety of the child, the therapist, the playroom, and the toys as well as reduce behaviors that interrupt the therapeutic process, such as frequently leaving the room, taking items from the playroom, socially inappropriate behaviors such as undressing and inappropriate attempts for affection, such as kissing the therapist or sitting on their lap (Landreth, (2023). Limits also maintain the here-and-now focus of therapy, anchoring the child to reality (Landreth, 1993, p. 24). This is especially important for children who have experienced complex trauma, as it is common for their play to trigger their past trauma. For example, a child who witnessed a shooting is likely to have a reaction to the toy gun in the playroom. If this is their only traumatic experience, they may simply verbalize, "That's what the guy had at the store," in which case the therapist would reflect, "Sounds like you remember seeing that at the store, when the guy was shooting." For a child who has experienced multiple traumatic events, however, the likelihood of having a fight, flight, or freeze response is high. A flight response may result in a child becoming aggressive and in need of reorientation to present time and space.

Landreth (2012) proposed the ACT model (acknowledge the child's desire, communicate the limit, and target an acceptable alternative) for limit setting and emphasized that the therapist must set limits with a calm demeanor, offering the opportunity for self-control rather than a focus on external control, all the while conveying acceptance of the child. A child with a flight response may try and leave the playroom, necessitating the need for the therapist to set a limit such as, "I know you want to leave the playroom, but our time is not up for today—we still have 15 minutes left." This offers a structuring limit, returning the child to the here and now. If the child appears fearful, this would be acknowledged, with a reminder that they are safe in the playroom. In extreme cases, where the child becomes dysregulated to the point of panic and wanting a parent, the CCPT therapist would acknowledge their feelings and they would go together to get the parent to ensure that the child feels safe and trusts their need to attune with the help of a capable parent. The same type of response may appear as the child dissociates by quickly stopping their play when they see the gun and moving to another type of play altogether. The therapist would simply acknowledge this—"Looks like you decided to do something different"—just as an observation and without judgment, believing the child will return to this work when they are emotionally ready to do so. A freeze response may include the child having the appearance of glazing over, or even suddenly lying down for a nap. Again, the therapist would trust the child and simply acknowledge this without judgment or directing them to do something else: "Looks like right now you feel so tired and just want to lie down."

As revealed above, the first step of the ACT model is to acknowledge the feelings and desires of the child verbally. The second step is for the therapist to communicate the limit, and then to target an acceptable behavior. The final step is to state the final choice (Landreth, 2012). Through the ACT model, the therapist conveys acceptance of the child while maintaining needed boundaries for physical and emotional safety, enabling the child to solve their own problems and gain a sense of self control.

Children who have experienced complex trauma are treated no differently than a child with other presenting problems, as the focus is always on the child and seeing the world through their eyes. However, because adults often are the source of children's traumatic experiences, it is common for therapeutic relationships to be tested. The CCPT therapist must be very patient as well as able to set firm and consistent limits. It is also common for dissociative behaviors to occur with complex trauma. When a child with a fight response demonstrates very aggressive behaviors toward themselves or the therapist, a therapeutic hold may be required. This should be a last resort and only utilized by a therapist who is trained to do so in a safe and caring manner. From a CCPT perspective, this would be used only if the child chooses to continue behaviors that could harm them or the therapist. The therapist could say, "I know you want to hurt yourself, but you are not for hurting. If you choose to keep hurting yourself, you choose for me to keep you safe." If the behavior continues, the CCPT therapist could say, "I can see that right now you are choosing for me to hold you until you are able to keep yourself safe." The CCPT therapist would maintain a calm, caring tone and demeanor during the therapeutic hold, rocking in a slow rhythmic manner to help soothe and regulate, and let the child know that they will keep them safe until they are able to do it for themselves. Once the behavior subsides, the therapist would acknowledge, "I can see you are choosing to keep yourself safe now," empowering the child with a facilitative response. It is crucial that the therapist not be angry or aggressive but continue to treat the child in a nurturing way. This can be difficult when the therapist is the target of anger and aggression, so it is important to remain grounded and focus on the needs of the child. The therapist does not want to convey a desire to overpower the child, as this can be retraumatizing, and thus they must communicate verbally and physically that their purpose is to keep the child safe until they are able to do so for themselves.

The CCPT therapist aligned with the basic principles and embracing the objectives of CCPT creates a warm, accepting, safe environment for the child, facilitating their feelings through the language of play. Limits are set on an as-needed basis in a firm but consistent manner with a calm, caring demeanor, enabling the child to develop self-control and feelings of empowerment, with the therapeutic relationship as the impetus for healing. The skilled CCPT therapist constantly asks themselves, "Is this my need or the child's?" as well as "What message am I sending if I set a limit, and what message am I sending if I don't set a limit?" to maintain the focus on the child and their needs.

Themes

As previously mentioned, the CCPT therapist recognizes themes in the child's play. Themes may include aggression, power and control, helplessness, safety and security, mastery, nurturing, death/loss, and sexuality (Bratton & Homeyer, 2002). Themes are derived from what the child chooses to play with and how the toy is utilized. The play is often repetitive with intensity and emotional energy (Landreth, 2023). Children who have experienced complex trauma will have play themes associated with their experience. For example, a child who has been sexually abused will likely physically act out this abuse in the playroom several times to cathartically reconcile what happened to them. Once this is done, their play themes are likely to transition to more nurturing themes such as caring for the doll or puppets with the medical kit or by cooking.

Summary

CCPT is a developmentally appropriate approach, meeting children where they are and seeing the world through their eyes. Children naturally have repetitive play after a traumatic experience; it is their attempt to reconcile and reorganize their experience, presenting ample opportunities to learn self-responsibility and build self-esteem. The CCPT therapist consistently responds by setting limits as needed and returning responsibility to ground the child in reality, and maintaining the safety of the playroom, therapist, and child. Through this process, new neural pathways are created, allowing the child to have healthy relationships outside the playroom as they learn to trust the therapeutic relationship and themselves.

CCPT Research

CCPT has a plethora of studies spanning the last 80 years that demonstrate the effectiveness in both school and clinical settings and with various populations (Lin & Bratton, 2015; Post et al., 2019; Ray et al., 2015; Schoonover & Perryman, 2022). As an evidenced-based approach, it has been given a scientific rating of three out of five for promising research evidence by the California Evidence-Based Clearinghouse for Child Welfare [CEBC] (2023). This includes research evidence for children three to ten years of age who are struggling with disruptive behaviors and anxiety, and those exposed to domestic/intimate partner violence in the home. Progress has been shown in as few as 12–16 sessions lasting 30 minutes, and several of these studies included play sessions two to three times weekly (Lin & Bratton, 2015; Ray et al., 2015). CCPT studies with positive outcomes include increases in self-esteem, expressive language in students with speech delay, academic achievement, and adaptive as well as overall behaviors (Blanco & Ray, 2011; Blanco et al., 2012, 2017; Danger & Landreth, 2005; Kot et al., 1998; Perryman & Bowers, 2018; Massengale & Perryman, 2021; Post et al., 2004).

CCPT research has included minoritized children and those from various diverse backgrounds (Lin & Bratton, 2015; Massengale & Perryman, 2021; Perryman et al., 2020; Taylor & Ray, 2021). Because CCPT is "sensitive to the uniqueness of the child," respectful of the relationship with unconditional positive regard, and seeks to fully understand the child's experiences in the world (Landreth, 2023, p. 99), it is an ideal approach to working with diverse children. Additionally, cultural awareness and humility on behalf of the therapist are crucial to the therapeutic relationship with diverse and minoritized children as well as their families. Through CCPT, the therapist demonstrates their genuine interest in their client, and this must include acknowledging client identities as well as existing limitations due to differences. This special way of being with children—seeing the world through their eyes with cultural awareness and humility—creates a safe environment for the children's self-expression. As such, CCPT is thoroughly researched with children with numerous presenting issues and from diverse backgrounds and has been shown as an effective approach.

CCPT Research with Children Experiencing Complex Trauma and Dissociation

CCPT is well researched with children exhibiting internalized and externalized behaviors as well as disruptive behaviors associated with trauma such as impulsivity and anxiety, and has shown positive results (Gutermann et al., 2016; Haas, 2017; Humble et al., 2019; Kram, 2019; Parker et al., 2021; Perryman et al., 2018, 2020; Ray et al., 2021; Schoonover & Perryman, 2022). In terms of trauma, some research has specifically focused on ACEs (Haas & Ray, 2022; Patterson et al., 2018; Ray et al., 2021; Schoonover & Perryman, 2022). While to this author's knowledge no articles currently exist on CCPT and complex trauma, there are studies that focus on CCPT with children who have multiple ACEs, which does indicate complex trauma (Ray et al., 2020, 2021; Schoonover & Perryman, 2022) and the effectiveness of the approach.

A study by Schottelkorb et al. (2012) compared trauma-focused cognitive-behavioral therapy, a widely used therapeutic treatment for children, with CCPT with children who were refugees and found both to be effective for decreasing symptoms. Ray et al. (2021) conducted a randomized control study with 112 participants, collecting data for over three years, and found that CCPT resulted in increased empathy, social competence, and self-regulation and caused a decrease in externalized behaviors. Schoonover and Perryman (2022) conducted a single-case design using 16 sessions of

CCPT with five children who had experienced multiple ACEs and were in a trauma-focused school. Findings included increased consistency in scores with 16 sessions, and a decrease in participants' externalized behaviors in the classroom while the intervention took place. These effects continued afterward with a stabilizing carry-over effect, showing CCPT as an effective treatment modality for children who have experienced ACEs. Conroy and Perryman (2022) suggested that CCPT is effective for addressing ACEs with children because it provides safety, engagement, co-regulation, understanding of self, regulatory expansion, and exploration (SECURE). Other studies have supported the decrease in symptoms for children who have experienced ACEs as well (Haas & Ray, 2020; Kot et al., 1998; Kram, 2019). As such, CCPT remains the most well-researched intervention in the play therapy field (Landreth, 2023) and has a relational emphasis that "better meets the developmental needs of children who experience ACEs" (Parker et al., 2021, p. 2). Additionally, it has clear aspects in place to assure the child of their safety through appropriate limit setting and repetition, empowering them to express themselves through their developmentally appropriate language of play.

Case Example and Conceptualization[1]

Six-year-old Damien was referred for counseling by the Children's Services Division after being removed from his home and placed in foster care due to abuse and neglect. Reported ACEs included sexual and physical abuse by a parent, as well as neglect. Presenting issues included severe speech and learning delays and behavioral issues at home and school. He was also blind in one eye due to physical abuse. His therapist was a licensed professional counselor (LPC) and a registered play therapist (RPT), aligned with a CCPT theoretical perspective.

The first meeting took place in the waiting room. There, Damien and his brother were jumping on furniture, throwing objects at the window, and yelling inaudible words as they waited for their therapists. Damien's therapist took him gently by the hand and sat on the floor at his level. Smiling, then introduced herself, stated her name, and let Damien know it was time to go to the playroom. They stood and began to walk toward the door, and Damien ran quickly past her to the playroom and continued the same destructive behaviors.

Weekly sessions focused on building a therapeutic relationship and establishing a safe environment, which involved a great deal of repetition. Several limits had to be set to ensure the safety of Damien, the playroom, and the therapist, and they were tested many times. Damien repeatedly attempted to tie up the therapist and stab her with the toy knife, yelling and cursing at her. As these behaviors emerged, the therapist calmly and consistently used the ACT model for limit setting to ensure both safety and opportunities to learn self-control with natural behavioral consequences. The therapist stated, "I know you really want to stab me, but I am not for stabbing. You can choose something else in the room to stab if you want to." This offered opportunities for Damien to take responsibility and control. At times, final limits had to be set, where the therapist stated: "If you choose to stab me, then you choose not to play with the knife today." This messaging assured him that the therapist would ensure safety and allowed Damien to make decisions for himself. When he persisted, the therapist acknowledged his continued desire to stab her, reiterating that she was not for hurting, and said, "I see you have chosen not to play with the knife today, so you can either give me the knife or you can put it on the shelf."

Patience and persistence on behalf of the therapist were important in order to establish a trusting relationship. It was also important that the knife be in the playroom for the following sessions so that Damien continued to have opportunities to gain self-control and make choices. Damien continued this play for several weeks but directed the play toward a doll, choosing to keep the knife. Slowly the repetitive violent play lessened, and some nurturing play began.

Damien additionally exhibited bossy behaviors toward the therapist, yelling at her to do things he was capable of doing for himself. The therapist would return power by stating, "I know you want me to _____ but that is something you can do yourself." These responses were met with frustration and anger, but slowly, Damien was observed to begin doing things more for himself. There were also sessions in which Damien wanted the therapist to tie him up and stab him, as this had been the way in which he was accustomed to experiencing connections with adults. The therapist set limits around this—of course, she would in no way want to reinforce this kind of abusive relationship. In doing so, the therapist stated: "I know you want me to tie you up, but I choose not to." This modeled expectations for the way he should be treated by an adult, but also showed that it is okay to say no.

There were times when the play scenario was so intense that Damien would withdraw suddenly from it and move to another area of the room, to explore a cash register, for example. This was viewed as his way of creating distance from these painful memories until he was ready to process them. The therapist did not question or try to get him to return to the play, trusting that he would return when emotionally ready to do so. Landreth (2023) refers to these moments as emotional blocks, and stresses the importance of respecting the child's process as they work to make meaning, as a young child does not developmentally have the verbal coping mechanisms to articulate their feelings.

During this kind of transition, there were instances of Damien attempting to hurt the therapist and then nurturing her with the medical kit or cooking for her afterward. Damien seemed to be attempting to internally resolve the abuse and neglect inflicted by an important adult in his life with his current experiences of safety, warmth, and consistency with the therapist to trust her and himself. Damien would become frustrated when he was unable to hurt the therapist because of her set limits and repeatedly attempted to get the therapist to follow his commands. The therapist remained calm and consistent with the limit. At one point, Damien asked, "But why not," to which the therapist responded, "I know you are frustrated because I won't hurt you, but children are for loving, not for hurting." Damien then stated angrily, "You don't tell me… my family can hurt me if they want to." The therapist reflected, "You want to make sure I know that your family can hurt you if they want to," and then added, "but you are not for hurting." This was a powerful statement and demonstrated his attempt to make sense of how he had been treated, while at the same time, feeling protective of his family. This illuminated Damien's confusion about how someone he loved and was his family could hurt him but also his developing reality of relationships and self-worth he was coming to be aware of from his work in the playroom as he worked toward self-actualization. This scenario was played out many times in numerous ways, requiring persistence and patience on the part of the therapist, but it eventually proved to be a turning point in Damien's therapeutic process.

As sessions progressed, Damien's aggressive play ceased, and he began to meet the developmental milestones that had been stunted because of abuse and neglect. His nurturing play became focused on himself; he cooked and ate his favorite foods, and looked after the doll. The therapist responded with esteem-building comments, such as, "You know just what that baby needs" and "You worked hard to make those noodles just the way you like them." His play became more spontaneous and freer, and he was observed to sing as he cooked, "Noodles are for loving." His speech became more intelligible, and he began making academic growth in school with fewer externalizing behaviors, leading to healthier social functioning.

Conclusion

This chapter discussed the incidence of childhood complex trauma in the United States and the repercussions for children and society. Evidence-based approaches for treating children who have experienced trauma and complex trauma in the form of multiple ACEs were reviewed, along with the requirements for evaluating therapeutic approaches. The needs of children suffering from trauma, specifically ACES, were discussed along with the current research supporting the use of CCPT as an evidence-based approach to meet these needs.

CCPT is a relationally focused, developmentally appropriate, evidence-based approach for addressing the needs of children who have experienced complex trauma. These children require warm, safe adults to help them heal and grow, which necessitates a strong therapeutic relationship with a skilled therapist who possesses developmental knowledge, cultural humility, and the ability to warmly and consistently respond to the repetitive needs of the child. CCPT focuses on meeting children at their developmental level and readily offers opportunities for addressing the lower brain needs of repetition. Play is the natural language of children, and children who have experienced complex trauma seek resolution through repetition in their play. The CCPT therapist uses facilitative responses to address these needs. They provide a safe and accepting therapeutic relationship as they track the child's play, reflecting content and feelings as they consistently facilitate decision making, return responsibility, offer esteem-building responses, and set limits.

This process of change is not a quick fix—again, the lower brain requires time and repetition, with some neurosystems taking more time than others. Early developmental trauma will take longer because the part of the brain impacted was organized by early experiences and not intended for change (Perry, 2006). CCPT follows the child's natural progression and nurtures feelings of security and empowerment in the child through co-regulatory relationships, creating new neural pathways for connection and ways of being beyond the playroom.

Note

1 This is a composite case and the client's real name has been changed.

References

Allen, F. (1942). *Psychotherapy with children*. W. W. Norton.
Association for Play Therapy (APT). (2023). Retrieved October 20, 2023, from https://www.a4pt.org/
Association for Play Therapy (APT). *About APT*. Retrieved October 20, 2023, from a4pt.org/page/AboutAPT
Association for Play Therapy (APT). *Education and training*. Retrieved October 20, 2023, from a4pt.org/page/EducationTraining
Association for Play Therapy (APT). *Publications*. Retrieved October 20, 2023, from a4pt.org/page/Publications
Axline, V. (1947). *Play therapy: The inner dynamics of childhood*. Read Books Ltd.
Badenoch, B. (2018). *The heart of trauma: Healing the embodied brain in the context of relationships*. W. W. Norton.
Baggerly, J., & Exum, H. A. (2007). Counseling children after natural disasters: Guidance for family therapists. *American Journal of Family Therapy, 36*(1), 79–93. https://doi.org/10.1080/ 01926180601057598
Bellis, M. A., Hughes, K., Ford, K., Ramos Rodriguez, G., Sethi, D., & Passmore, J. (2019). Life course health consequences and associated annual costs of adverse childhood experiences across Europe and North America: A systematic review and meta-analysis. *The Lancet: Public Health, 4*(10), e517–e528. https://doi.org/10.1016/S2468-2667(19)30145-8
Blanco, P. J., Holliman, R. P., Muro, J. H., Toland, S., & Farnam, J. L. (2017). Long term child-centered play therapy effects on academic achievement with normal functioning children. *Journal of Child and Family Studies, 26*, 1915–1922. https://doi.org/10.1007/s10826-017-0701-0
Blanco, P. J., & Ray, D. C. (2011). Play therapy in elementary schools: A best practice for improving academic achievement. *Journal of Counseling & Development, 89*, 235–243. https://doi.org/10.1002/j.1556-6678.2011.tb00083.x
Blanco, P. J., Ray, D. C., & Holliman, R. (2012). Long-term child centered play therapy and academic achievement of children: A follow-up study. *International Journal of Play Therapy, 21*(1), 1–13. https://doi.org/10.1037/a0026932
Bratton, S., & Homeyer, L. (2002). Play therapy session summary. University of North Texas—Department of Counseling, Development and Higher Education Counseling Program Clinical Services.

California Evidence-Based Clearinghouse for Child Welfare (CEBC). (2023). *Child-centered play therapy.* cebc4cw.org/program/child-centered-play-therapy-ccpt

Centers for Disease Control and Prevention. (2021, September 22). *Preventing Adverse Childhood Experiences: Data to Action (PACE:D2A).* Violence Prevention. cdc.gov/violenceprevention/aces/preventingace-datatoaction.html

Centers for Disease Control and Prevention. (2023, June 29). *Adverse Childhood Experiences (ACEs).* Violence Prevention. cdc.gov/violenceprevention/aces/index.html

Choi, K. R., Seng, J. S., Briggs-King, E. C., Munro-Kramer, M. L., Graham-Bermann, S. A., Lee, R., & Ford, J. D. (2017). The dissociative subtype of posttraumatic stress disorder (PTSD) among adolescents: Co-occurring PTSD, depersonalization/derealization, and other dissociation symptoms. *Journal of the American Academy of Child & Adolescent Psychiatry, 56*(12), 1062–1072. https://doi.org/10.1016/j.jaac.2017.09.425

Conroy, J., & Perryman, K. (2022). Treating trauma with child-centered play therapy through the SECURE lens of polyvagal theory. *International Journal of Play Therapy, 31*(3), 143–152. https://doi.org/10.1037/pla0000172

Cozolino, L. J. (2002). *The neuroscience of psychotherapy: Building and rebuilding the human brain.* W. W. Norton.

Cudzik, M., Soroka, E., & Olajossy, M. (2019). Dissociative identity disorder as a wide range of defense mechanisms in children with a history of early childhood trauma. *Current Problems of Psychiatry, 20*(2), 117–129. researchgate.net/publication/334589971_Dissociative_identity_disorder_as_a_wide_range_of_defense_mechanisms_in_children_with_a_history_of_early_childhood_trauma

Danger, S., & Landreth, G. (2005). Child-centered group play therapy with children with speech difficulties. *International Journal of Play Therapy, 14*(1), 81–102. https://doi.org/10.1037/h0088897

D'Elia, D., Carpinelli, L., & Savarese, G. (2022). Post-traumatic play in child victims of adverse childhood experiences: A pilot study with the MCAST-Manchester child attachment story task and the coding of PTCP markers. *Children (Basel, Switzerland), 9*(12), Article 1991. https://doi.org/10.3390/children9121991

Erikson, E. (1972). Play and actuality. In M. Piers (Ed.), *Play and development* (pp. 127–167). W. W. Norton.

Felitti, V. J., Anda, R. F., Nordenberg, D., Williamson, D. F., Spitz, A. M., Edwards, V., Koss, M. P., & Marks, J. S. (1998). Relationship of childhood abuse and household dysfunction to many of the leading causes of death in adults: The adverse childhood experiences (ACE) study. *American Journal of Preventive Medicine, 14*(4), 245–258. https://doi.org/10.1016/S0749-3797(98)00017-8

Freud, A. (1946). *The psychoanalytic treatment of children.* Imago.

Gaskill, R. (2022, June). Back to the future: The intersection between play therapy and science. *Play Therapy, 17*(2), 4–7.

Gaskill, R., & Brown, J. (2016, June). *NMT guided school based programs.* Proceedings of the 2nd International Neurosequential Model Symposium, Banff, Canada.

Gaskill, R., & Perry, B. D. (2017). A neurosequential therapeutics approach to guided play, play therapy, and activities for children who won't talk. In C. A. Malchodi & D. A. Crenshaw (Eds.), *What to do when children clam up in psychotherapy: Interventions to facilitate communication* (pp. 38–66). Guilford Press.

Gil, E. (2006). *Helping abused and traumatized children: Integrating directive and nondirective approaches.* Guilford Press.

Guerney, L. F. (1983). Client-centered (nondirective) play therapy. In C. Schaefer & K. O'Connor (Eds.), *Handbook of play therapy* (pp. 21–64). Wiley.

Gutermann, J., Schreiber, F., Matulis, S., Schwartzkopff, L., Deppe, J., & Steil, R. (2016). Psychological treatments for symptoms of posttraumatic stress disorder in children, adolescents, and young adults: A meta-analysis. *Clinical Child and Family Psychology Review, 19*(2), 77–93. https://doi.org/10.1007/s10567-016-0202-5

Haas, S. (2017). *Child-centered play therapy with children affected by adverse childhood experiences: A single case design.* [Unpublished doctoral dissertation]. University of North Texas.

Haas, S. C., & Ray, D. C., (2020). Child-centered play therapy with children affected by adverse childhood experiences: A single-case research design. *International Journal of Play Therapy, 29*(4), 223–236. https://doi.org/10.1037/pla0000135

Hambridge, G. (1955). Structured play therapy. *American Journal of Orthopsychiatry, 25*, 304–310.

Humble, J. J., Summers, N. L., Villarreal, V., Styck, K. M., Sullivan, J. R., Hechler, J. M., & Warren, B. S. (2019). Child-centered play therapy for youths who have experienced trauma: A systematic literature review. *Journal of Child & Adolescent Trauma, 12*(3), 365–375. https://doi.org/10.1007/s40653-018-0235-7

Klein, M. (1932). *The psycho-analysis of children.* Hogarth Press.

Kot, S., Landreth, G. L., & Giordano, M. (1998). Intensive child-centered play therapy with child witnesses of domestic violence. *International Journal of Play Therapy, 7*, 17–36. https://doi.org/10.1037/h0089421

Kram, K. (2019). *Child-centered play therapy and adverse childhood experiences: Effectiveness of impulsivity and inattention.* [Unpublished doctoral dissertation]. University of North Texas.

Landreth, G. (1991). *Play therapy: The art of the relationship.* Accelerated Development.

Landreth, G. (1993). Child-centered play therapy. *Elementary School Guidance & Counseling, 28*(1), 17–29. jstor.org/stable/42869126

Landreth, G. (2012). *Play therapy: The art of the relationship.* Routledge.

Landreth, G. (2023). *Play therapy: The art of the relationship* (4th ed.) Routledge.

Levine, P. (2015). *Trauma and memory: Brain and body in a search for the living past; a practical guide for understanding and working with traumatic memory.* North Atlantic Books.

Levy, D. (1938). Release therapy for young children. *Psychiatry, 1,* 387–389.

Lin, Y.-W., & Bratton, S. C. (2015). A meta-analytic review of child-centered play therapy approaches. *Journal of Counseling & Development, 93*(1), 45–58. https://doi.org/10.1002/j.1556-6676.2015.00180.x

Massengale, B., & Perryman, K. (2021). Child-centered play therapy's impact on academic achievement: A longitudinal examination in at-risk elementary school students. *International Journal of Play Therapy, 30*(2), 98–111. https://doi.org/10.1037/pla0000129

Merrick, M. T., Ford, D. C., Ports, K. A., & Guinn, A. S. (2018). Prevalence of adverse childhood experiences from the 2011–2014 behavioral risk factor surveillance system in 23 states. *JAMA Pediatrics, 172*(11), 1038–1044. https://doi.org/10.1001/jamapediatrics.2018.2537

National Child Traumatic Stress Network. (2023). *Effects.* Complex Trauma. nctsn.org/what-is-child-trauma/trauma-types/complex-trauma/effects

Panksepp, J., & Bevin, L. (2012). *Archaeology of the individual: Neuroevolutionary origins of human emotion.* W. W. Norton.

Parker, M. M., Hergenrather, K., Smelser, Q., & Kelly, C. T. (2021). Exploring child-centered play therapy and trauma: A systematic review of literature. *International Journal of Play Therapy, 30*(1), 2–13. https://doi.org/10.1037/pla0000136

Patterson, L., Stutey, D. M., & Dorsey, B. (2018). Play therapy with African American children exposed to adverse childhood experiences. *International Journal of Play Therapy, 27*(4), 215–226. https://doi.org/10.1037/pla0000080

Perry, B. D. (2001). The neuroarcheology of childhood treatment. The neurodevelopmental costs of adverse childhood events. In K. Franey, R. Geffner & R. Falconer (Eds.), *The cost of maltreatment: Who pays? We all do* (pp. 15–37). Family Violence and Sexual Assault Institute.

Perry, B. D. (2006). Applying principles of neurodevelopment to clinical work with maltreated and traumatized children: The neurosequential model of therapeutics. In N. B. Webb (Ed.), *Working with traumatized youth in child welfare* (pp. 27–52). Guilford Press.

Perry, B. D., Hambrick, E., & Perry, R. (2016). A neurodevelopmental perspective and clinical challenges. In *Transracial and intercountry adoptions* (pp. 126–153). Columbia University Press. https://doi.org/10.7312/fong17254-008

Perry, B. D., & Winfrey, O. (2021). *What happened to you? Conversations on trauma, resilience, and healing.* Flatiron Books.

Perry, L. (1988). *Play therapy behavior of maladjusted and adjusted children.* [Doctoral dissertation, University of North Texas]. UNT Digital Library. digital.library.unt.edu/ark:/67531/metadc331633

Perryman, K., Blisard, P., & Moss, R. (2019). Using creative arts in trauma therapy: The neuroscience of healing. *Journal of Mental Health Counseling, 41*(1), 80–94. https://doi.org/10.17744/mehc.41.1.07

Perryman, K., & Bowers, L. (2018). Turning the focus to behavioral, emotional, and social well-being: The impact of child-centered play therapy. *International Journal of Play Therapy, 27*(4), 227–241. https://doi.org/10.1037/pla0000078

Perryman, K., Robinson, S., Bowers, L., & Massengale, B. (2020). Child-centered play therapy and academic achievement: A prevention-based model. *International Journal for Play Therapy, 29*(2), 104–117. https://doi.org/10.1037/pla0000117

Piaget, J. (1972). Some aspects of operations. In M. Piers (Ed.), *Play and development* (pp. 15–27). W. W. Norton.

Porges, S. W. (2009). The polyvagal theory: New insights into adaptive reactions of the autonomic nervous system. *Cleveland Clinic Journal of Medicine, 76*(Suppl. 2), S86–S90. https://doi.org/10.3949/ccjm.76.s2.17

Post, P., McAllister, M., Sheely, A., Hess, B., & Flowers, C. (2004). Child-centered kinder training for teachers of pre-school children deemed at-risk. *International Journal of Play Therapy, 13*(2), 53–74. https://doi.org/10.1037/h0088890

Post, P. B., Phipps, C. B., Camp, A. C., & Grybush, A. L. (2019). Effectiveness of child-centered play therapy among marginalized children. *International Journal of Play Therapy, 28*(2), 88–97. https://doi.org/10.1037/pla0000096

Ray, D. (2018, March). The evidence-base determination: A moving target. *Play Therapy, 1*(13), p. 21.

Ray, D. C. (Ed.). (2016). *A therapist's guide to child development: The extraordinarily normal years.* Routledge/Taylor & Francis Group.

Ray, D. C., Angus, E., Robinson, H., Kram, K., Tucker, S., Haas, S., & McClintock, D. (2020). Relationship between adverse childhood experiences, social-emotional competencies, and problem behaviors among elementary-aged children. *Journal of Child and Adolescent Counseling, 6*(1), 1–13. https://doi.org/10.1080/23727810.2020.1719354

Ray, D. C., Armstrong, S. A., Balkin, R. S., & Jayne, K. M. (2015). Child-centered play therapy in the schools: Review and meta-analysis. *Psychology in the Schools, 52*(2), 107–123. https://doi.org/10.1002/pits.21798

Ray, D. C., Burgin, E., Gutierrez, D., Ceballos, P., & Lindo, N. (2021). Child-centered play therapy and adverse childhood experiences: A randomized controlled trial. *Journal of Counseling & Development, 100*(2), 134–145. https://doi.org/10.1002/jcad.12412

Rogers, C. R. (1961). *On becoming a person: A therapist's view of psychotherapy.* Boston: Houghton Mifflin.

Schaefer, C. E., & Drewes, A. A. (Eds.). (2014). *The therapeutic powers of play: 20 Core agents of change* (2nd ed.). Wiley.

Schoonover, T. J., & Perryman, K. (2022). Child-centered play therapy and adverse childhood experiences: A single-case research design. *Journal of Child and Adolescent Counseling, 9*(1), 1–20. https://doi.org/10.1080/23727810.2022.2138045

Schore, A. N. (2003). *Affect regulation and the repair of the self* (Vol. 2). W. W. Norton.

Schottelkorb, A. A., Doumas, D. M., & Garcia, R. (2012). Treatment for childhood refugee trauma: A randomized, controlled trial. *International Journal of Play Therapy, 21*(2), 57–73. https://doi.org/ 10.1037/a0027430

Shusta-Hochberg, S. R. (2003). Therapeutic hazards of treating child alters as real children in dissociative identity disorder. *Journal of Trauma & Dissociation, 5*(1), 13–27. https://doi.org/10.1300/J229v05n01_02

Siegel, D. (2010). *The mindful therapist.* W. W. Norton.

Substance Abuse and Mental Health Services Administration (SAMSHA01) (2017). *National registry of evidence-based programs and practices.* Retrieved from samhsa.gov

Substance Abuse and Mental Health Services Administration (SAMSHA) (2023, March 17). *Understanding child trauma.* SAMSHA. samhsa.gov/child-trauma/understanding-child-trauma.

Taft, J. (1933). *The dynamics of therapy in a controlled relationship.* Macmillan.

Taylor, L., & Ray, D. C. (2021). Child-centered play therapy and social–emotional competencies of African American children: A randomized controlled trial. *International Journal of Play Therapy, 30*(2), 74–85. https://doi.org/10.1037/pla0000152

van der Kolk, B. (2014). *The body keeps the score: Brain, mind, and body in the healing of trauma.* Penguin Books.

van der Kolk, B. A., & Fisler, R. E. (1994). Childhood abuse and neglect and loss of self-regulation. *Bulletin of the Menninger Clinic, 58*(2), 145–168.

Waiess, E. A. (2006). Treatment of dissociative identity disorder: "Tortured Child Syndrome." *Psychoanalytic Review, 93*(3), 477–500. https://doi.org/10.1521/prev.2006.93.3.477

28
TRAUMAPLAY™
An Integrative Play Therapy Model

Paris Goodyear-Brown and Eleah Hyatt

Introduction

Origins and Development

The evolution of TraumaPlay began as an attempt to make sense of disparate theories of change within the fields of child trauma and play therapy. A therapeutic preschool program and several inner-city elementary schools became the real-world laboratory in which core components of the model were tested and integrated. These learning environments consisted of children aged 5–12 seeking support services for disruptive and dysregulated behaviors. Upon further assessment, it was found that the children with the biggest behaviors also had complex trauma histories often accompanied by dissociation. While the level of dissociation ranged from mild to severe, almost all of the child clients had at least one identifiable dissociative symptom. Some had endured chronic traumatization at critical periods of development including multiple attachment disruptions. Others had experienced the in utero injuries of alcohol or drug use, or the toxic effects of massive cortisol releases that accompany domestic violence. Many of these children were forced to remain below window level while at home due to the drive-by shootings that happened without warning in their neighborhoods.

Many of the children referred for counseling had three or more adverse childhood experiences (ACES) (sexual abuse, physical abuse, domestic violence, incarceration of a parent, substance use of a parent, parental mental illness, etc.). At the time, the therapies embraced by the school system were behavioral therapy and trauma-focused cognitive behavioral therapy (TF-CBT) (Cohen & Mannarino, 2015; Cohen et al., 2018). While these approaches were helpful with some children, many others remained entrenched in complex trauma symptoms of dissociation and avoidance or cycles of hyperarousal and collapse. Teachers interpreted these symptoms as hyperactivity, "zoning out," school phobia, or a disdain for learning. Dissatisfied with the limitations of the available treatments, I (Paris) turned to the field of play therapy and pursued training in child-centered play therapy (CCPT) (Axline, 1947; Landreth, 2012), a foundational, evidenced-based play therapy approach (Bratton et al., 2005, 2013; Garza & Bratton, 2005; Ray et al., 2022) in addition to Theraplay®[1], an attachment-focused, therapist-directed play therapy approach with its own evidence base (Booth & Jernberg, 2009; Money et al., 2021; Salo et al., 2020; Siu, 2009, 2014).

As I therapeutically engaged these disparate methods, a typology of sorts emerged. A first group of children responded well to TF-CBT. A second group made great strides with CCPT. A third group responded well to an attachment-based approach. A fourth group emerged that did not respond to one specific treatment but needed a combination of all of the above. The fourth group, those who represent four or more ACES, who presented with complex trauma and dissociation, became the fertile soil out of which the TraumaPlay model grew.

The question of what it was about the ACES that lead to such devastating effects on a child's development revealed to me that each ACE robbed the child of an attuned, responsive caregiver, one who delights in the child while engaging in thousands of repetitions of serve-and-return communications over critical periods of development. Lower-order processes, such as regulation of the autonomic nervous system, precede higher-order processes, and our neurobiological understandings of bottom-up brain development (Perry et al., 1995) frame the interruptions that van der Kolk (2009) labeled developmental trauma disorder.

Wrestling with the above disparities illuminated the value of an attuned, responsive caregiver in a child's healing process and gave rise to the model's guiding principle: *following the child's need*. Human needs change based on signals our bodies give us from the inside out (interoception), signals our bodies receive from the world around us (exteroception), and how we make sense of situational variables like relational ruptures and repairs, the crisis of the week, and so on. The neurochemical boxing match often raging between cortisol and oxytocin/dopamine informs moment-to-moment treatment choices. Neurobiological understandings anchor the TraumaPlay model in cross-hemispheric work, moving between left and right brain ways of knowing, while also working from a bottom-up neuro-scaffolding perspective (Gaskill & Perry, 2014; Schore, 2019). The child's need, as it is showing up in their big behaviors, emotional extremes, or cognitive distortions, clearly requires that a bottom-up framework be used as the scaffolding for intervention.

Therapeutic Influences and Best Practices

In the last 20 years, the seminal play therapy theories—child-centered, filial therapy (including child-parent relationship therapy), Adlerian, cognitive behavioral, Gestalt, and Jungian—have been joined by a host of emerging play therapy models that are integrating new developments in the fields of complex trauma, relational neuroscience, neurodivergencies, embodied health, the science of resiliency, and more. An explosion in the fields of neuroscience and interpersonal neurobiology and new integrations, such as the neurosequential nature of brain development and its facilitation through play (Perry, 2006; Gaskill & Perry, 2014; Stewart et al., 2016), somatic experiencing (Levine, 1997; Payne et al., 2015), and polyvagal theory (Porges, 2015; Porges & Dana, 2018, Chapter 4) have added greatly to our understanding of underlying processes at work in TraumaPlay.

Attachment theory, beginning with Bowlby and inclusive of the Circle of Security Protocol (Cooper et al., 2011; Kim et al., 2018) and other holistic models like trust-based relational intervention (TBRI) (Purvis et al., 2007), have informed the construction of the TraumaPlay model, particularly in regards to the following components: enhancing safety and security, soothing the physiology, and parents as partners. TF-CBT and eye movement desensitization and reprocessing (EMDR) (Beer, 2018; Shapiro, 2017) have uniquely influenced the TraumaPlay components related to gradual exposure, addressing the thought life, and cross-hemispheric engagement.

TraumaPlay pays homage to the seminal models that have come before while leaning into the question of *when* in a continuum of treatment (assessment phase, working phase, termination phase), *with whom* (child, caregiver, parent-child dyad, or whole family), and *to what end* (with which specific population or clinical presentation) each way of working in the broader field of play therapy is most efficacious (Drewes et al., 2011; Kaduson et al., 2019; Schaefer & Drewes, 2015). Our answer is that it all depends on the following: What can the system hold collectively? What is the window of tolerance for each therapeutic participant? Where is the most effective point of change? What is the therapist's scope of practice or clinical expertise? And is the clinician willing and able to come alongside the chaos of the family system while providing an anchoring presence?

The Framework

TraumaPlay is a comprehensive, components-based approach to play therapy with traumatized and attachment-disturbed children and their caregiving systems. Developed for children with complex trauma and dissociation, TraumaPlay, formerly known as Flexibly Sequential Play Therapy, is steeped in an understanding of the neurobiology of play and the neurobiology of trauma as well as the power of one to heal the other. Play is the natural language of children (Landreth, 2012) and the digestive enzyme that allows traumatic material to be metabolized (Goodyear-Brown, 2009). Foundational to the model is an appreciation of the therapeutic powers of play and the belief that play is not merely a vehicle for delivering treatment but *is* the change mechanism with many healing qualities in and of itself (Schaefer & Drewes, 2013). These authors organized a series of 20 core agents of change into four categories (facilitates communication, fosters emotional wellness, increases personal strengths, and enhances social relationships) that continue to guide our understanding of the power of play therapy (see Figure 28.1).

Play is an integral part of a child's expression of self and a window into their world (Oaklander, 1978; Vijay Sagar, 2011). Grounded in attachment theory, the TraumaPlay model equips the therapist to meet the child or family moment-to-moment as therapeutic needs are assessed. The sequential framework of therapeutic treatment goals serves as the guiding structure under which clinicians have freedom to employ a variety of interventions. Components include enhancing safety and security, assessing current coping and augmenting adaptive coping, soothing the physiology (which includes sub-goals of enhancing self-regulation and offering parents as soothing partners), increasing emotional literacy, play-based gradual exposure/post-traumatic play (which encompasses the continuum

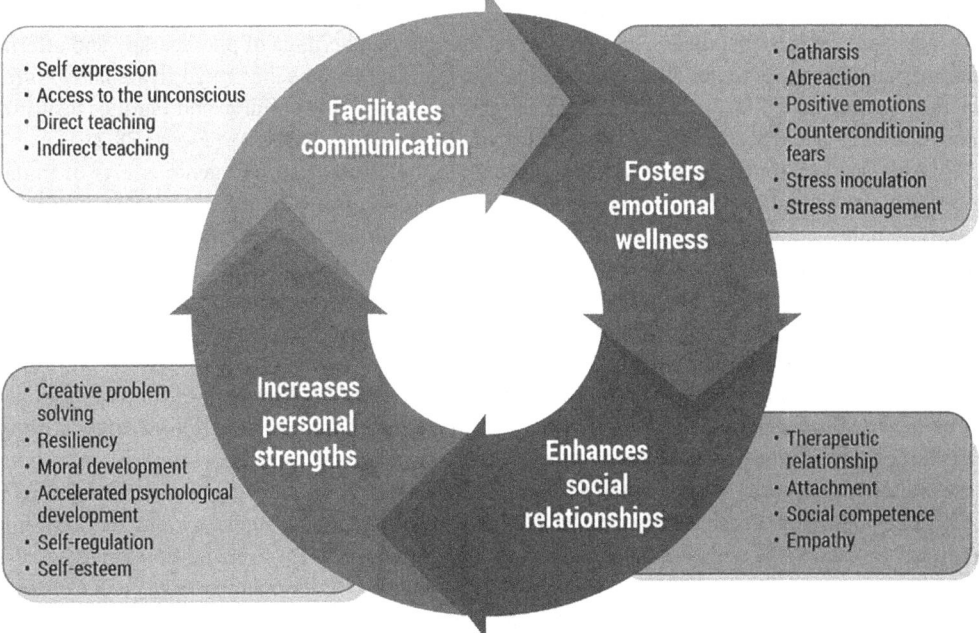

Figure 28.1 Therapeutic Powers of Play. Copyright Judi Parson. Reproduced with Permission.

The Handbook of Complex Trauma and Dissociation in Children

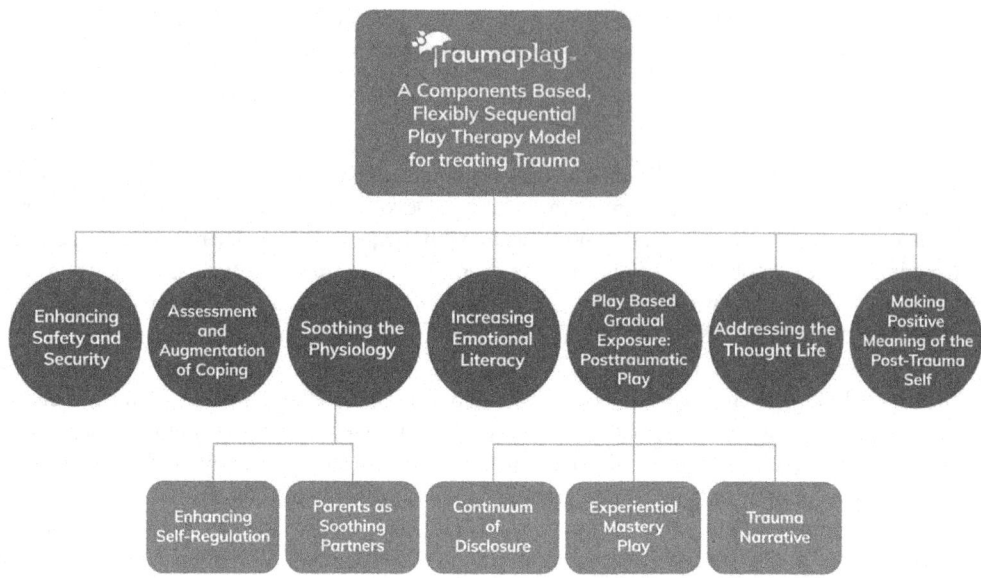

Figure 28.2 The TraumaPlay Flowchart. Copyright @Paris Goodyear-Brown. Reproduced with Permission.

of disclosure, experiential mastery play, and trauma narrative work), addressing the thought life, and making positive meaning of the post-trauma self.

All components can be pursued with a client individually or with the involvement of available caregivers, although building coherent shared narrative in family work requires advanced training in the model. The best-practice, evidence-informed treatment goals provide the scaffolding for a wide range of clinically sound, creative and engaging play-based interventions that offer developmentally sensitive approaches to therapeutic growth. Harnessing the rich heritage of play therapy and offering nuanced pathways for both nondirective and directive approaches to be integrated, TraumaPlay offers a clinically nuanced, child-focused, need-driven approach to helping children and families heal from complex trauma and dissociation (Goodyear-Brown, 2009, 2019a, 2021a; see Figure 28.2).

The sequence of components is aimed at protecting the client from iatrogenic effects of trauma processing. For example, clinicians need to know how a child copes with difficult content prior to approaching trauma content in a more formalized way. When chronic traumatization has occurred at the hands of caregivers during critical periods in a child's development, relational safety may comprise months of therapeutic work. The role of parents as eventual story keepers for their children guides the decision to focus on enhancing the attachment relationships between parents and children prior to entering any targeted trauma processing.

The framework is also meant to offer flexibility both in terms of the length of time spent in pursuit of each goal (some clients may experience an almost immediate neuroception of safety with the play therapist in the playroom, while others may need six months to develop a sense of safety in the space and/or in their relationship with their therapist) and whether or not every goal in the framework needs to be addressed. Some clients may have experienced a discrete traumatic event and have high emotional literacy skills and attuned caregivers, making it unnecessary to spend time on the goal of increasing emotional literacy. Children with complex trauma and dissociation may be out of touch with the signals their body is sending them that emotion is present and may have no experience of affect regulation in relationship with another (Schore & Schore, 2008), and therefore need extended time expanding their feelings vocabulary and nuancing emotional granularity.

The framework offers a guide to the treatment of complex trauma and dissociation while serving as a scaffold that encourages clinicians to say "yes & yes" to integrating multiple mediums and modalities. It should be clearly stated here that the integration of any play therapy method requires an immersion in learning and practice by trained practitioners in that method. TraumaPlay is a model of reconciliation aimed at helping play therapists triage when and how to integrate disparate play therapy methods. It will be most useful to advanced practitioners. Therefore, foundational training in specific theoretical orientations and play therapy modalities helps lay the groundwork for TraumaPlay.

An Explanation of Each TraumaPlay Component

Enhancing Safety and Security

Child clients and their parents must feel safe with the therapist and within the therapeutic space (Goodyear-Brown and Yasenik, in press) before any other treatment goals can be pursued. While the neuroception of safety is a full-body process that happens in the blink of an eye and is outside our conscious awareness, it is made up, at least in part, of our interoception (our perception of what is happening within our bodies) and our exteroception (our perception of environmental stimuli). Therefore, TraumaPlay therapists value the therapeutic relationship and understand the critical importance of *being with*—that is, presenting as attuned and present (Crenshaw & Kenney-Noziska, 2014; Geller & Porges, 2014). The therapeutic space itself runs a close second in importance, as the specifically chosen toys and tools and the maintenance of a predictable arrangement of the play space all together function as a co-therapist in the healing of the child (Goodyear-Brown, 2021a).

Assessment and Augmentation of Coping

It is both best practice and clinical wisdom to assess for the coping repertoires of the child and the parent (Amnie, 2018; Gruhn & Compas, 2020; Vernhet et al., 2019) in relation to stressful experiences prior to addressing historically stressful experiences together. Specific interventions are focused on revealing the entirety of the child's or teen's current coping repertoire, whether the coping strategies are adaptive or maladaptive (Sandler et al., 2000). When maladaptive strategies are identified, there is a natural tendency to highlight the difficulties with these strategies (Folkman & Moskowitz, 2004). TraumaPlay therapists instead work to augment adaptive coping strategies through playful practice during sessions that reinforce psychoeducation around healthy ingredients used in adaptive coping responses (Goodyear-Brown, 2009, 2022).

Soothing the Physiology

Children who have experienced chronic traumatization at critical periods early in development may wrestle with disorganization of their reptilian brain stem and subsequent interruption in the neurosequential development of other brain structures that are directly tied to a child's functional sense of competence (Perry et al., 1995; Gaskill & Perry, 2014). As self-regulation is always preceded by co-regulation, this component is further broken down into strategies for enhancing self-regulation and a focus on including parents as soothing partners.

Enhancing Self-Regulation

This sub-goal of soothing the physiology involves discrete skill-building areas such as breath work, mindfulness, biofeedback somatic soothing techniques, guided imagery, and role-based embodiment of extreme states in play ... such as a child choosing to be a snail in his shell followed by the same child turning into a roaring lion. TraumaPlay therapists view the cycles of up-and-down regulation in play therapy to be a primary mechanism, mediated by the social engagement with the play therapist, for expanding the child's window of tolerance for distress and excitation.

Parents as Partners

It is well established that parent involvement in play therapy amplifies the treatment effects (Bratton et al., 2005; Dowell & Ogles, 2010; Goodyear-Brown, 2019b, 2021b; LeBlanc & Ritchie, 2001; Lin & Bratton, 2015). When attachment ruptures have occurred during critical periods of development, or when a child has experienced chronic traumatization, abuse, or neglect at the hands of their caregiver, parents (or other available caregivers) become necessary partners in treatment and will provide the bulk of reparative doses of serve-and-return communications. Parent coaching follows the parent's need, paralleling the way the play therapist follows the child's need, throughout the continuum of treatment. Each parent and family system is unique and will require a finessed treatment plan. The TraumaPlay Assessment Phase includes a Nurture House Dyadic Assessment (NHDA) that is completed with the client and each available caregiver. The information gleaned from the NHDA is used to nuance the treatment goals that involve the parent.

Some parents may have a high degree of integration and self-awareness when they enter treatment and may immediately absorb any psychoeducation offered, achieving important paradigm shifts with the right dose of honed information. One such shift might be from the parent seeing the child's behaviors as purposeful—*he is choosing to defy me*—to seeing the child's behavior as a legitimate and potentially unmet need or dysregulation that requires the co-regulation of the caregiver. Some parents may need to be taught specific co-regulation skills, have the therapist model the skills and give the parent supported practice, first in the playroom and then generalized for other environments. Parents can be partners in creating nuanced narratives with children who are missing important pieces of information, but they may need therapeutic support to tell the truth to their children in a developmentally sensitive manner.

When the clinician has offered all of the above and the parent continues to feel stuck, they may need any of the following: guided exploration of their own "shoulds" because these generate shame and get in the way of positive shift; deepening awareness of their own negative activation when their child behaves in certain ways; and cross-hemispheric reflective attachment work to help the parent understand their own early attachment relationships (Goodyear-Brown, 2021b). Indeed, TraumaPlay clinicians triage the treatment needs of the parent, classifying the parent's therapeutic needs in one of eight categories (Goodyear-Brown, in press). Additionally, more is caught than taught and all parents benefit from being attributed with positive intentionality and receiving the play therapist's genuine delight in them throughout treatment.

Increasing Emotional Literacy

Many children exposed to chronic traumatization who come for TraumaPlay treatment have a restricted emotional vocabulary or may struggle with knowing how to manage their emotions without being overcome by dissociative tendencies. When a client has limited emotional literacy, it may be helpful to expand the client's feelings vocabulary, their ability to understand emotional granularity, or their capacity to use their own body's cues to interpret the emotion they are experiencing (Oksuz, 2016; Thornback & Muller, 2015) to support their healing work. Children with complex trauma and dissociation will need significant time spent honing their interoception prior to being able to name emotions at all. The adaptive brilliance of children who dissociate during terrifying or overwhelmingly painful experiences can also create an inability for that child to feel their body's signals that emotion is present. This work can be slow-going and often requires nonverbal, play-based activities that support a child's ability to work kinesthetically with symbols that represent emotion while learning to read what their bodies are telling them.

Play-Based Gradual Exposure/Post-Traumatic Play

Continuum of Disclosure

TraumaPlay conceptualizes three separate processes by which child clients might approach their trauma content. The first is called the *continuum of disclosure* and honors the glimpses and snapshots of the trauma that the child risks showing as the therapist follows the child's lead in play. Play is the language of children and the toys are their words (Landreth, 2012). There may be no words accessible to the child, especially if their trauma occurred prelinguistically. Complex trauma is often encoded somatically and iconically, in our bodies and in imagery, making it most natural for children to articulate their traumatic experiences more eloquently in their play than through their words. Additionally, play encourages symbolic expression, accesses both left and right brain ways of knowing (Gil, 2016), and invites implicit memories to be activated in the playroom. When an implicit memory is activated, it is not accompanied by an experience of remembering (Squire & Dede, 2015). These glimpses can look like behavioral choices or dysregulated activation, but they are often implicit memories. For example, a four-year-old boy enters the playroom. He sees a 2-foot-long plastic dinosaur and eagerly takes it down off the shelf. He unscrews the tail from the backside of the dinosaur so that a gaping hole is exposed. He moves over to the play kitchen area, picks up the play mixing blades, and begins to jam them into what looks like the anus of the dinosaur. Each thrust of the beaters into the hole is accompanied by sexual grunting noises. The child is in a dissociative state as this glimpse of the trauma is shared. The therapist's main job in this process is to become the child's story keeper and communicate an acceptance of the glimpse or fleeting expression of the trauma content, amplifying the message, *I see what you are showing me and you can show me more.*

Experiential Mastery Play

Experiential mastery play is the second process by which play-based gradual exposure occurs. Chronic interpersonal traumatization, especially if it involved a primary caregiver, may require a child to wrestle with betrayal trauma dynamics while also struggling with disempowerment. Many children use the playroom to approach the complexity of their relationship with their abusers by choosing perpetrator symbols. For example, a child chooses the Two-Face character from the Batman series to represent his abuser. One side of the figure is a charming, approachable gentleman. The other side is monstrous and scary. This figure represents the child's struggle to show the dichotomous experience of the real-life caregiver. He puts the figure in jail or buries it in the sand, experiencing mastery over the symbolic content.

Children with complex trauma may not be able to experience nurture directly from the therapist at first and may choose self-objects and watch how the therapist cares for them, receiving nurture vicariously from these therapist-symbol interactions while the therapist earns the right to nurture the client more directly. Clinicians also offer experiential mastery play when they pair their approach to trauma content with competency surges for the child. This may involve offering the child big body engagement, such as swinging or climbing, paired with exploration of the hard thing that happened. The embodied belief "I can do it" mitigates the child's approach to scary stuff. The child who does not want to look at his own adoption story instead asks to play a game that requires scrambling up to the top of a stack of slipper pillows. At first glance, this may look like distraction or noncompliance, but it is often the child's internal wisdom seeking a way to feel competent and good before approaching the hard thing. It is the wise therapist who will dance with the child toward and away from the trauma content, reflecting attunement and honor of their present need.

Trauma Narrative

The third process is specific to cases in which the child or teen is so mired in avoidance symptoms of PTSD that it impacts their functioning in one or more developmental arenas. When a child is entrenched in an embodied belief that avoiding any thoughts, feelings, people, places, or things related to the traumatic event is the only way to stay safe, but they are continuing to experience intrusive symptoms such as nightmares, flashbacks, recurring images, or phobic behaviors, they need the help of a story keeper to move toward integration. These clients may need more structure from the therapist as they work together to create an integrated coherent trauma narrative (Key & Newland, 2020). Creating a coherent narrative involves combining the facts of what happened with the thoughts, feelings, and somatic experiences that are inextricably tied to the trauma. In these cases, offering expressive mediums consistent with the child's developmental level and shared power is of paramount importance (Goodyear-Brown, 2009). TraumaPlay asserts that "choice amplifies voice," so clients are offered a choice as to *when* (in two or four more sessions) they want to play through the story and *how* they want to play out the story (in the sand tray or with art, clay, puppets, etc.). Clients are always provided with the power to let the therapist know when they need to stop or pause. When this third process is active, the TraumaPlay therapist is very conscious about titrating the dose of exposure and intentionally offers child-led playtime at the end of the session. This allows co-regulation and self-regulation to occur through the developmentally sensitive process of nondirective play.

Addressing the Thought Life

This component of treatment is embedded in the final phase of the TraumaPlay treatment framework, not because it is unimportant but because it is so important (Cohen et al., 2016) and it can be difficult to access early in the treatment process. As discussed previously bottom-up brain development and the embodied experience of complex trauma necessitates a neurodevelopmental and right brain focus on healing, especially in early phases of treatment. In many cases, it may be difficult to access the child client's core cognitive distortions until a post-traumatic play process or trauma narrative process has occurred (Knell, 1998). Often, the child's false attributions—for example, beliefs such as "I was raped because I wore a short skirt"—are not accessible to the clinician until integrative trauma narrative work has begun. Addressing the thought life is like the act of sweeping, coming behind the other components to clean up any cognitive distortions that may still remain. The process helps identify negative self-talk and create more compassionate, kinder ways for clients to speak to themselves.

Making Positive Meaning of the Post-Trauma Self

This final component of TraumaPlay is meant to ensure that the emotional toxicity has been leeched out of the traumatic event (in single-incident trauma) so that the client can place the trauma within a larger life narrative without it causing negative activation (Tedeschi & Calhoun, 2004). In complex trauma cases, the goal is to help the client celebrate new integration of previously dissociated parts into a more unified sense of self. These children also need deep understanding of the risks they are taking when they trust their caregivers and ask for help. The courage needed to move from a control foundation to a trust foundation with caregivers can be celebrated. During this phase of treatment, the client's hard work, new learning or integrations, and the therapeutic relationship are all celebrated, and a meaningful goodbye is achieved (Gil & Crenshaw, 2015; Goodyear-Brown, 2009).

Dissociation

Dissociation exists on a continuum, and while we have certainly seen children who present with fully disparate personalities, we are much more likely to see children who have split off parts of the self in a variety of developmental arenas. Complex trauma cases may present with compartmentalized or exiled younger, highly traumatized parts or amplified protective or aggressive parts that are now problematic for them. Parts work and the playful integration of parts can be invited in each of the core components of TraumaPlay. When aspects of the chronically traumatized child show up in some relationships and hide in others, we dive deep into parents as partners, post-traumatic play, and trauma narrative components. When fragmented emotions need exploration and synthesis, we move into soothing the physiology to increase interoception and then into increasing emotional literacy. When disjointed or contradictory self-talk is present, we come alongside the child to address the thought life. When polarized somatic states are activated, we move into soothing the physiology and offer competency surges that dance on the edges of polarized states. TraumaPlay therapists are ready to work with dissociative symptoms as they present in any of the core components and may use playful mediums such as nesting dolls, puzzles, sand tray creations, and creative image cards that support the exploration of a child's inner world. Novelty is paired with the integration of fragmented parts in the areas of the somatic, emotional, cognitive, and relational self, which ultimately seeks to help the child develop a coherent and congruent self-concept.

Therapist Roles and the Cascade of Care

The Cascade of Care in the TraumaPlay model describes the mechanism by which TraumaPlay therapists embody certain roles based on attachment principles and the neurodevelopmental needs of children and teens, which then supports the client's caregivers' ability to grow into these roles themselves. The triad of therapist roles include safe boss, nurturer, and story keeper (Goodyear-Brown, 2021b).

Safe Boss

Clinicians and caregivers shift in and out of these roles based on moment-to-moment answers to the TraumaPlay guiding question: What is the underlying need of this child right now? (see Figure 28.2). The brain stem, which mitigates the autonomic nervous system, is always asking the question, "Am I safe?" When clients need help regulating this lower brain region, the clinician moves into the role of safe boss, offering co-regulation, predictability, structure, and routine in the physical environment and setting boundaries as needed around safety issues. It is a seminal belief in TraumaPlay that children feel safer when they know where the boundaries are. They also feel safer when they understand that their caregiver can enforce the boundaries in a way that is "bigger, stronger, wiser, and kind" (Cooper et al., 2011; Kim et al., 2018).

Nurturer

The role of nurturer is meant to meet the needs of the mid-brain, the limbic system, which is often asking the question, "Am I loved?" In the role of nurturer, the therapist delights in the child, or parent, or both, reinforcing the child's sense of self as being precious, worthy, and enough. Theraplay and trust-based relational intervention (TBRI) are heavily relied on when the child needs the nurturer, and The Circle of Security® Parenting™ program can help expand a parent's understanding of this role. Therapist activities might involve delighting in the child's freckles or facilitating an in vivo experience of supporting the parent-child dyad as a powerful team as they stick together.

Story Keeper

Working bottom-up, the neocortex is always asking, "What can I learn from this?" It is only online if the lower brain region questions "Am I safe?" and "Am I loved?" have been answered with a resounding affirmative. The story keeper role involves threading the needle backward from the child's current big behaviors all the way to their earliest experiences, if needed. Story keepers are focused on figuring out the most integrated and organic way for each client presentation to make sense of their story.

Case Conceptualization

Case conceptualization in TraumaPlay is systemic and begins with an invitation to the clinician to slow down the assessment phase and more intentionally understand the impact of complex trauma on the child's development in each developmental arena. Therapists are equally focused on understanding the quality of the attachment relationship (including any consequences resulting from intergenerational trauma) between each primary caregiver and the child. Current parenting paradigms and practices are also assessed. The therapist remains curious about the child's developing self-concept as well as their inner working models of relationships throughout the assessment phase.

The first session is for parents or caregivers only, as the therapist begins establishing the roles of the parent as safe boss, nurturer, and story keeper. If the child is present, the parent may present with strong negative activation in response to their child's behaviors, and if the therapist even nods in an attempt to communicate, "I hear you" to the exasperated parent, the child may perceive the therapist as colluding with the parent regarding the child's badness. Parents need to have their felt sense of their relationship with their child (even if this is disgust or exhaustion) held without judgment before they can enter into the sort of reflections that lead to paradigm shifts. One of the TraumaPlay maxims is, "You can give only what you have received," so providing exhausted and shame-ridden parents a safe and nonjudgmental space for holding their story becomes paramount in their ability to embody this story-keeping role themselves and provide the same for their children.

In each of the next two sessions, the NHDA is completed with the parent (or available caregiver) and child together. The child's first exposure to treatment is a version of special playtime with each parent. This de-pathologizes the child, who is often seen by the system as the identified patient and shifts the focus of treatment to the larger family system.

The parent-child dyad is invited into a playroom and the therapist explains that they will have five minutes of child-directed playtime, followed by five minutes of parent-directed playtime, followed by parent-directed cleanup (similar structure to the Dyadic Parent-Child Interaction Coding System (DPICS) within parent-child interaction therapy [PCIT]). The parent will then move to specific prompts written on cards designed to give the therapist glimpses into how the dyad approaches a variety of tasks (many are taken from the Marschak Interaction Method [MIM] from Theraplay). While much data is being recorded throughout the NHDA, including how many questions, criticisms, reflections, and so on are present, as well as how the dynamics of structure, engagement, nurture, and challenge look within this dyad, there are two questions that the therapist remains continuously curious about during the assessment: (1) What is it like to be the parent of this child? and (2) What is it like to be the child of this parent?

Prompts that explore how the dyad approaches stressful things are also embedded in the assessment (Goodyear-Brown, 2021), as are the therapist's observations of the dyad outside the playroom. The autonomic nervous systems of both the parent and the child are reacting to each other, to the therapist, and to the new environment simultaneously. It is clinically useful for the therapist to experience the energy in the room while providing a tether if things become uncomfortable.

One of the most interesting prompts in the NHDA is the Baby Story prompt, which reads, "Adult tells the child a story about when the child was a little baby, beginning with the words, 'When you were a little baby.'" TraumaPlay therapists understand that the stories we are told are the stories we become ... until we learn a new story. Whether or not a new story is needed, how it could be told and who can tell it are among the key elements in case conceptualization.

After the dyadic assessments have been completed, the child client meets with their therapist for two or three individual sessions. Part of each session is child-led, and the therapist is using child-centered responses and entering the child's world as they move into a new space. The focus of the therapist during this time is simply *being with* the child. This phrase, *being with*, is shorthand for entering the phenomenological field of the child, the felt reality of the child.

The second half of each session is a more directive play therapy assessment aimed at understanding the client's current emotional literacy, their current coping repertoire, and their perception of the family dynamics. Several cross-hemispheric tools may be used during this time. The Family Play Geno-Story (Gil, 2014; Goodyear-Brown, 2019a, 2022) invites clients to choose miniatures to represent each of their family members, to arrange them in the sand tray, and then to tell a story about the characters. The Color-Your-Heart (Goodyear-Brown, 2002, 2022) invites the child into a cross-hemispheric exploration of their current emotional life and the situations that engender these emotions. Other assessments are chosen based on specific presenting symptoms (e.g., anxiety or anger). The fifth or sixth session is typically a parent-only feedback session in which the therapist is able to lay out a systemic case conceptualization and engage in collaborative treatment planning that will likely include a combination of individual and dyadic work with the child and their available caregivers.

Case conceptualization and the guiding TraumaPlay principle of "co-regulation always precedes self-regulation" scaffolds clinical decision-making regarding how long core components might take and helps the clinician decide which components will be included in a treatment plan. For example, a client presents with an acute trauma, such as a car accident. After the assessment phase, it is clear that this client has high emotional literacy already and parents who are supportive, attuned attachment figures. It might be decided that little treatment time needs to be spent in increasing emotional literacy or equipping parents as partners. Contrast this example with that of a child with an ACES score of four, who is in their fourth foster home. This complex trauma presentation may include dissociation, fragmentation of self, self-sabotaging interpersonal patterns, and more. That child may need extended time in each component and may need four months of enhancing safety and security before any other goals can be pursued. The TraumaPlay Mapping Tool was created to help clinicians track their treatment choices (Goodyear-Brown, 2021b; see Figure 28.3).

A pinball machine serves as a metaphor for the fluid, dynamic process of following the child's need. Clinicians who feel stuck with a client use this tool to map how many sessions have been spent working with the child and/or parent in each component. For example, a client might have spent the first six working-phase sessions enhancing safety and security. The clinician would write "1–6" above the part of the machine labeled "Enhancing Safety and Security." Tracking sessions (how many and which ones) spent in each treatment goal helps practitioners reflect on the therapeutic dance and see the whole continuum of treatment to date. They may realize that they have missed a component—perhaps they have not incorporated parents as partners—or they may perceive that they moved to play-based gradual exposure too quickly and need to bump back up to augmenting adaptive coping.

Miles and Mom: Case Example

Miles was born addicted to methamphetamines. His mother had already chosen an adoptive family for him, and his adoptive mother was present in the hospital from the moment of his birth. Miles is black and his adoptive parents are white. The family lives in the American South, where many people

The Handbook of Complex Trauma and Dissociation in Children

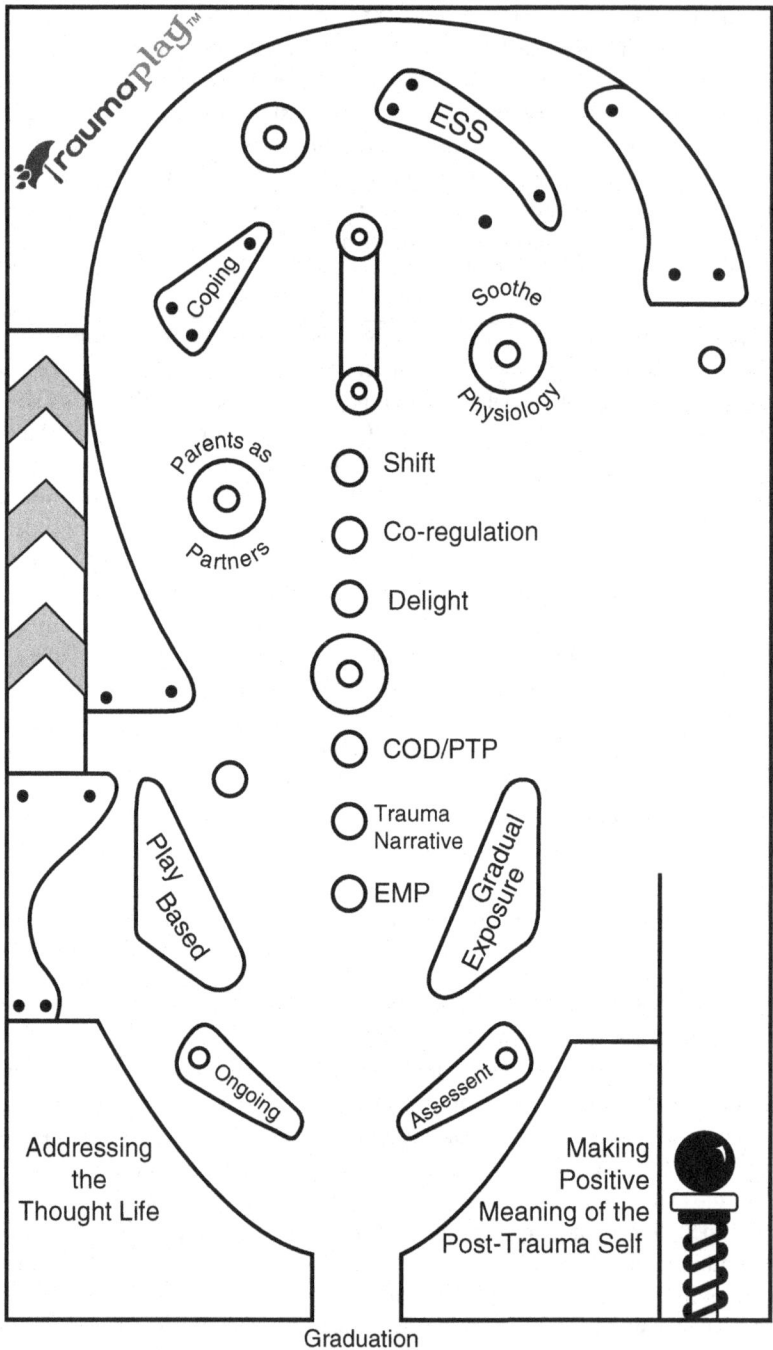

Figure 28.3 The TraumaPlay Mapping Tool. Copyright @Paris Goodyear-Brown. Reprinted with Permission.

claim, "I don't see color." Miles entered treatment at four years old. The presenting issues were intense dysregulation that showed up as hyperactivity, aggression, impulsivity, and inattention paired with an inhibited ability to accept nurturing care from his parents. He was well on his way to being diagnosed with ADHD and possibly ODD if the underlying threads of his story could not be woven together and held in the care and context of his forever family. A brief synopsis of how the dyad worked to bring integration in each component of the model follows.

Assessment Phase

The therapist greeted the adoptive parents, Molly and John, and used this first meeting to build rapport with the caregivers without Miles present. Through the TraumaPlay therapeutic role of story keeper, the therapist facilitated a safe space for the parents to share honestly and openly about the delights and stressors of welcoming their son home through adoption.

During the biopsychosocial interview, the therapist expressed a keen interest in Miles's earliest experiences, including the child's story about how and why he doesn't live with his biological family, and his parents' adoption narrative. The therapist asked open-ended questions that encouraged Molly and John to share information about any in utero threats (drugs, alcohol, additional stressors, medical issues) and their experiences of their first moments, first weeks, and first years parenting their son. Molly explained that she had known his birth mother prior to her becoming pregnant and had nurtured her through the delivery, acknowledged her grief, and respected the birth mom's choice to leave the hospital quickly. After the birth, Miles began to experience his first withdrawal symptoms from the methamphetamine that was in his system. The nurses told Molly that his was the most intense case of withdrawal that they had ever seen. Up to this point, Molly had been offering the therapist only factual information. But when the therapist leaned in and gently asked, "What was it like for you to be holding this little one who was in such distress?" Molly began to cry as she described the intensity of his withdrawal symptoms. She described holding him as he relentlessly cried and screamed. She would hold him as he seized and shook and passed out. She would hold him in his fevers and sweats, and then it would start all over again. At no time during the first couple of months would he mold to her or sigh and relax into her shoulder as her biological children had done. Nothing she could do would soothe him. In the toddler years, Miles was described as being very energetic, was sometimes hyperkinetic, and was highly independent, rarely seeking nurturing care.

During the NHDAs, Miles moved excitedly from toy to toy in the playroom, unable to settle into an elaborated play theme. He did not invite Mom into his play and often acted as if she were not present. Mom tracked well with him and stayed physically close as he moved around the room. Miles was not as kinetic in his session with Dad but resisted the nurture-driven tasks with similar vigor in both assessments.

The therapist then met with him individually for three sessions. In each initial session, the therapist offered child-led play therapy for half the session and invited Miles to complete a play-based assessment activity for the other half, including a Family Play Genogram, a Color-Your-Heart, and a self-portrait. Miles drew a self-portrait that depicted himself as a stick figure sitting alone in the driver's seat of a massive alien spaceship shaped like a creature with legs. In the illustration, he is surrounded by giant creatures attacking him. Alligator-type creatures are chewing at the legs of the spaceship. His face is turned toward the onlooker, includes a pronounced frown and looks a little panicky. While he is in the driver's seat of the alien body, there are no controls (no buttons, no steering wheel, nothing) inside (see Figure 28.4).

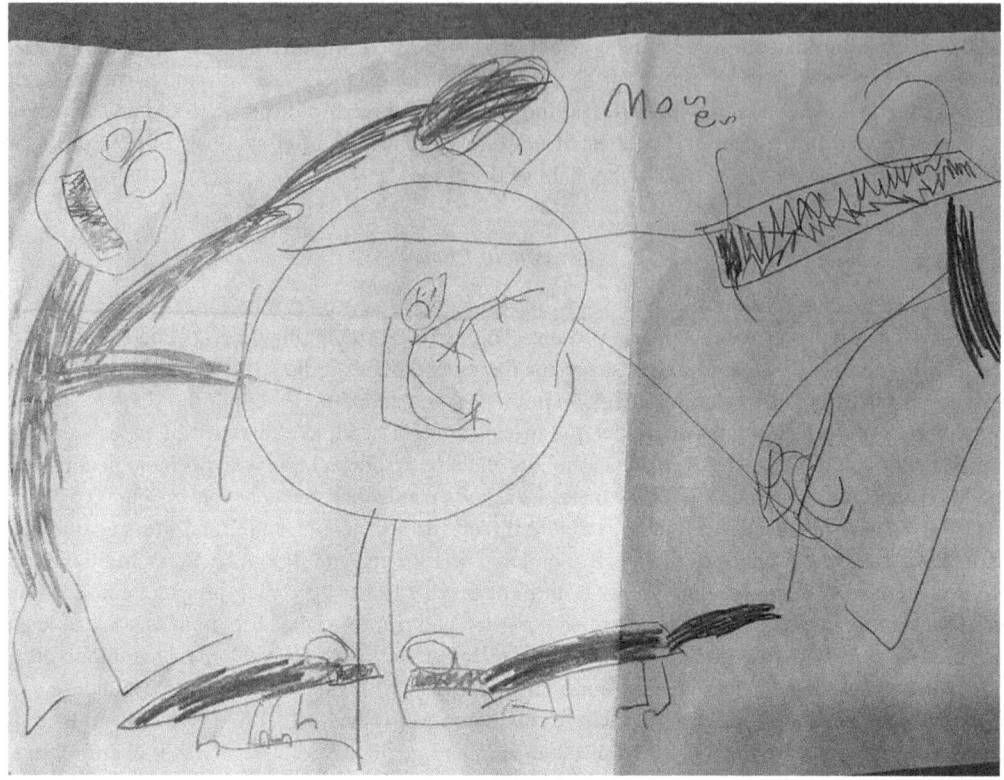

Figure 28.4 Miles alone While Alien's Attack. This Is an Image of a Child's Pencil Drawing of a Self-Portrait Completed during the Assessment Phase of Treatment.

The assessment phase suggested an underlying need for a repatterning of his nervous system, which could be achieved through reparative doses of serve-and-return communications from a strengthened relationship with his caregiver while building a new sense of competence as they co-created new connecting experiences together.

Enhancing Safety and Security

The first few treatment sessions were a combination of child-led play and Theraplay activities as the therapist got to know the dyad. Molly watched as the therapist responded to Miles over the course of the first few child-led sessions. Molly began to use the language and to shift in and out of the safe boss and nurturer roles. She practiced the skills of child-led responding and worked alongside the therapist in the first several sessions to reflect, describe, and track Miles's play. During each session, Miles would become dysregulated in some way and the therapist would model, "Your body is letting me know that you need …" and offer a change of activity, closer physical proximity, a change in environment from inside to outside or from bigness to smallness of space, food, drink, or a boundary setting prompt. Hide and Seek Gummy Worms was a favorite nurturing game for Miles and his mother. Molly would close her eyes while the therapist placed gummies in different parts of the client's clothing. Then she would look for the gummies and when she found one, she would make loving eye contact with Miles while feeding it to him. At first, it was hard for him to be fed and he would grab for the gummies, but after several weeks, Miles began to ask for this game and sat very still with his mouth wide open while being fed.

Throughout these early sessions, Molly was also taught how to tell "delighting in" stories, and these became part of every session. Miles, Molly, and the therapist would settle into a nurturing nook and have a snack while Molly would tell a story about something cute he had done that week, or some new competency he had achieved, like climbing to the top of the monkey bars. The therapist began referring to mom as a safe boss and supporting Molly by acting, at all times, as a safe boss of the space for both parent and child.

On several occasions, Miles chose scary or aggressive action figures and contained or manipulated these toys in various ways, gaining a sense of experiential mastery during this kind of play and experiencing competency surges, a full-body sense of "I am strong. I am able. I can handle this." At the end of each session, Miles would choose a vulnerable creature, usually a miniature puppy, and insist that the therapist put it somewhere safe until he returned. This vicarious nurture of the self-object further enhanced the neuroception of safety for Miles.

Around session six of the treatment phase, the 12th session in total, the therapist introduced the Boo Boo routine from Theraplay. In TraumaPlay, narrative work is combined with nurturing care, so when the therapist noticed the scrape on Miles's knee, she asked out loud how Miles had gotten the scrape. Mom and Miles were both equally engaged in telling the story of how he had been running down the driveway when he fell and scuffed his knee. The therapist wondered out loud if they could put a Band-Aid on the scar now to mark the hurt then and how Mom took care of it. When Miles saw the Band-Aid, he jerked away and began to scream, "No!" and pushed away from Mom. People who didn't know his story might think he was throwing a tantrum or actively rejecting his mother. Moving into the story keeping role, the therapist quickly passed Miles a soft blanket as a gesture of comfort, which he quickly grabbed and pulled over his head, covering his whole body with it. The therapist said,

> You know, Mom, I remember about Miles that his birth mom had some yucky stuff in her body that was hurting her and when he was born he still had some of that yucky stuff inside his body. It took a while for his body to get rid of the yucky stuff, and there were a lot of days when he was just a baby that his body hurt. I wonder if baby Miles believed that sometimes you just have to hurt, and his baby brain thought that no one could help him feel better. Mom, I know that although you held him, rocked him, and soothed him, his body kept hurting until all the yucky stuff was gone. Now ... he's almost 5 years old, and maybe big boy Miles is learning that you can help him feel better when he is feeling yucky, and that there is help available when he hurts.

Just then, Miles slowly extended his knee from underneath the blanket and placed it in his mother's lap. Embodying the story keeping role in that moment meant understanding and narrating the big behavior by threading the needle all the way back to his earliest experience in the hospital.

Assessing for and Augmenting Coping

The therapist saw early on that the client's coping strategies often involved moving into his own world or responding to a neuroception of danger, including friendly overtures from Mom, with a fight response. Miles and Molly created a Coping Tree (Goodyear-Brown, 2022), reflecting both his adaptive and maladaptive coping strategies. It became clear that Miles preferred coping responses that helped him feel strong and in control. The therapist reframed this in the context of his early disempowerment and current need for a sense of competency. It became clear that stretching Miles's very narrow window of tolerance (WOT) (Siegel, 1999) for distress would be easier to achieve if relational risks that required vulnerability (a potential felt sense of weakness for him) were accompanied by a competency surge. Molly also began to shift her paradigm to understanding that her own adaptive coping would require her to recognize when she was outside of her own WOT and to learn how to get back to her optimal arousal window as fast as she could.

Soothing the Physiology

When Miles was a newborn and chronically overwhelmed with painful full-body withdrawal symptoms, he harnessed the genius of the disembodied self, disconnecting his mind from his body for self-protection. Somatic grounding activities included a host of deep-breathing exercises, play-based mindfulness practice, and expanding circles of excitation and calming in play. Miles particularly liked engaging in challenge-based activities where he would test his body with Mom as his cheerleader. Miles and his mother would create obstacle courses in the backyard and move through them together. These upregulating games were quickly followed with down-regulating exercises, like balancing a peacock feather, humming with Humbug Rocks (Goodyear-Brown, 2022), or engaging in yoga poses together.

Parents as Soothing Partners

As Miles built his sense of self-efficacy and competency, he began to take bigger risks. He and Mom painted each other's hands and made a beautiful butterfly together. Mom's hands were the large top wings of the butterfly and Miles's hands made the bottom wings. They talked about how all the wings were needed for the butterfly to fly. The therapist asked if they wanted to name it, and they decided to title it Hope.

Miles became aware of the slack line in the backyard of Nurture House and asked if we could play outside. He ran over to the slackline, jumped on top of it, balanced his body as he took three steps along the slackline, and then fell off. He landed on his feet and jumped right back up to try again. The therapist moved into story keeper role again, saying,

> I am remembering how much you like to do things by yourself. Mom, he really wants to get as far along on this slackline as he can … will you just go and stand nearby? Mom will be right there, sticking together with you, and your body will know when you need her.

Mom obliged and walked beside him as he moved across the first 5 feet of the line.
When he reached out and grabbed Mom's hand, the therapist said,

> His body was letting you know he needed some help to balance. Wow! You guys are moving quickly together … you're almost there … you did it! When you stick together, you can do amazing things!

Both Molly and Miles were smiling, beaming from ear to ear. Miles then did something surprising. He said, "Hey, Mom, I wanna jump on it. Will you help me?" Miles held Mom's hand as they moved back to the middle of the line. He turned sideways, held both of his mother's hands in both of his, and leaned almost his whole weight on his mom's arms while jumping up and down on the line (see Figure 28.5).

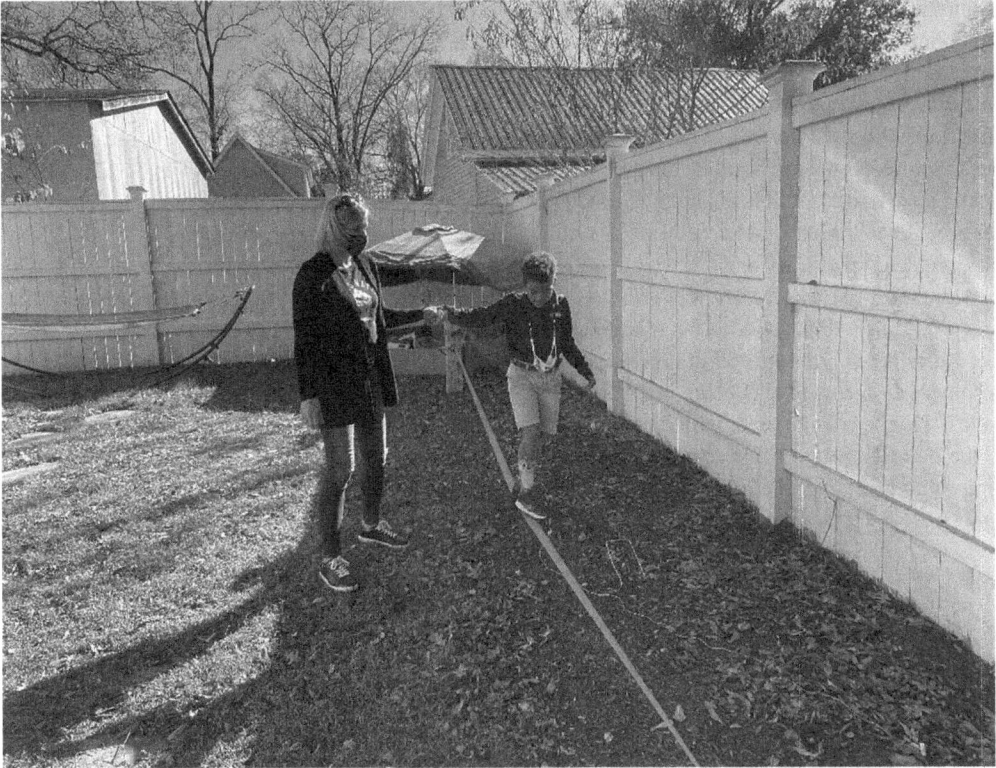

Figure 28.5 Miles Lets Mom Help.

Increasing Emotional Literacy

Miles and Molly started developing a shared emotional lexicon in their first session with their therapist. Molly was asked to invest in a set of emotion-specific cards, and Molly and Miles began to lay out their feeling faces after difficult moments at home. The therapist played games aimed at nonverbal identification of each other's feelings in session. The mother-son dyad read bibliotherapy resources about feelings while snuggled in a nurturing nook, and Molly was actively coached on how to name and validate Miles's feelings without judgment. Part of their termination process involved Miles and his mom making multicolored sand art bottles. Each layer of sand represented a feeling expressed by Miles and held by his mom over the course of treatment. These small matching bottles were placed on strings and became matching necklaces that served as transitional objects for both parent and child from the safety of the playroom to their home.

Play-Based Gradual Exposure/Trauma Narrative Work

The therapist had been weaving the task of story keeping throughout the therapeutic process, beginning with Miles's withdrawal symptoms as a baby, offering small, titrated doses of exposure to the hardest parts of his story. After around 20 sessions or so, Miles began to ask for more details about his birth story. Molly had been meeting collaterally with the therapist for trauma-informed parent coaching, and both agreed that Miles was ready to have the story of his birth told, but in the contained environment of the sand tray. The story was enacted, with spontaneous participation from Miles throughout the process. Mom began by narrating and acting out her arrival at the hospital just before his birth. As her miniature figure burst into the hospital room we had created in the sand, Miles blurted out the question, "Where was Dad?" Molly said, "Good question! He was at home with the other kids, but as soon as you were born, he got into a car and drove through the night to get to us." Miles wanted to find a car and a dad figure and play out Dad's mad dash to the hospital. Molly then offered, "After we brought you home, if I couldn't be holding you, Daddy would have you strapped to his chest." Miles looked up quickly and focused intently on his mom. "He did?" asked Miles. The therapist realized that most of the integration of narrative surrounding Mom and Miles had been created, and Miles was now shifting his focus to his relationship with his adoptive father. The therapist said, "It seems like Miles is really interested in this idea that his dad kept him strapped to his chest. Wonder if there is some way for us to show this in the sand tray?" Miles piped up and said, "Do you have a rubber band?" He spent some time, with intense energy, strapping the "baby" who represented his self-object to the dad figure that had been used in the nurturing narration. Miles put this creation of Dad and himself strapped together with a rubber band on a shelf in the sand tray room as he left the session.

Addressing the Thought Life

Miles had been in treatment for at least seven months and had his fifth birthday before the work of addressing his thought life began. This component of treatment includes an exploration of the client's core beliefs, his current negative self-talk, and his cognitive distortions. However, Miles's developmental capacities had to be understood to maximize treatment gains. According to Piaget (1950), Miles would be in the preoperational stage of cognitive development. According to Erikson (1965), he would be straddling the divide between two developmental stages: initiative versus guilt and industry versus inferiority. When adoptive children straddle multiple developmental levels, it is most protective to focus the therapeutic work on remediating the earlier developmental task. Erikson would say that the key question Miles is answering in this stage of his development is: Am I good or bad? During this stage, children are beginning to assert control and power over their environment. If the child exerts the right amount of power, they experience competency. If they exert too much power, they experience disapproval, an experience Miles had repeatedly in his preschool years.

Making Positive Meaning of the Post-Trauma Self

The age at which Miles's treatment occurred (late four-year-old self to early six-year-old self) necessitated that this cognitive work be contextualized in relationship with his co-regulating caregivers. The core cognitive distortions carried by many of our traumatized children are, "I am bad; I am unworthy of love; I am unable to get my needs met." Normalizing the safe, nurturing care that all little ones should receive became an important theme in Miles's treatment. During one session, Miles chose a baby bear sand tray miniature and put it in the sand tray. The therapist wondered out loud what the baby bear might need to feel safe and grow. Miles scurried about, finding water, food, and a cave for shelter. Mom found a mama bear and added it to the sand tray, saying she didn't want the baby bear to be all alone. Miles looked at the tray for a moment and then tucked the baby bear right next to the mama bear, and said, "Now they can snuggle whenever the baby is cold or scared ... like we do."

Conclusion

TraumaPlay is an attachment-based, neurobiologically informed, flexibly sequential play therapy model for treating traumatized children and their families. TraumaPlay's key components serve as an umbrella framework that invites integration of several evidence-based play and child therapy approaches. TraumaPlay therapists embrace the core principle of following the child's need on a moment-to-moment basis throughout the continuum of treatment while fluidly embodying the roles of safe boss, nurturer, and story keeper, and helping the caregivers of traumatized children do the same.

Note

1 Theraplay® is a registered service mark of The Theraplay® Institute, Chicago, IL, USA.

References

Amnie, A. G. (2018). Emerging themes in coping with lifetime stress and implication for stress management education. *SAGE Open Medicine, 6*, Article 2050312118782545. https://doi.org/10.1177/2050312118782545

Axline, V. (1947). *Play therapy*. Ballantine.

Beer, R. (2018). Efficacy of EMDR therapy for children with PTSD: A review of the literature. *Journal of EMDR Practice and Research, 12*(4), 177–195.

Booth, P. B., & Jernberg, A. M. (2009). *Theraplay: Helping parents and children build better relationships through attachment-based play*. John Wiley & Sons.

Bratton, S. C., Ceballos, P. L., Sheely-Moore, A. I., Meany-Walen, K., Pronchenko, Y., & Jones, L. D. (2013). Head start early mental health intervention: Effects of child-centered play therapy on disruptive behaviors. *International Journal of Play Therapy, 22*(1), 28–42.

Bratton, S. C., Ray, D., Rhine, T., & Jones, L. (2005). The efficacy of play therapy with children: A meta-analytic review of treatment outcomes. *Professional Psychology: Research and Practice, 36*(4), 376–390.

Cohen, J. A., Deblinger, E., & Mannarino, A. P. (2018). Trauma-focused cognitive behavioral therapy for children and families. *Psychotherapy Research, 28*(1), 47–57.

Cohen, J. A., & Mannarino, A. P. (2015). Trauma-focused cognitive behavior therapy for traumatized children and families. *Child and Adolescent Psychiatric Clinics, 24*(3), Article 557570. https://doi.org/10.1016/j.chc.2015.02.005

Cohen, J. A., Mannarino, A. P., & Deblinger, E. (2016). *Treating trauma and traumatic grief in children and adolescents*. Guilford Publications.

Cooper, G., Hoffman, K., Powell, B., & Marvin, R. (2011). The circle of security intervention: Using the therapeutic relationship to ameliorate attachment security in disorganized dyads. In J. Solomon & C. George (Eds.), *Disorganized attachment and caregiving* (p. 318). Guilford Press.

Crenshaw, D. A., & Kenney-Noziska, S. (2014). Therapeutic presence in play therapy. *International Journal of Play Therapy, 23*(1), 31.

Dowell, K. A., & Ogles, B. M. (2010). The effects of parent participation on child psychotherapy outcome: A meta-analytic review. *Journal of Clinical Child & Adolescent Psychology, 39*(2), 151–162. https://doi.org/10.1080/15374410903532585

Drewes, A. A., Bratton, S. C., & Schaefer, C. E. (2011). *Integrative play therapy*. John Wiley & Sons.

Erikson, E. H. (1965). *Childhood and Society* (Revised ed.). Penguin Books.

Folkman, S., & Moskowitz, J. T. (2004). Coping: Pitfalls and promise. *Annual Review of Psychology, 55*, 745–774. https://doi.org/10.1146/annurev.psych.55.090902.141456

Garza, Y., & Bratton, S. C. (2005). School-based child-centered play therapy with Hispanic children: Outcomes and cultural consideration. *International Journal of Play Therapy, 14*(1), 51.

Gaskill, R. L., & Perry, B. (2014). The neurobiological power of play: Using the neurosequential model of therapeutics to guide play in the healing process. In C. A. Malchiodi & D. A. Crenshaw (Eds.), *Creative arts and play therapy for attachment problems* (pp. 178–194). Guilford Press.

Geller, S. M., & Porges, S. W. (2014). Therapeutic presence: Neurophysiological mechanisms mediating feeling safe in therapeutic relationships. *Journal of Psychotherapy Integration, 24*(3), 178. https://doi.org/10.1037/a0037511

Gil, E. (2014). *Play in family therapy*. Guilford Press.

Gil, E. (2016). *Posttraumatic play in children: What clinicians need to know*. Guilford Press.

Gil, E., & Crenshaw, D. A. (2015). *Termination challenges in child psychotherapy*. Guilford Press.

Goodyear-Brown, P. (2002). *Digging for buried treasure: 52 prop-based play therapy interventions for treating the problems of childhood*. Author.

Goodyear-Brown, P. (2009). *Play therapy with traumatized children: A prescriptive approach*. Wiley.

Goodyear-Brown, P. (2019a). *Trauma and play therapy: Helping children heal*. Routledge.

Goodyear-Brown, P. (2019b). Parents as partners: Enhancing co-regulation and coherence though an integration of play therapy and EMDR. *Go With That, 24*(1), 28–33.

Goodyear-Brown, P. (2021a). Integrating the therapeutic powers of play in traditional clinical practice settings. In E. Prendiville & J. Parson (Eds.), *Clinical applications of the therapeutic powers of play* (pp. 29–45). Routledge.

Goodyear-Brown, P. (2021b). *Parents as partners in child therapy: A clinician's guide*. Guilford Press

Goodyear-Brown, P. (2022). *Big behaviors in small containers: 131 Trauma-informed interventions for disorders of dysregulation*. PESI Publishing.

Goodyear-Brown, P., & Yasenik, L. (in press). *Polyvagal power in the playroom: A guide for play therapists*. Routledge.

Gruhn, M. A., & Compas, B. E. (2020). Effects of maltreatment on coping and emotion regulation in childhood and adolescence: A meta-analytic review. *Child Abuse & Neglect, 103*. https://doi.org/10.1016/j.chiabu.2020.104446

Kaduson, H. G., Cangelosi, D. M., & Schaefer, C. E. (Eds.). (2019). *Prescriptive play therapy: Tailoring interventions for specific childhood problems*. Guilford Press.

Key, D., & Newland, R. (2020). Creating trauma narratives for young children. The Brown University Child and Adolescent Behavior Letter, *36*(10), 1–6. https://doi.org/10.1002/cbl.30493

Kim, M., Woodhouse, S. S., & Dai, C. (2018). Learning to provide children with a secure base and a safe haven: The Circle of Security-Parenting (COS-P) group intervention. *Journal of Clinical Psychology, 74*(8), 1319–1332. https://doi.org/10.1002/jclp.22643

Knell, S. (1998). Cognitive-behavioral play therapy. *Journal of Clinical Child Psychology, 27*(1), 28–33. https://doi.org/10.1207/s15374424jccp2701_3

Landreth, G. L. (2012). *Play therapy: The art of the relationship*. Routledge.

LeBlanc, M., & Ritchie, M. (2001). A meta-analysis of play therapy outcomes. *Counselling Psychology Quarterly, 14*(2), 149–163. https://doi.org/10.1080/09515070110059142

Levine, P. A. (1997). *Waking the tiger: Healing trauma: The innate capacity to transform overwhelming experiences*. North Atlantic Books.

Lin, Y. W., & Bratton, S. C. (2015). A meta-analytic review of child-centered play therapy approaches. *Journal of Counseling & Development, 93*(1), 45–58. https://doi.org/10.1002/j.1556-6676.2015.00180.x

Money, R., Wilde, S., & Dawson, D. (2021). The effectiveness of Theraplay for children under 12: A systematic literature review. *Child and Adolescent Mental Health, 26*(3), 238–251. https://doi.org/10.1111/camh.12416

Oaklander, V. (1978). *Windows to our children: A Gestalt therapy approach to children and adolescents*. Real People Press.

Oksuz, Y. (2016). Evaluation of emotional literacy activities: A phenomenological study. *Journal of Education and Practice, 7*(36), 34–39.

Payne, P., Levine, P. A., & Crane-Godreau, M. A. (2015). Somatic experiencing: Using interoception and proprioception as core elements of trauma therapy. *Frontiers in Psychology, 6*, 93. https://doi.org/10.3389/fpsyg.2015.00093

Perry, B. D. (2006). The Neurosequential Model of Therapeutics: Applying principles of neuroscience to clinical work with traumatized and maltreated children. In N. B. Webb (Ed.), *Working with traumatized youth in child welfare* (pp. 27–52). Guilford.

Perry, B. D., Pollard, R. A., Blakley, T. L., Baker, W. L., & Vigilante, D. (1995). Childhood trauma, the neurobiology of adaptation, and "use-dependent" development of the brain: How "states" become "traits." *Infant Maternal Health Journal, 16*, 271–291. https://doi.org/10.1002/1097-0355(199524)16:4<271::AID-IMHJ2280160404>3.0.CO;2-B

Piaget, J. (1950). *The psychology of intelligence*. Routledge.

Porges, S. W. (2015). Play as neural exercise: Insights from the polyvagal theory. *The Power of Play for Mind Brain Health. Mindgains.org, GAINS*, 3–7.

Porges, S. W., & Dana, D. (Eds.). (2018). *Clinical applications of the polyvagal theory: The emergence of polyvagal-informed therapies*. W. W. Norton.

Purvis, K. B., Cross, D. R., & Sunshine, W. L. (2007). *The connected child: Bring hope and healing to your adoptive family*. McGraw-Hill.

Ray, D. C., Burgin, E., Gutierrez, D., Ceballos, P., & Lindo, N. (2022). Child-centered play therapy and adverse childhood experiences: A randomized controlled trial. *Journal of Counseling & Development, 100*(2), 134–145.

Salo, S., Flykt, M., Mäkelä, J., Lassenius-Panula, L., Korja, R., Lindaman, S., & Punamäki, R. L. (2020). The impact of Theraplay therapy on parent-child interaction and child psychiatric symptoms: A pilot study. *International Journal of Play, 9*(3), 331–352. https://doi.org/10.1080/21594937.2020.1806500

Sandler, I. N., Tein, J.Y., Mehta, P., Wolchik, S., & Ayers, T. (2000). Coping efficacy and psychological problems of children of divorce. *Child Development, 71*(4), 1099–1118. https://doi.org/10.1111/1467-8624.00212

Schaefer, C. E., & Drewes, A. A. (2013). *The therapeutic powers of play: 20 Core agents of change*. Wiley.

Schaefer, C. E., & Drewes, A. A. (2015). Prescriptive play therapy. In Charles E. Schaefer and Athena A. Drewes (Eds.), *Handbook of play therapy* (pp. 227–240). Wiley

Schore, A. N. (2019). *Right brain psychotherapy*. W. W. Norton.

Schore, J. R., & Schore, A. N. (2008). Modern attachment theory: The central role of affect regulation in development and treatment. *Clinical Social Work Journal, 36*(1), 9–20. https://doi.org/10.1007/s10615-007-0111-7

Shapiro, F. (2017). *Eye movement desensitization and reprocessing (EMDR) therapy: Basic principles, protocols, and procedures*. Guilford Press.

Siegel, D. J. (1999). *The developing mind: Toward a neurobiology of interpersonal experience*. Guilford Press.

Siu, A. F. (2009). Theraplay in the Chinese world: An intervention program for Hong Kong children with internalizing problems. *International Journal of Play Therapy, 18*(1), 1.

Siu, A. F. (2014). Effectiveness of Group Theraplay® on enhancing social skills among children with developmental disabilities. *International Journal of Play Therapy, 23*(4), 187.

Squire, L. R., & Dede, A. J. (2015). Conscious and unconscious memory systems. *Cold Spring Harbor Perspectives in Biology, 7*(3), Article a021667. https://doi.org/10.1101/cshperspect.a021667

Stewart, A. L., Field, T. A., & Echterling, L. G. (2016). Neuroscience and the magic of play therapy. *International Journal of Play Therapy, 25*(1), 4. https://doi.org/10.1037/pla0000016

Tedeschi, R. G., & Calhoun, L. G. (2004). Target article: Posttraumatic growth: Conceptual foundations and empirical evidence. *Psychological Inquiry, 15*(1), 1–18. https://doi.org/10.1207/s15327965pli1501_01

Thornback, K., & Muller, R. T. (2015). Relationships among emotion regulation and symptoms during trauma-focused CBT for school-aged children. *Child Abuse & Neglect, 50*, 182–192. https://doi.org/10.1016/j.chiabu.2015.09.011

van der Kolk, B. A. (2009). Developmental trauma disorder: Towards a rational diagnosis for chronically traumatized children. *Praxis der Kinderpsychologie und Kinderpsychiatrie, 58*(8), 572–586. https://doi.org/10.13109/prkk.2009.58.8.572

Vernhet, C., Dellapiazza, F., Blanc, N., Cousson-Gélie, F., Miot, S., Roeyers, H., & Baghdadli, A. (2019). Coping strategies of parents of children with autism spectrum disorder: A systematic review. *European Child & Adolescent Psychiatry, 28*(6), 747–758. https://doi.org/10.1007/s00787-018-1183-3

Vijay Sagar, K. J. (2011). Play therapy: A window into the child's world. *Andhra Pradesh Journal of Psychological Medicine, 12*(1), 7–9.

29
THERAPLAY AND PARTS WORK

Karen Andor and Dafna Lender

Introduction

Theraplay is a parent-child psychotherapy that was created by Ann Jernberg and Phyllis Booth in 1968 (Booth & Jernberg, 2010). Faced with the challenge of how to meet the psychological needs of Chicago Head Start children, they developed an innovative treatment program where lively, attuned volunteers played interactive, fun, and nurturing activities with troubled preschoolers, and the preschoolers' troublesome behavior improved. In the 1970s, Jernberg and Booth translated the model to focus on the parent and child relationship in a clinical setting. The result of this collaboration was Theraplay.

Theraplay is based on the types of activities, communications, and interactions that healthy parents intuitively have with their babies. At their heart, the activities focus on face-to-face, playful, nurturing interactions like peekaboo and patty-cake. But Theraplay is not for infants only. In fact, most clients who are treated with and benefit from Theraplay are 3–12 years old. The spirit and essence of the young parent-infant activities are modified to fit the developmental level of the child. The activities emphasize all the nonverbal behaviors that, in a split second, tell a child they're safe and that there is joy in connection: the rhythmic, prosodic voice; the curious, open face; the smooth, coordinated gestures; the touch and playfulness, rather than cognitive, verbal, or imaginary games. Theraplay offers a vehicle for creating the fun and lighthearted moments that enable nonverbal connection and facilitate the soothing and caring interactions that promote attachment. What Theraplay does *not* do for healing attachment trauma is explicitly invite the child to bring up and talk about traumatic memories. Theraplay does not focus on explicit memory (creating a more coherent autobiographical narrative through developing a story of the past trauma) but rather works on the level of procedural memory (nonconscious, bodily feeling of lack of safety vs. safety, disconnection vs. connection).

Children with complex trauma have many acute but also many chronic relational events that are traumatic (for example, being severely yelled at, cursed at, sent away to isolation for long periods, humiliation, or being forced to participate in activities that are frightening or cruel), during the crucial time when their brain and personality are still developing. Additionally, because they are still children and therefore dependent on their caregivers, they are forced to adapt to the caregiver's mode of relating, even if it is cruel, neglectful, or severely misattuned. When the attachment and traumatic stress become too intense, a child may fight or run away. Frequently, because they feel trapped and do not have the tools to cope or defend against the parent's injurious behavior, they will collapse and withdraw. All of these responses are dissociative coping behaviors. These responses may manifest in what is perceived by adults as willful misbehavior on the part of the child, such as such as chaotically running around and "acting silly."

In Theraplay, the therapist helps the parent engage in healthy types of interactions in a way that is attuned and responsive, thereby creating a new, healthier experience for the child. When, inevitably, the child displays dissociative behaviors, which according to Nijenhuis (2017) are always part of trauma, the therapist and parent (with the help of the therapist's guidance) respond to the child with empathy and modify the activity to show the child attunement and make overtures of repair with them. If a child becomes angry or dysregulated or withdraws, the therapist and parent actively support the child's responses by both acknowledging the child's need to respond in this way and showing that they are not angry and have not given up on the relationship. This leads to the child eventually recovering from the perceived rupture in the relationship and learning that they can reengage and return to the connection with their trusted adult. This repeated pattern of attuned connection, rupture, and repair (along with regular parent-only sessions to help parents integrate the new experiences and apply them at home) is the main mechanism that helps children with complex trauma heal and earn secure attachment (Siegel, 1999).

Theraplay is often sufficient for improving both the symptoms of the child and the relationship between parent and child. However, there are certain children who require the additional support of explicit understanding of their attachment trauma story. In these cases, an additional modality can be easily combined with Theraplay. In this chapter, we will outline a useful intervention, TIST for children, developed by Karen Andor (2023), for helping a child integrate and process their attachment trauma and understand their dissociative behavior on an explicit level.

Case Conceptualization

Case conceptualization is the first, very important step in the Theraplay process. It informs how the therapist will structure their therapy sessions in order to support the child (Norris et al., 2020). It also provides an opportunity to determine if the child is dissociating.

Standardized questionnaires—such as the Behavior Assessment System for Children, Third Edition (BASC-3) and the Parenting Relationship Questionnaire (PRQ)—about the child's behaviors and parents' attitudes are completed by the caregivers before the intake interview. These questionnaires are then explored in an initial intake interview with the child's caregivers, where they have an opportunity to discuss the history and current functioning of the family. Caregivers are also asked about the child's behaviors as well as their functioning at school and in other environments (Norris et al., 2020). Careful reading of the intake questionnaires and an understanding of dissociation while conducting the carer interviews will assist the therapist in determining if and how the child is dissociating.

After the intake interview, the caregivers and the child attend an assessment session called the Marschak Interaction Method (MIM) (Norris et al., 2020). This is a structured observation technique for which the caregivers are given nine simple tasks to complete with their child. It provides a further opportunity to determine if the child and/or their caregiver are dissociating. The MIM provides information about the quality and nature of the relationship between the child and each of their caregivers. The MIM is videoed, and this provides the therapist with an opportunity to analyze the parent-child interactions.

Dissociative behaviors can be observed in the MIM assessment. The child may dissociate to activate a submissive part who is very compliant with all the activities. Afterward, the caregiver may comment that that was unusual behavior, as the child tends to be oppositional at home. The child may dissociate to an attachment cry defense state who, when the parent reenters the room, may cling to them, continue to cry, and cannot be soothed. More extreme dissociative behaviors may also be observed. For example, the child may find the intimacy and eye contact from the caregiver so threatening within the unfamiliar setting of the therapy room that it may trigger a dorsal vagal collapse and the child may collapse to the floor and become unresponsive. (When a child triggers into dorsal vagal collapse in a Theraplay session, they can be regulated by reading a picture book to them using a storytelling tone of voice.)

There are a number of caregiver behaviors that can lead to children dissociating that may also be observed in the MIM. Lyons-Ruth et al. (2006) gave examples of a number of caregiver behaviors that are frightening or frightened. One example is of the caregiver who provides contradictory cues to their child, such as inviting the child to approach verbally, but at the same time physically withdrawing by turning to look away from the child or pulling their bodies back. Another example is when the caregiver expects the child to meet their emotional needs—they may have an unconscious expectation that the child take care of them rather than them taking care of the child's emotional needs. These frightening or frightened behaviors communicate to the immature infant that the caregiver is both the source of comfort and the source of distress. Since the infant's cognitive and emotional development are immature, and as they have a limited range of behavioral responses, they are entirely dependent on their caregivers to determine the degree of threat in the environment and take appropriate action to soothe or protect them (Lyons-Ruth et al., 2006; Liotti, 2022; please see Chapter 4 on disorganized attachment). This is why these frightened or frightening caregiver behaviors have such a significant effect on a child's ability to cope.

Therapists may also find it useful to use checklists for dissociative symptoms while viewing and analyzing the MIM. This will help them to make decisions regarding the quality of the child's attachment and if and how they are dissociating. For information on checklists and how to do this, please see Chapters 21–23, which will guide therapists in what somatic markers to look for when assessing whether or not a child is dissociating.

The MIM is followed up by a feedback session with the caregivers who were involved in the MIM sessions. This provides an opportunity to discuss interactions between the child and the caregiver(s). Since the MIM is videotaped, the therapist has the opportunity to discuss interactions between the caregiver and the child in a way that is understandable and observable to the caregiver. The therapist discusses the caregiver-child interactions with empathy and understanding around any difficulties. The therapist will also focus on the positives in the interactions—moments of joy, smiles, eye contact, and warmth. If Theraplay treatment is recommended and if the caregivers decide that they would like to proceed with the therapy, then an agreement is made on how many sessions the family is likely to need, depending on the severity of the presenting problem.

The MIM provides an opportunity to determine the course of Theraplay sessions, but also whether Theraplay that includes the caregiver is the most appropriate course of treatment for the child. If the caregiver has the appropriate resources within themselves and they are open to growth, self-reflection, and working on their own trauma and attachment histories, then it is possible to include them. However, if caregivers have personality disorder traits or are abusive, it may not be appropriate to include them in the Theraplay sessions. In fact, it is likely that Theraplay will increase the disorganized attachment within the child. Theraplay is an attachment-based therapy designed to develop appropriate attachment within the child toward their caregiver, but if the caregiver is the source of threat for that child, the child's defensive system, and subsequently their dissociation, will only be strengthened (see Chapter 40 on Liotti's work).

Some therapists will work individually in Theraplay with children who have no attachment caregiver available. While this is not an ideal situation and every attempt should be made to include an attachment figure in therapy, in reality, certain children, like those who live in children's homes where there is no parent figure and there is a shortage of childcare workers, the therapist can use Theraplay with the child alone. In these cases, it is recommended that the therapist be experienced and under the supervision of a certified Theraplay supervisor. This is because the bond that may develop between therapist and child could be even stronger than if the therapist uses less experiential therapies; therefore, the therapist would need to be mindful of their own countertransferential processes to be sure that they are acting in ways that are meeting the child's needs. Furthermore, the therapist should modify the Theraplay activities to involve the least amount of direct caregiving and physical proximity while still meeting the child's needs for nurture. For example, the child and therapist can share a snack and the therapist can enjoy the child's enjoyment of the snack, but the therapist may not feed the child directly, as is sometimes done in Theraplay with a parent present.

Case conceptualization in Theraplay is initially formulated around the MIM assessment and subsequent caregiver feedback session. However, case conceptualization is not a one-off initial process that determines the entire course of Theraplay treatment. After every session, the Theraplay therapist determines whether they need to continue with the same activities or if they need to make adjustments to better meet the child's needs based on what happened in the previous session. In this way, the therapist is always endeavoring to meet the child's needs as they evolve and change.

Caregivers who are more capable should always be part of this process, and also participate in a caregiver feedback session with the therapist after every four Theraplay sessions. This is so the caregiver is able to develop their skills, expand their understanding of their child, and ultimately meet the child's needs independently and appropriately. As Rothschild (2017) points out, clients come to therapy for only one hour a week. They need to cope between sessions, and for this reason, it is essential that parents are part of the therapy process, from intake to end, in order to facilitate their ability to transfer what has been learned in Theraplay sessions into real-life situations. Furthermore, the child (Brish, 2022) needs consistent co-regulation in order to change their attachment style, and this needs to go beyond what the therapist can offer in a one-hour session once a week. As part of Theraplay, activities are given to parents to do at home on their own when they and their child are in a position to do so.

If a parent's symptoms are significant and they need their own help in order to consistently and predictably do the activities at home, the Theraplay therapist should hold off on prescribing this "homework." Instead, they can increase the frequency of parent-only sessions (standard frequency is once every three dyadic sessions) to once every two dyadic sessions or even sooner. During the parent-only sessions, the therapist should practice the activities with the parent, process how the parent feels during the activities, and address any attachment-related trauma memories that the parent has as a result of playing the activities (Lender, 2023). For example, a parent may be overly competitive because they were severely shamed as a child. Therefore, in a simple activity like the basket toss with their child, they get stressed and therefore critical and controlling when their child "makes a mistake" and doesn't throw the ball on the "right" cue word. The therapist would then explore and support the parent in how they were parented during similar situations. The therapist would demonstrate compassion and empathy for the parent's own experience and then encourage them to separate their own reactions from what is going on with their child in the "here and now."

The Core Elements of Theraplay

Theraplay is one of the few play therapies that helps clients process procedurally learned implicit memories. According to Fisher (2017), procedural memory encodes survival habits such as avoiding eye contact, withdrawing when approached, dislike of physical contact, and not asking for help when distressed. These are often learned within the early attachment relationship and as a result are preverbal and not accessible to consciousness. These may not necessarily be directly related to an abusive traumatic event, though they might be. They are very often learned as a result of the day-in, day-out subtle interactions with a caregiver who may be misattuned, depressed, frightened, or frightening.

Perhaps because of a parent's weak attunement or inability or unwillingness to co-regulate, the child's implicit relational knowing assumes their parent is not a source of safety and connection.

Theraplay specifically processes these implicit procedurally learned memories through a series of interactive, playful, face-to-face activities. Although these activities are fun, fun is not the goal. Theraplay creates interpersonal experiences that are noncongruent with a child's insecure internal working model. This challenges their brain to develop new, healthier implicit relational knowledge of what it is like to be in a relationship with their caregiver. The child therefore also begins to learn what it is like to be in connected relationships more generally. Theraplay also supports caregivers to meet their child's needs by lending their whole self to their child. This, in turn, helps the child modulate and organize their experiences with and expectations of trusted others. Through repeated, predictable patterns of play, a child learns, perhaps for the first time, to interact with their parent in a trusting way. This helps activate and strengthen the connection between parent and child. The relationship between the parent and child no longer triggers disorganized attachment. As a result, the child does not dissociate into fragmented survival defenses and the child's nonconscious expectations of what happens when they interact with others is reset.

Because it is a right-brain, somatic, and nonverbal therapy, Theraplay does not have specific strategies to help process traumatic memories. If a child is still triggered by, for example, a certain phrase or color despite making good progress through Theraplay sessions—and by good progress, we mean that the child is much happier, has developed better relationships with caregivers, family, and peers, is more regulated, and is able to engage in school—then the child would need specific trauma-informed support to process their memories around the trigger. If the Theraplay therapist has this type of training, they can now start helping the child process those memories within the sessions. If not, the best course of action would be for Theraplay therapy to end and for the child to be referred to a trauma therapist who has specific training in therapies that can process this trauma, such as EMDR, somatic experiencing, or sensorimotor psychotherapy. Alternatively, the Theraplay therapist can work in parallel with a trauma therapist to help reduce the child's activation and to keep the child more regulated while they are processing trauma. If this were to happen the Theraplay therapist and the trauma therapist need to liaise on a regular basis.

The MIM analysis informs the therapist on how they are going to structure the treatment sessions in terms of the child's needs. The MIM is analyzed using the concept of the Four Dimensions of Theraplay, which are Structure, Engagement, Nurture, and Challenge. The Four Dimensions are one of the core concepts around which Theraplay is organized. These dimensions are based on the kind of interactions that a healthy parent provides for their infant in a secure attachment.

Structure is the element of good caregiving that forms the foundation for all the other dimensions. "Good enough" caregivers are trustworthy and predictable, and they help define and clarify the child's experience. The caregiver sets boundaries to ensure the child's safety and helps the child understand the world in which they live.

Children who have experienced trauma have also often been subject to structure that was overly rigid, nonexistent (in the case of neglect or poor parenting), or chaotic and inconsistent. This affects the child's ability to have an internal sense of stability in their environment as well a sense that relationships are predictable, safe, and consistent. Traumatized children will fight against structure, as they have learned to either cope on their own or do not trust adults to support them with an attuned, supportive, and consistent structure. The therapist's role is to introduce structure in a way that is fun and playful, but always consistent. This might mean that the therapist uses the same set of activities in every session to support the child. Although this may appear to be a very boring way of doing Theraplay when there are more than 160 activities to choose from, the great variety may be too much for the traumatized child to cope with, as it introduces too much inconsistency. As the child progresses in sessions, the therapist can introduce a little bit of variety with the introduction of one of a set of four new activities per session. A different one can be introduced per week, while all the other activities stay the same. This helps the child learn to tolerate new activities in small amounts within the safety of a well-established routine.

Engagement relates to the way the parent entices the child into connection using excitement, surprise, and stimulation in order to maintain maximal level of alertness and engagement. They also soothe and calm the child when necessary so that the child is again available for engagement. These efforts to engage the child are regulating and must be appropriate to the child's emotional state, developmental level, and needs. Regarding difficulties in the dimension of engagement, the therapist might observe the following behaviors: a child or parent avoiding eye contact, the inability of the parent and child to "get into sync" or sustain intersubjectivity or a play sequence. Social engagement is an essential component of communicating to the system that it is safe. Fisher (2017) encourages therapists to use their social engagement system at all times to support the client's social engagement system to come online through mirroring the therapist. Therapists must be able to keep their social engagement system activated even when the child or caregiver is hostile or rejecting them. In order to achieve this, the therapist needs to feel confident within themselves so they are not triggered by the child or caregiver.

Nurture is the warm, tender, soothing, calming, and comforting behavior that a parent provides for a child. The dimension of Nurture helps a child down-regulate when they dysregulate into hyperactivity. The consistent comforting and available presence of the adult over time helps the child develop the capacity to take over these functions for themself. Some caregivers find it difficult to offer gentle, warm, attuned nurturance to their child. Some children have suffered abuse, endured medical procedures, or have had frightened or frightening parents, and so do not feel comfortable with or comforted by this dimension of Theraplay. In this case, the therapist will structure sessions to help the child accept nurturing and to support the caregiver to provide appropriate nurturing for the child's needs.

The *Challenge* dimension consists of behaviors that caregivers engage in to stimulate development, encourage progress, set developmentally appropriate expectations, and take pleasure in the child's achievement. Experience with appropriate challenges gives the child a sense of mastery and develops realistic self-expectations. The child feels competence and has confidence. Some caregivers find it difficult to determine how to appropriately challenge children and how to provide positive reinforcement for their successes. Some children have had a number of difficulties and as a result have low self-esteem and low self-efficacy. Challenge is very important for traumatized children, as they often believe they have no worth or they are bad at their core. Challenge gives them an experiential opportunity to see that they are able to achieve amazing things and to experience the delight and pride of the therapist and caregivers, emotions with which they may have had little experience. It is very important for the therapist to guide the caregiver in the sessions when challenge activities are taking place, to help them react appropriately to their child's failed attempts and successes.

It is very common for a child to have needs that are greater in more than one of these four areas and lesser in others. If this is the case, the therapist will design sessions that take this into account. They will focus on areas where the child has needs, but also take into consideration the child's ability to tolerate these experiences.

The Child in Theraplay

Five-year-old Cleo and her mother, Nina, are in a Theraplay session. In the intake, Nina described Cleo as oppositional and controlling. At home, Nina feels frustrated that even simple requests such as "Don't play with the ball inside the house" are met with resistance. Nina stated feeling like her daughter is disobeying her on purpose.

In the session, Cleo is sitting on a cushion on the floor with her legs folded, facing the Theraplay practitioner. The practitioner asks warmly, "Did you bring all ten toes in your shoes today?" while gently putting her hand on Cleo's foot. Cleo frowns and pushes the Theraplay practitioner away with her legs. This is likely the result of an implicit memory that touch is not soothing, and so Cleo defends against this feeling by pushing the therapist away from her. Rather than tell her, "No, in here we don't kick," the practitioner takes Cleo's feet in her hands and says, "Boy, you've got strong legs! Wow! I bet you can't push me over with these legs, on the count of three!" The practitioner holds Cleo's feet in the palms of her hands, counts to three, and then, when Cleo pushes again, the practitioner rocks backward with a big "Ooohhh!" sound. When the practitioner sits back up, the look on Cleo's face has changed from unhappiness to proud delight.

What just happened here? The practitioner attuned to the child's bodily tension, offered a cooperative way of co-regulating the tension by creating a game of "push me over," and then came back up to reconnect with Cleo. This created an intersubjective moment for Cleo. Games like these, the hallmark of Theraplay, help reframe and organize a child's ambivalent feelings (*I am interested and wary at the same time*) into a moment of reciprocal play, giving the child an opportunity to experience themselves as strong and—most importantly—connected to a supportive adult, rather than as bad, rejected, and isolated from the adult. In this way, a Theraplay practitioner can give a child new meaning to being themselves in the context of a safe and pleasurable relationship as it occurs within the therapy session. Theraplay can challenge the child's—and the parent's—relational knowledge as it happens in real time within the session, and this is a powerful way to process trauma and dissociation (Fisher, 2017; Rothschild, 2017).

In the example of Cleo, the Theraplay activity was enough in and of itself to provide her with a positive experience, which her neurobiological system was able to embrace and process. There are some children who are very triggered by Theraplay. This will be discussed later in the chapter.

Working with Parents in Sessions

Working with parents where possible in Theraplay is crucial for the child's progress, as discussed earlier in the chapter. Caregivers are usually included in sessions, first to observe the therapist working with their child, so that the therapist can model how to regulate and attune to the child. As time goes by and the child becomes more regulated and the parent's skills develop through regular feedback sessions, the therapist can help guide the parent to regulate, understand, and attune to their child's needs themselves. This is empowering for caregivers and helps the child develop a secure attachment to their parents.

Let's go back to the case of Cleo. In a session with Cleo's mother, Nina, the Theraplay practitioner has cued up the video to show Nina the moment when Cleo kicked her foot and the practitioner turned it into a "push me over" game. The practitioner asks Nina a series of questions that promote parental self-reflection like: What might Cleo be feeling in this moment? Why do you think Cleo behaved the way she did? When Nina watches the video, she sees that the way the practitioner responded to Cleo's kicking changed Cleo's unhappy demeanor to one of pride and interest. Nina and the practitioner wonder aloud what the underlying reason was for Cleo to kick her feet to begin with. Nina's first thought is that Cleo wanted to be in charge, and because the practitioner, not she, had come up with the "counting toes" game, she opposed it. The practitioner that while that is one possibility, another possibility is that Cleo felt uneasy and weary of the practitioner's intentions, so she pushed away with her feet to get some distance and protect herself. Nina responds that she has never thought about Cleo's behavior in this way. Together, Nina and the practitioner reflect on why Cleo may feel mistrusting of playful, adult-led interactions. Nina reflects on the possible reasons for her daughter's behavior, as well as on the influence of the attuned structure and playful reframing the practitioner did, and becomes aware of how she can also respond to Cleo in a similar way at home when Cleo seems oppositional.

Ideally, parents are able to work together with the therapist to change their perceptions of their child's behavior and participate in Theraplay sessions in order to support their child. However, this is not always the case. Parents bring their own attachment histories and traumas to Theraplay sessions. Therapists need to be mindful of this and assess the caregiver's ability to participate in sessions in a way that promotes the child's mental health. The therapist also needs to be observant and to reflect on each session from the initial intake interview and throughout the course of therapy to determine whether or not the parent is an adequately positive force in the therapy.

Let's look at the case of Mary and Emily. Mary was the single parent of two boys and a girl. Mary confided that she was unable to hug Emily, her ten-year-old daughter. She was very comfortable hugging her sons, who were often boisterous and aggressive. Mary disclosed that Emily made her skin crawl. In the intake, Mary shared that she had been sexually abused as a child. All she could manage with Emily was to hold Emily's hand and keep as much physical distance between them as possible while doing this. Emily expressed feeling ugly and isolating herself from other kids during school playtimes, and it was posited that Mary's physical rejection of Emily was at the root of Emily's poor self-esteem and low self-confidence.

The therapist adapted the Theraplay sessions for this situation. She had weekly feedback sessions with Mary to support her with what was evoked for her in Theraplay sessions. She also started Theraplay sessions by having Mary sit as far away from her and Emily as the room allowed. Mary's only job was to observe. As the therapy progressed, Mary started to feel more comfortable and curious. She wanted to participate in the sessions too and join in the fun. She saw that the therapist was comfortable being physically close to Emily. By the time therapy was terminated, Mary felt very comfortable cuddling with and kissing Emily, which this little girl very much needed.

Mary was also able to process some of the sexual abuse memories through the Theraplay treatment process, as she realized that she saw herself as a little girl reflected in Emily. They were both quiet and compliant. Mary learned that these were not bad qualities that had caused her to be abused. Instead, these were just her qualities and the qualities of her little girl who needed to be cherished.

In this case, the therapist may have decided that working with them together in the same room would have been too triggering for both of them. This may have been the correct call to make if the therapy had not progressed in a positive forward direction. There are other cases when it would not be advisable to work with the parent and child together.

Nine-year-old Andrew's mother, Sheila, struggled with alcohol addiction. She was not able to stay sober for any length of time. She was a single parent, like Mary. Her ex-husband had been very violent toward her and their children, and as a result, he was not permitted to have contact with her or the children, by court order.

The initial interview and the MIM analysis provided enough information for the therapist to determine that Sheila was not able to work in a manner that would support Andrew's trauma processing and attachment needs. Sheila presented as "out of it" much of the time, sometimes slurring her words, sometimes having tangential thoughts and staring into space for brief periods of time. There was a possibly dissociated side to Sheila that came out periodically; she would make nasty, disparaging comments to Andrew about what he was doing in the MIM. For example, when Andrew briefly put the comb to his mouth during the "Adult and child comb each other's hair" task, Sheila barked, "Don't put the comb in your stinky mouth and then try to use it on me!" Andrew froze briefly and then jumped toward his mom with the comb in his hand, trying to touch it to her hair. She pulled away in disgust while Andrew laughed in an uncomfortable, high-pitched tone.

Sheila was not open to the feedback from the MIM, becoming defensive over any perceived criticism. The therapist felt that Sheila would not benefit from participating in Theraplay sessions at that time. Andrew, however, needed support with regulation, as his behavior was becoming more and more violent, and he was hurting his classmates.

Andrew had an experienced key adult who was assigned to him. Theraplay sessions focused on regulating him and supporting his key adult to do Theraplay activities with him in class when needed. While this intervention was not enough to help Andrew with the attachment trauma he had experienced or to help him process all of the physical trauma he had suffered, it did support him to be able to access more of his lessons and seek support when he was upset by his peers, instead of lashing out at them.

The case of Andrew and Sheila demonstrates why each case needs to be treated on an individual basis, and why it is so important to get a thorough background history, meet with caregivers, and complete the MIM assessment. Both the cases of Emily and Andrew demonstrate how therapy sessions need to be monitored and evaluated on an ongoing basis in order to determine how best to support the child and their caregivers where possible.

The Therapist in Theraplay

The cases of Cleo, Emily, and Andrew provide a glimpse into how key the therapist is in sessions and show that the therapist plays a big role in managing both the child and the caregiver. The therapist needs to be able to attune to their clients and facilitate the caregiver to develop this skill too. The therapist also needs to be able to co-regulate their child clients and possibly the parent clients too, and to use touch in a manner that is appropriate and that allows touch to communicate attunement and co-regulation for the child clients.

The ability to engage both the caregiver and child in these natural interactions that promote the child's ability to self-regulate are clearly important for a child's mental health. But it requires a therapist who is able to attune to the child's and caregiver's needs, feelings, and inner worlds. The therapist must be able to regulate their own nervous system—this is essential for Theraplay to be effective. For instance, a dysregulated, anxious therapist may appear frightened of the child and caregiver. The therapist may be tentative when interacting with a child who has dissociated into a fight response, and as a result, this may be more triggering for that fight part, as it may perceive that what the therapist is doing is threatening, since they are anxious about what they are attempting. An anxious therapist may cause caregivers to undermine them if they pick up the lack of confidence in the therapist.

We all bring our attachment histories with us into our practice as therapists. If we struggle to attune to others because we did not experience their trauma ourselves, this will impact the effectiveness of our sessions with highly traumatized children and caregivers. Our difficulties with attunement are likely to reinforce the misattuned experiences the child has already had with their caregivers and this will serve only to reinforce the disorganized attachment and heighten the resultant dissociative response.

If we are not comfortable with touch due to our own implicit memories of our experience of touch with our parents, we will communicate this to our child clients through our awkwardness, discomfort with closeness, or our desire to be overly tactile without taking into account how the child's nervous system may be feeling overwhelmed by this.

Theraplay more than most play therapies requires more of the therapist as a person. In psychodynamic play therapy, for instance, the therapy requires the therapist to be attuned and regulated, but the therapist also sits at a distance from the child, which supports the therapist to be able to feel more regulated and gives them more time to think. The Theraplay therapist who actively participates in sessions needs to be able to nonverbally regulate the child with their own regulated nervous system at all times throughout the therapy session.

Theraplay is a very rewarding therapy when it is used effectively, but it does require us to do our own work on our trauma and attachment histories as well as to understand the social and cultural environments that informed our early years in order for us to be effective in dealing with traumatized and dissociative children and their caregivers.

Levels of Integrative Work

Theraplay has always advocated for and promoted integration with other therapies in order for children to receive the most effective therapeutic support. The reason for this is that Theraplay has always been aware of the limitations within the model as well as the strengths. The goal of Theraplay therapists is always to support the child's growth and healing. There are some difficulties that can arise in Theraplay sessions, particularly when supporting highly traumatized children who are dissociating.

In order to manage this more effectively, Karen Andor (2023) adapted Janina Fisher's (2017) Trauma-Informed Stabilization Treatment (TIST), a therapeutic model specifically for working with dissociation in adults (based on the Structural Dissociation model and internal family systems therapy), to work with children in Theraplay sessions. Andor found the combination of Theraplay with TIST for children to be a very effective treatment for children who dissociate both within therapy sessions and at home and school. It can be used for children aged 4 and up.

The Structural Dissociation model developed by van der Hart et al. (2006) views the personality as naturally divided in all of us, but under the conditions of trauma, the part of the personality in the left hemisphere, which is responsible for functioning in daily life, is cut off from the survival defensive parts, which exist in the right hemisphere and are always anticipating danger (Fisher, 2017). These two parts function independently of each other (van der Hart et al., 2006; also please see Chapter 6). This is because the child developmentally does not have the skills needed to regulate overwhelming internal and relational experiences, which develop only from being appropriately cared for. The child will therefore have a part that is able to function in daily life and an emotional part based in their trauma. This is known as primary structural dissociation. Most of the children who attend Theraplay sessions have primary structural dissociation, as in Cleo's case. They respond very well to the Theraplay model, which tends to resolve this primary dissociation in a way that allows children to enjoy more functional relationships and be less triggered and more regulated in daily life.

However, when trauma is ongoing, as it pervades the fabric of daily life through interactions with frightened or frightening, misattuned, or abusive parents, the emotional part splits off into the survival defenses of fight, flight, freeze, or submit (van der Hart et al., 2006) and attachment cry (Fisher, 2017). This is characterized by a lack of cohesion and coordination between these systems, and as a result, each of these survival defenses takes on its own autonomous functioning in service of protecting the child from harm. This is termed "secondary structural dissociation." Tertiary structural dissociation is rarer (van der Hart et al., 2006) and occurs within the milieu of extreme ongoing abuse. This ultimately leads to a diagnosis of dissociative identity disorder and is characterized by survival defenses that have become more elaborated and autonomous and the formation of several parts that function in daily life. Dissociation is therefore on a continuum (van der Hart et al., 2006).

Andor adapted Janina Fisher's TIST model to work with secondary dissociation in children, but it can also be used for tertiary dissociation. Andor added in shame and control as additional dissociated emotional parts based on the work of psychologists Dan Hughes and Karlen Lyons-Ruth. Children tend to feel shame because of their difficulties with dissociation and not having had their attachment needs met appropriately. This can become an unconscious dissociated defense that protects the child from doing something "wrong" again. Children also tend to take control when they do not trust adults (Lyons-Ruth et al., 2006); this can become dissociative, with the part wanting to be in control at all times to protect the child.

The effect of all defenses needs to be lessened because they are destabilizing (Fisher, 2017; Rothschild, 2017; van der Hart et al., 2006) and impact the child's ability to cope in day-to-day life. Many of the techniques in Theraplay can be used together with TIST to help stabilize the dissociative child—for instance, the newspaper punch activity can be used to down-regulate the fight part if this part is activated and needs to punch. For this reason, this approach fits well with Theraplay, as will become clear in the case of Alfie, described later in this chapter. Only Theraplay therapists with trauma-informed training should do this kind of treatment.

Fisher (2017) argued that all therapeutic relationships trigger the attachment system, which in turn triggers the dissociated defensive system. Andor argued that Theraplay is even more triggering for children with secondary and tertiary dissociation, as not only does the child form an attachment to the therapist, as they would in any therapy, which triggers the defensive system, but also Theraplay is a therapeutic approach that specifically works on developing healthy attachment and includes the significant attachment figure in the therapy room. Without a specific approach to managing dissociation in therapy sessions, this results in the child decompensating and dissociating. TIST for children is one effective way to address this issue, as it offers the therapist and therefore the child and their caregivers not only an understanding of what is happening, but also, and more importantly, specific strategies to process this.

Here is an example: Alfie, who is eight years old, was not able to manage school, and as a result, he was being home-educated by his single mother, Victoria, who had been doing this since the COVID-19 lockdowns. Alfie would often refuse to go to school before the lockdowns, but Victoria was able to coax him in each morning. However, after the lockdowns, Alfie adamantly refused to go to school. Victoria, at her wits' end, sought out Theraplay for him. After her initial interview, where she talked about Alfie's history, Victoria attended the MIM assessment together with Alfie.

Alfie and Victoria interacted fairly well in the MIM assessment. There was eye contact and moments when they shared a laugh. As often happens in the MIM, Victoria did not prepare Alfie appropriately for the "leaving the room" task. She just said she would be back in a minute and left the room. Alfie busied himself during this time by pulling faces at the camera and laughing. Occasionally, he looked at the door to see if his mother would come back in again. When she returned, they happily played a game of thumb-wars together.

Alfie was on his best behavior during the MIM, showing a submissive state. Sometimes, Victoria found it difficult to keep a consistent structure, which Alfie's dissociated controlling part responded to by taking over the task from her. It was possible to see this was a controlling part because at no time did this part relinquish control, as would often happen if the child was in a more unified state.

Andor (2023) uses the MIM combined with her training in the TIST model to determine whether or not a child is dissociating (but other methods can be used); she also monitors the child in each session to determine if dissociation is occurring. Andor finds that when a child is dissociating into parts, the behavior of these parts is out of proportion to the situation; they are unable to be reasoned with and are extreme and persistent. It is very difficult to down-regulate them without somatic interventions such as those that Theraplay offers. If the child is not dissociating into parts but rather pushing limits, then the child is able to see reason, but they may refuse to engage with it. The behavior, not out of proportion or extreme in its intensity, typically has a clear cause that can easily be picked up by the therapist.

Before the sessions with Alfie and Victoria began, the therapist went through the MIM assessment with Victoria. It was agreed that Alfie would benefit from more support in terms of having consistent structure and that he would need more support whenever Victoria left him. Even though he appeared to cope well when she left him for a short period of time, he did feel anxious, and this may also have caused his issues with separation anxiety at school.

It is common for children to be quite compliant and curious when they first start Theraplay sessions, but this is certainly not always the case. Some children may enter the therapy room for the first time in a highly activated fight or flight state. Children who are in a submissive state may appear to enjoy the fun games and activities. They appear to like interacting with their caregiver and the therapist. They may also seem to benefit from having the attention from the therapist and their caregiver focused solely on them. This is the honeymoon phase, which is typically observed in the initial stages of Theraplay treatment. However, after a few sessions, other dissociated parts may be triggered as the attachment system starts to receive the healthy attunement and regulation it needs. This is when impasses in Theraplay are encountered.

The initial sessions appeared to be enjoyable experiences for Alfie and Victoria. Alfie responded well to having more structure, and at home, he was engaging more in his homeschooling, whereas before there had been some resistance. Victoria shared that she was trying out more structure at home and, having observed how the therapist was interacting with Alfie, was feeling more confident about it. She was feeling optimistic about the sessions and was very pleased with the progress Alfie was making.

Then, from what appeared to be out of the blue, Alfie started to decompensate in sessions. He refused to engage in one session, instead sitting under a table and crying. The therapist and Victoria tried to engage him by reassuring him, normalizing how he was feeling and playing a fun game of "keep up" with a balloon near him to signal that he was safe. Every now and then the therapist would allow the balloon to drift down near Alfie to allow him an opportunity to engage in the game if he wanted to. Instead, Alfie angrily shouted, "No!" and smacked the balloon away before retreating back under his table and crying.

Alfie's attachment needs had been met through the Theraplay sessions, and this had in turn had triggered his defensive system (this typically happens five to ten sessions into Theraplay). His flight state had driven him under the table, and when the balloon drifted near him, his defensive fight part had been triggered, which smacked the balloon away. Both parts were protecting him from being hurt, fearing that his attachment needs might not be adequately met.

Alfie eventually slithered out from under the table, lay on his back with his arms outstretched and cried out, "Mommy! Mommy! Mommy!" repeatedly. Victoria, feeling her son's desperation, responded immediately and went to him to pick him up and cuddle him. As soon as she neared him, Alfie kicked her viciously away. Victoria looked very uncertain and vacillated between moving toward Alfie and retreating out of harm's way. This caused Alfie to kick harder and cry out for her louder. The therapist felt for both Alfie and Victoria, caught in Alfie's ongoing disorganized attachment cycle. Victoria's frightened and uncertain behavior further exacerbated this cycle, as it communicated to Alfie's defensive system that she was a source of alarm. Alfie was in the throes of his fight and attachment cry parts trying to unsuccessfully manage his dysregulation, and at that point his prefrontal cortex was offline.

Why was this all happening now? Victoria had experienced domestic violence while she was pregnant with Alfie and for a few months after he was born, before she bravely made the decision to leave Alfie's father and parent Alfie on her own. Victoria disclosed that she had been physically assaulted on several occasions by her ex-partner, but that this had never happened in front of Alfie, and she also believed that Alfie was too young to remember anyway. The therapist explained to Victoria that Alfie was indeed too young to understand what was happening; however, he would have picked up the signals from her that she was upset, sad, anxious, and frightened, and this would have triggered his defensive system. The time after leaving her partner was also very stressful for Victoria, as she had nowhere to live. She'd had to find a women's shelter, where she shared accommodation with two other women and their children before finding her own place to live. This was a very stressful time for her; she had little support, and this too would have resulted in her being a frightened and frightening figure for Alfie at a time when his nervous system was too immature to process this properly.

This was now all coming to the fore in Theraplay sessions as Alfie's defenses were triggered by his developing closeness to the therapist and his mother. The therapist used TIST for children to explain to Alfie and Victoria what was happening. She used Andor's DIDDY parts doll[1] to demonstrate to Alfie which survival parts were protecting him and how. Using a narrative approach with the doll, the therapist explained to Alfie how the parts were being triggered in sessions and at home, where they were in his body, and what they were thinking and feeling. DIDDY is used to help bring the parts to life for the child in a sensitive and attuned manner. It is easier for children to see an external representation of their internal world rather than trying to imagine it and hold it in mind, especially when they have completely dissociated into a survival part. Both Alfie and Victoria felt immense relief; they immediately understood the model, and it made sense and offered hope to them.

The therapist then used Theraplay activities to help regulate Alfie's parts as they manifested themselves in sessions. For instance, in one session, Alfie triggered into both his attachment cry part and his fight state and jumped on his mother. He was trying to push her backward. Victoria responded with a cry of alarm and pain. She was concerned that she and Alfie would tip over backward and they would both be hurt, and the pressure of Alfie's body weight pressing down onto her crossed legs hurt her. She reprimanded Alfie, which only served to escalate his behavior. The therapist intervened using the "push me over, pull me up" game with Victoria and Alfie. The therapist engaged Alfie by saying she had a great idea for a game and quickly helped him step off his mother's legs and get into position to play the game. Alfie responded to this immediately—he understood at this stage that the therapist would help regulate his dissociated parts.

The therapist structured the game for Victoria and Alfie to make sure it was regulated and safe. At the same time, using Andor's DIDDY doll, she explained how Alfie's fight part needed to push his mother away while his attach cry part wanted to pull her close and cuddle with her. With time, Alfie started to become more regulated. Afterward, the therapist used the DIDDY doll to demonstrate how the parts were activated in Alfie's body. She showed him how the attach part was in his arms, wanting to pull his mom closer to him for a cuddle, and at the same time his fight part was in his arms and legs, which were pushing her away. She helped him to understand what was happening and to feel empathy and gratitude for how amazing these parts were at protecting him. The therapist did this by speaking to the parts in the doll and demonstrating that she was not scared of or anxious about them.

As his defensive parts down-regulated and his prefrontal cortex came back online, Alfie was able to articulate that he was anxious that his mother would not be able to protect him when he restarted school. Victoria and the therapist were able to explain step-by-step how Victoria would make sure that school would support Alfie better this time. He felt relaxed, heard, and understood, and he was able to snuggle into his mother's arms and receive the soothing, love, and comfort he so desperately needed and which his dissociated defensive system had been protecting him from getting.

It is important that when working with dissociation, the therapist promotes compassion and acceptance of the dissociated parts at a pace tolerable to the child. It takes time, repetition, and practice for the child to understand that the parts are trying to help and protect them rather than purposefully get them into trouble or make life difficult for them. The therapist models this by showing empathy toward and understanding of each part's function, and regulating each part through Theraplay activities to demonstrate that safety can be established. The therapist also models for the child that they are accepting of each part, and gives them similar attention. In this case, the therapist supported Alfie's attach and fight parts equally. All parts need to find safety in order for the child to heal from trauma, and integration requires that the parts be differentiated and understood individually before they can be linked to each other. This needs to be repeated for the client many times in order to alter their implicit procedural learning (Fisher, 2017).

By the end of therapy, Alfie was able to successfully and confidently return to school. He did not trigger into his dissociated defensive parts very often—only when he encountered a new and unfamiliar situation, and even then, he was able to quickly regulate himself or ask for support from his teachers or his mother. Victoria accessed her own therapy for the trauma she had experienced. This further contributed to the success of the therapy.

Conclusion

Theraplay is a therapeutic modality that has much to offer children who are traumatized and dissociated, especially when combined with Andor's TIST for children. Many therapies for children focus on analyzing the child's thoughts and psychological processes and work with narratives the child recalls of traumatic events. These therapies offer valuable support for children, but they often do not offer the opportunity to work with sequelae of trauma and dissociation as they play out in the therapy room in relation to the child's significant attachment figure.

Theraplay on its own, or combined with TIST for children for more severe cases, sets up a situation where the child is interacting with their attachment figure throughout the session and where healthy attachment is gently nurtured. It is within this milieu that the child's trauma manifests itself, as most trauma stems from ruptures in our early attachment relationships, which are not repaired; from unintentional misattunement on the part of the caregiver; from frightened or frightening caregiver behaviors; or from the experience of abuse and neglect within those early attachment relationships. It is widely understood that with post-traumatic stress disorder, stimuli that remind the survivor unconsciously of the traumatic event will trigger trauma responses. So too do the day-to-day relationships within a child's life trigger implicit memories and subsequent trauma reactions, and implicit memory flashbacks and subsequent dissociative responses to cope with this. These are not necessarily narratives that can be recalled and processed somatically or cognitively only. These often need to be processed nonverbally and relationally within the child's relationship to their attachment figure(s).

Theraplay offers an opportunity to build healthy parent-child interactions and to develop parents' abilities to nurture, regulate, and attune to their children in order to appropriately meet their needs so that children do not need to carry the legacy of attachment trauma into their future lives as adults, suffering difficulties in their personal and work relationships and ultimately passing on this attachment trauma to their own children.

Note

1 See karenandor.com/diddy-doll.

References

Andor, K. (2023). *Training and workshops*. karenandor.com.
Booth, P. B., & Jernberg, A. M. (2010). *Theraplay: Helping parents and children build better relationships through attachment-based play*. John Wiley & Sons.
Brish, K. H. (2022). Attachment and dissociation. In V. Sinason & R. Potgieter Marks (Eds.), *Treating children with dissociative disorders: Attachment, trauma, theory and practice* (pp. 7–9). Routledge.
Fisher, J. (2017). *Healing the fragmented selves of trauma survivors: Overcoming internal self-alienation*. Routledge.
Lender, D. (2023). *Integrative attachment family therapy*. PESI Publishing.
Liotti, G. (2022). Infant attachment and dissociative psychopathology: An approach based on the evolutionary theory of multiple motivational systems. In V. Sinason & R. Potgieter Marks (Eds.), *Treating children with dissociative disorders: Attachment, trauma, theory and practice* (pp. 10–26). Routledge.

Lyons-Ruth, K., Dutra, L., Schuder, M., & Bianchi, I. (2006). From infant attachment disorganization to adult dissociation: Relational adaptations or traumatic experiences. *Psychiatric Clinics of North America, 29*(1), 63–86. https://doi.org/10.1016/j.psc.2005.10.011

Nijenhuis, E. (2017). Ten reasons for conceiving and classifying post-traumatic stress disorder as a dissociative disorder. *European Journal of Trauma and Dissociation, 1*(1), 47–61. https://doi.org/10.1016/j.ejtd.2017.01.001

Norris, V., Lender, D., & Booth, P. (2020). *Theraplay: The practitioner's guide*. Jessica Kingsley Publishers.

Rothschild, B. (2017). *The body remembers: Volume 2*. W. W. Norton.

Siegel, D. (1999). *The developing mind: Towards a neurobiology of interpersonal experience*. Guilford Press.

van der Hart, O., Nijenhuis, E., & Steele, K. (2006). *The haunted self: Structural dissociation and the treatment of chronic traumatization*. W. W. Norton.

30
A SYNERGETIC PLAY THERAPY APPROACH

Lisa Dion

Introduction

Synergetics, a word first coined by scientist Buckminster Fuller in 1975, is the study of systems in transformation, with an emphasis on overall system behavior that is unpredictably anticipated by the behavior of any individual components. The term itself beautifully reflects what is going on in the therapeutic relationship between the therapist and the child and how integration and healing take place.

As the therapist and child interact, a union of systems emerges as the therapist attunes to their own internal systems and subsequently to the child's internal systems. A synergy emerges from this connection, allowing for co-regulation. In this deeply connected interpersonal space, as the therapist and the child enter a "synergetic field" in which right hemisphere to right hemisphere communication arises, the child borrows the therapist's regulatory capacity, making it safer for the child to be able to move toward the difficult thoughts, feelings, and sensations they would not have been able to move toward as readily on their own. This process allows for integration and transformation of even the most complex trauma and dissociative patterns.

This chapter explores how Synergetic Play Therapy (SPT)'s tenets and philosophy can be used to help treat children with complex trauma and dissociation. A focus will be on the therapist's role as the child's external regulator for trauma integration using a non-directive approach. An exploration of dissociation as a homeostatic mechanism in the mind and a case study are also presented to support the understanding. In addition, several composite cases will be presented and discussed throughout the chapter.

Synergetic Play Therapy

SPT was first created in 2009. It is a research-informed model of play therapy bridging the therapeutic power of play with nervous system regulation, interpersonal neurobiology, physics, attachment theory, mindfulness, and therapist authenticity. Its primary play therapy influences are Child-Centered, experiential, and Gestalt theories. Although SPT is a model of play therapy, it is frequently referred to as a "way of being" with self and other, allowing its tenets to be applied to any model of play therapy or any model of play therapy being able to be applied to it. Its application as a model is both non-directive and directive (Dion, 2018; Simmons, 2020).

The overarching goals of SPT are to support the integration of the challenging thoughts, feelings, and sensations a child is holding, repatterning the protective patterns of activation of the autonomic nervous system, and to support the child in being able to attach to self (Dion, 2018; Simmons, 2020; Townsend et al., 2021). The concept of attaching to self will be explored later in this chapter, as it is an integral part of working with complex trauma and dissociation. To achieve these goals, a brief overview of how SPT views dissociation is offered, followed by an introduction to the model's nine primary tenets. Special attention to dissociation is woven throughout each of the tenets.

Dissociation

SPT looks at dissociative states as an adaptive strategy for self-preservation and protection existing across a continuum, but also as part of a homeostatic mechanism in the mind. In mild dissociation, the mind "zones out" or drifts off into daydreams. In more extreme cases, a feeling of not being real or out of one's own body (depersonalization) or switching into other protective personas that exist in other realities (self-state changes) can emerge. Whatever the case, the mind is attempting to deal with a perceived challenge, while both the mind and body are in an on-going process of attempting to achieve homeostasis.

Synergetic Play Therapy Tenets

The Child's Symptoms Are Understood as Expressions of the Activation of the Autonomic Nervous System

SPT recognizes that whatever the child's symptoms are, they are related to the conscious and unconscious perceptions the child is having or has had regarding their life experiences. When a threat or challenge is perceived, the mind and body quickly move into their protective responses to deal with the situation. In these moments, the autonomic nervous system is designed to rev up into a sympathetic fight or flight response to take on the challenge or shut down into a parasympathetic dorsal response, moving toward immobilization for protection (please see the chapter on polyvagal theory in this book for a more in-depth discussion on this process). During situations where the perception of the challenge is too great, the mind will dissociate as a way to put the individual in a state where they are able to feel separate from their thoughts, feelings, and sensations, thus creating a psychological escape when a physical escape is not possible. It is important to understand that dissociation can occur during all states of activation and is not just limited to a parasympathetic dorsal response. A blackout rage, as an example, is a form of dissociation that occurs during sympathetic arousal.

All expressions of the autonomic nervous system and patterns in the mind are viewed as the innate wisdom of the child, and therefore, no behavior is viewed as dysfunctional. Looking through the lens of nervous system, activation allows the therapist to recognize that the symptoms are the child's attempt to communicate how they are managing the thoughts, feelings, and sensations they are currently experiencing internally. In situations of complex trauma, a child may have adapted multiple protective strategies and responses, and therefore display a variety of symptoms of dysregulation, both in and out of the therapy sessions. It is also important to understand that as children play, tell their stories, and recall the experiences in their lives, they simultaneously activate the corresponding patterns of nervous system activation and protective patterns associated with the conscious and unconscious perceptions that are arising. In other words, a child's dysregulation will naturally emerge when unresolved memories and/or disowned parts are activated in the therapeutic process. This means that in session as the child plays, the child's dissociative patterns will emerge into the playroom, creating the opportunity for integration.

A Synergetic Play Therapy Approach

The Child Projects Their Inner World onto the Toys and the Therapist, Setting the Therapist up to Experience the Child's Perception of What It Feels Like to Be Them

When children enter the playroom, they set the stage for the possibility of the therapist becoming aware of what it feels like to be the child. Through their body language, words, actions, and play, the child engages with both the toys and the therapist, setting them up to experience what it feels like to be them. In the field of play therapy, it is understood that children project their inner worlds onto the toys. As an example, if a child holds the perception that they were trapped and scared with no escape and this is a primary challenge they are working through, the child may recreate play where a toy is trapped and scared in some way. SPT goes one step further to understand that this same projective process is happening with the therapist. For example, the child may attempt to trap the therapist, telling the therapist not to move or they will get hurt or creating a play scenario where the therapist is trapped in a room with a monster with no escape. The purpose of these interactions is for the therapist to be offered an opportunity to experience what it feels like to be trapped with no escape and thus understand the child's experience. This is true whether the therapist is an active participant in the play or is asked to observe the play. It is also true for all other emotions and experiences. The child will use whatever means necessary or available to set the toys and therapist up to feel anxious, not good enough, scared, overwhelmed, helpless, or whatever the challenge is that the child is attempting to work through. This "Set Up," as it is referred to in SPT, is not a manipulative process; rather, it is an "offering" of essential information between client and therapist.

In addition to the above, the discovery of mirror neurons in the 1990s at the University of Parma helped reveal that when people observe each other, their brains build a detailed simulation of what they are seeing, including the motor components. In these moments, the brain tries to feel what the other person is feeling, and it interprets what is being seen and heard as a shared experience with others (Iacoboni, 2008). The clinical significance of this is that when the therapist is listening, engaging in, or observing the child's play and stories, the therapist's body and mirror neurons are picking up on all of the child's nonverbal and verbal cues. These cues, which include the states of activation of the autonomic nervous system, influence the somatic shifts that occur inside the therapist and support the therapist to feel what it is like inside the child. In cases of dissociation, the therapist will also be set up to feel the dissociative tendencies. Karen Hoppenwasser refers to this phenomenon as "dissociative attunement," which can be further explored in her chapter in this book. This process occurs whether the therapist wants to feel the setup or not, as it is part of the resonance field and communication system that occurs between individuals.

As Iacoboni (2008) wrote:

Our mirror neurons fire when we see others expressing their emotions, as if we were making those facial expressions ourselves. By means of this firing, the neurons also send signals to emotional brain centers in the limbic system to make us feel what other people feel.

(p. 119)

The Therapist's Ability to Use Mindfulness to Attune to Themselves and the Child Is an Essential Component for Co-Regulation

In order for the therapist to attune to the child, they must be open to their own bodily and emotional states (Schore, 2019; Siegel, 2010). This requires mindfulness, which can be described as the ability to become aware of what is (Wolf & Serpa, 2015). When the therapist is not willing or is unable to feel the shifts that are occurring inside of themselves during the play, they will instinctively move away from those particular emotions or body sensations, denying their existence, shutting them down in some way, emotionally flooding, and even dissociating them from mindful awareness. In these moments, the therapist is unable to attune to the child and the child is potentially left feeling unsafe and unseen (Siegel, 2010). Dales and Jerry (2008) describe the importance of the therapist moving toward difficult and intense states in order to attune like this:

> Much like the mother who is implicitly modeling for the child her own struggles to regulate her own dysregulated state, the therapist must be able to resonate empathically with the clients, psychobiologically feeling their difficult, intense states. Without this ability to self-manage, the therapist cannot help the client to regulate.
>
> *(p. 300)*

Allan Schore (2019) also explains that the therapist's ability to pick up and attune to both the child's distress and negative emotional states, as well as their positive emotional states (Bullard, 2015; Schore, 2019), is necessary to regulate the child's arousal states. This means that for attunement to occur, therapists must be capable of mindfully feeling in their bodies the full range of what the child is feeling and move toward those internal experiences.

Attunement is also essential for titration, which means to continually adjust the balance. As children work through their challenges, they will naturally be in and out of their window of tolerance. The window of tolerance is described as the optimal zone of arousal that allows a person to integrate information (Ogden et al., 2006; Siegel, 1999). During play therapy sessions, both the therapist's and the child's windows of tolerance are changing moment to moment as they each respond to their inner and outer environments. Through mindful attunement, the therapist is able to recognize and respond to what is needed in the moment for both to stay within their capacity for integration. For children with complex trauma and dissociative tendencies, mindful attunement and titration are even more important as the child brings the challenging components of their experiences and protective patterns into the playroom. As the therapist and child relive the trauma together, the therapist's ability to titrate the intensity is paramount.

Attunement also allows the therapist to sense the child's emotional age, which is likely different from their chronological age in sessions. This level of mindful attunement is significant; in connecting to it, the therapist is better able to be present with the child in their regression as the child works through their challenges, allowing for more resonant responses and reflections on the part of the therapist. Tracking the absence of regression into younger emotional ages and states is also viewed as a demonstration that the child has integrated the challenge from their memory network to the present. Regression as part of dissociation will be explored later in this chapter, in the case study.

The Therapist Becomes the External Regulator Modeling and Co-Regulating the Child for Integration and Re-Patterning of the Autonomic Nervous System

Becoming the child's external regulator for trauma integration is the most important role of the therapist in SPT (Dion, 2018; Townsend et al., 2021). As the challenging thoughts, feelings, and sensations enter the play, precipitated by the child client, the attuned therapist opens up to the internal feelings and sensations arising and is then able to begin to modulate the intensity through the use of authentic dialogue describing cognitive, emotional, and sensorimotor states, along with modeling regulation of bodily sensations through breath and movement (Badenoch, 2008; Dion & Gray, 2014).

Because the mirror neuron system allows children to understand meaning and intention behind actions and learn via observation, prior neural programming and patterns of activation of the autonomic nervous system can be disrupted when the child observes the therapist regulating in the midst of the dysregulation that arises through the child's play and stories (Bandura, 1977; Heyes, 2009).

As the therapist mindfully and consciously feels the activation and moves toward the uncomfortable thoughts, feelings, and sensations, they model to the child that it's okay for them to also move toward their experiences instead of running away from them (Ogden et al., 2005, 2006; Siegel, 2010). What was once perceived as too much or too challenging can now be processed and integrated. For example, when the child sets the therapist up to feel trapped with no escape, the therapist's ability to mindfully regulate themselves in the intensity models to the child that it is okay to also move toward the intensity, for integration. It is at this point that the therapist can co-regulate with the child—the child in a sense borrows the therapist's regulatory capacity, which supports their ability to move toward their own challenging physical and emotional internal states, and shifting the need for dissociation, if that was their present strategy for managing the intensity. The result is that new brain connections can be formed, patterns of activation can be rewired, and new neural organization can be achieved (Edelman, 1987; Tyson, 2002; Dion & Gray, 2014).

In SPT, the metaphor of "rocking the baby" is often used to describe this process, as it mimics the dance that takes place between a caregiver and an infant as they move in and out of synchronicity, laying down an imprint for the child's ability to regulate (Dion, 2018).

The Therapist's Ability to Be Congruent and Authentic in Language and Nonverbal Signals Allows the Child to Feel Safe in the Relationship and Engage in Reflective Awareness

When a therapist is experiencing emotions such as grief, anger, fear, or anxiety in session and attempts to disguise their feelings in some way, the child is able to pick up on the therapist's nonverbal and verbal cues (Dion, 2018). In these moments, the cues are letting the child know that the therapist is being incongruent. As the brain is primed for tracking incongruence in the environment as a possible sign of lack of safety, it is essential that the therapist work toward developing congruence and authenticity in language and nonverbal signals. When a child's brain registers incongruence in the environment, the child will naturally focus on the incongruence to try and make sense of it, rather than engage in "reflective awareness," which can be understood as turning the mind's attention back on itself. The capacity for "reflective awareness" is an important component of the mind necessary for integration. In Carl Rogers', 1995 book, *A Way of Being*, he shares the importance of being authentic and congruent in the therapeutic relationship this way:

> The more the therapist is himself or herself in the relationship, putting up no professional front or personal facade, the greater the likelihood that the client will change and grow in a constructive manner. This means that the therapist is openly being the feelings and attitudes that are flowing within at the moment. The term *transparent* catches the flavor of this condition: the therapist makes himself or herself transparent to the client; the client can see right through what the therapist is in the relationship; the client experiences no holding back on the part of the therapist.
>
> *(p. 115)*

Authenticity is essential in teaching children how to regulate their nervous systems and rewire their brain activity (Dion & Gray, 2014; Townsend et al., 2021). When the child's mirror neuron system is activated, the therapist's mindfulness and authentic expression can trigger new brain activity that can become associated with the feelings in the neural nets of memories, ultimately helping rewire the child's neural network, as Badenoch (2008) and Siegel (1999) explain.

In SPT, authenticity is carried into the play itself. In addition to tracking the child's play using observational statements, the Synergetic Play therapist responds authentically to the child's own initiated play and stories as the child sets up the therapist to feel what it is like to be the child. This response is different from pretending in a role or acting. For example, a child uses a dragon puppet to pretend to bite and scare a small kitty puppet. As the therapist observes this play, they respond with observation statements such as, "The dragon is scaring the kitty." In addition, the therapist also provides a genuine and authentic response to the play, saying, "I feel scared that the kitty is not safe and might get hurt." In the example of the therapist being set up to feel trapped in a room with a monster, the therapist authentically responds with, "I am trapped and scared. I have no way to protect myself or escape." The therapist's ability to reflect within to make sense of their own inner experience and share it with the child is incredibly powerful, as it is often these types of statements that help the child feel *felt* and *known*. When the therapist tracks the play with observational statements and responds to the child's initiated play and stories in an authentic and congruent way, the child is able to see and hear themselves reflected back, providing an opportunity to engage in reflective awareness. This process supports the shifting of the child's attention from outside of themselves to looking within, as well as bringing the child into the present moment.

The Therapist Supports the Child in Integrating Their Perceptions of the Perceived Challenging Events and Thoughts in Their Lives

Children enter therapy with various perceptions about themselves and the challenging events that have occurred in their lives. These perceptions are both conscious and unconscious and become the drivers behind the child's behaviors, protective patterns, and view of themselves and the world. As children play out and share stories about their challenges, the therapist supports the child in making meaning of their experiences, thereby helping the child integrate their perceptions into a cohesive narrative and integrated view of the self.

As explored in the first tenet, the child's perceptions are also linked to their nervous system states and protective patterns. In therapy, as the child learns that it is safe to move toward their challenging thoughts, feelings, and sensations for integration, new beliefs and possibilities emerge within them. In situations where the child has developed a pattern of dissociation as a means for protection, they begin to recognize that the challenges that prompted the need to leave the present moment and disconnect from the intensity are now within their window of tolerance. As such, their nervous system activation and protective patterns also begin to shift. For example, a child who developed a protective strategy of dissociating each time she was physically hit by her grandmother comes to play therapy. Even though she no longer has contact with her grandmother, she still dissociates by zoning out and disconnecting from the present moment each time she hears her grandmother's name and her mind quickly recalls the painful memories. In her sessions, she recreates play scenes indicative of the painful experiences she had with her grandmother. As she does, the therapist co-regulates and titrates her through the intensity, helping her stay more mindfully present with herself. As her ability to stay present with the challenge increases, so do themes of safety and connection in her play, thereby shifting her perception of the intensity. The result is an increased sense of safety and a decrease in her need to zone out when her grandmother's name is mentioned.

The Therapist Supports the Child in Getting in Touch with Their Authentic Self—Who They Truly Are Rather Than Who They Think They Should Be

Children often enter therapy holding on to messages and beliefs about who they should be instead of who they are. These "shoulds" influence children's behavior patterns as they strive to be someone other than who they are, yet are not able to be successful in the attempt. This incongruence in their inner environment creates an inner conflict between their authentic self and the fantasies in their heads about who they "should" be. The result is activation of the autonomic nervous system as the child revs up into fight or flight or shuts down against their own internal beliefs. It can also result in patterns of dissociation when the pain of not being able to be authentic is too great.

In the play therapy process, the therapist becomes curious about what is most meaningful to the child, noticing what the child gravitates toward in the play and conversation. This also includes the therapist becoming curious about the child's identities and unique profile. In the therapy process, the therapist supports the child in becoming empowered within themselves to make their own choices, discover their own interests, and embody who they authentically are. The therapist also works to help the child's caregivers recognize their child's uniqueness and authenticity. The therapist understands that when a child has permission to be themselves, they have the highest probability of developing self-love and increased self-worth, leading to less dysregulation and activation, less need for dissociation, and an increase in purpose and sense of self.

An important consideration is that the concept of the self is complex, as it implies some experience of a unified sense of identity, which for some children with early trauma and complex trauma may have been compromised. When it is formed is a contested topic, in that some believe that the self already exists, while others believe the self develops over time after birth. What the self actually is also remains up for debate. Some describe the self as an innate essence or consciousness itself. Others believe that the experience of self is simply an experience of parts.

Whatever the beliefs, for many individuals, their experience of the self is described as a felt sense of inner connectedness, mindful awareness, and groundedness. From a physiological perspective, there seems to be less dysregulation, less inner brain noise, and a higher capacity for mindfulness when the self is being connected to. Being a complex area of study with many perspectives, it is an essential area to explore as the mental health field continues to deepen its understanding and appreciation for how healing occurs.

The Therapist Is the Most Important Toy in the Playroom

The most essential toy in the playroom is the therapist, as in SPT, toys and language are not required. The rest of the toys are secondary and are used to facilitate the children's perception of the challenging experiences they are processing, their relationship to themselves, and the relationship with the therapist. Toys are used in both non-directive and directive play. From an SPT perspective, toys can be anything the child uses to facilitate their process, and are not limited to the traditional Western idea of what a toy is. The specific toys used are also not the focus in SPT. The focus instead is on *how the child plays with the toys*, as this is what gives rise to the feelings and nervous system activation. For example, if a child is setting up the therapist to feel anxious or hypervigilant, the child might ask the therapist to sit on the floor while they build a tall block tower in front of them. Each time another block is added, the tower slightly wobbles with the possibility of crashing down on top of the therapist, creating the felt sense of anxiety, or the child might ask the therapist to sit quietly as they place a leaf on their legs, telling them it is a spider, again creating the felt sense of anxiety. In both scenarios, the main focus is the processing of the anxiety or hypervigilance, not the meaning of the blocks or the spiders.

It is also understood that without toys and language, healing through play is still possible, as the therapist and child co-regulate together in their interactions much like the way an attuned caregiver plays with an infant. Not relying on specific toys and spoken language allows SPT to be used with children whose words don't come easily, are nonverbal, or who speak a language different from that of the therapist.

The Synergy between the Therapist's Authenticity, Attunement, Congruence, and Nervous System Regulation Supports the Child in Learning How to Attach to Self, the Cornerstone of All Healing

The concept of attachment to self in SPT is a cornerstone understanding for integration and the ultimate goal for all children. It implies the ability to mindfully connect with the self in the midst of challenging thoughts, feelings, and sensations.

Helping a child find an internal sense of safety by attaching to self is key for integrating dissociation in children, as the trauma is able to integrate when the child can mindfully move toward the activation in their system and then move through it. For this reason, not only does SPT focus on helping the child attach to self, but also in many cases the work is focused on helping the child develop a unified sense of identity to attach to. This is incredibly significant for children with histories of complex trauma and dissociative tendencies, as they had to detach from themselves for survival and likely have a distorted sense of self or never learned how to attach to self in the first place.

From an SPT perspective, as children explore their challenges and experience the dysregulated activation inside of themselves, with the support of the therapist they simultaneously learn how to regulate through it, allowing them to be present in the activation without moving away from it. This ability to *be with* is the integrative force as the child learns how to access a sense of safety within. It is also from this place that a child learns to sense their own boundaries and window of tolerance, and how to titrate the intensity of their own experiences.

From this perspective, it is also understood that regulation does not mean being calm, but rather describes a process of connection. It is the ability to have a moment of mindful awareness and engage in ventral vagal activation to modulate the intensity of the activation of the sympathetic or dorsal parasympathetic protective responses. This ability to connect within and attach to self in the midst of the disturbance allows the child to adjust the intensity.

This same process of attaching to self is a core therapist skill in SPT training, recognizing that as the therapist enters the synergetic field with the child, they must be able to connect inward as they are asked to relive the child's trauma *together*. The therapist must be able to be in the felt sense of the child's world without getting lost in it. In SPT, this is described as the ability to be in it and not in it simultaneously, attuning to the realness of the play while knowing that it is the child's play and stories. Teresa Kestly (2014) defines it as the ability to monitor the felt sense (right hemisphere) while being able to track and maintain conscious awareness (left hemisphere). The ability of the therapist to attach to self creates the synergy for their authenticity, attunement, congruence, and nervous system regulation to support the child in feeling safe enough to come back into presence with themselves.

Recognizing that the therapist's ability to mindfully feel their own internal shifts and consciously modulate and adjust is a fundamental part of being able to co-regulate with their client, attention is given to strengthening the therapist's interoceptive sense during SPT training. The interoceptive system is the body-to-brain axis of signals and receptors that exist throughout the body, including internal organs, bones, muscles, and skin. These receptors send information to the brain, which uses it to determine how the body is doing and what needs to be adjusted to ensure homeostasis (Mahler, 2015; Tsakiris & De Preester, 2018). The concept of homeostasis will be elaborated on later in the chapter. As therapists learn how to feel, attune, and attach to themselves in the midst of their dysregulation, they simultaneously widen their capacity to hold both their own and the child's activation, creating safety for the child.

In summary, Badenoch (2011) beautifully describes the dance of interpersonal regulation like this:

> When the relationship is experienced as safe enough, dissociative experiences will begin to come into conscious awareness. As we resonate together, the activation will amplify and, if our

window of tolerance is broad enough to contain this energy and information, our patient will also experience a widening of his or her window. In the research of Carl Marci and Helen Reiss (2005), these moments of autonomic synchrony were subjectively experienced as empathetically rich interpersonal joining. This research showed that within the session, nervous systems flow into, out of, and back into synchrony many times. This rhythm is parallel to the dance of mother and infant as they move from attunement to rupture and back to repair over and over, laying the foundation for security and resilience.

(p. 195)

Dissociation as a Homeostatic Mechanism

Homeostasis can be defined as any self-regulating process by which systems attempt to maintain balance, equilibrium, and stability. This stability exists in a state of dynamic equilibrium, where built in regulatory systems continuously respond to conditions attempting to bring the system back to a state of stability ("Homeostasis," 2023).

The concept of homeostasis was first explored in 1849 by French physiologist Claude Bernard. Later, in 1963, physician Walter Cannon described in his book *The Wisdom of the Body* how the human body contains homeostatic mechanisms to help the body stay in maximum wellness. These homeostatic mechanisms include, but are not limited to, maintaining a steady level of temperature, water, salt, sugar, protein, fat, calcium, and oxygen contents of the blood. His work also included coining the term "fight or flight" to describe what happens in response to perceived threat, asserting that homeostasis also occurs within the body during times of trauma and psychological emergencies. Cannon (1963) asserted that the homeostasis occurring in the body does not happen by chance, but rather as the result of organized self-government.

Current research continues to illuminate the homeostatic mechanisms that exist throughout the body as well as in the brain as systems continually adapt to maintain stable and balanced dynamics. One example in the brain is how the neuronal networks in the brain self-organize toward excitation/inhibition balance (EI ratios) via changes in connectivity (Sukenik et al., 2021). Feedback systems seem to exist on all scales from the individual neurons to synapses to multiple neurons with synchronized entanglements of chemistry, electronics, photonics, and quantum entanglement throughout (Demartini, personal communication, May 10, 2023).

To understand how dissociation is part of homeostasis in the mind, it is helpful to explore physics, one of SPT's influences. There exists a symmetry law in quantum physics that doesn't allow for any isolated half-quantum states (one particle) without an anti-half-quantum state (an equal yet opposite mass and charge particle) somewhere else to balance it out. According to quantum physics, all phenomena are universally full quantum, meaning that nothing exists without its equal opposite ("Antiparticle," 2023; Demartini, 2022; Siegel, 2018). In his groundbreaking work, Dr. John Demartini, human behavior expert, demonstrates how the mind always maintains a full-quantum state by creating simultaneous conscious/unconscious splits, or, in physics terminology, simultaneous complementary pairs of positive and negative particles (Demartini, 2002). This discovery was further verified by the research of H. C. Barron et al. in 2016, when they discovered that at the same time a memory is created, an anti-memory is simultaneously created and stored unconsciously. In other words, as an individual perceives an experience, the mind splits the experience into positive and negative charges, where one stays conscious and the other goes unconscious as it filters information through the senses and associations with what is being perceived. To further understand, if a positive valence is given to an experience, the negative aspects of the experience go unconscious, or vice versa: if a negative valence is given to an experience, the positive aspects of the experience go unconscious. This conscious/unconscious split then drives the experience of emotions, activation of the autonomic nervous system, behaviors, and protective patterns, including dissociation. When a person perceives reality as not safe and too overwhelming, their brain will simultaneously create a counterbalanced virtual positive reality to hold the mind in homeostasis (Demartini, 2002, 2022). As an individual dissociates, where they go in their dissociative state is also not random. The content of their dissociation is the reciprocal or complementary opposite of what is being perceived in the individual's reality, also drawing from past associations. From this understanding, dissociation is not viewed solely as a survival mechanism to avoid pain, but rather also part of the mechanism designed to keep the mind in homeostasis and in a full-quantum state. This insight has the ability to offer new possibilities for integration and understanding on how to work with complex trauma and dissociation.

To explore this further, let's look at an example. Lauren, age 5, developed an imaginary friend named Tony. Her mother noticed that Tony had emerged a year prior to therapy, a few months after Lauren's father unexpectedly passed away. Lauren and her father were very close. They would spend a lot of time together playing and having what they called "adventures." These adventures would involve scavenger hunts in the backyard, building elaborate forts in the living room, and going on bike rides through their nearby forests. Lauren, an only child, viewed playtime with her dad as very important, and it was one of the things she perceived she most missed when he passed away. In the session, when Lauren introduced Tony to her therapist, she said that Tony was her best friend, and asked if they could all play in the sand tray together. During the play, Lauren (and Tony) would bury treasures in the sand tray and ask the therapist to find them. This example is significant, as it demonstrates Lauren's dissociative experience of creating an imaginary friend (positive charge) to fill the void of losing her father (negative charge). The characteristics of the imaginary friend were also the exact traits that she perceived to now be missing, and therefore were not random. In Lauren's mind, Tony was real, and when they played together, she didn't have to feel the pain of losing the playmate and "adventures" she had with her dad. We can see that the creation of her imaginary friend was the mind maintaining a full quantum state so that nothing was inherently missing, and the perceived pain of losing experiences with her father was counterbalanced by the positive experiences with her imaginary friend.

To tie this into SPT, we can also see that Lauren set up the therapist to feel what it was like to want to be connected to something she could no longer see. When the therapist was asked to find the buried treasures, they were also being asked to feel the longing of wanting to find something important while wondering if they were ever going to be able to find it. And to further heighten the feelings, as Lauren talked to Tony, the therapist felt the sadness and confusion of wanting to see and talk to someone who was there but couldn't be seen.

Maya's case is another example of how dissociation is a homeostatic mechanism in the mind. Maya's parents divorced when she was 6. By age 10, she primarily lived with her mother but would visit her dad occasionally on weekends. She was brought to therapy because her mother was concerned about some of her "strange" behaviors and language. Her mother would see Maya wandering around the house talking to herself but wasn't fully able to understand what Maya was saying. When Maya was asked who she was talking to, she shared with her mother that she was given an extraordinary gift: she could foresee people's deaths and could prevent their suffering. Maya also shared that it was the moon that gave her this gift and that she had been told she would be the greatest psychic on the planet.

During an SPT session, Maya created a play scenario where the therapist was told that they had to go hide in a corner. As the therapist hid, Maya turned off the lights, explaining that a scary man was yelling and they needed to be very, very quiet, so he didn't come after them. As they were hiding in the corner, the therapist noticed a change in Maya's body and eyes. Her eyes seemed to wander off as her body became incredibly still. Moments later, Maya turned the light on and proceeded to pull out the art supplies. Very quietly, she drew a picture of a girl walking freely in a meadow. The moon was in the sky illuminating a pathway for the girl to walk.

Without understanding how dissociation is a homeostatic mechanism of the mind and that the content within a dissociative state is not random, the connection between Maya's play and her drawing might easily be missed. In her play, Maya brought to life the negative charge, which was the felt sense of being trapped in the dark, hypervigilant while unable to predict whether they were going to get hurt, and fear of a scary man representing the masculine. In her drawing, she drew the counterbalanced positive charge (where she had gone in her dissociative state when her mind drifted in the play): the moon, representing the feminine, illuminated the dark sky, providing a feeling of safety. The little girl could freely walk through the meadow, not trapped, under the moonlight. With the pathway lit, she could predict the way out. It was later learned that she didn't like going to her dad's house because "he yells and is scary," and that often she would go hide in the dark in the bathroom, hoping he wouldn't come after her and yell at her. Maya was able to share that it was during one of these times that the moon granted her the psychic gift of being able to predict people's deaths so she could prevent their suffering.

From these two examples, we can see how the content of the dissociation was created to balance out the perception that was being experienced in reality. An important question for therapists to also explore is how the homeostatic mechanisms of the mind are also occurring during perceived positive experiences. According to quantum physics, the counterbalanced negative anti-memory must also exist in the mind.

Synergetic Play Therapy and Dissociation

As the therapist facilitates the child's play and dissociative states, it is not essential that they understand the details of what is occurring in the child's mind in order to facilitate the integration of their experiences. The therapist's primary role is to follow the tenets outlined in SPT to become the child's external regulator to help integrate the challenges, keeping in mind that as the child recalls their painful thoughts, feelings, and sensation, their protective patterns will naturally simultaneously arise. This means that for children who have dissociation as a strategy, the tendency to dissociate while they process their trauma is high and normal. It also means that as the attuned therapist is set up to feel what is happening inside of the child, the therapist will also sense the urge to dissociate. In the example of Maya, as the therapist co-regulated her in the sensation of feeling trapped and hypervigilant, they not only saw a shift in Maya's eyes and body but also felt an energetic shift within their own body, providing another clue that Maya had just dissociated.

It is also important to note that with the overarching goal of helping the child attach to themselves in the present moment, part of the focus must be on strengthening the child's interoceptive sense. Through both directive and non-directive strategies, the therapist scaffolds building the child's interoceptive awareness at a pace that is best for the child and allows the child to stay at the edge of their window of tolerance. Strategies include mindfulness practices, body checks/exploration, feeling games, sensory games, breathwork, artwork, the therapist's own naming of their inner experience, and bringing attention to a particular part of the body.

As the child's ability to safely sense what is happening inside of themselves increases, they increase their ability to stay more present and connected to their body. For children who have dissociative symptoms, this is an incredibly important part of treatment. As the child learns how to feel their sensations, access their own ventral state, and mindfully be with the intensity, the mind no longer needs to escape the present moment to find safety in a virtual reality.

Complex Trauma and Dissociation Case Study

Johnny, age 4, was brought to play therapy with a Synergetic Play therapist for concerns related to aggressive outbursts and animalistic behaviors such as growling and biting. During the intake, his mother shared that while pregnant with Johnny, she was in a domestic violence situation, often fearful for her own life and the life of her unborn baby. She reported that as a baby Johnny would look off into the distance, and sometimes it would be challenging to regain his attention. He was also described as often not easy to soothe. As he got older and became mobile, she described him crawling on the floor growling like an animal when he became agitated. She reported that his "growling and staring off into the distance behaviors" had continued to the present day. Following how a Synergetic Play therapist would begin to conceptualize this case, the therapist became curious about how early complex and developmental trauma might have affected his ability to regulate, contributing to the behaviors described by his mother. The therapist also became curious about Johnny's ability to regulate through the states of activation in his autonomic nervous system when agitated, supporting his ability to stay connected to himself and others in the present moment. The description of animal-like behaviors and "staring off into the distance" also created curiosity about the possibility of dissociation being a significant part of what was happening for Johnny.

During his first session, the therapist immediately noticed the hyper-aroused movements in his body as he moved from play scene to play scene with little ability to settle. Each scene was filled with themes of lack of safety and unpredictability with no spoken word, only hyper-aroused breathing patterns. As the therapist observed his movements and play, she began to tune into her own body, feeling a simultaneous quickening in her own system along with the fear and hypervigilance he was bringing to life and setting her up to experience alongside him.

As he brought his inner world to life, setting up the toys and her to feel how he was feeling, she began the process of becoming his external regulator to help him more easily move toward his challenging thoughts, feelings, and sensations. When he grabbed a young-looking boy puppet and shook it vigorously, she responded with, "The doll is being shaken and it looks like it is getting hurt." As Johnny continued to shake the doll, the therapist continued making observational statements to let him know she was understanding what he was trying to say. Noticing her own sympathetic arousal intensifying, she used her own mindful awareness to begin to regulate herself through deeper breaths and energetically anchoring her own body into the floor to stay grounded. As she held dual awareness of the activation of her ventral state in the midst of the sympathetic arousal, she created a neuroception of safety inside herself, allowing her to stay deeply present and connected to Johnny. These moments of "rocking the baby" were incredibly significant for integrating Johnny's early developmental trauma. As they co-regulated together, moving in and out of the intensity, he was able to begin to borrow her regulatory capacity to move toward the challenge for integration.

Johnny continued with the same play for a few more moments, and sensing that she was able to be present with him in the intensity, he quickly stopped and dropped to all fours. He began to growl, looking around the room for things to put into his mouth. Recognizing his need for something to be in his mouth, she quickly grabbed a soft stuffed animal to bring to him, knowing she could wash it later.

She understood that Johnny had just regressed to a much younger emotional age. She also understood that his embodiment of the animal-like behaviors was a key indicator that there was some level of dissociation occurring and that he was also responding from much more primitive and impulsive parts of his brain. During highly charged perceptions, that state can become, in a sense, frozen in time, and sometimes at several points in time. These frozen moments in time have embedded within them the beliefs, physiology, emotions, sensory data, and behavior responses taken in during the imprint experience (Shapiro, 2017). Age regression is a form of dissociation from the present as the individual returns to the stored state in an attempt to integrate it.

Dissociation in age regression also occurs on a continuum. For some, they may feel like themselves, but not feel the right age. In these moments, they may talk in a more childlike voice and behave in more childlike ways. Some may have a sense they have regressed, while others may not at all be aware they have regressed. In either case, the individual deviates from their "normal" developmental stage (Demartini, 2022).

In Johnny's case, when he dropped to all fours and began to growl, he went into a full dissociated regressed experience. From this, it can be understood that in his early development, he experienced a shock or perception of extreme pain. Although in the specific moment of the play the details of the content of his conscious/unconscious split were unknown, the therapist understood that somewhere in his mind he had stored the anti-memory to the pain and lack of safety he perceived in his reality. This is a significant moment in the therapy, as it is here that Johnny can integrate his perceptions of the pain and challenges he experienced as well as repattern his pattern of protection.

A few sessions later, during another moment of regression, he crawled up onto the couch and positioned himself behind the cushions, trying to get comfortable, but he couldn't. His agitated body was struggling to settle. A few seconds later, his body collapsed into stillness as he stared off into the distance, seemingly unable to move. The therapist quietly rocked back and forth reflecting, "I see you. I see you there. I am here and you are there." When he came back to the present moment, he crawled off the couch and crawled into her lap and for a few seconds she was able to literally "rock the baby," helping him repattern his ability to rest while in a feeling of safety.

Over the following sessions, each time Johnny's play intensified and his dissociated protective patterns arose, his therapist allowed herself to attune to herself so that she could attune to him and he could borrow her regulatory capacity, disrupting his neural network and bringing about the potential for repatterning his protective patterns. Over their sessions together, as he continued to sense her ability to attach to herself in the intensity, he allowed himself to go deeper and deeper into his trauma. In one particular session, he grabbed a dragon puppet and quickly moved toward her, having the dragon breathe fire all over her body, pretending to burn her. Moving toward the play, she authentically and congruently responded, "Ouch! My body is on fire. It is hurting. I am being hurt!" while simultaneously hugging herself, modeling attaching to herself in the midst of the intensity. Understanding that his mirror neuron system was tracking her and observing what she was modeling, she continued to work toward responding in authentic and congruent ways while modeling that it was safe to connect inward. As this continued, he intensified the play, moving the felt sense beyond fear and hypervigilance to terror. In SPT, if the intensity is too much for the therapist and their own protective patterns begin to emerge, they can set a boundary by acknowledging and redirecting the play into an expression that allows them to continue to stay present and connected. In this instance, the therapist was able to continue to stay present in the intensity.

In another instance, Johnny went over to the sand tray and began to pour the sand into containers. At one point, the sand spilled out of one of the containers, covering his hands, initiating another collapse and dissociative response. As the sand touched his skin, it was too much for his sensory and interoceptive system, and he emotionally flooded. As his body moved into stillness and his mind drifted away, his therapist stayed present with him, anchoring into her own ventral state, allowing some part of him to borrow her regulatory capacity to come back to the present moment. She observed his feet moving back and forth and followed his body's lead. "Left, right. Left, right," she quietly said, enhancing his own bilateral input for integration.

In each instance, she allowed his dissociative protective pattern to emerge as she gently helped him sense it was safe to return to the present moment and himself. Again, it is important to remember that his therapist didn't need to understand why this was happening or what the trauma was that dissociated him from his body in such a significant way. She only needed to stay attuned, mindfully present and connected to herself, while allowing his trauma to unfold.

As Johnny continued to work through his early trauma in the subsequent sessions, the therapist remained committed to being his external regulator and "rocking the baby." She noticed that his ability to settle increased. His dissociative protective pattern began to integrate, including his regression into animal-like behaviors, and the themes in his play moved from fear and hypervigilance to safety and comfort, indicators that his trauma was integrating. Other indicators that he was experiencing safety within and attaching to himself emerged as he began to seek out comfort by curling up next to her and gently making physical contact by touching her hair or arm. The same puppet that was used to chew on was later protected, soothed, and cared for in the play, and by the end of their journey together, Johnny was talking in full sentences and their time in session was spent making art together. Johnny had arrived back to himself and was now more fully anchored in the present moment and his chronological age.

The final piece of treatment was supporting his mother, as the therapist recognized his mother's own trauma history was impacting her ability to be his external regulator. Through coaching, joint play sessions, and having the therapist as her external regulator to help repattern her system, Johnny's mom was able to slowly also learn how to "rock the baby."

Conclusion

The therapist, becoming the external regulator, creates a neuroception of safety so the child is able to rock within the embrace of their ventral state, leading to faster and deeper transformation. It is the synergy of the therapist's authenticity, attunement, congruence, and nervous system regulation that supports the child to continue to safely move toward the thoughts, feelings, and sensations that prompted the need to disconnect from the present moment and create safety in a virtual reality. The end result is the ability to find safety in the present moment and in the body as the child's protective responses are repatterned and the child learns that it is okay to attach to themselves. This synergy also allows the tenets of SPT to be easily intertwined with other helpful healing modalities and theories.

References

Antiparticle. (2023, April 25). *Wikipedia.* en.wikipedia.org/wiki/Antiparticle

Badenoch, B. (2008). *Being a brain-wise therapist: A practical guide to interpersonal neurobiology.* W. W. Norton.

Badenoch, B. (2011). *The Brain-Savvy Therapist's Workbook: A companion to being a brain-wise therapist.* W. W. Norton.

Bandura, A. (1977). *Social learning theory.* Prentice Hall.

Barron, H. C., Vogels, T. P., Emir, U. E., Jbabdi, S., Dolan, R. J., & Behrens, T. E. J. (2016). Unmasking latent inhibitory connections in the human cortex to reveal dormant cortical memories. *Neuron, 90*(1), 191–203. cell.com/neuron/fulltext/S0896-6273(16)00168-9

Bullard, D. (2015). Allan Schore on the science of the art of psychotherapy. *Psychotherapy.net.* psychotherapy.net/interview/allan-schore-neuroscience-psychotherapy

Cannon, W. (1963). *The wisdom of the body.* W. W. Norton.

Dales, S., & Jerry, P. (2008). Attachment, affect regulation and mutual synchrony in adult psychotherapy. *American Journal of Psychotherapy, 62*(3), 283–312. https://doi.org/10.1176/appi.psychotherapy.2008.62.3.283

Demartini, J. (2002). *The breakthrough experience.* Hay House.

Demartini, J. (2022). *Prophecy I* [Class handout]. Demartini Institute.

Dion, L. (2018). *Aggression in play therapy: A neurobiological approach for integrating intensity.* W. W. Norton.

Dion, L., & Gray, K. (2014). Impact of therapist authentic expression on emotional tolerance in synergetic play therapy. *International Journal of Play Therapy, 23,* 55–67. https://doi.org/10.1037/a0035495

Edelman, G. M. (1987). *Neural Darwinism.* Basic Books.

Heyes, C. (2009). Evolution, development and intentional control of imitation. *Philosophical Transactions of the Royal Society B, 364*(1528), 2293–2298. https://doi.org/10.1098/rstb.2009.0049

Homeostasis. (2023). *In Encyclopedia britannica*. britannica.com/science/homeostasis.
Iacoboni, M. (2008). *Mirroring people: The new science of how we connect with others*. Farrar, Straus and Giroux.
Kestly, T. (2014). *The interpersonal neurobiology of play: Brain-building interventions for emotional well-being*. W. W. Norton.
Mahler, K. (2015). *Interoception: The 8th sensory system*. AAPC Publishing.
Marci, C. D., & Reiss, H. (2005). The clinical relevance of psychophysiology: Support for the psychobiology of empathy and psychodynamic process. *American Journal of Psychotherapy, 259*(3), 213–226. https://doi.org/10.1176/appi.psychotherapy.2005.59.3.213
Ogden, P., Minton, K., & Pain, C. (2006). *Trauma and the body: A sensorimotor approach to psychotherapy*. W. W. Norton.
Ogden, P., Pain, C., Minton, K., & Fisher, J. (2005). Including the body in mainstream psychotherapy for traumatized individuals. *Psychologist-Psychoanalyst, 25*(4), 19–24.
Rogers, C. (1995). *A way of being*. Mariner's Publishing.
Schore, A. N. (2019). *Right brain psychotherapy*. W. W. Norton.
Shapiro, F. (2017). *Eye movement desensitization and reprocessing (EMDR) therapy: Basic principles, protocols, and procedures*. Guilford Press.
Siegel, D. J. (1999). *The developing mind: How relationships and the brain interact to shape who we are*. Guilford Press.
Siegel, D. J. (2010). *The mindful therapist: A clinician's guide to mindsight and neural integration*. W. W. Norton.
Siegel, D. J. (2018). *Aware: The science and practice of presence*. TarcherPerigee Publishing.
Simmons, J. (2020). Moving toward regulation using synergetic play therapy. *Canadian Journal of Counselling and Psychotherapy, 54*(3), 242–258.
Sukenik, N., Vinogradov, O., Weinreb, E., & Moses, E. (2021). Neuronal circuits overcome imbalance in excitation and inhibition by adjusting connection numbers. *PNAS, 118*(12), Article e2018459118. https://doi.org/10.1073/pnas.2018459118
Townsend, B., Ishman, L., Dion, L., & Carnes-Holt, K. (2021). An examination of child-centered play therapy and synergetic play therapy. *Journal of Child and Adolescent Counseling, 7*(3), 193–206. https://doi.org/10.1080/23727810.2021.1964931
Tsakiris, M., & De Preester, H. (2018). *The interoceptive mind: From homeostasis to awareness*. Oxford Academic.
Tyson, P. (2002). The challenges of psychoanalytic developmental theory. *Journal of the American Psychoanalytic Association, 50*(1), 19–52. https://doi.org/10.1177/00030651020500011301
Wolf, C., & Serpa, G. (2015). *A clinician's guide to teaching mindfulness: The comprehensive session-by-session program for mental health professionals and health care providers*. New Harbinger Publications.

31
AN INTEGRATIVE AND PHASE-ORIENTED APPROACH TO SANDTRAY THERAPY

Ana M. Gómez and Marshall Lyles

Introduction

As we reach a greater understanding of the effects of chronic and complex traumatization on children's neurodevelopment and identity formation, the practice of sandtray therapy must also expand to meet the needs of this population. This chapter proposes and delineates a phase-oriented approach to treatment, encompassing the integration of models such as polyvagal theory, regulation theories, attachment theory, dissociation theory, information processing, interpersonal neurobiology (IPNB), and memory reconsolidation theory. Offering practical sandtray strategies guided by case conceptualization and intentional moment-to-moment decision-making, the following sections provide novel ways in which the sandtray process can kindle, invite, regulate, contain, and repattern the child's nervous system while also expanding their field of awareness. This chapter honors and actively embraces the historical influences and traditions of sandtray therapy while offering possibilities and expansions of how we deliver sandtray therapy to the children most impacted by trauma. This chapter also provides several composite cases that illustrate therapeutic strategies and clinical conceptualization.

History: The Past and Present of Sand-Based Therapies

Over the last 100 years, sandtray therapy has evolved to include diverse therapeutic approaches that utilize the same basic materials of sand, a tray, water, and miniature figures (Homeyer & Sweeney, 2023). Within the greater body of trauma-informed (Malchiodi, 2020), attachment-sensitive (Gil, 2014; Homeyer & Lyles, 2022; Lyles, 2021), expressive, and play-based approaches to healing, sandtray therapy is consistently discussed as a modality well-matched with trauma healing (Homeyer & Lyles, 2022).

In truth, the use of sand, symbols, and stories in healing rituals dates back to much earlier periods than the last 100 years of formalized use within professional therapy. Indigenous healers, throughout time and across multiple continents (Something Curated, 2021), have harnessed the power of these elements in rituals and ceremonies to address a variety of afflictions. Once psychotherapy was formalized as a profession, the origins of modern-day sandtray therapy developed within the context of World War I and worldwide trauma (Unwin & Hood-Williams, 1988). Dr. Margaret Lowenfeld, a pediatrician and pioneer in child psychotherapy who worked in relief aid in Poland after World War I (Dr Margaret Lowenfeld Trust, n.d.), returned to London and saw the same devastation in children's faces that she saw in adults during her post-war medical service overseas (Homeyer & Sweeney, 2023). Lowenfeld saw a need to bring the therapy to a developmentally appropriate level for children and established the Clinic for Nervous and Difficult Children in the late 1920s (Homeyer, n.d.).

Without the benefit of relational neuroscience data, Lowenfeld used observational skills to develop a platform for children's psycho-emotional healing that could tap into and support the integration of fragmented implicit memory networks (Badenoch, 2018; Grayson, 2022). Lowenfeld's primitive beginning with a few sensory toys blossomed into a well-established expressive approach to healing that empowers those with inner wounds to make new meaning of their experiences through metaphor-rich, concrete worlds (Unwin & Hood-Williams, 1988) and quickly began to spread into theory-specific applications like the much acclaimed Jungian approach of sandplay popularized by Dora Kalff (2003). Present-day sandtray therapists are extending this approach and establishing core competencies that will allow the work to develop for years to come (Homeyer & Stone, 2023).

Sand-Based Therapies Research

Research utilizing sand-based therapies shows promising results; however, studies on the subject matter do not specify the presence of PTSD, complex trauma, or dissociation. Multiple studies present quantitative and qualitative data supporting sandtray therapy's effectiveness (Flahive & Ray, 2007; Kern Popejoy et al., 2020). Creative methods and storytelling that include sandtray interventions have been documented as effective in resolving reported clinical symptoms (Desmond et al., 2015; Knoetze, 2013; Scaletti & Hocking, 2010). In addition, sandtray therapy has been used effectively as a cross-cultural therapeutic intervention that can bridge language and cultural differences. We hope this chapter ignites interest and mobilizes the field to address and study the best ways sand-based therapies can be implemented and delivered to support the healing of children most impacted by trauma.

An Integrative and Phase-Oriented Approach to Sandtray Therapy

Over the last two decades, multiple authors have proposed a variety of models for a phase-oriented approach, initially proposed by Pierre Janet (1859–1947), to the treatment of complex trauma (Courtois & Ford, 2013; van der Hart et al., 2019), which the International Society for the Study of Trauma and Dissociation (ISSTD) has established as a gold standard (2004, in press). Three phases have been recommended: phase one, dedicated to establishing safety, stabilization and capacity building; phase two, focused on integrating trauma memories, as well as tapping into multiple domains of integration (Siegel, 2020); and phase three, directed to the integration of states and identity in the emerging personality of the child. Though a phased-oriented approach is organized sequentially, we propose that the movement and advancements through the phases are dictated by the longings and rhythms of the child's embodied and relational mind. A circular instead of linear movement often occurs in children exposed to severe traumatization, where the child may return to the initial phases of treatment after a short visit to the trauma processing phase (Gomez, 2023). Each phase invites and touches the mind and the nervous system of both the child and the clinician in unique ways. As the clinician accompanies the child through multiple layers of the self, serving as a witness, companion, and external regulator, the child achieves sensorimotor and relational completions, as well as integration across the nine domains outlined by Siegel (2020).

Within the phases, a sandtray therapist benefits from the wisdom provided by multiple relational neuroscience theories that explore the needed components for moving toward neural integration. These include the polyvagal theory (Porges, 2011), which speaks to the connection between body and brain in the processing of safety and threat; interpersonal neurobiology (Siegel, 2020) and the neurosequential model of development, which provide a description of the ingredients needed for reestablishing vertical integration (Perry, 2014); Schore's (2019) and McGilchrist's (2009) teachings about accomplishing horizontal integration during trauma healing; Ecker's (2015) discussion of reconsolidating trauma-fractured memory networks; Shapiro's (2018) adaptive information model; and, finally, trauma-sensitive play therapy methodologies (Gil, 2016).

We take a comprehensive approach that unites the foundational theories and approaches to sandtray therapy while expanding with new developments and therapeutic tendencies. However, the connective tissue and organizing entity is the clinician's intentional mind that holds the knowledge, theories, and understandings while also holding space to receive data from the child and the intersubjective field. We place great emphasis on the clinician's capacities for mentalization, case conceptualization, and intentional moment-to-moment decision-making to organize all the models and hands-on strategies we propose. The clinician dances with the data emerging from the child's embodied mind, adapting to meet each moment's demands for safety. Even though the therapeutic process in sandtray therapy is more about *being* with the child than *doing*, the sandtray clinician holds a myriad of tangible and intangible therapeutic tools. They are utilized while guided by the clinician's capacity to hold the child's mind in mind, be interoceptive, and receive inner data while remaining connected to themselves and their nervous system. The therapeutic companionship invites moment-to-moment adjustments to meet the child in the places where corrections, repair, and completions are possible.

Phase 1: Safety and Stabilization for Children with Complex Trauma and Dissociation

Creating a Safe Space: Tangibles and Intangibles

Safety is a relational and biological imperative (Porges, 2021). The restoration of safety is a relational, sensory-based experience that invites social engagement and connection and is co-created throughout the therapeutic process and the three phases of treatment. Safety can be delicate and confusing for survivors of complex trauma and those with trauma-related dissociation. Therapists understand that clients need to feel safe in the physical spaces where therapy occurs as well as within the therapeutic relationship to find integration at multiple levels. However, nervous systems that have been repeatedly hurt in relationships often perceive safety as existing only in self-protective states such as fight, flight, or collapse. These complex views of safety must be well navigated by the sandtray therapist so that clients come to experience the healing potential of relational security in their own time (Badenoch, 2018; Dana, 2018).

One of the benefits of sandtray therapy for a client holding unprocessed trauma is that safety might be found in sandtray materials even before the client feels a sense of relational safety with the therapist (Badenoch, 2008; Homeyer & Lyles, 2022). This is due, in part, to the highly symbolic nature held by each of the sandtray therapy supplies that allow a client as much distance from the concrete realities of the wounding that they may require in order to make new meaning of the internalized pain. Additionally, working in a sand tray allows a client to maneuver between bottom-up and top-down neurological processes in the rhythm they find tolerable (Freedle, 2019).

Child clients need to test that both the room and the person of the therapist are equally competent containers for their pain (Gil, 2016), and they need space for playfulness and safe exploration (Leader, 2022). Victims of complex trauma often have varying sensory needs; some may desire sensory activation, while others may be more sensory avoidant. Additionally, some self-states may hold conflicting needs for activation and avoidance simultaneously. Sandtray office spaces need to allow

An Integrative and Phase-Oriented Approach to Sandtray Therapy

child clients empowerment through increasing or decreasing sensory stimulation as the work unfolds. They should also provide the space to hold the polarities of competing and diverging needs so these can enter consciousness.

An example of this type of dynamic work comes from Jack, a ten-year-old, who had been working through attempts at internalizing relational safety for several sessions. He would experiment with creating worlds in the sand that had fortified shelters, protective figures that were both strong and nurturing, and stories that tested the "realness" of how new figures might handle intrusions. At times, the content in the tray would become overly activating, and Jack would need to put on a cape and use his whole body to act out a stance of protection. He would sprint about the room and use "powers" to prevent danger from entering the story. Other times during work with these safety-themed trays, Jack would suddenly tire and need to rest under a blanket. The therapist offered sensory-rich transitions, like smelling an essential oil "potion" as Jack was ready to return to the tray, to gently provide an option for Jack to return to contact with his body. Jack needed to pendulate from his work in the sand tray to other parts of the room where his nervous system could demonstrate his body-mind reactions to the offering of safety. The room and therapist supported these swings, and Jack was eventually able to maintain longer contact with his created worlds and resulting physiological states (Figure 31.1).

Additional small trays, even homemade or inexpensively sourced ones, can offer the child with complex trauma and dissociation the freedom to move between a standard option, a smaller version, or grouping small trays for expansion. Additionally, having multiple trays can allow clients to pendulate between worlds of dramatically different tones as they experiment with widening their tolerance of affective material (Homeyer & Lyles, 2022). Kate, an eight-year-old, fell into a pattern

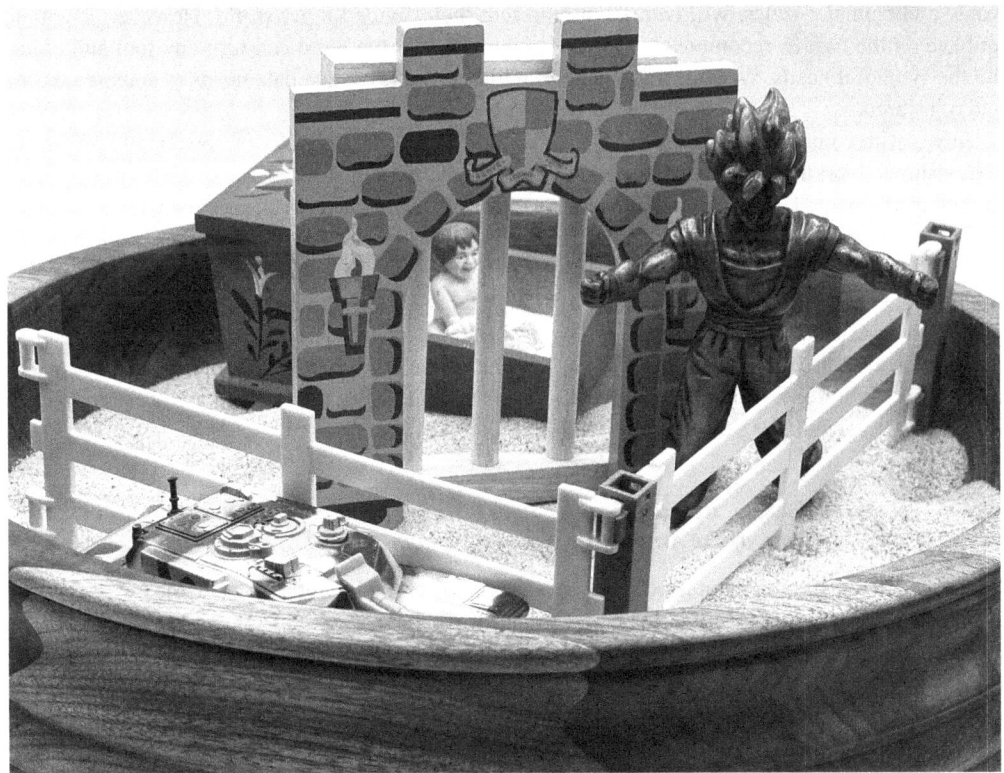

Figure 31.1 Jack: Baby Sheltered Behind a Fortified Wall with Many Levels of Protection in Front.

593

of creating elaborate and complex worlds in the traditionally sized rectangle tray. However, when the main character in the story encountered a difficult moment, that figure would need to momentarily leave the world and visit the heart-shaped or body-shaped tray. Kate would then construct a smaller world that could meet the character's needs in a tray congruent with the integration attempt, and the renewed character could return to the original story with a new state of mind. Kate used the different trays to safely experiment with creating new meanings, carrying that awareness back into the complexity.

A sandtray therapist's miniature collection often becomes a focal point in their developing sandtray practice. Some additional types of materials and figures can be helpful to traumatized clients. Cloth for covering trays that become too painful or dysregulating (some transparent or translucent and some opaque), container-type figures that can hold or hide other miniatures, and a variety of nesting dolls are just some items that can become specifically supportive to clients working through trauma narratives (Gomez, in press; Homeyer & Sweeney, 2023). Additionally, sandtray therapists must remember the tremendous importance of having a variety of shadow figures (Liu et al., 2021), as well as figures depicting grief, pain, and a wide range of human emotions as they support the expression and validation of the often terrifying imprints left in the child's inner world by trauma. Considering that children affected by trauma bring significant developmental deficits and unmet needs, the miniature collection should have abundant figures that support the child in meeting unmet needs, such as music boxes and musical instruments, food, baby bottles, small blankets, baby rattles, rocking chairs, ribbons and cords (to represent connection if needed), rubber bands (to hold figures together), binoculars (to titrate by zooming in or out or focus on a specific area of the tray). For children with an internal dissociative organization, figures depicting diversity within, such as three-dimensional people and animal puzzles, will help them represent their divided inner world. However, if you do not have all the figures recommended, please remember that the mind can turn any tool and object into the symbol it needs. We trust that the mind will find its way when data needs to emerge into the field of awareness.

Clients with complex trauma histories and symptoms of dissociation live a specifically protective relationship to working memory that is non-consciously functioning to divert experiences away from activating fragmented, wounded memories. The symbols in sandtray work create an anchor that allows clients to experience a sense of distance from charged implicit material as they work with the impact of these memories (Fleet, 2023; Gomez, 2019, in press). Traumatized clients are sensitized to pick up on the agendas of others. Even if a sandtray therapist's agenda is intended to encourage freedom for the client, those with histories of complex trauma can sense any agenda as increasing pressure and attempts at control, dynamics likely familiar in the formation of the trauma memories. The sandtray therapist needs to let go of expectations for how the work may unfold and what completed worlds may involve in the sand (Badenoch, 2022).

Stabilization, Resourcing, Capacity Building, and the Repatterning of the Autonomic Nervous System in the Tray

When working with children affected by chronic traumatization, the initial work in the tray is focused on building safety and capacities for connection, affect regulation, and tolerance. The rhythm in which the child moves along the initial phases of treatment is subjected to the pace established by the child, which can vary from session to session and even from moment to moment (Homeyer & Lyles, 2022). Initially, the tray is utilized to touch, contain, soothe, and work with the primary regulating system of the child and expand the boundaries of affect tolerance. Interoceptive and exteroceptive awareness-building is supported and often encouraged as the child engages with their own stories. The sand and miniature collection join in to become tools and "avatars" to the minds they touch and

An Integrative and Phase-Oriented Approach to Sandtray Therapy

invite (Gomez, 2019, in press). The clinician moves within a continuum of directive to non-directive approaches, making active invitations for world creations, offering moments of silent presence, utilizing reflective communication and mirroring, asking questions, and becoming curious as ways to expand meaning or bring information into the child's field of consciousness. The clinician as a co-regulator and co-organizer may pendulate and invite the child's embodied mind to move into or away from any emerging material, honoring the demands of the moment for correction, repair, witnessing, completions, or safety. The clinician also stays in awareness to observe their own inner callings and remains open to the field of possibilities that exist in the moment and the unknown. Spontaneously emerging, planned, and directive resources are invited and welcomed in the tray. If we look closely, most sand worlds have hidden implicit or explicit resources in need of connection to the conscious mind. Morgan, a ten-year-old, created a sandtray world colored by the shadows of an evil dragon that had trapped a princess. On the other side of the tray, a friend and supporter of the princess, Wonder Woman, had defeated a much larger dragon. In the middle, an eye lived inside a castle and witnessed the occurrences in the tray. The princess lived in complete hopelessness and powerlessness despite the triumph of her companion, Wonder Woman. Morgan had been severely bullied by her sibling and several children at school. She also had a very supportive family and friends in her neighborhood. However, she felt perpetually disempowered, alone, and helpless. The clinician supporting the expansion of meaning and integration, reflected on the polarities in the tray and the hidden treasures by wondering out loud if the eye could hold the two realities in the tray and the assets that the princess and Wonder Woman possessed. Eventually, Wonder Woman and the princess faced the dragon and won the battle. Morgan replaced the dragon with a much smaller figure (Figures 31.2 and 31.3).

Children have multiple ways of relating to their sand worlds (Homeyer & Sweeney, 2023; Rae, 2013). They may interact with characters and avatars while remaining in the refuge of the metaphor, or they can witness their own life story and observe what is emerging in their bodies as their nervous systems are kindled by their sand worlds. After observing and spending time with the moment of triumph in her story, Morgan, the ten-year-old in the case above, was invited to move from object to self and notice how it was for her to be a witness to her sand world. While stimulating interoceptive awareness, the clinician invited Morgan to connect to her body and watch what was happening or what the body wanted to say or do. Morgan grabbed a sword and began to run around the tray and the

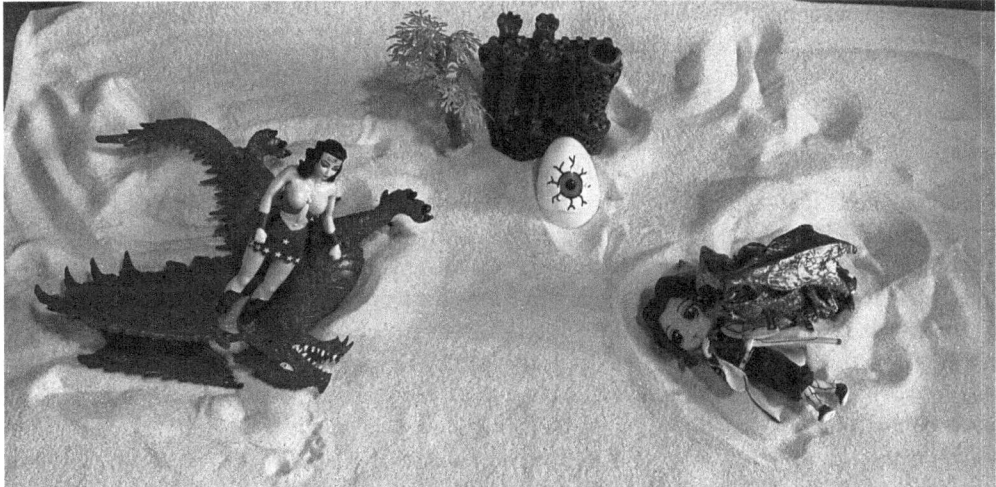

Figure 31.2 Morgan 1: Wonder Woman Defeated a Giant Dragon, and a Smaller Dragon Overpowers the Princess.

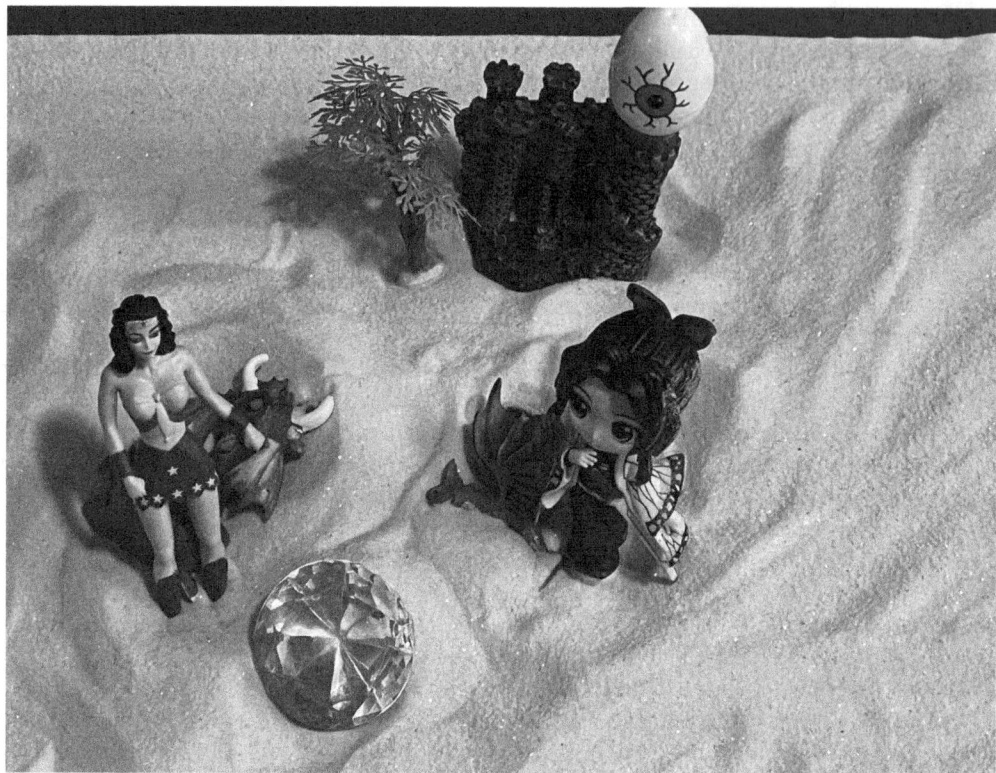

Figure 31.3 Morgan 2: The Princess, with the Help of Wonder Woman, Defeats the Evil Dragon.

playroom while yelling out loud that she was feeling powerful too, just like Wonder Woman and the princess. While remaining in the refuge of the metaphor, the child can still experience and receive the avatar's offerings as a witness (Gomez, in press). The avatar's triumphs and the resulting affective states begin to repair previously ruptured autonomic states. The child does not have to own the story told by the sand characters to receive its offerings.

Systemic and Dyadic Sandtray Work

The labor in the tray is often accompanied by active and parallel work with the caregiver, as the lives of these children exposed to chronic traumatization are often colored by impaired caregiving, parental trauma, and addictions that result in abandonment and abuse. Acts of commission and omission tinted their early life, and as such, the caregiver's involvement is paramount in their healing journeys. Sandtray therapists welcome caregivers into the sand work to exponentially impact the growth of reflective functioning within the child's system (Ensink et al., 2016; Gomez, 2013; Homeyer & Lyles, 2022; Lyles, 2021). Sand stories co-constructed by the parent and child may yield relational patterns that need healing. During the initial phases and throughout treatment, the clinician supports the restoration of the parent's role as the bigger and wiser co-regulator and co-organizer of the child's system. In these cases, treatment may be delivered by a team of clinicians to the child and the parent individually and systemically. Sandtray therapy can be effectively provided to adults with trauma histories (Kern Popejoy et al., 2020) and families (Lyles, 2020). If the parent needs and accepts individual sandtray therapy, there are many possibilities in which the parent can explore their relational tendencies, internal representations, meta-perceptions, and traumas that now become activated by their child, affecting their meaning-making and the resulting parental behaviors.

Children with complex trauma often have a depleted resource reservoir that needs fulfillment and nurturance. Inquiries or reflections that support the child and parent in finding the missing experiences and developmental ruptures of the "little hurt self" (Gomez, 2013; Wesselmann et al., 2018) initiate the recognition of the acts of omission and unmet needs. Dyadic interventions in the tray delivered by the caregiver and guided by the clinician that repair, validate, accompany, witness, protect, and mirror create opportunities for the child to experience the world, the caregivers, and themselves in new ways (Gomez, 2013, 2023). Titration is often necessary for the child who has become phobic of their longings. The sand characters and avatars serve as the vehicle for the child to gradually begin to experience the forces of connection, nurturance, protection, and regulation before they can be the direct recipients. Caregivers can speak to, sing lullabies to, rock, and hold the sand characters or the child themselves and their divided inner world in the tray and allow them to experience the love and resonance they never did before. The child's fractionated inner world now has the opportunity to be physicalized, witnessed, and felt as a whole through the eyes of the parent and the clinician. In the case of an institutionalized child with an absent or wounding caregiving system, the clinician's mind and the sand tray with all its companions serve as the vessel and the mirror in which the child can begin to see the self within the possibility for wholeness.

Phase 2: Integration of Trauma Memories

The movement from capacity building and stabilization into trauma processing and integration may happen organically and be more circular than linear in progression (Gomez, in press). The child may migrate from capacity building into accessing traumatogenic material and back into resource development and regulation in a nonlinear fashion. The embodied mind of the child will move in the direction of its callings, and as such, the use of a phase-oriented treatment is fluid and flexible. Memories of trauma may surface spontaneously without the therapist's direction (Homeyer & Lyles, 2022). Over time, the trauma may emerge with greater clarity while still hidden under the metaphor and the characters of the sand world. It is important to clarify that integration occurs at multiple domains and levels (Siegel, 2010) throughout the three phases.

After playing with fire, Sarah, a ten-year-old, burned her home, and her dog died. Due to her parents' drug addiction and frequent physical abuse, Sarah was removed from her home and placed in foster care. During therapy, Sarah created worlds in the sand depicting an alligator that killed anything and anyone who came in contact with her. She never acknowledged or talked about her life story or any emerging emotions. However, the alligator frequently expressed anger and the desire to destroy the world around her. Multiple trays often depicted the same acts of aggression and violence. One day, Sarah announced that she was no longer playing with the alligator; instead, she began to bring people into her sand stories. One of her sand worlds depicted a fire inside a house where two children and a dog were living. Parents were absent; however, Sarah brought a wizard who rescued all the children and their dog from the burning home. Despite the resemblance of the sand world to Sarah's life story, there was no ownership or acknowledgment yet. She made references to "the children" and the "fire" with no conscious involvement of the self in the tray. However, the protective barriers that grew out of survival in Sarah's mind were gradually eroding and becoming more permeable, allowing Sarah's inner story to become increasingly available to her conscious mind. Eventually, Sarah began to talk about the actual fire and her feelings, and the clinician invited the story to make itself visible to Sarah in the tray in any way it wanted to be seen and felt.

Sandtray therapy offers titration and a gradual entrance into material that otherwise would overwhelm the child's system. When processing trauma memories in the tray with conscious ownership and recognition, the inner system of parts needs to be involved in deciding when, how, and what will be processed in the tray (Steele et al., 2017). The inner system decides the memory they want to visit, how much and what parts of the experience they are ready to see, know, and interact with, and how the trauma story will be represented in the tray. Parts are invited into the tray in a way that honors them. Some parts or elements of memory may long to be seen, witnessed, and known in their totality, while others may want to be hidden under the sand, a tray covering, or under another figure (Gomez, in press).

When processing trauma in the tray, children can execute new actions that could not be performed during the traumatic event and complete truncated nervous system responses when ready. If a fight or flight response surfaces in the tray carried out by a character or the child, movement may be invited or supported when emerging organically; the clinician can also observe and track somatic reactions in both the character's body and the child's. The clinician dances with directive and non-directive approaches that support the repatterning and resetting of the nervous system stuck in the threat response cycle and the reconsolidation, assimilation, and integration of trauma memories. Additionally, vertical, horizontal, temporal, interpersonal, narrative, and state integration as well as integration of consciousness are at play, which portray healing as a journey instead of a task to accomplish and attain. Ecker and Bridges (2020) discussed integration through the lens of memory reconsolidation (MR). MR research brought forward the hopeful awareness that past emotional learning from wounded and fractured memories can be updated and reframed. After a target memory is safely and relationally awakened, and the internalized schema (emotional learning) is activated, a person can practice experiencing the old emotional learning while simultaneously witnessing a new possibility—another reality.

Children processing their traumas through sand worlds present in varied states and all of their creations contain therapeutic potential. Some may create intensely dynamic scenes, and others' sand worlds may be largely empty. Their narratives may be elaborate or nonexistent. Their emotional states could appear regulated, hyper-aroused, or hypo-aroused. The trauma-aware sand therapist does not "need" the client to create a particular world with a specific energy to see the value in every presentation. They meet the client and their needs in every emerging moment. For example, Charlie, age 11, struggled to work with themes of nurture and protection in his sand work for many sessions. His background as a child in foster care with multiple placements before adoptive parents offered permanency left him suspicious of recognizing and settling into relational safety. These early sessions brought a variety of emotional fireworks. However, as Charlie stabilized, his sand worlds featured stories closely matching his past experiences. He began to be able to sink into these stories with increasing connection and coherence and less emotion. Charlie let himself witness his past through these externalized images and narratives while introducing new possibilities and endings. The emotional lessons embedded in his created worlds now included new awareness and not just old learning.

Sandtray therapy welcomes the potential of integrating previously fragmented memories in an empowering manner. Children with complex trauma deserve to experience a therapist and therapeutic process that offer the gentle meeting of needs-lined memories that were formerly harmed, neglected, or exploited. As a series of worlds are made in sandtray sessions, these children get to pace their integration of these memories consistent with their unique presentations and abilities to unlearn and relearn what safe relationships can offer.

Working with Caregivers during the Processing Phase

Directive strategies can be used to invite the child in the parent's companionship to co-construct adverse life stories in the sand. The child can verbally and nonverbally process the experiences of abandonment, abuse, and loss. Through explicit storytelling or story-making, the caregiver can become an active companion in the tray. Implicit and explicit imprints left in the brain and the nervous system can now be accessed, allowing completion, integration, and social engagement. The implicit accessing of memories of trauma also holds the colors and gamut of past wounding experiences (Gomez, 2017). For example, the parent may help rescue a doggie from the hands of a monster or protect a baby in danger, allowing for relational repair and restorative experiences. Either way, the child's mind and nervous system are receiving the offerings of the story and acts of triumph. When the doggie completes a truncated defensive response and finds freedom, it is felt and experienced by the child's nervous system. Both the child and the caregiver may extend the movement beyond the vortex of the sand tray as they both run while holding the rescued doggie. Dissociative parts or ego states may show up in the tray, allowing the parent to display compassion, validation, nurturance, and love while under the clinician's guidance and companionship.

Phase 3: Integration of Identity

Attachment theory asserts that who humans think they are has been shaped by what key relationships taught them to be. Terrifying and/or unavailable caregivers unleash a torrent of necessary self-protective states in a developing child's nervous system. Living in these relationships and states of mind harmfully impacts identity development over time. However, when all parts of a traumatized nervous system feel permitted to stop functioning independently in self-protection and resume their cooperative and connected rhythms, a sense of belonging and positive identity development comes back online for children. This process comes in response to the experience of co-regulated and internalized safety and the healing of fragmented memory networks.

After the early phases of healing from complex trauma in children occur with the assistance of sandtray therapy, these clients often demonstrate a sense of empowered self-leadership in their remaining sand work. Identities rooted in an awareness of the innate possession of goodness and strength know how to explore and return for moments of nurturing in their created sand images and narratives. Seven-year-old Anika experienced early life medical trauma exacerbated by a neglectful home environment. She spent many sessions in sandtray therapy, creating disjointed worlds that were largely incoherent and defended before beginning to organically include safe resources. As this shift occurred, Anika demonstrated a capacity to recreate elements of her story, even preverbal elements, through metaphor. Her demeanor soothed and her body relaxed as she experimented with alternative and peaceful endings to worlds once dominated by struggle. One day, in response to a world she created about a wounded unicorn who was abandoned and rescued and who grew into a leader of the unicorns, Anika declared, "I think I have magic just like the unicorns!" (Figure 31.4).

When fragmented memories find integration, a child has a solid base for exploring a sense of self in a more integrated manner. In the sandtray, this is often reflected in the spontaneous inclusion of resilient elements in the created worlds: an injured figure gains access to a medical kit, a perilous river gets a bridge for safe crossing, or a perpetrator figure gets caged. While the previous phases of treatment may have found these elements included, this might have required processing and the therapist's support. The identity integration phase may see these developments as spontaneous and less cumbersome steps a child makes of their own volition. Parts that had remained trapped in trauma time now show greater temporal orientation, as they are finally free from the burden of being custodians of their painful stories. These parts are now free to join in the tapestry of a unified self. However, integration would occur in diverse and unique ways for each child.

Working with Caregivers during the Integration of Identity Phase

From an attachment theory perspective, when caregivers support this process, children most easily root in a secure identity. This means that caregivers of children with complex trauma must make room within themselves to see their children in light of their healing identities and not just the wounded

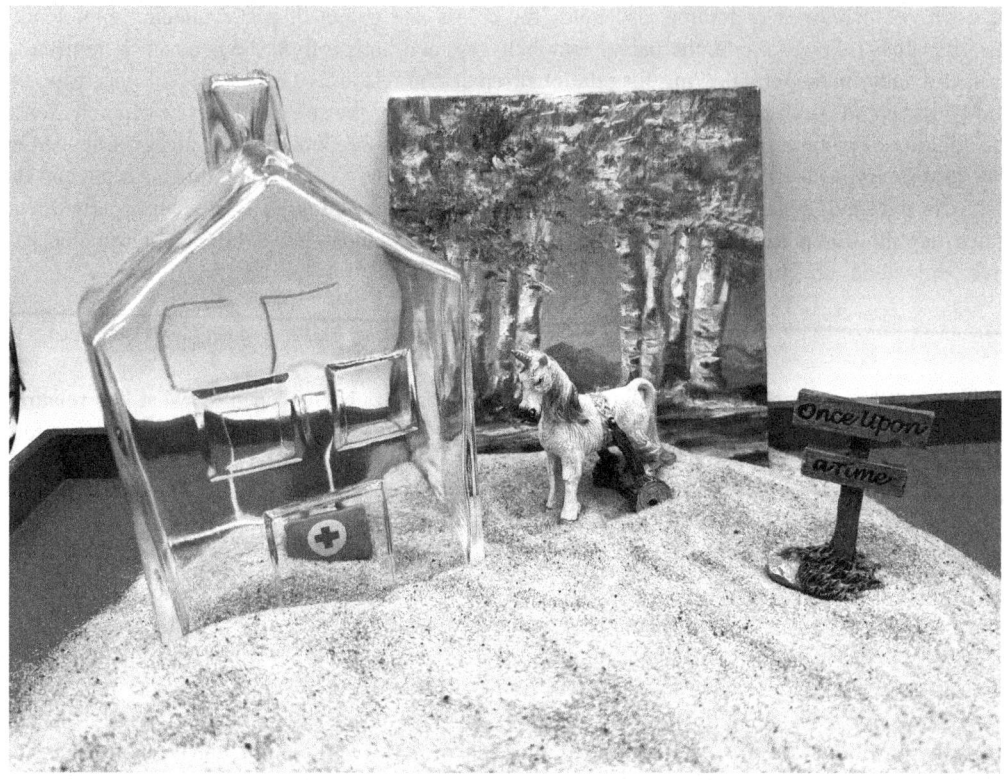

Figure 31.4 Anika: Unicorn in Medical Recovery Stands in Forest Ready to Tell Their Magical Story.

ones. Caregivers safely included in their children's sandtray work help scaffold children toward new meaning-making while internalizing their concrete markers of children's internal movements. Trauma-formed patterns of autonomic activation held by a dissociative part begin to release the rigid walls holding on to high mobilization, dorsal collapse, and several other states. They are finally liberated from the prisons imposed by trauma. The divisions in autobiographical memory begin to dissolve as the sense of a unified self emerges. However, integration represents a unique combination and recipe for each human mind. For many children, renegotiating their identities will be a lifelong journey that may require new work to reattune to the self. The self will be redefined repeatedly throughout development, and through these voyages, the work in the sand tray will continue to be a faithful companion (Gomez, in press).

Advanced Tray Exploration and Processing in Children with Complex Traumatization

Sandtray Therapy for Treating Dissociative Children

When working with children affected by chronic traumatization, the work in the tray should be part of a comprehensive and ongoing assessment of dissociation throughout the three phases of treatment. While there are potentially helpful standardized instruments available, the presence of dissociation can emerge at any moment, especially as children start to explore aspects of their story that approach their wounded and well-protected inner dissociative structure. Even if a formal assessment revealed no chronic dissociation patterns during an early phase of treatment, this does not indicate that dissociation would never manifest during sandtray sessions. An attuned sandtray therapist will remain aware of all streams of data provided by the child and welcomes any dissociation with the attuned care the child deserves.

Dissociative processes, whether mild, moderate, or severe, surface in the sand worlds and the child's nonverbal and body-based communication. The inner world of dissociative children is often nuanced with radical polarizations, fragmentations, and differential accessibility to autobiographical memory (Putnam, 1997). The child's capacity to integrate affective and body-based data with stimuli generated from their external world has been diminished by occurrences of chronic traumatization (Hill, 2015). Sandtray play provides a safe space for the child's mind to express and connect with internally and externally generated data even in the presence of trauma-related phobias, such as those of memories, emotions, and ultimately their inner world. The play in the sand invites the interoceptive and proprioceptive systems to restore the coherence ruptured by trauma, while providing refuge through distance and containment.

Sandtray work provides distance from what otherwise may be consuming and overwhelming (Homeyer & Lyles, 2022) and embraces the full dissociative spectrum, from mild to moderate to severe. It offers the dissociative child sensory stimulation, regulation, presence, storytelling, and connection to the body through movement in multiple forms. Children who create worlds in the sand that contain pockets of dissociation may lose awareness of their body (for example, becoming very still or spilling sand), lose access to speech and provide little or no narrative, or show surprise at the time remaining in a session. Each presentation allows the attuned sandtray therapist to become a reliable co-organizer of chaotic implicit material. These moments are less about having novel sandtray tools or techniques and instead can be compassionately met through a soft, strong presence, humility about the ease of ruptures in these moments, and gently paced reflections.

For children on the more severe side of the dissociative spectrum, the sand tray and the miniatures offer a refuge, a safe space, and a channel of expression to the compartmentalized system. Dissociative parts may make a full and explicit entrance into the tray, where there is acknowledgment and recognition of such parts, or they may enter quietly and implicitly, hidden under the characters' costumes that give an entrance and a route into the outer world. At times, the energy and data emerging in the sand stories extend beyond the physical boundaries of the tray as the child moves from object to self to engage in sensory-based explorations and the execution of movements that the body longs to complete.

Children presenting with dissociative tendencies and symptoms may become immersed and absorbed in fantasy as a coping method. They may not have had adequate experiences that allow them to develop a clear line between real and pretend. However, the clinician and sandtray work in the therapeutic session provide the bio-emotional regulation that helps the child's nervous system stay grounded in the present safety, preventing absorption and immersive trauma-based states. This will ultimately allow the child to interact with their own stories while held by the clinician's engagement system. In addition, the play in the sand tray embraces the subjectivities of the child's mind and uses one of the correctives to dissociation: curiosity (Gomez, 2019). The clinician's reflective and curious mind actively accompanies the child, gently promoting the movement toward realization, integration, and expansion of awareness. Through amplifying metaphors without a push for interpretation (Gil, 2014), children get to experiment with multiple possible meanings and states of mind and practice curiosity without threat. Curiosity allows for holding more than one meaning at a time and for practicing response flexibility. Sandtray therapists bring into the therapeutic relationship their skills of mirroring (Fonagy et al., 2018), tracking, reflecting, and witnessing the organization of developing sand worlds. Combined with the attachment-sensitive skill of repairing ruptures from moments of misattunement in understanding the created worlds, clients are supported in becoming more reflective and less reactive (Dana, 2018). Holding a safe relational space, the clinician keeps the child's mind within its frontiers of tolerance while accessing ingrained incongruencies, trauma-based reenactments, and fantasies. The clinician utilizes the child's natural developmental capacities for play and later developed symbolism to access what otherwise would be intolerable to the child's system. In the safety of the relationship with the clinician and the caregiver, the child can move into knowing, feeling, and realizing their own story (somatic, emotional, cognitive and behavioral) while promoting interpersonal/intrapersonal synergy and neuro-affective growth.

Interpersonal rhythms and sustained resonance are challenging for dissociative children with chronically wounded relational needs. The sand tray's concrete tools and natural bi-hemispheric processes related to movement, sensation, imagery, and narrative allow this co-created dance to have the dimensionality necessary for presence, integration, and healing. Sandtray therapy allows for engagement through as much distance as necessary (Gomez, 2013, 2017), such as when a child represents an offender through an animal or inanimate object instead of a human figure. The sand tray gives room for the child to keep sharing their cognitive, sensory-based, and affective stories and to feel witnessed even when words are not available, such as when a young one stops verbally narrating their world of demonstrated cruelty while continuing to manipulate figures through burying, caging, or hiding. Sandtray work supports the ability to practice holding two things together in a concrete manner that can be developmentally complicated, especially for children whose developing minds have been impacted by ongoing trauma and dissociation. The tools organic to sandtray therapy can move to meet the changing developmental needs of a healing child's mind. However, these tools work best when held within an alive, flexible relational connection.

Dissociative Parts and Inner Relational Dynamics in the Tray

When we work with highly dissociative children, uncertainty and ambiguity are frequent visitors and companions. When the child plays with the sand tray and miniatures, they may show moments of disengagement or enter a trance-like, freeze, or collapse state. Their play may become rigid and trauma-focused (Gil, 2016). However, sandtray therapy's often dynamic process—touching the sand, moving around, going to the shelves to grab new figures—can keep the child engaged, present, and connected to their bodies. Movement and engagement with the sand and the figures can kindle the social engagement system. The presence of the ventral vagal circuit of the autonomic nervous system (ANS) can inhibit the neural pathways that promote mobilization and collapse responses (Porges, 2011), as play functions as a neural exercise that can down-regulate fight or flight states (Porges, 2021).

Self-states and parts exist on an integration-dissociation continuum, from emerging ego states that share co-consciousness to dissociative parts that coexist between dissociative walls and barriers (van der Hart & Dorahy, 2009). The compartmentalization of experience and identity represents the child's best attempt to survive; each part has a story to tell, and the sand tray becomes a safe and contained vessel to hold space for them. The child's inner system may be invited to unblend how they want to be witnessed into the tray. Fraser's dissociative table technique (1991) has been adapted to the work in the sand tray (Gomez, in press; Lyles, 2021; Monaco, 2021) as a directive protocol to access dissociative parts that are ready to be seen, acknowledged, and recognized. Beyond accessing the child's parts and exploring their shifting moment to moment, relational dynamics will also reveal the child's inner organization. A system holding high polarizations and inner conflict will exacerbate symptoms, so a way of increasing stability and balance is by addressing the inner conflict and their power differences (Steele et al., 2017). When parts surface implicitly, hidden under sand stories and characters, it may be challenging to know whether an ego state that does not signal division in the child's emerging personality or a dissociative part formed and compartmentalized due to trauma is surfacing. The therapist holds the overall clinical landscape, dissociation-specific data, and the child's history to provide context to the sand world's moment-to-moment emerging stories and characters. The clinician may gently invite interoceptive intelligence and curiosity about how the sand world and each character interact with the child's inner world.

When working with children with compartmentalized identities and a fragmented sense of the world, inviting resources that promote safety may bring significant challenges and dilemmas. One dissociative part may find safety where another part finds panic. The inner system and its differences and conflicts may be acknowledged when inviting the child to create directive resources in the tray. Gomez (2019, in press) suggested invitations to have "inside visits" and to "check inside agreements and disagreements," as well as to have "moments of curiosity" to dialogue with the inner system of parts before completing a sand world that is holding a resource. This is not only stimulating interoceptive awareness but increasing co-consciousness among parts. For instance, when creating a safe or happy place or a team of companions in the tray during the initial phase of treatment, the child is invited to engage with the "inside world" and the different sides of them when deciding on what figures to bring into the tray. Once the happy world is created, the inner system is consulted before deciding if it feels complete. Disagreements and dilemmas may be represented in the tray. As they enter the sand, they also enter the child's nervous system and field of awareness, even without any verbalizations. When working with non-directive and implicit worlds, the clinician can acknowledge that different parts of the child may have different feelings or reactions to what is unfolding and emerging in the tray (Gomez, 2019). When the inner system is ready to a direct travel through traumatic memories, the trauma may emerge in the sand spontaneously or as a result of an invitation from the clinician. The memory is encouraged to emerge in the sand in whatever way it chooses to be revealed and witnessed. It may appear hidden, covered, or fully open. Titration and distance, whether offered organically by the sand story or intentionally tendered by the clinician, are intricately woven throughout treatment. Hence, information enters the embodied mind of the child at a rhythm and pace that supports integration and repair. The inner configuration of parts may appear disorganized to their witnesses, yet it holds internal consistency and structure that has significance and function for each child. With permission, the therapist enters the road into exploring the inner system in the tray with humility and respect.

Nervous System States in Sandtray Work

Multiple manifestations of the nervous system will surface in the tray throughout the different phases of treatment. The nervous system will make its presence known gently or rowdily in the tray. It may seek refuge, safety, and the expansion of its capacities during the initial phases of treatment, or it may seek the completion and execution of a truncated defense response during the processing phases. Nevertheless, the nervous system travels circularly throughout the phases, seeking wholeness, integration, homeostasis and regulation.

When focusing on the material inside a created sand world, the complex trauma-sensitive therapist will hold in mind that both explicit and implicit material is revealed through the chosen metaphors. These metaphors exist in individual miniatures, but even more complex metaphors are alive in the space between these figures. For example, 11-year-old Mark may choose chickens, a chicken coop, and a wolf to place in a section of the sand tray. Each piece has metaphoric potential. The metaphor becomes more enlivened as the wolf is placed in a hiding spot behind the coop where the chickens cannot see it. It would reveal an entirely different metaphor and nervous system state if the chickens buried the wolf under their coop and they were celebrating in their safe home. However, miniatures alone are only one clue to a client's inner world, and co-creating meaning safely will include hearing the greater story of the figures and "listening" to the client's body.

The sandtray therapist invites a narrative for the sand world, which may or may not be something the client can or needs to share. When a story is told, important information for understanding the client's connection to their states of mind comes through the contextualization of the chosen miniatures and through the verbal and nonverbal language patterns accompanying each piece of the narrative. As exemplified by the Adult Attachment Interview (AAI) (George et al., 1996), people's use of language shifts as their states of mind shift throughout sharing personal material. Mark's chickens may be sharing freely about their coop, and he could speak easily and coherently. Then, when the wolf is introduced into the story, Mark's language might shift. He could mix up verb tenses, start "forgetting" parts of the story, become emotional, or even stop talking. These are just a few examples of the many possibilities for attuning to the underlying states that are revealed through how a narrative is told. Again, the client remains in charge of how much they can notice, reveal, and receive. The sandtray therapist tracks, reflects, and asks questions congruent with the treatment phase and the client's receptivity and capacities.

Mark's connection to his own body is another source of information about his implicit world. Mark may become clumsy or hyper-focused as he selects and arranges the figures. Mark could be unaware of spilling sand from the tray or spend 30 minutes carefully sweeping away sand from one spot under the chicken coop. A client's connection to and use of their body offers critical information that supports possibilities for attunement and resonance.

Mark may have some explicit awareness of abstractly illustrated memories, or all of the work can be implicit. Clients can work with and heal complex trauma in sandtray therapy at either level. The sandtray therapist internally organizes what they are noticing and hearing in the trays that clients create (as well as in the client's bodily expressions) and assesses whether they are working to stabilize, integrate, or move forward through re-engagement with life. If Mark were in the stabilization phase, the sandtray therapist may notice the chosen miniatures and arrangement of that hiding wolf and reflect, "There is danger lurking, and the chickens do not seem to know. I wonder how we keep them safe." The therapist could also say, "It feels really scary to see unprotected chickens. I wonder if there is a protector figure that might be needed." If Mark were further into the phase of treatment and working on integration, the figures could be dynamically acting out violence and/or self-protection. The sandtray therapist may model big sighs and say something like, "I am noticing that my hands, and maybe even your hands, got tight when the wolf became aggressive!" In this phase, the therapist might add, "The chickens can say anything they want to the wolf in this tray when ready. You are in charge of this world." When working with a dissociative matrix or entrenched and polarized ego states, the clinician may acknowledge emerging differences and polarizations: "Sometimes we may feel and want different things to happen in the tray. One side may wish for the protection of the chickens, while another may want to support the wolf." For the client using these figures in a late phase of treatment, the therapist might add, "You have figured out how to tell this story in new ways! I wonder what the chickens need to do now."

Patterns of autonomic activation become evident and depicted in the worlds of children with complex trauma and symptoms of dissociation (Lyles & Homeyer, 2024). Mobilization and the participation of the rambunctious sympathetic system with its accompanying fight or flight responses make their entrance into the tray through battles and grievances among characters. Parts holding these defensive strategies may show up to tell their stories, offering an opportunity to witness and co-regulate previously ruptured autonomic states. With or without ownership, the child and clinician can dance with the energy emerging in the tray. The parasympathetic nervous system, with its various paradoxes and gamut of submission and collapse and the parts that hold them, enters sand stories with its slower pace and lower energy.

In some cases, the tone of the tray is completely overtaken by collapse, stagnation, and lack of movement. The tray as the mirror of the mind will often show, just like a kaleidoscope, the moment-to-moment changes occurring in the child's inner world (Gomez, in press). Through shared moments of coherence and mirroring, the forces of the ventral vagal system are brought into the tray, creating new opportunities to experience the self within the safety of a relationship with another. Invitations to represent and physicalize new connections, moments of expansion, and meaning-making will further support new internalizations in the child's representational system and the synaptic architecture of the child's mind. Autonomic activation patterns do not always show up in a linear and organized manner; instead, the process may be messy, as is our human existence. Sometimes, moments of realization and integration occur in quietness and stillness, while other times, they happen in the middle of chaos, noise, rambunctiousness, and disorderliness. However, as companions and witnesses, we remain present, at times in the unknown, ambiguity, and uncertainty. Our nervous systems are also influenced and attuned to the child's felt and experienced patterns of activation as we witness their rhythms in the tray. As we connect and pay attention to our embodied minds, our resonance circuits will touch and record our clients' actions, feelings, and intentions (Badenoch, 2008).

Amanda, a 12-year-old who spent her first five years in an orphanage, suffered severe neglect and abuse from her caregivers and orphanage workers. Amanda's recounts of her life were scattered, and the events of her days were fragmented and sometimes absent. Her initial trays were incredibly lonely, with very few figures and people. The pace of her voice was slow, and the characters and stories depicted in the tray were colored by a deep loneliness, shame, and fear. During one of her sessions, Amanda displayed a different energy, demeanor, and the world she created was distinct. The clinician curiously explored the tray, wondering aloud what was different this time. Amanda stated, "She is not playing in the tray today." Using reflective communication, expanding meaning, and promoting linkages and integration, the clinician stated, "I see there is a different side of you playing in the tray today. These two sides of you play and tell stories quite differently." Amanda nodded and stated that she (the other part) was very sad. One part of Amanda held her accounts of neglect, loneliness, and invisibility, while the other reflected her rambunctious, playful, and sometimes aggressive self. They both held different patterns of autonomic activation and were linked to different memory neural networks. They both created the space to hold pieces of the story that Amanda's conscious mind could not yet hold in its totality, all in the service of survival.

In sandtray therapy, the clinician accompanies the child through the nonverbal, affect-rich, brain-generated material and then makes invitations to the linear-verbal left brain (Badenoch, 2008). As co-organizer and co-creator of meaning, the clinician can gently lable or support the child in naming and representing the experience and data unfolding in the tray. In the case of Amanda, the clinician began to name the divisions not to fix them, but to bring them into the child's field of awareness so her mind could begin the process of assimilation and integration. As Amanda and her therapist co-constructed greater levels of safety, additional parts emerged in the tray—sometimes quietly and hidden, and other times loudly and abruptly. Parts also began to address their differences and conflicts, and worked to negotiate how their needs, emotions, and challenges could coexist in one self. The gradual work in the tray began to soften dissociative barriers, reducing inner conflict and increasing cooperation among parts, which resulted in greater regulation of Amanda's nervous system. With greater stability and homeostasis, the stories of trauma and adversity emerged more freely, seeking recognition, validation, and integration. Amanda began to realize and recognize the parts emerging in the tray as her own, and even beyond that, she began to see herself as a whole.

Attachment Patterns and Tendencies in the Tray

The child's play in the sand can give clues to the clinician about relational material and the child's inner attachment world (Homeyer & Lyles, 2022) throughout the different phases of treatment. Attachment patterns are sensory-motor and body-based memory schemas that are known without being thought of (Cozolino, 2014). These memory systems become the foundation for predicting how others respond and behave relationally (Siegel, 2010, 2020). The work in the sand permits the repair of ruptures in the bonding process while using symbols, metaphors, and right brain–generated material. Sandtray therapy creates a portal into the implicit and explicit mind so these attachment tendencies can be seen, explored, witnessed, and integrated. This is paramount, considering that children exposed to chronic trauma present with deep attachment injuries, unfulfilled needs, and developmental interruptions that demand witnessing, acknowledgment, and recognition. These wounds of attachment and insecure internal representations may be observed through characters depicting relational patterns shaped by preoccupation, anxiety, or fear of separation. During the initial phases of treatment, the caregiving system (anyone in the tray with a caregiving role) will begin to show up in the sand worlds of these children, exhibiting inconsistent and unpredictable patterns of care. Characters representing parents or authority figures may show dysregulated anger, criticism, and frightened or frightening features and characteristics. Relationships among characters in the tray may be distant and disengaged; on the contrary, they may be symbiotically connected and enmeshed. The child may create stories with characters portraying a high activation of the attachment system and attachment cry.

A four-year-old coming to therapy because of severe anxiety created in every session a similar world in which a baby monkey was searching for her parents. Every time the baby monkey found Mom or Dad, adversity would follow: a storm, an accident, or an evil character would take the baby away, and at the end of every session, she would find Mom and Dad, only to begin this odyssey again and again. The information emerging from the tray showed high preoccupation around the child's relationships with her parents and activation of the attachment system. The responsibility of finding, connecting, and staying "in relationship" with the parents fell exclusively into the hands of the baby monkey. As the clinician began to explore the parent-child relationship in greater depth, it became evident that the child's real-life interpersonal dynamics were not much different from those unfolding in the tray.

Sometimes, the relational environment in the tray surrounding characters shows disengagement and detachment. Figures may be placed away from each other instead of facing each other (Homeyer & Lyles, 2022). The characters in the tray may depict relationships colored by unavailability, distance, and absence. The lack of protection from protective and nurturing figures may show a dismissing caregiving tendency. Characters attempting to elicit care can also speak about the child's deep and rooted adaptations and developmental interruptions. Characters may follow their caretakers constantly or, on the contrary, portray patterns of self-sufficiency, never asking for help or relying on others.

Trauma bonds and idealization of wounding attachment figures may also appear in the tray. Severe traumatization and exposure to interpersonal trauma and violence may lead to the fragmentation of experience and internalization of oppression, patterns of violence and betrayal, and misuse of power and domination. The unmetabolized trauma in the child's mind is compartmentalized and disconnected (Shapiro, 2018). Dissociative adaptations to trauma become rigid and entrenched in children with a dissociative matrix, where multiple versions of the self coexist. The dilemmas and paradoxes in connection to the perpetrator, especially if they are important attachment figures, surface in the sand as well as polarization and ambivalence surrounding these characters. A character may be simultaneously loved and hated in the same world. Throughout multiple sessions, the worlds may oscillate from stories of alliance and loyalty to ones of hatred and animosity toward the "bad" characters. In the tray, the child can show and work through their most profound conflicts with the actual and the internalized perpetrators.

The play in the tray helps the child work through and resolve inner conflicts while updating their autobiographical consciousness. When clinicians reflect on and offer inquiries about these perpetrator characters, we begin to see the reverse responsibility transferred from the victim to the perpetrator. Jose, a nine-year-old with a history of abandonment and ritualistic and torturing abuse at the hands of his uncle and father, created worlds where the main character was a monster who killed, abused, and tortured animals and children. When the clinician was wondering and reflecting out loud about how the monster was killing and hurting others, Jose stated that he and the monster enjoyed their suffering. He stated that he deeply loved the monster. Jose enacted the perpetrator's behaviors, emotions, and ambitions for several sessions, remaining entirely and utterly loyal to him.

Jose was reenacting the victim and the perpetrator dynamics as they both had been internalized. In his real life, Jose would victimize animals while showing no remorse yet simultaneously feeling a paralyzing fear of the memories of his own victimization. In these cases, clinicians taking sides will not help the child resolve and integrate these enormous dilemmas and polarizations, especially if they exist within a dissociative matrix. Parts within the dissociative milieu will protect each polarity to its ultimate consequences, increasing the internal conflict instead of ameliorating it. Supporting the child in bringing the two polarities together while witnessing with curiosity may start the integration and expansion of consciousness. Sandtray therapists may bring the polarities together as the two coexist in the child's mind: the perpetrator and the powerless victim. For example, the therapist may say,

> I see that the monster kills and hurts and enjoys the suffering he is observing; I also see the animals that suffer, and feel so powerless and without a choice. They both have their side of the story and their feelings.

The clinician brings both the victim's and the perpetrator's polarity into the child's field of consciousness and their perspective and emotions to support integration. A protective character may also surface, giving the child the full trauma spectrum in the tray. The clinician follows as the child's consciousness dances with these polarities, experiencing all of the shades of each as they all coexist in the child's mind. This opens up a field of possibilities for the embodied mind of the child to experience the ever-flowing rhythms of expansion and constriction that occur in the healing of trauma-formed polarizations.

Interoception and patterns of nervous system activation may be explored through the characters and avatars. The therapist may say, "As the animals notice the monster, what do they feel? What happens in their bodies? What parts of their bodies want to move, and which want to remain still? What is different in the body of the monster?" The child's body may also be explored while remaining connected to the metaphor and story, to promote interoceptive intelligence. As the child expands their window of tolerance and borrows empowerment, ventral vagal intelligence, and safety from the clinician, expansions and movement begin to overtake the tray and the child's psychobiological systems.

In the work with Jose, curiosity was invited: Was the monster always powerful? The clinician also reflected on the victims as they were being submissive and pleasing to the monster. Staying with the metaphor, the clinician began to wonder if loving the monster had been their only survival choice, since the monster was bigger and stronger: "I wonder if they are doing the very best they can to survive." Through the avatars, the clinician began to name Jose's idealization and attachment to the perpetrator as his only form of self-protection. It took several trays for Jose to feel empowered to oppose the monster. During one of the sessions in later phases of treatment, Jose brought a lion into the tray that, while asleep, could be a powerful contender to the monster. First, the lion entered quietly, but it became stronger as the sessions progressed. The clinician reflected on the lion's growing strength and wondered if the animals victimized by the monster knew about the potential ally they possessed within the tray. As the lion began to wake up to a new state of empowerment, Jose moved out of his survival adaptations into greater ventral vagal efficacy. Jose's nervous system began to find new ways of interacting with others and the world through the stories and worlds, along with the clinician's presence, witnessing, mirroring, and co-regulating forces. New meanings were also co-created as the trauma was metabolized and integrated. Corrective relational experiences and completions began to penetrate dissociative barriers, rearranging autobiographical memory and Jose's relationship with his internalized oppressor. The nine domains of integration (Siegel, 2010) began to emerge, giving Jose a connection to himself with a greater sense of harmony among parts that were previously in conflict.

A Developmental Perspective on Sandtray Therapy

With all its richness, sandtray work adapts well to various stages of development. The child can use and mold their sand stories as they please and as their minds and nervous systems demand. Children as young as three years of age affected by complex trauma and dissociation can benefit from the offerings of sandtray therapy. Their play and interactions with the tray are marked by their unique developmental needs and capacities. Considering that sand worlds and stories do not rely solely on verbal narratives, the young child with limited verbal capacities finds ample possibilities of expression in the sand tray with miniatures.

Young children may approach the sand tray with a developmentally appropriate dynamic, which often looks like the creation of a puppet show or engagement in dollhouse play inside the tray. One opportunity sandtray therapy offers through this type of play is the added containment that comes through working in a boundaried space and the sensory grounding of the sand. This can be especially important for young children impacted by complex trauma. The sandtray therapist can use their traditional sand skills but may need to offer tracking statements and reflections during the creation of worlds, as young children may never "finish the scene" and sit to process it.

Repetitive and rigid play in the tray may occur as the young child reenacts trauma. Andrew, a three-year-old, repetitively trapped animals in boxes without the possibility of escape. Andrew would become silent and disconnected from his surroundings, including his therapist. Every so often, the time dedicated to sand tray work was titrated, so Andrew sometimes played in the sand tray for only a few minutes before needing distance, rest, or containment. While witnessing and accompanying the reenactment, the clinician also made moment-to-moment micro adaptations to the intonation of her voice, facial expressions, and physical proximity to match the child's needs for safety, reassurance, and companionship. She remained connected to the signals of her nervous system to convey her presence, stimulate the child's social engagement, and provide a corrective experience. She gently reflected on Andrew's actions and, at times, wondered out loud what was happening to the trapped animals and the trapper. The clinician's mind began to hold and contain Andrew's dysregulated autonomic rhythms. The clinician's therapeutic use of self provided a holding space for Andrew, where the intolerable became tolerable and integration a possibility. Andrew started to express his fear for the animals as well as the power of the trapper. The clinician delivered invitations to see possibilities and access resources. Andrew's father joined the sessions and became another avatar in his young child's mind. Andrew would direct his dad to push the trapper and save the animals inside the cages. Andrew would play both the trapped and the trapper and sometimes switch roles with his father. Over multiple sand worlds, Andrew's mastery grew, and with it, his sense of empowerment and agency that, according to his father, extended beyond the boundaries of the sand tray. As the animals were becoming more assertive, so was Andrew.

Older children straddle the developmental line between holding the playfulness of younger children and the emergence of abstract thinking about metaphors. They may become younger in their presentation as they attempt to complete a sand world, especially one that holds charge around attempting to hold safety or a representation of a trauma wound. This can be especially true when severe dissociation is active. A trauma-sensitive sandtray therapist can offer processing options that meet the young child's parts while staying engaged with the present-day older child. This might look like "comic book processing," where there is a game of finding six moments to take pictures of a shifting sand world (Lyles, 2021). This can be printed onto a single page and captioned. In so doing, the child embodies mentalization practice but still benefits from active, dynamic work.

Conclusion

Sandtray therapy, when facilitated by a trained provider, offers multiple relational opportunities for trauma repair. From sensory-rich expressive materials to metaphor-forward processing of created worlds, the externalization of wounded narratives can be safely updated over time, providing a foundation for strength-based identity reclamation. The organic sensitivity to nonlinear, phased treatment inherent to sandtray therapy can be an effective platform for welcoming dissociatively held states into relational awareness, states that have protectively distanced parts of self from elements of memory networks holding complex trauma. The sandtray therapist who partners well with caregivers to adapt these materials and processes in a developmentally sensitive manner will experience deep clinical work, where child clients' courage and resilience lead them into much-deserved healing.

References

Badenoch, B. (2008). *Being a brain-wise therapist: A practical guide to interpersonal neurobiology*. W. W. Norton.

Badenoch, B. (2018). *The heart of trauma: Healing the embodied brain in the context of relationships*. W. W. Norton.

Badenoch, B. (2022). Sandtray with a mind of its own: Developing trust in the wisdom of the process. In R. Grayson & T. Fraser (Eds.), *The embodied brain and sandtray therapy: Stories of healing and transformation* (pp. 209–221). Routledge. https://doi.org/10.4324/9781003055808-15

Courtois, C. A., & Ford, J. D. (Eds.). (2013). *Treatment of complex PTSD: Scientific foundations and therapeutic models* (2nd ed.). Guilford Press.

Cozolino, L. J. (2014). *The neuroscience of human relationships: Attachment and the developing social brain*. W. W. Norton.

Dana, D. (2018). *The polyvagal theory in therapy: Engaging the rhythm of regulation*. W. W. Norton.

Desmond, K., Kindsvatter, A., Stahl, S., & Smith, H. (2015). Using creative techniques with children who have experienced trauma. *Journal of Creativity in Mental Health, 10*(4), 439–455. https://doi.org/10.1080/15401383.2015.1040938

Dr Margaret Lowenfeld Trust. (n.d.). About Lowenfeld. Retrieved March 14, 2023, from lowenfeld.org/about-lowenfeld

Ecker, B. (2015). Memory reconsolidation understood and misunderstood. *International Journal of Neuropsychotherapy, 3*(1), 2–46. https://doi.org/10.12744/ijnpt.2015.0002-0046

Ecker, B., & Bridges, S. K. (2020). How the science of memory reconsolidation advances the effectiveness and unification of psychotherapy. *Clinical Social Work Journal, 48*(3), 287–300.

Ensink, K., Bégin, M., Normandin, L., & Fonagy, P. (2016). Maternal and child reflective functioning in the context of child sexual abuse: Pathways to depression and externalising difficulties. *European Journal of Psychotraumatology, 7*(1), Article 30611. https://doi.org/10.3402/ejpt.v7.30611

Flahive, M., & Ray, D. (2007). Effect of group sandtray therapy with preadolescents. *Journal for Specialists in Group Work, 32*(4), 362–382. https://doi.org/10.1080/01933920701476706

Fleet, D. (2023). *Pluralistic sand-tray therapy: Humanistic principles for working creatively with adult clients*. Routledge.

Fonagy, P., Gergely, G., & Jurist, E. L. (Eds.). (2018). *Affect regulation, mentalization and the development of the self*. Routledge.

Fraser, G. A. (1991). The dissociative table technique: A strategy for working with ego states and dissociative disorders and ego-state therapy. *Dissociation, 4*(4), 205–213.

Freedle, L. R. (2019). Making connections: Sandplay therapy and the neurosequential model of therapeutics. *Journal of Sandplay Therapy, 28*(1), 91–109.

George, C., Kaplan, N., & Main, M. (1996). *Adult attachment interview* (3rd ed.). Unpublished manuscript, Berkeley: Department of Psychology, University of California.

Gil, E. (2014). The creative use of metaphor in play and art therapy with attachment problems. In C. A. Malchiodi & D. A. Crenshaw (Eds.), *Creative arts and play therapy for attachment problems* (pp. 159–177). Guilford Press.

Gil, E. (2016). *Posttraumatic play in children: What clinicians need to know*. Guilford Press.

Gomez, A. M. (2013). *EMDR therapy and adjunct approaches with children: Complex trauma, attachment, and dissociation.* Springer Publishing Company.

Gomez, A. M. (2017). *EMDR-sandtray-based therapy training manual.* Unpublished manuscript.

Gomez, A. M. (2019). The world of stories and symbols: The EMDR-sandtray protocol. *Go With That Magazine, 24*(1), 35–39. emdria.org/course/the-world-of-stories-and-symbols-an-introduction-to-the-emdr-sandtray-protocol-with-complex-and-developmental-trauma

Gomez, A. M. (2019). The world of stories and symbols: The EMDR-sandtray protocol. *Go With That Magazine, 24*(1), 35–39. https://emdria.org/course/the-world-of-stories-and-symbols-an-introduction-to-the-emdr-sandtray-protocol-with-complex-and-developmental-trauma

Gomez, A. M. (2023). *EMDR therapy basic training manual.* Unpublished manuscript.

Gomez, A. M. (in press). *EMDR–sandtray-based therapy: Healing complex trauma and dissociation across the lifespan.* W. W. Norton.

Grayson, R. (2022). Healing the embodied brain: The neurobiology of sandtray therapy. In R. Grayson & T. Fraser (Eds.), *The embodied brain and sandtray therapy: Stories of healing and transformation* (pp. 28–53). Routledge.

Hill, D. (2015). *Affect regulation theory: A clinical model.* W.W. Norton.

Homeyer, L. E. (n.d.). *The history of sand therapy.* World Association of Sand Therapy Professionals. worldsandtherapy.org/page/history

Homeyer, L. E., & Lyles, M. N. (2022). *Advanced sandtray therapy: Digging deeper into clinical practice.* Routledge.

Homeyer, L. E., & Stone, J. (2023). Sand therapy standards: Views from the field. *World Journal for Sand Therapy Practice, 1*(1). https://doi.org/10.58997/wjstp.v1i1.4

Homeyer, L. E., & Sweeney, D. S. (2023). *Sandtray therapy: A practical manual.* Routledge.

International Society for the Study of Dissociation Taskforce (ISSTD). (in press). Guidelines for the evaluation and treatment of dissociative symptoms in children and adolescents. *Journal of Trauma and Dissociation.*

Kalff, D. M. (2003). *Sandplay: A psychotherapeutic approach to the psyche.* Temenos Press.

Kern Popejoy, E., Perryman, K., & Broadwater, A. (2020). Processing military combat trauma through sandtray therapy: A phenomenological study. *Journal of Creativity in Mental Health, 16*(2), 196–211. https://doi.org/10.1080/15401383.2020.1761499

Knoetze, J. (2013). Sandworlds, storymaking, and letter writing: The therapeutic sandstory method. *South African Journal of Psychology, 43*(4), 459–469. https://doi.org/10.1177/0081246313506663

Leader, C. J. (2022). Through the eyes of a child: Sandtray therapy with children. In R. Grayson & T. Fraser (Eds.), *The embodied brain and sandtray therapy: Stories of healing and transformation* (pp. 107–121). Routledge.

Liu, Y. Y., Li, K., Bin, T., Tan, J. F., Wang, Z. D., Wang, J. X., & Shen, H. Y. (2021). Psychological symptoms and the use of shadow miniatures in sandplay therapy. *The Arts in Psychotherapy, 75*, Article 101834. https://doi.org/10.1016/j.aip.2021.101834

Lyles, M. (2021). Room for everyone: Family-based play therapy in the sandtray. In A. Beckley-Forest & A. Monaco (Eds.), *EMDR with children in the play therapy room: An integrated approach* (pp. 75–108). Springer.

Lyles, M., & Homeyer, L. (2024). Safety in sand and symbols: Polyvagal shifts in the sand tray. In P. Goodyear-Brown & L. Yasenik (Eds.), *Polyvagal power in the playroom.* Routledge.

Malchiodi, C. A. (2020). *Trauma and expressive arts therapy: Brain, body & imagination in the healing process.* Guilford Press.

McGilchrist, I. (2009). *The master and his emissary.* Yale University Press.

Monaco, A. (2021). Understanding and responding to dissociation. In A. Beckley-Forest & A. Monaco (Eds.), *EMDR with children in the play therapy room: An integrated approach* (pp. 251–290). Springer.

Perry, B. D. (2014). The neurosequential model of therapeutics in young children. In K. Brandt, B. D. Perry, S. Seligman & E. Tronick (Eds.), *Infant and early childhood mental health* (pp. 21–47). American Psychiatric Press.

Porges, S. W. (2011). *The polyvagal theory: Neurophysiological foundations of emotions, attachment, communication, and self-regulation.* W. W. Norton.

Porges, S. W. (2021). *Polyvagal safety: Attachment, communication, self-regulation.* W. W. Norton.

Putnam, F. W. (1997). *Dissociation in children and adolescents: A developmental perspective.* Guilford Press.

Rae, R. (2013). *Sandtray: Playing to heal, recover, and grow.* Rowman & Littlefield.

Scaletti, R., & Hocking, C. (2010). Healing through story telling: An integrated approach for children experiencing grief and loss. *New Zealand Journal of Occupational Therapy, 57*(2), 66–71.

Schore, A. N. (2019). *Right brain psychotherapy*. W. W. Norton.

Shapiro, F. (2018). *Eye movement desensitization and reprocessing. Basic principles, protocols, and procedures* (3rd ed.). Guilford Press.

Siegel, D. J. (2010). *Mindsight: The new science of personal transformation*. Bantam Books.

Siegel, D. J. (2020). *The developing mind: How relationships and the brain interact to shape who we are* (3rd ed.). W. W. Norton.

Something Curated. (2021, November 19). *Stories in the sand: A history of the indigenous painting form*. Retrieved March 13, 2023, from somethingcurated.com/2021/11/19/stories-in-the-sand-a-history-of-the-indigenous-painting-form

Steele, K., Boon, S., & van der Hart, O. (2017). *Treating trauma-related dissociation: A practical integrative approach*. W. W. Norton.

Unwin, C., & Hood-Williams, J. (1988). *Child psychotherapy, war and the normal child: selected papers of Margaret Lowenfeld*. Sussex Academic Press.

van der Hart, O., Brown, P., & van der kolk, B. (2019). Pierre's Janet treatment of posttraumatic stress. In G. Craparo, F. Ortu & O. van der Hart (Eds.), *Trauma, dissociation and a new context for psychoanalysis* (pp. 75–108). Routledge.

van der Hart, O., & Dorahy, M. J. (2009). History of the concept of dissociation. In P. Dell & J. O'Neill (Eds.), *Dissociation and the dissociative disorders: DSM-V and beyond* (pp. 3–26). Routledge.

Wesselmann, D., Armstrong, S., Schweitzer, C., Davidson, M., & Potter, A. (2018). An integrative EMDR and family therapy model for treating attachment trauma in children: A case series. *Journal of EMDR Practice and Research, 12*(4), 196–207. https://doi.org/10.1891/1933-3196.12.4.196

32
ART THERAPY

Elizabeth Davis

Introduction

Basic to any learning is the ability to meaningfully reflect on one's lived experience; when experiences can be reflected on, meaningful understandings can be garnered to meet future challenges. Problems in learning from experiences emerge when events are too emotionally overwhelming to reflect on, as in traumatic experiences (Bateman & Fonagy, 2019; Stavropoulos & Elliott, 2022). Traumatic experiences essentially create a psychic overload and the need to implement innate survival-based defenses (such as fight, flight, or freeze) to escape (Bateman & Fonagy, 2019). The resulting memories then go unreviewed due to avoidance strategies and meaning making and learning stops. Traumatic memories then remain poorly understood and attached to survival-based defenses.

Prolonged and chronic exposure in early childhood to traumatic experiences can have a cascading impact on a child's ability to navigate life's stressors and develop meaningful knowledge of themselves and others. Overwhelmed by chronic trauma, the child must erect dissociative defenses as default strategies for escape, which relieve them of intolerable emotions. But these default dissociative strategies, necessary for the child to manage chronic trauma exposure in childhood, can impede the development of critical knowledge and skills that form the foundation for making coherent sense out of life and managing emotions in the future (Linde-Krieger et al., 2023; Liotti, 1999). Without the development of foundational knowledge and skills, a child's emotional, behavioral, interpersonal, neurobiological, and cognitive development (Linde-Krieger et al., 2023) can be impacted. The child then experiences escalating trauma symptoms. With more symptoms, stress, and trauma, the reliance on dissociation increases to ever greater degrees (Schore, 2023). The result of this developmental impact is a complex set of symptoms alongside missing knowledge and skills to meet the challenges of life, presenting even more significant hurdles for the child as they grow.

Complications in Treating Developmental Trauma

Clinicians tasked with helping children recover, need skills and approaches to face the complex difficulties that developmental trauma presents. Trauma experiences held by children elicit ongoing fear and dysregulated emotions that continue to repel inward reflection; yet, looking inward is where the skills to manage and recover from symptoms can be found and developed. Additionally, the clinician is tasked with addressing the dissociative defenses that are rooted in the trauma experience encoded at the child's developmental age when learning stopped and dissociative strategies took over. Therefore, the clinician must be mindful of their client's limited developmental capacities and not assume that because the child is older, they have the skills typical of their age group (Bateman & Fonagy, 2004).

Further challenges in treatment arise due to the difficult task of forming a therapeutic relationship. A child's experience of distrust in others due to insecure and disorganized attachment—because they have not experienced a trustworthy caregiver who can aid them under stress—teaches them that others are not helpful at best and potentially harmful at worst (Lorenzini et al., 2019). The innate response for the child who experiences their caregivers as unhelpful, absent, or abusive is to shut off from their caregiver's mind, as a defense (Bateman & Fonagy, 2019). This leaves the child in a distrustful state, which Anthony Bateman and Peter Fonagy of the Anna Freud Centre for Children and Families in London, researchers in the field of theory of mind and attachment in children, call *epistemic distrust*. In *epistemic distrust*, the flow of knowledge between the child and caregiver is blocked and the child is siloed off from the exchange of beneficial information needed to acquire the skills and capacities to manage interpersonal life. Treatment approaches for developmental trauma therefore need to address complicated relational barriers of distrust that have impeded the flow of knowledge in the past, in addition to compromised emotional regulation and dissociative defenses. Although clinicians are tasked with a complicated set of goals to help their clients heal, many researchers and therapists have documented and studied what has been successful for them. Working within a community of other therapists who confront the same challenges is vitally important for the clinician to grow skills and insight into how to help their clients recover.

Treatment Recommendations

The guidelines set out by the International Society for the Study of Trauma and Dissociation (ISSTD) Child Trauma Task Force (Silberg, 2004) are one of the few sources available for working with children who present with dissociation. The ISSTD is currently in the process of updating their recommendations in 2023, but approaches are still largely based on a three-phase model that goes back over a century to Pierre Janet, one of the founding fathers in the field of trauma studies. In 2012, the International Society for Traumatic Stress Studies formed a Complex Trauma Task Force (Cloitre et al., 2012) endorsing the triphase model as still the safest approach for the treatment of complex trauma in adults (Silberg & Dallam, 2023).

The triphasic model, or phase-based approach to treatment, phase one begins with assessment, stabilization, skill building, and establishing a therapeutic alliance. Following stabilization, in phase two, the client confronts the task of the reappraisal of traumatic memories to reorganize and make a meaningful understanding from the experience. In phase three, and vitally important for the client to maintain gains from previous phases, the task is to address the behaviors, habits, and reflexive defenses that formed around traumatic experiences and subsequent trauma reminders that are no longer adaptive, and limit future growth (Cloitre et al., 2012).

However, research with children has largely been based on anecdotal evidence and in small clinical trials within residential treatment settings. Approaches have endorsed bolstering resiliency through emphasis on empathic structure, sensory-based approaches, and addressing environmental and attachment issues in a structured sequential process (see Kagan & Spinazzola, 2013; Perry, 2009; Purvis & Cross, 2013). Approaches such as those proposed by Joyanna Silberg and Frances Waters recommend working systemically to address family relationships, and the systems in which the child is imbedded, as well as providing psychoeducation and trauma memory reprocessing, alongside the phased model mentioned above (Silberg & Dallam, 2023).

Art therapy can be effectively integrated into these clinical approaches as an adjunct or singular method of engaging children in residential treatment, inpatient, community wraparound, and individual therapy. Below, I offer the integration of art therapy as a treatment modality to address some of the complex issues that children with developmental trauma present with. The art therapy methods I employ follow the triphase model of trauma treatment, emphasizing the power of creative approaches for developing stabilization skills and resources, building a therapeutic alliance, enhancing psychoeducation success, bolstering mentalization skills and meaning making, aiding the reprocessing of traumatic memories, and supporting the development of new behaviors and skills to meet future challenges.

Cautions and Considerations Working with Children

Working with children who present with developmental trauma is a team effort. The young child, school-aged child, or even adolescent does not present alone but within systems such as their family of origin, foster care, residential facilities, schools, child protection, and their community at large. My previous experience working with children has largely been part of integrated wraparound services offered through county and state programs to address children at risk for juvenile justice, inpatient settings, and placement in residential care. I have additional years of experience working in residential and day treatment facilities for children with emotional disturbances, as well as in foster care and inner-city clinics. These experiences have taught me that the child is only one part of the system that the therapist must attempt to engage. Parent and caregiver education on trauma, parent training, parent-and-child therapy, and at times referrals for parents or caregivers to engage in therapy themselves is often part of the process. Additionally, working with schools, teachers, committees that provide special education services, child protective services, foster agencies, facility support staff, and natural supports such as siblings, relatives, and neighbors may be necessary to help the child heal and meet their therapeutic goals. When a child is still in a home experiencing abuse, treatment is limited to support and education to address crisis and safety (Silberg & Dallam, 2023). A child's dissociative defensive structure has developed to survive in the environments that have been overwhelming for them. A safe environment is a prerequisite for addressing trauma processing; without systemic and environmental change, the therapist's efforts to aid the child's healing may jeopardize their ability to cope. However, early treatment for children who present with developmental trauma can prevent the cascade of issues that follow, including increased complexity of treatment, more accumulated trauma, and prevention of further trauma for the generation that follows.

Precautions Using Art Therapy and Art Media

Working with creative arts materials may initially appear straightforward. Many therapists can recall working with paints and markers as children in an uncomplicated way. However, art therapists undertake special training to understand the nature of the experience of utilizing creative media and directives specifically with persons who struggle with trauma and other mental health concerns. This training allows for safety, containment, attunement, and the unfolding of expansive possibilities. For the non-art therapist, experience is needed to understand how a specific media may elicit sensory memory or be technically frustrating to use, especially for clients with trauma histories. Knowing the potential risks of and skills for utilizing art media can prevent retriggering or creating frustration and overwhelm for clients. Some of the pitfalls non-art therapists fall into are offering directives that come off as a canned approach or are given prescriptively, rather than addressing the individual client's needs to be creative and innovative. Or the therapist may overinterpret their client's creations, which can be intrusive for the client as well as inaccurate. Some therapists who are personally proficient in an art medium may overemphasize technique, acting more like an art teacher than a therapist supporting their client's own investigatory process. Therapists who use art media therefore need to understand not just the technical use of the art materials but also the approach with their specific client to avoid creating frustration, igniting feelings of shame, and inhibiting free expression. For the non-art therapist, having a creative arts therapist who specializes in trauma treatment as a consultant is advised to learn to approach the use of arts media appropriately and effectively. A creative arts therapist as a consultant can help the non-art therapist grow skillfully, learn the pitfalls, understand their client's art expressions, and suggest approaches or media that might benefit specific clients the most.

Art Making in the Therapeutic Relationship

The therapeutic relationship is vitally important for healing relational trauma and holds the potential for providing new experiences of another person perhaps dissimilar from what the client has previously experienced. When effective, the therapeutic relationship allows space for the client to rework and revise their self-beliefs, and offers a place where skills can be practiced, and problems solved for managing interpersonal experience. According to Daniel Brown, associate clinical professor of psychology at Harvard Medical School, and David Elliott, clinical psychologist and faculty at the International School of Psychotherapy, Counseling, and Group Leadership, children by the age of three and four years old begin to develop relational belief systems and schemas regarding what to expect and how to navigate relationships (2016). This means that even a very young child who presents with developmental trauma brings with them the complicated and often disorganized relational patterns and schemas indicative of their traumatic early relationships. In therapy, this can mean the child can be triggered by the very source of where they are seeking help, as their expectations in relationships with adults may be to receive abuse, neglect, and exploitation.

For some children, the challenge of the relationship may override the advantages that therapy promises to offer. This is where art therapy can be a valuable approach, as it opens another place to meet that is less threatening than direct interpersonal exchange. When I was working in a residential setting, and with youth at risk for placement in inpatient hospitalization, I was often brought to cases due to the difficult engagement issues previous therapists had encountered. The advantage, as an art therapist, was the ability to engage youth in this other arena and with an external focus that could potentially could be fun. This potential other focus offered youth a sense of control over their level of engagement in the interpersonal sphere.

In addition to an alternate interpersonal meeting place, art therapy may provide a form of indirect mirroring through the creation of the art form. In their work at the Oxford College of Arts and Therapies, Springham and Huet (2018) developed a biopsychosocial model of art therapy that may help explain the benefits of using creative arts therapies to communicate indirectly when direct exchange feels too threatening. They suggest that the act of paying joint attention to the art and the client as the client creates allows for a mirroring experience through the art object. Essentially, the therapist "marks" the expressive form through their reaction to the art object, then mirrors back to the client their understanding of the form and, in doing so, mirrors the client indirectly. This indirect mirroring allows more space for the relationally fearful client to manage the intensity of the relational exchange while also providing the client with the feeling of being seen. With clients who present with disorganized attachment, having the indirect option of being seen may provide more tolerance for the process of expression as therapy progresses.

A few guidelines when using art as part of therapy are important to keep in mind. Fundamental to inviting a client into an art experience is the understanding of art media (as noted above). Offering creative options that exceed what feels manageable can result in a relational rupture or misattunement, a feeling on the part of the client that their experience is not understood, and they are not understood. A therapist mindful and skilled in the use of art media can anticipate the potential feelings, sensory implications, and frustrations a client may experience. When the client feels confident that the therapist will have their back, then they are secure enough to undertake risks and explore. Another rule that art therapists learn, but therapists who have their own art practices may be unaware of, is the need to treat one's own art process as private information. In this case, the unaware therapist may influence the client by offering their own art preferences and media approaches, or even have their personal art displayed in their office. Many survivors of interpersonal trauma have learned to hyper-attune to others to stay safe, which carries over to therapeutic relationships. In the case of the therapist sharing their own artwork, the client may idolize the therapist as an artist, or alternatively feel intimidated and envious. The therapist should therefore generally treat their own artworks and preferences as personal information.

A final point for clinicians to keep in mind is that creatively producing an art object in therapy is a collaborative endeavor. The process involves multiple shared experiences, such as joining in a vision, joint problem-solving, and taking concrete actions together, all leading to the creation of an art object reminiscent of the shared experience. This experience is a collaborative and connected one where the therapist facilitates the experience and offers options and assistance where needed. For the client with developmental trauma and symptoms of dissociation, the art object then can serve a special function, evoking this ongoing connection and collaboration to the therapist between sessions. Art objects, therefore, hold meaning beyond the mere process. They can hold the potential to keep the relational experience alive and active long after the session is over. As Winnicott (2005/1971) describes, transitional phenomena act in the "intermediate area of experience," embodying both "creative activity and projection of what already has been introjected" (pp. 2–3). The art object, as a transitional container of relational experience and projected meaning, can support the security of the therapeutic relationship.

Art Therapy Integrated into Phase-Oriented Treatment-Phase One

The beginning of treatment is a time of uncertainty. A child with developmental trauma is likely with their caregivers or system advocates who are initiating the treatment due to specific behaviors or symptoms. The child may find therapy confusing initially and the focus on them difficult to manage. In these stressful first encounters, art making may help mitigate stress for the child. Research on art making and stress reduction has come a long way in the past decade. While it may be common sense to many who use crafts or other creative pastimes for relaxation, there is now ample evidence that creating art does have the potential to lower cortisol levels (Kaimal et al., 2016; Martin et al., 2018). Integrating creative arts early on can potentially relieve some of the client's initial stress.

Although art therapists may begin treatment with specific drawing-based assessments, these directives require training and experience, especially with clients presenting with trauma and dissociation. For those therapists who are not specifically trained in art therapy assessment, approaching the integration of art experience in a playful way and with sensitivity to performance anxiety is recommended. The therapist may start with a menu of choices, such as inviting the child to draw their favorite landscape or animal, make a mandala, or draw a scribble or doodle. Initially avoiding directives that might ignite strong emotional states, such as mask making, family drawings, use of messy art materials that can be challenging to use or that have strong sensory components (such as clay, paint, or chalky pastels), will allow the child to wade into the process, increasing the likelihood of a positive experience.

Media that the child chooses can also be important for understanding the child's tolerance and preferences. Some children may be initially intimidated by art materials that are unfamiliar. Having an assortment of simple art media such as crayons, oil pastels, markers, colored pencils, collage materials, an assortment of beads and string, outlines or coloring sheets, and natural materials can provide a good array of choices. Some school-aged children, those who particularly struggle with

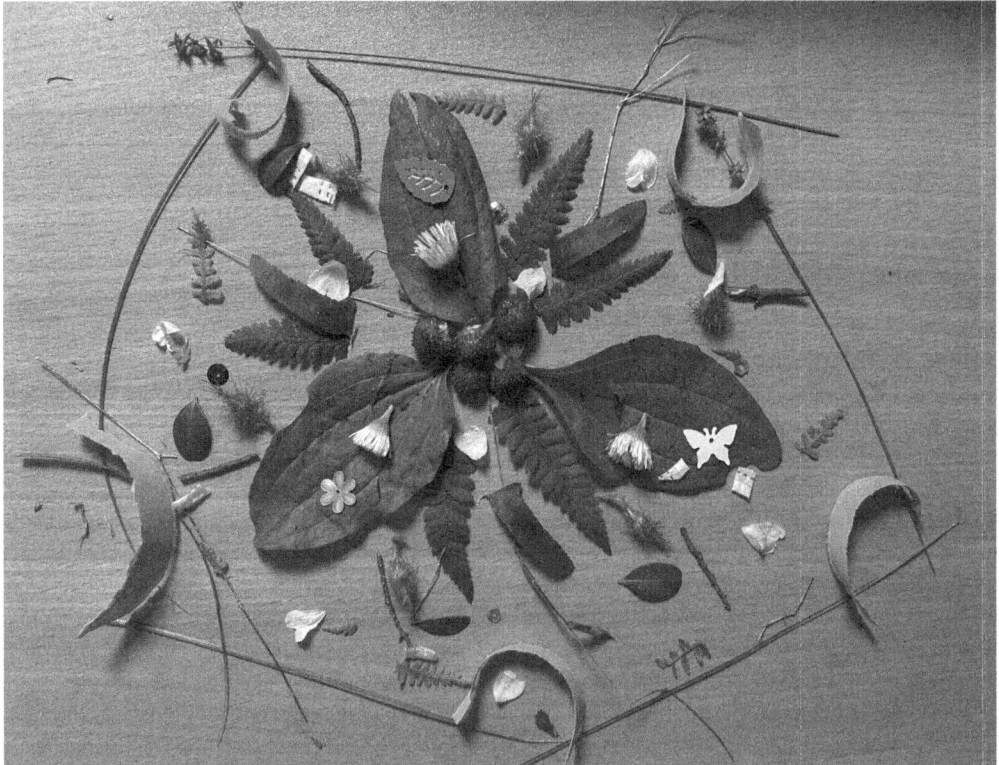

Figure 32.1 Loose Parts Mandala.

perfectionism around their art creations, are inhibited to express initially and may be more comfortable with collage materials or a *loose parts* approach (Flannigan & Dietze, 2018), using objects found in nature, craft materials, or objects found in the typical household (beans, rice, paper clips, buttons, etc.) to create a design on any surface (see illustration of *loose parts* mandala) (Figure 32.1).

History-Gathering

Exposure to the past can elicit negative emotions, and even dissociation, with children who present with developmental trauma and dissociation. Being creative from the beginning of history-gathering helps promote a mindful, playful engagement with the past that facilitates containment and a reflective stance, with the added calming benefit of art making. When taking a history, the therapist should be mindful to include focus on positive and resourceful moments, not just negative ones, like experiences of pride, mastery, joy, and calm, as well as past challenges. These experiences form the foundation for building skills of self-regulation and can help the client identify and solidify internal resources in later sessions. Additionally, children who are particularly avoidant of reflecting inward can feel less threatened by the process when positive moments are initially the focus. For children who are preoccupied with emotions and overwhelming past experiences, the focus on positive moments can help them find a more balanced perspective that serves as information to counter negative self-beliefs.

There are endless ways of engaging creativity while taking a history. The approach I often give at the onset is "How would you like to represent the journey of your life so far?" I may offer a menu, if needed, based on the media they like. The traditional road metaphor is often discussed as an option, or the Tree of Life metaphor. Children have chosen bridges as well to represent their journey moving away from a traumatic past. Most important to this process is the child's felt sense of choice in how they represent their story.

Below are descriptions of an approach to history-gathering that incorporates containment strategies, which are often needed when working with children who present with developmental trauma. Keep in mind that with each client the process should be open, not emulative, and spark innovation, which allows for an accurate metaphor that reflects their unique experiences.

Container Timelines

Container timelines provide an opportunity for the child to contain aspects of their history, leaving only the part that is being discussed and explored open visually and concretely. Bethany Brand et al. (2022), in their work *Finding Solid Ground*, an evidence-based approach for trauma survivors diagnosed with dissociative disorder, identified containment as one of the core skills for recovery. When traumatic material can be effectively contained, the client is better prepared to separate the past from the present, regulate themselves, manage their current needs, and engage in meaningful reflection. These skills are essential during history-gathering given the potential for destabilization and loss of present orientation.

Many common objects can act as containers for timelines. Some favorites are condiment cups, envelopes, pockets, accordion folders (especially ones made for coupons), baby food jars, folded napkins (with each folded section representing a different time period), and even scrolls (paper simply rolled up in the form of a scroll). When using condiment cups, presenting each cup as a "time capsule" can be helpful because it helps the client visually separate and organize different periods of time. I invite the child to choose several cups and label them in the phases or time frames that make sense for them. For the young child, this might take the form of one cup for each year of their life, for example, a five-year-old child may have five cups and then an extra cup for what they hope to do in the future. The child is then invited to free associate about their past while choosing from scrapbook bits, images, craft materials, and cut-out pictures, which they then place into the corresponding time frame cups. The approach is intended to spark their memories and thoughts about their past experiences. For example, they may choose a picture of a bottle to represent being bottle fed, or a toy image to represent a memory of receiving a special stuffie. Having images relieves the young child from finding the words and therefore allows for more effective history-taking with children who cannot easily dictate the story of their life chronologically but are able, if prompted, to remember different events that both supported and challenged them.

Case Example: Sophia[1]

Sophia is a nine-year-old who was brought into therapy by her foster mom, Barbara, who explained that Sophia had been in her home for four years and that she was in the final stages of adopting her. Barbara, as well as Sophia's caseworker, related Sophia's history of severe abuse and neglect, including the loss of both parents—one to addiction, one to abandonment—placement at two-years-old in the custody of her uncle, who was suspected of sexually and physically abusing her, and subsequent placement in foster care at four, where she was initially in an emergency placement. She was described by Barbara as unpredictable, loving, and clingy, then angry and violent. She presented with tantrums, aggression toward her foster mom, and oppositional behaviors. Barbara was struggling with her choice to adopt her, and desperate to find effective treatment.

When Sophia began therapy, she seemed performative, often taking on the persona of a much older youth. As therapy progressed, however, Sophia revealed another mode or self-state that seemed regressed, more like a three-year-old. Using a phase-based approach, work focused initially on emotional literacy and regulation, parenting strategies, and building reflective skills. The phase-based trauma treatment approach was discussed with Barbara, and she was enlisted as a partner in the healing and recovery process. Goals for Sophia followed the phases—to learn to manage her emotions and grow insight, reprocess previous traumatic memories, and learn new ways of behaving in relationships that would help her meet future challenges.

In Sophia's second session, I introduced the container timeline as an approach to history-taking, building an understanding of how Sophia understood herself and past experiences. Sophia presented initially as very reluctant to discuss the past, but utilizing condiment containers and lots of bits and pieces of scrapbook and craft materials, she seemed to relax and approached the process playfully. She created a "container tower" using a wooden heart as a base; each container represented a year of her life. She placed sand, words, stickers, and objects in the containers to signify experiences that she remembered, beliefs she held about herself, and strengths she had discovered. Sophia placed a large green dragon sticker near the top of the container tower to symbolize how difficult it was adjusting to life with her foster mom. Sophia expressed pride in her creation and picked out a special hiding place in the therapy room (on top of a cabinet out of sight) to keep it safe (Figure 32.2).

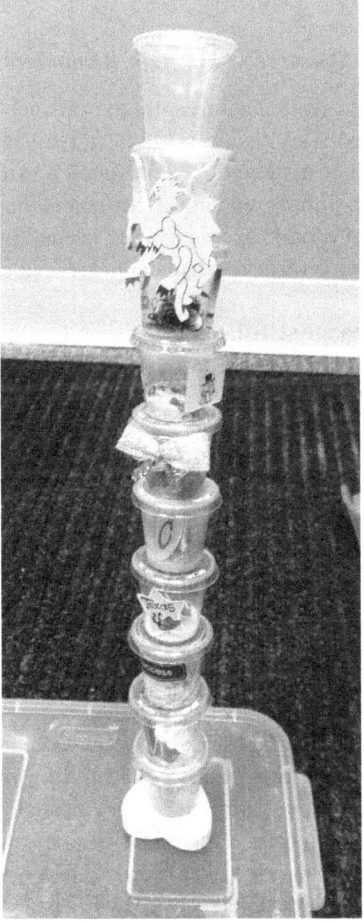

Figure 32.2 Time Capsules.

Developing Strengths and Resources

A child's ability to eventually manage trauma processing rests on finding their strengths, including their internal capacities such as abilities and talents, as well as resources such as family, friends, community, and nature. All children come with strengths that, if utilized when needed, can help them better regulate to manage distress and navigate through challenges. Internal strengths can often be identified when taking a history by asking the child or their caregivers about what they feel they are good at, or identifying what challenges they have overcome and what others have said about them. External strengths may be accounted for by assessing their current circumstances at home, school, and in their wider community. When finding strengths, it is often important to link them concretely to the child's experience. Children who have experienced trauma may have difficulty believing they possess or have access to strengths and resources. By linking strengths to concrete experience, the child is merely asked to review the evidence, not just accept it on face value (Greenwald, 2007). Compassion, honesty, openness, forgiveness, kindness, perseverance, generosity, commitment, gratitude, friendship, care from others, intelligence, positive affiliation with others, abilities, empathy, strength, control, energy, nature, animals, creativity, spiritual connection, courage, and assertiveness are but a few strengths that I have handy on a list for children and families to help them identify these foundational tools for the journey of healing.

Resource or Strength Reminders

Offering children a creative way to symbolize strengths expressively can help them concretely access and remember them when needed. Very young children (three-year-olds) may be better at remembering an internal representation of a strength when offered a symbolic external representation as a reminder (Fonagy et al., 2004). Simply creating an art object that can act as a symbolic reminder of the internal strength can help the child access it when needed in a challenging situation. A child may make a bracelet, token, or amulet that acts like the proverbial rabbit's foot to help the child stay connected.

Children who present with separate self-states may also utilize this approach to identify the special survival qualities that self-states have offered in the past. This can recast self-states as possessing strengths utilized to meet overwhelming challenges. Understanding that a self-state may have developed a quality to meet the needs of surviving trauma helps the child see themselves as a survivor, addressing shame and increasing their capacity to connect with parts of themselves with compassion.

Case Example: Sophia

As a part of exploring her inner strengths, Sophia identified several self-states, one of which was like a child who would become hyper and engage in risk-taking—often approaching strangers, climbing on furniture in the waiting room, taking off from her foster mom in a store, and getting out of her seat at school. Sophia had received frequent negative feedback due to this part's behavior and made her foster mom very nervous for her safety at times. When discussing this self-state, Sophia was invited to think of the qualities this part processed, noting its survival strengths. Sophia identified the part as having energy, boldness, and courage. She expressed identifying with a character in the movie *The Incredibles 2*, Jack-Jack, who is a baby with powers they cannot yet control (Bird, 2018). Sophia expressed appreciation that her hyper part had tried to help her manage her stress, with its energy and courage to approach strangers and engage in risky behaviors. However, as a baby-like part, her hyper part still needed help from her older, wiser self as well as her foster mom to learn to use her powers wisely. "Baby," as she came to refer to this self-state, could now be seen as special, in the process of

Art Therapy

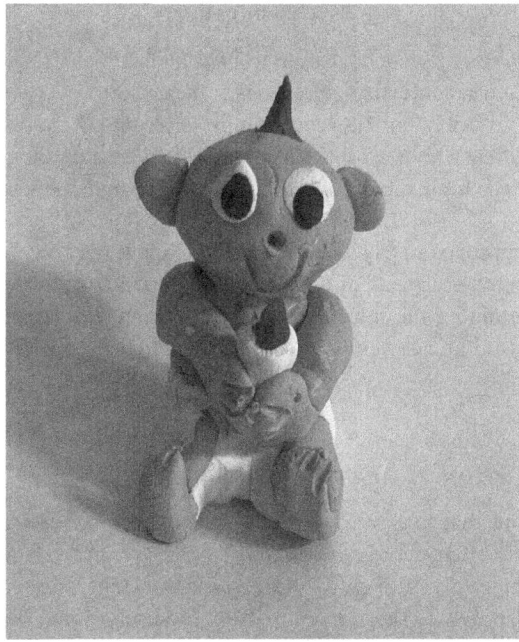

Figure 32.3 Resource Reminder: "Baby."

learning to develop control over her powers of energy and courage for good. Making a polymer clay version of this part in the likeness of Jack-Jack helped Sophia stay aware of and hold a more balanced and reflective relationship with this part (Figure 32.3).

Suggested Procedure for Creating a Strength or Resource Reminder

Suggested questions to identify strengths and resources with caregivers and children include: *How have you managed to get through challenging situations in the past? What have you noticed you* [or alternatively a self-state] *are good at? What have others said that they enjoy or appreciate about you? What ways have you helped others or animals?* [If a child struggles to find a strength, then get creative. The child, even by showing up and engaging in therapy, has demonstrated strengths such as willingness to try something new.]

Now link the resource or strength to the evidence and repeat back to the child. For example, "I've learned some good things about you [or a self-state], such as, you are caring, because when your friend was hurt, you helped them."

Now identify a creative symbol for the strength or resource. Ask questions such as: *If ____ was an animal, word, thing, or symbol, what might it look like? What color or shape would it be? Take a moment to imagine ____. What would you like to name or label it?* [Now invite the child to create.] *Would you like to create ____ using the art materials?* [After the child creates the reminder, ask if they would like to reflect again.] *Now take a moment to test your ___. Can you imagine using it in a future situation? Is anything else needed to make it even stronger?* [If finished, invite the child to connect deeper with their creation.] *Imagine all the positive feelings, thoughts, and beliefs that ___ brings up. How was that?*

Psychoeducation

The therapist traditionally uses psychoeducation to help clients make sense of their symptoms and behaviors, to normalize and recontextualize responses they had to overwhelming experiences, and acquire missing adaptive information. However, simply offering psychoeducation through teaching may fail to motivate children who need the information delivered on their developmental level. In addition, the child may have limited capacity to reflect inward and connect the information to their personal experience.

Below, I describe an approach to psychoeducation to explain the "compass of shame" by Daniel Nathanson (1992). Many other aspects of treatment may also be useful to teach in a creative way to aid in meaningfully retaining the information. Approaching psychoeducation in these creative ways can often put the child at ease, allowing them to explore the information in a hands/on and concrete way.

Shame Psychoeducation

Toxic shame is the shame that overwhelms and does not resolve, and can leave the individual chronically feeling small, often depressed, anxious, or angry and vigilant in relation to others. Beliefs of being unlovable, ugly, broken, worthless, incompetent, stupid, and so on are common shame-based beliefs that prevent clients from trusting themselves and others. These feelings and beliefs lie at the core of developmental trauma, alongside the experiences of betrayal by those whom the child depended on for survival. (See Chapter 39 to further explore the role of shame in developmental trauma.)

The goal of shame education is to address both the dysregulating feeling of shame and the source and true purpose of its existence for the client. Psychoeducation can help recontextualize shame as an emotional process that occurred so they could survive trauma. Uncoupling shame from the attachment to the shaming caregiver may involve education on healthy attachment as well as an understanding of shame's purpose as a protective emotion when no other alternative existed. It is important to keep in mind that any ongoing shaming experiences that may be happening within the child's family system preclude addressing shame directly. Additionally, caregivers who do not understand the function of shame (such as foster parents, adoptive parents, other family members, and residential facility staff) may benefit from shame education to prevent unwittingly disciplining children in a way that reinforces shame beliefs. Helping caregivers and supports approach discipline in a way that holds the child's internal world and worthiness as separate from identified negative behaviors is vitally important for the child to recover.

In his seminal work, *Shame and Pride: Affect, Sex, and the Birth of the Self*, Nathanson (1992) identified four basic patterns of defense used to manage the overwhelm of shame. He constructed a model for illustrating this in the form of a compass, with the identified patterns at each pole: *avoidance, withdrawal, attack self,* and *attack others*. These reaction patterns are interpersonal defenses that are enacted when shame is felt, similar to fight, flight, freeze, and shutdown. For example, to escape shame, one may enact a fight response—*attack other*—externalizing anger onto another person. In *attack other* mode, they may verbally or physically attack, bully, assault, or act aggressively to prevent holding the feeling of shame. Or the individual may alternatively *attack self*, a fight response turned inward, which can manifest as self-criticism, self-harm, or even attempting suicide. Individuals who *withdraw* may hide from the world, shut down, avert their gaze in sessions, avoid interaction with others, and feel fearful interpersonally. *Avoid* behaviors manifest as a form of flight, distancing from internal experience. They may use drugs or alcohol, seek distractions, and engage in intense fantasy to escape shame.

Art Therapy

Since addressing shame is central for recovery from developmental trauma, exploring the purpose of shame using a model such as Nathanson's compass of shame can be especially useful. Below is a creative and sensorial way to help children identify and develop reflective awareness of shame.

Compass of Shame in the Sand

Incorporating natural materials such as sand and rocks with a paper plate provides a simple structure for teaching the compass of shame model. I label the plate rim with the four poles of the compass: *avoid, withdrawal, attack self,* and *attack other,* pour some sand into the plate, and offer stones to explore the weight that shame feels like. The sand is used as a natural concrete boundary for obtaining emotional distance, which can allow for more reflective engagement.

I begin by providing an explanation of shame, based on Nathanson's approach above, using examples from my own experience that help normalize shame. Being playful and allowing for some laughter when discussing shame can help in this exercise, as even the word "shame" may evoke the emotion. However, a comical discussion that allows for laughter can relax the child and even make the experience of exploring shame fun (Figure 32.4).

Following the discussion, I invite the child to explore shame by providing an example from their own life, if they are within their window of tolerance to do so. The therapist, using their clinical judgment, may alternatively ask the child to choose an example from a movie, book, or TV show where the child felt the protagonist experienced shame. Having a few storybooks available on shame may be useful if the client struggles to find an example. I then invite the child to draw on a small slip of paper an image or a few words to signify the experience and then bury the paper in the sand to get some distance from it. Following that, I invite the child to use the stones, to place them at whichever four poles of the compass signify the emotional and behavioral reactions they observed in reaction to shame. Stones feel heavy, as does shame, and the child can use the weight of the stones as a sensorial signifier.

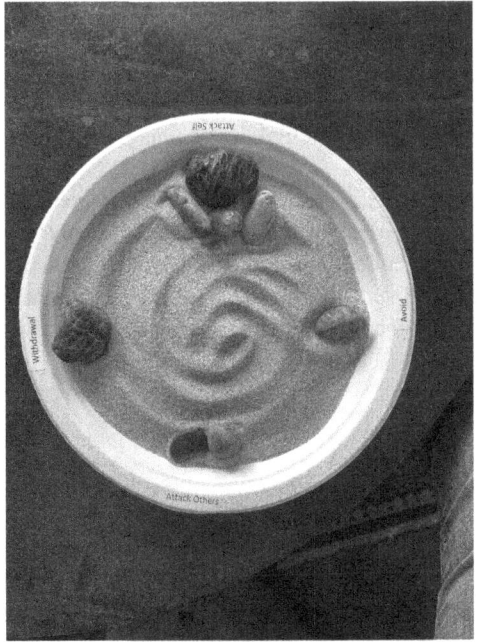

Figure 32.4 Shame Compass in the Sand with Stones: Part One.

After placing the stones at the poles, I invite the child to retrieve the note and offer compassionate resources to the experience of shame in the form of wise or soothing sand tray figures, words, or gifts in the form of stickers or drawings. Alternatively, the child may want to put the note in a container if it is about their own experience. This part of the education is important for closure, as the child may need compassion and containment if they shared their own example, or desire to give compassion to the protagonist in the story.

Case Example: Sophia

Sophia came to therapy with her foster mom, and both were invited to report a good thing and then something that was challenging from the week. Mom reported an incident where Sophia had a "meltdown" and refused to follow instructions to put her book bag away. The refusal led to Sophia shutting down and hiding in her closet, refusing to come out or talk. Mom eventually called the caseworker to help her deescalate Sophia, who appeared regressed and frozen. The choice to explore this incident using the shame compass was determined based on both Sophia's and Mom's agreement, their level of trust established in previous conversations in therapy, and their previous successful working through of the incident with the caseworker.

Sophia began by first drawing on a small piece of paper how she felt when her mom asked her to put her book bag away. Sophia drew a sad face, then folded it up and buried it under the sand. Sophia was then invited to place stones at the poles of the compass, indicating how she had responded. Sophia placed most of the stones on the *withdrawal* pole but some on *attack other* and *attack self*. She was then asked if she wanted to talk about how she responded. Sophia shared that she was feeling rejected and that she was a disappointment to her mom, which she said were triggered by the tone of her foster mother's voice. Mom was then invited to give her response to the experience. Mom also drew a sad face, buried it under the sand and placed stones primarily at the *attack self* pole, but a few at *attack other*. She expressed feeling helpless. After the exercise, both acknowledged their awareness of shame-based beliefs that come up when they are in conflict and discussed ways they could communicate their feelings using a feeling chart placed in a common area of the home. This exercise was followed by both being invited to choose sand tray figures from the shelf to bring wisdom and compassion to the parts of them that had gotten overwhelmed in the experience. Sophia picked an elephant, one of her favorite animals, and a lifeboat. Sophia's foster mom chose a wise Buddha-like figure and a mother figure for advice.

When working dyadically, the therapist should approach this exercise with care and discernment, making sure that there is enough trust for the two to share openly. Caregivers and children who are locked in epistemic distrust may default into non-mentalizing modes with each other, and then learning from the experience will stall. But in the case of a parent and child who have some trust, the experience can work to increase mentalization between them and the ability to repair ruptures (Figure 32.5).

Suggested Script for Compass of Shame in Sand

Would you like to explore a memory to see how the compass of shame works? [If yes, continue by asking the child for a minor experience where they might have experienced shame]. *Recall a memory where you felt hurt, vulnerable, or angry in reaction to the words or actions of another person.* [Alternatively, offer this directive:] *Recall a movie, book, or TV character who you think experienced shame. Draw a quick image or write down what the experience was on the paper provided, and then fold it.* [The child is then invited to bury the note.] *Place the paper in the middle of the compass and bury it in the sand. Now reflect on how you* [or the character in the story] *reacted to the experience.*

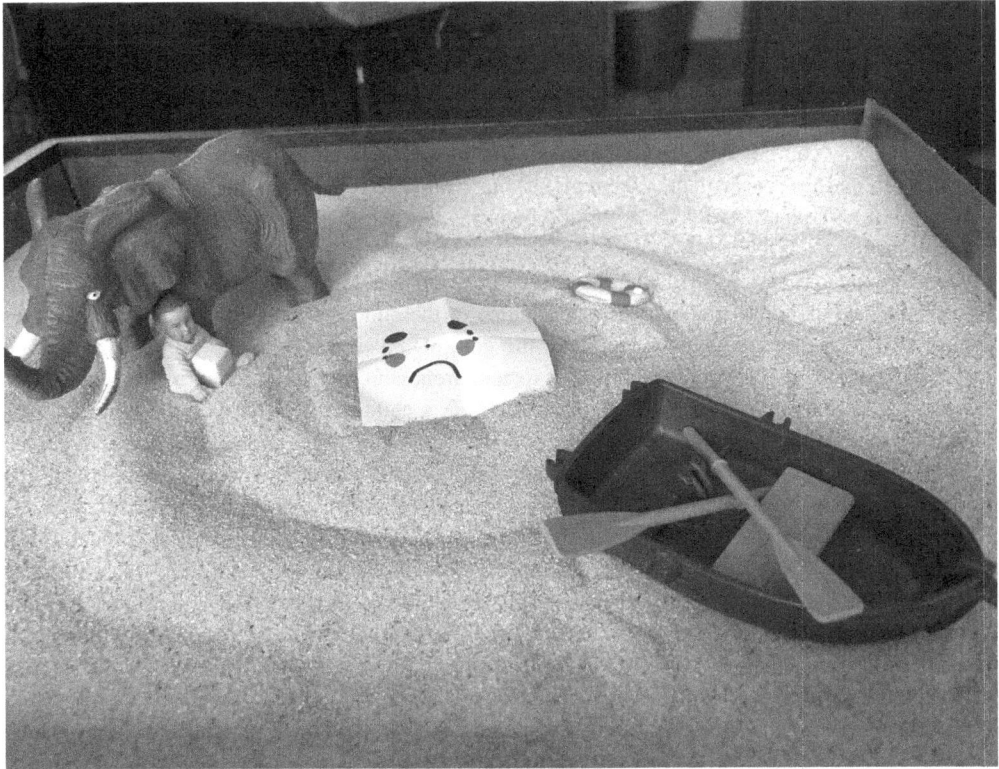

Figure 32.5 Shame Compass in the Sand with Figures: Part Two.

Use as many stones as you like to show how you [or the protagonist] *experienced shame, placing them at the four poles, attack self, attack other, withdraw, avoid.*

[Following the stone placement, invite the child to retrieve the note and offer resources such as words or gifts of compassion to the experiencer.] *Now retrieve the note from the middle. Would you like to offer some support to yourself* [or the protagonist]*? You can use sand tray figures if you like that may bring comfort or wisdom. You can use playful stickers or draw an image to help.* [If needed, offer containment:] *You may even want to put the note in a box for safe keeping.*

Exploring Attachment

Helping the client develop an understanding of healthy attachment is one core component of treatment for developmental trauma in phase one (Brown & Elliott, 2016). Clients' early attachment experiences often tell them that they must be needless to survive, or that their needs are too much to handle. The fact that everyone has needs, not just physically but emotionally, often comes as new information to them. Adults with attachment trauma may engage in resource narratives—such as those found in the work of Daniel Brown & David Elliott (the Ideal Parent Figure method, 2016), Ricky Greenwald (Developing Secure Attachment, 2013), and Philip Manfield (Dyadic Resourcing, 2010)—that help them connect with a model of healthy attachment through imaginal rehearsal. But for children, these approaches often exceed their developmental capacities and present difficulties in implementation. The developmental needs timeline takes a concrete approach that offers distance and the creative potential of playful expressive arts to engage the child in the activity.

Developmental Needs Timeline

In this exercise, I offer the child polymer clay with which to create figurative representations at different developmental ages. The mini figures are molded, using the wide array of colors polymer clay comes in, to represent the different stages of development such as baby self, toddler self, school-aged self, etc. The clay can be cooked in any standard oven on a low temperature so that the figures can be made hard and feel permanent. When embarking on this activity, the clinician should have some knowledge of and experience with using polymer clay, so that they can effectively assist the child with their creations.

If appropriate and desired by the child, I invite the parent or caregiver into sessions to assist with this activity. The caregiver can act as an apprentice to the child, helping them create their figures. Additionally, when the caregiver is included, the goal of the activity can address their attachment relationship with the child. For the adoptive or foster parent who is providing a permanent placement, the opportunity to express what they would provide for a child at different ages can ignite positive feelings of connection. When presenting this activity with a biological parent, who may have a history of trauma and conflict, I discuss the intention of the activity with them ahead of time and how they may engage with their child to achieve possible repair and increase attachment security.

Before beginning this activity, I offer a short explanation of the procedure and offer a few tips on using polymer clay. Many clay tools are available at craft stores, such as molds, clay cutters, sculpting knives, and shape cutters, and can expand the possibilities of the activity. However, a simple plastic knife and a round marker to use as a rolling pin can be enough. Then I invite the child to make figurative representations at different ages, such as baby, toddler, school-aged, teen, and so on. After each figure is made, I ask the child to explore what they believe is needed for a child of that age. For example, for the baby self, I may ask generally what they believe babies might want, like a bottle, teddy bear, a special person, a comfy bed, or being held. The identified items or symbols to represent needs are created out of clay and offered to the representation. Psychoeducation around needs can be provided at each age to fill in missing information. For example, for a toddler, the therapist may suggest they need to explore, or might begin to test limits, and yet need their caregiver nearby; with an older child, the therapist might discuss the need for friends and feeling included, and developing skills.

When engaging in this directive, the therapist should keep in mind that the focus is not on the child's actual history of development but on exploring developmental needs. Focus on the child's actual history may emerge naturally as the subject matter is explored, and the activity does have the potential to ignite feelings concerning neglect and trauma, absence of connection, and grief. However, the therapist who frames the activity as an exploration of healthy development and an opportunity for imaginative and playful exploration of needs can guide the experience.

Occasionally, a child will be hesitant to engage in creating any human form or may struggle with the idea of equating this to their own history of development. In these instances, I offer the alternative directive of exploring an animal's development. The child will then be offered the option to create an animal of their choosing as a baby, toddler equivalent, and so on. An example is a newborn puppy, young puppy, and older puppy. Children then are offered the same developmental information but through the distance an animal metaphor provides.

Case Example: Sophia

Sophia explored developmental needs using panda bears. She worked with her foster mom and me, apprentices helping her explore and create. Her foster mom was able to offer her feelings about what she would give a baby panda, a toddler panda, and an older child panda. Baby panda was given a bed to sleep in and a doll to play with. Sophia also made an animal keeper that resembled her foster mom,

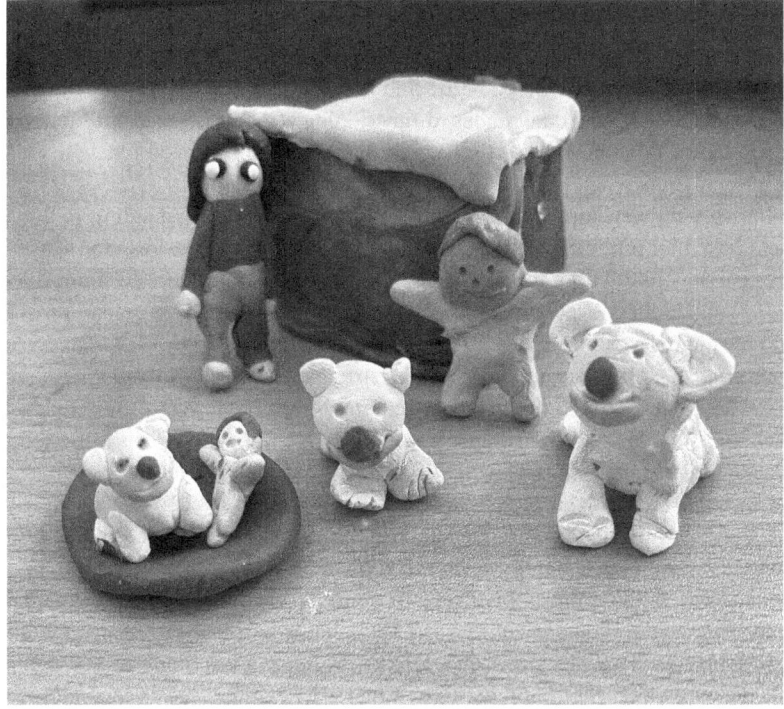

Figure 32.6 Developmental Bear Figures: Baby, Toddler, and School Age.

and a house. The toddler panda was given Sophia's favorite meal: tacos. Older child panda was given a computer to play on. Although the activity used animal figures, it equally mirrored the needs and discussion of humans (Figure 32.6).

Suggested Script for Growing Needs Timeline

Create clay models of a person [or an animal] *as they grow up.* [If needed, add.] *You may want to create a newborn, toddler, older child, teenager, and even an adult. Imagine what each need* [or the chosen animal] *at these various stages of growing up. Create out of clay what is needed and give it to the figure* [or animal figure]. *Imagine the figures receiving what was needed.*

Art Therapy Integrated into Phase-Oriented Treatment-Phase Two

In phase two of treatment the therapist and client have a relationship that provides enough safety to move toward exploring the source of the symptoms that brought the client into treatment. Skills, resources and information have been identified in phase one that will help the client to proceed to phase two, where fears, phobias, and trauma can begin to be explored more directly. Therapists may find entry into phase two returns to phase one often as trauma exploration may unearth new memories and fears around attachment and loss. The therapist should be prepared to follow the client's regulation capacity and not stick with a ridged linear idea of treatment progression as the phases themselves overlap. New psychoeducation or revisiting skill development may be needed as the layers of trauma are explored. Art therapy can provide a flexible and organic approach for a client who can use art materials both for their regulating and soothing qualities as well as expressive potential to engage past trauma experience.

Repairing the Psychic Split and Finding Meaning

According to Fonagy et al. (2004), a child cannot maintain the unbearable state of uncertainty, fear, and isolation that results from childhood abuse and neglect, and as a result, they are forced to "split their ego functioning to maintain dual modes of functioning" (p. 266). In a "split" self, the child finds relief from uncertainty, no longer aware of the emotional ambiguity that results with child abuse and neglect. The chronic experience of having split off from the ambiguities inherent in life experience, however, can disrupt the development of mentalization skills (an understanding of the intentions of self and others based an internal representation of feelings, beliefs, desires, and reason). The split state may provide the child with a feeling of certainty, a kind of hiding place from the overwhelming ambiguities and conflicts experienced in childhood, but it leaves them reliant on childlike ways of understanding themselves and others. The child whose mentalizing skills have not been fully formed and become stuck in *prementalizing modes* struggles as they grow older with processing the complexities of past interpersonal traumas that require an understanding of themselves, others and perspective taking. Helping the child enhance and develop mentalization skills is therefore critical for processing past interpersonal trauma as well as meeting the demand of future challenges relationally.

Fonagy et al. (2004) identified key types of prementalizing modes that are naturally part of early development, where a child's capacity to mentalize has not been fully formed. These states are *psych equivalent, pretend mode, and teleological*. Psych equivalent is identified by feelings being given the same weight as reality without the ambivalence of doubt. For example, in the early stages of working with Sophia she would often present in a self-state that would insist on crawling under my desk, expressing she felt safer there. Even though a threat was not present (and even though a part of her could logically acknowledge this), her feelings of threat were experienced as equivalent to reality, and therefore she felt the need to seek protection.

In teleological mode, the actions of others are understood as the sole evidence of reality, without the accompanying understanding of the other having an internal world of feelings, beliefs, desires, and intentions that may motivate their behavior. For example, in teleological mode, Sophia would read the actions of her foster mom telling her to do something in a stern voice as proof she was not loved or lovable, because her mom's voice did not sound loving at the time. Sophia struggled to account for her foster mother's overall intentions and desires.

In pretend mode, the child creates an invulnerable silo of defenses protecting their internal pretend world where they can feel safe from life's uncertainties and ambiguities. Pretend mode draws its name from pretend play, a suspension of the real-world in favor of the imaginary. In this imaginary world the child can have the illusion of power over the forces of the past and challenges of the present by discounting, splitting off, or dissociating away any incongruities. When Sophia was in pretend mode, I experienced her as indifferent and discounting in reaction to my perspective if it did not match hers, even seeming to not hear what she was uncomfortable with, like, for example, the session coming to an end. She could also often talk about her day in a distant, matter-of-fact way that did not seem connected to her emotions or others—for example: "Yes, I got in trouble at school today, but that was not my fault. The teachers are stupid, and I don't need that school anyway."

Art and expressive therapies hold specific qualities that are ideal for addressing mentalization deficits resulting from the psychic split in childhood. Fonagy (2012) has been a supporter of the potential of art therapy to address deficits of mentalization: "Art therapy has the key or perhaps a key to our understanding of the mechanisms underpinning change in all kinds of psychological treatments" (p. 90). Additionally, art therapy "allows the internal to be expressed externally so that it can be verbalized at a distance through an alternative medium and from a different perspective" (Bateman & Fonagy, 2004, p. 172). Bateman and Fonagy (2004) went on to state, "Under these circumstances mentalizing becomes conscious, verbal, deliberate, and reflective" (p. 172). Art therapy, therefore, holds the potential as a form of mentalization therapy, that can aid trauma processing. The distance, containment, perspective, and the natural regulating qualities that art expression embodies can help the child step into phase two. The child can use expressive media as an interactive, (with both the self and the therapist), and reflective process for self-discovery enabling the child to make meaningful understandings out of past experiences.

Below, I explore a few approaches of how to address the split in consciousness. However, there are a couple of cautions to keep in mind when working with children who are struggling in *prementalizing modes*. First is the sensorial power of art media to trigger flashbacks or flooding for those who experience the sensory quality of art materials as too real. I have heard clients refer to wet clay, for example, as disgusting, with little capacity to separate a sensation from their emotional reaction, as in "The clay is disgusting" as opposed to "I think the clay feels disgusting." Some clients also may not tolerate certain colors of paint or odors of media—even pencils were intolerable for one client. When a client is in psych equivalent mode, the experience of the media can be as if it is a real threat.

Second, clients may engage with the materials in a regressive way that can potentially ignite dissociation. For the clinician, it is important to keep in mind that regression can happen quickly, and a child may seem 12 one minute and then present more as three or four years old if a perceived trigger arises. For the clinician, understanding how to time-orient and ground their client when they lose orientation is critical (Martin, 2016). If the clinician is well attuned and mindful of their client's window of tolerance, understands the sensorial and technical challenges of using the art media they offer, and is able to offer grounding assistance and orienting strategies, they can help their client utilize the benefits of art expression.

Art Expression and Implicit Mentalization

Inviting children to express themselves when feelings feel too real can result in implicit unconscious art expressions that may be experienced as cathartic—as one child expressed, "like throwing up on paper." Splashes of paint and brush strokes that may have been intended to produce a precalculated image can merge with feelings without a felt sense of separation. A metaphorical buffer may be absent to mediate the experience between feeling and expression. The expression is the feeling and the feeling the expression. When children are asked to reflect on their creations, the process of mentalizing begins. The therapist may suggest to the child questions that are grounding so that the child can orient to the here and now, such as, "Tell me about your art," "What was it like for you to make these lines, shapes and images?" "What would you like to do with your art?" These questions bring the child back to the present and promote reflection on the process. If the child is present and open to reflecting verbally, then noticing what emotions, and meaning the work holds can be explored. Most important for the therapist to keep in mind is to remain attuned with their client, which reinforces a connection in the present moment as well as enhancing the feeling of being seen for the client.

Case Example: Sophia

Sophia's interpretation of the red paint was that it was "bad." She used her hands and smeared the red paint all over the paper. When asked to reflect on the picture, she expressed needing to use black paint to "box in the bad." She used black to surround the red paint and keep it contained. The way Sophia used her hands and emoted characterized her experience where the paint was equivalent to an internal experience of "bad" feelings. She expressed relief after painting and was offered play time and conversation about some of her favorite activities following the art experience (Figure 32.7).

When children are in pretend mode, art products tend to reflect little overt expressive emotion, and the art piece may present more as a pretend self than an authentic self. However, often, these

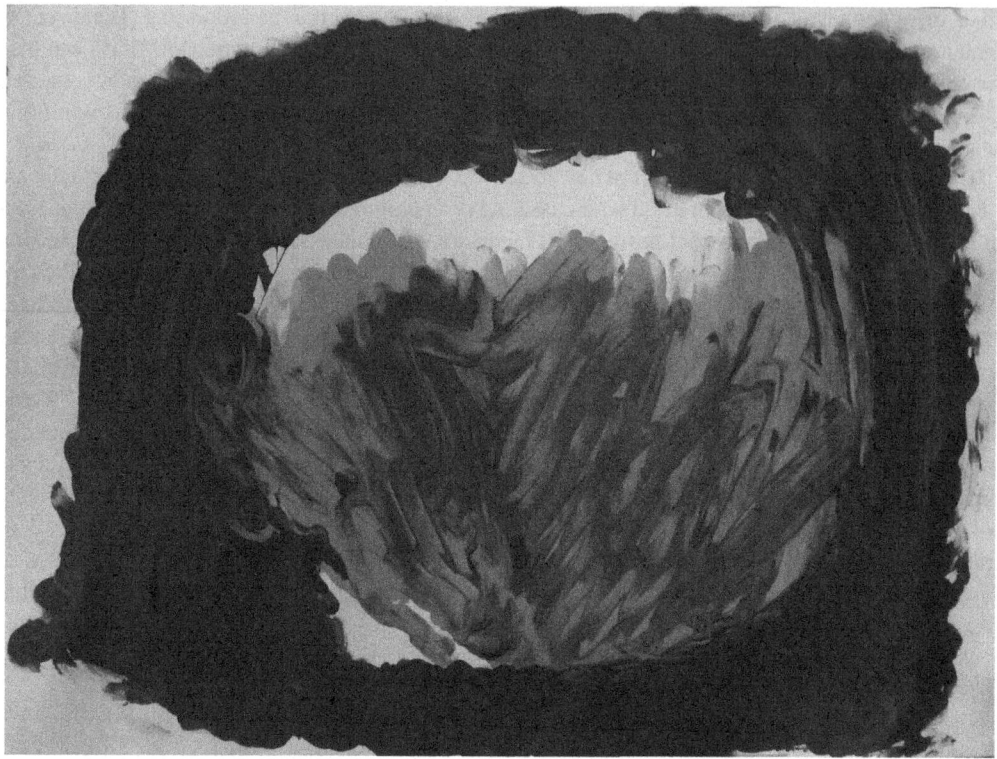

Figure 32.7 Smeared Red Paint with Black Border.

expressions carry unconscious and more hidden emotional elements in the artistic expression. Aspects of the expression may appear missing, for example, or overemphasized, or there may be unusual, exaggerated details. When emotions are disguised, the therapist may be mindful of the child's need to keep them that way. Asking the child for their emotions about their art piece may ignite defenses instead of insight. The therapist may in these cases use art experience as a means for indirect connection with feelings that are held unconsciously. The therapist's questions may nudge the child to notice in a gentle manner: "What do you like/dislike about your artwork?" "What inspired your design?" or "What does your artwork remind you of?" These questions allow for distance from emotions but also encourage reflection on the process and the larger world.

Case Example: Sophia

In this portrait, Sophia presents an older-looking self with exaggerated features. Although the face depicts a smile, the lips and eyes tell a different story. According to Sophia, the portrait depicts a cool person, popular and fashionable. Sophia indicated this was an ideal of what she wanted to look like and be like. However, the image also offers contradictions to this cool and ideal portrayal. The girl's shirt displays tears and a broken heart. The eyes seem more pessimistic or guarded than happy or proud. The large head and tiny neck with a coiled choker portray a bound and constricted experience for the viewer. These implicit metaphorical elements may be initially well camouflaged. When looking at art that may be created by a client in pretend mode, the therapist might approach their client's creations by emotionally checking in with the elements of the picture and noting the feelings that arise. Incoherence between the client's overt expression and the therapist's felt sense when exploring the image more deeply may inform the therapist of the client's conflicts, struggle, and underlying emotions which are not ready to be voiced.

Art Expression and Explicit Mentalization

As children become more comfortable with art making and identifying emotions, their ability to express themselves in their artwork can emerge more intentionally. Art expression may involve the use of explicit metaphors to depict states of consciousness, beliefs, desires, experiences, and feelings. Using metaphors can allow for a level of pretending and yet hold the very raw experience. Additionally, metaphors aid in perspective taking and understanding abstract concepts such as emotions and thoughts that are often hard for children to articulate verbally (Casasanto & Gijssels, 2015). Reflection on the metaphorical content of the artwork may lead to increased capacity to identify feelings and beliefs more consciously which can aid in processing trauma. This more explicit and intentional use of art expression can allow a child a way of talking about difficult experiences and feelings that are hard to express verbally.

When a child is ready to address the conflicts resulting from traumatic experience through art, trauma resolution approaches such as EMDR (Eye Movement Desensitization and Reprocessing) may be an option (for those therapists trained in this trauma resolution method) to integrate with art therapy and phase two treatment (Davis et al., 2022). Expressive representations of trauma material can aid EMDR by both helping the client contain traumatic content, as well as offering needed psychological distance to maintain dual attention (present oriented while focused on past trauma). Artwork can help contain trauma material by symbolizing aspects of the traumatic experience within the expressive forms. The meaning of the artwork then can act as a placeholder for the trauma itself. The child can look upon their art as an object they have power over, can react to, and can destroy if desired. As a placeholder for the trauma, the artwork can be physically kept at a distance from the mind. Just as many EMDR trained therapists offer their clients distance from a trauma memory by instructing them to watch it as if they were watching a movie (Shapiro, 2018, p. 166), artwork can hold the experience of trauma at a distance, but also in a concrete way. With the utilization of art expression bolstering the child's capacities to contain and have distance, more energy to engage mentalization capacities may be available to resolve traumatic memories. Especially with children who may operate often on a concrete level as well as struggle with emotional regulation, scaffolding the trauma processing phase in this way may be especially beneficial.

Case Example: Sophia

As part of exploring her reaction to the "Me Too" movement and as a way to engage her own sexual abuse history, Sophia created "Me Too." Using hot glue (in black, clear, and pink colors), beads, and buttons Sophia worked with my assistance to envision a way to metaphorically express a state of feeling frozen, violated, and caught between her biological family and her safety. Her artwork depicts a central generic female body outline traced from a bathroom sign. The body outline is filled in with globs of clear hot glue and embedded buttons. Surrounding the female figure Sophia used globs of hot glue (like thick paint) to create a black area on the figure's left side and a pink area on the figure's right. The split black and pink image with the central female figure filled in with clear glue and embedded buttons creates the illusion of a child caught between dark and light forces, frozen in milky goo. Sophia was able to talk about the image as symbolic of her experience and how dissociation felt for her. Following the art creation Sophia was able to begin processing the memories of molestation with EMDR using her art creation as a container and reminder of her experience. Sophia indicated following processing that she could see the memories more in the past and better understand the part of herself that freezes.

Art Therapy: Advocacy and Meaning Making, Phase Three

A client's creations, when used as a way to document and validate their experiences of trauma can hold the potential to transcend dissociation on more than a personal scale. The power of art to confront societal dissociation for those who are oppressed and suffer injustices has been demonstrated repeatedly over the course of human history. The work of Pablo Picasso, Eugene Delacroix, Frida Kahlo, Cindy Sherman, and countless others represent artists whose objects changed societal awareness by holding the psychic reality of those who were oppressed. Nan Goldin, American photographer and activist for LGBTQ2IA+ rights, demonstrates the power of art and the artist as a social agent. In *All the Beauty and the Bloodshed* (Poitras, 2022) Goldin stated, "Photography was always a way to walk through fear." Her photographs hold the reality that a dissociated society has denied. For Goldin, her art became a way of holding on to the reality that her psyche could not bear to hold alone in a society that could not be trusted to even acknowledge it. With her work exploring HIV/AIDS and the opioid epidemic, Goldin portrayed that reality as a means of not forgetting or dissociating the reality away. As she states, "How do you show the world that you did experience that, …? …that is the reason I take pictures."

In the same way, art therapy has the potential to help the complexly traumatized child find their larger voice for both them and the larger world. This step of risking to create an authentic expression of the self can be engaged in art therapy by helping the client imagine themselves going out into the world. How will the discovery of the past inform their future? What challenges do they feel they will face? The client carries the gains from processing trauma forward. In phase three of trauma treatment this may mean the task of discovering new ways of engaging in relationships as well as figuring out how to step into life with wholeness and authenticity. Phase three is vitally important for healing with developmental trauma and dissociation as this phase may represent a novel experience of life that the client finds unfamiliar. New behaviors are needed to supplant the often reflexive old behaviors learned under trauma conditions. Instead of just surviving the child begins the journey to explore their true feelings, beliefs, desires and intentions, perhaps for the first time, and with the understanding of life as uncertain and full of future challenges.

Case Example

The youth in this example depicted themselves facing their future after working through trauma memories in phase two. Challenges they will encounter are symbolized as bubble forms. Leaves in the picture represent their positive connection to nature as well as the passing of time. They expressed their artwork reminds them to stay grounded, not forget but not be bound by the traumas of the past, and to use the courage they found through recovery to accomplish their goals. The city background represents their home and holds the perspective of being a part of a much larger whole. For them this perspective represented being a part of a larger world and not separated or alone.

Conclusion

The potential of art therapy as a front-line approach for treating developmental trauma and dissociation in children offers the special advantages of addressing the client's fear of connection and their deficits in skills, alternative ways of approaching psychoeducation, and the enhancement of mentalization and containment enhancing opportunities for self-discovery and making meaning. Art experience for the child who has been denied the rights of safety and security can serve to empower their capacities to confront the split within. When words are too threatening and too difficult to find or form, voice can be restored through expression. At the core of art therapies' advantages lie the creative experience and corresponding object, created in an interpersonal sphere, that allows for a revitalization of agency and the space to make meaning out of experience. This approach offered to a child with developmental trauma has the potential to empower them as an advocate for themselves as they navigate their lives through their developmental pathway and toward new relationships and connection with the world at large.

Note

1 All details of "Sophia," including all associated artwork, are representative of clinical cases and Sophia is not an actual client.

References

Bateman, A., & Fonagy, P. (2004). *Psychotherapy for borderline personality disorder: Mentalization-based treatment*. Oxford University Press.

Bateman, A., & Fonagy, P. (2019). *Handbook of mentalizing in mental health practice*. American Psychiatric Association Publishing.

Bird, B. (Director). (2018). *The Incredibles 2* [Film]. Buena Vista Pictures.

Brand, B. L., Schielke, H. J., Schiavone, F., & Lanius, R. A. (2022). *Finding solid ground: Overcoming obstacles in trauma treatment*. Oxford University Press.

Brown, D. P., & Elliott, D. S. (2016). *Attachment disturbances in adults: Treatment for comprehensive repair*. W. W. Norton.

Casasanto, D., & Gijssels, T. (2015). What makes a metaphor an embodied metaphor?. *Linguistics Vanguard, 1*(1), 327–337. https://doi.org/10.1515/lingvan-2014-1015

Cloitre, M., Courtois, C. A., Ford, J. D., Green, B. L., Alexander, P., Briere, J., Herman, J. L., Lanius, R., Stolbach, B. C., Spinazzola, J., van der Kolk, B. A., & van der Hart, O. (2012). The ISTSS expert consensus treatment guidelines for complex PTSD in adults. https://istss.org/clinical-resources/trauma-treatment/new-istss-prevention-and-treatment-guidelines/

Davis, E., Fitzgerald, J., Jacobs, S., & Marchand, J. (Eds.). (2022). *EMDR and creative arts therapies* (1st ed.). Routledge. https://doi.org/10.4324/9781003156932

Flannigan, C., & Dietze, B. (2018). Children, outdoor play, and loose parts. *Journal of Childhood Studies, 42*(4), 53–60. https://doi.org/10.18357/jcs.v42i4.18103

Fonagy, P. (2012). Art therapy and personality disorder. *International Journal of Art Therapy, 17*(3), 90. https://doi.org/10.1080/17454832.2012.740866

Fonagy, P., Gergely, G., Jurist, E., & Target, M. E. (2004). *Affect regulation, mentalization, and the development of the self*. Other Press (Original work published in 2002).

Greenwald, R. (2007). *EMDR within a phase model of trauma-informed treatment*. Routledge.

Greenwald, R. (2013). *Progressive counting within a phase model of trauma-informed treatment*. Routledge.

Kagan, R., & Spinazzola, J. (2013). Real life heroes: Application of a developmental, resilience- centered treatment model for children in residential treatment. *Journal of Family Violence, 28*, 705–715. https://doi.org/10.1007/s10896-013-9537-6

Kaimal, G., Ray, K., & Muniz, J. (2016). Reduction of cortisol levels and participants' responses following art making. *Art Therapy: Journal of the American Art Therapy Association, 33*(2), 74–80. https://doi.org/10.1080/07421656.2016.1166832

Linde-Krieger, L., Yates, T., & Carlson, E. (2023). A developmental pathways model of dissociation. In M. Dorahy, S. Gold & J. O'Neil (Eds.), *Dissociation and the dissociative disorders* (pp. 149–160). Routledge.

Liotti, G. (1999). Disorganization of attachment as a model for understanding dissociative psychopathology. In J. Solomon & C. George (Eds.), *Attachment disorganization* (pp. 39–70). Guildford Press.

Lorenzini, N., Campbell, C., & Fonagy, P. (2019). Mentalization and its role in processing trauma. In B. Huppertz (Ed.), *Approaches to psychic trauma* (pp. 403–422). Rowan & Littlefield.

Manfield, P. (2010). *Dyadic resourcing: Creating a foundation for processing trauma*. Create Space Independent Publishing.

Martin, K. (2016). *EMDR & structural dissociation theory*. Webinar series, January–March.

Martin, L., Oepen, R., Bauer, K., Nottensteiner, A., Mergheim, K., Gruber, H., & Koch, S. C. (2018). Creative arts interventions for stress management and prevention: A systematic review. *Behavioral Sciences (Basel, Switzerland), 8*(2), Article 28. https://doi.org/10.3390/bs8020028

Nathanson, D. (1992). *Shame and pride: Affect, sex and the birth of the self*. W.W. Norton.

Perry, B. (2009). Examining child maltreatment through a neurodevelopmental lens: Clinical applications of the neurosequential model of therapeutics. *Journal of Loss and Trauma, 14*(4), 240–255. https://doi.org/10.1080/15325020903004350

Poitras, L. (Director, Producer). (2022). *All the beauty and the bloodshed* [Film]. Praxis Films.

Purvis, K., Cross D., Dansereau D., & Parris S. (2013). Trust-based relational intervention (TBRI): A systemic approach to complex developmental trauma. *Child & Youth Services, 34*(4), 360–386. https://doi.org/10.1080/0145935X.2013.859906

Schore, A. (2023). Attachment and the developing right brain. In M. Dorahy, S. Gold & J. O'Neil (Eds.), *Dissociation and the dissociative disorders* (pp. 177–208). Routledge.

Shapiro, F. (2018). *Eye movement desensitization and reprocessing (EMDR) therapy: Basic principles, protocols, and procedures* (3rd ed.). Guilford Press.

Silberg, J. (2004). Guidelines for the evaluation and treatment of dissociative symptoms in children and adolescents. *Journal of Trauma & Dissociation, 5*(3), 119–150. https://doi.org/10.1300/J229v05n03_09

Silberg, J., & Dallam, S. (2023). Dissociative disorders in children and adolescents. In M. Dorahy, S. Gold & J. O'Neil (Eds.), *Dissociation and the dissociative disorders* (pp. 434–447). Routledge.

Springham, N., & Huet, V. (2018). Art as relational encounter: An ostensive communication theory of art therapy. *Journal of the American Art Therapy Association, 35*(1), 4–10. https://doi.org/10.1080/07421656.2018.1460103

Stavropoulos, P., & Elliot, D. (2022). Controversies in the treatment of traumatic dissociation. In M. Dorahy, S. Gold & J. O'Neil (Eds.), *Dissociation and the dissociative disorders* (pp. 713–727). Routledge.

Winnicott, D. W. (2005). *Playing and reality*. Routledge (Originally published in 1971).

PART 4

Important Treatment Considerations

33
THE THERAPEUTIC RELATIONSHIP

Jillian Hosey and Eva Teirstein Young

Introduction

A relationship-based approach to child trauma therapy considers the important roles of bonding, attachment, and early development, using the relationship as the vehicle to bring development back on track (Gil, 2010; Pearlman & Courtois, 2005; Agarwal et al., 2019; Silberg, 2001). It proposes that healing from trauma happens within the context of a close and bonded therapeutic relationship (Courtois & Ford, 2016; Cronin et al., 2014; ISSTD, 2004, in press; Norcross & Wampold, 2019), and that relationships can help "protect from and heal following stress, distress, and trauma" (Perry, 2009). It is within the relational landscape that we attend to (re)experiencing the internal experience of safety, inviting a child's spontaneous expression and embracing their imagination; this becomes the fluid thread that is woven through the co-occurring treatment-related tasks of both "doing" (based on intervention) and "being with" (based on being with the process and what emerges). For children with chronic traumatic experiences, the therapeutic relationship is often the first invitation to engage in authentic, safe, and attuned play alongside a grown-up who is accepting and interested in what is being shared and created, inviting spontaneity and following the child's lead. The therapist who collaborates, while not interfering, in the child's process of play begins to attend to important aspects of being in safe "togetherness," while providing a space in which the client can "create health" (Tuber, 2008, p. 1; Winnicott, 1945). When a child's development is disrupted by relational trauma, it is the therapeutic relationship that facilitates restoration of the developmental trajectory. This may include the (re)development of both co-regulation and self-regulation capacities (Silberg & Dallam, 2023); the identification, expression, and modulation of feelings (Gil, 2016); and collaborating with the child to dynamically revise Internal Working Models (Pearlman & Courtois, 2005) or attachment schemas (Cappas et al., 2005; Cozolino, 2014).

Due to the complex symptom constellation complexly traumatized child clients present with, clinicians may find themselves attending to multiple treatment tasks simultaneously; therapists serve as a child's external *psychobiological regulator* (Gil, 2010; Schore, 2003). Using "right-brain to right-brain therapeutic interaction" (Schore, 2016), therapists facilitate change for child clients, mirroring nonverbal communication that supports growth in the therapeutic relationship and the parent-child relationship. In this multifaceted role, the therapist provides a holding environment (Slochower, 2018; Winnicott, 1971), containment (Bion, 1962), titrating the various potentially conflicting feelings arising from connectedness and developing regulatory capacities to internalize the thing they need—an Other (Gil, 2010). Within this process, "the therapist is called on to provide complex trauma survivors with an alternative attachment model" (Courtois & Ford, 2016, p. 275), through which children may (re)experience safety and (re)build regulation and self-soothing skills while discovering and exploring their wishes, desires, and self-agency. Through the therapeutic relationship, children and caregivers are invited to enter an environment that offers increased opportunities for post-traumatic growth (Tedeschi & Calhoun, 2004).

The therapeutic relationship is truly unique; it facilitates discovery and self-expression. Its relevance and impact transcends modality or intervention. The therapeutic relationship has been found to contribute to improved outcomes and reduced symptomatology (Ellis et al., 2018; Norcross & Wampold, 2019; Shirk & Karver, 2003), and is a predictor of greater adherence to and engagement in treatment (Keller et al., 2010). According to Manassis (2014), the alliance between the child and therapist is "the cornerstone for any successful treatment" (p. 208). However, data about the predictive nature of childhood trauma, treatment outcomes, and the quality of alliance within the therapeutic relationship continues to remain limited in work with children.

This volume offers the reader the opportunity to explore a variety of theories, approaches, and modalities pertaining to the identification and treatment of children with histories of complex trauma and dissociative symptoms. Each chapter focuses on a different aspect of treatment, including the therapeutic relationship, honoring the inherent complexity in each clinical approach. Interestingly, different modalities present different conceptualizations of the therapeutic relationship—more specifically, what it means, how it unfolds, and its level of importance to treatment outcomes (Shirk & Karver, 2003). Despite a lack of consensus in this area, social neuroscience research and clinical experience support the link between therapeutic success and the therapeutic relationship "regardless of the theoretical orientation of the therapist or whether the therapist considers the relationship to be an active aspect of the change process" (Cozolino, 2014, p. 397).

The focus of this chapter is the centrality of the therapeutic relationship to treatment with children with histories of complex trauma and dissociation. The chapter takes a psychodynamic perspective recognizing the impact of complex trauma on the nervous system, the use of implicit relational communication to support repatterning, and the incorporation of a Winnicottian conceptualization of child development, framing the therapeutic relationship as *the core facet* of therapeutic work with complexly traumatized and dissociative children. Winnicottian tenets were chosen to provide a way to discuss the nuanced relationship of self, other, and self-in-relation-to an Other through a bidirectional process, whereby the grown-up caregiver and the child, or the therapist and child client, influence each other through the natural language of play (Gil, 2017). Psychoanalyst Donald Winnicott (1971) believed that play is a creative activity in which the child uses the "whole personality" (p. 54) and discovers the self, as the therapist becomes attuned to and follows the spontaneous gestures (Winnicott, 1965) of the child. Winnicott emphasized the child's individual, innate potential in contrast to the focus on unconscious drives (Slochower, 2018), and believed in the centrality of the protective maternal holding environment that would provide a setting, protected from environmental impingements, in which the infant could develop ego-strengths via a "continuity of being" (Winnicott, 1965, p. 52). To illustrate these concepts and provide readers with fundamental treatment-related information, this chapter will first explore notions of the therapeutic relationship and some key concepts, the impact of early attachment disruptions on the capacity to connect and play, themes related to countertransference, and common relational challenges that arise during the hard work of play with dissociative children and their caregivers. This is followed by relational considerations and some strategies to promote the development of cohesion within the evolving relational environment. Case composite examples will be provided throughout.

The Multiple Layers of the Therapeutic Relationship

Schore (2019) shared that

> the human brain develops within the context of an emotion-regulating relationship with another human being ... The relationship between the therapist and client is called the therapeutic alliance, and unless it is strong enough, it cannot provide a growth-facilitating environment for the complex trauma patient's underdeveloped right brain.
>
> *(p. 242)*

Within this context, the therapist becomes a relational bridge, inviting states of being into the holding environment of therapy with empathy and lack of judgment, allowing the child's internal world to reveal itself in their own time and at their own pace. Winnicott (1971) stated that, while honoring play as the natural language of the child (Gil, 2017; Gomez, 2012), "psychotherapy takes place at the overlap of two areas of play, that of the patient and that of the therapist. Psychotherapy has to do with two people playing together" (p. 38). It is within this milieu that "the repair, restoration or creation of effective working models of attachment, and the application of these models to current interpersonal relationships, including the therapeutic alliance" can occur (Cook et al., 2005, p. 394; Silberg, 2021). In treatment sessions with children, we integrate materials and techniques that engage the whole brain and all the different ways of being emerging through the childs play. This facilitates meaning and experience to unfold as the therapeutic relationship develops. The therapeutic relationship can strengthen disrupted areas of growth, supporting redevelopment of social-emotional skills and metacognition. It is through this process that therapists support the restoration of the child's developmental trajectory.

All Behavior Is Communication

Within the relationship, all behavior is considered communication (ISSTD, 2004, in press; Silberg, 2021), and there is always a feeling that precedes a behavior. Emotionally attuned therapists are available to perceive information transmitted in wordless ways, supporting the development and expansion of more coherent representations of self and other (Gil, 2010). Via "right-brain processes that are reciprocally activated on both sides of the therapeutic alliance ... right brain interactions 'beneath the words' nonverbally communicate essential, nonconscious bodily based affective relational information about the inner world of the patient (and therapist)" (Ford & Courtois, 2020, p. 26). Gil (2010) stressed developmental research and expert consensus that "implicit communication is as important to creating transformative changes in psychotherapy as is explicit communication." Furthermore, "since dissociation, by its very nature, is nonverbalized, the importance of the analyst's being attuned to implicit communication cannot be overstated" (p. 3).

Responsive and reflective mirroring can offer corrective experiences of attunement and empathic acceptance while providing nurturance and *collaborative* relating (Ford & Courtois, 2020; Forner, 2019; Siegel, 2001). Children "learn to represent internal experiences because these experiences are first made real by another's recognition of them" (Slade, 1994, p. 95). The therapist notices and reflects feelings as they become available, joining the child, at times in a wordless manner. This type of wordless communication serves "as the foundation of creating new neuronal pathways that contribute to actual development of the brain and of heretofore implicit self, which contributes to change and healing" (Ford & Courtois, 2020, p. 94). Other authors have referred to such engagement as "Attuned Communication" (Forner, 2019) and "Empathic Attunement" (Hopenwasser, 2008). The therapeutic environment is a holding environment (Winnicott, 1965) that can be viewed as a container (Bion, 1962), holding the dissociated feelings and expressions for the child. The meaning of those expressions reveal themselves in time, sometimes taking years.

In an initial session, a precocious, friendly, and enthusiastic ten-year-old boy drew two pictures while sharing, with much bravado, that he misbehaved at school, got in fights, competently traveled around the city by himself, often forgot things, and had not had contact with his mother since he was four years old. As he talked about his older siblings and powerful father, a small cat with a bright red tongue and wide-open eyes emerged in one drawing; the other drawing that followed portrayed a very sad and disoriented-looking small puppy. The therapist observed disorganization in the drawing and noticed aloud how these little creatures looked sad, alone, and somewhat confused. These observations were ignored. The therapist, noticing a shift in the boy's enthusiastic engagement, did not push further, recognizing that the client sets the pace. Eleven years later, the now 21-year-old client asked for a consultation. He had found his mother, and they were going to meet. He wanted to return to the therapist to discuss disturbing feelings that were arising and causing much distress. He began to talk about the frustrating family dynamics related to his desire to see his mother. His siblings and father were angry; he was sad. The therapist rose from her chair and walked to the shelves on the other side of the room where the two pictures he'd drawn years ago remained. The client held the small pictures in his hands, stunned and grateful that the therapist had "held on to them for all these years." Noting that his emotions were now more available, the therapist suggested that his feelings were not new, but perhaps they had been out of his awareness since he was a child. Perhaps, these were the feelings that motivated the "misbehavior," forgetfulness, and disorientation he had experienced as a child. The therapist's respect, validation of the child, and recognition of the feelings projected onto the drawings helped the now emerging adult make his previously unformulated experience of a tumultuous, chaotic childhood thinkable and knowable (Stern, 2010). With this new, empathic understanding of himself as a child, accompanied by the knowledge that his therapist has held his artwork on her shelf and held him in her mind (Fonagy et al., 2019) he was then able to stay connected to his own thoughts and feelings when he finally reunited with his mother.

According to Winnicott (1994), the therapist who works with dysregulated children may be the first adult to supply an environment that is responsive and devoted to the child's individual needs. In this way, the therapist displays

> all the patience and tolerance and reliability of a mother devoted to her infant, has to recognize the patient's wishes as needs, has to put aside other interests in order to be available and to be punctual, and objective, and has to seem to want to give what is really only given because of the patient's needs.
>
> (p. 356)

This provides what Winnicott (1994) termed an "ordinary environment," where essential needs are met and hold more importance than any content that arises in a session. It is here that the child client is invited to be themselves, which is a complicated process for traumatized and dissociative children.

The (Re)development of a Felt Sense of Safety and Trust

We endeavor to build a sense of safety in the therapeutic environment. Childhood experiences of complex trauma compromise the capacity for connection, mutuality, safety, and trust, as the associated relationship functions as the source of both trauma and safety. According to Gómez et al. (2016), "The experience of being rendered powerless by betrayal, within a relationship on which an individual depends, challenges one of the most basic human survival mechanisms—one's orientation toward connection with others" (pp. 167–168). Building a sense of internal safety in a relationship is a titrated, mindful, and recursive process, individualized to each child and their caregiving system. This process is one that includes progressions and regressions, relational disruptions and repairs, and corrective experiences as part of the re-scaffolding of internal and external relational safety. During all phases of treatment, focus is on developing a sense safety, following the child's pace, while enhancing relational capacities and what Fonagy et al. (2019) called "epistemic trust." As you may have already come to conclude, achieving this in therapy with children with histories of complex trauma and dissociation can be challenging and complicated. Many children come to therapy with early experiences of harm and abuse, sometimes ongoing, that frame their internal schemas of others, themselves, and relationships. When early relationships have been problematic or harmful, there is a procedurally learned expectation that it will happen again (Cozolino, 2014). According to Schore (2016), "experiences of relational trauma and attachment dysregulation are expressed in the therapeutic alliance" (p. 17).

Ideally, the therapist consistently and predictably endeavors to be seen and experienced by the child as a new type of grown-up, one who offers an alternative experience to previous relationships. This new type of grown-up is one that is not punitive, is respectful and curious about the motivations behind behaviors that lead to interpersonal conflicts, who invites the child to set the pace, and creates the foundations for safety. This new type of child-adult relationship forms the basis of the therapeutic collaboration, the experience of trust and positive rapport (Silberg, 2021), and an imaginal container through which a child can heal.

However, developing trust frequently presents a challenge to building the therapeutic alliance with dissociative children (Putnam, 1997). Perry (2009) noted that

> the presence of new and unfamiliar individuals can actually activate the already sensitized stress-response systems in these children, making them more symptomatic and less capable of benefiting from our efforts to comfort and heal. Our well-intended interventions often result in relational impermanence for the child.
>
> *(p. 248)*

As such, the development of the therapeutic relationship can be expected to take time and be fraught with challenges, as learning to feel safe both within oneself and in the presence of another, is a learning process. As part of the redevelopment of a felt sense of safety and trust, children who have been betrayed by those upon whom they depend are quite wise to observe, test, and distrust their therapist. Repeated validation of this relational dilemma, along with an inviting, permissive stance, may help a child "buy in" to the idea that playing with this person might be worth a try (Silberg, 2021). This approach aligns with Perry's (2009) assertion that "patterned, repetitive activities shape the brain in patterned ways, while chaotic experiences create chaotic dysfunctional organization" (p. 252).

While external pressures may lead to shared anxieties and urgency related to treatment pace and trajectory, Kluft (1992) cautions therapists that moving too quickly can lead to crisis and extend the length of therapy, stating, "Often, slower proves to be faster" (p. 145). A successful therapeutic relationship grows and develops within an environment that respects and tolerates the child's apprehension and lack of relational trust. Remedying this is slow and requires the therapist to tolerate their own discomfort or eagerness to succeed. This can be challenging when faced with the reality that "many chronically traumatized clients have learned to 'read' and respond to the signals of others—especially abusers and anyone else in a position of power" (Courtois & Ford, 2016, p. 92). As such, the relational field is often fraught with a minefield of terror-derived triggers that activate disavowed, disowned, dissociated behavior, affect, knowledge, sensation, and memory that have become imprinted on the child (Braun, 1988). Therapists may therefore anticipate that the treatment relationship is highly likely to activate the child's feelings and emotions related to their past experiences, which recruit the strategies of trauma-derived multi-motivational systems (Liotti, 2016, 2017).

Affect Scripts

Bringing together Putnam's theory of discrete behavioral states, attachment theory, affect theory, and interpersonal neurobiology, Silberg's (2021) affect avoidance theory offers an organizational structure for understanding the emergence of dissociative coping and disorganized attachment strategies that may emerge in a therapy session. According to Silberg (2021), these emergent strategies represent patterns of behavior that shape and manage the interpersonal environment and become more rigid and inflexible the more they are utilized. While this may seem like a challenge to building the therapeutic alliance, affect avoidance theory reconceptualizes such challenges as adaptive strategies for self-preservation in the face of trauma-related affect such as terror, humiliation, or grief. These strategies provide important data about a child client's relational experiences, attachment models or schemas, and corresponding learned and reinforced affect scripts (Silberg, 2021). According to Silberg, affect scripts are described as "collections of learned associations between affect, what stimulated them, and behaviors that provide useful responses to these affects" (p. 27). When associated with trauma, they may become autonomous and confused with the original source of danger. Thus, the therapeutic relationship inadvertently activates "fear-based states" linked to trauma-derived, state-dependent memories of Internal Working Models of other, self, and relationships.

How affect scripts emerge in the therapy session is unique to the child and their experiences. They may vary from attack to avoidance, reflecting the approach and retreat behaviors of the child displaying disorganized attachment patterns and strategies (Main & Solomon, 1986), and may include mobilizing or immobilizing strategies (please see Chapter 10) to manage the autonomic responses that ensue. In applying affect avoidance theory, a therapist who understands the protective motivations of activated affect scripts responds by noticing, being curious, naming, and differentiating past and present experiences, all while validating the motivation to support a slow and gentle softening of fear-based states and outdated models and representations. Together as play partners, the child and therapist create new adaptive experiences and strategies for maintaining connection within the relationship.

As an example, a young child, whom we will call Ben, was in therapy for two years due to a history of sadistic abuse and terrorization, and was now being bullied by an older boy at day camp. Ben identified that when being threatened by the bully, he "felt like fog because only fog can escape." Upon further exploration of other times in his life when he had felt like fog, it became clear that the dissociative strategy that was activated in the play space (Young, 2022) is what helped him survive the abuse that had occurred two years prior. However, now, in the present, this strategy did not serve him: when the bully approached Ben, he became immobilized and was unable to get the help that was available. Once the therapist and Ben had identified this strategy and script, the therapist was able to support Ben to discern "then" from "now" (Silberg, 2021), and he and his father were able to problem solve and identify current resources at day camp. When the bully approached him the next day, Ben got away and advocated for the help that he needed instead of becoming immobilized, and the bigger child was held accountable.

Play and the Development of the Relational Self

The role of play as a relational language is of the utmost importance to facilitate the child's expression and exploration. To support inter- and intrapersonal post-traumatic development, the safe enough, attuned caregiver navigates the needs of the infant and the simultaneous demands and impingements of the environment, watching for danger and tending to daily needs and care. It is within this container of safety that the healthy child is free to explore the self and negotiate the environment at their own pace, on their own terms, through spontaneous, impulsive gestures of playing. Unstructured, spontaneous free play is essential to child development. It is through play that curiosities are explored, feelings are expressed, and thoughts are revealed. Through play, children develop executive competence and confidence, as well as social and emotional awareness. Through this process, primary caregivers mirror and hold, allowing for the true self to be revealed and organized.

Winnicott's (1960) concept of human development identifies the *true self* as the authentic core of the personality. He believed that this begins with potential, stating, "Periodically, the infant's gesture gives expression to a spontaneous impulse; the source of the gesture is the True Self, and the gesture signifies the existence of a potential True Self" (Winnicott, 1965, p. 145). Environmental impingements, however, require the child to protect the true self by developing a false self, which allows a child to comply with the daily demands of the environment. "Trauma necessitates the premature maturation of a 'false' self that rigidifies and obscures more spontaneous, authentic experience (Winnicott, 1965, 1971)" (Carlson et al., 2009, p. 2). Through play, children engage in a creative process through which a path to themselves, as well as to others, is revealed.

Tuber (2008) offered a wonderful example of the "unique realness" of the spontaneous gesture and its potential for expression and connection. A toddler is playing with a small toy lion while sitting contently in a stroller, pushed by his mother. A man walks by and catches the toddler's eye. Immediately, the little child points the lion toward the stranger, letting out a playful roar. The stranger smiles and maybe even chuckles. The child returns to his solitary play in the stroller. Content after the moment of related play while perched in the safety of the stroller, the mother and toddler continue on their way.

Play as a Relational Tool for Healing

The role of play as a relational language is of the utmost importance to facilitate expression and exploration for children. Winnicott believed that one's individual play holds intrinsic therapeutic value that promotes self-healing. This optimistic thread runs through Winnicott's work (Lenormand, 2018), and is compatible with Silberg's (2021) treatment principle related to a therapist's "intense belief in the possibility to heal and the potential for future thriving" (p. 70). This stance of hope cannot be performative in relationship, as traumatized children are quite sensitive to neurocepting inauthenticity or a lack of sincerity. In therapy, a cohesive environment supports the development of a cohesive sense of self across behavioral states, as a child comes to know who they are through the eyes of a safe enough organizing play partner. Through play, children explore their internal and external worlds and engage in a creative process through which a path to themselves, as well as to others, is revealed.

It is within an attuned, developmentally appropriate, and consistent environment that fertile ground is laid for cohesive development, whereby the infant can rely on the felt sense that there is someone focusing on the infant's environmental, physical, and emotional needs. It is within this world of safety that the infant/child explores, and the self emerges (Ehrensaft & Cohen, 2012). Within the cohesive environment of therapy a child may engage in free expression and exploration of the self, experiencing, discovering, and making sense of their range of feelings and affects (Young, 2022) and developing mentalizing capacities (Gomez, 2012). Mentalization refers to reflective functioning, and it enables children to think about the thoughts, feelings, and beliefs of themselves and others. It is critical for developing capacities for regulation, impulse control, and the experience of self-agency. Exploring the meaning of the behavior and actions of others contributes to the child's capacity to discover the meaning of their own experiences (Fonagy, 2001).

For example, as Ben's treatment relationship deepened, he said, "Things are in order in [my therapist's] office." He was not referring to how the toys were organized. He was referring to the reliability, predictability, and safety of the therapeutic relationship, which invites the child's ways of being—and parents and caregivers, when appropriate—to play. This unique relationship is held by a room that can endure what it takes to hold the feelings, behaviors, and toxic experiences waiting to be recognized.

Play(ing) in the Therapeutic Relationship

Children who have had adverse experiences that cause reliance on dissociation often have difficulty experiencing gratification from their play, whether it be solitary or with others. Some children may become absorbed in their own play, whereas other children cannot engage in successful play, much less become absorbed in their internal world (Slade, 1994). Slade (1994) noticed gaps in the dissociated child's narrative, shifts in voice tone, lapses in play, and disrupted structure and organization. However, rather than shifting into a verbal interpretation, she found that when the therapist played alongside the disorganized child, becoming an enhancing play partner, play capacities develop, facilitating the child's capacity to discover and express connection and meaning to the self. Therapists are encouraged to suspend interpretation and play freely, becoming "organizing, enhacing and engaged play partners" (p. 81), which helps promote relational bonds and emotional resilience (Ginsburg & Committee, 2007).

Before a child can play by themselves or with others, they must have had the experience of playing in the presence of someone (Winnicott, 1958). This may be the very first aspect of treatment we focus on, building the tolerance to even consider being in a relationship that may display caring. A child cannot relax dissociative defenses in order to become absorbed in their own creative process unless they feel cared for and protected. It is when one feels cared for and protected, and experiences a felt sense of safety (Waters, 2016), that one is free to relax vigilance, be themselves, and become absorbed in fantasies and explorations that provide paths to their internal world. For example, when we consider the child's history and the unique function of a symptom through a trauma and dissociation lens, silence in session, rather than an act of resistance, may be reconceptualized as a developmental achievement that signals a child's growing ability to be in the presence and safety of an "other" (the therapist) while also absorbed in their own self (Winnicott, 1958).

In the play space of therapy, treatment is individualized for each child, and the development of play in each child is recognized and honored, allowing for organic transitions from play in the presence of someone, to playing with someone, to building the capacity for playing alone (Winnicott, 1958). Within this context, the child takes the lead, and the therapist, often alongside the caregiving system, collaborates with the child while attuning to the emergence of dissociative symptoms and phenomena, including self-states that emerge in play. This process includes anticipating and exploring transference and countertransference themes and reactions as they arise within the relationship (for further information on transference and countertransference, please see further in this chapter, as well as the Chapter 17).

For example, Ben called the perpetrators of his abuse "the terrible people." His parents often attended the sessions, sometimes sitting quietly, sometimes being loving, soothing parents, sometimes playing and problem solving with their child and the therapist. In one particular session, Ben was exploring the incident with the bully described above. Because of their tendency to become disoriented, dissociative children often experience further victimization, for example, in the form of bullying. The "bigger boy" at Ben's day camp liked to make him do things he did not want to do. On this day, the older boy told him to throw a toy at a camp counselor. Ben did throw the toy and was sent to the camp director's office. When his therapist told him that his mother had told her about the incident, he immediately began drawing the incident with markers. He carefully drew tables and chairs, and included the initials of students at each desk. While drawing a picture of the toy in the air, he said, "Then the toy went flying towards the camp counselor." The therapist responded, "The toy just flew towards the camp counselor?" At this moment, the therapist noticed a magnifying glass that had been left on the table. Trusting her own capacity for authentic, spontaneous play, she picked up the magnifier and said to Ben, "The toy just flew across the room? Can we get a closer look at that?" What followed was a series of drawings in which Ben and the therapist used the magnifying glass to safely move closer and closer to the affective experience.

The therapist helps the child discover safe, effective ways of communicating through play, modeling for the caregiver new ways of engagement that may be translated outside of the therapy room into day-to-day life. When Ben, in describing symptoms of depersonalization, shared that when the bully threatened him, he felt like fog, powerful feelings of shame emerged alongside an impulse to disappear, causing him to withdraw from the therapist. Ben moved naturally to his father's lap and rested quietly as the father provided comfort. As Ben connected to his father, the therapist invited playful movement. This allowed for reengagement with the therapist. As eye contact was made again, the therapist decided to reflect on Ben's predicament curiously. He could have refused to throw the toy and be hurt by the bigger boy, or he could be in trouble for throwing the toy at the counselor. This was a predicament that needed to be named. Using the magnifying glass allowed him to have creative control over how close or distant he was to the distressing feelings and memories. He realized that the big kid at day camp was not the terrible guy from a long time ago. While father and son collaborated on naming practical solutions to these predicaments, the therapist drew a picture of Ben speaking with his camp counselor, asking for help, reflecting all they discussed. Before leaving the session, Ben drew a magnifying glass in the shape of a heart on a picture he had drawn of himself, and wrote, "No more predicaments." When he arrived at his next session, Ben reported that the bigger boy had been at it again, but this time he remembered that the terrible people from a long time ago were far away and he was able to escape from the bigger boy and get the help he needed.

The essential point to hold in mind is that there are two aspects of play, authenticity and a space for transition and play. Any therapeutic relationship, like all relationships, cannot always be perfect. Relationships are subject to errors in judgement, lapses in attentiveness, bad timing, etc. What is essential is the development of the child's capacity to tolerate moments of missattunement and ruptures while learning the process of repair.

The Developing Therapeutic Relationship: Why Is This So Difficult?

Disorganized Attachment

Liotti (2022) defined disorganized attachment as a "relational conflict between the attachment system and the defense system" (p. 17), suggesting that disorganized attachment predicts the possibility of dissociation later in life, more so than remembered reports of traumatic events (Liotti, 2017; please see Chapter 4). Young children cannot effectively handle fear or remove themselves from danger. In such situations, attachment needs become paramount as the child may be bewildered, hypervigilant, and unable to comprehend why they are not being rescued (Silberg, 2021). What becomes more challenging is when the attachment system is both the source of safety and the source of danger, and simultaneous impulses to approach and avoid are activated (Main & Hesse, 1990). When the attachment figure's behavior is frightening, frightened, or always changing (Kobak et al., 2015), the infant cannot develop effective ways to reach out to establish safety. Thus, because the caregiver is not focused on the infant's needs, the infant ends up focusing all their attention on the caregiver's behavior, which leaves them alone to fend for themselves—there is no help in navigating, learning, and adapting to their environment or developing a sense of themselves. For these children, any perceived threat will activate both the survival/fear system and the attachment system, which are intrinsically intertwined (Liotti, 2017).

The attachment system is the infant's first line of protection against real or perceived threat, and the traumatized child's attachment system is wired for perceiving danger. Subtle changes on a caregiver's face can alert a protective self-state to intervene; this process alerts the fear system, which activates the attachment system, which reactivates the fear, reactivating the attachment needs ... and the cycle repeats. Both fear and attachment systems are motivated for survival, creating confusion and disorientation in the child (Silberg, 2021). The conflict between the desire to approach and the impulse to flee the frightening, much-needed attachment figure triggers the perpetrator/protector self-state, pulling everyone into the helpless, solutionless pattern of approach and retreat (Hesse & Main, 1990; Potgieter-Marks, 2012). This very process lends to the formation of affect scripts, which become activated in the therapy relationship and other relational environments. The child and the family may be unaware of the presence of these scripts that can cause perplexing shifts in behavior and affect (Silberg, 2021; please see Chapter 3). Caregivers may react with anger and confusion to the child's aggressive and volatile behavior, misunderstanding the protective motivations of shifting self-states.

Returning to Ben, when his mother had a baby, his father accompanied him to therapy sessions. At this time, the family was managing a self-state, Thrash, who is always mad and is all red. Thrash can do "bad things," like overflowing the bathroom sink or threatening his mother with a knife or to kick the new baby. When this happens, it seems like Mommy is mad or scared, and this makes Ben think that Mommy is one of the terrible people. Ben becomes unable to think, stuck in the solutionless predicament of feeling threatened by his mother's reaction to his behavior while needing her for soothing and regulation at the same time. This is when Thrash emerges to protect Ben from perceived dangers and intense feelings, especially shame (Young, 2022).

In session, Ben drew a picture of Thrash. Despite his descriptive verbalizations, he did not include the color red in the drawing. The therapist invited Ben to show her what it was like to be this way of being Ben. He clenched his fists, growled, scrunched up his face, stomped around the room, and yelled, "I'm a great person, I'm not a terrible person!" His father was invited to join the play, clenching his fists and stomping around the room. Father and child roared and played in the presence of the therapist. Within the holding environment of the therapeutic relationship, Ben was beginning to repair "the dissociative split between his mind and his body" (Young, 2022, p. 188). When the session was about to end and Ben went to the door, he was observed to quickly return to the drawing and color Thrash in red.

Disorganized Play

Children with disorganized attachment histories and strategies may have difficulty engaging in successful play. Early in her career, Slade (1994) described children who presented with play that "was highly disorganized, vague, and primitive; at other times, they couldn't make believe at all. Instead, they immersed themselves in barren repetitive play that made any attempt at discussion or interpretation impossible" (p. 81). Since creative play leads to self-discovery, the first order of business with a child who cannot successfully explore through play is to bring the child "from a state of not being able to play into a state of being able to play" (Winnicott, 1971, p. 38). Disorganized children in treatment will typically need a therapist who can patiently and safely help the child engage in symbolic play and use symbolic language to create cohesive narratives about their emotional experiences (Slade, 1994).

The traumatized, disorganized child cannot create a coherent sense of self without the help of a co-organizing "other." Within this process, therapists are keen to attune to the emergence of alternating Internal Working Models (Bowlby, 1973), which may make the child appear irrational or manipulative. Disorganized children may have difficulty remembering events, including their own daily thoughts and feelings; lack the ability to speak coherently; repeat unchangeable and sometimes grim scenarios in their play; shift states rapidly; and find themselves in one solutionless relational predicament after another (Terr, 1990; Young, 2022), as they attempt to achieve and restore safety and connection. The child client may feel out of control or frightened, while the therapist feels disoriented, incompetent, or exasperated. According to Trevarthen and Aitken (2001), "violence and cruelty is always accompanied, or preceded, by disruption to the affective patterns of caregiver-child or caregiver-infant interaction, and these psychosocial or psychiatric aspects should be taken into account in planning intervention" (p. 26). Brisch (2022) stated: "These children live in a sort of dissociated attachment state that seems to be highly resistant to external influence" (p. 8), such as a new, intimate, therapeutic relationship.

Disorganization in the Developing Therapeutic Relationship

Because of a lack of control over behavior and memory, dissociative, disorganized, and disoriented children are often reprimanded and judged, which serves to increase already intense feelings of shame and adds to their distress, compelling the child to utilize coping strategies that were developed when in a state of chronic fear and terror. It is important to articulate the message that the therapist maintains an "attitude of deep respect for the wisdom of individual coping techniques" (Silberg, 2021, p. 70), and that they understand that the child's choices of action or inaction seemed to be the only option at the time. Approaching a child in this way, with no judgment or accusations is crucial, especially when confronted with destructive behaviors and subsequent needs to establish safety-related boundaries and limits. Sharing one's understanding and respect for the child's mind that chose a particular way of coping with distress and pain can be quite a relief for a child who has experienced relational trauma, as shame about their symptoms and behaviors contributes to feelings of hopelessness (Silberg, 2021).

Therapists, like the children they work with, have their own relational history. Both therapist and client have developed representations of self and other within the context of early relational experiences that can influence reactions and responses in sessions. These early psychological representations can impact various clinician competencies, including the capacity to tolerate stress and distress, as well as to communicate needs and desires effectively (Cook et al., 2005). The ways in which the child's attachment history intersects with that of the therapist can cause anxiety, questions, and a sense of futility in the therapist (Sachs, 2017) that need to be explored in clinical supervision/consultation. It is important that therapists remember that the child's behaviors are communications of how the child feels at that precise moment—the child is projecting their feelings of fright and disorientation onto the therapist, who, if not anticipating these complicated moments, can also become frightened and out of control, leading to enactments of the disorganized attachment dynamic that can destabilize the therapeutic relationship.

Common Relational Challenges That Arise in Working with Children and Their Caregiving Systems

The development of a constructive, healing relationship between a therapist and a child with a history of complex trauma is … complex. Hopenwasser (2008) described the attuned therapist as a "microtonal tuning fork" (p. 349) that resonates directly and indirectly with mind-body shifts that emerge throughout a therapy session. Therapists can be "drawn into attunements with the rhythms and moods of others often without knowing it or without knowing why" (Howell, 2011, p. 232). The therapist endeavors to be predictable, punctual, available, and preoccupied with the client in front of them. Yet, we cannot dismiss the fact that the therapist also has nuanced Internal Working Models, strategies, fears, and defenses. After all, mental health is all a matter of degree, and as Sullivan (1966) stated, "we are all more simply human than otherwise, be we happy, contented and detached, miserable and mentally disordered, or whatever" (p. 7). It is within this realm that we attune to the roles of transference, countertransference, enactment, and reenactment as essential aspects of relational treatment.

Transference and Countertransference

According to Howell (2011), traumatic transference may present in a covert manner and "refers to the patient's expectation that he or she will be abused and exploitatively used as a narcissistic extension of the therapist" (p. 225). It is considered the most basic type of transference in clients with dissociative identity disorder. Countertransference is a phenomenon in which feelings from the therapist's own personal history become activated, sometimes in reaction to the client's transference toward the therapist. Schowalter (1986) stated:

> If the therapist's response is not based solely on the child client's influence, but is at least partially defensive and based on his or her own unconscious needs or feelings of early deprivation, the reaction crosses over into the realm of what is considered countertransference.
>
> *(p. 43)*

Countertransference is often unconscious, outside of the therapist's awareness, where it can remain unrecognized, unexplored, or unmanaged until it is addressed. Personal exploration and consistent consultation with a mentor experienced in working with child dissociation is crucial to one's capacity for sustaining engagement and maintaining a professional, grounded stance. When explored and understood, countertransference reactions can provide the therapist with useful information about their client's attachment style, dependency needs, and safety considerations. However, when left unattended, countertransference has the potential to be a catalyst for co-created conflicts or predicaments that enact historical dynamics. These ruptures in treatment can be quite difficult to tolerate. Yet, a therapist who can play can also share with their client, "I wonder why I did that," demonstrating an understanding of the value of countertransference material as it arises in a session.

Schowalter (1986) offered the example of a young psychiatric supervisee who was conflicted about labeling a child with the specific diagnosis of which the child clearly met criteria. The more the therapist was questioned, the more reluctant to diagnose he became. Finally, he was asked if there might be any personal reasons for his reluctance. The young therapist then recalled that he had been labeled as a troublemaker when a young child and that this had always felt unfair. The supervisee and supervisor were then able to include the therapist's now conscious over-identification with his patient in their discussion of the diagnosis.

Countertransference reactions may be more likely to arise in work with children than with adults (Abbate, 1964; Schowalter, 1986). Typically, in treatment with adults, there is more talk than action. It is the opposite in child treatment, where play and action are the natural activity in which children relate to themselves and others (Gil, 2017). In child treatment, libidinal and aggressive communications that are played out directly in real time are likely to provoke personal reactions from the therapist. Some patients even seem to induce identical reactions in almost everyone who works with them. Schowalter (1986) referred to Berta Bornstein's (1948) emphasis on the frequent pulls for regression when a therapist is continually confronted with these impulses in a young child. Bornstein suspected that this could be a contributing factor in why some clinicians stop working with children. Sometimes a client is the same age as the therapist's child, or may have similar conflicts as a therapist's child or the therapist themself. Some therapists become aware through experience that certain types of clients induce behaviors in them that interfere with the success of the treatment. Schowalter (1986) also acknowledged that young therapists might become therapists to process their own experiences and/or rework their own developmental dependency themes. With good consultation and a therapist's willingness to explore their own psychodynamics, it is possible that these liabilities will become a therapist's strength.

Working with children also includes working with parents. Working with children and their families often brings up complex and confusing feelings that are quite different from those when working with adults, which can influence clinical judgment and therapist behavior (Rasic, 2010). For example, a therapist might believe they could manage the child better than the parent, or perhaps the therapist has an internalized need to prove that the parents are wrong. The idea that a therapist needs to maintain an alignment or positive relationship to a child's caregiver can be the source of conflict for a therapist who feels competition with parents or has over-identified with the part of the child that did not receive or is not receiving appropriate care from the caregivers, for whatever reason. It is also common for a therapist to feel protective of the caregivers' feelings, eliciting concern about hurting the parents. These concerns can cause a therapist to become overly cautious, inhibiting the capacity to collaborate successfully with a parent. It can be helpful to keep in mind that in child treatment, we are always working toward the goal of helping the parent of the disorganized child develop the skills to appropriately soothe, manage, and care for their distressed child, as a child will not be in therapy forever (Wieland, 2017).

The therapist who is ready to work with children who have experienced the most disorganized and disorienting attachments (1) is prepared for the intensity of need and conflicting and perplexing changes of affect and relatedness, (2) embraces the chaos, fear, love, creativity, and playfulness, and (3) must be grounded in a sense of their own identity and defensive strategies. Supervision and consultation with a knowledgeable clinician will help differentiate reactions that relate to the therapist's past relational experiences. Understanding the dynamics underlying one's personal and emotional responses to a client can be quite informative and reveal clues to the child's attachment style, strengths, and weaknesses, contributing to case conceptualization and treatment planning. It can also be helpful in mitigating enactments.

Enactments and Reenactments

Countertransference brings to life the dynamics of the client's and therapist's internal worlds (Dalenberg, 2004), which can lead to enactments. According to Bromberg (2011), enactments occur within the relationship between a client and therapist, and create an interpersonal dynamic in which a destabilizing feeling is felt and responded to *by the dyad*. Enactments will often emerge in play and behavior, bringing aspects of the trauma into the play space, thereby externalizing worries and fears (Gil, 2017). Enactments differ from reenactments, which emerge as a *client's* repetitive attempts to achieve mastery of an event or experience, whether metaphorically or directly. Both enactments and reenactments are unconscious until made conscious, and both have the potential to be either re-traumatizing or healing (for further information on enactments and reenactments, readers are encouraged to see Case, 2008).

Instinctual drives and defenses (please see Chapter 40) will appear in treatment in much the same way as they come into play between a child and the mother. Powerful instincts may be communicated with aggression, hate, and anger in the face of frustration. Sometimes, a child's need and love can feel dangerous, manifesting in "a natural sequence of ruthless love, aggressive attack, guilt feeling, sense of concern, sadness, and a desire to mend and build and give" (Winnicott, 1964, p. 109). For children to integrate all the aspects of their experience, the therapist and engaged caregiving system are tasked with being present, reliable, and consistent in their survival of the chaotic and sometimes dangerous behavior, intervening with necessary limits that regulate and provide safety (Winnicott, 1964). The attuned therapist, like the good enough mother, is responsive and adaptive to the child's needs (Winnicott, 1971) and understands that all behavior is communication (ISSTD, 2004; Silberg, 2021; Waters, 2016), no matter what this may activate in the therapist.

Attuning to and identifying relational patterns as they emerge in treatment are essential as part of supporting children to develop a felt sense of trust and safety within the therapeutic relationship. When a therapist grounds themselves in the adage "know thyself," not only will they feel competent in the play space of treatment, but they will also experience the rewards of engaging in this specialized work. Developing a safe community for consultation, whether group or individual, will provide the therapist with a consistent and predictable environment of their own in which to explore and reflect on the intimate feelings that develop in the therapeutic relationship with a child with a history of complex trauma and dissociation. To ensure that the therapy is focused on the client's needs and not those of the therapist, the therapist must take responsibility for their own personal growth, self-awareness, and self-care.

Practical Considerations and Strategies for Working with Relational Nuances

To address how to work with the nuanced relational challenges described above, we suggest an initial grounding in the knowledge that transference, countertransference, enactments, and reenactments cannot be avoided, and that instead, these are sources of important clinical information about both our client and the therapy. According to Trevarthen and Aitken (2001), all human beings are

> sensitive at some level to the communicative expressions of other persons, and to the motives and emotions behind them. All humans can detect rhythmic impulses and qualities of other persons' behaviours that are contingent upon and related emotionally to their own expressions.
>
> *(p. 31)*

Therapists are encouraged to anticipate a range of both subjective and objective feelings and emotions in response to interactions in therapy with children with complex trauma and dissociation. Understanding the dynamics underlying one's personal and emotional responses to a client can be quite informative, revealing clues to the child's attachment style, strengths, and weaknesses, contributing to case conceptualization and treatment plan. This includes knowing one's limits and their capacity to tolerate mess in their office, and engaging in ongoing self-care. This in turn supports clinicians to use themself in the therapeutic space in ways that are attuned to the unique relational nuances as they arise, and ensures that the therapy is meeting the needs of the client rather than those of the therapist (Winnicott, 1994).

Therapists' Use of Self in Relationship

As we come to better know and understand ourselves, we can more authentically show up in relationship and attune to the unique and nuanced relational needs and schemas of traumatized and dissociative children and their caregiving systems. According to Shewfelt (2018), this is described as "right brain to right brain presence" in therapy or

> the therapist's capacity and sensitivity to notice the subtle cues from the client's tone of voice and prosody, body language, facial cues, and so forth, which convey the moment-to-moment emergence of the client's unconscious experience. This involves the therapist's capacity to

respond with accuracy and sensitivity in a well-timed attuned response, so that the client can feel emotionally accompanied and engaged.

(p. 65)

We may notice clients fall silent, avoid eye contact, say "I don't know," turn off the camera in virtual sessions, disengage through video games or electronic devices, leave the room, cease talking, hide or turn away, or become angry and aggressive, and treatment feels stuck. How we understand these unique expressions and then respond matters, as these responses can serve as corrective and reparative relational experiences. Silberg (2021) proposed helpful therapeutic stances that state: "I can accept you no matter how terrible you think you are"; "I deeply want you to get well, but it is ultimately completely within your own control"; "I can accept your anger and disappointment (even in me) and not reject you"; "You can abandon me; I can't/won't abandon you"; and "You don't have to do anything to please me. I am here for you" (pp. 74–76). Briere and Lanktree (2011) provided examples of therapist behaviors that can support the development of the therapeutic relationship, even amid the challenges, which include the use of attunement, empathy, acceptance, understanding, and curiosity.

The therapist who works with anyone with trauma-related dissociation must be able to sit with all that cannot be known. Tronick (2009) spoke about "therapist unknowables" as meaning-making processes that shape one's way of being and responding that are simply outside of what can be known and brought into awareness. The therapist who can tolerate not knowing what cannot be known facilitates the dynamic process of co-creating meaning. As the therapist attunes to only what is being communicated with or without words, they also begin to listen and interact on a level that "implicitly processes moment-to-moment attachment communications and socioemotional information at levels beneath awareness" (Schore, 2019, pp. 28–29). This level of attunement lends a synchronicity with the child that promotes the growth of the therapeutic alliance and contributes to building positive transference and adaptive relational experiences for the child, as well as a model for caregiving systems (Waters, 2016). According to Hopenwasser (2008), "attunement is a rhythmic encounter that is entirely dependent on being present in the moment" (p. 357), and is essential between a therapist and a child client in order to heal lower brainstem disorganization and repattern the nervous system (Dion, n.d.).

Despite the importance of attunement, misattunement and relational rupture will occur, and "the key is not in the misattunement, but in the interactive repair" (Schore, 2019, p. 279). The therapist is called upon to accept the inevitability of relational discord as part of the therapy rather than as an indication of therapeutic failure or impasse. Therapists must master the ability to apologize and acknowledge errors and mistakes authentically without defensiveness (Silberg, 2021).

Operationalizing Right-Brain to Right-Brain Communication (with or without Play)

According to Schore (2019),

the patient's right brain needs to feel that it is seen, so although a therapist's left brain must listen to the words created by the patient's left brain in order to form an objective assessment of the patient's problem, the therapist must be sensitive enough to pick up on, and empathize with, what is going on implicitly within the client's right brain and body.

(p. 242)

Howell (2021) observed that this level of "intersubjective affective responsiveness" is communicated via "body rhythms, somatic states and facial expressions" (p. 231), and is aligned with how dissociated traumatic memory is implicitly stored and then communicated nonverbally. A cognitive evolutionist perspective to case formulation premises paying attention to the attachment system and the ways it may intersect with the development of a safe enough therapeutic relationship, as "the reactivation of implicitly traumatic relational memories in the therapeutic relationship can cause difficulties or prevent the use of, at least in the first phase of treatment, the techniques and operating methods" (Farina, 2021, p. 184).

Use of attunement, presence, and resonance provides cues related to relational needs and deficits, supports choices around the use of language, and facilitates the conditions for exploring option and choice within safe and healthy boundaries. This, in turn, supports the building and rebuilding of epistemic trust within relationships and facilitates more mindful attachment (Siegel, 2009). This is not a onetime intervention, and it is repeated in a manner that is layered across all phases of treatment to help build predictability and opportunities to experience relationships within which safety can be assessed and agency can be exercised. Frequent repetition of intervention, rather than duration length, leads the brain to respond with *more gusto* and supports the creation of new synaptic connections (Siegel, 2009).

To be engaged in such a *communicative musicality* that "carries emotion from one to the other" (Malloch, 1999, p. 48), therapists' awareness of their own affective states is essential as part of mindful awareness related to self-expression, communication, and sensory matches or mismatches across words, body language, facial expression, and prosody/tone. Applying Trevarthen's (1974) theory of innate intersubjectivity here considers that infants are "born with awareness specifically receptive to subjective states in other persons" (Trevarthen & Aitken, 2001, p. 4); thus, we can assume children have had procedural learning in constantly attuning to the states of the other.

Facial expression, body posture, and prosody/tone of voice impact the autonomic nervous system and can contribute to the activation of survival states in the therapy room. In this way, the therapist is attending to themselves from the inside out, being mindful of how each moment intersects with their own internal working models and how this may lead to incongruence. A moment that calls for melodic prosody may not be appropriate if another state emerges that cannot yet tolerate safety, internally or externally, in the room with the therapist—we are thus engaged in a dance, closely following the client. Such use of language is not static, but moves in coordination with the client as their affective states shift. We thus shift with them, offering open-ended invitations to collaborative, curious, and creative meaning making of all that could not be simultaneously known and survived.

Language

In addition to attending to the process of communication, the corresponding words and how we say those words matters. More explicit forms of language used in play predict challenges and proactively allows for preparation, is invitational rather than demanding, and communicates choices. Preparatory language may include offering a step-by-step overview of what to expect or what comes next, and is collapsed and fractionated according to needs. In doing this, the therapist is concerned with the impact of complex trauma on relational needs across all states of the child, and responds by supporting transitions and micro changes, and creating predictability. Invitational language is open and collaborative and involves asking, rather than telling. This may include offering opportunities for the child to decide when things start and stop in the play space, to practice giving and revoking consent or permission within the relationship, or to share when the therapist gets it wrong. Choice-based language provides options, rather than demanding or telling (*see Trauma-Sensitive Yoga*, Emerson et al., 2009), and does so using wonder and curiosity. It may include offering contained options to exercise "choosing" and exercising back power and control in helpful ways, which includes the right to refuse.

Attunement and language interact across all phases of treatment. In the initial phase of treatment, which focuses on assessment and stabilization, clinicians may use language to attune to what happened relationally just before defensive adaptations emerged, to manage states of fear and offer to the child curious opportunities to use the therapist as a safe container, to practice co-regulating. In the phase of treatment that focuses on memory work, new relational mastery experiences may be used as adaptive information that offers time orientation and bridges "then" and "now." In the final phase of treatment, which focuses on reconnection and moving forward, attuned language supports the navigation of termination dynamics, integrating new experiences into a new future template as the self and self-agency is built across the different phases of development and life transitions, and creating the opportunity to have a "good" goodbye. It is important to note, however, that there is a dearth of research specific to language-related phenomena that contribute to an understanding of the role of language in the effectiveness of psychotherapy (Farina et al., 2023).

Conclusion

Nearing his final session, Ben's mom said, "Did you share what you told me yesterday?"

"I can draw it," Ben answered. When he finished, the left side of the paper was titled "US ME." Under the title was a drawing of Ben and his therapist. He was saying to his therapist, "I have parts." On the right side of the paper was the title THE ME. Under that title was a drawing of Ben and his mother. Here, Ben was saying, "Mommy, I am the me." This is exactly what we are striving for in therapy with dissociative children. Our role is not ongoing forever. The hope is that the work done within the therapeutic relationship will have provided enough regulation and integration that the child believes in themselves, so that every new experience, moving forward, is not tainted by the past experiences of trauma (Wieland, 2017). As a result, the child gets to go on being and growing as a child.

Bringing together psychoanalytic, attachment, attunement, relational, and neurobiological concepts, this chapter sought to highlight the centrality of the therapeutic relationship to healing from complex trauma and dissociation. To illustrate the complexity of this relationship, attachment dynamics and the use of implicit communication was explored and illustrated via the use of case examples. We recognize that this chapter barely skims the surface of all that entails the therapy relationship, or the depth of Winnicott's work and legacy. We hope that despite these limits, that this chapter generates interest and begins to shed light on aspects of the work that are not modality specific, but instead encompasses all that it means to be human and in relationship. Furthermore, we hope that this is a starting point for a journey into the psychodynamics of relationship and intersubjectivity (Stolorow & Atwood, 2014).

References

Abbate, G. M. (1964). Child analysis a different developmental stages. *Journal of the American Psychoanalytic Association, 12*, 135–150.

Agarwal, V., Sitholey, P., & Srivastava, C. (2019). Clinical practice guidelines for the management of dissociative disorders in children and adolescents. *Indian Journal of Psychiatry, 61*(Suppl 2), 247.

Bion, W. (1962). *Learning from experience*. Heinemann.

Bornstein, B. (1948). Emotional barriers in the understanding and treatment of young children. *American Journal of Orthopsychiatry, 18*(4), 691–697. https://doi.org/10.1111/j.1939-0025.1948.tb05131.x

Bowlby, J. (1973). *Attachment and loss: Vol. 2. Separation: Anxiety and anger*. Basic Books.

Braun, B. G. (1988). The BASK model of dissociation. *Dissociation: Progress in the Dissociation Disorders, 1*(1), 4–23.

Briere, J., & Lanktree, C. B. (2011). *Treating complex trauma in adolescents and young adults*. Sage Publications.

Brisch, K. H. (2022). Attachment and dissociation. In V. Sinason & R. Potgetier-Marks (Eds.), *Treating children with dissociative disorders: Attachment, trauma, theory and practice* (pp. 7–9). Routledge.

Bromberg, P. (2011). *The shadow of the tsunami and the growth of the relational mind.* Routledge.

Cappas, N. M., Andres-Hyman, R., & Davidson, L. (2005). What psychotherapists can begin to learn from neuroscience: Seven principles of a brain-based psychotherapy. *Psychotherapy: Theory, Research, Practice, Training, 42*(3), 374–383. https://doi.org/10.1037/0033-3204.42.3.374

Carlson, E. A., Yates, T. M., & Sroufe, L. A. (2009). *Development of dissociation and development of the self. Dissociation and the dissociative disorders.* Routledge.

Case, C. (2008). Action, enactment and moments of meeting in therapy with children. In D. Mann & V. Cunningham (Eds.), *The past in the present* (pp. 116–129). Routledge.

Cook, A., Spinazzola, J., Ford, J., Lanktree, C., Blaustein, M., Cloitre, M., & van der Kolk, B. (2005). Complex trauma in children and adolescents. *Psychiatric Annals, 35*(5), 390–398. https://doi.org/10.3928/00485713-20050501-05

Courtois, C. A., & Ford, J. (2016). *Treatment of complex trauma: A sequenced, relationship-based approach.* Guilford Press.

Cozolino, L. (2014). *The neuroscience of human relationships: Attachment and the developing social brain* (2nd ed.). W. W. Norton.

Cronin, E., Brand, B. L., & Mattanah, J. F. (2014). The impact of the therapeutic alliance on treatment outcome in patients with dissociative disorders. *European Journal of Psychotraumatology, 5*(1), Article 22676. https://doi.org/10.3402/ejpt.v5.22676

Dalenberg, C. J. (2004). Maintaining the safe and effective therapeutic relationship in the context of distrust and anger: Countertransference and complex trauma. *Psychotherapy: Theory, Research, Practice, Training, 41*(4), 438–447. https://doi.org/10.1037/0033-3204.41.4.438

Dion, L. (n.d.). *Tenets of synergistic play therapy.* Synergetic Play Therapy Institute. synergeticplaytherapy.com/synergetic-play-therapy.

Ehrensaft, M. K., & Cohen, P. (2012). Contribution of family violence to the intergenerational transmission of externalizing behavior. *Prevention Science, 13*, 370–383. https://doi.org/10.1007/s11121-011-0223-8

Ellis, A. E., Simiola, V., Brown, L., Courtois, C., & Cook, J. M. (2018). The role of evidence-based therapy relationships on treatment outcome for adults with trauma: A systematic review. *Journal of Trauma & Dissociation, 19*(2), 185–213. https://doi.org/10.1080/15299732.2017.1329771

Emerson, D., Sharma, R., Chaudry, S., & Turner, J. (2009). Trauma-sensitive yoga: Principles, practice, and research. *International Journal of Yoga Therapy, 19*, 123–128. https://doi.org/10.17761/ijyt.19.1.h6476p8084l22160

Farina, B. (2021). The role of trauma in psychotherapeutic complications and the worth of Giovanni Liotti's cognitive-evolutionist perspective (CEP): Commentary on chapter "Strengths and limitations of case formulation in constructivist cognitive behavioral therapies." In G. M. Ruggiero, G. Caselli & S. Sassaroli (Eds.), *CBT case formulation as therapeutic process* (pp. 177–189). Springer Nature. https://doi.org/10.1007/978-3-030-63587-9_18

Farina, B., Liotti, M., Imperatori, C., Tombolini, L., Gasperini, E., Mallozzi, P., Russo, M., Malucelli, G. S., & Monticelli, F. (2023). Cooperation within the therapeutic relationship improves metacognitive functioning: Preliminary findings. *Research in Psychotherapy: Psychopathology, Process and Outcome, 26*(3), 712. https://doi.org/10.4081/ripppo.2023.712

Fonagy, P. (2001). *Attachment theory and psychoanalysis.* Routledge.

Fonagy, P., Luyten, P., Allison, E., & Campbell, C. (2019). Mentalizing, epistemic trust and the phenomenology of psychotherapy. *Psychopathology, 52*(2), 94–103. https://doi.org/10.1159/000501526

Ford, J. D., & Courtois, C. A. (2020). Defining and understanding complex trauma and complex traumatic stress disorders. In J. Ford & C. A. Courtois (Eds.), *Treating complex traumatic stress disorders in adults: Scientific foundations and therapeutic models* (2nd ed., pp. 3–34). Guilford Press.

Forner, C. (2019). What mindfulness can learn about dissociation and what dissociation can learn from mindfulness. *Journal of Trauma & Dissociation, 20*(1), 1–15. https://doi.org/10.1080/15299732.2018.1502568

Gil, E. (2010). *Working with children to heal interpersonal trauma: The power of play.* New York: Guilford Press.

Gil, E. (2017). *Posttraumatic play in children: What clinicians need to know.* Guilford Press.

Gil, E. M. (2016). Using integrated directive and nondirective play interventions for abused and traumatized children. In L. A. Reddy, T. M. Files-Hall & C. E. Schaefer (Eds.), *Empirically based play interventions for children* (pp. 95–113). American Psychological Association. https://doi.org/10.1037/14730-006

Ginsburg, K. R., & Committee on Psychosocial Aspects of Child and Family Health. (2007). The importance of play in promoting healthy child development and maintaining strong parent-child bonds. *Pediatrics, 119*(1), 182–191. https://doi.org/10.1542/peds.2006-2697

Gomez, A. M. (2012). *EMDR therapy and adjunct approaches with children: Complex trauma, attachment, and dissociation*. Springer Publishing Company.

Gómez, J. M., Lewis, J. K., Noll, L. K., Smidt, A. M., & Birrell, P. J. (2016). Shifting the focus: Nonpathologizing approaches to healing from betrayal trauma through an emphasis on relational care. *Journal of Trauma & Dissociation, 17*(2), 165–185. https://doi.org/10.1080/15299732.2016.1103104

Hopenwasser, K. (2008). Being in rhythm: Dissociative attunement in therapeutic process. *Journal of Trauma & Dissociation, 9*(3), 349–367. https://doi.org/10.1080/15299730802139212

Howell, E. F. (2011). *Understanding and treating dissociative identity disorder: A relational approach* (Vol. 49). Routledge.

International Society for the Study of Dissociation. (in press). Guidelines for the evaluation and treatment of dissociative symptoms in children and adolescents. *Journal of Trauma & Dissociation*.

International Society for the Study of Dissociation, Task Force on Children and Adolescents. (2004). Guidelines for the evaluation and treatment of dissociative symptoms in children and adolescents. *Journal of Trauma & Dissociation, 5*(3), 119–150. https://doi.org/10.1300/J229v05n03_09

Keller, S. M., Zoellner, L. A., & Feeny, N. C. (2010). Understanding factors associated with early therapeutic alliance in PTSD treatment: Adherence, childhood sexual abuse history, and social support. *Journal of Consulting and Clinical Psychology, 78*(6), 974–979. https://doi.org/10.1037/a0020758

Kluft, R. P. (1992). The initial stages of psychotherapy in the treatment of multiple personality disorder patients. *Dissociation, 6*(2), 145–161. Presented at the Amsterdam Meetings of the ISSMP&D.

Kobak, R., Cassidy, J., Lyons-Ruth, K., & Ziv, Y. (2015). Attachment, stress, and psychopathology: A developmental pathways model. In D. Cicchetti & D. J. Cohen (Eds.), *Developmental psychopathology: Theory and method* (2nd ed., pp. 333–369). John Wiley & Sons.

Lenormand, M. (2018). Winnicott's theory of playing: A reconsideration. *International Journal of Psychoanalysis, 99*(1), 82–102.

Liotti, G. (2016). Infant attachment and the origins of dissociative processes: An approach based on the evolutionary theory of multiple motivational systems. *Attachment, 10*(1), 20–36.

Liotti, G. (2017). Conflicts between motivational systems related to attachment trauma: Key to understanding the intra-family relationship between abused children and their abusers. *Journal of Trauma & Dissociation, 18*(3), 304–318. https://doi.org/10.1080/15299732.2017.1295392

Liotti, G. (2022). Infant attachment and dissociative psychopathology: An approach based on the evolutionary theory of multiple motivational systems. In V. Sinason & R. Potgetier-Marks (Eds.), *Treating children with dissociative disorders: Attachment, trauma, theory and practice* (pp. 10–26). Routledge.

Main, M., & Hesse, E. (1990). Parents' unresolved traumatic experiences are related to infant disorganized attachment status: Is frightened and/or frightening parental behavior the linking mechanism? In M. T. Greenberg, D. Cicchetti & E. M. Cummings (Eds.), *Attachment in the preschool years: Theory, research, and intervention* (pp. 161–182). University of Chicago Press.

Main, M., & Solomon, J. (1986). Discovery of a new, insecure-disorganized/disoriented attachment pattern. In M. Yogman & T. B. Brazelton (Eds.), *Affective development in infancy* (pp. 95–124). Ablex Publishing.

Malloch, S. N. (1999). Mothers and infants and communicative musicality. *Musicae Scientiae, 3*(1), 29–57. https://doi.org/10.1177/10298649000030S104

Manassis, K. (2014). *Case formulation with children and adolescents*. Guilford Press.

Norcross, J. C., & Wampold, B. E. (2019). Relationships and responsiveness in the psychological treatment of trauma: The tragedy of the APA Clinical Practice Guideline. *Psychotherapy, 56*(3), 391–399. https://doi.org/10.1037/pst0000228

Pearlman, L. A., & Courtois, C. A. (2005). Clinical applications of the attachment framework: Relational treatment of complex trauma. *Journal of Traumatic Stress: Official Publication of the International Society for Traumatic Stress Studies, 18*(5), 449–459. https://doi.org/10.1002/jts.20052

Perry, B. D. (2009). Examining child maltreatment through a neurodevelopmental lens: Clinical applications of the neurosequential model of therapeutics. *Journal of Loss and Trauma, 14*(4), 240–255. https://doi.org/10.1080/15325020903004350

Potgieter-Marks, R. (2012). When the sleeping tiger roars: Perpetrator introjects in children. In R. Vogt (Ed.), *Perpetrator introjects: Psychotherapeutic diagnostics and treatment models* (pp. 87–110). Asanger.

Putnam, F. W. (1997). *Dissociation in children and adolescents: A developmental perspective*. Guilford Press.
Rasic, D. (2010). Countertransference in child and adolescent psychiatry—A forgotten concept? *Journal of the Canadian Academy of Child & Adolescent Psychiatry, 19*(4), 249–254.
Sachs, A. (2017). Through the lens of attachment relationship: Stable DID, active DID and other trauma-based mental disorders. *Journal of Trauma and Dissociation, 18*(3), 319–339. https://doi.org/10.1080/15299732.2017.1295400
Schore, A. (2003). *Affect regulation and the repair of the self*. W. W. Norton.
Schore, A. N. (2016). Relational trauma, brain development and dissociation. In J. D. Ford & C. A. Courtois (Eds.), *Treating complex post-traumatic stress disorders in children and adolescents: Scientific foundations and therapeutic models* (pp. 3–23). Guilford Press.
Schore, A. N. (2019). *Right brain psychotherapy*. W.W. Norton.
Schowalter, J. (1986). Countertransference in work with children. Review of a neglected concept. *Journal of the American Academy of Child Psychiatry, 25*(1), pp. 40–45. https://doi.org/10.1016/S0002-7138(09)60597-5
Shewfelt, M. (2018). The relationship is the therapy: Applying interpersonal neurobiology in psychotherapy. *The Neuropsychotherapist, 6*(12), 62–71.
Shirk, S. R., & Karver, M. (2003). Prediction of treatment outcome from relationship variables in child and adolescent therapy: A meta-analytic review. *Journal of Consulting and Clinical Psychology, 71*(3), 452–464. https://doi.org/10.1037/0022-006X.71.3.452
Siegel, D. J. (2001). Toward an interpersonal neurobiology of the developing mind: Attachment relationships, "mindsight," and neural integration. *Infant Mental Health Journal: Official Publication of the World Association for Infant Mental Health, 22*(1–2), 67–94.
Siegel, D. J. (2009). Mindful awareness, mindsight, and neural integration. *The Humanistic Psychologist, 37*(2), 137.
Silberg, J. L. (2001). Dissociative disorders. In H. Overvaschel, M. Hersen, & J. Faust (Eds.), *Handbook of conceptualization and treatment of child psychopathology* (pp. 449–474). Pergamon.
Silberg, J. L. (2021). *The child survivor: Healing developmental trauma and dissociation* (2nd ed.). Routledge.
Silberg, J., & Dallam, S. (2023). Dissociative disorders in children and adolescents. In M. J. Dorahy, S. N. Gold & J. A. O'Neil (Eds.), *Dissociation and the dissociative disorders: Past, present, future* (2nd ed., pp. 433–447). Routledge.
Slade, A. (1994). Making meaning and making believe: Their role in the clinical process. In A. Slade & D. P. Wolf (Eds.), *Children at play: Clinical and developmental approaches to meaning and representation* (pp. 81–107). Oxford University Press.
Slochower, J. (2018). D.W. Winnicott: Holding, playing and moving toward mutuality. In M. Charles (Ed.), *Introduction to contemporary psychoanalysis: Defining terms and building bridges* (pp. 97–117). Routledge/Taylor & Francis Group. https://doi.org/10.4324/9781315180120-5
Stern, D. B. (2010). *Partners in thought: Working with unformulated experience, dissociation and enactment*. Routledge.
Stolorow, R. D., & Atwood, G. E. (2014). *Contexts of being: The intersubjective foundations of psychological life*. Routledge.
Sullivan, H. (1966). *Conceptions of modern psychiatry*. W. W. Norton.
Tedeschi, R. G., & Calhoun, L. G. (2004). A clinical approach to posttraumatic growth. In P. A. Linley & S. Joseph (Eds.), *Positive psychology in practice* (pp. 405–419). John Wiley & Sons. https://doi.org/10.1002/9780470939338.ch25
Terr, L. (1990). *Too scared to cry: Psychic trauma in childhood*. Harper & Row.
Trevarthen, C. (1974). The psychobiology of speech development. In E. H. Lenneberg (Ed.), *Language and brain: Developmental aspects: Neurosciences research program bulletin* (Vol. 12, pp. 570–585). Neuroscience Research Program.
Trevarthen, C., & Aitken, K. J. (2001). Infant intersubjectivity: Research, theory, and clinical applications. *Journal of Child Psychology and Psychiatry and Allied Disciplines, 42*(1), 3–48.
Tronick, E. (2009). Multilevel meaning making and dyadic expansion of consciousness theory: The emotional and the polymorphic polysemic flow of meaning. In D. Fosha, D. J. Siegel & M. F. Solomon (Eds.), *The healing power of emotion: Affective neuroscience, development & clinical practice* (pp. 86–111). W. W. Norton.
Tuber, S. (2008). *Attachment, play, and authenticity: A Winnicott primer*. Jason Aronson, Incorporated.
Waters, F. S. (2016). *Healing the fractured child: Diagnosis and treatment of youth with dissociation*. Springer.
Wieland, S. (2017). *Parents are our other client: Ideas for therapists, social workers, support workers, and teachers*. Routledge.

Winnicott, D. W. (1945). Primitive emotional development. *The International Journal of Psychoanalysis,* 26, 137–143.

Winnicott, D. W. (1958). The capacity to be alone. *International Journal of Psychoanalysis,* 39, 416–420.

Winnicott, D. W. (1960). Ego distortion in terms of true and false self. In D. W. Winnicott (Ed.), *The maturational processes and the facilitating environment: Studies in the theory of emotional development* (pp. 140–152). Karnac Books.

Winnicott, D. W. (1964). *The child, the family and the outside world.* Penguin Books.

Winnicott, D. W. (1965). *The maturational processes and the facilitating environment: Studies in the theory of emotional development.* International Universities Press.

Winnicott, D. W. (1971). *Playing and reality.* Tavistock Publications.

Winnicott, D. W. (1992). *Through paediatrics to psychoanalysis: Collected papers.* Brunner/Mazel.

Winnicott, D. W. (1994). Hate in the counter-transference. *Journal of Psychotherapy Practice and Research,* 3(4), 348–356.

Young, E. T. (2022). I didn't know where you were: In the play space of treatment with a young dissociative boy. In V. Sinason & R. Potgetier-Marks (Eds.), *Treating children with dissociative disorders: Attachment, trauma, theory and practice* (pp. 180–197). Routledge.

34
BOUNDARIES AND ETHICS

David S. Prescott

Introduction

Boundaries and ethics play an important role in understanding, assessing, and treating children with histories of complex trauma and dissociation. This chapter argues that in order to best serve people with histories of severe and repeated trauma, professionals[1] need to look beyond the language of the existing ethical codes of professional organizations and examine how best to maintain the highest standards of behavior with clients who have historically been treated unethically (at best) and had their boundaries violated.

It may help to start with an illustration of how boundary crossings and violations may occur under common circumstances.[2] From there, practitioners should consider ethics and boundaries as they apply in the therapeutic relationship.

Illustration

Darnell, a clinician of several years' experience, participated in implementing an empirically supported treatment model for treating trauma. The implementation project was stringent, involving several days of training and several months of periodic fidelity monitoring. Within the United States, the larger project reflected a statewide attempt to provide trauma-informed care to adolescents who were under the supervision of the state's Department of Child and Family Welfare (DOCFW). Of note was that the treatment method itself had been developed and found to be effective with a different population (adult females) from where it was now being applied (adolescent males and females).

In order to ensure that clinicians practiced with fidelity to the model, each session was recorded on video. The camera was focused on the clinician and not the client, and the recordings were confined to a secured information channel. Under these conditions, it seemed that little could go wrong. From the perspective of the developers, their consultant/trainer, and administrators at the DOCFW, the primary threat to the model's fidelity was the clinicians administering it. Like countless others involved in implementation, they had experienced situations where clinicians strayed from the manual and improvised in sessions, thereby potentially undermining the treatment fidelity. During the training, and in subsequent consultation calls with the clinicians, the consultant/trainer and developers emphasized the importance of taking no liberties with the curriculum and recording each session.

Darnell scheduled a first session with Sam, an 11-year-old male with a horrific history of sexual abuse, who had recently been referred after his stepfather was convicted of a drug offense. Atop other sequelae of sexual abuse, Sam was expressing confusion about his gender and his mother and school counselor were describing dissociative symptoms.

Darnell explained the video-recording process and that a review team would be assessing his work but nothing having to do with Sam, who responded immediately with, "Yes, I'll be happy do that for you." Darnell thanked Sam and explained it wouldn't be necessary after all. Darnell noticed that Sam seemed to become more present and engaged after this. They completed the first session with little difficulty.

Darnell called his supervisor after the session: "I know that everyone wants every session recorded," he said.

> Please try to understand; this is a child whose entire survival has depended on making adults happy. For all we know, Sam was video recorded during the abuse he experienced. He goes along with what adults want from him because when he was younger it would have been much worse for him if he didn't. This wasn't informed consent; it was a symptom of the very trauma I was trying to help with. I couldn't in good conscience go forward, even though he appeared to be consenting. Worse, I had reason to believe he may have been dissociating during the consent process.

The supervisor understood and said she would handle the inevitable fallout from those in charge of the implementation. The fallout that did occur took the form of warnings: "Yes, we understand, and it was the right decision. However, don't forget that we've seen our share of clinicians who didn't want to submit videos, so our expectation is that this won't happen again." The dynamics left the treatment team on edge and worried about the possible consequences of standing up to the consultant and DOCFW administration again.

Perhaps the biggest lesson from this situation is how nuanced working with complex trauma can be. Understanding how abuse dynamics might play out in very subtle ways, as Darnell did, is an important first step. Ultimately, among the most effective questions professionals can ask is whether—and how—a given action is in a client's short- and long-term best interests, or whether the action considered serves the needs of others.

Other questions arise from this situation as well. Among them are: What considerations should practitioners give when applying a method or model developed for one population to a different demographic? In this case, the model was developed and validated with adults and some adolescents and was now being used with children. In what ways might this practice resemble the off-label use of medications? Children are, after all, more dependent on the adults around them than adolescents and emerging adults. Viewing them as younger versions of older people can be the first step to misapplied treatment and failed therapeutic alliances.

Questions remain. What dual relationships exist when a large agency such as a child welfare agency or school department essentially mandates a treatment? In this instance, the DOCFW administration's motivation was based on the realization that people who come under their supervision have typically experienced trauma. However, the DOCFW, like other agencies, holds considerable power over its charges. To what extent does a referral to treatment appear as a demand to participate against one's will? To what extent is the modality assessed as appropriate for the person being treated? Where does informed consent begin and end under these circumstances? Taking this point a step further, what are the ethics of assigning a single, specific treatment to a client without discussing other options?

A central challenge for practitioners, one that may not be apparent in a cursory review of the codes of ethics of the helping professions, is the lived experience of our clients, which has too often translated as, "You must, or I'll hurt you." Just as no one has the right to say this to others, our clients' experiences remind us that a primary obligation practitioners have is to refrain from replicating this dynamic and the environments in which it has appeared.

What Are Ethics?

The definitions of and reasons for adopting codes of ethics have received considerable attention elsewhere in the literature (Pope et al., 2021) and require little further discussion here. Codes of ethics exist in numerous areas of professional practice, including those of doctors, nurses, social workers, psychologists, and certified counselors. As of 2008, 25 states have required ongoing training in boundaries and ethics as part of professionals' license renewals (Association of Social Work Boards [ASWB], 2008).

In a recent paper, Watts (2021) focused on the elements that make ethics training more and less effective, including areas such as knowledge of ethics and practical application of ethical decision-making. Training in ethics itself presents a dilemma: on the one hand, this author is aware of little if any evidence concluding that ongoing training in ethics for the purpose of license renewal actually improves the behavior of trainees. On the other hand, it seems unconscionable not to maintain an ongoing focus on ethics as a subject of professional attention. In the end, adhering to codes of ethics protects both the client and professional alike. The client is protected from harm or exploitation while the professional is protected from even the appearance of causing harm.

In the author's experience, definitions of ethics for various professions have centered on the moral correctness of professional conduct, with the intention of doing no harm, and performing one's work in the spirit of justice. Sawyer and Prescott (2010) noted that professional ethics are typically founded on underlying values such as:

- Clients are, by definition, vulnerable when receiving mental health services.
- Professionals have varying degrees of perceived or real power and authority (and this is especially true when clients are mandated by the courts or social service agencies into treatment).
- There is an essential need for physical and psychological safety for clients who receive mental health services (p. 2).

Likewise, Sawyer and Prescott (2010, p. 4) also noted that common elements of ethical codes include:

- upholding the dignity of the person
- avoiding discrimination
- preventing harm
- informed consent
- preventing conflicts of interest
- avoiding multiple or dual relationships
- engaging in no sexual relationships or intimacies
- engaging in no sexual harassment
- protecting privacy
- refraining from unnecessary physical contact

In recent years, professional organizations such as the American Psychological Association and the National Association of Social Workers have added professional self-care to discussions of ethical considerations (Abramson, 2021). While it may seem sad that this needs to be codified, its importance in effective mental health practice should be obvious. When professionals are not rested and at peace with themselves, clients may suffer the consequences, particularly those with histories of complex trauma and dissociation. A client (who is a friend and gave permission to share this) of another therapist recently shared with the author that there are several areas of her life she does not share with her therapist because the therapist already has much happening in her own life, and she doesn't want to upset her further. This is particularly concerning when in the adult psychotherapy literature, one study found that over 90% of adult psychotherapy patients report having lied to their therapists (Blanchard & Farber, 2015). One has to wonder about how therapists are interacting with clients to elicit these kinds of responses. Given the subtleties of complex trauma and dissociation, it is all the more helpful to use measures that examine trauma symptoms and dissociation lest they be missed in clinical sessions or misidentified as behavioral issues.

What Are Boundaries?

Boundaries are the structural and interpersonal aspects of a relationship that make therapy possible. It is always the responsibility of the professional to ensure that boundaries are clear. Structural boundaries include considerations such as clarity and agreement about the time and place for services; interpersonal boundaries include the limits of relationships, such as gift-giving, explicit expectations that there will be no sexual contact, and agreement on the nature of any physical contact (such as handshakes, fist bumps, occasional pats on the shoulder), all depending on the circumstances in which treatment takes place.

At their core, effective interpersonal and professional boundaries leave each person feeling *protected* and *connected*. Although these are simple enough to describe, questions and seemingly unpredictable answers can arise quickly. For example:

A therapist working with a client to explore music playlists to assist in self-regulation finds that the client also has knowledge of older music that the therapist's family has listened to. Acknowledging their shared interest could potentially help their mutual understanding of each other. However, it could lead to boundary issues if it were to lead to family conversations about the therapist and their musical tastes.

A therapist in the same treatment setting elects not to wear a wedding ring because he wishes to protect his privacy. In this setting, the direct care staff freely share their relationship status. Questions arise as to whether this should be a personal decision or if the administration should develop a policy so that no one is placed in an awkward situation.

The answers to these questions can often be answered by exploring what is in the clients' *long-term* best interests. In the first example, there are other ways to forge a strong therapeutic alliance that don't hinge on risky personal disclosures. In the second example, the concern might best be addressed by providing guidance to all employees about how to respond to personal questions in a manner that leaves clients feeling protected and connected.

Why Should We Care?

In a classic article on professional boundaries, Smith and Fitzpatrick (1995) emphasized the need for professionals to *abstain from personal gain, remain neutral, and foster independence and autonomy*. Certainly, the first of these, abstaining from personal gain, can be relatively easy to accomplish with firm structural boundaries around occurrences such as gift-giving, or avoiding dual relationships. Professionals will occasionally need to be on guard against interpersonal gain, such as receiving gratification from being an important person in the life of the client or viewing themselves as a savior of children.

The second of the above principles, neutrality, can also be accomplished under other circumstances. However, professionals will want to be on guard against interpersonal values, attitudes, and beliefs entering the therapeutic arena. It has long been noted by professionals that traumatized people can have an eerily accurate sixth sense about what people around them may be thinking or feeling. It is not uncommon for professionals to have attitudes and beliefs that they refrain from sharing with clients. In fact, many professionals have attempted to appear neutral in discussing a client's relationship while secretly thinking to themselves, "Leave him! Leave him now! He's obviously no good for you and could become violent again with the least provocation." Unfortunately, clients with histories of complex trauma and dissociation can often sense that the person they are talking to is thinking things that are different from what they are saying, and can be acutely sensitive to indications that the professional is not saying what they are really thinking. This can be highly unnerving for the client and professional alike, since it can sometimes replicate the environments in which abuse occurred (for example, the home where everyone knew that abuse occurred, but no one dared to talk about it). At the same time, however, it can also be vital to clarify that there are some topics one does not remain neutral on, such as safety and freedom from abuse for all.

It can be useful for professionals to consider their own values, attitudes, and beliefs outside of sessions by exploring hypothetical situations. Given that professionals are expected to be neutral unless there are compelling reasons not to be (for example, when dealing with client disclosures that require a mandatory report to a child protective services agency), here is a sample of possible situations to consider the bounds of neutrality:

- A girl with a history of complex trauma and dissociation enters treatment and is thinking about who she wants to be in the future and what she might do for a living. Do you have a strong opinion about this? On its surface, it seems to be a deeply personal decision that only she can make; you may have a role in helping her to clarify her decision.
- Treatment is guided in large part by the client's sensitivities around abuse dynamics. Almost beyond their awareness, the therapist is steering the child's treatment away from those areas that are close to their own unresolved issues or internal cues that function as echoes of their own trauma. Where would your neutrality begin and end here?
- A therapist avoids strong affect and feelings based on their own limited capacities rather than on the needs of the child. They may tell themselves they are looking out for the best interests of the child, who might continue to experience these feelings after the session but does not explore this in supervision.
- A therapist works only with those elements of trauma and dissociation that they feel comfortable with, perhaps feeling a strong urge to "fix" things in the client's life before fully understanding the child and the context of their life.

Some of these scenarios are more difficult than others, mirroring the decisions professionals must make in mental health settings. For professionals providing direct services, the temptation to fix clients' problems and provide solutions can be very strong. This can easily lead to bypassing professional neutrality along the way.

The examples provided immediately above also speak to the third principle discussed by Smith and Fitzpatrick (1995), that of *independence and autonomy*. This principle is particularly important, since so much of what constitutes trauma involves violating another's independence and autonomy. It can be easy to think of independence and autonomy as it pertains to broader life issues, such as changes in relationship status (e.g., supporting the person who is leaving an abusive marriage), supporting a client's efforts to pursue gender-affirming care, or helping the client who has been molested by a family member to live free and apart from those who harmed them. Of course, for clients with histories of complex trauma and dissociation, questions of independence and autonomy can surface in the daily routines of life, even in the lives of children. Having a role in deciding what to eat, what to wear, and when to do which activity can take on a special meaning for each client.

For these reasons, supporting client independence and autonomy should be at the top of every professional's mind. Examples from the author's practice (in primarily inpatient treatment settings) of how well-intended professionals can do harm include the therapist saying:

- "With your trauma history, you really need to do [a specific form of trauma therapy]," without discussion of what type of therapeutic work the client would find helpful.
- "I can make a referral to your medication prescriber, but I can tell you that you'll need to be on those medications for the rest of your life. They're helping you manage your behavior."
- "We're here to work on your trauma, and here's how we're going to deal with it."

In contrast, a psychologist colleague outside the United States was once asked to conduct an evaluation on an Indigenous adolescent who had just been arrested. He had a long history of abuse and neglect, all in the context of massive cultural trauma. He was on probation, and one evening while his mother was drunk at home, she told him to go to a nearby pub to borrow money to buy more alcohol. He was arrested for a violation of his community supervision rules as he left the pub and headed home. The psychologist, feeling that the arrest was itself unjust, decided that she could at least give the young client every opportunity to explain who he was and why he did what he did so that she could write the fairest report for the court. She later said, "Given how counter-therapeutic the entire situation was, I could at least be the professional who offered a choice when all other choices had been taken away."

While the three principles set forward by Smith and Fitzpatrick (1995) are of obvious importance, several other considerations fall outside their bounds. The first is the obligation to impart accurate information. On more than one occasion, the author has heard professionals state to the client or in their presence that they have been "scarred for life" by the abuse they have suffered. Often, this has happened in the context of clients testifying in cases against the people who abused them. While there is no question that traumatized people often carry the physical and metaphorical scars of their victimization for the rest of their lives (and most of them are all too aware of this without being reminded), it is also true that a significant number of those who survive complex traumas can rebuild their lives (Fuller-Thomson et al., 2016). Telling someone they are scarred for life can produce an unintended iatrogenic effect, and ethical and boundary concerns can follow. Ethical and boundary concerns follow when we tell someone, potentially very inaccurately, that they are the one thing they don't want them to be.

A final boundary consideration that has received very little discussion has to do with empathy, validation, and shame. It is well established in clinical research that empathy is a central feature of any effective therapy or therapist (Moyers & Miller, 2013). However, in working with clients with histories of complex trauma and dissociation, it can be vital to remember that empathy has often been weaponized against them. Often, this has taken the form of someone using knowledge of their vulnerabilities against them. This is not an entirely new idea; it's long been known that the most effective hunters are those who can understand and predict the internal mindset of their prey. Likewise, truly sadistic individuals can inflict additional harm because of their understanding of the inner world of the people they victimize. As a result, professionals need to be cautious in how they use empathy. Too much can replicate abusive environments where the client's needs for connection and coregulation were never met; too much empathy at once may leave clients exposed and vulnerable. As commonly occurs with therapeutic processes, there is no single way to balance the amount of empathy expressed, and the most effective way to ensure one isn't having a negative effect is to check in with the client directly and frequently. Further suggestions are provided below.

Boundary Crossings

Sawyer and Prescott (2010), Smith and Fitzpatrick (1995), and others have distinguished between *boundary crossings* and *boundary violations*. The former describes departures from common practice that may or may not benefit the client. Professionals working with groups of children, for example, might occasionally bring in snacks knowing that offerings of food are a nearly universal signal of goodwill and that those who have had a snack can often focus better within treatment sessions. In other settings, this would not be considered acceptable. Boundary violations, however, are departures from accepted practices that pose an unacceptable risk to the client or therapeutic processes.

Pope and Keith-Spiegel (2008) identified seven cognitive errors by clinicians that can contribute to boundary crossings and violations:

1. What happens outside the psychotherapy session has nothing to do with the therapy.
2. Crossing a boundary with a therapy client has the same meaning as doing the same thing with someone who is not a client.
3. Our understanding of a boundary crossing is also the client's understanding of the boundary crossing.
4. A boundary crossing that is therapeutic for one client will also be therapeutic for another client.
5. A boundary crossing is a static, isolated event.
6. If we ourselves don't see any self-interest, problems, conflicts of interest, unintended consequences, major risks, or potential downsides to crossing a particular boundary, then there aren't any.
7. Self-disclosure is, per se, always therapeutic because it shows authenticity, transparency, and trust.

These incorrect assumptions can serve as a useful checklist for professionals engaged in the day-to-day work of tailoring their treatment approach to meet the needs of their clients.

Considerations for Paraprofessionals

A couple of additional points are worth considering for those engaged in residential/group care, case managers, and the like.

First, although it might seem obvious, it is worth remembering as well as training and retraining staff that any form of sexual behavior with clients is unethical and non-consensual by nature. It is illegal and will always be harmful to clients who are entrusted to the care of others. There are no exceptions to this. It is particularly important to note in child complex trauma cases because clients in group care can often behave differently from other children. Male staff might perceive a female client acting in a seemingly seductive fashion. Should staff members believe that a client is flirting with them, it is imperative to view this as a trauma symptom. The behaviors that seem flirtatious can, in fact, be a strategy for survival; in essence, the child is testing the staff member as if to say, "Let's see how you behave when I flirt with you. If you flirt back or otherwise approach me, I will know that you can't be trusted." In some cases, flirtation may occur because it is the only way that a traumatized client knows how to interact with adults, primarily men, who hold power and authority over them. Maintaining professional boundaries in the face of this interactive style is fundamental to preventing harm to both clients and the adults who care for them.

Second, it is often crucial to remember that hypervigilance and being quick to anger are primary survival skills for children and adolescents with histories of complex trauma and dissociation. In fact, fighting back against power and authority has often served them well in the past, no matter how much it appears inappropriate outside of the abusive environments they've endured. The most ethical and effective approach is to stay within boundaries marked by a calm and soothing approach. When a client becomes irate, moving closer to them (as if preparing to take physical action) or raising the rate, pitch, or volume of one's speech virtually guarantees retraumatization for the client. In group care, the most effective front-line staff are those who can always display a calm and soothing demeanor. One residential program for justice-involved youth reduced the number of physical restraints of clients to the extent that they became very rare events. Chief among their techniques was to form a human shield when one resident would attempt to attack another, to prevent both the attack and the staff becoming physically aggressive with traumatized adolescents.

Digging Deeper: The "Big Four" Ethical Principles

Having examined ethics and boundaries, this section looks deeper at the foundation of ethical and effective professional practice. Varkey (2021) emphasized four principles that are staples of professional codes of ethics. Although the language can vary from one profession to the next, these are beneficence, nonmaleficence, autonomy, and justice. Autonomy is discussed earlier and is mentioned again here not for its role in helping professionals stay on track (as above) with best practices, but rather, because its role as a fundamental cornerstone of professional ethics serves as a reminder that solo practitioners and agencies alike should maintain an explicit focus on helping clients to achieve and uphold autonomy at every turn. While most professionals define their work as helping traumatized people recover, this principle reminds us that *how* we attempt to help is vitally important. Agency policies, interventions, and therapist styles that unnecessarily restrict client autonomy will almost certainly not succeed in the long run.

Autonomy can become complicated when professionals are working with children in the context of their families. Privileging autonomy with young people in a family context can vary from one culture to the next and depend on the constellation of family members. There are no blanket solutions for every case; rather, professionals should actively ask themselves how they can best support each client's autonomy in the circumstances that they exist. Often, this might mean privileging the family's autonomy as well as the child's. An example of this is provided later in this chapter.

Justice as an ethical principle makes sense and appears completely reasonable. With complex trauma and dissociation, however, matters become more complicated. Often, children and adolescents with histories of complex trauma have had direct or indirect involvement with the legal or child welfare systems. Matters can become particularly complicated when the client with complex trauma has close ties to the person who abused them or others. While many of these situations are addressed in the literature, it can be all too easy for professionals to give the appearance of taking sides and disparaging the person who caused harm unnecessarily or gratuitously.

Obviously, no professionals tolerate abuse or serious wrongdoing by caregivers; framing the message to children and adolescents is important. "Your father is in a place where he will get help and be prevented from harming others" is different from statements indicating that he is a bad person. The first type upholds justice, while the second may appear to uphold justice, but does so at the expense of supporting the client in autonomously forming their own conclusions about their father. After all, those who abuse have often also been beloved by those whom they hurt and whose conclusions may be complicated. These nuanced boundaries and ethical applications are in no way tolerant of abuse. Instead, professionals can use these principles to form statements and interventions that will be the most beneficial to the client from the greatest number of perspectives over the long term.

Beneficence—being kind, charitable, or benevolent—is a straightforward principle. In the author's experience, it has been misused primarily in situations where other principles, and even common sense, were not adhered to. In one instance, a detention facility for juveniles experienced considerable difficulties due to its stance on trauma-informed care. Believing that the adolescents in their care were behaving badly due to their trauma histories (which was an accurate appraisal), they elected not to impose any kinds of sanctions on misconduct. The well-intentioned thought was that since this aggression was a trauma symptom, it should be addressed in treatment (also accurate, but insufficient to create a safe environment), and that formal responses to problem behavior should be reserved only for other kinds of clients. Unchecked, these behaviors quickly escalated in this environment, with the result that clients and staff members suffered injury because of escalating violence within an environment which had, ironically, become traumagenic.

In another example, a client with a significant history of complex trauma and an autism spectrum disorder sexually touched another client while improperly supervised in a self-contained special education treatment program. The supervising clinician refused to report this breach of supervision policy to the necessary authorities. This was because he believed that the behavior was simply symptomatic of complex trauma and autism and therefore did not constitute a failure of the program to supervise the children in its care. This person did not remain in their position for long after this, having defied the law and ignored the potential harms to each child as well as the program. While each of the above examples may seem unlikely to happen in one's own environment, they were the result of seasoned professionals' actions, taken in the belief that they were upholding beneficence, but ignoring other aspects of professional boundaries and ethics.

The final of the "big four," nonmaleficence (refraining from causing harm or neglect), may well be the most important. Every professional endorses nonmaleficence, but not all notice when they are engaged in it. In most cases, actions that constitute maleficence are easy to identify. The picture is less clear when complex trauma and dissociation is involved, as the examples in this chapter show. Rather than review examples, it may be better for professionals to review their practice and ask:

- In what small ways might I be causing harm to clients? This could include anything from disparaging remarks made about family members to the use of sarcasm in one's humor.
- In what small ways might I be neglecting clients or their presenting symptoms? This could include not being fully present in sessions, not engaging in appropriate screening and assessment, or not ensuring that one is talking about goals and topics that are personally relevant and meaningful to the client. Because dissociation is all about keeping secrets inside, if we don't ask, a child (or person of any age) won't disclose these experiences. Thus, we miss a lot and are no longer providing attuned, ethical treatment.
- Have I taken any actions in the course of any client's treatment that have served my needs or that of my agency that were not in client's long-term best interests and that might have resulted in harms, no matter how small?
- In what ways might I be engaging in nonmaleficence by not adequately upholding the other "big four" ethical principles in a balanced fashion?

It is worth reiterating that very few professionals don't believe they live up to these ethical principles. However, the application of these principles requires closer scrutiny when considering children and adolescents with complex trauma and dissociation, especially when professionals can never entirely know when an action intended to be therapeutic ends up retraumatizing a client. Finally, in cases of complex trauma, the literature has never, to the author's knowledge, discussed the fact that adhering to each of these ethical principles can sometimes require considerable nuance and balance on the part of the professional.

Steps in Ethical Decision-Making

In those moments when professionals, paraprofessionals, and administrators are faced with ethical quandaries, there are few things more helpful than having a checklist to follow. Pope and colleagues

(2021) assembled a list of steps for decision-making that is worth mentioning. They have written extensively on this topic, though the steps are only summarized here:

1. State the question, dilemma, or concern as clearly as possible.
2. Anticipate who will be affected by the decision.
3. Figure out who, if anyone, is the client.
4. Assess whether your areas of competence—and of missing knowledge, skills, experience, or expertise—are a good fit for this situation.
5. Review relevant formal ethical standards.
6. Review relevant legal standards.
7. Review the relevant research and theory.
8. Consider whether personal feelings, biases, or self-interest might affect your ethical judgment.
9. Consider whether social, cultural, religious, or similar factors affect the situation and the search for the best response.
10. Consider consultation.
11. Develop alternative courses of action.
12. Think through the alternative courses of action.
13. Try to adopt the perspective of each person who will be affected.
14. Decide what to do, review or reconsider it, and take action.
15. Document the process and assess the results.
16. Assume personal responsibility for the consequences.
17. Consider implications for preparation, planning, and prevention.

As a case example, let's return to the circumstances of our first illustration in this chapter. In it, Darnell worked as part of a team implementing an empirically supported treatment for trauma as part of a collaboration between his mental health agency and the DOCFW. In this instance, a teenage girl had been referred for treatment by her DOCFW case manager. She vehemently insisted she did not want this treatment and told her case manager, who suggested she talk with Darnell. However, when she spoke with her parents, they were adamant that she should stay in treatment because this was what the case manager, an agent of the state, wanted. Whether it really was a requirement or a recommendation remains unclear, but in the client's eyes, the entire process was intrusive and against her will. One day, Darnell found out that the girl had fought back against her parents so strongly that her father physically restrained her while her mother drove the car to the office. Darnell immediately canceled the curriculum portion of the session, explained his intent that this be a safe space for her, allowed her to cool off, and eventually just had a conversation with her for the balance of the time.

Darnell, his supervisor, and the agency director then contacted the DOCFW administration, requesting a meeting with all of those in charge of the implementation, including the consultant. The DOCFW administration was sympathetic, while the consultant, obviously invested in the implementation efforts, said that Darnell should work harder to engage the young woman. Meanwhile, the agency did not want to harm their relationship with either the DOCFW or the consultant.

The agency team met and reviewed the basics. They had an ethical obligation to the client (the teenage girl) and only a contractual obligation to the DOCFW. The young girl was the person most affected by the appearance of being forced against her will into treatment. The team recognized that by continuing to provide treatment, none of the "big four" ethical principles (autonomy, beneficence, nonmaleficence, and justice) were being served. They recognized that despite the best intentions of all, there were compromised boundaries and potential conflicts of interest across the board, with the result that the teenage girl felt neither protected nor connected. Further, if the structural boundaries were compromised (by the dual relationship of the DOCFW's providing both probation conditions and monitoring closely their contracted mental health treatment), the interpersonal boundaries were unacceptable, since the client trusted no one involved.

Compared to the harm of continuing with her in treatment, the harm to the agency of terminating the contract appeared quite small. Adopting the perspective of all involved, the agency team wrote a letter explaining the potential harms of continuing with treatment. After all, they possessed the greatest expertise on trauma treatment in general and on their clients specifically. They ensured that the DOCFW and consultant knew that it was their decision to terminate services and they bore complete responsibility. After exchanging viewpoints, the agency and DOCFW decided to terminate the contract altogether. Subsequent follow-up assessment by the agency's board of directors affirmed for them that this had been the right decision and neither the agency nor the DOCFW ever engaged in this type of collaboration again. What had started as a good idea ended up hopelessly conflicted and misapplied through practically no fault of any one individual.

Best Ways to Prevent Boundary and Ethical Problems

There are several models in psychotherapy that align themselves, directly or indirectly, with elements of effective ethical practice as well as helping ensure excellent professional boundaries. All professionals are encouraged to familiarize themselves with them, since they are evidence-based, and practicing them can build one's interpersonal skills with clients and colleagues alike.

The first, Motivational Interviewing, is a person-centered counseling style that addresses the common problem of ambivalence about change (Miller & Rollnick, 2013, in press). It is centered on a foundational spirit of delivery that includes partnership, acceptance, compassion, and (in the most recent edition, in press at this writing) empowerment. Each of these spirit factors supports a professional approach that upholds beneficence, autonomy, justice, and nonmaleficence.

As examples, if a professional is conducting each issue in a spirit of partnership, in which they are essentially on an equal footing with the client, it can be easier to uphold these four ethical principles than if professionals view themselves as the experts in the room whose job it is to build a better life for their client (which is more in line with a physician-patient relationship). Partnership in this context involves the belief that while the professional may possess expertise in complex trauma and dissociation, only the client is the expert on their own lives. Professionals who work in partnership with their clients are more likely to be experienced as abstaining from any personal benefit in treatment or to be operating with a conflict of interest. These professionals are also more likely to provide a balanced sense of being both protected and connected to their clients. Further, this kind of approach, through its ongoing model of healthy communication, is one way professionals can support normative child development. Perhaps most importantly, partnership lends itself to a sense of autonomy and adheres to nonmaleficence.

Likewise, the client who feels accepted by the professional is more likely to experience treatment as beneficent and supporting their autonomy in an environment of nonmaleficence. Accordingly, practicing with priorities of compassion and empowerment can uphold all four of the primary ethical principles. What is most fundamental in this way of working is its assurance that the client and professional are equal, willing partners in change.

Another element of Motivational Interviewing is its emphasis on exploring and resolving ambivalence about change. Becoming expert on understanding how people with histories of complex trauma and dissociation can feel two or more ways about elements of their life is extremely helpful to the client who feels stuck and unable to move forward with their life. Here are three examples, framed as double-sided reflective statements:

- "On one hand, you really want to feel better about your life, and on the other hand, there is a part of you that is really uncertain."

- "On one hand, you want to focus on your future, and on the other hand, it's like you're always needing to be on the lookout so that you don't get hurt in the here and now."
- "You're really feeling two ways about being here. Part of you wants to be safe and do well at home and in school, and part of you just wants to be left alone."

With each of these statements, it would be tempting to add that this experience is normal, to be expected, or otherwise completely understandable. In Motivational Interviewing, however, best practice is to ask permission of the client before sharing one's feedback or advice.

Ultimately, an aim of Motivational Interviewing is to allow each client to explore their own internal desires, abilities, reasons, and needs to make changes. By exploring and reflecting back these motivations, practitioners can help clients make the changes that are right for them, in an atmosphere that feels empowering, thus adhering to the ethical principles of effective practice, as well as upholding boundaries that contribute to client safety. Crucial to successful Motivational Interviewing is that its style and principles be adapted to the individual characteristics of each client. Motivational Interviewing occurs differently depending on the age and personal characteristics and culture of every person.

Another approach that can uphold ethical principles and maintains boundaries is Feedback-Informed Treatment (FIT) (Prescott et al., 2017, 2023). FIT is a transtheoretical approach that uses ongoing administration of outcome and alliance measures to collect real-time client feedback about their experience in therapy. "Transtheoretical" means that FIT can be applied across disciplines, no matter what treatment approach the therapist is using. Although FIT can improve the effectiveness of professionals over time, it is mentioned here because of its established capacity to improve client outcomes. Some measures and norms for its use have been adapted for children, and it can be used with caregiving systems as well (Valla & Prescott, 2019).

Central to FIT is its focus on collecting feedback from the client on measures of well-being and the therapeutic/working alliance. Of particular interest in working with complex trauma, FIT ensures that the client has a voice in treatment at every step. Within this method, it is vital that professionals:

- Create a culture of feedback in which clients are free and encouraged to rate and discuss their experiences without fear of retribution or complication, and with the hope of having an active role in the course of their own treatment.
- Demonstrate that they have strongly considered that feedback and have taken action accordingly. This can take different forms. One client once noted that his therapist's office needed more artwork on the walls and was delighted to return the following week to find that his therapist had agreed and hung more paintings. Another client once told the author to ask more pointed questions and to challenge him more, and he became more involved when this happened in subsequent sessions.

Getting heartfelt, honest, and actionable feedback from clients requires considerable skill. For professionals who are more accustomed to an expert-driven approach (in which the professional is the expert whose approach is better left unchallenged), it can require rejecting erstwhile approaches, attitudes, and beliefs about clients and treatment processes. Nonetheless, by viewing the client's input into treatment services as meaningful and requiring consideration, professionals are more likely to practice with nonmaleficence, justice, autonomy, and beneficence.

For clients with histories of complex trauma and dissociation, inviting feedback on the alliance can reverse patterns of deferring to others who have more power; this is one reason it can be so difficult to elicit the client's voice. In essence, the professional is asking:

- "How well am I listening to you?"
- "Is what we're doing important to you?"

- "Do you like what we've done today?"
- "Do you hope to do the same kinds of things next time?"

One professional who participated in a study and was found to be among the most effective therapists studied once remarked privately, "What I've learned is that I need feedback not because I'm a great therapist; I'm not. Rather, if I don't get feedback, all of my assumptions and approaches will be wrong more often than they're right."

Going Upstream

As a brief thought exercise for upholding excellent boundaries and ethics, consider: What is one thing any child client with a history of complex trauma and dissociation might want right now? It can be as simple as to enjoy a trip to the park (or as complex as having multiple competing wants and needs). Then ask: If they had that in their lives right now, then what would they have? For example, the client who wants to enjoy a trip to the park may feel that they are able to do something effectively. If they could do something effectively, then what else would they have in their life? It may be that this sense of effectiveness means they can make decisions for themselves based on what they want and not on what others want from them. And upstream from making their own decisions is independence and autonomy.

By continually exploring what is upstream from a particular issue or behavior, practitioners can better align with what is personally meaningful and relevant to the client. Through this alignment, professionals can become better attuned and display more effective empathy and compassion. By doing each of these, professionals can better uphold beneficence, autonomy, justice, and nonmaleficence. It can be useful to remember that upstream from every situation are broader goals the professional can connect with. The client's search for autonomy, independence, and justice in their lives may be just beyond otherwise challenging behaviors such as opposition, defiance, or refusing to participate. By respecting the larger goals, professionals are in a better position to help their clients.

A Meditation on Boundaries[3]

Complex trauma and dissociation typically stems from abuse and broken boundaries. This means professionals need to guard against leaving clients feeling unprotected or unconnected or creating boundaries that are blurred or diffuse. Among the best ways to prevent blurred, diffuse boundaries is to contemplate how they work in one's life. To that end, professionals and clients alike may benefit from a contemplative exercise to explore the nature of one's boundaries.

Take a moment to relax where you are. You may be standing, sitting, or even lying down. If you like, you can feel your body connecting with both the ground below and the atmosphere above you. If you like, you can relax your shoulders and slow your breathing. You can relax the muscles in your face and let go of any tension in your hips or legs. You can also let go of any thoughts that might have been troubling you or put them to one side as you go through this activity.

As you relax and feel yourself becoming centered, you can start to sense where your boundaries are. Boundaries can change shape and size or vary from what you say to others to how you allow others' actions to affect you. Some people feel more like they are surrounded by little walls when they are on a city bus, while others feel as though they have more expansive boundaries when out in nature. Where are yours right now?

There are those who experience their boundaries as a sort of egg shape around their body, while others feel boundaries as a kind of energy shield roughly the same shape as their bodies. Everyone is different. Where do you feel yours?

As you explore your boundaries, you might look at them from the outside. What colors are your boundaries? How do the colors change in different circumstances? What do your boundaries look like and feel like from the outside?

Next, you might imagine touching the inside of your boundaries with your fingers. What do your boundaries feel like? What do they look like on the inside? Do things inside your boundaries sound different from outside them? Some people have even been curious to see if they can smell or taste their boundaries, but this is all up to you.

As you explore your own boundaries in this way, are there any places where they've been damaged or need repair? If so, how can you best attend to these places? Is there someone or something that can help you? Have there been events in your life that caused you not to attend to these boundaries? As you work on bringing them back to full strength, how might you continue to maintain them? How often would you like to check in on your boundaries to make sure you are protected and connected, and can best be of service to yourself and others?

As you reflect on your own boundaries, you can also consider what you may need in order to look after them in your daily life in the most effective ways, and plan accordingly.

Conclusion

Thinking of boundaries and ethics as ongoing processes involving different steps, approaches, and skills can protect both the client and the professional. The most ethical practices support client autonomy, provide beneficence and justice, and uphold nonmaleficence. Clients who feel protected and connected will always be more positively affected by interventions. The most skilled professionals, and the safest agencies, work to uphold these principles every day.

Notes

1. Because this chapter is intended to be relevant for all who work in the helping professionals, it uses the term "professionals." This term includes people with backgrounds in psychology, social work, counseling, administration, education, and criminal justice.
2. All cases have been modified to protect the privacy and confidentiality of everyone involved.
3. I am grateful to author Langston Kahn (2021) for his work in this area, on which this exercise is based.

References

Abramson, A. (2021). The ethical imperative of self-care. *Monitor on Psychology, 52*, 47. apa.org/monitor/2021/04/feature-imperative-self-care

Association of Social Work Boards (ASWB) (2008). Continuing education requirements. Retrieved May 18, 2010, from ASWB.org

Blanchard, M., & Farber, B. (2015). Lying in psychotherapy: Why and what clients don't tell their therapist about therapy and their relationship. *Counselling Psychology Quarterly, 29*, 1–23. https://doi.org/10.1080/09515070.2015.1085365

Fuller-Thomson, E., Baird, S. L., Dhrodia, R., & Brennenstuhl, S. (2016). The association between adverse childhood experiences (ACEs) and suicide attempts in a population-based study. *Child: Care, Health and Development, 42*(5), 725–734. https://doi.org/10.1111/cch.12351

Kahn, L. (2021). *Deep liberation: Shamanic tools for reclaiming wholeness in a culture of trauma*. North Atlantic Books.

Miller, W. R., & Rollnick, S. (2013). *Motivational interviewing: Helping people change* (3rd ed.). Guilford Press.

Miller, W. R., & Rollnick, S. (in press). *Motivational interviewing* (4th ed.). Guilford Press.

Moyers, T. B., & Miller, W. R. (2013). Is low therapist empathy toxic? *Psychology of Addictive Behaviors, 27*, 878–884. https://doi.org/10.1037/a0030274

Pope, K. S., & Keith-Spiegel, P. (2008). A practical approach to boundaries in psychotherapy: Making decisions, bypassing blunders, and mending fences. *Journal of Clinical Psychology, 64*(5), 638–652. https://doi.org/10.1002/jclp.20477

Pope, K. S., Vasquez, M. J. T., Chavez-Dueñas, N. Y., & Adames, H. Y. (2021). *Ethics in psychotherapy and counseling: A practical guide* (6th ed.). John Wiley & Sons.

Prescott, D. S., Maeschalck, C. M., & Miller, S. D. (2017). *Feedback-informed treatment in clinical practice: Reaching for excellence*. American Psychological Association.

Prescott, D. S., Maeschalck, C. M., & Miller, S. D. (2023). Feedback-informed treatment. In R. Fulmer (Ed.), *Counseling and psychotherapy: Theory and beyond* (pp. 342–366). Cognella.

Sawyer, S., & Prescott, D. (2010). Boundaries and dual relationships. *Sexual Abuse: A Journal of Research and Treatment, 23*(3), 365–380. https://doi.org/10.1177/1079063210381411

Smith, D., & Fitzpatrick, M. (1995). Patient-therapist boundary issues: An integrative review of theory and research. *Professional Psychology: Research and Practice, 26*(5), 499–506. https://doi.org/10.1037/0735-7028.26.5.499

Valla, B., & Prescott, D. S. (2019). *Beyond best practice: How mental health services can be better.* Routledge.

Varkey, B. (2021). Principles of clinical ethics and their application to practice. *Medical Principles and Practice, 30*(1), 17–28. https://doi.org/10.1159/000509119

Watts, L. L. (2021). Benefits of effective ethics training. In L. Watts, K. Medeiros, T. McIntosh & T. Mulhearn (Eds.), *Ethics training for managers: Best practices and techniques* (pp. 33–46). Routledge.

35
SOCIOCULTURAL DETERMINANTS, ANTI-OPPRESSIVE AND CULTURALLY RESPONSIVE PRACTICES

LaKaavia Taylor and Krystal K. Turner

Introduction

Adverse childhood experiences (ACEs) are potentially traumatic experiences and events encountered by children (Boullier & Blair, 2018). While around 45% of the child population experience at least one ACE, African American and Latine children are impacted significantly by ACEs: an estimated 61% of African American children and 51% of Latine children have experienced at least one ACE (Sacks & Murphey, 2016). When the trauma becomes complex, it leads to further distress. Complex trauma entails exposure to multiple or repeated traumas over time, such as chronic abuse, neglect, and family violence (Complex Trauma Treatment Network of the National Child Traumatic Stress Network, 2016b). Current literature indicates the association between complex trauma and dissociation (Kruger, 2020; Pierorazio et al., 2023; Rhoades, 2005). Similar to the experiences of ACEs, complex trauma disproportionately impacts children and youth from minoritized backgrounds. More specifically, children from Black, Indigenous, and people of color (BIPOC) backgrounds experience elevated experiences of traumatization and trauma-related disorders in comparison to children from white and European groups (Pumariega et al., 2022). Themes in the literature suggest trauma impacts a child across the lifespan with a higher probability of health problems, mental health diagnoses, and substance abuse (Crouch et al., 2017; Ray et al., 2022a). Additionally, the themes consistently show that higher ACE scores correlate with reduced academic performance, prevalence of behavioral disorders, and decreased social-emotional development.

In response to complex childhood trauma, children will make attempts to regain physical safety and security (Complex Trauma Treatment Network of the National Child Traumatic Stress Network, 2016a). When faced with difficulties with physical safety, children often retreat emotionally and psychologically, which may result in dissociation. The experience of dissociation is an adaptive phenomenon that disconnects one from their thoughts, feelings, bodily responses, and environment (Choi et al., 2018). As we have seen in other chapters in this volume, responses to dissociative experiences can range from mild to severe. The greatest capacity for using dissociation as a defense is in childhood, suggesting susceptibility in early development. However, when a child experiences complex trauma and dissociative behaviors, it does not happen in isolation from the child's culture and environment. A holistic and cultural approach is vital to understand, assess, and intervene. The clinician has many sociocultural factors to consider and infuse into treatment. In this chapter, we will discuss the sociocultural determinants of complex trauma and dissociation; anti-oppressive and culturally responsive strategies and approaches; and case approaches to provide examples of application.

Sociocultural Determinants of Complex Trauma & Dissociation

Dissociation manifests in many forms, with behavioral indicators and experiences related to memory, concentration, perception, and identity (Choi et al., 2018). Specifically, children can experience forgetfulness, dazed states, and altered identities (Myrick & Green, 2014). While these are common indicators, culture has a significant influence on how dissociation and complex trauma manifests in children and families. Therefore, how dissociation is experienced, the meaning assigned, the expression or symptoms, and familial responses are highly impacted by social-cultural determinants (e.g., gender, race, socioeconomic status, and language) (Gopalkrishnan, 2018). Dissociation may help children cope culturally in a society where messages about their self-worth and identity can be devalued. In continued times of social unrest, discrimination, hate crime, racism, inequality, marginalization, misogyny, and oppression are influential in the trauma trajectories and mental health history of culturally diverse groups (Gómez et al., 2021). While there is consensus in the literature regarding sociocultural influences on complex trauma and dissociation, research is challenging and limited in general regarding this area, specifically with children from different cultural groups (Pierorazio et al., 2023). We know much about dissociation from the lenses of Western, middle-class, male-focused, and adult populations (Sholevar & Joshi, 2017). Furthermore, available research centers on interpersonal causes of dissociative behaviors, neglecting sociocultural factors (Gómez et al., 2021).

Most often, there is an underrepresentation of children from different cultural groups in trauma research related to dissociation, especially with cultural populations in which research shows susceptibility. For example, dissociation is a symptom often correlated to a history of physical and sexual abuse in childhood (Moore et al., 2015). Children from minoritized groups have a higher susceptibility to physical and sexual abuse (Pumariega et al., 2022). An estimated 90,000 children experience sexual abuse a year (Moore et al., 2015). Of the 90,000, around 20% are African American children. Studies that address therapeutic interventions for sexual abuse with African Americans are additionally limited, as well as similar findings with Asian, Latine, and American Indian child populations. Considering scholars' role in disseminating knowledge and strategies through literature, clinicians may struggle to identify tools needed to assess and work with dissociation in children from diverse cultural backgrounds. The high rates of ACES experienced by children from BIPOC groups appear to be impacted by the combination of culture along with historical, intergenerational, and racial trauma. Dissociation appears to serve as an attempt to grapple with the different forms of trauma experienced by BIPOC children and their caregivers.

Cultural Views & Mental Health

In many cultures, there is a stigma around mental health (Rössler, 2016). Often, mental health challenges are considered a weakness and a private concern. In some cases, it can be psychologically damaging or bring shame to a family to seek help. Furthermore, for some populations with a BIPOC background, there is a collectivistic value in that help-seeking is from within the family. Despite this, families might not handle or even understand the complexity of trauma responses such as dissociation. It is critical to look beyond the child as an individual and understand their cultural context. Culture influences how children and families understand and cope with mental health struggles (Rosmarin & Koenig, 2020). There is literary support that indicates BIPOC and immigrant populations are more likely to report physical rather than psychological symptoms (Marsella & Yamada, 2000).

These factors indicate the possibility of internalized psychosocial distress along with overlooked symptoms of mental health.

Culture influences the expression of mental health challenges and beliefs about what causes them to manifest (Rosmarin & Koenig, 2020). Individuals from BIPOC populations may attribute the cause of mental health beliefs as having origins beyond scientific causes. Literature provides evidence regarding the spiritual and religious impacts on mental health (Exline & Wilt, 2023). A mental health struggle can serve as deeper spiritual learning or spiritual punishment (Rosmarin & Koenig, 2020). Thus, supernatural and spiritual experiences may be considered as sources of coping with or causing further mental health challenges. Spirituality can provide a sense of meaning, emotional resilience, and reducing stress. However, while spirituality has many known benefits, it can be a source of distress (Marsella & Yamada, 2000).

Due to the experiences of BIPOC populations in the United States, it is not uncommon for communities of color to have suspicion toward mainstream culture in society. This phenomenon is called *cultural mistrust*, which derives from the inequalities and historical events experienced by BIPOC populations in health care (Fortuna et al., 2022). For example, Whaley (2001) found that cultural mistrust attitudes and behaviors are reported by African Americans in psychosocial settings and mental health settings. Similarly, Kim et al. (2017) indicated that higher experiences of microaggressions increased the experience of cultural mistrust in Asian cultures. While these studies focus on adults, they provide context to what caregivers and family members of child clients are experiencing. Considering the familial impact on mental health and historical influence on children, these studies promote the importance of assessing the cultural experiences of a child's family.

Intergenerational Trauma

When children and families seek therapy, they are not just carrying with them the present trauma, but also bringing with them the emotional weight of generations before them. Children learn how to respond and adapt to traumatic experiences based on familial and environmental responses (Bray, 2023). These processes are called *intergenerational trauma*, which occurs when unresolved trauma in one generation affects subsequent generations until reconciled (Fortuna et al., 2022). The effects of the trauma become embedded in the cultural narratives across generations. Intergenerational trauma can predispose children to further psychological distress and challenges with mental well-being (Isobel et al., 2019). Due to these factors, scholars urge clinicians and mental health professionals to consider intergenerational trauma in interventions (Bray, 2023). This is especially critical considering that dissociation can complicate the identification of trauma.

Isobel and colleagues (2019) explained that dissociation connected to intergenerational trauma is often embedded in collective silence, partial processing, or denial that the trauma that occurred. In marginalized and minoritized families, intergenerational trauma is often the result of widespread and continuous violence, abuse, and oppression, such as disenfranchisement in society, police brutality, and lack of accessibility to cultural care. These forms of disparities promote the idea that the experiences of marginalized children and families are not valid. Therefore, intergenerational trauma impacts the mental and physical health of culturally diverse children and families across the lifespan. Research indicates the intergenerational association between ACEs encountered by BIPOC caregivers and trauma-related symptomology in their children. For example, Leslie et al. (2023) found that higher PTSD scores in children are associated with caregiver ACEs. Leslie and colleagues (2023) thus emphasize the importance of assessing caregiver ACEs at intake and as part of family focused trauma interventions. Similarly, Ochoa et al. (2022) found that parent ACEs are associated with increased externalizing behaviors in Latine youth. These studies suggest the need for family based approaches to trauma and dissociation.

Racial Trauma

BIPOC and marginalized children commonly experience racial incidents connected to discrimination, racism, and microaggressions (Cénat, 2023). The harmful effects on the physical and emotional well-being of BIPOC children have been documented in the literature. For example, Savell et al. (2019) found a correlation between witnessing parental discrimination in early childhood and displaying disruptive behaviors in adolescent development. The experience of racial stress and trauma can lead to low academic performance, a decrease in self-esteem, and early school dropout for BIPOC families (Wei et al., 2011). Clinicians are urged to understand that constant racial incidences are in addition to the harm of other ACEs (e.g., violence, minority stress, and oppression) common in BIPOC populations. Furthermore, the encounters are not limited to individual experience, but are also across institutions and systems. The challenge with racial trauma is that the experience feels confusing, uncontrollable, and, most of all, reoccurring (Polanco-Roman et al., 2016). The resulting coping mechanisms for racial trauma include altered thinking, negative mood, avoidance, and emotional reactivity, which are often common in trauma-related disorders.

Race-based trauma affects many aspects of a child's life. Experiences of trauma can cause feelings of hopelessness and powerlessness, threatening their view of a just and safe world. Furthermore, a child's developmental level impacts how children respond to racial trauma (Complex Trauma Treatment Network of the National Child Traumatic Stress Network, 2016b). For example, young children who experience racial trauma such as exposure to social injustices in media may process the information literally (Goodman, 2020). This literal interpretation may cause behaviors such as hypervigilance, replaying the event repeatedly, and sleep problems. Older children have increasing racial awareness with an ability to understand societal perspectives regarding race (Gil & Drewes, 2021). The greater their understanding, the more impactful racial trauma manifests. Therefore, children in this age group tend to question and worry about whether similar racially motivated experiences will happen to them. Moreover, their senses of safety, comfort, and identity are altered. For example, children from BIPOC populations may develop racial mistrust, displaying signs of guardedness and suspicion toward those from different racial groups (Comas-Díaz et al., 2019). Children may also internalize the racism they experience by adopting the negative stereotypes of their racial group.

Comas-Díaz et al. (2019) described the impact of racial trauma as the equivalent of psychological scars, indicating the lasting impact. The complexity of racial trauma intensifies if the trauma is not acknowledged or validated. Furthermore, sharing experiences of racism and racially charged events can feel incredibly exposing and vulnerable (Williams et al., 2018). Therefore, many of those who experience racial trauma have not had an opportunity to process their experience due to stigma. As a result, the individual may engage in passive actions to cope with the racial trauma, such as internally replaying the experience, accepting it, and keeping it to themselves (Polanco-Roman et al., 2016). Considering how much dissociation impacts cognitive appraisal, coping skills related to cultural identity can serve as a buffer.

Lenses to Understand Complex Trauma, Dissociation, and Culture

Due to lived experiences of diverse child populations, clinicians have a commitment to understand trauma and dissociations through the anti-oppressive, intersectionality, and family lenses. In the following section, we will discuss the framework and cultural lenses for understanding complex trauma and disassociation.

The Anti-Oppressive Lens

The field of mental health is still relatively new to incorporating culture. Even when culture is addressed in trauma-focused mental health with children, often matters of racism, discrimination, and oppression are not considered in evaluation and diagnoses (Corneau & Stergiopoulos, 2012). Anti-oppressive practice entails recognizing multiple forms of oppression that occur at the individual, institutional, and societal levels (Medlock et al., 2018). The focus is on how levels of systems and organizations create and maintain inequitable power imbalances and conditions between clients and mental health professionals, and society. More specifically, anti-oppressive practices entail removing barriers to equal access, opportunities, and resources from social and cultural disparities.

An anti-oppressive lens is necessary to understand complex trauma because most models of child mental health focus on individualistic factors rather than the interrelated cultural, structural, and societal influences (Abbott & Taylor, 2013). For example, if a BIPOC child is experiencing dissociation from trauma, a traditional approach is addressing related triggers. While the traditional approach is helpful, a therapist operating from an anti-oppressive lens must first acknowledge the impact of societal and cultural norms related to trauma, additionally exploring what trauma and dissociative behaviors mean to the child and their family. These aspects are imperative because cultural beliefs and socialization influence the child's subjective perception and meaning of the trauma. Therefore, an anti-oppressive stance invites the family and child to share their lived experiences and perspectives verbally or through expressive mediums, which will play a prominent role in assessment and treatment.

The Intersectionality Lens

An intersectionality framework is a critical lens for understanding complex trauma in children. Kimberle Crenshaw (1989) coined and defined *intersectionality* as the multiple facets of an individual's identity that intersect and impact their experiences of power, status, and privilege. The premise of intersectionality is that an individual's social position is shaped by overlapping identities such as race, ability status, language, gender, culture, and religion (Collins & Bilge, 2021). Therefore, because a child's cultural identities are experienced simultaneously, an intersectionality framework is essential. Clinicians can promote culturally responsive care by considering children's cultural identifiers with the trauma experienced. This is especially important because the combination of a child's identities is crucial to understanding how symptoms of complex trauma and dissociation, behaviors, and distress emerge and manifest. Children with more oppressive intersectional identities (e.g., race, ethnicity, gender, socioeconomic status, and spiritual) may have increased exposure to trauma with magnified effects due to lived experiences. A child's lived experiences can interfere with their ability to engage in or utilize coping skills. For example, consider an Asian American child experiencing sexual abuse. Coupled with the experience of abuse, they may experience microaggressions related to their gender and race. Thus, the intersection of their identifiers could intensify their symptoms of worry and low self-confidence connected to the sexual abuse trauma.

Utilizing an intersectionality framework when addressing trauma considers how the child's sociopolitical environment is influencing their overall well-being. It promotes focusing on the interaction between biological and social factors that may produce or be the product of complex trauma. For example, consider a child who is Native Hawaiian and is experiencing dissociative symptoms because of severe physical neglect. To approach the complex trauma from an intersectionality perspective, it would be necessary for clinicians first to understand that Native Hawaiian children are likely to experience anxiety because of intergenerational trauma, have limited access to healthcare, and are more likely to seek support from healers. Based on the combination of these factors, it would be necessary for the clinician to assess if aspects of immigration are impacting the emotional and physical toll on the family and compounding the complex trauma. Furthermore, focus on how the child and family are describing the trauma symptoms is essential, since internalization of emotions is often the result of intergenerational trauma. Lastly, working to promote cultural safety with the child and family, consider that Native Hawaiian families may prefer seeking support from natural healers. These examples promote the importance of utilizing an intersectional framework to ensure all components of the child's life are considered, for more holistic and culturally responsive care.

The Family Lens

A family framework is necessary to understand complex trauma in children. According to Daniels and Bryan (2021), when children encounter trauma, it impacts the family. Each member of the family system influences how the family responds and adapts to the trauma. Family responses will depend on each member's age, developmental level, history of trauma, relationship to the child, and familial culture. These responses are essential for clinicians to consider how a family will recover from the trauma. A healthy and cohesive family structure with bonded relationships positively impacts how a family will cope. Ultimately, limited resources and difficulties with addressing the trauma can cause traumatic stress, which impedes healthy family functioning.

Complex trauma also impacts child attachment relationships (Kliethermes et al., 2014). Families may experience a continuum of psychological, physical, behavioral, and cognitive reactions, from mild to severe, in response to a child experiencing trauma in the family. Psychological responses may include reactions such as anger, hypervigilance, guilt, anxiety, and fear. Family members' physical responses may manifest in fatigue, headaches, and sleep difficulties. Cognitively, a family may show difficulties concentrating, replay thoughts about the events, and avoid memories of the experience. Behavioral reactions can include over-protection of family members, decline in performance (academic, job, extracurricular), and self-destructive behaviors.

When a child member of the family experiences trauma, it can either bring families together or complicate family relations (Kliethermes et al., 2014). For some families, the trauma draws families closer as they work together to heal. In this case, the family develops a greater appreciation of its own functioning. Regarding parent-child relationships, parents may readjust their parenting behaviors, such as increased nurturing and empathic responses, to ensure their child's safety. How a parent responds following the trauma significantly affects how children respond and their functioning after the trauma. Some families may face disruption due to the different ways each member reacts to trauma. Due to heightened emotionality and stress, communication breakdowns can occur in the family. Furthermore, family responsibilities and roles might be blurred. The family may also lose sight of what the family needs to keep everyone safe and secure. For parent-child relationships, parents may become emotionally unavailable due to the overwhelm of the trauma. Additionally, increased parental stress may cause the parent to isolate and withdraw due to feeling helpless and unable to address the emotional toll of a child experiencing trauma.

Proposed Approaches and Therapeutic Strategies

As previously mentioned, complex trauma impacts minoritized children at a higher rate than their white counterparts (Pumariega et al., 2022). As the prevalence of trauma continues to rise among BIPOC children and children with varying marginalized identities, mental health professionals search for culturally informed, evidence-based practices to help support healthy development and coping skills. While a dearth of research exists specifically observing children diagnosed with dissociative disorders, researchers work to learn how ACEs, complex trauma, and various forms of abuse are correlated with the development of dissociative disorders in adulthood (Nesbit et al., 2022).

Still, while mental health professionals continue to work toward finding accessible solutions to mitigate the impact of complex trauma, it is paramount that those specializing in working with children with trauma displaying early signs of dissociative behaviors find culturally inclusive ways to best support the child and their families. The following sections provide readers with commonly used, culturally informed, therapeutic modalities that can potentially offset factors and symptomology resulting from complex trauma and high ACE scores that could potentially lead to dissociative symptoms.

Culturally Responsive Framework & Orientation

To tailor trauma-informed approaches, clinicians must be culturally attuned to aspects of the child's cultural identity and experiences. Therapists are encouraged to focus on assessing and exploring matters around intersectionality, such as the child's and family's race, ethnicity, gender, and immigration status when assessing trauma symptomology (McIntosh, 2019). To focus on cultural responsiveness, therapists must adopt a multicultural orientation (MCO). An MCO entails (1) cultural humility, (2) cultural opportunities, and (3) cultural comfort (Owen et al., 2016).

Cultural humility is "an interpersonal stance that is other-oriented rather than self-focused regarding the cultural background and experience of the client" (Hook et al., 2017, p. 9). Embodying cultural humility is centered on awareness and exploration of self and clients. Therapists should be aware that without awareness and exploration, it will be challenging to facilitate the child client in a culturally congruent manner while they process their trauma. Thus, clinicians are encouraged to identify and explore the client's cultural identities, beliefs, values, and biases through mediums such as a cultural collage, journaling, drawing, or sand tray.

Considering the role of power and privilege in the experience and severity of the trauma, clinicians are urged to explore personal aspects of power, privilege, and oppression (Gopalkrishnan, 2018). When they do not direct their attention to matters of power, they run the risk of implicit biases and microaggressions. Therefore, when clinicians engage in processes to explore their identities, they are encouraged to acknowledge and address any challenges. They can engage in this process through an exercise such as the "power flower activity" (Arnold et al., 1991). This activity invites the clinician to label identities on the inner petals of a flower and the identifiers of power on the outer petals. The individual's identifiers are then color-coded to distinguish those with power and those with oppression. Exploring privilege and oppression allows the clinician to understand the impact and processes of power more effectively.

Cultural Opportunities

Cultural opportunities are a subset of cultural humility and entail seeking moments to explore the child's and family's cultural identities (Owen et al., 2016). This can occur when a child nonverbally or verbally expresses culturally related content. For example, consider a child verbalizing negative gender identity comments. Instead of the clinician rescuing the client from experiencing their difficult emotions by saying "You are perfect just how you are," they use this moment as a cultural opportunity. Therefore, they convey to the child that the topic is safe to discuss by reflecting on a statement such as "You feel confused about your gender and body." The clinician might ask the child to create a song or draw a picture about their gender, or use gender-expansive toys to allow safe processing of their emotions. To further address the cultural opportunity and better understand the client's distress, the clinician could explore the family's views and values about gender. Furthermore, the clinician could examine and explore with the child's family any gender-related experiences the client might have encountered. Inviting cultural opportunities can facilitate cultural trust and relationship building between the child, family, and therapist (Ray et al., 2022c). Considering the turbulent history of culturally diverse groups in mental health, attending to cultural opportunities is incredibly important (Fortuna et al., 2022).

Cultural Comfort

Cultural comfort is the behavioral disposition of ease and openness when a child client and their family directly or indirectly express one or more salient parts of their cultural identity (Ray et al., 2022c). It involves the utilization of cultural humility once the cultural opportunity is identified. Cultural comfort helps children decipher the level of safety in exploring cultural topics (Pérez-Rojas et al., 2019). For example, the clinician might reflect to the child, "Your *abuela* shared that you are afraid to speak Spanish at school because you think students will judge you. You can choose to speak English, Spanish, or both during our time together."

Cultural Attunement to the Physiological Impact of Trauma

Trauma symptoms and culture are interrelated (Pumariega et al., 2022). Furthermore, children from diverse families tend to hold trauma physically, resulting in bodily reactions in the form of psychosomatic responses (Marsella & Yamada, 2000). Clinicians can misinterpret or overlook the cultural manifestation of trauma in children. Therefore, they should pay particular attention to physiological symptoms the child or parent reports, such as headaches, stomachaches, and sleep problems. These symptoms can be indicators of underlying traumatic distress related to aspects of a child's race, ethnicity, gender, or immigration experiences (Gopalkrishnan, 2018). For example, consider an immigrant child who has experienced violence in their home country and reports to the therapist frequent physical complaints. The physical symptoms provide greater context to the severity of the trauma. Gutierrez (2018) powerfully described immigrant children as having emotional scars from immigration that manifest physically if left unaddressed. Considering culture and development, clinicians can assess the physical impact of trauma using a body scan or mindfulness activity to help the child identify and become aware of bodily sensations. Cultural considerations include using culturally related terminology or a prerecorded prompt led by someone from the child's cultural group, available on platforms such as YouTube. Additionally, assessing the child's physical safety is important to consider. The clinician can engage the child in an expressive arts activity, such as a safe-space activity in which the child is asked to create a visual or artistic representation of what provides safety. The clinician can use this assessment to determine the child's sense of safety and security from their perspective. Observing physical symptoms helps prompt cultural intentionality.

Often, a child's culture is filled with rules and expectations about the expression of distress (Rosmarin & Koenig, 2020). These expectations can be spoken or unspoken rules or standards. Therefore, when assessing trauma, the therapist must identify the cultural patterns of emotions and behaviors connected to the trauma (Farrelly-Rosch, 2018). It is integral for the therapist to understand and gain knowledge about the cultural expressions of trauma within the family. Once the understanding is developed, clinicians are encouraged to attend to the trauma with consideration to how the child and family define it—for example, using the child's language and words along with materials (e.g., papers, dolls, and puppets) that are congruent with their identifiers when addressing trauma. This can be accomplished with different methods, such as the child drawing how their body feels when experiencing traumatic memories, or making movements or sounds to represent their trauma emotions. The examples used are also developmentally appropriate, considering children have difficulty verbalizing their symptoms, and a more expressive and creative medium can make it safe for cultural expression (Gil & Drewes, 2021).

Culturally Informed and Responsive Exploration of Intersectionality

Trauma impacts a child's sense of self, and considering that the self-structure encompasses sociocultural factors, clinicians are tasked with helping children understand their intersecting identities (Gómez et al., 2021). Before exploring the client's intersecting identities, clinicians are encouraged to dedicate time to exploring their own intersectionality and the role it plays in their life. One method they can use to do this is to complete a written or an audio journal describing different aspects of their identity and beliefs about how those experiences influence how they view themselves and others. Exploring their intersectionality allows therapists to experience their thoughts, feelings, and reactions. Clinicians who do not explore their own intersectionality are at risk of making biased interpretations and stereotyping child clients and their families. Furthermore, exploring intersectionality increases a therapist's attunement to cultural opportunities, increasing cultural safety and inclusivity. Therefore, clinicians are tasked with exploring how their intersectionality may serve as the source of strengths and obstacles.

In addition to clinicians exploring their intersectionality and researching other groups, acknowledging the intersecting identities of children is critical to facilitating cultural safety and inclusivity. The ADDRESSING framework can aid clinicians in exploring salient sociocultural identifiers to consider when understanding the cultural identity of children and families (Hays, 2008). ADDRESSING stands for age and generational influences, development, disability status, religion and spiritual orientation, ethnicity and race, socioeconomic status, sexual orientation, Indigenous heritage, national origin, and gender identity. This framework is not an exhaustive list but a starting point for exploring identities. Clinicians are encouraged to consider the child's age in describing intersectionality and to determine a need for psychoeducation (Gil & Drewes, 2021). Children's books on intersectionality can help clinicians process this concept with children in developmentally appropriate ways. For example, the book *Intersection Allies: We Make Room for All* covers intersectionality in a child-friendly manner with inclusive language. Once the child has understood the concept, the clinician is encouraged to invite the child to spot cultural identifiers (e.g., race, gender, sexuality, spirituality, and nationality) that are important to them. Creative mediums can facilitate this process for children. The therapist can invite the client to use figures, drawings, or dolls to represent the different identifiers. Possible discussion points with the child include described feelings and thoughts, what makes the identifiers vital to them, what they want people to know about their identities, and any confusion or concerns around the named identifiers.

Culturally Informed and Responsive Treatment Planning

Culturally responsive treatment planning is collaborative, emphasizing the family's and child's treatment and healing practices. When developing goals for the child, the clinician can explore with the child and family what values the clinician should consider. Child clients benefit when the clinician is familiar with the customs, traditions, and rituals that families practice. Obtaining the family's input is crucial to aligning treatment goals culturally. When developing goals for the child, ask the child and their family about beliefs to consider in healing and what experiences aid in implementing strategies toward their defined view of healthy functioning. Another helpful question to ask is how the family knows when their needs and expectations are met, based on previous experiences with professionals. The family's cultural values are the foundation of the treatment plan. For example, if communal support is a strong cultural value in a child's family, the clinician could include goals around fostering social connections and support in helping the child reduce physiological arousal related to trauma triggers. If the family values spiritual or religious practices, encouraging participation in spiritual activities to support the healthy expression of distressing emotions related to the trauma would be helpful. Respecting the child and encouraging participation throughout the process increases involvement and retention. Therefore, clinicians are tasked with exploring factors such as the family's and child's concept of wellness and distress, current healing practices, and cultural views of the problem. When therapists create respectful and inclusive spaces, it increases cultural intentionality with children from different cultural backgrounds. For example, a therapist working with a child from an East Asian culture who is exhibiting disruptive behaviors may consider a standard value of *filial piety*, which entails respect for parents and elders (Tanqueco & Patel, 2020).

Working with Caregivers

Brown and colleagues (2020) discussed the importance of caregiver involvement in the child's therapeutic process. They noted that when providing trauma-informed care, involving parents can help the child begin to see their parent as a source of support. To meet this particular need, interventions that focus on the parent-child relationship with built-in parental support have shown great success in working with children with trauma symptoms (Brown et al., 2020; Landreth & Bratton, 2019; Messer et al., 2022). These interventions that monitor parental stress allow parents to process their own experiences, and their concerns and insecurities as parents. This aspect is critical because caregivers' and families' responses to the trauma impact the trajectory of the child. The therapist should be aware that caregivers are working to help their child heal alongside the impact of cultural identifiers such as ethnicity, gender, and disability status. Therefore, clinicians are encouraged to discuss their cultural beliefs, values, and customs in working to understand and address the child's trauma. Parent consultations offer time to focus on parenting skills and explore the family's cultural history. In this way, clinicians can implement the family's cultural values into the therapeutic strategies the caregivers are taught to use with their children. For clinicians working with families with children coping with dissociative behaviors, understanding the family's culture can help with better tailoring training, consultations, and treatment goals sensitive to the family's unique cultural makeup. Therefore, it is helpful for the clinician to ask sociocultural questions such as how the family identifies, how the child and family view trauma, what are family values, and what are the reactions to the child attending therapy. Focusing on the child's and family's strengths is incredibly important, as this aspect can be an overlooked cultural factor. Any skills taught should include the values and beliefs discovered from the sociocultural history and focus on the parent as the change agent, to empower their parenting strengths. Strategies that rely on the parents as the change agents are culturally inclusive because they provide natural opportunities for caregivers to implement their cultural values.

Multicultural Toys and Materials

When working from any therapeutic approach to address trauma, the child therapist needs to create therapeutic spaces that are culturally inclusive and inviting for children with varying identities (Ray et al., 2022b). This starts before the child enters the therapy room, such as by representing diversity on websites, paperwork, office decor, and in the makeup of counselors and staff (Gil, 2021). Regarding the therapy space, child therapists must carefully select toys, materials, and mediums to help children engage in direct or metaphorical expressions that are culturally congruent with their background. When therapy toys and materials reflect a child's background, it promotes valuing their culture and identity. As a result, children will be more interested and engaged in communicating their experiences verbally or nonverbally. Therefore, child clinicians must demonstrate cultural humility and intentionality in selecting items to address the child's trauma.

In the therapeutic space, dolls, puppets, and miniatures should include different ethnicities and body sizes, physical features, gender expansion, functions, and roles. Clinicians should include items with more realistic qualities to prevent them from promoting cultural microaggressions and stereotypes. Dolls and miniatures representing various identities can be beneficial to encourage cultural self-expression and daily life experiences for matters that complicate trauma, such as racial identity, gender, and family concerns (Codrington, 2021). These items allow for flexibility for self-directed or directed play, allowing the child the freedom to express themselves in various ways. Gender-neutral dress-up and imaginative clothing can help with flexibility in expression and reduce the child's feeling of restrictions to be themselves.

Culturally focused books are another culturally responsive medium to address trauma. Books promote free emotional expressions and creative thoughts as well. They can facilitate questions, conversations, and unique interpretations when the characters and plots are congruent with the child's identities. Furthermore, these types of books can provide opportunities for child therapists to introduce a trauma-focused concept or coping skill in a developmentally appropriate manner, which can increase overall social-emotional competence. When children experience trauma, they often feel alone in their experiences and question their self-worth. Therefore, books with identifiers connected with the child can foster cultural pride and a sense of connection, providing an overall sense of empowerment to heal.

Artistic materials such as clay, paints, fabrics, multicultural colors, beads, and paper should be considered when working toward cultural intentionality. Considering the complexity of trauma and the intersectionality of culture, culturally focused artistic materials allow for a wide range of cultural and ethnic explorations. More specifically, art materials facilitate the processing of emotions in a non-threatening manner. Therefore, it is a culturally responsive avenue to identify internal emotions and thoughts connected to the child's trauma.

Expressive-Based Techniques

Since children are not always able to articulate their emotions or experiences, providing a therapeutic avenue for them to communicate is essential (Gil & Briere, 2011; Landreth, 2023). For children experiencing dissociative symptoms, verbalizing their processing maybe especially difficult. Approaches that do not rely on verbalizations exist to help children lean into more natural forms of communication, such as play, music, art, and other abstract forms of communication to make sense of their world. For children with complex trauma, therapists want to be careful not to retraumatize them by encouraging them to relive the experience in their real world (Evans, 2021). Puppet play, art therapy, bibliotherapy, and sandtray therapy are modalities that allow children to project their experiences, which may help them process them in a comfortable way.

Puppet play can be a culturally inclusive way for children to explore complex emotions and difficult experiences. The ability to project their thoughts, feelings, and cultural identity onto the puppets can provide a healthy way for them to make meaning of themselves and of difficult situations. The sand tray is a medium that allows children to create versions of their world, including their experiences and cultural identities, using miniature figurines and sand. Because children are not required to verbally discuss a harrowing event, they are free to symbolically process their worldview in their own way. Using a prompt such as "create the world you are in, in the sand" can provide a link between the child's conscious and unconscious (Gil & Briere, 2011). Similarly, the same prompt can be used for art therapy. The therapist can ask the child to draw a picture of their world, providing the child the materials to create how they see their world. This use of free association can provide the therapist with insight into the child's perceptions.

These expressive-based strategies' use of projection can be a therapeutic tool for children with complex trauma and dissociative symptoms. Allowing the child the opportunity to externalize through these techniques by endowing external items with their thoughts and feelings may provide a degree of removal that may be more manageable for the child to process. While many interventions exist for children with complex trauma, additional research is needed on culturally inclusive modalities that are developmentally appropriate for children.

The Case of Tishena

The following fictional case study addresses a combination of the proposed strategies and approaches discussed earlier in the chapter. The case is not meant to be a blueprint of what should occur in therapy but rather is to provide examples of how utilizing the understanding of sociocultural influences and infusing anti-oppressive and culturally responsive practices can promote healing.

Identifying Information

Tishena is nine years old and in the fourth grade. She is African and Asian American and bilingual, and resides with her biological mother (African American), Ms. William-Zhang, paternal grandmother (Asian American), and two older brothers. Tishena's biological father died of a terminal illness when she was seven years old.

Presenting Concerns

Ms. Williams-Zhang sought therapy for her daughter due to concerns related to Tishena's anxiousness, distractibility, low self-worth, and withdrawal after she revealed ongoing sexual abuse by an adult family friend. Ms. Williams-Zhang reported that Tishena is "triggered" each time she hears someone with the name of the relative who abused her. Additionally, Ms. Williams-Zhang reported she was very concerned about Tishena appearing to "zone out" and "freeze" at home and school. Tishena has lost interest in peer relationships, family activities, and academic tasks.

Culturally Conscious Intake

During the intake and initial parent consultation, the therapist recognized that demographic factors such as ethnicity, language, gender, and socioeconomic status impacted how Tishena and Ms. Williams-Zhang related to her and the mental health treatment. Thus, the therapist first explored Ms. Williams-Zhang's beliefs, goals, and expectations about seeking care, especially considering that the mother viewed it as misaligned with her cultural values and desired a natural healer. The therapist specifically made note of myths and stigma held by Ms. Williams-Zhang. Following this, to understand the family better, the therapist gained insight into how the family identified culturally and linguistically. The therapist understood how views of trauma differ across cultures; thus, Ms. Williams-Zhang was asked how she believed aspects of culture were connected to the symptomatology related to Tishena's sexual abuse. The therapist intentionally communicated to Ms. William-Zhang that Tishena's symptoms were to be expected, individually and culturally, considering what she had experienced. Furthermore, the therapist explored family strengths and values, which Ms. Williams-Zhang reported were family bonds, faith, and perseverance.

Anti-Oppressive Practices

To infuse anti-oppressive practices, the therapist acknowledged that she was not the expert on Tishena's life. Instead, she recognized that her social identity and values impacted how she conceptualized Tishena and her family. To prevent further retraumatizing and oppressing the family, she created a sand tray representing her own values and those she had learned about the family from the intake. The therapist reflected on her strengths and areas of growth. While she has worked with BIPOC children in the past, she acknowledged her limited awareness of oppression faced by multiracial and linguistically diverse children and families. Therefore, she identified books, resources, and training to support her work with Tishena.

In the initial sessions, Tishena presented as hesitant and anxious. The therapist used this phase to build the relationship by facilitating cultural safety, and engaged in the process by sharing her identities and inviting Tishena to share hers through painting. Tishena created a painting to represent her biracial identity, hair texture, and gender identity. The therapist used this to broach similarities and differences in their identities.

During the early phase of therapy, the therapist also promoted shared power and relationship building due to the roles safety and security play in trauma and reducing oppression. The therapist intentionally provided consistent choices and opportunities for Tishena to collaborate on activities to build and promote the child-therapist relationship. To increase Tishena's comfort with the expression necessary to process the trauma, the therapist focused on reflecting sensitive emotions and content. Additionally, she collaborated with Tishena to solve challenges by returning responsibility and setting limits. In this phase of therapy, Tishena primarily engaged in independent tasks and activities with limited verbalizations. The therapist interpreted this to indicate Tishena's readiness to find ways to increase security and comfort in therapy, which is instrumental in working to heal trauma.

Focusing on cultural responsiveness, the therapist gathered information about Tishena's sociocultural environment to develop hypotheses and tailor interventions. To infuse intersectionality, the therapist acknowledged that sociocultural influences impacted the expression and manifestation of Tishena's sexual trauma and dissociative symptomology. She invited all members of Tishena's family to engage in creating a family sand tray to gain a sociocultural understanding of Tishena's sexual abuse. Tishena identified themes of fear and hesitancy in a rabbit miniature that hid from being attacked by a lion. The therapist believed the theme represented her symptoms of freezing, zoning out, and isolating after the sexual abuse. Tishena seemed to be struggling with motivation and trust in her abilities, conveying the need for coping in this area. Her engagement with therapy materials indicated repetition with an elevated level of intensity. She primarily displayed escape, safety, culture, and control themes, which appeared to be her metaphorically responding to sexual abuse. Due to the themes, the therapist used a safe-space expressive arts activity as an assessment to identify Tishena's sense of safety and support.

The therapist focused the session on helping Tishena gain insight into how her trauma was connected to her social concerns, fears, and self-motivation. Furthermore, it was vital for Tishena to identify her maladaptive beliefs about herself, others, and the world. Tishena appeared to operate from the beliefs that she was helpless, she should not trust others, and the world is a scary place. The therapist theorized that her beliefs could be connected to dissociative behaviors used to cope. Expressive arts and bibliotherapy with a cultural focus were used to help Tishena gain a greater understanding of her beliefs. The combination of reflections, expressive arts, and bibliotherapy increased insight into her emotions, behaviors, and thinking about her experiences. She showed greater initiation of engagement with the therapist and increased engagement in activities. She also responded more positively to returning responsibility and encouragement. The therapist met with Tishena's mother and grandmother to share themes in Tishena's insight, along with teaching skills (encouragement and reflection of feelings) and activities to build family connections.

In the final phase of therapy, the therapist focused on helping Tishena and her family identify alternative behaviors and skills for use outside the playroom. The therapist used multicultural books to introduce concepts to Tishena and then utilized puppets to help Tishena role-play self-regulation skills to lessen the trauma and dissociative symptoms. The therapist also reviewed these strategies with the family and taught them how to initiate these activities with Tishena at home.

Conclusion

As diverse cultural groups continue to populate the United States, movement toward culturally responsive and anti-oppressive practices is imperative. Specifically, anti-oppressive and culturally responsive practices are necessary to validate and include sociocultural influences in the treatment of traumatized children and families. When sociocultural influences are attended to, children's cultural safety is allowed to heal from trauma. The complexity of trauma and dissociation can cause intense turmoil for children. Children from BIPOC and marginalized populations are increasingly vulnerable to the turmoil caused by various types of ACEs. Adlerian play therapy, child-centered play therapy, and expressive-based, play-based, and family approaches are interventions well-suited to address dissociation. These interventions may be able to counteract symptoms and factors brought on by complex trauma and high ACE scores, which may otherwise contribute to dissociative symptoms.

References

Abbott, C., & Taylor, P. (2013). Anti-discriminatory practice and antioppressive practice. In S. Keen & K. Brown (Eds.), *Action learning in social work* (pp. 67–78). SAGE Publications. https://doi.org/10.4135/9781526401519.n6

Arnold, R., Burke, B., James, C., Martin, D., & Thomas, B. (1991). *Educating for a change*. Doris Martin Institute for Education and Action/Between the Lines.

Boullier, M., & Blair, M. (2018). Adverse childhood experiences. *Pediatrics and Child Health, 28*(3), 132–137. https://doi.org/10.1016/j.paed.2017.12.008

Bray, B. (2023, January 25). Generational trauma: Uncovering and interrupting the cycle. *Counseling Today*. https://www.counseling.org/publications/counseling-today-magazine/article-archive/article/legacy/generational-trauma-uncovering-and-interrupting-the-cycle

Brown, E. J., Cohen, J. A., & Mannarino, A. P. (2020). Trauma-focused cognitive-behavioral therapy: The role of caregivers. *Journal of Affective Disorders, 277*, 39–45. https://doi.org/10.1016/j.jad.2020.07.123

Cénat, J. M. (2023). Complex racial trauma: Evidence, theory, assessment, and treatment. *Perspectives on Psychological Science, 18*(3), 675–687. https://doi.org/10.1177/17456916221120428

Choi, K. R., Seng, J. S., Briggs, E. C., Munro-Kramer, M. L., Graham-Bermann, S. A., Lee, R., & Ford, J. D. (2018). Data at-a-glance. Dissociation and PTSD: What parents should know. National Child Traumatic Stress Network. nctsn.org/sites/default/files/resources/fact-sheet/data_at_a_glance_dissociation_and_ptsd_parents.pdf

Codrington, J. (2021). Culturally and racially attuned play therapy: Toward a social justice approach. In E. Gil & A. A. Drewes (Eds.), *Cultural issues in play therapy* (2nd ed., pp. 58–74). Guilford Press.

Collins, H. P., & Bilge, S. (2021). *Intersectionality*. Polity Press.

Comas-Díaz, L., Hall, G. N., & Neville, H. A. (2019). Racial trauma: Theory, research, and healing. Introduction to the special issue. *American Psychologist, 74*(1), 1–5. https://doi.org/10.1037/amp0000442

Complex Trauma Treatment Network of the National Child Traumatic Stress Network. (2016a). Complex trauma: In urban African-American children, youth, and families. nctsn.org/resources/complex-trauma-urban-african-american-children-youth-and-families

Complex Trauma Treatment Network of the National Child Traumatic Stress Network. (2016b). Complex trauma: Facts for treatment staff in residential settings. nctsn.org/resources/complex-trauma-facts-treatment-staff-residential-settings

Corneau, S., & Stergiopoulos, V. (2012). More than being against it: Anti-racism and anti-oppression in mental health services. *Transcultural Psychiatry, 49*(2), 261–282. https://doi.org/10.1177/1363461512441594

Crenshaw, K. (1989). Demarginalizing the intersection of race and sex: A Black feminist critique of antidiscrimination doctrine, feminist theory and antiracist politics. *University of Chicago Legal Forum, 1989*(1), Article 8. chicagounbound.uchicago.edu/uclf/vol1989/iss1/8

Crouch, E., Strompolis, M., Bennett, K. J., Morse, M., & Radcliff, E. (2017). Assessing the interrelatedness of multiple types of adverse childhood experiences and odds for poor health in South Carolina adults. *Child Abuse & Neglect, 65*, 204–211. https://doi.org/10.1016/j.chiabu.2017.02.007

Daniels, A. D., & Bryan, J. (2021). Resilience despite complex trauma: Family environment and family cohesion as protective factors. *Family Journal, 29*(3), 336–345. https://doi.org/10.1177/10664807211000719

Evans, C. (2021). Trauma-informed Adlerian play therapy: A case study. *Journal of Individual Psychology, 77*(3), 362–373. https://doi.org/10.1353/jip.2021.0025

Exline, J. J., & Wilt, J. A. (2023). Supernatural attributions: Seeing God, the devil, demons, spirits, fate, and karma as causes of events. *Annual Review of Clinical Psychology, 19*(1), 461–487. https://doi.org/10.1146/annurev-clinpsy-080921-081114

Farrelly-Rosch, A. (2018). *Dissociation and trauma in young people.* National Centre of Excellence in Youth Mental Health. orygen.org.au/Training/Resources/Trauma/Fact-sheets/Dissociation-trauma

Fortuna, L. R., Tobón, A. L., Anglero, Y. L., Postlethwaite, A., Porche, M. V., & Rothe, E. M. (2022). Focusing on racial, historical and intergenerational trauma, and resilience: A paradigm to better serving children and families. *Child and Adolescent Psychiatric Clinics of North America, 31*(2), 237–250. https://doi.org/10.1016/j.chc.2021.11.004

Gil, E. (2021). White privilege, anti-racism, and promoting positive change in therapy. In E. Gil & A. A. Drewes (Eds.), *Cultural issues in play therapy* (2nd ed., pp. 32–58). Guilford Press.

Gil, E., & Briere, J. (2011). *Helping abused and traumatized children: Integrating directive and Nondirective Approaches.* Guilford Press.

Gil, E., & Drewes, A. A. (2021). *Cultural issues in play therapy* (2nd ed). Guilford Press.

Gómez, J. M., Gobin, R. L., & Barnes, M. L. (2021). Discrimination, violence, & healing within marginalized communities. *Journal of Trauma & Dissociation, 22*(2), 135–140. https://doi.org/10.1080/15299732.2021.1869059

Goodman, B. (2020, December 27). *Children notice race several years before adults want to talk about it.* American Psychological Association. apa.org/news/press/releases/2020/08/children-notice-race

Gopalkrishnan, N. (2018). Cultural diversity and mental health: Considerations for policy and practice. *Frontiers in Public Health, 6*. https://doi.org/10.3389/fpubh.2018.00179

Gutierrez, B. (2018, August 3). *Trauma of immigrant children linked to physical ailments.* University of Miami News and Events. news.miami.edu/stories/2018/08/trauma-of-immigrant-children-linked-to-physical-ailments.html

Hays, P. A. (2008). *Addressing cultural complexities in practice: Assessment, diagnosis, and therapy* (2nd ed.). American Psychological Association. https://doi.org/10.1037/11650-000

Hook, J., Davis, D., Owen, J., & Deblaere, C. (2017). *Cultural humility: Engaging diverse identities in therapy.* American Psychological Association. apa.org/pubs/books/4317453

Isobel, S., Goodyear, M., Furness, T., & Foster, K. (2019). Preventing intergenerational trauma transmission: A critical interpretive synthesis. *Journal of Clinical Nursing, 28*(7–8), 1100–1113. https://doi.org/10.1111/jocn.14735

Kim, P. Y., Kendall, D. L., & Cheon, H.-S. (2017). Racial microaggressions, cultural mistrust, and mental health outcomes among Asian American college students. *American Journal of Orthopsychiatry, 87*(6), 663–670. https://doi.org/10.1037/ort0000203

Kliethermes, M., Schacht, M., & Drewry, K. (2014). Complex trauma. *Child and Adolescent Psychiatric Clinics of North America, 23*(2), 339–361. https://doi.org/10.1016/j.chc.2013.12.009

Kruger, C. (2020). Culture, trauma, dissociation: A broadening perspective for our field. *Journal of Trauma & Dissociation, 21*(1), 1–13. https://doi.org/10.1080/15299732.2020.1675134

Landreth, G. L. (2023). *Play therapy: The art of the relationship.* Routledge.

Landreth, G. L., & Bratton, S. C. (2019). *Child parent relationship therapy (CPRT): A 10-session filial therapy model.* Routledge.

Leslie, C. E., Walsh, C. S., & Sullivan, T. N. (2023). Implications of intergenerational trauma: Associations between caregiver ACEs and child internalizing symptoms in an urban African American sample. *Psychological Trauma: Theory, Research, Practice, and Policy, 15*(5), 877–887. https://doi.org/10.1037/tra0001334

Marsella, A. J., & Yamada, A. M. (2000). Culture and mental health: An introduction and overview of foundations, concepts, and issues. In I. Cuéllar & F. A. Paniagua (Eds.), *Handbook of multicultural mental health* (pp. 3–24). Academic Press. https://doi.org/10.1016/B978-012199370-2/50002-X

McIntosh, L. M. (2019). Compound fractures: Healing the intersectionality of racism, classism and trauma in schools with a trauma-informed approach as part of a social justice framework. *Journal of Educational Leadership and Policy Studies, 3*(1). files.eric.ed.gov/fulltext/EJ1226938.pdf

Medlock, M. M., Shtasel, D., Trinh, N. T., & Williams, D. R. (Eds.). (2018). *Racism and psychiatry: Contemporary issues and interventions*. Springer International Publishing.

Messer, E. P., Eismann, E. A., Folger, A. T., Grass, A., Bemerer, J., & Bensman, H. (2022). Comparative effectiveness of parent-child interaction therapy based on trauma exposure and attrition. *Psychological Trauma: Theory, Research, Practice, and Policy*. Advance online publication. https://doi.org/10.1037/tra0001259

Moore, S. E., Robinson, M. A., Dailey, A., & Thompson, C. (2015). Suffering in silence: Child sexual molestation and the Black church: If God don't help me who can I turn to? *Journal of Human Behavior in the Social Environment, 25*(2), 147–157. https://doi.org/10.1080/10911359.2014.956962

Myrick, A. C., & Green, E. J. (2014). Establishing safety and stabilization in traumatized youth: Clinical implications for play therapists. *International Journal of Play Therapy, 23*(2), 100–113. https://doi.org/10.1037/a0036397

Nesbit, A., Dorahy, M. J., Palmer, R., Middleton, W., Seager, L., & Hanna, D. (2022). Dissociation as a mediator between childhood abuse and hallucinations: An exploratory investigation using dissociative identity disorder and schizophrenia spectrum disorders. *Journal of Trauma & Dissociation, 23*(5), 521–538. https://doi.org/10.1080/15299732.2022.2064579

Ochoa, L. G., Fernandez, A., Lee, T. K., Estrada, Y., & Prado, G. (2022). The intergenerational impact of adverse childhood experiences on Hispanic families: The mediational roles of parental depression and parent–adolescent communication. *Family Process, 61*(1), 422–435. https://doi.org/10.1111/famp.12652

Owen, J., Tao, K. W., Drinane, J. M., Hook, J., Davis, D. E., & Kune, N. F. (2016). Client perceptions of therapists' multicultural orientation: Cultural (missed) opportunities and cultural humility. *Professional Psychology, Research and Practice, 47*(1), 30–37. https://doi.org/10.1037/pro0000046

Pérez-Rojas, A. E., Brown, R., Cervantes, A., Valente, T., & Pereira, S. R. (2019). "Alguien abrió la puerta": The phenomenology of bilingual Latinx clients' use of Spanish and English in psychotherapy. *Psychotherapy, 56*(2), 241–253. https://doi.org/10.1037/pst0000224

Pierorazio, N. A., Nester, M. S., Shandler, G., & Brand, B. L. (2023). "This 'prison' where I cannot heal": Interactions of culture, dissociation, and treatment among individuals who dissociate. *European Journal of Trauma and Dissociation, 7*(2), Article 100325. https://doi.org/10.1016/j.ejtd.2023.100325

Polanco-Roman, L., Danies, A., & Anglin, D. M. (2016). Racial discrimination as race-based trauma, coping strategies, and dissociative symptoms among emerging adults. *Psychological Trauma: Theory, Research, Practice, and Policy, 8*(5), 609–617. https://doi.org/10.1037/tra0000125

Pumariega, A. J., Jo, Y., Beck, B., & Rahmani, M. (2022). Trauma and US minority children and youth. *Current Psychiatry Reports, 24*(4), 285–295. https://doi.org/10.1007/s11920-022-01336-1

Ray, D. C., Burgin, E., Gutierrez, D., Ceballos, P., & Lindo, N. (2022a). Child-centered play therapy and adverse childhood experiences: A randomized controlled trial. *Journal of Counseling and Development, 100*(2), 134–145. https://doi.org/10.1002/jcad.12412

Ray, D. C., Chung, R. K., Turner, K. K., & Aguilar, E. V. (2022b). The multicultural playroom: A Delphi study. In D. C. Ray, Y. Ogawa & Y.-J. Cheng (Eds.), *Multicultural play therapy: Making the most of cultural opportunities with children* (pp. 279–299). Routledge.

Ray, D. C., Ogawa, Y., & Cheng, Y.-J. (2022c). *Multicultural play therapy: Making the most of cultural opportunities with children*. Routledge, Taylor & Francis Group.

Rhoades Jr., G. F. (2005). Cross-cultural aspects of trauma and dissociation. *Journal of Trauma Practice, 4*(1–2), 21–33. https://doi.org/10.1300/J189v04n01_03

Rosmarin, D. H., & Koenig, H. G. (Eds.). (2020). *Handbook of spirituality, religion, and mental health*. Elsevier Science & Technology.

Rössler, W. (2016). The stigma of mental disorders: A millennia-long history of social exclusion and prejudices. *EMBO Reports, 17*(9), 1250–1253. https://doi.org/10.15252/embr.201643041

Sacks, V., & Murphey, D. (2016). *The prevalence of adverse childhood experiences, nationally, by state, and by race or ethnicity*. ChildTrends. childtrends.org/publications/prevalence-adverse-childhood-experiences-nationally-state-race-ethnicity

Savell, S. M., Womack, S. R., Wilson, M. N., Shaw, D. S., & Dishion, T. J. (2019). Considering the role of early discrimination experiences and the parent–child relationship in the development of disruptive behaviors in adolescence. *Infant Mental Health Journal, 40*(1), 98–112. https://doi.org/10.1002/imhj.21752

Sholevar, G. P., & Joshi, S. V. (2017). Cultural child and adolescent psychiatry. In A. Martin, F. R. Volkmar & M. H. Bloch (Eds.), *Lewis's child and adolescent psychiatry: A comprehensive textbook* (pp. 319–349). Wolters Kluwer.

Tanqueco, R., & Patel, S. (2020). *Mental health facts for Asian Americans/Pacific Islanders*. American Psychiatric Association. psychiatry.org/File%20Library/Psychiatrists/Cultural-Competency/Mental-Health-Disparities/Mental-Health-Facts-for-Asian-Americans-Pacific-Islanders.pdf

Wei, M., Ku, T. Y., & Liao, K. Y. (2011). Minority stress and college persistence attitudes among African American, Asian American, and Latino students: Perception of university environment as a mediator. *Cultural Diversity & Ethnic Minority Psychology, 17*(2), 195–203. https://doi.org/10.1037/a0023359

Whaley, A. L. (2001). Cultural mistrust: An important psychological construct for diagnosis and treatment of African Americans. *Professional Psychology: Research and Practice, 32*(6), 555–562. https://doi.org/10.1037/0735-7028.32.6.555

Williams, M. T., Metzger, I. W., Leins, C., & DeLapp, C. (2018). Assessing racial trauma within a DSM-5 framework: The UConn Racial/Ethnic Stress & Trauma Survey. *Practice Innovations, 3*(4), 242–260. https://doi.org/10.1037/pri0000076

36
PRENATAL REFORM
Complex Trauma, Dissociation, and Bonding with the Calming Womb Model

Rosita Cortizo

Introduction

The Calming Womb Family Therapy Model (CWFTM) was conceptualized after more than 30 years of prenatal and perinatal psychotherapy and collaboration with pregnant women and their families. For the purposes of this chapter, the following definitions are applied: *womb baby* refers to the infant from conception and the evolving emotional attunement of the client to their baby in the womb; *bonding* is defined as the unilateral attunement of the mother toward her womb baby during pregnancy (Cortizo, 2019); and *attachment* means the relationship the child forms with the parents after birth (Deneault et al., 2023). All situations and clinical dilemmas in the chapter have been mixed, combined, and changed, and the names have no relation to persons' names. The clinical events discussed, though mixed, altered, and unidentifiable, are real. The path into chronic traumatization for many children begins in the first years of life. As a result, interventions that directly work on preparing the caregiver's embodied mind to attune, resonate, and participate in mutual regulation with their infants are paramount.

A person's life events impact the experience of preconception, conception, pregnancy, and birthing. Incidents of distress, trauma, and loss as a child or adult may have created lasting patterns of response to the environment and to the emotions felt or avoided somatically. Although preconception will be briefly discussed, as it is a critical lifespan leading to conception, this chapter will focus on pregnancy and the CWFTM.

Preconception: Critical Lifespan Opportunity

Preconception refers to the awareness and health of every person across the lifespan before the years they can have a child, prior to a potential pregnancy (Toivonen et al., 2017), and focuses on providing preventive education, and in doing so, taking necessary steps to protect the health of the parents they might be and the baby they might have sometime in the future. The aim of community-based preconception education is to universally and proactively teach and prepare those before their prenatal readiness with age-appropriate health and psychological information and support. Preconception precedes pregnancy and is the earliest phase of life for humans and a time of significant transition, adjustment, and changes. Therefore, it is imperative that those of age to conceive are provided *timely* preconception health information and become actively educated about prenatal health, family planning choices, and affective wellness by their parents, pediatricians, and nurses even if they are not yet ready for conception, as this is associated with a healthier lifestyle of women during the preconception period.

There is a high prevalence of high-risk health behaviors in persons able to conceive and actively preparing to achieve pregnancy immediately. Preconception health promotion and interventions should be a key component for those in reproductive-age populations and as part of a life course approach to optimizing public health. Dennis et al.'s (2022) study outcomes demonstrated adaptable targets for preconception programs and factors that can be used to identify at-risk groups requiring intervention. Individual-level interventions require societal changes that promote healthy behaviors through better health policies and strong public health messaging. Poels et al.'s (2017) research showed that despite a high level of pregnancy planning, only a quarter of women sought a prenatal healthcare consult. However, 60% of women acquired preconception health information by themselves. Poels et al. (2017) concluded that gathering preconception information, either by women themselves or by means of a preconception health consult, increases the likelihood of women positively changing their lifestyle prior to pregnancy recognition. These results are highly indicative of the social need for both further research and policy making with special attention to underage and younger populations who are of childrearing age, and ensuring their communities are prepared for such an endeavor.

Conception

Conception, pregnancy, and gestation are a great source of delight, hope, and anticipation for most clients with great potential for healing and transformation; however, they may also cause anxiety, distress, depression, trauma, and feelings of ambiguity (Talley, 2013). Parenting, maternal bonding, and biological effects on fetal development begin before birthing (Daglar & Nur, 2018; Glover & Capron, 2017). Even though pregnancy is a major phase of life for adults or teenagers and their families, prenatal psychotherapeutic treatment and interventions are frequently overlooked. Dubber et al.'s (2015) study supported the hypothesized a negative relationship between mother and womb baby bonding and post-birthing maternal attachment impairment, as well as the role of postpartum depressive symptoms. In the CWFTM early identification of bonding impairment during the prenatal assessment, and postpartum depression/anxiety/psychosis/trauma/birth-trauma identification in mothers or carrying persons, plays an important role for the prevention of potential attachment impairment in the early post-birthing period. In their research, Reck et al. (2016) observed that the maternal relationship seems to shield the negative impact of postpartum depression on parenting stress, and suggested interventions to strengthen maternal bonding and mother-infant interaction in order to prevent impairment of the mother-child relationship. The CWFTM assesses, provides psychoeducation, and enhances bonding practices in sessions and systemically. Pregnancy represents a vital time to interrupt the pattern of intergenerational transmission and repetition of abuse and psychiatric vulnerability (Seng et al., 2013). Prenatal early interventions support vulnerable mothers who have preexisting trauma or who may be at high risk for prenatal stress.

Reducing mothers' intense fear of and emotional reactivity to childbirth, or tokophobia, while increasing their preparedness for labor, predicts an increase in positive maternal bonding (Klabbers et al., 2016). Daglar and Nur (2018) observed that as the prenatal bonding level increases, so does the level of post-birthing attachment. While childhood trauma was not found to be predictive of postpartum depression, both past depression and gestational depression at 12 weeks post-birthing convincingly were (De Venter et al., 2016). Collaborating with pregnant clients and their womb babies from conception through the first year after birth and beyond is the mission of the CWFTM.

Pregnancy: A Pivotal Phase of Life

Aitina became pregnant as she was preparing to go to college. Unfortunately, she could not become a stay-at-home mother after her brief maternity leave due to the couple's financial constraints.

Laila, a teenager, discovered she was pregnant after her boyfriend broke up with her. She felt distraught, lonely, ashamed, unprepared and had severe postpartum depression that required psychiatric care.

Prenatal psychotherapy to support mothers affected by trauma is crucial and often overlooked. In particular, since prenatal dissociated trauma could be activated, this period offers enormous opportunity for intervention and hope for parents, particularly if either or both are survivors of extreme, chronic abuse (Guyon-Harris et al., 2020).

Complex chronic trauma-enduring pregnant women may lack prenatal medical and emotional social supports as they start to fulfill their mothering role (Delker et al., 2020). The goal of the CWFTM is to evaluate, treat dissociative phenomena, and provide trauma-informed support and resources to decrease the pregnant client's toxic stress morbidity, improve the experience of prenatal care, and positively impact the outcomes for the parent and infant. Making sense of the past creates space for prenatal bonding and post-birthing attachment (Cortizo, 2019, 2021). Pregnancy is a pivotal phase of life and a time when a client's own traumatic experiences, psychophysiology, bonding, and attachment deficits can be assessed and treated; it is also when intergenerational transmission of dysfunctional patterns can be prevented. Prenatal trauma therapy must be titrated and adapted to the needs of the client, including increasing the capacity of affect tolerance and the vulnerability for antenatal conditions.

The comprehensive CWFTM approach provides family therapy and addresses the repercussions of pregnancy on the partner and siblings. Partners must also adjust to the client having diminished sexual interest after birthing due to many hormonal and other medical factors (Rupert, 2016). Having to take a relational secondary seat may activate traumatic distress in a previously abused or abandoned partner. To begin to address these issues early, partners are brought into the CWFTM during the second pre-perinatal visit. During the six months post-delivery, parents often experience physical strain, sleep disruption, fatigue, irritability, difficulty concentrating, lower functionality at work, and more (Chiorino et al., 2016). Frequently, there are also financial and medical access challenges. Siblings are similarly challenged when a new baby comes home. Their academic performance sometimes suffers for a period. The youngest sibling typically experiences significant fear of being displaced or replaced, especially if still a toddler. It is crucial that parents attend to such concerns for siblings throughout their pregnancy and when the baby comes home. A major focus of CWFTM is to help the mother or carrying person maintain a state of calm in addressing the family's needs.

Unexpected Challenges

While there may be ongoing moments of bliss and welcome bonding that pave the way for a glorious pregnancy, educating and empowering mothers to self-soothe and remain both present and positive throughout the multiple unplanned events is both helpful and necessary.

The pre-perinatal treating team, support staff, and caregivers will also benefit from being educated and sensitized about some of the most common psychological pre-perinatal complications, the significant numbers of high-risk or failed pregnancies, pre-perinatal myths, and other untold stories.

In the spirit of assisting the client and baby and their supportive pre-perinatal team, I have compiled a list of the many unforeseen emotional difficulties and physical symptoms a pregnant client may experience, be exposed to, and suffer.

Some of the psychological pre-perinatal complications are:

- Prenatal dysphoria and anxiety
- Hormone induced affect/mood shifts accompanied by increased sensitivity
- Preexisting anxiety
- Preexisting depression
- Developmental, adult post-traumatic stress disorder (PTSD), dissociative phenomena
- Acute stress
- Incest resulting in pregnancy
- Sexual assault resulting in pregnancy
- Bodily triggered traumatic memories
- Multiple coexisting psychological disorders (e.g., Bipolar I-II, ADHD)
- Substance abuse
- Exacerbated chronic pain
- Failed prenatal attempts including in vitro fertilization (IVF)
- Maladaptive body image
- Unexpected weight gain
- Recent romantic relational rupture
- Past or ongoing domestic violence with current flashbacks
- Unplanned teen or adult pregnancy
- Abortion indecision leading to shame
- Adoption ambivalence and guilt
- Lack of social and familial supports
- Partner's dismissiveness and lack of involvement
- Loved one's over-involvement resulting in stress
- Financial limitations
- Unemployment
- Homelessness, or at risk of, due to pregnancy
- Laboratory abnormalities resulting in fear and affect dysregulation
- Medical complications (e.g., preeclampsia, placenta previa, and gestational diabetes)
- Planned, or unplanned cesarean section

Often, expectant mothers experiencing the above medical and psychological difficulties are initially hesitant to be referred to a pre-perinatal psychotherapist. The reasons many clients may refuse therapy include prenatal mood swings, feeling overwhelmed, fatigue, dysphoric mood, familial stigma, financial limitations, cultural biases, religious beliefs, not wanting to be perceived as "damaged goods," or past limited benefits from such services. Introducing the CWFTM early on as a part of the integrated and comprehensive pre-perinatal routine of preventive care reduces such discomfort and stigma. Despite the reluctance of a few mothers or carrying persons, most pregnant clients are receptive to receiving services if these enhance or provide womb-parenting skills, developmental education, and tools to become an attentive parent. Overall, expectant clients embrace the opportunity to attend couple's therapy, hypnobirthing groups (Phillips, 2020) and health educational classes with their significant others. Parental developmental attachment wounds and deficits are important reasons to heal in the psychotherapy situation. Often, mothers or carrying persons who coped with difficult life situations prior to becoming pregnant have a difficult time once pregnant due to various added pressures. Thus, current prenatal stresses and preexisting difficulties frequently become the port of entry to the CWFTM.

High-Risk Conditions

Pregnant clients who experience homelessness, PTSD, Bipolar I-II disorder, and/or suicidal thoughts; who have a domestic violence history, and/or are actively dissociated, substance dependent, chronically medically ill, or recently separated; and who experience current or chronic symptoms of emotional dysregulation exacerbated by the current pregnancy and or other factors, need to be educated, encouraged, and referred in a timely manner for pre-perinatal therapy. Pervasive multi-intergenerational maladaptive patterns; adverse childhood events (Anda et al., 2020); environmental stresses; intrapersonal incongruences or conflict caused by unresolved trauma; relational conflicts; developmental or adult PTSDs; acute stress disorders; prenatal medical concerns; or unplanned pregnancies are common roadblocks to wellness and need to be assessed and treated promptly.

A CWFTM comprehensive early assessment is needed to identify and evaluate psychosocial pre-existing disturbances, current worries, and unresolved losses before the baby's birthing and through the first year of life. Distressing circumstances include unplanned and unwanted pregnancies, unexpected maternal separations from loved ones, abandonment by partners, family illnesses, financial difficulties, and family deaths. Prenatal psychotherapy can help prevent complications and inform mothers about important steps they can take to protect their womb baby and ensure a healthy pregnancy. It is essential to provide multidisciplinary and multiphased treatment to support the expectant client (Weinstein, 2016) and womb baby.

Disempowerment

Inadvertently, perinatal medical staff may focus on the medical aspects of the pregnancy at the expense of the mother's emotional experience, causing unsettling emotions to be dismissed, unexpressed, and denied. Healthy pregnant clients who were self-directed and capable of making their own decisions before their pregnancy unexpectedly find themselves responding passively and losing efficacy. This passive response oftentimes is enabled by their health providers, partners, and close relatives, who take it upon themselves to make decisions for the pregnant woman or carrying person.

Prenatal Humiliation

The practice of expectant clients "keeping their pregnancy a secret" from others is common, often due to previous traumatic loss, unresolved grief, previous life experiences, shame, fear, powerlessness, confusion, and guilt (Caldwell et al., 2024). Stigma regarding unplanned and unwanted pregnancies has diminished due to changes in gender norms. This has also led to greater awareness of the emotional impact of pregnancy on the mental state of the mother and the possible effects of their distress on the womb baby. These unexpressed and painful unresolved feelings may "freeze" into traumatic memories over time (Dana, 2018; Porges, 2021).

Hormonal-Physiological Shifts

Complications and affect dysregulation caused by hormonal changes during the first trimester could trigger existing involuntary traumatic stress processes and have a distressing impact on the life of the parents, and more specifically on the expectant client (Madhavanprabhakaran et al., 2015).

Stress

Stress becomes maladaptive when coping mechanisms fail. It is during periods of overstimulation of the sympathetic system that the ventral vagal system is inhibited. Its inhibition, which usually results in flight-or-fight responses in a person, does not bode well for a pregnant mother's unborn child (Verny, 2018). *Atypically high and prolonged* concentrations of the stress hormone cortisol have harmful effects on the developing baby (McGowan & Matthews, 2018). In cases of severe traumatization, the mother may move into dorsal vagal shutdown, immobility, and hopelessness. Trauma-informed treatments such as eye movement desensitization and reprocessing (EMDR) therapy, which increase internal and external resources; upregulation as well as down regulation; and self-soothing practices (Phase 2) and holistic mind-body-spirit approaches such as mindfulness (Siegel, 2018), prenatal yoga, and meditation early on in therapy (van der Kolk et al., 2014) are beneficial to both the mother or carrying person and womb baby during the early parenting periods. Supportive interventions that increase felt sense of safety and regulated internal environments is especially beneficial for prenatal clients with preexisting histories of trauma, unresolved grief, and traumatic stress symptoms (Weinstein, 2016).

Anxiety

Pregnancy-related anticipatory anxiety can impact the overall health of the woman or carrying person. The incidence of prenatal anticipatory anxiety is between 14% and 54% (Madhavanprabhakaran et al., 2015), increasing the likelihood of bonding difficulty, preterm labor complications, lengthy birthing, Caesarian section, low birth weight, attachment, and lactation challenges (Chiorino et al., 2016). Childbirth anxiety for women with a previous stillbirth is understandably common yet treatable (Zolghadr et al., 2019).

Hidden Trauma, Dissociative Phenomena, and Pregnancy

The implications and consequences of untreated childhood mistreatment, neglect prevalence, complex trauma, and dissociation and their impact on prenatal wellness have been extensively addressed.

According to Seng et al. (2009), child abuse history seems to be the greatest risk factor for PTSD criteria in pregnancy. In another analysis, Seng et al. (2010) confirmed that PTSD symptom rates are higher in prenatal samples than in the general female population (6%–8% versus 4%–5%), perhaps due to exacerbations of preexisting PTSD, which is often chronic or recurring. This finding has been linked with physical illness across a lifetime. The researchers estimated that the overall rate of lifetime PTSD was 20.2%; 17% in the predominantly private-payer settings, and 23% in the predominantly public-payer settings. Links between gestational PTSD and both lower birth weight and shorter pregnancy were stronger for women whose PTSD occurred after abuse. PTSD in pregnancy, or coexisting with depression, is associated with postpartum dysphoria, while postpartum depression alone or simultaneous with post-traumatic stress was linked with impaired bonding (Seng et al., 2011). Seng et al. (2013) documented that one in three women reports a history of sexual or physical abuse and that 1 in 12 expectant mothers is affected by PTSD.

Historical untreated trauma and internalized oppression can have a deleterious effect on prenatal and parenting experiences: obstetric and gynecological (OB-GYN) procedures may dysregulate the autonomic nervous system (ANS) (Ogden, 2021) of clients. Pregnant clients who have experienced childhood sexual abuse may find that trauma symptoms are activated during their pelvic examinations, prenatal care exams, labor, birth, and procedures that require them to remain motionless and in vulnerable positions. Waiting in a gown, on an exam table in a cold medical exam room, even without physical contact, may trigger re-experiencing of past traumatic incidents accompanied by freeze, fight or flight, collapse, or dissociative responses (Seng et al., 2008). The clients' own developmental trauma and PTSD symptoms may be triggered during early postnatal interactions with their newborn (Fraiberg, 1980). For example, a woman who experienced frequent pain growing up may reject her infant girl. Alternatively, the girl child may trigger trauma reminders in the mother, who unconsciously withdraws or shuts down based on the prospects of raising a female who the mother anticipates will similarly experience the pain and trauma she did growing up. This projection can lead in this case to infant rejection and poor bonding.

It is at this pivotal stage, after identifying trauma or other preexisting psychological conditions, that pregnant clients must be referred by their treating medical teams to trauma-informed psychotherapists for further assessment, screening, and prenatal trauma treatment.

Experiencing dissociation during labor predicts worsened outcomes. Pregnancy is a crossing opportunity between generations, and it seems essential to address complex trauma and dissociative phenomena prior to birthing or during the childbearing years. Kruger and Fletcher's (2017) study suggested that childhood emotional neglect by biological parents or siblings and later emotional abuse by partners predicted dissociative disorder (DD), and developmental neglect supports maladaptive attachment-based cycles of abuse in adulthood. Taking a routine childhood history of emotional neglect by parents or siblings and screening adult emotional abuse by partners may facilitate timely identification of DD in adulthood.

To make good use of the above prenatal research information, the CWFTM provider nurtures a clinical grasp of the client's subjective experience of developmental trauma and treats all presentations within the trauma–dissociation continuum with empathic curiosity (Chefetz, 2015). The existence and authenticity of developmental trauma memories, as well as their avoidance, has been at the core of complex professional deliberations and disputes. The definition and context of memory lapses, amnesia, or suppression have been so historically controversial that it is easy to conceptualize the delay in our understanding of hidden memories and dissociative processes (Collin-Vézina et al., 2015). Recently, van der Kolk (2022) reported that regardless of the subjects' age at which the complex trauma was experienced, a survivor who forgets childhood abuse may have memory that manifests psycho-biologically in other ways, such as through phobias, difficulty learning and focusing, speechless terror, and shameful self-perceptions. Stress that overwhelms the organism affects people's neurobiological functioning, involving a large variety of brain structures, neurotransmitter systems, and hormonal responses.

Sexual molestation, trafficking, abduction, infant/child traumatic programming, and rape are common causes of PTSD and dissociative phenomena. Being betrayed or violated by a person who is important or in a position of authority disrupts basic trust. The closer the child is to the abuser, the more profound the betrayal, and often the less likely the chances of escape (Harsey & Freyd, 2020). Memory avoidance, traumatic amnesia, and dissociation are ways of forgetting that which one cannot bear. Disbelief, self-doubt, denial, memory confusion, and recall disorganization are some of the frequent dissociation culprits, but betrayal is the main source. The amnesia rate for sexual abuse incest survivors is higher than for other sexual abuses. Throughout the past 30 years, forgetting childhood sexual abuse and dissociating painful material prevalence have been well documented (Alaggia et al., 2017). Complex trauma is emotionally devastating, implausible, and intolerable, with dissociative phenomena likely occurring as a protective mind-body savior. Pregnant clients who present with developmental, relational complex trauma may require that we hold the incongruence of an unbearable past in the present, along with a reasonably stable and consistent present. The foundation of the field of complex trauma and dissociation, and all the harm that comes from infant attachment-trauma injuries (Khoury et al., 2020), is this very problem—not caring for pregnant clients and their womb babies early enough or during conception.

Swales et al. (2018) findings suggested that the effects of childhood exposure to traumatic events remained after accounting for more proximal traumatic events in adulthood and concluded that there could be consequences for the baby from *sustained* maternal cortisol elevation, and that the relationship between adult trauma and prenatal cortisol is moderated by childhood trauma. While discussing each prenatal barrier to bonding is beyond the scope of this chapter, identifying pre-birth broken

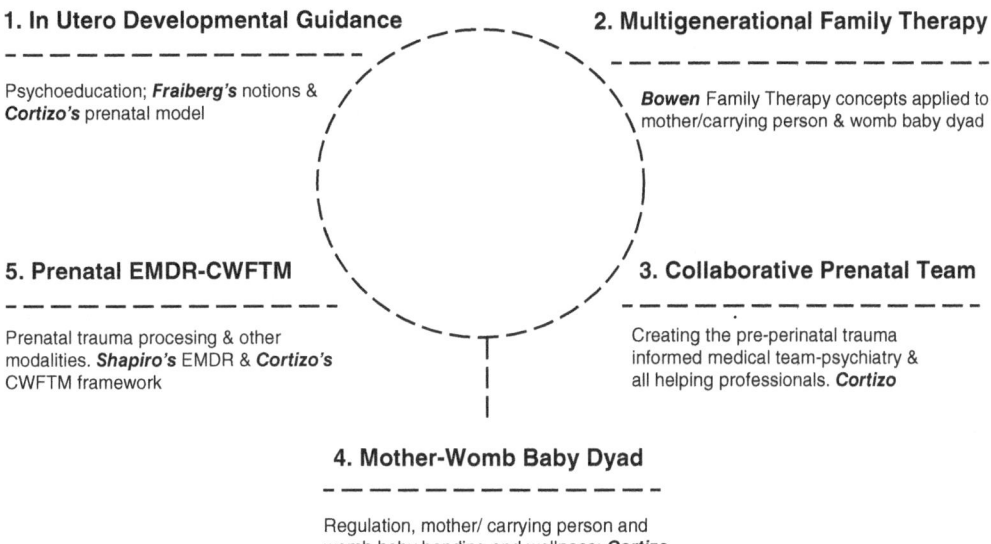

Figure 36.1 The Calming Womb Family Therapy Model (CWFTM).

bonds is of outmost significance and value for the purposes of assessment, treatment, and prevention. Treating trauma in the earliest lifespan stage is the CWFTM's optimal goal (Figure 36.1).

The Calming Womb Family Therapy Model (CWFTM): Five Pillars

The CWFTM promptly assesses, treats, and prevents traumatic transference, enactments, and intergenerational traumatic bonding, and enhances the pregnant client's internal resources. The concurrently titrated and contained practice of the CWFTM and EMDR therapy promotes pregnant clients and their womb babies' wellness and connectedness. Much attention needs to be paid to dissociated trauma responses, specifically since confusion and avoidance of hurt and humiliation can be prenatal bonding barriers. The model provides the pregnant client with intrapersonal and interpersonal psychoeducation, experiential insights, behavioral and emotional programming modification, and practical tools for symptom reduction and self-regulation throughout their prenatal care and a year postnatally.

In the next section, the five pillars that inform this model will be explained, as well as how each of these concepts serves as a building block. *Psychotherapists not trained in EMDR therapy can substitute Pillar 5 for a preferred trauma-informed narrative model. The CWFTM can be practiced alongside any therapy model. While the pillars work well together, these can be practiced individually, and in the clinical sequence warranted.*

Pillars 1: In Utero Developmental Guidance

Definition and Practice

The term *in utero developmental guidance* refers to the early prenatal education of the parent that is integrated in psychotherapeutic work. In utero guidance is a form of psychoeducation informed by the pregnant client's gestational trimester, personal doubts, and individual psychological needs, and provided by the pre-perinatal psychotherapist. This psychoeducation includes in-session bibliotherapy, videotherapy, conjoint sessions with the medical team, and interventions with family members. In utero developmental guidance is adapted to alleviate the expectant client's and womb baby's chronic external pressures, emotional distress, and the impact that the attendant anguish places on the bonding and relationship with the in utero baby. What is addressed in therapy is what the client brings to therapy, including the psychological conflicts that are already distorting their relationship to the womb baby (e.g., a crisis at the time of conception, or grief during gestation). In utero developmental guidance must enhance and promote the client–womb baby bond, educate the parent in understanding fetal development, and assist the parents in doing their own healing before the child's birthing. Finding new, nurturing, child-rearing approaches will facilitate optimal development in every stage of the baby's existence.

In utero developmental guidance identifies the importance of providing the earliest and most up-to-date prenatal psychoeducation to the client and their partner. For this purpose, I have educational books on embryo development readily available and in utero and infant neurobiological developmental posters in my office, and I offer bibliotherapy on topics such as the effects of hormonal changes on mood and the senses (e.g., smell, touch). This intermediation is adapted to alleviate the expectant client's and womb baby's chronic external pressures and emotional dysregulation. The way a client was nurtured and reared in their own infancy and childhood affects how they parent and interacts with others. Addressing the client's doubts, providing in utero developmental psychoeducation, enhancing their womb baby bonding, clarifying the couple's relational misconceptions, and healing multi-intergenerational dysfunctional patterns are critical at this stage. Fraiberg (1980) did not directly address dissociative phenomena or "prenatal" developmental guidance in her seminal developmental guidance work with babies, but she did inspire an outline for the CWFTM ten-month prenatal experience-dependent in utero developmental guidance that is contingent on and concordant with maternal regulation practices and highlights the importance of supporting mothers during their prenatal care. Prenatal psychotherapy gains and achievements may be more readily transmitted to subsequent generations.

Prenatal Therapeutic Alliance

A warm and attentive therapeutic relationship and kind tone are essential to the CWFTM. Since the onset of the COVID-19 pandemic, videotherapy and telehealth have facilitated the attendance of prenatal psychotherapy sessions by pregnant clients from the convenience of their own homes, without concerns about transportation, babysitting, or being observed or stigmatized. Those clients who prefer videotherapy or telehealth over the in-person format often cite feeling "less scrutinized" and having enhanced opportunities for self-expression, connection, and intimacy. This more neutral therapeutic space provides clients with novel opportunities for self-awareness, creative experience, and collaboration, with potentially a greater sense of agency over their experience (Simpson et al., 2020).

However, when impediments to the alliance occur, the therapist will do well to view this barrier as a possible manifestation of negative transference. Negative transference is considered a defense against hurtful feelings and memories that are being transferred and re-experienced with the treating therapist. As soon as these transference reenactments and painful feelings are validated and given space, and broken alliances are repaired (Eubanks et al., 2019), the mother can find new, more adaptive responses to old struggles. Parenting a female womb baby, for example, may trigger many of the mother's unhealed wounds; hence the wisdom of practicing EMDR therapy, which focuses on healing the traumas of expectant mothers.

Pillar 2: Multigenerational Family Therapy

Bowen Theory and Application

Foundational to Bowen's (1976) systemic approach is a conceptualization of families as interactive systems rather than individuals. This model identifies and systemically treats the multi-intergenerational dysfunctional family patterns, viewing the family as an *emotional unit* with complex interfaces. It is the nature of a family that its members are intensely connected emotionally. *Multigenerational transmission* is the process of family patterns repeating through generations. Specific roles and *triangles* reappear. Examples are the scapegoat-superstar sibling dyad, depression, substance abuse, or secrecy.

The concept of *differentiation of the self* is the cornerstone in the theory. It is the ability to separate feelings and thoughts. Undifferentiated people cannot separate feelings and thoughts; when asked to think, they are flooded with feelings and have difficulty thinking logically and basing their responses on that. Further, they have difficulty separating their own from other's feelings; they look to family to define how they think about issues, feel about people, and interpret their experiences. This defines people according to the degree of fusion between the emotional and intellectual functioning of the individual.

Family projection is a process by which the primary parents transmit their immaturity, lack of differentiation, and emotional problems to their children. The projection process can impair the functioning of one or more children and increase their vulnerability to clinical symptoms. Children inherit many types of problems, as well as strengths, through the relationships with their parents. The child who is the object of the projection process becomes the one most attached to the parents positively or negatively and the one with the least differentiation of the self. When the mother is the primary caretaker and especially during pregnancy, they are more prone than the partner to excessive emotional involvement with the womb baby or with one or more of the children. For example, a mother may perceive their womb baby girl to be in danger because of their own traumatic past, and repeatedly react with fear and worry as the child grows up, until the child's sense of safety becomes dependent on the mother's constant protection. The partner typically occupies the outside position in the parental triangle, except during periods of heightened tension in the mother-child relationship. Couples who reduce their tensions with their family by *cutting off* their ties to them risk making themselves too dependent on each other and their child. Bowen believed that children develop certain personality characteristics based on the *sibling position* in their families. Sibling position and knowledge of general family characteristics is helpful in predicting what part a child will play in the family emotional process, and in predicting family patterns in the next generation.

Bowen's *family therapy with one person* seeks to work with the most motivated family member, especially when many are unavailable or remain unmotivated. A single highly motivated person, such as a pregnant client in the case of the CWFTM, can be the pivot for changing an entire family system.

Other Key Family Enactments

Traumatic Transference

Negative transference in the therapeutic situation is a defense against hurtful feelings that are being transferred and re-experienced with the treating therapist. This enactment offers the psychotherapist an opportunity to assist the client in acknowledging and working through similar patterns in the client's relationships with others (Harvey, 2020). When these are validated and explored, the client can find new responses to old conflicts. Prenatal and perinatal transference is a protective defense.

An example of an expectant client transferring negative feelings to their womb baby is a woman who experienced frequent sexual abuse growing up and who later rejects or constantly fears for her infant girl. Alternatively, the girl child may continue to trigger trauma memories in the mother, who may become dismissive and indifferent toward her child due to the fear of nurturing a girl who may relive and enact her childhood pain. If the womb baby is male, the mother may fear or have difficulty feeling loving toward him if she experienced paternal abuse.

Gender Preference and Expectations

In many cultures, male offspring are desired in order to inherit property and carry on the family name. In a 2011 survey (Guilmoto, 2015), American parents favored boys by a 28–40% margin. Likewise, in many countries, parents prefer sons over daughters, as evidenced by the sex ratios of children in various countries. Although biologically the sex ratio of children is around 95 girls to every 100 boys, this number generally evens out due to the higher infant mortality rate of boy infants (Seager, 2018). Scholars argue that the expected birth sex ratio in a normal population is in the range of 103 males to 107 females at birth.

The problem is particularly severe in China and India. The preference for sons over daughters can be connected to several reasons. In these countries, it is argued that son preference is linked to factors including economics, religion, and culture. In India, having a son ensures that families are more economically secure by not having to provide but rather receiving dowry payments. In China, the past one-child policy has contributed to the sex imbalance. Furthermore, in countries where there are discriminatory practices regarding women inheriting, owning, or controlling land by law, having a son ensures that the family will not have to worry about the legal aftermath if something were to happen to them. It can also be argued that parents in these countries are aware of the potential hardship their daughter would endure in her lifetime, and therefore prefer to have a son in order not to see their daughter suffer. Often, this son preference results in female feticide and prenatal sex selection (Das Gupta, 2020).

Noticeably, in South Korea, where there was once a strong, traditional son preference, the trend has recently shifted to a greater preference for daughters, or no preference. The drop in son predilection reflects shifts in intergenerational relations, financial and societal changes that have redefined the meaning and value of children in the context of economic uncertainties, very low fertility, and population aging (Seo et al., 2022).

Given the previously presented reports, it is important to consider the cultural, religious, and familial gender expectations and to assist the client in identifying their own anticipated wishes. Embracing the gender of the baby openly and unconditionally is the ultimate pre-perinatal treatment objective.

Pillar 3: Collaborative Pre-Perinatal Trauma-Informed Team Approach

The pre-perinatal psychotherapist needs to develop a close working relationship with the client's OB-GYN team. This includes regular and ongoing conversations and meetings with the OB pre-perinatal medical doctors, midwives, pre-perinatal support staff, medical assistants, psychiatrist, primary care provider (PCP), coordinators, nutritionists, lactation specialists, health educators, gestational diabetes (GDM) personnel, and front-desk receptionists.

The trauma-informed pre-perinatal psychotherapist needs to provide ongoing psychoeducation to the client's OB-GYN team. These psychoeducational collaterals could be in person or via video conferences, provided to the individual or the whole pre-perinatal team. EMDR pamphlets, virtual video links, and online sites with EMDR education are some of the many readily available educational tools.

Pillar 4: Client and Womb Baby Dyad Wellness

Prenatal Bonding

The CWFTM treats the client and womb baby as a family dyad. Prenatal bonding and emotional wellness are at the core of the CWFTM. In this model, parental bonding is uniquely characterized by the unilateral feelings of the client and the womb baby, *before birthing*. Bonding paves the way for *post-birthing* healthy attachment. Additionally, the CWFTM program provides couples or family bonding psychoeducation, and addresses the impact pregnancy and prenatal bonding have on the partner and the baby's siblings. Family members and the partner are welcome to attend sporadic or ongoing conjoint sessions throughout the client's care, if the client wishes, but ultimately the expectant client and womb baby remain the identified clients. It is well documented that the way a person was cared for and nurtured in infancy and childhood affects the parenting and interaction with others (Moog et al., 2023). Bowlby (1979) observed and documented how a parent's own childhood nurturing and mothering experiences become an internalized model of future parenting. Thus, it is imperative to nurture bonding between client and womb baby from the moment prenatal care begins.

Pre-perinatal Self-Regulation

Pre-perinatal self-regulation, self-care, and emotional wellness are fundamental to the CWFTM. Understanding prenatal stress, developmental complex trauma, and dissociative phenomena and their direct impact on the developing fetus can inform psychotherapeutic treatment decisions, especially when treating pregnant clients who are severely distressed, dissociative, and unable to bond.

The pregnant client's sense of emotional mastery, in utero development knowledge, and physical calmness are crucial to womb baby bonding. Throughout the pre-perinatal care therapy sessions, the client will learn and practice multiple state-change interventions such as somatic relaxing exercises, trauma-informed mindfulness (Forner, 2019), and grounding practices that enhance their sense of wellness, reduce their emotional distress, and increase their sense of self-mastery and prenatal tranquility. Trauma-informed treatments such as EMDR therapy that increase internal and external resources are beneficial to both the client and the womb baby during the early parenting periods. Supporting paced interventions that increase the client's and womb baby's felt sense of safety and regulated internal environments is especially beneficial for those with preexisting histories of trauma, unresolved grief, and traumatic stress symptoms (Weinstein, 2016).

The importance of the client's acknowledgment of the baby's presence from conception and self-regulating reflectively are essential to the CWFTM bonding and maternal attunement. Interrupted prenatal bonding and parental interactions in early infancy are associated with deficient child outcomes; hence the benefits of identifying early risk factors for such disrupted interactions. Nyström-Hansen et al.'s (2019) recent study pointed to the prospect of third-trimester high cortisol concentrations (HCC) being a possible indicator for upcoming parenting difficulties and deficits in expectant mothers with severe mental illness and histories of adverse childhood experiences. Such a finding may expedite timely prenatal interventions to support and treat pregnant maternal deficits that may result in adaptive maternal interactions in early infancy. Most recently, Khoury et al. (2020) reported study results that reflect the importance of measuring the effects of high levels of HCC and depression on pregnant clients. According to the findings, both HCC and depressive symptoms interacted to predict both maternal withdrawing (high depressive symptoms with HCC) and inappropriate or intrusive interaction (low depressive symptoms with HCC), both of which are deleterious for infant development.

During therapy, the pregnant client discusses and practices multiple state-change interventions that benefit their sense of wellness, reduce emotional discomfort, and increase a sense of self-mastery and prenatal calmness. The client learns to regulate their affect, remain within a window of tolerance by modulating the arousal (Ogden, 2021), enhance dual awareness (Schubert et al., 2011), practice relaxation exercises (van der Kolk et al., 2014), role-play limit setting (Knell & Dasari, 2011), and rehearse grounding practices (Siegel, 2018). All these activities will positively impact client and womb baby bonding. Learning the above self-care practices is part of EMDR therapy's Phase 2, preparation for trauma treatment (Shapiro, 2018).

Pillar 5: Prenatal EMDR-CWFTM Framework

While this chapter focuses on the integration of EMDR therapy, and the CWFTM, other therapeutic techniques, such as hypnosis, narrative models, and somatic interventions, may also prove effective, but those were not included in the development of this protocol.

The purpose of the CWFTM application is to carefully evaluate, treat, and prevent traumatic bonding and maladaptive repetitions, and to increase the pregnant client's wellness. The simultaneous and contained practice of the CWFTM and EMDR therapy supports pregnant clients and their womb babies' attunement and bonding. Dissociation phenomena in response to trauma can interfere with prenatal bonding when the client is not able to be in touch and feels the shame, grief, fear, or pain caused by an event or multiple past traumatic incidents.

The CWFTM is a comprehensive early trauma-intervention approach for the assessment and treatment of client and their womb babies throughout their prenatal care and a year after birthing. It provides in utero developmental psychoeducation and facilitates collateral support and collaboration with the medical services to the client. Multi-intergenerational maladaptive enactments, projections, and unwarranted transferences are identified and treated in a timely manner within a comprehensive model that respects and values clients' family beliefs.

EMDR therapy is based on adaptive information processing (AIP), which proposes that conditions are often the result of maladaptive encoding or incomplete processing of traumatic life experiences. This interferes with the client's ability to integrate these experiences in a functional way. The eight-phase, three-pronged process of EMDR enables the continuation of normal information processing and integration. EMDR therapy targeting past experiences, current triggers, and future potential challenges results in the alleviation of presenting symptoms, a decrease or elimination of distress from the disturbing memory, and an improved view of the self, others, world, and/or future. Consequently, EMDR therapy is the approach of choice for the CWFTM. From the initial stages of prenatal care, EMDR therapy is informed by the CMFTM; both are used concurrently.

Prenatal Complex Trauma and Dissociative Phenomena Methodology

Over two decades of prenatal-perinatal EMDR therapy practice have provided evidence-based clinical observations, conclusions, and trauma-informed interventions. It is interesting to note that when a pregnant client is suitably ready and is treated by a prenatal trauma-dissociation-informed psychotherapist, prenatal EMDR-CWFTM therapy has consistently resulted in symptom reduction, traumatic experience processing-resolution, and trait change. Disturbing past incidents causing gestational distress, interfering with prenatal bonding, and affecting the prospect of the infant's secure attachment must be treated in a timely manner. If therapeutic resources are limited, consultation is advised. To enhance robust outcomes and team collaboration, the CWFTM recommends that the OB-GYN medical doctor or midwife are trauma- and EMDR-educated prior to treatment. Medical consent to initiate EMDR therapy is optional and recommended.

The use of EMDR therapy's eight phases and standard procedures are informed by the CWFTM's gestational recommendations. EMDR-CWFTM recommendations include **Phase 1:** completing a paced psychosocial, bonding, attachment, and birth history of the pregnant client; individualized treatment planning; trauma and dissociation screening (Cortizo, 2020b, 2020a); in utero guidance education; and EMDR instruction; and **Phase 2:** extensive resourcing; symptom stabilization; and mindfulness (Forner, 2019); and gestational relaxation practices and preparation. **Phases 3–8:** are the same as the EMDR standard protocol with particular emphasis on gestational somatic attunement and maternal bodily regulation and containment.

Cultivating and increasing the pregnant client's stability, sense of safety, and competency for processing complex trauma and dissociative material requires a clinician that is attuned, synchronic, that can hold the mother's mind in mind, contingent and compassionate who can help titrate the activating material and regulate the pace of psychotherapy and the client's participation in it. Somatic attunement to both the pregnant client's and therapist's experience is a fundamental therapeutic process that strengthens the treatment. Prenatal EMDR therapists must nurture the collaborative frame of the therapy and establish an empowering relationship capable of coregulating the client's state during both resource development and trauma processing. These functions can be enhanced by regularly evaluating, supporting, and looking for opportunities to strengthen affect regulation, resources and competencies, and by staying attentive to empathic opportunities, relational repairs, and countertransference. Choices that transform and guide the treatment process and affect its pacing derive from the therapist's self-awareness, the client's readiness, the therapeutic alliance, and an understanding of complex trauma, dissociative processes, the therapeutic process, and CWFTM-EMDR.

Prenatal EMDR-CWFTM Discussion

Critical to prenatal treatment are common anecdotal myths that can impact early treatment access and affect prenatal bonding outcomes.

Prenatal Treatment Common Myths and Clarifications

"The pregnant client should initiate trauma processing and EMDR therapy during the second trimester." This depends on the client's unique prenatal situation, not on the gestational count alone. In addition, most expectant clients enter therapy by their eighth gestational week. By the time EMDR Phases 1 and 2 are completed, including thorough trauma and dissociation assessments, questionnaires, an attachment genogram, and an EMDR treatment plan, most likely the client is in the second gestational trimester. Postponing or starting treatment needs to be directly related to the client's clinical assessment, readiness, obstetric advice, and gestational stability. Pregnant clients need to be cautiously assessed for trauma and dissociative processes, but delaying healing solely because the client is pregnant is unwarranted.

EMDR therapy must be offered to pregnant clients as soon as the client is ready and the obstetric team consents.

"The womb baby may be affected by the influx of cortisol during reprocessing traumata." Although the womb baby may be exposed to cortisol levels during pregnancy in addition to trauma processing, the important goal is to reduce the prenatal chronic stress. Resourcing, containment, and self-care practices are all necessary abilities. Precautions include installing resources, pacing or slowing down trauma processing material, and processing present triggers first.

Pacing traumatic material allows the client to participate with their therapist in determining how much will be processed in every session. This active collaboration allows the expectant client to replace traumatic stress and helplessness with empowerment. The trauma- and dissociative-phenomena-informed EMDR prenatal clinician needs to keep the client from re-experiencing marked disturbance, but there is no need to postpone health restoration.

"**Ask the OB-GYNs, midwives, psychiatrists, and other medical treating professionals for permission to proceed with EMDR or other trauma prenatal therapy.**" This is an important practice, but unfortunately, often gynecologists, obstetricians, midwives, psychiatrists, and medical providers lack information about complex trauma–dissociative processes, and how EMDR therapy can assist their prenatal clients.

It is the function and role of the EMDR therapist to educate such providers. In-services, psychoeducation, EMDRIA pamphlets, bibliography, and the distribution of virtual materials are crucial.

Cautions

When a pregnant mother is experiencing drastic hormonal shifts, feels constant physical pain, is at high risk of premature labor or childbirth, has a history of complex trauma and dissociative processes or declines EMDR therapy Phases 3–6, the best course of treatment is to focus on EMDR Phases 1–2 and 7–8, specifically Phase 2, including relaxation practices, in utero developmental guidance, pre-perinatal bibliotherapy/videotherapy, and EMDR resourcing.

Recommendations

Further research by prenatal and perinatal EMDR-trained clinicians is needed, specifically while the pregnant client is attached to a fetal monitor during EMDR therapy. Such procedure is currently uncommon due to the providers' time constraints and clients' privacy protocols. To demonstrate the efficacy of the model, replication of the EMDR protocol along with the CWFTM to a wider prenatal population is recommended.

This discussion and these findings significantly underscore the importance of:

1. Early child abuse interventions and the screening of dissociative processes starting in infancy
2. Trauma and dissociation assessments and preconception treatment
3. Prenatal screening, psychosocial assessments, and the treatment of preexisting PTSD, dissociative phenomena, anxiety, depression, and other disorders
4. Establishing universal requirements for assessing antepartum pre-treatment baselines and post-treatment outcomes
5. Evaluating both resiliency and maladaptive intergenerational patterns at the beginning of prenatal psychotherapy
6. Further research studying the impact of dissociative processes on prenatal care
7. Prenatal secondary and tertiary treatment for the parents, and primary prevention for the womb baby
8. Concurrent practice of CWFTM-EMDR therapy and other somatic, hypnotic, narrative interventions to support pregnant clients' and their womb babies' attunement and bonding
9. Quantitative prenatal EMDR therapy research to identify best bonding practices
10. Pacing trauma processing to prevent potentially destabilizing pregnant clients
11. The mother being able to initiate paced and contained pre-perinatal EMDR therapy—once the obstetric provider has given treatment authorization, and the expectant client has been screened and assessed for trauma and dissociation and informed about the benefits, contraindications, and possible risks, and given her informed consent
12. A revision of the ISSTD guidelines prior to trauma and dissociation treatment
13. Prenatal interventions and research developed, tested, and measured for effects.

Complex Presentations

Unperceived pregnancy is defined as the inability to recognize gestation until the 20th week of conception. In the case of total denial, the pregnancy goes unrecognized until birthing. This condition can result in a traumatic birthing, medical and psychiatric complications, the loss of the newborn, traumatic stress, and forensic consequences (Sar et al., 2017). Unfortunately, the phenomenon has not attracted sufficient attention in psychological and psychiatric literature despite the existing epidemiological research on it. EMDR therapy can reduce the shame, guilt, and traumatic stress caused by this condition.

Tokophobia, first described in literature by Knauer in 1897, is the severe fear of pregnancy and/or childbirth, and can lead to avoidance of childbirth as well as cesarean section requests or demands. It can be classified as primary or secondary. Primary is the morbid fear of childbirth in a client who has no previous experience of pregnancy. Secondary is the morbid fear of childbirth, developing after a traumatic obstetric event in a previous pregnancy. Most pregnant clients can cope with such fears and anxieties through self-help efforts, social support, and medical help. However, when it becomes pathological dread, it is treated as tokophobia. The EMDR standard protocol with a focus on processing the present fear of childbirth can reduce a client's distress.

CMFTM Post-Birthing

While many clients have wonderful post-birthing support and experiences, others will encounter unforeseen medical or emotional challenges. Most expect to hold their babies soon after delivery, to be discharged home with their newborns, and to hold their babies in the comfort of their home. However, many will not be able to do so. As much as clients may have been educated and prepared by their health educators and lactation specialists, unplanned cesarean sections and lactation challenges occur.

Frequent post-birthing challenges include moderate to severe postpartum depression, anxiety, psychosis, acute stress, trauma, and stress disorder, which could appear within two to four weeks or over time.

Whether through rape or birth trauma, mothers who lose a child pre- or postnatally have high rates of depression and anxiety and receive limited treatment for these conditions, if any. Post-birthing emotional dysregulation often interferes with the parent-child's attachment, and prompt intervention is critical.

Conclusion

Reversing Prenatal Inertia

The goals of the CWFTM practice are to assess early on any prenatal trauma and dissociative processes; provide trauma-informed adapted interventions; increase client and baby dyad bonding; repair broken bonds; involve all medical and psychotherapy teams; and increase the pregnant client's internal resources. Because expectant clients with a history of developmental or adult maltreatment, complex trauma, and dissociative adaptation are at risk of being retraumatized or overwhelmed by birthing, and of dissociating, it is recommended that trauma-informed clinicians universally and comprehensively assess for dissociative coping during pregnancy. Such potential for integral resilience, harmony, and healing is associated with reduced psychopathology, improved well-being, and the multi-intergenerational transmission of health. The CWFTM's ultimate objective is to support and facilitate the conception and nurture of healthy infants by promoting bonding, providing prenatal developmental education and guidance internationally, and to heal trauma in the earliest lifespan stages.

References

Alaggia, R., Collin-Vézina, D., & Lateef, R. (2017). Facilitators and barriers to child sexual abuse (CSA) disclosures: A research update (2000–2016). *Sage Journals, 20*(2), 260–283. https://doi.org/10.1177/1524838017697312

Anda, R., Porter, L., & Brown, D. (2020). Inside the adverse childhood experience score: Strengths, applications and misapplications. *American Journal of Preventive Medicine, 59*(2), 293–295. https://doi.org/10.1016/j.amepre.2020.01.009

Bowen, M. (1976). *Family therapy: Theory and practice therapy.* Gardner Press.

Bowlby, J. (1979). On knowing what you are not supposed to know and feeling what you are not supposed to feel. *The Canadian Journal of Psychiatry. 24*(5), 403–408. https://doi.org/10.1177/070674377902400506

Caldwell, J., Meredith, P., Whittingham, K., Ziviani, J., & Wilson, T. (2024). Women pregnant after previous perinatal loss: Relationships between adult attachment, shame, and prenatal psychological outcomes. *Journal of Reproductive and Infant Psychology, 42*(4), 653–667. https://doi.org/10.1080/02646838.2023.2180142

Chiorino, V., Roveraro, S., Cattaneo, M., Salerno, R., Macchi, E., Bertolucci, G., Mosca, F., & Fernandez, I. (2016). A model of clinical intervention in the maternity ward: The breastfeeding and bonding EMDR protocol. *Journal of EMDR Practice and Research, 10*(4), 275–292. https://doi.org/10.1891/1933-3196.10.4.275

Collin-Vézina, D., Sablonni, D. L., Palmer, A. M., & Milne, L. (2015). A preliminary mapping of individual, relational, and social factors that impede disclosure of childhood sexual abuse. *Child Abuse & Neglect, 43*, 123–134. https://doi.org/10.1016/j.chiabu.2015.03.010

Cortizo, R. (2019). The calming womb family therapy model: Bonding mother and baby from pregnancy forward. *Journal of Prenatal and Perinatal Psychology and Health, 33*(3), 207–220. birthpsychology.com/wp-content/uploads/journal/published_paper/volume-33/issue-3/lUJHZoyP.pdf

Cortizo, R. (2020a). Prenatal and perinatal EMDR therapy: Early family intervention. *Journal of EMDR Practice and Research, 14*(2), 104–115. https://doi.org/10.1891/EMDR-D-19-00046

Cortizo, R. (2020b). Hidden trauma, dissociation, and prenatal assessment within the calming womb model. *Journal of Prenatal and Perinatal Psychology and Health, 34*(6), 469–481. birthpsychology.com/wp-content/uploads/journal/published_paper/volume-34/issue- 6/NNRsuErB.pdf

Cortizo, R. (2021). Prenatal broken bonds: Trauma, dissociation and the calming womb model. *Journal of Trauma and Dissociation, 22*(1), 1–10. https://doi.org/10.1080/15299732.2021.1834300

Chefetz, R. (2015). *Intensive psychotherapy for persistent dissociative processes: The fear of feeling real.* W. W. Norton & Company.

Daglar, G., & Nur, N. (2018). Level of mother-baby bonding and influencing factors during pregnancy and postpartum period. *Psychiatria Danubina, 30*(4), 433–440. https://doi.org/10.24869/psyd.2018.433

Dana, D. (2018). *The polyvagal theory in therapy: Engaging the rhythm of regulation.* W.W. Norton & Company.

Das Gupta, M. (2020). What hypotheses can research on son preference in Asia offer for European historical demographic research? *The History of the Family, 27*(4), 791–800. https://doi.org/10.1080/1081602X.2022.2129417

Delker, B., Van Scoyoc, A., & Noll, L. (2020). Contextual influences on the perception of pregnant women who use drugs: Information about women's childhood trauma history reduces punitive attitudes. *Journal of Trauma & Dissociation, 21*(1), 103–123.

Deneault, A., Hammond, S., & Madigan, S. (2023). A meta-analysis of child–parent attachment in early childhood and prosociality. *Developmental Psychology, 59*(2), 236–255. https://doi.org/10.1037/dev0001484

Dennis, C., Brennenstuhl, S., Brown, H., Bell, R., Marini, F., & Birken, C. (2022). High-risk health behaviours of pregnancy-planning women and men: Is there a need for preconception care? *Midwifery, 106*, Article 103244. https://doi.org/10.1016/j.midw.2021.103244

De Venter, M., Smets, J., Raes, F., Wouters, K., Franck, E., Hanssens, M., Jacquemyn, Y., Sabbe, B. G. C., & Van Den Eede, F. (2016). Impact of childhood trauma on postpartum depression: A prospective study. *Archives of Women's Mental Health, 19*, 337–342. https://doi.org/10.1007/s00737-015-0550-z

Dubber, S., Reck, C., Muller, M., & Gawlik, S. (2015). Postpartum bonding: The role of perinatal depression, anxiety and maternal-fetal bonding during pregnancy. *Archives of Women's Mental Health, 18*, 187–195. https://doi.org/10.1007/s00737-014-0445-4

Eubanks, C. F., Muran, J. C., & Safran, J. D. (2019). Repairing alliance ruptures. In J. C. Norcross & M. J. Lambert (Eds.), *Psychotherapy relationships that work: Evidence-based therapist contributions* (pp. 549–579). Oxford University Press. https://doi.org/10.1093/med-psych/9780190843953.003.0016

Forner, C. (2019). What mindfulness can learn about dissociation and what dissociation can learn from mindfulness. *Journal of Trauma and Dissociation, 20*(1), 1–15. https://doi.org/10.1080/15299732.2018.1502568

Fraiberg, S. (1980). *Clinical studies in infant mental health: The first year of life.* Basic Books.

Glover, V., & Capron, L. (2017). Prenatal parenting. *Current Opinion in Psychology, 15*, 66–70. https://doi.org/10.1016/j.copsyc.2017.02.007

Guilmoto, C. Z. (2015). The masculinization of births: Overview and current knowledge. (J. Trove, Trans.), *Population, 70*(2), 185–243, cairn-int.info/article.php?ID_ARTICLE=E_POPU_1502_0201

Guyon-Harris, K., Madigan, S., Bronfman, E., Romero, G., & Huth-Bocks, A. (2020). Prenatal identification of risk for later disrupted parenting behavior using latent profiles of childhood maltreatment. *Journal of Interpersonal Violence, 36* (23–24). https://doi.org/10.1177/0886260520906175

Harvey, M. (2020). Traumatic transference. *The Hearing Journal, 73*(1), 29, https://doi.org/10.1097/01.HJ.0000651548.37119.ad

Harsey, S., & Freyd, J. (2020). Deny, attack, and reverse victim and offender (DARVO): What is the influence on perceived perpetrator and victim credibility? *Journal of Aggression, Maltreatment & Trauma, 9*(8), 897–916. https://doi.org/10.1080/10926771.2020.1774695

Khoury, J. E., Bosquet Enlow, M., Patwa, M. C., & Lyons-Ruth, K. (2020). Hair cortisol in pregnancy interacts with maternal depressive symptoms to predict maternal disrupted interaction with her infant at 4 months. *Developmental Psychobiology, 62*(6), 768–782. https://doi.org/10.1002/dev.21950

Klabbers, G., van Bakel, H., van den Heuvel, M., & Vingerhoets, A. (2016). Severe fear of childbirth: Its features, assessment, prevalence, determinants, consequences and possible treatments. *Psychological Topics, 25*(1), 107–127. hrcak.srce.hr/file/230452

Knell, S., & Dasari, M. (2011). *Play in clinical practice: Evidence-based approaches.* Guilford Press.

Kossak, M. (2015). *Attunement in expressive arts therapy.* Charles C. Thomas, Publisher.

Kruger, C., & Fletcher, L. (2017). Predicting a dissociative disorder from type of childhood maltreatment and abuser-abused relational type. *Journal of Trauma and Dissociation, 18*(3), 356–372. https://doi.org/10.1080/15299732.2017.1295420

Madhavanprabhakaran, G. K., D'Souza, M. S., & Nairy, K. S. (2015). Prevalence of pregnancy anxiety and associated factors. *International Journal of Africa Nursing Sciences, 3*, 1–7. https://doi.org/10.1016/j.ijans.2015.06.002

McGowan, P., & Matthews, S. (2018). Prenatal stress, glucocorticoids, and developmental programming of the stress response. *Endocrinology, 159*(1), 69–82. https://doi.org/10.1210/en.2017-00896

Moog, N., Cummings, P. D., Jackson, K. L., Aschner, J. L., Barrett, E. S., Bastain, T. M., Blackwell, C. K., Bosquet Enlow, M., Breton, C. V., Deoni, S. C. L., Duarte, C. S., Ferrara, A., Grant, T. L., Hipwell, A. E., Jones, K., Leve, L. D., Lovinsky-Desir, S., & Miller, R. K. (2023). Intergenerational transmission of the effects of maternal exposure to childhood maltreatment in the USA: A retrospective cohort study. *Lancet Public Health, 8*(3), 226–237. https://doi.org/10.1016/S2468-2667(23)00025-700025-7

Nyström-Hansen, M., Andersen, M. S., Khoury, J., Davidsen, K., Gumley, A., Lyons-Ruth, K., MacBeth, A., & Harder, S. (2019). Hair cortisol in the perinatal period mediates associations between maternal adversity and disrupted maternal interaction in early infancy. *Developmental Psychobiology, 61*(4), 543–556. https://doi.org/10.1002/dev.21833

Ogden, P. (2021). The different impact of trauma and relational stress on physiology, posture, and movement: Implications for treatment. *European Journal of Trauma & Dissociation, 5*(4). Article 100172. https://doi.org/10.1016/j.ejtd.2020.100172

Phillips, B. (2020). Hypnosis in the clinical setting. *Journal of the American Association of Nurse Practitioners, 32*(5), 351–353. https://doi.org/10.1097/JXX.0000000000000422

Poels, M., van Stel, H. F., Franx, A., & Koster, M. (2017). Actively preparing for pregnancy is associated with healthier lifestyle of women during the preconception period. *Midwifery, 50*, 228–234. https://doi.org/10.1016/j.midw.2017.04.015

Porges, S. (2021). Polyvagal theory: A biobehavioral journey to sociality. *Psychoneuroendocrinology, 7.* Article 100069. https://doi.org/10.1016/j.cpnec.2021.100069

Reck, C., Zietlow, A. L., Müller, M., & Dubber, S. (2016). Perceived parenting stress in the course of postpartum depression: The buffering effect of maternal bonding. *Archives Women's Mental Health, 19*, 473–482. https://doi.org/10.1007/s00737-015-0590-4

Rupert, F. (2016). *Early trauma: Pregnancy, birth and first years of life.* Green Balloon Publishing.

Sar, V., Aydin, N., van der Hart, O., Frankel, S., Sar, M., & Omay, O. (2017). Acute dissociative reaction to spontaneous delivery in a case of total denial of pregnancy: Diagnostic and forensic aspects. *Journal of Trauma and Dissociation, 18*(5), 710–719. https://doi.org/10.1080/15299732.20161267685

Schubert, S., Lee, C., & Drummond, P. (2011). The efficacy and psychophysiological correlates of dual-attention tasks in eye movement desensitization and reprocessing (EMDR). *Journal of Anxiety Disorders, 25*(1), 1–11. https://doi.org/10.1016/j.janxdis.2010.06.024

Seager, J. (2018). *The women's atlas.* Penguin Group.

Seng, J., Low, L., Sperlich, M., Ronis, D., & Liberzon, I. (2009). Prevalence, trauma history and risk of posttraumatic stress disorder among nulliparous women in maternity care. *Obstetrics and Gynecology, 114*(4), 839–847. https://doi.org/10.1097/AOG.0b013e3181b8f8a2

Seng, J., Low, L., Sperlich, M., Ronis, D., & Liberzon, I. (2011). Posttraumatic stress disorder, child abuse history, birth weight, and gestational age: A prospective cohort study. *BJOG: An International Journal of Obstetrics and Gynaecology,* 1329–1339. https://doi.org/10.1111j.1471-0528.2011.03071.x

Seng, J., Rauch, S., Resnick, H., Reed, C., King, A., Low, L., McPherson, M., Muzik, M., Abelson, J., & Liberzon, I. (2010). Exploring posttraumatic stress disorder symptom profile among pregnant women. *Journal of Psychosomatic Obstetrics & Gynecology, 31*(3), 176–187. https://doi.org/10.3109/0167482X.2010.486453

Seng, J. S., Sperlich, M., & Low, L. K. (2008). Mental health, demographic, and risk behavior profiles of pregnant survivors of childhood and adult abuse. *Journal of Midwifery & Women's Health, 53*(6), 511–521.

Seng, J., Sperlich, M., Low, L., Ronis, D., Muzik, M., & Liberzon, I. (2013). Childhood abuse history, posttraumatic stress disorder, postpartum mental health and bonding: A prospective cohort study. *Journal of Midwifery and Women's Health, 58*(1), 57–68. https://doi.org/101111/j.1542–2011.2012.00237.x

Seo, G., Koropeckyj-Cox, T., & Kim, S. (2022). Correlates of contemporary gender preference for children in South Korea. *Population and Development Review, 48*(1), 161–188. https://doi.org/10.1111/padr.12458

Shapiro, F. (2018). *Eye movement desensitization and reprocessing (EMDR) therapy: Basic principles, protocols, and procedures.* Guilford Press.

Siegel, D. (2018). *Aware: The science and practice of presence.* Penguin Random House.

Simpson, S., Richardson, L., Pietrabissa, G., Castelnuovo, G., & Reid, C. (2020). Videotherapy and therapeutic alliance in the age of COVID-19. *Clinical Psychology & Psychotherapy, 28*(2), 409–421. https://doi.org/10.1002/cpp.2521

Swales, D., Stout-Oswald, S., Glynn, L., Sandman, C., Wing, D., & Poggi, E. (2018). Exposure to traumatic events in childhood predicts cortisol production among high risk pregnant women. *Biological Psychology, 139,* 186–192. https://doi.org/10.1016/j.biopsycho.2018.10.006

Talley, L. (2013). Stress management in pregnancy. *International Journal of Childbirth Education, 28*(1), 43–45.

Toivonen, K., Oinonen, K., & Duchene, K. (2017). Preconception health behaviours: A scoping review. *Preventive Medicine, 96,* 1–15. https://doi.org/10.1016/j.ypmed.2016.11.022

van der Kolk, B. (2022). Posttraumatic stress disorder and the nature of trauma. *Dialogues in Clinical Neuroscience, 2*(1), 7–22. https://doi.org/10.31887/DCNS.2000.2.1/bvdkolk

van der Kolk, B., Stone, L., West, J., Rhodes, A., Emerson, D., Suvak, M., & Spinazzola, J. (2014). Yoga as an adjunctive treatment for post-traumatic stress disorder: A randomized controlled trail. *Journal of Clinical Psychiatry, 75*(6), 3559–3565. https://doi.org/10.4088/JCP.13m08561

Verny, T. (2018). *Prenatal psychology 100 years: A journey in decoding how our prenatal experience shapes who we become.* Cosmoanelixis.

Weinstein, A. D. (2016). *Prenatal development and parents' lived experiences: How early events shape our psychophysiology and relationships.* W.W. Norton & Company.

Zolghadr, N., Khoshnazar, A., MoradiBaglooei, M., & Alimoradi, Z. (2019). The effect of EMDR on childbirth anxiety of women with previous stillbirth. *Journal of EMDR Practice and Research, 13*(1), 10–19. https://doi.org/10.1891/1933-3196.13.1.10

37
FRACTURED BONDS
Healing Trauma in the Caregiving System

Maria Zaccagnino, Martina Cussino and Cristina Civilotti

Introduction

According to research published in the literature, the evolutionary dimension of attachment and caregiving is thought to play an essential role in triggering and maintaining traumatic experiences. Indeed, maltreatment and physical abuse appear to be transmitted to subsequent generations due to negative and dysfunctional caregiving methods that create an emotional vulnerability in future relationships (Liotti & Farina, 2011). In the clinical context of working with children and parents, when moving into the most central areas of distress, the therapist may encounter situations where the adaptive reappraisal process is not easily activated or is blocked due to the patient's difficulties and defense mechanisms. These difficulties may manifest themselves, for example, in the emergence of dissociated, protective parts that have precisely the task of protecting the patient from accessing traumatic material that is excessively painful. Additionally, the transmission of unresolved transgenerational trauma does indeed occur in various ways through the caregiving system, including nonverbal ways such as gestures and glances. When a parent experiences trauma, they may develop one or more defense mechanisms to survive through strategies such as numbing, minimizing, or avoiding the trauma. The transgenerational transmission of an unresolved trauma through the caregiving system thus preserves both the traces of the trauma and the defense mechanisms that the parent developed to deal with the original event.

Some forms of traumatization and associated dissociative disorders are thought to be caused by the transfer of traumatic content from the parent to the child (Kostova & Matanova, 2024; Yehuda & Lehrner, 2018). This process is known as intergenerational transmission of trauma. It is as if these defense mechanisms live on at the time of the trauma, protecting the child and/or the entire family relationship system with the same strategies. When a triggering event occurs in the child's life, the parent's traces and defense mechanisms are reactivated in relation to the child's challenges. For this reason, children's symptoms may not regress, and therapists may find themselves feeling stuck in therapy.

In the initial stages of traumatic content interventions, it is essential to work with the parent to develop knowledge about the different aspects of their self that may be involved in maintaining the child's symptoms. Parent-centered intervention makes it possible to address the child's difficulties and promote their well-being while preventing the families themselves from being thrown off track.

We argue that our first goal as clinicians must be to integrate the parent's parts that get activated in relation to the child's symptoms. This chapter describes the use of EMDR therapy as an intervention that supports integrating the parts of the self. However, this work with parents can be integrated into different psychotherapeutic orientations.

The Attachment and Caregiving Systems: A Brief Theoretical Consideration

"Attachment" refers to the intimate emotional bond that individuals develop with the important people in their lives, usually parents or primary caregivers. Attachment is a fundamental element in an individual's socio-emotional development and influences how they perceive themselves, others, and the world around them. Attachment also provides a child with a sense of security and influences their future ability to form relationships (Bowlby, 1969, 1973). The caregiving system has a primary function of providing parental protection to children, and it is closely linked to the attachment system, which is under constant development.

Bowlby (1969, 1973) devoted much time to discerning activating and deactivating elements of the child's attachment system. These elements are recognized through internal and external stimuli that have become associated with situations that trigger anxiety or stress in the child and require a parent's help. As soon as the attachment signals are activated, it is up to the parents to use attuned and appropriate responses that achieve the protective goal (i.e., physical proximity to the child, holding the child in their arms, looking at them, comforting them, calling them to them, and smiling). The adult's behavioral responses, however, depend on the assessment of the sources of information involved. The most important are the type of signals sent by the child and his own perception of danger or threat (Cassidy & Shaver, 1999). This last consideration illustrates the extent to which the parent's story is intertwined with that of their child since the interpretative framework of the stimuli proposed by the child always passes through the lens with which the parents view them.

The attachment theory framework provides a clear explanation and understanding of these processes. Bowlby (1969) states that an intrinsic attachment behavioral system governs the child's proximity-seeking behaviors. This system aims to seek the care and protection of the caregiver—also known as the attachment figure—in response to perceived or actual stress or danger. The most critical component influencing the development of the attachment relationship is the reciprocal pattern of influence between the infant's behavior and that of the caregiver (Ainsworth et al., 1978a; Bowlby, 1969, 1973; De Wolff & van Ijzendoorn, 1997). At the same time, the attachment and caregiving systems develop in parallel, as previously mentioned. As the child creates an Internal Working Model (IWM) of the caregiver, the parent creates a unique and distinct image of caregiving that differs from other models. According to George and Solomon (1996), this representation is critical to the control and growth of parental behavior aimed at providing nurturance and protection. The mother's representation of her attachment experiences and her current relationship with the child work together to shape her ability to form coherent, positive, and flexible representations of her child, as well as her relationship with them and their feelings (Bowlby, 1969; Button et al., 2001; Cassidy, 1988; George & Solomon, 1996; Slade, 1999).

Essentially, every human develops an attachment system (based on the IWM of closeness) and a caregiving system (to fulfill the needs of others). Unresolved trauma and/or grief that a caregiver has previously experienced and are dysfunctionally stored in memory systems (e.g., adults categorized as "Unresolved" in terms of trauma and/or grief in the Adult Attachment Interview [AAI] [George et al., 1985]) may be reactivated during caregiving. In response to their child's desire for attachment, a parent may experience painful, unresolved traumatic memories that can simultaneously activate their attachment and caregiving systems. The attachment mechanism is activated and evokes strong feelings of fear and/or anger when no caregivers are nearby to soothe the parent's distress.

Therefore, while the baby is crying, "unmanaged" parents may unintentionally and abruptly express fear or anger (stemming from the parent's attachment system) to soothe their baby (a simultaneous attempt stemming from the parent's caregiving system). In other words, a traumatized primary parent may have difficulty effectively responding to the child's demands due to a variety of factors that influence their ability to bond with the child (Hesse & Main, 1999, 2000, 2006).

Traumatic interference may occur when a primary parent feels an emotion so intensely that it overrides and gets in the way of attachment emotions, in turn leading to emotional disconnection. When a baby cries, the primary parent may inadvertently isolate or react with worry, fear, anger, sadness, or resentment instead of responding in a loving and caring way that is attuned to the needs of their baby. The infant may suffer physiological and psychological effects if the primary parent regularly responds in this way (Hesse & Main, 1999, 2000, 2006; Iyengar et al., 2014; Jacobvitz et al., 2006; Kim et al., 2014; Lyons-Ruth et al., 2005; Madigan et al., 2006; Madrid et al., 2006; Saunders et al., 2011; Siegel, 1999). A child is placed in an irreversible paradox by any parental behavior that directly frightens them. The caregiver is both the cause and the solution to the child's alarm, resulting in an unresolved terror without a solution (Liotti & Farina, 2011; Hesse & Main, 1999). These infants are thus unable to develop a coherent behavioral strategy to deal with this incongruent, emotional difficulty, which consists of a vicious cycle of increasing anxiety and conflicting goals, or approach and avoidance (Schore, 2002; Liotti, 2004; Schore & Schore, 2008; Farina & Liotti, 2013). A parent's unresolved emotional states may cause unresolved anxiety and dissociative reactions in the child, even if the parent's behavior does not constitute actual abuse. Examples may be parents who persistently respond to the child's cries with an absent and impassive gaze or parents who seek their own sense of safety through the child, reversing the attachment relationship.

It is important to emphasize that early attachment disorders or disruptions, while a significant risk factor, do not automatically predict the development of dissociative disorders or susceptibility to symptoms of post-traumatic stress (Damis, 2022; Farina & Imperatori, 2023). Empirical evidence suggests that changes in attachment style are possible, although there is growing evidence that the attachment style formed in infancy remains relatively stable (Bar-Haim et al., 2000; Girme et al., 2021; Gruda et al., 2022; McConnell & Moss, 2011; Moss et al., 2005; Waters et al., 2000). Bowlby (1973) suggested that attachment style is significantly associated with a person's development over time and with positive and negative life events (e.g., psychotherapy) (Civilotti et al., 2019; Connors, 2011; Daniel, 2006; Mair, 2021; Mallinckrodt, 2010; Saunders et al., 2011; Zaccagnino et al., 2014). In three case studies, Wesselmann and Potter (2009) showed how using EMDR therapy as an intervention and support in processing early relationship memories could improve a client's access to adaptive information about distressing memories while reducing associated negative beliefs about vulnerability, self-worth, and helplessness.

Attachment, Trauma, and Dissociation

The research contributions of Main et al. (1985) on adult attachment initially explored the phenomenon of intergenerational transmission of attachment and, more recently, with traumatic content that has not been processed in the attachment figure. Traditional attachment research assumes that a parent's mental representations of the attachment experiences they had in childhood strongly influence their caregiving behaviors and thus also influence the quality and characteristics of their child's attachment. This influence explains the correlation found between the attachment models observed in the Strange Situation (Ainsworth et al., 1978b) and the linguistic and narrative styles that characterize parents' descriptions of their attachment experiences in the AAI (Ainsworth et al., 1978a; Kondo-Ikemura et al., 2018; Lee Raby et al., 2013; Weinfield et al., 2004). When present, frozen traumatic content is often passed on as non-declarative, somatoform content or as material that remains indecipherable within the child's experience. The child engages with it without understanding its meaning and may attribute its parts of suffering to one—if not several—past generations (Booker et al., 2020; Crespo & Fernández-Lansac, 2016; McNally, 2022; Moulds & Bryant, 2005; Risan et al., 2020).

Since attachment insecurity is a central experience in adults with many types of disorders, it is crucial to focus on the analysis of a caregiver's ability to mentalize and narrate traumatic content when parenting a dissociative child. It is essential to remember that the development of mentalization (the ability to hold another's mind in mind) is closely linked to the quality of early attachment experiences that form the relational matrix within which this capacity is structured (Fonagy & Campbell, 2016; Fonagy & Target, 1997; Schwarzer et al., 2021). Fonagy and Bateman (2008) state that insecure attachment experiences and/or unfavorable traumatic situations in the relationship with caregivers hinder the development of the ability to mentalize and impair the development of a coherent self-structure and the ability to regulate emotions, exposing the individual to significant vulnerability to psychopathology.

According to the DSM-5 (American Psychiatric Association, 2013), trauma is primarily associated with post-traumatic stress disorder (PTSD) and acute stress disorder. Trauma can be the result of a single event with strong physical and/or psychological effects (as described in the DSM-V), or it can be the result of long-lasting experiences of abuse, neglect, or violence. In the first instance of abuse-related trauma, we often speak of trauma with a capital "T" (or major trauma). In the second instance of neglect, we often speak of attachment-related trauma associated with attachment-related dissociation, sometimes referred to as small "t" traumas (or relational trauma). In contrast to the former, traumas with a small "t" are not characterized by major traumatic experiences but by an extreme perception of danger and as a chronic trait. Liotti (2004, 2006) hypothesized that a child who is exposed to the care of an abusive or frightening caregiver and a series of microtraumas (or small "t" traumas) that are repeated over time is likely to develop disorganized attachment and complex PTSD. Disorganized attachment occurs when the child interacts with an adult who is perceived as both a source of danger and protection (Liotti & Farina, 2011), who behaves unpredictably and frightens the child so that he or she is unable to develop a coherent attachment strategy.

Peterson and Seligman (1983) emphasize two characteristics that are associated with traumatization and lead to dissociation: the state of helplessness and subjective perception of the impossibility of changing or escaping the situation (inescapability) and the lack of control (powerlessness). The first characteristic expresses the lack of control over an external danger or an imminent threat (i.e., the impossibility of confronting it and acting). This concerns both the physiological reaction of the central nervous system and the subjective perception of one's own inability. The second aspect underlines the lack of control over one's own emotional and cognitive states (i.e., the psychobiological, emotional, cognitive, and behavioral functions [Schore & Schore, 2008; van der Kolk et al., 2009]). Thus, the traumatic experience is a complex phenomenon characterized by different dimensions that lead to dysregulation and the emotional, cognitive, and behavioral aspects that characterize it (Liotti & Farina, 2011).

When working with an abusive parent in clinical practice, we may be dealing with high levels of traumatization in the parent that manifest in overt violent behavior or in more subtle ways that allow the trauma to take hold in the child's psyche. These are the dissociated memories that first emerge that we focus on processing and integrating into the parental narrative to prevent them from further affecting the child or the relationship with the child. To understand how trauma affects the parent and child's regulatory systems, we must consider the etiopathogenesis of dissociation and dissociative disorders in the context of a complex multifactorial framework. As we have learned in the previous chapters of this volume, trauma-related dissociation and dissociative disorders in their multiple manifestations represent highly complex clinical conditions. This complexity takes on even more elusive forms when the perspective shifts to the longitudinal level, that is, when one focuses on the intergenerational transmission between parent and child (Lanius et al., 2014; Lev–Wiesel, 2007; Liotti & Farina, 2011; Yehuda & Lehrner, 2018).

An attachment disorder rooted in the relationship with an attachment figure with an "unresolved" history leads to dissociation and a breakdown of the integrative functions of consciousness that are typical of dissociative experiences. The unintegrated content is kept away from the person's consciousness so they can live their life without the pain associated with the traumatic event becoming overwhelming. Dissociated parts of the self can emerge from these initial wounds to keep incompatible aspects separate and thus be able to confront them (Forgash & Copeley, 2014; van der Hart et al., 2011). At the same time, it is possible that parts present at the time of the traumatic event(s) form alongside injured parts to protect them. To this end, parts of the self develop adaptive strategies and behaviors necessary for the individual's survival at the time of the trauma. For example, we may observe attempts to numb the pain, to remove some painful fragments of the lived experience, to explore one's past reluctantly or not at all, dissociative states in sessions, self-harming acts, or anti-conservative acts. These strategies initially enable the child, and later the adult, to survive and deal with emotions that would otherwise be perceived as overwhelming. During a child's development, these defense mechanisms in the parent are reactivated whenever the injured parts feel in danger or in situations in which the individual could re-experience the pain of the trauma.

Vicarious Trauma and Dissociation in the Context of the Parental Relationship

As we have discussed so far, exposure to dissociative content originating from the parent has devastating effects on the child, as it impairs the formation of a secure attachment between the child and their caregiver. Lack of secure attachment may also lead to the loss of primary self-regulation and interpersonal relationship skills (Cook et al., 2005). It is not so much the discomfort of the caregiver that harms the child, but rather the distress of the adult that can override or distract from the child's needs and negatively impact the child. Children may respond to this distress by avoiding or suppressing their feelings or behaviors, withdrawing from the caregiver, or focusing on the parent to alleviate the parent's distress. A caregiver who denies the child's experiences may cause a child to act as if the trauma did not occur, learn not to trust the primary caregiver, or fail to learn to use language to cope with obstacles. The concept of "complex trauma" in this perspective encompasses not only exposure to multiple traumatic experiences but also the impact of these experiences on short- and long-term outcomes (Herman, 1997). Traumatic experiences are not just about abuse or neglect but also other types of events, such as witnessing domestic violence, ethnic cleansing, or war. In recent years, several other clinical hypotheses have emerged that envision the transmission of dissociated traumatic content between parents and children in an implicit manner (Salberg, 2016; Bradfield, 2013). It has become increasingly clear that children's regulatory functions and stress response systems are closely linked to the relationship with the primary caregiver (Scheeringa & Zeanah, 2001).

So what happens when the parent is dissociative and the traumatic content of their life has not been integrated? How does this affect the child's adaptation to stress? If we use the model proposed by Scheeringa and Zeanah (2001), we may conceptualize the impact through moderation and compound effects. Regarding the moderation effect, a mother's relationship with the child, including her ability to interpret their signals and respond effectively to their needs, moderates the strength of the association between the distressing event (i.e., the independent variable) and the symptomatic reactions (or the dependent variable). Thus, we recognize an a priori expected negative effect between the traumatic event and the child's dissociative symptoms because the child directly experienced the event. However, the magnitude of the dissociative effect may be increased or decreased by the mother's reactions to the child. We also speak of "traumatization and vicarious dissociation" regarding a parent-child relationship in which the mother has usually been exposed to a traumatic event, which she then dissociates, but the child does not. Indeed, the mother's relationship with the child explains the impact of the traumatic event (which the child did not directly experience) and the child's symptoms. In this case, the specific impact on the child depends on the nature of the impact on the caregiver. Thus, without the parent-child relationship, there would be no impact of the trauma on the child.

The "compound effect" focuses on a combination of the moderation effect and the effect of traumatization and vicarious dissociation when both the caregiver and the child are traumatized and the dissociative behavior of one exacerbates that of the other. Children are directly affected by both the traumatic event and the impaired reactivity of the caregiver, in turn exacerbating symptomatology. In this case, reading their child's signals, understanding their behavior, and responding appropriately are impacted, and three specific patterns may emerge. The first is the withdrawn/unresponsive/unavailable response, so defined because acute or chronic PTSD can cause traumatized adults to be significantly less available to their children due to their own struggles. A child's dissociative response or symptoms may be due to a relatively recent event, while the parent's trauma is either chronic or further in the past. This pattern is more common in primary parents who have suffered from previous trauma themselves and for whom their children's traumas evoke painful memories and emotions that are avoided as a defense. In this situation, their child's symptoms will likely worsen without clinical intervention.

The second pattern is an overprotective/restrictive response after a child has been exposed to trauma. In this response, a parent will become restrictive and overprotective for fear that the child will be re-traumatized. Although this model may manifest in cases where the parent is also present and traumatized by the same experience as the child, it is also possible for the caregiver to be traumatized even if they do not witness the experience. In addition, feelings of guilt may arise if a parent was not present during the traumatic event or able to protect the child. In these cases, the parent may reconstruct an imaginary scene of the traumatized child and then relive this vision in an intrusive state.

The final response pattern is that of re-experiencing danger and fear. Some adults respond to traumatic experiences by becoming overwhelmed by memories of the trauma. Thus, if a parent is traumatized and dissociates, this response may re-traumatize the child. In this sense, a parent may become so overly anxious that they can no longer control their dissociative expressions or behaviors to protect the child (Scheeringa & Zeanah, 2001).

To summarize, caregivers who have had dysfunctional or traumatic relationships with their own caregivers are highly susceptible to experiencing difficulties in raising their children. If they have experienced complex childhood trauma, they may use dissociation as a defense against their own pain, making it difficult for them to respond in a way that is appropriate to the child's emotional state. In addition, they may view a child's behavioral responses to trauma as a threat or personal provocation rather than a reenactment of what happened to the child or a behavioral representation of what the child cannot express in words. The simultaneous presence of the need for closeness and the fear of closeness to their traumatized child may also trigger memories of loss, rejection, or abuse of the caregiver, thus impairing their parenting skills (Cook et al., 2005).

Treatment Considerations

To attend to the transgenerational transmission of trauma in child treatment, we suggest working in parallel with the child and the affected parent as part of a team-based approach. According to our clinical observations, such an approach includes one therapist who works with the child and another who works with the parent(s). Using the same approach and method to treatment to maintain consistency, the therapists must simultaneously work on the meaning of the symptoms for the child and the associated transgenerational, unresolved trauma of the parent. Parental involvement and cooperation are essential from the earliest stages of treatment (i.e., when useful information is gathered to help the therapist create an effective plan for treating the child's symptoms). To this end, it is useful to ask the parents questions about traumatic aspects of their own history on a transgenerational level from the outset. This ideally includes a narrative of the major events in their lives, the attachment dynamics that shaped the relationship with their primary caregivers in childhood, any traumatic events such as grief, violence, abuse, etc., and the caregiving relationship with the child and any difficulties in this area.

For the purposes of this chapter, the Adaptive Information Processing (Shapiro, 2013, 2018) model will be used as the modality that frames treatment. This is consistent and aligned with attachment theory and the transgenerational transmission of trauma to provide a framework for case conceptualization and to process the traumatic events. This parallel processing is effective in resolving symptoms related to the parent's unresolved trauma (Zaccagnino & Cussino, 2013).

Assessing Caregiver Attachment and Parenting Styles

The aim of collecting data on a parent's personal history is to identify possible traumatic events in their history that could be directly related to the difficulties reported by the child. A detailed history of the client's main current relationships, problem areas, and associated distress must be taken to gather specific information about the family of origin. To this end, specific questions may be asked to explore the client's current mental state concerning past attachment experiences through a description of episodes related to the relationships with their key attachment figures in childhood.

Globally, the IWM of attachment and level of reflective functioning are measured using the aforementioned AAI (George et al., 1985; Cloitre et al., 2002; Fonagy & Target, 1997). The AAI is a semi-structured interview that assesses discursive representations of early attachment relationships through questions designed to help the parent reflect on how the early attachment relationships have affected their adult personality, what experiences may have been a barrier to their growth, and an explanation and reflection on the motivations that they believe may have triggered their parents' behavior toward them. A section of the interview is devoted to a detailed description of grief and episodes perceived as traumatic by the parents. It is imperative to ask the parent for an account of these issues to identify possible signs of unresolved issues.

Some questions from the AAI, which are publicly available, explore questions about the client's history in the following manner:

1 I would like you to choose five adjectives or words that reflect your relationship with your mother/father, as far back as you can remember from your early childhood. Can you think of a memory or event that illustrates why you consider your relationship as _____? (Insert adjective chosen by client.)
2 What did you do as a child when you were upset/worried/had emotional problems? How did your parents react? Can you tell me about a particular incident?
3 What happened when you were physically hurt? Can you remember a specific incident?
4 Can you remember the first time you were separated from your parents? How did you react? How did they react? Can you remember other significant separations?
5 Did you ever feel rejected as a child? How old were you when you felt that way, and what did you do? Why do you think your parents behaved this way? Do you think they knew how you felt?
6 Did you experience the loss of a parent or other loved one as a child? Can you tell me anything about it? How old were you? How did you react? Did you expect it, or was it a sudden loss? Can you remember your feelings at the time? Have your feelings about this death changed over time?
7 Are there other experiences that you consider potentially traumatic?

Direct questions about the parent's life and attachment histories are essential, as they help the parent become aware of the extent to which the parent-child dynamics have affected the child's ability to interact and cope with problem areas. By analyzing these aspects in depth, the therapist can identify which parts of the parent's relationship history are most associated with the symptoms reported by the child. Starting with the most painful aspects related to the child's difficulties, the links between these dynamics and the parent's experiences and attachment history can be adaptively resolved. This is important because it makes it possible to identify the transgenerational dynamics of vulnerability most related to the symptoms reported by the child. In this section of questions, it is essential to explore the presence of possible difficult and/or traumatic life events that have taken place in the parents' lives and have never been told to the child. This may represent an untold story within the family system and, as such, needs to be explored, processed, and told to the child in a developmentally appropriate manner.

To assess the effectiveness of the parental care system, the Parent Development Interview (PDI) (a semi-structured clinical interview consisting of 45 questions [Aber et al., 1985]) may be used to gather additional relevant information about a parent's ability to articulate their emotional experience of their relationship with a particular child in a fluent and coherent manner (Aber et al., 1999; Sleed et al., 2020). Henderson et al.'s (2007) PDI Coding system was developed based on Slade et al.'s (1993) PDI Coding System. The rating scales are used to code three main features of parental representations: parental representation of own affective experience, parental representation of their child's affective experience, and global codes and parental state of mind in relation to the child. According to a validation study, the PDI relates to several relevant criteria, including attachment in adults and children (Anis et al., 2020; Slade et al., 2005). The interview questions explore the areas of vulnerability in the relationship history with the child, focusing on how moments of vulnerability are handled. It is important to explore with the parents the most difficult moments in caring for the children to identify the lines in the parent's life story that are directly linked to these narratives. Some questions include:

1 Can you describe yourself as a parent?
2 What do you enjoy most about being the parent of (child's name)?
3 What causes you the most pain or difficulty as the parent of (child's name)?
4 When do you feel safe as the parent of (child's name)?

This investigation phase is critical because it allows the parent to focus on managing the normal dynamics of caring for their child without focusing solely on managing symptoms. By asking specific questions regarding how the parent cares for the child, you can learn which moments within the relationship might be more difficult. It is essential to help the parent understand and validate the negative emotions they experience at some moments when caring for their child. By starting from these moments, you can retrace the life events that contributed most to triggering these difficulties.

Before beginning an in-depth assessment of the child's symptoms as part of gathering history, it is crucial to have a detailed overview of the child's developmental history. For this reason, it is also helpful to ask parents specific questions about the child's conception, pregnancy, and birth history and to inquire about their developmental milestones. To understand how to gather relevant and detailed information about the history of the child's difficulties, with particular attention to the life events that contributed to the onset of the disorder, see Chapter 13 focused on screening, assessment, and clinical interviewing.

Another essential aspect to investigate with the parent is the onset and course of the symptoms reported by the child. The purpose of this is to try and understand the life events that have shaped the child's life and the lives of those around them, both before and after the emergence of symptoms, to gain a clearer view of the triggering event that leads to the onset of symptoms. It is useful to explore not only the specific characteristics of the child's difficulties with the parents but also the coping strategies used by the parent and the challenges experienced in this area. Specific questions may be asked about the presence of similar symptoms in the parent's family history across generations to gain a more detailed insight into the dynamics that structure the child's difficulties.

When working with parents, it is crucial to understand the emotions that get cued in the parents when the child's symptoms emerge. The areas where the child faces difficulties can elucidate important information about the role of parent-child dynamics and interactions. Questions may include the following:

1 What aspect is the most difficult for you when you are trying to deal with your child's symptoms? How do you usually behave when your child is showing these symptoms?
2 How do you feel when your child is behaving this way? What do you say about yourself then? What do you say when your child behaves like this?
3 If you imagine that your child is trying to communicate something by showing the symptom, what do you think they are trying to communicate?
4 What helps you most when your child's symptoms occur?
5 What causes you more difficulties in these moments instead? What would you need to cope with it?
6 What do you think could be useful for the child in these moments? What could help them in these moments? What makes it difficult for you to help them in these moments?

Based on this information, therapists may help the parent(s) better understand the areas of vulnerability in their life that are most associated with the child's symptoms using EMDR procedures and techniques designed to elicit early memory networks from which symptoms are manifesting. Therapists may also ask questions about specific factors that perpetuate symptoms within the larger family structure to better understand the meaning of the child's symptom within the family system. Some questions may include:

1 Why should your child keep the symptom?
2 What are you afraid of losing if your child gets better? Do you have any fears or worries?

Targeted psychoeducational work with the parent ideally follows to help parents better understand the deeper meaning of the child's symptoms and the extent to which they meet the parent's specific needs. This work is crucial in helping the child and their parents break the cycle perpetuating the symptom.

Treatment Planning with Parents

Starting with the areas of vulnerability arising from the parent's history, the relationship difficulties with the child, and the coping difficulties with their symptoms, we use EMDR therapy procedures to map the memories most directly related to each line in the parent's history. It is useful to dwell on the emotional experiences, the dysfunctional cognitive schemas, and the physical sensations experienced during these periods to stimulate the implicitly stored memory networks containing dysfunctionally stored trauma material. In this way, we can help the parent recognize analogies and connections between the past and the present. A therapeutic plan that works in partnership with parents must include two distinct phases: (1) understanding and processing, together with the parents, any difficult and/or traumatic memories related to the child's life history and the onset, history, and maintenance of the symptoms reported by the child, and (2) constructing narratives about the traumatic events in the parent's and child's lives that are more meaningful and related to the child's symptoms. The following guidelines should define the treatment plan:

1 **The precipitating event:** In therapeutic work with parents, it is crucial to address the precipitating event (if any) that triggered the onset of the symptoms in the child. It is essential to remember that the event that triggers the symptoms in the child can be found both in the parent's and child's life history. Therefore, it is helpful to start from the memories reported by the parents during the history-taking phase and to identify all related episodes in their life history. If it is not possible to identify the precipitating event, start from the parent's experience of the child's difficulties and use float back to identify any directly related targets in their life history.
3 **Big "T" Traumas:** If there are major traumas in the parent's or child's life history, you must first process these using the standard EMDR protocol.
4 **Small "t" traumas in the parent's life and the relationship history with the child:** In this phase of the therapy plan, it is essential to work on all the goals related to the difficult moments in the parent's attachment history. This is because they are directly related to the care modalities the parent can use in their relationship with the child. The traumas that are directly linked to the triggering event are then processed. All difficult moments in the parent's life history are then identified, the significance of which is usually linked to the critical core of the triggering event.
5 **Goals related to the symptoms or disorder:** At this point, all goals directly related to the child's difficulties must be addressed, as well as goals related to the impact of the difficulties on the relationship, following a chronological order until all goals related to the child's symptoms have been addressed.

Identification of Resources

The therapist's goal is to help parents identify the resources (especially relational resources) that can help them manage the relational dynamic with the child and their difficulties. It is essential to understand what may be useful for parents to manage the difficult moments and the moments when they also felt skilled in other areas of their lives or in managing the child's symptoms. These can be strengthened in appropriate ways. Some questions therapists may ask include:

1 Imagine that your child is feeling better. What would be the most important aspect for you?
2 What would help you support your child?
3 What were the positive moments when you were feeling well together?
4 What would you need to cope with your child's symptoms at this moment?

Working with Parts

The functioning of symptoms and the specific effects on the client's physical and mental health must be explored in depth. When we find ourselves stuck in the child's therapy, EMDR work with different parts of the parent's self is essential. Working with the parent in this way to develop knowledge about the different aspects of the self that may be involved in maintaining the child's symptoms is done in the Preparation Phase of EMDR therapy. It may include parent-centered interventions that support addressing the child's difficulties and promote well-being while preventing the families from dropping out of treatment. This includes explaining concepts to the client related to what "parts of the self" are and how parts of the self play a fundamental role in one's history and in the history of their child's disorder. To this end, the dysfunctional dynamics that characterize the difficulties reported by the parents in their relationship with their child must also be explained, analyzing in depth the dynamics of activation and deactivation of the attachment and care systems of both the parent and the child, and highlighting the role of possible traumatic events in the development of difficulties in this area. Psychoeducation is essential to enable the parents to increase awareness of their own functioning dynamics and to help them explore and apply new, more appropriate coping strategies for dealing with disruptive events. In addition, it is essential to explain to parents how the difficulties related to attachment/caregiving dynamics affect the quality of their caregiving and the possible occurrence of the symptoms so that they can reflect on these aspects. By helping parents understand what "intergenerational transmission of trauma" means, one can clarify the impact that some events in the parent's life may have had on the child's quality of life and the onset of the reported difficulties.

Developing a trusting relationship between the therapist and the client is essential for a parent to feel welcome and able to take in and establish a shared knowledge about the specific aspects of their functioning and symptoms that may play an important role in maintaining the child's symptoms. In some situations, however, working effectively with a parent may not be possible because their parts of self are so activated to protect that therapeutic work is prevented. It can be helpful to support the parent in reflecting on the meaning they have assigned to the symptom and if a part of them is trying to play a protective role toward the child and themselves in this way. When the caregiver talks about parts of the self that are activated, reference may be made, for example, to:

1 Parts that protect the parent from coming into contact with their traumatic memories through the child's symptom.
2 Parts that express the unspoken and delegitimized suffering of the parent through the child's symptom.
3 Parts that are maintaining a secondary advantage within the current family's system through the child's symptom.

When the presence of one or more parts of the parent is highlighted, the therapist must recognize them and work to understand the meaning behind these manifestations. These may appear dysfunctional, but they must be understood and accepted as attempts by the parent to protect themselves. The dissociative table/meeting place may be used to identify parts (Fraser, 1991; González & Mosquera, 2015; Zaccagnino, 2017, 2022). Once identified, interventions that offer Recognition, Approach, Acceptance, Visualization, Empathy/Attunement, Reassurance, Understanding, Legitimization, Validation, and Valorization may be used (Zaccagnino, 2022). Through this process, the therapist supports the client in connecting internally to their parts to engage in questioning and curiosity, alongside bilateral stimulation, as appropriate. The therapist must differentiate the objectives of the work, depending on the part activated, so that the interventions are as effective as possible. In particular, it is good to remember that we are trying to work toward a new frame of care and nurturing with wounded parts while developing cooperation and an alliance with protective parts (Zaccagnino, 2017, 2022). We endeavor to support the adult self to maintain orientation to the security of present time and space while working with the other parts of self, remembering that there is an adult that can overcome past traumas and build the skills to cope with everyday life in the present. The therapist working from a welcoming and non-judgmental stance will help the protective parts of the parents so they can feel accepted. Only after the work of co-awareness, welcoming, and acknowledgment can you ask these parts specific questions to understand their story. You can then ask each of them where they came from and where they learned to use this particular defense strategy. By asking specific questions about when the part has been present, you will get a clearer and more complete view of the precipitating factors underlying the child's symptoms. Some questions to probe this area are as follows:

1 Is there a part of you that wants to say something when your child is in trouble? What does this part want to say?
2 When did this part form? What was happening in your life at that moment?

In this way, parents can understand that the activation of this part is functional and that its goal is to maintain the child's symptom as a modality to protect the traumatized parts of the parent's self. To understand the role played by the part that is activated in these contexts, it is essential to start from the moment the child shows the symptom and ask the parents:

1 Is there a part that fears something if the child's symptom disappears?
2 Does this part feel that it can only communicate through the child's symptom?
3 Is there a part of you that finds it difficult to let go of the child's symptom? Is this part afraid of something? Why?
4 Is this part somehow protecting you and your child? Does it allow (you and your child) to act? Does it prevent (you and your child) from acting?

Please note: To help the protective part of the parent feel legitimate and welcome, it might be important to ask the part directly (through the adult part of the client) to tell their personal story from their perspective. In this way, you can access information that would not come up in any other way.

Conclusion

In summary, working with the parent's parts of self is of fundamental importance when working with traumatized and dissociative children or when the therapist encounters a blockage during the various phases of the child's therapy. In particular, it emphasizes the importance of welcoming, validating, and understanding the function of a parent's parts of self, their history, and their goals in order to integrate them and obtain help from them in processing traumas, starting with those related to attachment, which have generated suffering in the subject and can keep symptoms active (Zaccagnino, 2022).

References

Aber, J. L., Belsky, J., Slade, A., & Crnic, K. (1999). Stability and change in mothers' representations of their relationship with their toddlers. *Developmental Psychology, 35*(4), 1038.
Aber, J. L., Slade, A., Berger, B., Bresgi, I., & Kaplan, M. (1985). *The parent development interview* [Unpublished manuscript]. Barnard College.
Ainsworth, M. D. S., Blehar, M. C., Waters, E., & Wall, S. N. (1978a). *Patterns of attachment: A psychological study of the strange situation.* Lawrence Erlbaum.
Ainsworth, M. D. S., Blehar, M. C., Waters, E., & Wall, S. (1978b). *Patterns of attachment: A psychological study of the strange situation.* Psychology Press.
American Psychiatric Association. (2013). *Diagnostic and statistical manual of mental disorders* (5th ed.). American Psychiatric Association Publishing. https://doi.org/10.1176/appi.books.9780890425596
Anis, L., Perez, G., Benzies, K. M., Ewashen, C., Hart, M., & Letourneau, N. (2020). Convergent validity of three measures of reflective function: Parent development interview, parental reflective function questionnaire, and reflective function questionnaire. *Frontiers in Psychology, 11*, 574719. https://doi.org/10.3389/fpsyg.2020.574719
Bar-Haim, Y., Sutton, D. B., Fox, N. A., & Marvin, R. S. (2000). Stability and change of attachment at 14, 24, and 58 months of age: Behavior, representation, and life events. *Journal of Child Psychology and Psychiatry, 41*(3), 381–388. https://doi.org/10.1111/1469-7610.00622
Booker, J. A., Fivush, R., Graci, M. E., Heitz, H., Hudak, L. A., Jovanovic, T., Rothbaum, B. O., & Stevens, J. S. (2020). Longitudinal changes in trauma narratives over the first year and associations with coping and mental health. *Journal of Affective Disorders, 272*, 116–124. https://doi.org/10.1016/j.jad.2020.04.009
Bowlby, J. (1969). *Attachment and loss* (Vol. 1). Basic Books.
Bowlby, J. (1973). *Attachment and loss* (Vol. 2). Hogarth Press.
Bradfield, B. C. (2013). The intergenerational transmission of trauma as a disruption of the dialogical self. *Journal of Trauma & Dissociation, 14*(4), 390–403. https://doi.org/10.1080/15299732.2012.742480

Button, S., Pianta, R. C., & Marvin, R. S. (2001). Mothers' representations of relationships with their children: Relations with parenting behavior, mother characteristics, and child disability status. *Social Development, 10*(4), 455–472. https://doi.org/10.1111/1467-9507.00175

Cassidy, J. (1988). Child-mother attachment and the self in six-year-olds. *Child Development, 59*(1), 121–134. https://doi.org/10.2307/1130394

Cassidy, J., & Shaver, P. R. (Eds.). (1999). *Handbook of attachment: Theory, research, and clinical applications.* The Guilford Press.

Civilotti, C., Cussino, M., Callerame, C., Fernandez, I., & Zaccagnino, M. (2019). Changing the adult state of mind with respect to attachment: An exploratory study of the role of EMDR psychotherapy. *Journal of EMDR Practice and Research, 13*(3), 176–186. https://doi.org/10.1891/1933-3196.13.3.176

Cloitre, M., Koenen, K. C., Cohen, L. R., & Han, H. (2002). Skills training in affective and interpersonal regulation followed by exposure: A phase-based treatment for PTSD related to childhood abuse. *Journal of Consulting and Clinical Psychology, 70*(5), 1067–1074. https://doi.org/10.1037/0022-006X.70.5.1067

Connors, M. E. (2011). Attachment theory: A "secure base" for psychotherapy integration. *Journal of Psychotherapy Integration, 21*(3), 348–362. https://doi.org/10.1037/a0025460

Cook, A., Spinazzola, J., Ford, J., Lanktree, C., Blaustein, M., Cloitre, M., DeRosa, R., Hubbard, R., Kagan, R., Liautaud, J., Mallah, K., Olafson, E., & van der Kolk, B. (2005). Complex trauma in children and adolescents. *Psychiatric Annals, 35*(5), 390–398. https://doi.org/10.3928/00485713-20050501-05

Crespo, M., & Fernández-Lansac, V. (2016). Memory and narrative of traumatic events: A literature review. *Psychological Trauma: Theory, Research, Practice, and Policy, 8*(2), 149–156. https://doi.org/10.1037/tra0000041

Damis, L. F. (2022). The role of implicit memory in the development and recovery from trauma-related disorders. *NeuroSci, 3*(1), 63–88. https://doi.org/10.3390/neurosci3010005

Daniel, S. I. F. (2006). Adult attachment patterns and individual psychotherapy: A review. *Clinical Psychology Review, 26*(8), 968–984. https://doi.org/10.1016/j.cpr.2006.02.001

De Wolff, M. S., & van Ijzendoorn, M. H. (1997). Sensitivity and attachment: A meta-analysis on parental antecedents of infant attachment. *Child Development, 68*(4), 571–591. https://doi.org/10.1111/j.1467-8624.1997.tb04218.x

Farina, B., & Imperatori, C. (2023). Are traumatic disintegration, detachment, and dissociation separate pathogenic processes related to attachment trauma? A working hypothesis for clinicians and researchers. *Psychopathology*, 1–12. https://doi.org/10.1159/000535191

Farina, B. & Liotti, G. (2013). Does a dissociative psychopathological dimension exist? A review on dissociative processes and symptoms in developmental trauma spectrum disorders. *Clinical Neuropsychiatry, 10*(1), 11–18.

Fonagy, P., & Bateman, A. (2008). The development of borderline personality disorder—A mentalizing model. *Journal of Personality Disorders, 22*(1), 4–21. https://doi.org/10.1521/pedi.2008.22.1.4

Fonagy, P., & Campbell, C. (2016). Attachment theory and mentalization. In A. Elliot & J. Prager (Eds.), *The Routledge handbook of psychoanalysis in the social sciences and humanities* (pp. 115–131). Routledge.

Fonagy, P., & Target, M. (1997). Attachment and reflective function: Their role in self-organization. *Development and Psychopathology, 9*(4), 679–700. https://doi.org/10.1017/S0954579497001399

Forgash, C., & Copeley, M. (2014). *EMDR e ego state therapy: Il trattamento del trauma e della dissociazione* [EMDR and ego state therapy: The treatment of trauma and dissociation]. Ferrari Sinibaldi.

Fraser, G. A. (1991). The dissociative table technique: A strategy for working with ego states in dissociative disorders and ego-state therapy. *Dissociation, 4*(4), 205–213.

George, C., Kaplan, N., & Main, M. (1985). *The adult attachment interview* [Unpublished manuscript]. University of California at Berkeley.

George, C., & Solomon, J. (1996). Representational models of relationships: Links between caregiving and attachment. *Infant Mental Health Journal, 17*(3), 198–216. https://doi.org/10.1002/(SICI)1097-0355(199623)17:3<198::AID-IMHJ2>3.0.CO;2-L

Girme, Y. U., Jones, R. E., Fleck, C., Simpson, J. A., & Overall, N. C. (2021). Infants' attachment insecurity predicts attachment-relevant emotion regulation strategies in adulthood. *Emotion, 21*(2), 260–272. https://doi.org/10.1037/emo0000721

González, A., & Mosquera, D. (2015). *EMDR e dissociazione: L'approccio progressivo* [EMDR and dissociation: The progressive application]. Giovanni Fioriti editore.

Gruda, D., Berrios, R. A., Kafetsios, K. G., & McCleskey, J. A. (2022). Time after time: Attachment orientations and impression formation in initial and longer-term team interactions. *Frontiers in Psychology, 13*, 882162. https://doi.org/10.3389/fpsyg.2022.882162

Henderson, K., Steele, M., & Hillman, S. (2007). *Experience of parenting coding system (ExPI coding system)* [Unpublished manuscript]. Anna Freud Centre, University College London.

Herman, J. L. (1997). *Trauma and recovery: The aftermath of violence—From domestic abuse to political terror*. BasicBooks.

Hesse, E., & Main, M. (1999). Second-generation effects of unresolved trauma in nonmaltreating parents: Dissociated, frightened, and threatening parental behavior. *Psychoanalytic Inquiry, 19*(4), 481–540. https://doi.org/10.1080/07351699909534265

Hesse, E., & Main, M. (2000). Disorganized infant, child, and adult attachment: Collapse in behavioral and attentional strategies. *Journal of the American Psychoanalytic Association, 48*(4), 1097–1127. https://doi.org/10.1177/00030651000480041101

Hesse, E., & Main, M. (2006). Frightened, threatening, and dissociative parental behavior in low-risk samples: Description, discussion, and interpretations. *Development and Psychopathology, 18*(2), 309–343. https://doi.org/10.1017/S0954579406060172

Iyengar, U., Kim, S., Martinez, S., Fonagy, P., & Strathearn, L. (2014). Unresolved trauma in mothers: Intergenerational effects and the role of reorganization. *Frontiers in Psychology, 5*, 966. https://doi.org/10.3389/fpsyg.2014.00966

Jacobvitz, D., Leon, K., & Hazen, N. (2006). Does expectant mothers' unresolved trauma predict frightened/frightening maternal behavior? Risk and protective factors. *Development and Psychopathology, 18*(2), 363–379. https://doi.org/10.1017/S0954579406060196

Kim, S., Fonagy, P., Allen, J., & Strathearn, L. (2014). Mothers' unresolved trauma blunts amygdala response to infant distress. *Social Neuroscience, 9*(4), 352–363. https://doi.org/10.1080/17470919.2014.896287

Kondo-Ikemura, K., Behrens, K. Y., Umemura, T., & Nakano, S. (2018). Japanese mothers' prebirth Adult Attachment Interview predicts their infants' response to the Strange Situation Procedure: The strange situation in Japan revisited three decades later. *Developmental Psychology, 54*(11), 2007–2015. https://doi.org/10.1037/dev0000577

Kostova, Z., & Matanova, V. L. (2024). Transgenerational trauma and attachment. *Frontiers in Psychology, 15*, 1362561. https://doi.org/10.3389/fpsyg.2024.1362561

Lanius, U. F., Paulsen, S. L., & Corrigan, F. M. (Eds.). (2014). *Neurobiology and treatment of traumatic dissociation: Towards an embodied self*. Springer Publishing Company.

Lee Raby, K., Cicchetti, D., Carlson, E. A., Egeland, B., & Andrew Collins, W. (2013). Genetic contributions to continuity and change in attachment security: A prospective, longitudinal investigation from infancy to young adulthood. *The Journal of Child Psychology and Psychiatry, 54*(11), 1223–1230. https://doi.org/10.1111/jcpp.12093

Lev–Wiesel, R. (2007). Intergenerational transmission of trauma across three generations: A preliminary study. *Qualitative Social Work, 6*(1), 75–94. https://doi.org/10.1177/1473325007074167

Liotti, G. (2004). Trauma, dissociation, and disorganized attachment: Three strands of a single braid. *Psychotherapy: Theory, Research, Practice, Training, 41*(4), 472–486. https://doi.org/10.1037/0033-3204.41.4.472

Liotti, G. (2006). A model of dissociation based on attachment theory and research. *Journal of Trauma & Dissociation, 7*(4), 55–73. https://doi.org/10.1300/J229v07n04_04

Liotti, G., & Farina, B. (2011). *Sviluppi traumatici: Eziopatogenesi, clinica e terapia della dimensione dissociativa* [Traumatic developments: Etiopathogenesis, clinic and therapy of the dissociative dimension]. Raffaello Cortina Editore.

Lyons-Ruth, K., Yellin, C., Melnick, S., & Atwood, G. (2005). Expanding the concept of unresolved mental states: Hostile/helpless states of mind on the Adult Attachment Interview are associated with disrupted mother–infant communication and infant disorganization. *Development and Psychopathology, 17*(1), 1–23. https://doi.org/10.1017/S0954579405050017

Madigan, S., Moran, G., & Pederson, D. R. (2006). Unresolved states of mind, disorganized attachment relationships, and disrupted interactions of adolescent mothers and their infants. *Developmental Psychology, 42*(2), 293–304. https://doi.org/10.1037/0012-1649.42.2.293

Madrid, A., Skolek, S., & Shapiro, F. (2006). Repairing failures in bonding through EMDR. *Clinical Case Studies, 5*(4), 271–286. https://doi.org/10.1177/1534650104267403

Main, M., Kaplan, N., & Cassidy, J. (1985). Security in infancy, childhood, and adulthood: A move to the level of representation. *Monographs of the Society for Research in Child Development, 50*(1/2), 66–104. https://doi.org/10.2307/3333827

Mair, H. (2021). Attachment safety in psychotherapy. *Counselling and Psychotherapy Research, 21*(3), 710–718. https://doi.org/10.1002/capr.12370

Mallinckrodt, B. (2010). The psychotherapy relationship as attachment: Evidence and implications. *Journal of Social and Personal Relationships, 27*(2), 262–270. https://doi.org/10.1177/0265407509360905

McConnell, M., & Moss, E. (2011). Attachment across the life span: Factors that contribute to stability and change. *Australian Journal of Educational & Developmental Psychology, 11*, 60–77.

McNally, R. J. (2022). Are memories of sexual trauma fragmented? *Memory, 30*(1), 26–30. https://doi.org/10.1080/09658211.2020.1871023

Moss, E., Cyr, C., Bureau, J.-F., Tarabulsy, G. M., & Dubois-Comtois, K. (2005). Stability of attachment during the preschool period. *Developmental Psychology, 41*(5), 773–783. https://doi.org/10.1037/0012-1649.41.5.773

Moulds, M. L., & Bryant, R. A. (2005). Traumatic memories in acute stress disorder: An analysis of narratives before and after treatment. *Clinical Psychologist, 9*(1), 10–14. https://doi.org/10.1080/13284200500116971

Peterson, C., & Seligman, M. E. P. (1983). Learned helplessness and victimization. *Journal of Social Issues, 39*(2), 103–116. https://doi.org/10.1111/j.1540-4560.1983.tb00143.x

Risan, P., Milne, R., & Binder, P.-E. (2020). Trauma narratives: Recommendations for investigative interviewing. *Psychiatry, Psychology and Law, 27*(4), 678–694. https://doi.org/10.1080/13218719.2020.1742237

Salberg, J. (2016). The texture of traumatic attachment: Presence and ghostly absence in transgenerational transmission. In J. Salberg & S. Grand (Eds.), *Wounds of history* (pp. 97–120). Routledge. https://doi.org/10.4324/9781315751061

Saunders, R., Jacobvitz, D., Zaccagnino, M., Beverung, L. M., & Hazen, N. (2011). Pathways to earned-security: The role of alternative support figures. *Attachment & Human Development, 13*(4), 403–420. https://doi.org/10.1080/14616734.2011.584405

Scheeringa, M. S., & Zeanah, C. H. (2001). A relational perspective on PTSD in early childhood. *Journal of Traumatic Stress, 14*(4), 799–815. https://doi.org/10.1023/A:1013002507972

Schore, A. N. (2002). The neurobiology of attachment and early personality organization. *Journal of Prenatal & Perinatal Psychology & Health, 16*(3), 249–264.

Schore, J. R., & Schore, A. N. (2008). Modern attachment theory: The central role of affect regulation in development and treatment. *Clinical Social Work Journal, 36*(1), 9–20. https://doi.org/10.1007/s10615-007-0111-7

Schwarzer, N.-H., Nolte, T., Fonagy, P., & Gingelmaier, S. (2021). Mentalizing and emotion regulation: Evidence from a nonclinical sample. *International Forum of Psychoanalysis, 30*(1), 34–45. https://doi.org/10.1080/0803706X.2021.1873418

Shapiro, F. (2013). *Getting past your past: Take control of your life with self-help techniques from EMDR therapy*. Rodale Press.

Shapiro, F. (2018). *Eye movement desensitization and reprocessing (EMDR) therapy: Basic principles, protocols, and procedures* (3rd ed.). Guilford Press.

Siegel, D. J. (1999). *The developing mind: Toward a neurobiology of interpersonal experience*. Guilford Press.

Slade, A. (1999). Representation, symbolization, and affect regulation in the concomitant treatment of a mother and child: Attachment theory and child psychotherapy. *Psychoanalytic Inquiry, 19*(5), 797–830. https://doi.org/10.1080/07351699909534277

Slade, A., Aber, J. L., Cohen, L., Fiorello, J., Meyer, J., DeSear, P., & Waller, S. (1993). *Parent Development Interview coding system* [Unpublished manuscript]. University of New York.

Slade, A., Grienenberger, J., Bernbach, E., Levy, D., & Locker, A. (2005). Maternal reflective functioning, attachment, and the transmission gap: A preliminary study. *Attachment & Human Development, 7*(3), 283–298. https://doi.org/10.1080/14616730500245880

Sleed, M., Slade, A., & Fonagy, P. (2020). Reflective functioning on the Parent Development Interview: Validity and reliability in relation to socio-demographic factors. *Attachment & Human Development, 22*(3), 310–331. https://doi.org/10.1080/14616734.2018.1555603

van der Hart, O., Groenendijk, M., Gonzalez, A., Mosquera, D., & Solomon, R. (2013). Dissociation of the personality and EMDR therapy in complex trauma-related disorders: Applications in the stabilization phase. *Journal of EMDR Practice and Research, 7*(2), 81–94. https://doi.org/10.1891/1933-3196.7.2.81

van der Hart, O., Nijenhuis, E. R. S., & Steele, K. (2011). *Fantasmi nel sé: Trauma e trattamento della dissociazione strutturale* [Ghosts in the self: Trauma and the treatment of structural dissociation]. Raffaello Cortina Editore.

van der Kolk, B. A., Pynoos, R. S., Cicchetti, D., Cloitre, M., D'Andrea, W., Ford, J. D., Lieberman, A. F., Putnam, F. W., Saxe, G., Spinazzola, J., Stolbach, B. C., & Teicher, M. (2009). *Proposal to include a developmental trauma disorder diagnosis for children and adolescents in DSM-V* [Unpublished manuscript]. https://complextrauma.org/wp-content/uploads/2019/03/Complex-Trauma-Resource-3-Joseph-Spinazzola.pdf

Waters, E., Weinfield, N. S., & Hamilton, C. E. (2000). The stability of attachment security from infancy to adolescence and early adulthood: General discussion. *Child Development, 71*(3), 703–706. https://doi.org/10.1111/1467-8624.00179

Weinfield, N. S., Whaley, G. J. L., & Egeland, B. (2004). Continuity, discontinuity, and coherence in attachment from infancy to late adolescence: Sequelae of organization and disorganization. *Attachment & Human Development, 6*(1), 73–97. https://doi.org/10.1080/14616730310001659566

Wesselmann, D., & Potter, A. E. (2009). Change in adult attachment status following treatment with EMDR: Three case studies. *Journal of EMDR Practice and Research, 3*(3), 178–191. https://doi.org/10.1891/1933-3196.3.3.178

Yehuda, R., & Lehrner, A. (2018). Intergenerational transmission of trauma effects: Putative role of epigenetic mechanisms. *World Psychiatry, 17*(3), 243–257. https://doi.org/10.1002/wps.20568

Zaccagnino, M. (2017). *Nuove prospettive nella cura dei disturbi alimentari: Il ruolo dell'attaccamento nel lavoro clinico con EMDR* [New perspectives in the treatment of eating disorders: The role of attachment in clinical work with EMDR]. FrancoAngeli Editore.

Zaccagnino, M. (2022). *Terapia EMDR: Attaccamento, concettualizzazione del caso e lavoro con le parti del Sé* [EMDR therapy: Attachment, case conceptualization and working with the parts of the Self]. Erickson.

Zaccagnino M., & Cussino M. (2013). EMDR and parenting: A clinical case. *Journal of EMDR Practice and Research, 7*(3), 154–166. https://doi.org/10.1891/1933-3196.7.3.154

Zaccagnino, M., Cussino, M., Saunders, R., Jacobvitz, D., & Veglia, F. (2014). Alternative caregiving figures and their role on adult attachment representations. *Clinical Psychology & Psychotherapy, 21*(3), 276–287. https://doi.org/10.1002/cpp.1828

38
INTERSECTING TIMELINES
Generational Perspectives

Rebeca Chow

Introduction

Generations play a significant role in shaping the world in which children grow up. Through *intergenerational transmission*, each generation carries with it the experiences of the previous generation. Every cohort consists of unique social markers—a set of distinct cultural, historical, and societal influences that shape the attitudes, behaviors, and worldviews of each generation (Kalkhurst, 2018). To effectively meet clients' needs across generations, therapists need to acknowledge the significant impact of distinct values, experiences, and expectations that shape each generation's daily experiences.

Strauss and Howe's (1991) generational theory states that generations occur in a four-stage facing cycle called *turning*, a change in society and culture. As these turnings unfold, they shape the collective experiences of the generations that come of age during them, influencing the adoption of corresponding patterns within these unique cultural contexts. Many authors (Drugas, 2022; Strauss & Howe, 1991) identify four turnings: (1) high turning (the first of the generation with an established general consensus about the direction of society; currently baby boomers), (2) awakening (the generation that challenges the social order, looking for new authentic self; currently Gen X and millennials), (3) unraveling (the generation with strong development of individualism, currently Gen Z), and (4) crisis (the generation that establishes a new feeling of belonging to a large social group, currently Generation Alpha).

Families have evolved to encompass a remarkable span of five distinct generations, each contributing to the development of the next generation. Research identifies the current generations as baby boomers, Generation X, millennials, Generation Z, and Generation Alpha (McCrindle & Fell, 2021; Twenge, 2023). This expanded generational time frame indicates that contemporary families frequently encompass grandparents, parents, children, and grandchildren, all coexisting within the same familial structure. This multigenerational makeup offers a wealth of diverse experiences but also presents the challenge of navigating differences across generations, cultural traditions, and potentially traumatic experiences (Swanzen, 2018). According to the *Diagnostic and Statistical Manual of Mental Disorders 5-TR* (American Psychiatric Association, 2022), individuals can experience trauma in four ways: (1) by directly experiencing a traumatic event, (2) by witnessing a traumatic event, (3) by learning of a violent or accidental traumatic event that happened to a close family member, or (4) from extreme or repeated exposure to harsh details of a traumatic event. Thus, intergenerational transmission acknowledges that shared experiences are passed down from one generation to the next and serve as a cultural continuum that helps maintain and evolve societal norms (Narayan et al., 2021). However, it also means that the traumas, inequalities, and injustices endured by previous generations can leave lasting imprints on the collective consciousness of the next generation's mental health. Yet, research shows that not all generational groups will experience traumatic stress proportionately (Buffel et al., 2021). From this perspective, it is beneficial for therapists to recognize the distinct characteristics of each generation, social markers, mental health challenges, and parenting styles for tailoring interventions that are sensitive to the specific needs and cultural contexts of the individuals they are working with, ultimately fostering more effective and empathetic therapeutic relationships.

Baby Boomers

The baby boomer generation was born between 1946 and 1964 (Kalkhurst, 2018). Baby boomers grew up in a time of much social change and innovation, and an uncertain future (Twenge, 2023). Baby boomers represent most of the current grandparent population, and a large segment of this population is considering retirement or actively retiring (Fingerman et al., 2020). Some of the primary social markers for this generation are the Cold War, the Vietnam War, the Civil Rights Movement, the Women's Liberation Movement, and the anti-war protests of the 1960s and 1970s, which left a lasting impact on their internal sense of safety as they witnessed war, racial injustice, and political unrest (Kalkhurst, 2018). Research suggests that some baby boomers struggle with anxiety, depression, and post-traumatic stress disorder (PTSD) as a result of the traumas they have observed or personally endured, which negatively affected their parenting ability and increased the risk of transmitting the same mental health struggles to the next generation (Narayan et al., 2021).

Baby boomers were raised in households characterized by traditional family structures, and they frequently uphold values such as family unity, responsibility, and defined gender roles. These beliefs can sometimes lead to conflicts when connecting with their adult Gen Xer and millennial children, who may have different perspectives and expectations regarding these matters (Evrensel-İnanç et al., 2022).

One prominent aspect of baby boomers as parents was the strong emphasis on education. While this instilled a sense of ambition and drive for success, it also created pressure to meet high academic expectations. According to Narayan et al. (2021), Gen X and millennials report higher levels of professional stress anxiety, feelings of inadequacy, and fear of failure that are rooted in this childhood relationship. In addition, baby boomers, influenced by their own experiences of cultural revolution, often sought to create open and communicative family environments. This encouraged emotional expression and empathy among their children; however, current social trends like the use of social media and smartphones for connection create conflicts among generations (Reese et al., 2022). For instance, a baby boomer might become visibly angry or judgmental of their adult Gen X or millennial children choosing to use technology when connecting with their own Gen Zer or Alpha children. Something as simple as a text during a family dinner can lead to a tense exchange between the two generations, with the baby boomer feeling disrespected and dismissed and the adult child feeling anxious from a clash of values and expectations regarding family interactions in the digital age.

Generation X

Generation X was born between 1965 and 1980 (Kalkhurst, 2018). Generation X, often referred to as the "latchkey generation," "baby busters," Gen X, and/or Gen Xers, represents a large portion of the parents raising millennials, Gen Z, and Gen Alpha. This generation grew up in a rapidly changing world characterized by shifting family dynamics, economic volatility, and technological advancement (Fingerman et al., 2020). The social markers for this generation were the economic downturns, the AIDS epidemic, the fall of the Berlin Wall, and the end of the Vietnam War (Kalkhurst, 2018). These events resulted in fragmented family experiences, with some individuals grappling with the emotional toll of parental separation or disconnection (Kurz, 2020). Research suggests that Gen Xers postponed marriage and parenthood, opting for education and career development first, due to their upbringing in households affected by divorce and dual-income parenting (Marzilli et al., 2021). One common manifestation of this childhood experience in adults of this generation is difficulty forming and maintaining stable relationships for fear of abandonment, and withdrawing to protect themselves from potential hurt (Turkle, 2017). In addition, this generation is characterized by higher levels of anxiety, depression, and social comparison; as Gen Xers became digital adaptors, these levels increased further (Twenge, 2023).

Gen Xers, the first generation to grapple with the stressors of advancing technology, face unique challenges related to online privacy, screen time, and the intricacies of social media. These experiences, combined with their own attachment backgrounds, have shaped enduring patterns established during childhood, such as trust, emotional intimacy, and effective communication (Fingerman et al., 2020). Moreover, when Gen Xers struggle with complex trauma, these technological stressors and attachment-influenced relationship dynamics can further complicate their journey toward healing and recovery. For instance, as a generation, they value independence and self-sufficiency, which may stem from experiences of coming home to empty houses due to parents' work schedules. Understanding and addressing these intersections can assist in providing effective support and intervention for this generation.

As parents, Gen Xers opted to address their own childhood experiences of loneliness by ensuring their children did not grow up unsupervised or lacking support, often by tightly scheduling their activities (Narayan et al., 2021). This generational context, coupled with the challenges of modern life, has contributed to a concerning increase in mental health issues among Gen X parents, finding themselves juggling demanding careers, the pressures of raising families, and caring for aging parents, leading to high levels of stress and burnout (Twenge, 2023). Furthermore, they grew up in an era when mental health awareness was limited, which can make it difficult for some to seek help for themselves and/or their children.

Generation Y

Generation Y, often referred to as millennials, represents a dynamic and influential cohort born roughly between 1981 and 2000 (Kalkhurst, 2018). This generation is in the key family forming life state, raising the two latest generations, Gen Z and Gen Alpha. Gen Y has been shaped by the transformative forces of the digital age, witnessing the rise of the Internet, the proliferation of smartphones, and the social media craze. However, the most significant events that happened to them were the September 11 attacks, the Columbine Shooting, and Y2K (Twenge, 2017). While other generations also experienced these events, they did not occur during their formative years, as they did for millennials, and these social markers signified a loss of innocence and made them a truly global generation. Paradoxically, despite being connected through technology, millennials report higher levels of loneliness and isolation compared to previous generations (Evrensel-İnanç et al., 2022). Furthermore, millennials were raised in the midst of the self-esteem movement, with many being told that they deserved the best and could grow up to be anything they wanted to be, and were applauded for any accomplishment. Research suggests the influence of this movement impacted this generation to have unrealistically high expectations in their personal and professional lives (McGuire et al., 2021; Swanzen, 2018; Twenge, 2011).

It appears that for millennials, mental health challenges are a result of a combination of factors, including family instability, digital age stressors, economic pressures, mental health stigmatization, and changing family structures (Twenge, 2011). For instance, millennials, as the initial cohort to fully mature in the digital age, confront a distinctive set of challenges. The prevalence of cyberbullying, online harassment, exposure to explicit or violent content, and the perpetual connectivity and comparison fostered by social media platforms have led to elevated levels of anxiety, depression, and pervasive feelings of inadequacy within this generation, surpassing rates observed in prior generations (Kurz, 2020). Despite being more cognizant of the significance of mental health, millennials often endure their struggles quietly, postponing or sidestepping treatment for conditions such as anxiety, depression, and PTSD. This can intensify the impact of complex trauma, largely due to the enduring stigma surrounding mental health that they inherit from prior generations.

As caregivers, millennials tend to adopt more collaborative and child-centered parenting styles. They place a significant emphasis on positive reinforcement, open communication, and fostering their children's individuality (Swanzen, 2018). One notable aspect of millennial parenting is their eagerness to use technology to enhance their children's learning and development. They are likely to introduce educational apps, interactive online resources, artificial intelligence (i.e., Alexa, Google Home), and digital platforms that can complement traditional forms of education (Schwartz et al., 2017). This digital fluency also allows them to maintain close connections with their children in a world where communication often occurs through screens, as they actively engage with their kids' online interests and activities. Overall, millennials bring a mix of innovative parenting approaches and generational influences to the parenting landscape of the 21st century.

Generation Z

Generation Z comprises individuals born between 2001 and 2015 (Kalkhurst, 2018). Generation Z, often abbreviated as Gen Z or Gen Zers or iGens (Twenge, 2017), is the first generation to have grown up entirely in the 21st century, and they are considered the first true generation of digital natives, having grown up with smartphones, social media, and constant access to the Internet (Drugas, 2022). Gen Z is confronting a unique set of mental health challenges as they navigate the complexities of digital technology and social media. Growing up in a hyper-connected digital age, Gen Z faces constant exposure to curated online personas, cyberbullying, and unrealistic beauty standards, contributing to anxiety, depression, and feelings of isolation (Dorsey & Villa, 2020). According to Jean Twenge (2023), a stunning 41% of iGens report feeling left out or having an internalized sense of loneliness even though they show themselves as so happy online, making goofy faces on Snapchat, and smiling in their pictures on Instagram. It appears that the decline in in-person social interactions has a strong correlation with dissociation due to the increase in smartphone and social media interactions (Ford, 2021; Schwartz et al., 2017). With the proliferation of social media platforms and online communication tools, many iGens find themselves more comfortable interacting through screens than being face-to-face (Twenge, 2017), and manifest a decrease in the development of crucial interpersonal skills, such as nonverbal communication and active listening (Thomas & Madiya, 2020). Additionally, the attraction to virtual worlds and digital entertainment has been correlated to different levels of dissociation such as daydreaming and fantasy involving a temporary separation from other mental processes (Badura Brack et al., 2022). Turkle (2017) stated that this online presence often competes with opportunities for genuine social interaction in the physical world and establishing meaningful connections in both the Gen Zers' personal and professional spheres.

One distinguishing characteristic of this generation has been the COVID-19 pandemic. Many Gen Zers had to forsake certain rites of passage, such as school formals, graduation, and socializing with friends and family. According to Rider et al. (2021), one in three youths suffer from a diagnosed mental health condition related to anxiety, depression, and/or loneliness due to the uncertainty and fear surrounding the pandemic, along with concerns about personal health and social isolation. This underscores the importance of targeted interventions and strategies to help bridge this gap and foster healthy social development in this tech-savvy generation.

Generation Alpha

Generation Alpha, also called Gen Alpha, comprises individuals born in 2016 and after (McCrindle & Fell, 2021). Gen Alpha is the first generation to have been born and fully shaped by the social makers of the 21st century, and most of them will live to see the 22nd century. In their life so far, the social and cultural markers have been the COVID-19 pandemic, racially charged sociopolitical events, protests in major cities, mental health crises, and educational challenges (Rider et al., 2021). Some researchers have referred to Gen Alpha as "Gen C" or "Generation COVID" because they will be the first generation to grow up largely or entirely in a world touched by the COVID-19 pandemic and the response to it (Marzilli et al., 2021). This generation has struggled with the loss of family members during a pandemic, increased social isolation, adjustment to online schooling, more screen time, less exercise and prosocial activities (sports, hobbies, clubs), and reduced medical and mental health care (Rider et al., 2021). In addition, research findings suggest that the pandemic disproportionally affected this generation due to the lower quality of family relationships and limited social resources (Marzilli et al., 2021; Rider et al., 2021).

Gen Alpha has mostly millennial parents who are attempting to run their families as mini democracies, seeking consensus from partners, kids, and extended friend circles on even the smallest decisions. For instance, millennial parents are backing away from the overscheduled days of their youth, preferring a more responsive, less directorial approach to activities. And they're teaching their kids to be themselves and try new things—often unwittingly conditioning Gen Alpha to see experiences as things to be documented and shared with the world. It appears that Gen Alpha will be the most educated generation and will stay at home with their parents later than even their predecessors. This becomes particularly important because the role of parents will span a longer age range with many of these Gen Alphas likely to be still living at home into their late 20s (Drugas, 2022).

One defining feature of Gen Alpha is their status as true digital natives. They have been exposed to smartphones, tablets, the Internet, and artificial intelligence (i.e., Alexa, Google Home, Siri) from infancy, making them the first true "digital integrators" (Badura Brack et al., 2022; Twenge, 2023). This early introduction to advanced technology plays a foundational role in shaping their cognitive development, which is rewriting their brains and affecting their ability to flourish in the real world (Siegel, 2015). Recent findings indicate that youth depression and anxiety doubled in the past couple of years due to heightened technology use at the expense of traditional play and physical activities (Swanzen, 2018). While technology provides global connectivity and vast information access, it has the potential to impede face-to-face social skills and hinder the development of meaningful relationships. There's a genuine concern that excessive screen time could diminish opportunities for authentic social engagement, emotional connections, critical thinking, and problem-solving skills (McCrindle & Fell, 2021). Paradoxically, Gen Alpha finds empowerment through technology, transitioning from being passive consumers to being active content creators and embracing a more collectivist approach. Armed with devices, they wield asymmetrical power to influence brands, shape culture, seek mental health services, and even instigate policy changes. It is crucial for caregivers and therapists to be cognizant of these potential effects and to proactively find ways to balance technology with real-world experiences. Encouraging outdoor play, fostering face-to-face interactions, and promoting activities that stimulate critical thinking are all vital strategies to mitigate the risk of dissociation from technology. By providing a balanced approach to technology use, we can help Gen Alpha harness the full potential of the digital age while also fostering its holistic development and well-being.

Just as every generation reacts to its predecessor, the Alphas are no exception. For them, the pendulum of behavior is returning to the fiscal conservatism and practical social values reminiscent of the baby boomers. Unlike their parents (Gen X and millennials), who lived through periods of economic prosperity and carefree spending, this generation is growing up in an era marked by economic instability and soaring housing costs (Twenge, 2023). In times like these, saving becomes a valued trait, job stability takes precedence, and the spotlight once again shifts to the end goal, not just the journey. Dedication and resilience are held in high regard, and there's a renewed appreciation for thriftiness and sustainable practices.

Finally, this generation is growing up in an environment where discussions about race, ethnicity, gender identity, and other dimensions of diversity are becoming more prominent and normalized (Drugas, 2022). One significant marker of diversity and inclusion for Gen Alpha is the increased representation of diverse voices in media, entertainment, and literature. Unlike previous generations, Generation Alpha is being exposed to a wider range of characters and stories that reflect the rich tapestry of human experiences. This exposure helps foster empathy and understanding, as they see people from different backgrounds, cultures, and identities as integral parts of their global awareness. For instance, Gen Alpha has unprecedented access to a global community and can connect with peers from different parts of the world. This exposure helps break down geographical and cultural barriers, leading to a more inclusive mindset.

Gen Alpha Complex Trauma and Dissociation

While further research is essential to comprehensively grasp the intricacies of complex trauma and dissociation within the context of Gen Alpha, preliminary observations allow us to draw some initial insights. Prior studies have indicated that exposure to trauma can leave children vulnerable to a range of negative consequences and has the potential to impact several areas of functioning and development (Kisiel et al., 2017; Lawson & Akay-Sullivan, 2020; Siegel, 2015). For Gen Alpha, as in previous generations, complex trauma and dissociation encompass a spectrum of challenges, including issues in caregiver-child relationships, struggles with emotional regulation, and difficulties in forming a stable sense of self (Cook et al., 2005).

In the digital age, the role of technology in caregiver relationships is an evolving area of concern (Kildare & Middlemiss, 2017; Wong et al., 2020). Parent-child interactions marked by high parental sensitivity and responsiveness contribute to the likelihood of an infant identifying their caregiver as a secure base and aid in the development of secure attachment styles and later optimal developmental trajectories (Ainsworth, 1979). However, the increasing use of technology in caregiving practices for Gen Alpha introduces a potential challenge. Complex trauma, characterized by repeated exposure to distressing events, particularly within the context of caregiving relationships, can be exacerbated by a caregiver's reliance on technology as a means of interaction and connection with their children (Wong et al., 2020). For instance, during a crucial moment of bonding like playtime or a shared activity, a caregiver may be engrossed in their smartphone, responding to emails, or scrolling through social media. This divided attention can send a message to the child that the device holds greater importance than their immediate interaction. In addition, the prevalence of screens in daily life may inadvertently replace face-to-face interactions that are fundamental for building trust and emotional connections. When a child observes their caregiver consistently engaged in technology, they may internalize a sense of emotional unavailability or detachment from the parent (McDaniel, 2020). This can potentially lead to feelings of insecurity and an uncertain sense of trust in their caregiver.

For Gen Alpha, the ability to regulate intense negative emotions and emotional arousal is linked to the use of technology compared to previous generations (McCrindle & Fell, 2021). For example, younger Gen Alphas are used to throwing a tantrum at the grocery store and having a caregiver give them a phone or iPad to regulate their emotions and help them calm down while watching a YouTuber or playing with their favorite app. In older Gen Alphas, augmented reality (AR), virtual reality (VR), and social media platforms appear to offer the same type of distraction and a means to temporarily disconnect from their immediate reality to cope with intense emotions or engage in avoidance behaviors. Recent studies suggest that these technologies could offer an avenue for children to experience dissociation, including depersonalization (feeling detached from oneself) and derealization (feeling that the external world is unreal or distant) (Hollis et al., 2020; Usmani et al., 2022). Dependence on technology as a primary tool for children to regulate their emotions can significantly impede their overall well-being and the development of their internal coping mechanisms (Haselgruber et al., 2021).

Unlike previous generations, Gen Alpha is raised in an era when social media platforms play a prominent role in shaping personal identities, especially when it comes to complex trauma and dissociation. From a young age, constant interaction with digital devices can alter the traditional avenues through which children form their sense of self and manage their distress. Instead of relying solely on face-to-face interactions and tangible experiences, children may increasingly engage with virtual environments and online personas to process overwhelming feelings and dissociate from painful experiences (Drouin et al., 2020). The exposure to digital spaces, from carefully curated profiles to raw and unfiltered content, can lead to a heightened awareness of self-presentation and a desire to craft their own online personas (Mann & Blumberg, 2022). A Gen Alpha child, for instance, may observe influencers or content creators on platforms like YouTube or Instagram who frequently showcase specific lifestyles, talents, or interests, thereby influencing their own understanding of what is valued or admired in their online communities. Gen Alphas are more likely to form their self-perception in accordance with these perceived ideals, which could result in a more meticulously curated or performance-driven sense of self (McCrindle & Fell, 2021; Pescott, 2020). While the digital landscape offers unique opportunities for self-expression and exploration, it also poses challenges. Gen Alpha may grapple with issues of authenticity, comparison, and the pressure to conform to online trends or standards. Navigating these complexities can shape how they form and evolve their sense of self in a world where the boundaries between physical and digital realms are increasingly porous.

Limitations and Future Directions

Even though generational research appears to be a framework that can inform the treatment of complex trauma and dissociation in children, there are major challenges: heterogeneity within generations, overlap of traumatic events, and intergenerational transmission of trauma. First, generational research provides broad trends and characteristics, but it is important to remember that individuals within a generation have unique experiences and responses to trauma. Factors such as family dynamics, personal experiences, and cultural background can significantly influence how trauma is experienced and coped with. Second, traumatic events do not always neatly align with generational boundaries. For instance, events like economic recessions, natural disasters, or large-scale conflicts can impact multiple generations simultaneously. Understanding the specific impact on a particular generation requires a nuanced examination of the historical context and individual experiences. In addition, trauma can take many forms, ranging from personal experiences (i.e., abuse and neglect) to collective experiences (i.e., wars and pandemics). Different generations may have experienced different types of traumas, requiring tailored approaches to understanding and addressing their specific needs. Third, generations can be deeply affected by trauma experienced by previous generations.

This intergenerational transmission of trauma can influence family dynamics, coping strategies, and mental health outcomes. Recognizing and addressing these complex interplays is essential for effective trauma-informed care.

Future research should continue to explore the complex interplay between generational factors and children's mental health. With the rapid pace of technological and social change, new generations (like Gen Alpha) are growing up in vastly different environments compared with previous generations, which supports the need for ongoing research and interdisciplinary collaboration to understand the impact of generational markers in complex trauma.

Conclusion

Understanding the generational context is paramount when addressing complex trauma and dissociation. It provides crucial insights into the historical, social, and cultural factors that have shaped an individual's experiences and coping mechanisms. By recognizing how generational influences contribute to trauma responses, clinicians and caregivers can tailor interventions that are sensitive to the unique needs of each generation. This knowledge allows for more effective support, validation, and healing, ultimately fostering a stronger therapeutic alliance and promoting resilience in individuals navigating complex trauma and dissociation. Moreover, an understanding of generational dynamics can guide the development of prevention strategies and public policies aimed at breaking intergenerational cycles of trauma, thereby creating a more compassionate and inclusive society for future generations.

Generational research proves to be a valuable consideration when addressing complex trauma and dissociation in family dynamics. Understanding the distinct historical, cultural, and generational perspectives allows for a greater awareness of the unique challenges and strengths each generation brings to the table. Recognizing these differences provides a crucial foundation for tailoring therapeutic interventions and equips mental health professionals with a heightened sensitivity to the evolving sociocultural landscapes that shape their clients' narratives. This emphasis on generational considerations marks a vital stride toward comprehensive and holistic mental health care for all individuals affected by complex trauma and dissociation.

References

Ainsworth, M. S. (1979). Infant–mother attachment. *American Psychologist, 34*(10), 932–937. https://doi.org/10.1037/0003-066X.34.10.932

American Psychiatric Association. (2022). *Diagnostic and statistical manual of mental disorders* (5th ed., rev.). https://doi.org/10.1176/appi.books.9780890425787

Badura Brack, A. S., Marklin, M., Embury, C. M., Picci, G., Frenzel, M., Earl, A. K., Stephen, J., Wang, Y.-P., Calhoun, V., & Wilson, T. W. (2022). Neurostructural brain imaging study of trait dissociation in healthy children. *BJPsych Open, 8*(5), e172. https://doi.org/10.1192/bjo.2022.576

Buffel, T., Yarker, S., Phillipson, C., Lang, L., Lewis, C., Doran, P., & Goff M. (2021). Locked down by inequality: Older people and the COVID-19 pandemic. *Urban Studies, 60*(8), 1465–1482. https://doi.org/10.1177/00420980211041018

Cook, A., Spinazzola, J., Ford, J., Lanktree, C., Blaustein, M., Cloitre, M., DeRosa, R., Hubbard, R., Liautaud, J., Olafson, E., Kagan, R., Mallah, K., & van der Kolk, B. (2005). Complex trauma in children and adolescents. *Psychiatric Annals, 35,* 390–398. https://doi.org/10.3928/00485713-20050501-05

Dorsey, J. R., & Villa, D. (2020). *Zconomy: How Gen Z will change the future of business—And what to do about it*. Harper Business.

Drouin, M., McDaniel, B. T., Pater, J., & Toscos, T. (2020). How parents and their children used social media and technology at the beginning of the COVID-19 pandemic and associations with anxiety. *Cyberpsychology, Behavior, and Social Networking, 23*(11), 727–736. https://doi.org/10.1089/cyber.2020.0284

Drugas, M. (2022). Screenagers or "screamagers"? Current perspectives on generation alpha. *Psychological Thought, 15*(1), 1–11. https://doi.org/10.37708/psyct.v15i1.732

Evrensel-İnanç, E., Aydoğmuş, C., Metin-Camgöz, S., & Özdilek, E. (2022). For generation Z: What is the underlying reason between emotional intelligence and depression relationship? [Z Kuşağı İçin: Duygusal Zekâ Özelliği ve Depresyon İlişkisinin Arkasında Yatan Sebep Nedir?] *Sosyoekonomi, 30*(53), 27–48. https://doi.org/10.17233/sosyoekonomi.2022.03.02

Fingerman, K., Huo, M., & Birditt, K. S. (2020). A decade of research on intergenerational ties: Technological, economic, political, and demographic changes. *Journal of Marriage and Family, 82*(1), 383–403. https://doi.org/10.1111/jomf.12604

Ford, J. D. (2021). Progress and limitations in the treatment of complex PTSD and developmental trauma disorder. *Current Treatment Options in Psychiatry, 8*(1), 1–17. https://doi.org/10.1007/s40501-020-00236-6

Haselgruber, A., Knefel, M., Sölva, K., & Lueger-Schuster, B. (2021). Foster children's complex psychopathology in the context of cumulative childhood trauma: The interplay of ICD-11 complex PTSD, dissociation, depression, and emotion regulation. *Journal of Affective Disorders, 282*, 372–380. https://doi.org/10.1016/j.jad.2020.12.116

Hollis, C., Livingstone, S., & Sonuga-Barke, E. (2020). The role of digital technology in children and young people's mental health: A triple-edged sword? *Journal of Child Psychology and Psychiatry, 61*(8), 837–841. https://doi.org/10.1111/jcpp.13302

Kalkhurst, D. K. (2018). *Intergenerational engagement: Understanding the five generations in today's economy.* CreateSpace Independent Publishing.

Kildare, C. A., & Middlemiss, W. (2017). Impact of parents' mobile device use on parent-child interaction: A literature review. *Computers in Human Behavior, 75*, 579–593. https://doi.org/10.1016/j.chb.2017.06.003

Kisiel, C., Summersett-Ringgold, F., Weil, L. E. G., & McClelland, G. (2017). Understanding strengths in relation to complex trauma and mental health symptoms within child welfare. *Journal of Child and Family Studies, 26*(2), 437–451. https://doi.org/10.1007/s10826-016-0569-4

Kurz, C. (2020, February 12). Introducing are we there yet? Today's parents, tomorrow's kids. ViacomCBS. insights.viacomcbs.com/categories/research-studies/are-we-there-yet

Lawson, D. M., & Akay-Sullivan, S. (2020). Considerations of dissociation, betrayal trauma, and complex trauma in the treatment of incest. *Journal of Child Sexual Abuse, 29*(6), 677–696. https://doi.org/10.1080/10538712.2020.1751369

Mann, R. B., & Blumberg, F. (2022). Adolescents and social media: The effects of frequency of use, self-presentation, social comparison, and self esteem on possible self imagery. *Acta Psychologica, 228*, Article 103629. https://doi.org/10.1016/j.actpsy.2022.103629

Marzilli, E., Cerniglia, L., Tambelli, R., Trombini, E., De Pascalis, L., Babore, A., & Cimino, S. (2021). The COVID-19 pandemic and its impact on families' mental health: The role played by parenting stress, parents' past trauma, and resilience. *International Journal of Environmental Research and Public Health, 18*(21), Article 11450. https://doi.org/10.3390/ijerph182111450

McCrindle, M., & Fell, A. (2021). *Generation alpha: Understanding our children and helping them thrive.* Headline Publishing Group.

McDaniel, B. T. (2020). Technoference: Parent mobile device use and implications for children and parent-child relationships. *Zero to Three, 41*(2), 30.

McGuire, R., Hiller, R. M., Anke, E., Pasco, F., Meiser-Stedman, R., Sophie, L., & Halligan, S. L. (2021). A longitudinal investigation of children's trauma memory characteristics and their relationship with posttraumatic stress disorder symptoms. *Research on Child and Adolescent Psychopathology, 49*(6), 807–816. https://doi.org/10.1007/s10802-021-00773-5

Narayan, A. J., Lieberman, A. F., & Masten, A.S. (2021). Intergenerational transmission and prevention of adverse childhood experiences (ACEs). *Clinical Psychology Review, 85*, Article 101997. https://doi.org/10.1016/j.cpr.2021.101997

Pescott, C. K. (2020). "I wish I was wearing a filter right now": An exploration of identity formation and subjectivity of 10-and 11-year olds' social media use. *Social Media + Society, 6*(4). http://dx.doi.org/10.1177/2056305120965155

Reese, E. M., Barlow, M. J., Dillon, M., Villalon, S., Barnes, M. D., & Crandall, A. (2022). Intergenerational transmission of trauma: The mediating effects of family health. *International Journal of Environmental Research and Public Health, 19*(10), Article 5944. https://doi.org/10.3390/ijerph19105944

Rider, E. A., Ansari, E., Varrin, P. H., & Sparrow, J. (2021). Mental health and wellbeing of children and adolescents during the covid-19 pandemic. *BMJ: British Medical Journal (Online), 374*. https://doi.org/10.1136/bmj.n1730

Schwartz, O. S., Simmons, J. G., Whittle, S., Byrne, M. L., Yap, M. B. H., Sheeber, L. B., & Allen, N. B. (2017). Affective parenting behaviors, adolescent depression, and brain development: A review of findings from the orygen adolescent development study. *Child Development Perspectives, 11*, 90–96. https://doi.org/10.1111/cdep.12215

Siegel, D. J. (2015). *Brainstorm: The power and purpose of the teenage brain.* Penguin.

Strauss, W., & Howe, N. (1991). *Generations: The history of America's future 1584 to 2069.* William Morrow.

Swanzen, R. (2018). Facing the generation chasm: The parenting and teaching of Generations Y and Z. *International Journal of Child, Youth & Family Studies, 9*(2), 125–150. https://doi.org/10.18357/ijcyfs92201818216

Thomas, M. R., & Madiya, M. S. (2020). Customer profiling of alpha: The next generation marketing. *Ushus Journal of Business Management, 19*(1), 75–86. https://doi.org/10.12725/ujbm.50.5

Turkle, S. (2017). *Alone together: Why we expect more from technology and less from each other.* Basic Books.

Twenge, J. (2011). Generational differences in mental health: Are children and adolescents suffering more, or less? *American Journal of Orthopsychiatry, 81*(4), 469–472. https://doi.org/10.1111/j.1939-0025.2011.01115.x

Twenge, J. (2017). *iGen: Why today's super-connected kids are growing up less rebellious, more tolerant, less happy, and completely unprepared for adulthood.* Atria Books.

Twenge, J. (2023). *Generations: The real differences between Gen Z, millennials, Gen X, boomers and silents and what they mean for America's future.* Atria Books.

Usmani, S. S., Sharath, M., & Mehendale, M. (2022). Future of mental health in the metaverse. *General Psychiatry, 35*(4), e100825. https://doi.org/10.1136/gpsych-2022-100825

Wong, R. S., Tung, K. T., Rao, N., Leung, C., Hui, A. N., Tso, W. W., Fu, K.-W., Jiang, F., Zhao, J., & Ip, P. (2020). Parent technology use, parent–child interaction, child screen time, and child psychosocial problems among disadvantaged families. *Journal of Pediatrics, 226*, 258–265. https://doi.org/10.1016/j.jpeds.2020.07.006

39
SHAME AND GUILT

Paula Moreno and Sandra Baita

Introduction

Shame and guilt are self-conscious emotions that arise in toddlerhood and continue to develop through childhood and adolescence (Thompson et al., 2006). Around the age of 5, children understand their own expression of these emotions, and by adolescence they are able to understand these same emotions in others. Whether these two emotions can be distinguished by the child when they emerge remains unclear (Luby et al., 2009), and a blend between the two of them seems to be a common experience, as shown by the research done by Tangney and Dearing (2002). These two authors also found that the terms "guilt" and "shame" are commonly interchangeably used.

Both emotions require capacity for self-appraisal of one's own actions and behaviors, but there is a consensus to differentiate guilt, as focused on negative aspects of one's own *behavior*, from shame, as focused on negative aspects of *self* (Kochanska et al., 2002; Tracy & Robins, 2006).

The experiences of both shame and guilt are influenced by social, cultural, religious, and family factors. There is an increased acknowledgement of the harm caused to children who are raised in unequal, racist, discriminative, and oppressive environments. Their alleged "defectiveness" is attributed to their gender, religion, economic status, sexual orientation, or other such factors. Societal rejection becomes a powerful amplifier of shame-based thoughts about self, and the lack of policies addressing their needs can make them feel invisible and unworthy. If these children feel they need to hide or do something to change their defectiveness in order to be accepted, their sense of guilt and shame can become a feature of their identity. Both emotions seem to have an adaptive purpose, and guilt has been associated with pro-social values and reparation (Bafunno & Camodeca, 2013). However, they can also become maladaptive and lead to both internalizing and externalizing problems (Muris, 2015; Muris et al., 2016). Although there is an increasing interest in understanding and treating shame in adult clients who suffered early interpersonal trauma, less focus has been given to the same issue in complexly traumatized children.

In our experience, children who have suffered abuse and neglect from their caregivers are prone to feeling guilty because their parents usually held them responsible for the abuse. It is our hypothesis that a pervasive sense of core shame grows underneath the internalization of guilt and responsibility for the suffered abuse, and that reaching shame and working with its toxic effects should be a primary therapeutic goal.

Research and Current Literature on Shame and Guilt in Child Complex Trauma and Dissociation Work

As developing human beings, children are particularly vulnerable to developing intense feelings of shame as a consequence of trauma. For better or worse, the building of their sense of self and self-attribution highly depends on both the implicit and explicit interpersonal exchanges with their caregivers. When the caregiving relationship is charged with high amounts of aggression toward the child, the child's developing sense of self and self-attribution will be compromised by the internalization of negative messages.

There is an important amount of research linking shame and self-blame with child sexual abuse. Some of these studies have found a significant relationship between shame and self-blame and the development of depression, PTSD, maladaptive coping strategies, and suicidal ideation (Alix et al., 2017; Feiring et al., 2002a, 2002b).

McElvaney and colleagues (2014) found that both shame and self-blame are key barriers to the disclosure of child sexual abuse, leading to important consequences not only for therapy but also especially for the investigation process and protection. Children feel ashamed and blame themselves for what happened (the abuse); for not telling, not preventing, or not stopping the abuse; and for the consequences that abuse disclosure causes for their family. This may be reinforced through explicit and/or implicit messaging by abusers and explicit blaming from non-offending caregivers either for not having disclosed earlier or for the consequences of their disclosure, including jail for the offender and financial burden for the family, as the most common.

However, child sexual abuse is not the only traumatic interpersonal event capable of inducing shame and self-blame in children.

Parisette-Sparks et al. (2017) referred to different studies that link parental harshness, rejection, indifference, and unresponsiveness to the development of maladaptive shame and guilt in children. Even if the authors do not refer explicitly to child abuse, we know that all these parental characteristics are features of abuse and neglect toward children, events that lie at the heart of developmental trauma and dissociation.

In the clinical literature, Silberg (2022) refers to "stuck thoughts" holding the painful meaning that traumatic events carry about how the child views themself. According to Silberg, these stuck thoughts are shame-based ideas where "the child survivor may engage in cycles of self-punishment as if to blame themselves for the trauma they suffered because of the perceived shameful characteristics of the self" (2022, p. 231). This view is coherent with our hypothesis: the child takes responsibility for the abuse and links this responsibility with a perceived negative feature of self. This cycle is reinforced by the explicit messages and implicit messaging from abusive caregivers, whereby the child does something bad in the eyes of the parent (like spilling a glass of water), and the parent batters the child and "explains" why he is doing so (*I punch you because you spilled the water*, and thus the child internalizes their responsibility for the punching), adding a label about the child's self (*I punched you because you spilled the water, and you spilled it because you are stupid, clumsy, and useless*). The child cannot confront or reject the caregiver's statement because it would be dangerous at least in two ways: on the one hand, it could bring more abuse. But on the other, confronting the caregiver would mean assuming it is the parent who is to blame (*I am not stupid, clumsy, or useless; rather, you are bad because you are punching me*), and if the child assumes the parent is "the bad guy" in the picture, then who would take care of them? Accepting responsibility for their behavior as the cause of abuse seems the most convenient solution. Of course, the cost is too high: the ongoing repetition of this cycle leads the child to internalize a message that holds together self-blame and shame: *I did something wrong because there is something wrong with me*. By internalizing these messages, the child can also keep the illusion of connection with her caregivers, even if they are abusive: *They are not bad, I am bad*.

Affective and behavioral dysregulation as manifestations of the pervasive trauma children have suffered, when not linked to the traumatic events themselves by the external observers (foster parents, schools, friends), become another source of reinforcement of these shame-based thoughts (Deblinger & Runyon, 2005). In our experience, this is especially the case of children who engage in sexualized behaviors and are labeled by their caregivers as potential abusers, or of those who steal either money or food and are labeled as thieves. Some children may also present themselves to the therapist with an identity built by their symptoms: *I come to see you because I am a liar; I must go to therapy because I am a thief.* When children introduce themselves to us clinicians in such sad ways, we are facing the core of the child's shameful experience about themself.

Different Lenses through Which We Can Understand Shame and Guilt in Child Complex Trauma and Dissociation

From an evolutionary perspective, shame can be *adaptive*, as a way of regulating social relationships within a group of people, and both shame and guilt arise within the interpersonal relationship of a child with their parents. Around the second year of life, even normal parental limits to a child's exploration can lead to a disruption in the emotional communication within the dyad. The child's joy in painting the walls with crayons is interrupted by the upset mother discovering this new "adventure." The child learns by their mother's face, tone of voice, and gestures that something in their connection is missed: a sense of embarrassment arises. The child blushes, lowers their head, and withdraws (Baita, 2022a). However, anytime this disruption is repaired by the attachment figure, adaptive shame starts to shape: the child learns what they can or cannot do, where, and under what circumstances. Schore (2019) refers to the child's disappointment when facing the maternal response; however, as long as the maternal response doesn't imply a continued disruption of the bond and is properly repaired, self-regulation is not endangered.

However, in the interpersonal scenario in which children with developmental trauma and dissociation grow up, the environment is filled with persistent overwhelmingly negative experiences with attachment figures without further repair. Such a context is the seed of the development of a *maladaptive* sense of shame, referred to as "core shame" (Cozolino, 2014), or "chronic" or "toxic shame" (Young, 2015). A child who grows up with constant offenses toward them might develop a shameful identity and pervasive feelings of inadequacy, leading to dysregulation and feeling and behaving outside of their window of tolerance, with extreme reactions that range from hyper-arousal (attacking others, or fleeing as self-defense) to hypo-arousal (withdrawal, avoiding eye gaze, curling inward or hunching—as ways of not being seen). In any case, the social engagement system (Porges, 2021) is shut down and connection with others fails (Steele et al., 2017).

Shame may inhibit the experience of other emotions such as enthusiasm, curiosity, and joy, as well as thoughts and behaviors related to them. Shame may also inhibit the expression of emotion such as anger or even the need for connection, with the child predicting they will be rejected or regarded as unacceptable by others (Steele et al., 2017).

When a child's needs for closeness and protection are met with a caregiver's distance and absence, the child is left feeling unseen and abandoned, which triggers a deep feeling of shame, as if an inherent defectiveness of the child is the cause of the caregiver's abandonment (*I'm not good enough to be seen/to be loved*). In turn, the child will develop a self-loathing stance that becomes the foundation of negative cognitions about themself. More often than not, the adult's lack of understanding and their judgment of the child reinforces this shameful dynamic, as well as the shameful belief about self (*There is something wrong with me*). We have repeatedly seen this symptom manifestation, especially in children who were adopted and returned to the system later. What we might call a "failed adoption" is what the child will see as a failure of themselves: it was not the system or the parents who failed to provide them with good and appropriate understanding and care; rather, it was their unlovability. Even though this dynamic prevents the child from connecting with others, shame itself functions to protect and hide their alleged "defectiveness" (*If others can't see my defectiveness, then I won't be rejected*).

Dissociation may be understood as a way of dealing with shame, where a dissociative state might hold the shameful experiences outside of conscious knowing, while another state might, in turn, reject it, creating internal conflict and phobic avoidance of inner experience. This dynamic shows our clients' deep lack of compassion toward themselves and their dissociated states, which forms the basis for introducing and practicing compassion in therapeutic work with clients of all ages. In order to reach the shame held within dissociative states, the clinician will need to process phobic avoidance (Steele et al., 2017) while working with compassion and self-compassion with the child. Compassion is a key element in helping the child engage in a curious exploration of their inner world. This is further discussed later in this chapter.

The child might create different states that help with avoiding contact with the states holding shame: if the dissociated shame is linked to an unbearable experience of helplessness, the child might develop another state that will act in a reckless way to show both how strong and brave they are and disdain for anything that looks weak or vulnerable. If the dissociated shame is linked to an experience of being constantly insulted and physically abused, the child might create a pleasing state whose job will be to satisfy others' needs. If shame is held in a dissociative state holding experiences of not being fed or taken care, the child might create a dissociative part in charge of providing all they want or need, which most of the time leads to externalized behaviors such as stealing. Most of the times, the way in which dissociative states created to deal with shame express themselves will give the therapist a clue about the experience the child is avoiding.

Education about how trauma affects us and how dissociation can help a person deal with unbearable feelings is an important step, right from the beginning of treatment (Silberg, 2022). Therapists should share the same information with caregivers in order to help them understand their child and become active participants in the therapeutic process, practicing new strategies to respond to their child's behaviors and prevent the reinforcement of shame.

Acknowledgment and praise of all aspects of the child—including the rejected aspects—by both therapist and caregivers is a fundamental step in working with shame. Shame is fueled by rejection, from both outside and inside, and without true acceptance from the adult's world, processing shame will be almost impossible for the child. Children expect from others the same rejection they have of their dissociated shameful states, and this is a powerful reason to reinforce their phobic avoidance. Acceptance can be a challenge, especially when the child presents with externalizing behaviors such as stealing, sexualized problems, or aggression toward others, and adult reactions toward these behaviors might reinforce the circuit of shame and rejection (Baita, 2022b). The therapist's curiosity about the reasons behind these behaviors is an adult reaction completely new and unexpected for the child and most of the time is the key to opening the door to the exploration of the inner world and paving the way to self-compassion.

Proposed Approaches and Therapeutic Strategies in Working with Shame and Guilt

Chronic shame is relational. The guilt derived from assuming responsibility for abuse and the consequent shaping of a shameful self are born within a repetitively disruptive relationship with what Young (2015) calls "a disintegrating" caregiver, and permeate the ways in which clients navigate relationships with themselves, others, and the world. Clinicians working with adult clients agree that no therapeutic approach will succeed without considering and addressing the chronic shame and guilt that also arises within the therapeutic relationship.

Traumatized children often have negative learned and internalized beliefs about themselves that they are mean, inadequate, not good enough, and accountable for what they have suffered and for the consequences of the intervention to protect them. Many of their symptoms are triggered within relationships, especially with their caregivers. Many parents describe their children as "provoking" them with misbehavior. When working with children, it is essential that we work with their caregivers as well: caregivers represent the most important relationship for our little clients, despite the fact that they often also inadvertently reinforce the shame-guilt circuit. When parents react harshly to a child's behavior, old scripts around relating inadvertently reinforce a sense of disconnection, as well as deep feelings of guilt and chronic shame within the child. As such, caregivers must be engaged and worked with as those who must repair the disruption in communication and bonding with the child and develop new predictable and consistent ways of engaging. This can be challenging if caregivers bring a child to therapy to have the therapist "fix" their behavior, as the work of therapy instead focuses on reaching and healing the heart of disconnection, which lies within the parent-child relationship.

Two approaches will now be introduced as ways of working with children and parents: compassion-focused therapy (CFT), adapted for children (Moreno, 2023), and eye movement desensitization and reprocessing (EMDR) with parents (Baita, 2022b).

Compassion-Focused Therapy (Adapted for Children)

CFT was developed by Paul Gilbert in 1980, integrating developmental psychology, affective neuroscience, attachment and cognitive-behavioral therapy, and mindfulness and compassion (Kolts, 2016). Gilbert (2009) developed this approach to work with clients who had a tendency toward shame, self-criticism, and self-loathing, by using compassion practices as a key tool to develop sensibility to suffering and a motivation to alleviate it.

Gilbert (2010) suggests that a self-critical mind is a mind focused on threat, and is often associated with feelings of inadequacy. It manifests through a deep self-hatred, especially in contexts where there has been severe abuse. In extreme cases, shame leads patients to avoid knowing their own inner world. Like adults, children may also reject their inner world, reinforcing the sense of shame and conditions for dissociation from this inner world and its components. Shame, self-criticism, and avoidance are strongly intertwined. Gilbert (2010) argues that the cultivation of self-compassionate ways of seeing oneself and addressing difficulties is a central goal of therapy.

Gilbert (2009) refers to three regulatory systems clients work through in therapy to develop a felt sense of safety and confidence as they approach traumatic material: the threat and self-protection system (threat system); the achievement, incentive, and resource-seeking system (drive system); and the calming, relaxation, and satisfaction system (soothing system).

The threat system includes emotions such as anger, rage, anxiety, and disgust. It helps us detect threats, activates the feelings that guide us toward them, and mobilizes and motivates us to act through fight, flight, or freeze responses. The drive system is associated with feelings such as enthusiasm, desire, and ambition. It is our primary source of resources. The soothing system is related to feelings of well-being, calm, safety, and peace. These are the emotions that help provide some balance when there are no active threats against which to defend. These feelings are associated with experiences of affection, acceptance, kindness, and affiliation. These three systems ideally function in balance, and if they become imbalanced, suffering arises. The work aimed at restoring balance lays the foundation for establishing the necessary safety to work with shame.

A place to start is to consider the role of warmth in the therapeutic process, as it provides verbal and nonverbal signals of interest, care, and kindness that are comforting. It also involves sharing positive affection between individuals, which stimulates bonding, affection, and feelings of connection, in contrast to indifference, avoidance, or attack. However, warmth is more likely to occur and be felt when individuals feel safe and trust each other. Warmth paves the way for positive feelings of tranquility, calmness, and being comforted and can counter defensive emotions such as anger, anxiety, and sadness, as well as defensive behaviors such as aggression or avoidance (Gilbert, 2010). Helping children experience warmth also cultivates internal experiences that counteract shame, such as security, calmness, warmth, and trust. Complexly traumatized children can react with distancing behaviors in response to the therapist's approach; they cannot find calm sensations because they have never experienced them.

Both mindfulness and compassion practices (calm breathing, compassionate imagery, building a calm imaginary place) are highly useful in helping clients focus on building self-compassion, tolerating closeness and warmth, generating strategies to cope with self-criticism, developing broader awareness to observe their own inner world, and generating ways of avoiding automatic post-traumatic responses, thus enabling the ability to choose how to respond. This discernment is achieved through mindfulness practices that invite the patient to notice different aspects of experience, specifically emotion, thought, and physical sensation. In this way, the patient is aided in improving interrelational connections.

Self-compassion refers to the ability to recognize one's own suffering and take action to alleviate it. In children, this can translate as recognizing their inner world and valuing and making sense of their emotions for the purpose of regulation. Self-compassion also promotes resilience, attenuating feelings of shame and disconnection from others. According to Neff (2012), the three elements of self-compassion—mindfulness, common humanity, and kindness—act as antidotes to shame. Mindfulness prevents over-identification with our mistakes; the notion of common humanity counters feelings of isolation from others; and kindness allows us to feel our worth despite our imperfections. In clients with unmet needs of love, connection, justice, respect, and safety, self-compassion serves a role of self-protection, respect, consideration, and safety that may not have been received from others (Neff, 2012). When we talk about common humanity, we integrate the concept that every human being who has gone through a traumatic experience can develop the same symptoms, emotions, and physical reactions. This concept, applied in therapy, generates feelings of calm that counteract the loneliness often caused by trauma (Moreno & Véliz Araya, 2022). Lastly, introducing experiences of loving-kindness to these children, who have been denigrated and emotionally and physically abused, does not come without great challenge, and as such, building loving-kindness is gradually offered both in the therapeutic relationship and through concrete therapeutic practices.

In therapy, we work by practicing and offering each of these components to the child to provide them with tools to cope with shame resulting from their lived experiences. Without the component of mindfulness, it would be impossible for the child to develop self-observation and discriminate against the elements of their experience. This also helps children discover triggers of emotions and behaviors, as well as find ways to regulate them. An example of how to engage children in the process of fostering resilience in this way is to help them create practices where they learn to explore their internal experience and view it with loving, non-judgmental eyes. We know that children who have experienced trauma may hold belief systems such as "I am not good enough to be loved," "I am in danger," "I did something wrong," "I am damaged," or "I cannot trust anyone." Establishing practices through mindfulness, compassion, and self-compassion helps children deal with these trauma-stuck belief systems in new and different ways.

Both mindfulness and compassion-based approaches, as well as Gilbert's CFT, assist the patient in seeking internal safety, regulating their emotions and physiological states, and replacing self-criticism with a more loving way of treating oneself and others. Both approaches highlight the importance of working with shame in the therapeutic relationship, with the therapist, through their own practice, being able to provide loving qualities in the relationship. To achieve these goals, the following practices are employed:

- Mindfulness (helps the patient pay attention to different parts of the internal and external experience)
- Compassionate imagery (through imagery work, the patient is helped to cultivate compassionate qualities such as loving-kindness, patience, wisdom, strength, kindness, and courage)
- Imaginary place of calm (imagery practices to activate the calm emotional response system)

These approaches can be integrated with other approaches, such as EMDR therapy and somatosensory approaches. Working from this approach attends to:

- Building a therapeutic relationship based on unconditional acceptance
- Enabling the child to learn emotional self-regulation and co-regulation with others
- Facilitating physiological self-regulation in the child
- Working with shame to reduce self-criticism
- Addressing avoidance used to manage the feelings of shame (e.g., encourages observation rather than avoidance of internal experience)

In practice, the CFT approach consists of the following stages, which includes child specific adaptations and considerations:

1 Establishment of therapeutic relationship/psychoeducation
2 Recognition of emotional regulation systems
3 Development of self-regulation skills
4 Exploration and coping with shame.

Establishment of Therapeutic Relationship/Psychoeducation

When working with children, the first consideration is whether the necessary conditions of safety are in place to begin therapeutic work. If the child is a victim of ongoing abuse, involvement of relevant and competent authorities is the primary method of initial intervention to effectively protect the child from harm. Once this consideration has been attended to, we turn toward building a relationship to support healing the effects of shame, as healing occurs in connection with others. For this reason, working from a relational or family perspective is fundamental, as well as modeling healthy relationships. We are engaged in observation and modeling curiosity, exploring shame-based manifestations in the therapist space. Like other emotions, shame also manifests in the body. When we observe a body-based cue or signal (e.g., head or back posture, tone of voice, and avoidance of eye contact), we should not let it pass by. This is an invitation to explore and understand the signals in detail, to understand what they are telling us. To assist in this process, Moreno (2023) developed a set of dragons that represent the fundamental aspects of CFT, as well as two puppet brains. One is the therapeutic brain, which contains the three emotional regulation systems inside; these can be taken out or hidden depending on which one is activated or needs to be activated. The second one is a primitive brain that accounts for the state of regulation that connects us with an evolutionarily ancient response mode. The dragons form a community and work together, and both the dragons and the brains are used from the beginning of therapy to help with psychoeducation and support the establishment of a therapeutic bond.

The first dragon embodies a compassionate ideal, holding within it the qualities of bravery, courage, kindness, strength, and tenderness. It has antennae that allow it to detect suffering, and it can lean on our bodies with its paws. Children can easily connect with it. Its gaze was designed to convey warmth, and the paws that rest on our shoulders provide strength. In this way, the possibility of approaching these qualities to connect them with one's own becomes more encouraging and easier to accept. This dragon does not live alone but is accompanied by three more dragons. Each one tells a different story. These stories are tied to the different places where we can position ourselves in relation to the activation of our central nervous system.

The second dragon is large and has a very intense color, and tells the story of its ability to dive into the deep depths of the sea. Unlike the first dragon, this one has very large wings and a very long tail to be able to emerge from those dark places that, at the same time, need to be explored. Children are offered this dragon to hold and invited to imagine exploring that suffering. This dragon has a baby dragon next to it, symbolizing suffering. The proposal is to hold it in cupped hands and observe it, rock it, feed it, sing to it, and keep it warm.

When the child shows dissociative symptoms, the dragons are used following the premises of the work framed in the theory of structural dissociation.

It is possible to carry out the practices explained in this chapter but working with the different dissociated aspects of the personality. Dragons can function as a loving bridge in the creation of awareness of these aspects, the installation of resources, or the emotional regulation of each of these parts. The dragons allow the child's loving gaze to work on their own internal world and each of their parts.

Through mindfulness, we can guide this approach, helping the child feel the subtleties of physical sensations and the emotions and thoughts that arise. If there is resistance to approaching this second or any other dragon, we can work with EMDR therapy to desensitize any phobia contributing to resistance-related symptoms. Depending on the stage of work we are in, it is also possible to reprocess traumatic material, but we must always consider that the offering of these practices must be careful and gradual, and the client does not necessarily have to practice them until there is readiness to do so. Helping clients feel love for themselves, their internal world, and their behaviors, can be counterproductive if the child does not feel ready for it yet.

Finally, there is the third dragon, a shameful one, which can hide its head inside its body and cover itself with its wings, and its tail shrinks when it takes its head out of its body. Experimenting with the dragon's body and its different postures opens the door to working with the child's body so they can recognize how certain postures communicate something about shame.

It is important to allow the child to choose which dragon will safeguard the work of the day in each session, allowing for a constant renewal of the intention to approach their internal world.

All dragons can be used from the first therapeutic encounter. The child can begin to approach them gradually, and the therapist determines the right moment to use the one that corresponds. It is possible to use them in all age groups. In family interviews, they are also very effective when it comes to psychoeducation and to carry out family mindfulness practices.

Recognition of Emotional Regulation Systems

It is almost impossible to separate the first phase of work from the ones that follow, as they integrate with each other. Shame involves the activation of very intense and extreme physiological responses in its manifestations, including hiding, curling up, covering oneself so there is no possible social connection, or hostile and aggressive behaviors. By establishing the therapeutic bond from the outset, we create a safe enough container that supports the recognition of emotional regulation systems, the triggers that activate each one, and the exploration and practice of different regulatory strategies.

For children with dissociative states, the use of dragons can facilitate approaching the states and creating awareness of their existence.

Development of Self-Regulation Skills

As the therapist gradually accompanies the child in exploring their internal world with the help of the dragons, the dragons can be used both as resources for regulation and to teach skills the child may not have developed. At this stage, tolerance for distress and connection with pleasant emotions become the focus of clinical work, serving as an important antidote against shame. Through this process, the therapist begins to get a glimpse of the function of shame in the child's life. To facilitate inner connection and communication, children can be invited to write letters from one dragon to another; for example, when a child needs courage, the dragon embodying the compassionate ideal can write a courageous letter to the dragon that is fearful under the sea.

The same resource can be used in approaching dissociated states: working with letters between the states and the dragons can be beneficial both for creating awareness of the internal world and for offering a resource that a certain state may need. For example, if a child aspect needs the development of patience, we can offer, through a dragon, to write to that state and give it ideas on how to practice patience. It is also possible to ask questions of that state in the dragon's letter. These questions also serve the goal of regulating the child, helping them become acquainted with their internal world, expanding their awareness of it, and acquiring resources. For the letter writing, Moreno (2023) has developed an "ancient papyrus" that invites children to explore different "mysterious" writing techniques, such as invisible ink or lemon-made ink to later uncover what is written. These letters from one state to another also help create co-awareness and share internal resources. Furthermore, practicing standing in the shoes of one dragon and then another enhances psychological flexibility, mentalizing capacities, and empathy.

Exploration and Coping with Shame

Working with textures is very helpful when encouraging the exploration of shame with children. Many children use their skin as a shield to protect themselves from what they consider shameful, and inviting the child to pet the "skins" of the different dragons (as they are very different in color, texture, roughness, smoothness, etc.) and compare the feel of them to what they notice on their own skin can be effective. Perhaps they can discover a scar and explore it, for example. Sometimes the skin is a good doorway to working on shame.

Some children describe their skin as having many layers that they can hide in. Their true self is hidden inside those layers that allow them to cover up what they feel is shameful. Other children say that if they have very thick skin, they can prevent their emotions from coming out from within or even from occurring. This avoidance causes their internal world to become isolated and unknown to them. They may feel ashamed of this world. If the dragons become skillful means to investigate what material each layer of skin is made of, what resources to use to explore it, the child will be able to gradually get closer to having a loving look at themselves.

Sometimes, children say they feel that their skin is full of scars or that they feel a wound that is visible, and that stigmatizes them. Exploring these wounds and looking for ways to heal them through the skins of the dragons first and then themselves is an important achievement to overcome the shame of their own wounds. Many times, we use "magical creams" or the "sacred fire" of the dragons to heal them.

Imagery is additionally used in CFT, with the aim of progressively supporting the development of compassion for one's own suffering. One practice adapted for children by Moreno (2023) is self-compassion. In this practice, one of the dragons represents the compassionate qualities that would be beneficial to cultivate in the child. These qualities include kindness, courage, wisdom, bravery, and love. Through a mindfulness practice, the therapist narrates a story, through the voice of the dragon, and reveals how as a guide, it can offer these qualities to the child. The compassionate dragon conveys those qualities through "sacred fire," made of colored fabrics and wires that allow it to move like fire. Receiving warmth in their hearts, generating a loving guidance in response to that reception of warm love, predisposes the child toward tenderness and kindness. That same transmitting fire can be for their own interior and for them to share with others. The therapist must be very attentive to manifestations of shame that may arise in the child and help them look at it and offer alternatives. It is also possible to play with different poses with the dragons to work on more gentle body postures that become resources against postures of shame.

EMDR Therapy in Work with Parents

According to Baita (2022b), parents of children who have suffered interpersonal trauma can be divided into three major groups: (1) parents who were actively involved in the traumatization (an abusive mother), (2) parents who suffered the same traumatic events along with the child (a mother abused by her husband who was, in turn, abusive toward their children), and (3) parents who were not involved in the traumatization of the child, or involved in the same traumatization suffered by the child. Within this third group there are two sub-categories: (3.1) parents who suffered early interpersonal trauma in their childhood, and (3.2) parents who didn't. In case 1, clinicians need to be sure whether or not the child is still at risk of further maltreatment, in which case the first action is to involve child protective services in order to provide environmental safety for the child. In case 2, clinicians need to know if the parent was exposed to trauma along with the child, and if the parent processed their own traumatic experiences. In case 3, the clinician needs to know whether the parent has processed their own early traumatic experiences, since the child's experiences can trigger the parent's own memories of abuse and neglect. In addition, research has shown that adoptive parents can be traumatized by knowing the preadoptive history of their children (Skandrani et al., 2019).

In Baita's experience, many parents are also traumatized by the ongoing repetition of disruptive behaviors and affective dysregulation of their children, especially when the children have received previous treatments that failed. Caregivers might engage in rumination about their "flaws" as parents, catastrophic thoughts about their child's future, and, in the most severe cases, blatant rejection of their children, including the thought or even the intention of returning them to the system if they were adopted (Baita, 2022b). As a rule of thumb, caregivers of traumatized children should process their own traumatic experiences; however, sometimes they feel overtaken by their child's actual problems and difficulties and struggle with starting a therapeutic process themselves. Other parents may be actively in therapy but with a non-trauma-informed clinician, leaving their own trauma unresolved. In these specific situations, the authors suggest the integration of a short EMDR-focused intervention with the parent, done either by the child's therapist in case there are no resources available in the therapist's community, or, in the best-case scenario, by another EMDR clinician with expertise in complex trauma and dissociation (Baita, 2022b). When the child therapist is in charge of offering this short intervention, which is not meant to be therapy for the parent, they will need to consider whether the specific rules and practice laws in their community/state/country allow them to provide brief interventions to their client's parents. Every time it is possible, working within a clinical team—with both the child's therapist and the parent's—is advisable. The goals for this intervention are to process any traumatic information that might be blocking the caregiver's capacity to connect with the child, and to support the caregiver to make an effective connection with the traumatic history of the child as the source of the current suffering. It is important to note that only trained EMDR therapists should be using this intervention.

Important conditions and steps to consider in this intervention include:

a A good alliance between caregiver and therapist. The caregiver needs to feel safe and comfortable in the relationship to disclose their own feelings and concerns, which sometimes can be harsh and painful. The therapist needs to be aware of the caregiver's potential fear of being misjudged for expressing anger, fear, or rejection toward the child and/or their behavior, and must be able to undertake a compassionate mindset, without overlooking the child's safety within the relationship with their caregiver.
b Suggesting the intervention to desensitize the caregiver's suffering when facing the child's current problems.
c If the provider of this intervention is the child's therapist, the clinician must be clear in explaining the limits and boundaries involved (no more than three sessions), and that this is not a replacement of the caregiver's own therapy or a therapeutic process the clinician will conduct alongside the child's therapy.
d This intervention is not suggested for parents who are highly dysregulated, dismiss any kind of help for themselves (including parents with psychiatric conditions who don't receive any sort of treatment), or have expressed strong thoughts about returning the child back to the system.

When parents are in a state of hopelessness and despair about their child's potential for change, which is often rooted in a year-long struggle with affective and behavioral dysregulation, or when they expect this dysregulation to repeat even after a day or two of calmness, our suggestion is to frame the intervention from the perspective of ongoing traumatic stress. For these cases, an EMDR recent event–related protocol such as the PRECI protocol (Jarero & Artigas, 2018) provides a good framework for the intervention. This protocol conceptualizes the "continuum of prolonged adverse experiences [which] creates a cumulative trauma exposure memory network of linked pathogenic memories with similar emotional, somatic, sensorial, and cognitive information that does not give the cumulative state-dependent traumatic memory network sufficient time to consolidate into an integrated whole" (Jimenez et al., 2020, p. 44).

There are cases in which the affective and behavioral dysregulation of the child causes a state of constant alarm, and caregivers express catastrophic fears about the near or distant future, in which either they (*the child will kill us*) or the child (*they will end up in jail if they keep stealing*) are in danger. The caregiver's hypervigilance and overreaction pervade the bond with the child, creating a state in which neither feels safe in the presence of the other. From the child's perspective, the disconnection from their caregiver is felt as rejection, fueling the internal sense of being worthless and not lovable, which is the heart of core shame. For these cases in which the reflective capacities of parents seem overcome by their fears, the Flashforward EMDR Protocol (Logie & de Jongh, 2014, 2016) can be helpful in decreasing their distress, as will be shown by the following case example. The Flashforward Protocol is based on research showing that "mental representations about potential future catastrophes can be processed in the same way as past events" (Logie & de Jongh, 2016, p. 81). The authors of this procedure recommend using it only when clients have processed past traumatic memories, although they also state that it can be used "when a future feared event is so disruptive to normal life that the client is either not sufficiently motivated to consider past events or is incapable of doing so" (Logie & de Jongh, 2016, p. 82). This is many times the case of caregivers of children with complex trauma and dissociation, especially when their dysregulation is extremely disruptive and threatens to harm or break the bonding between the child and their caregivers.

Case Example[1]

Bea is a ten-year-old-child who was separated from her biological parents at the age of 5 due to physical and sexual abuse and severe neglect. She spent five years in foster care until her adoption by Tomás and Marta. Previously, Bea underwent two failed adoption processes, and the moment in which she met Tomás and Marta, she said this would be the last attempt for her. While in foster care, Bea would engage in constant rage outbursts followed by periods of extreme withdrawal, during which she could stay in a dazed, trance-like state for hours. Her symptoms worsened when she went to live with Tomás and Marta; she claimed that she heard a voice commanding her to hurt her adoptive mother, which she did a couple of times.

Marta and Tomás's attitude toward Bea was kind and affectionate during the first months, but by the time of consultation, they were exhausted and in despair. Marta claimed to feel in danger with her daughter and rejected by her, and expressed feelings of rejection in turn toward her. She said these feelings were fueled by Bea claiming she would be better in foster care. Tomás presented as more patient and understanding than his wife, and more capable of helping Bea self-regulate. However, this was also creating distress within their relationship and they discussed divorce as a possibility for the first time. The cycle of attack from Bea and rejection from Marta was creating a huge obstacle to the development of a bond between them. Based on her former experiences of abuse at her birth home and later failed adoptions, Bea was acting from a shame-based thought of not being good enough to be loved by her adoptive mom. And Marta's rejection toward her daughter was fueled by her fear of being attacked by Bea, which was reinforcing shame-based thoughts. Working from a CFT framework adapted for children, the following process explains the work carried out with this family in three of the four stages explained in the previous paragraphs.

Establishment of Therapeutic Bond/Psychoeducation

Bea was observed to be highly reactive toward the therapist initially, and the familiar element of sharing a snack was used to establish a connection between them. Sharing a snack with Bea was a way to start building a bond. Initially, the therapist would bring the snack tray close, but the girl wouldn't touch it. On one occasion, the therapist asked if she didn't like what had been served, to which the girl responded, "I thought it was only for you. That I couldn't eat anything from there," as if she didn't have the right or was invisible to the therapist's eyes. This exchange allowed them to start playing with the image reflected in the coffee cup with milk. Both began to see themselves reflected in the cup, and this was the first time they could approach the feeling of shame.

Working with Emotional Regulation Systems—Introducing Each of the Dragons

Bea showed curiosity and attentiveness to the stories of each dragon, which allowed her to explore her reactions to her adoptive parents, as well as what triggered her anger, and this allowed them to start practicing regulation exercises, as follows:

Bea: [*holding the shame dragon puppet*] This happens in my head. I feel like I need to tuck it inside my body. [*She makes a gesture with the puppet hiding its head*] I feel like my body is like this, all red.

Therapist: If you close your eyes and imagine that you are the dragon... could you tell me where you feel those urges to hide? Have you felt them before?

Bea:	Here, in my face and throat. My current parents leave me out of their conversations. I'm alone.
Therapist:	Do you think you can bring the dragon and lean it against that part of your body?
Bea:	Yes.
Therapist:	Can we find a word or gesture to soothe that sensation?
Bea:	No, I can't. I get so angry that I want to hit. She doesn't understand that I feel lonely.
Therapist:	Do you think it's appropriate for me to offer you that gesture to calm it down?
Bea:	Yes.

The therapist brings the dragon's fire closer and gently rests it on Bea's throat while saying, "May you be calm, may you become aware of the anger and do something to calm it down without hurting anyone." At the same time, the therapist offers resources for Bea to use when feeling angry.

Working with Emotional Regulation Systems—Physiological Regulation

In several sessions, Bea displayed verbal hostility toward the therapist.

Therapist:	Did you come in today feeling very angry?
Bea:	I don't want to talk to you.
Therapist:	I understand. Can we do some breathing exercises to start?
	Bea reluctantly agrees.
Therapist:	Dad told me it was a difficult week. Can we draw the worst part?
	Bea draws a scene of shopping with her mother.
Therapist:	I'm going to get the smallest dragon. Remember that it can hold everything that makes us suffer inside?
	Bea agrees to have it close to her.
Therapist:	Can I ask the dragon what it needs right now?
Bea:	I don't know.
Therapist:	Let's look together. Maybe we can sing to it, rock it gently, maybe it's hungry.
Bea:	A song.

Together, Bea and the therapist sing to the small dragon that holds her anger. The therapist helps Bea calm this emotion before continuing the session, offering a corrective experience around unmet developmental needs.

Development of Self-Regulation Skills: Use of Compassionate Self as a Regulation Strategy

Bea expressed on several occasions that she didn't feel pleasant emotions. In a session, the therapist suggested she draw the outline of her body. Bea drew five ovals representing different layers of her skin, varying in thickness, and in the middle, a very small girl, covering her face and in a fetal position. Being able to go through each layer of skin and understand its function allowed for a gradual approach to that girl Bea described as being "hurt."

Therapist:	What does that skin of yours need to feel emotions of love, calmness, joy?
Bea:	My skin hurts a lot, I can't touch it.
Therapist:	Do you think we can ask for help from Amarú [the dragon representing compassionate ideal]?

	Bea takes the dragon and places it on her arms with its antennae toward her chest.
Therapist:	I have an idea. Let's ask Amarú to use his wisdom to find a healing cream so we can gradually heal that skin.
	Bea was very excited about the idea. This process took place over several sessions and at the end of each session, she made a drawing on her skin. After some time, Bea finally managed to draw her healthy skin and was able to practice with her therapist and the dragon Amarú how it feels to experience emotions of joy, calmness, and love. As the sessions progressed, Bea was able to explore not only her feelings of shame but also the motivations behind the attacks toward her adoptive mother, which decreased simultaneously with the work done with both her and her parents.

Simultaneous to Bea's therapy, Marta worked with a therapist through an EMDR model of treatment to process her intense feelings of rejection after she disclosed her pain about being attacked by her daughter at night. Marta had been in psychoanalytic therapy since the time in which her infertility was diagnosed, and she had a strong bond with her therapist and didn't want to make any changes. However, she agreed to do a brief EMDR-related intervention with the hope of releasing her hypervigilance and anxiety related to vivid images of her daughter attacking her and accompanying feelings of sadness and embarrassment. Whenever she had the thought of her daughter attacking her, she would distract herself by going out for a run.

Bea's therapist had explained to her the connection between the girl's traumatic past and her present behavior toward her mom, and this explanation made sense to Marta. However, she felt it wasn't enough for her to decrease the distress. After working on a few grounding exercises, the EMDR therapist explained to Marta the aim of the Flashforward Protocol and the procedure they would use. She was instructed to stop if she felt overwhelmed by her feelings, sensations, or images. Marta suddenly found the most catastrophic scenario she could imagine: Bea killing her. The worst part of this scenario was Bea's enraged face and her hands going after Marta's throat. Marta felt terror, and her body trembled. Below there is an excerpt of her processing. The symbol "//" replaces the instruction to keep processing given by the clinician:

Marta:	I recall I've asked the social worker why the previous family sent Bea back to the system. She said they couldn't handle her. I recall I told my husband, "There is something wrong about this child they don't want us to know." He said I was exaggerating. // I felt very miserable for this thought because Bea was so sweet at the beginning... // I recall the first time I felt afraid of being alone with her... I am ashamed of myself... // I couldn't even talk to my therapist about this... I was sure I was doing everything wrong. // I can't relax when I am with her... I feel like everything can change all of a sudden... // I shouldn't have these awful thoughts... I am not a good mother... [*As the procedure goes on, Marta seems stuck with negative thoughts about her parenting skills*]
Therapist:	What do you think a good mother for Bea should look like?
Marta:	Loving...
Therapist:	What does a loving mother do for her child?
Marta:	Take good care of her... // I do take good care of her... I do my best... // Sometimes we can enjoy being together... I wish everything could stay this way... // I wish she could trust me; I wish she could feel I will never hurt her in any possible way... //
Therapist:	If you go back to the picture of Bea killing you, tell me what comes out...
Marta:	[*smiles*] Can a child throwing a spoon or pushing you become a killer? [*the two ways in which Bea attacked her mother*] // Sometimes I feel so frustrated... I wish I could know what should I do not to trigger her...

The session ended with psychoeducation regarding how difficult it is for any parent to know exactly what to do and discussing how she was instructed by Bea's therapist to identify possible triggers. During the second session, the therapist resumed the Flashforward Protocol:

Therapist: I want you to go back to the picture in which you see Bea killing you and tell me what comes out.
Marta: I see a helpless little child afraid of being hurt.
Therapist: Look at any feeling, sensations, or words arising with this picture right now.
Marta: Who on earth could be so bad as to hurt a little child? How is it even possible? // I feel so sorry for her... I wish I could have known her before... // Bea's therapist taught us some resources to calm her down, but sometimes I am afraid of approaching her... // My husband knows how to cuddle her... I probably don't have this skill...
Therapist: Can you imagine yourself hugging and cuddling Bea?
M: [*closes her eyes and shakes*] I think I'm scared... // How could she feel safe with me if I'm scared of her? // I see myself petting her... I can do this... //
Therapist: Look at yourself cuddling her and tell me how does your body feel right now?
Marta: It's a warm sensation... she likes me cuddling her... [*smiles*] // Sometimes she falls asleep while I'm cuddling her... // She used to ask me to hug her when we were on the couch watching TV... I did but I rushed to undo the hug... // She probably felt unloved... [*sobs*]... // I don't want to make her feel unloved... she is my daughter...
Therapist: Go back to the moment in which you cuddle her...
Marta: It's still warm... // I wish I could have cuddled her as a baby... // She doesn't deserve to feel unloved... [*The connection with Bea as a child who was hurt and deserved to feel loved kept growing*]
Therapist: If you now go back to the picture of Bea killing you, what comes out?
Marta: [*shaking her head*] She won't, I know that... // I have been avoiding her since the time she threw [a spoon at me]... and even before that... // I probably felt responsible for not being able to understand or do things better... // It's not my fault what happened to her... I'm just trying to fix all the damage others did to her... and I must keep working until she realizes she deserves to be loved...
Therapist: I would like you to go to the picture of yourself petting her... [*Marta closes her eyes, smiles, and nods*] try to feel the warmth of this moment... notice how Bea feels safe with you... so safe that she is even able to fall asleep on your lap... What words would go better with this picture right now?
Marta: Sometimes I can make mistakes, but I will never hurt you, Bea...
Therapist: If you go one more time to the picture of Bea killing you, tell me what comes out...
Marta: Nothing... the picture is gone... I can only see my daughter afraid of being hurt... We won't hurt her...
Therapist: Can you imagine yourself telling Bea to tell her little voice inside that you will take good care of her and everything she has inside?
Marta: I find it funny... but I think I can....

By the end of the second and last session Marta was discussing ways in which she could have reacted the times in which Bea tried to attack her, realizing that her fear was so intense she reacted from a place of belief that she was in actual danger. On a follow-up a month later, Marta reported she no longer had any intrusive images and thoughts about being killed by Bea.

In turn, Bea became less reactive with her mother, and this allowed for a reinforcement of their bonding. Later in therapy, Bea invited both parents in so she could show them the dragons, and played with them, teaching what she had learned. Dyadic and/or family work is encouraged only when the child feels safe enough to share her internal world with parents, and when parents are self-regulated.

This comprehensive approach that seeks to intervene with children and family together allows for regulation and creates both individual and family resources to increase connection and communication. Without this work, Bea's recovery would have been impossible. Children's shame is born within a relationship and causes disconnection. This disconnection needs to be repaired within the relationship, for which the therapist is just a vehicle. If parents can understand how their child's behavior is rooted in this deep feeling of shame, they can hold all their child's suffering and learn strategies to respond instead of react when shame-based behaviors arise.

Conclusion

Experiencing shame leaves a person depleted of energy and feeling devastated, and is felt throughout the body—hence the importance of not only identifying the ways in which shame manifests, but also seeking external and internal contexts of safety to counteract it. In working with children, this involves including their families as well as understanding how shame is expressed within the therapeutic relationship, since the therapeutic relationship, like other interpersonal connections, can trigger shame. Even the simple gaze of a kind and empathetic therapist can activate it. This does not mean that therapists should not possess these qualities, but rather that we will need to tap into our creativity to uncover the threads of shame and not shy away from working with it. We may envision shame as torn and frayed fabric, where we can see only some threads. These threads can be observed through the body, through gazes, gestures, postures, silences, and breaths, as well as in the dynamics of the child's interpersonal relationships and in the space between the therapist and the child who comes for therapy. The therapist's ability to attune to the relational disconnections resulting from the activation of shame and to support their reparation is crucial in reinforcing development and reversing the core belief of inadequacy and defectiveness.

Note

1 All case examples in this chapter are composites.

References

Alix, S., Cossette, L., Hébert, M., Cyr, M., & Frappier, J. (2017). Posttraumatic stress disorder and suicidal ideation among sexually abused adolescent girls: The mediating role of shame. *Journal of Child Sexual Abuse, 26*(2), 158–174. https://doi.org/10.1080/10538712.2017.1280577

Bafunno, D., & Camodeca, M. (2013). Shame and guilt development in preschoolers: The role of context, audience and individual characteristics. *European Journal of Developmental Psychology, 10*(2), 128–143. https://doi.org/10.1080/17405629.2013.765796

Baita, S. (2022a). El circuito de la vergüenza nuclear y el rechazo en el trauma interpersonal temprano. Online workshop. Asociación EMDR Perú. September 30–October 1, 2022.

Baita, S. (2022b). Tratamiento del trauma del desarrollo y la disociación traumática en la infancia y adolescencia. Workshop. Asociación EMDR España, Madrid, November 11–13, 2022.

Cozolino, L. (2014). *The neuroscience of human relationship: Attachment and the developing social brain* (2nd ed.). W. W. Norton.

Deblinger, E., & Runyon, M. K. (2005). Understanding and treating feelings of shame in children who have experienced maltreatment. *Child Maltreatment, 11*(4), 364–376. https://doi.org/10.1177/1077559505279306

Feiring, C., Taska, L., & Chen, K. (2002a). Trying to understand why horrible things happen: Attribution, shame, and symptom development following sexual abuse. *Child Maltreatment, 7*(1), 25–39. https://doi.org/10.1177/1077559502007001003

Feiring, C., Taska, L., & Lewis, M. (2002b). Adjustment following sexual abuse discovery: The role of shame and attributional style. *Developmental Psychology, 38*(1), 79–92. https://doi.org/10.1037/0012-1649.38.1.79

Gilbert, P. (2009). *The compassionate mind*. Constable & Robinson.

Gilbert, P. (2010). *Compassion focused therapy*. Routledge.

Jarero, I., & Artigas, L. (2018). AIP model-based acute trauma and ongoing traumatic stress theoretical conceptualization. *Iberoamerican Journal of Psychotraumatology and Dissociation, 10*(1), 1–10. revibapst.com/volumen-10-numero-1-2018-2019

Jimenez, G., Becker, Y., Varela, C., García, P., Nuño, M. A., Perez, M. C., Osorio, A., Jarero, I., & Givaudan, M. (2020). Multicenter randomized controlled trial on the provision of the EMDR-PRECI to female minors victims of sexual and/or physical violence and related PTSD diagnosis. *American Journal of Applied Psychology, 9*(2), 42–51. https://doi.org/10.11648/j.ajap.20200902.12

Kochanska, G., Gross, J., Lin, M., & Nichols, K. (2002). Guilt in young children: development, determinants and relations with a broader system of standards. *Child Development, 73*, 461–482. https://doi.org/10.1111/1467-8624.00418

Kolts, R. L. (2016). *CFT made simple: A clinician's guide to practicing compassion-focused therapy*. New Harbinger Publications.

Logie, R., & de Jongh, A. (2014). The flashforward procedure: Confronting the catastrophe. *Journal of EMDR Practice and Research, 8*(1), 25–32. https://doi.org/10.1891/1933-3196.8.1.25

Logie, R., & de Jongh, A. (2016). The flashforward procedure. In M. Luber (Ed.), *EMDR therapy: Scripted protocols and summary sheets; treating anxiety, obsessive-compulsive and mood-related disorders* (pp. 81–90). Springer.

Luby, J., Belden, A., Sullivan, J., & Hayen, R. (2009). Shame and guilt in preschool depression: Evidence for elevation in self-conscious emotions in depression as early as age 3. *Journal of Child Psychology and Psychiatry, 50*(9), 1156–1166. https://doi.org/10.1111/j.1469-7610.2009.02077.x

McElvaney, R., Greene, S., & Hogan, D. (2014). To tell or not to tell? Factors influencing young people's informal disclosures of child sexual abuse. *Journal of Interpersonal Violence, 29*(5), 928–947. https://doi.org/10.1177/0886260513506281

Moreno, P. (2023). Dragones compasivos. Una adaptación de intervenciones basadas en CFT para la infancia. https://www.paulamoreno.org/post/dragones-compasivos-una-adaptaci%C3%B3n-de-intervenciones-basadas-en-cft-para-la-infancia

Moreno, P., & Véliz Araya, C. (2022). La humanidad compartida como parte de la intervención en niños y niñas que han sufrido traumas relacionales. *Revista de Psicotraumatología y Disociación, 11*(1), 7. revibapst.com/_files/ugd/c70085_5431cc5feb8d4f8d88d0c2f3c66dbb69.pdf

Muris, P. (2015). Guilt, shame, and psychopathology in children and adolescents. *Child Psychiatry and Human Development, 46*(2), 177–179. https://doi.org/10.1007/s10578-014-0488-9

Muris, P., Meesters, C., Heijmans, J., van Hulten, S., Kaanen, L., Oerlemans, B., Stikkelbroeck, T., & Tielemans. T. (2016). Lack of guilt, guilt, and shame: A multi-informant study on the relations between self-conscious emotions and psychopathology in clinically referred children and adolescents. *European Society of Child and Adolescent Psychiatry, 25*(4), 383–396. https://doi.org/10.1007/s00787-015-0749-6

Neff, K. (2012). *Self-compassion: The proven power of being kind to yourself*. HarperCollins.

Parisette-Sparks, A., Bufferd, S. J., & Klein, D. (2017). Parental predictors of children's shame and guilt at age 6 in a multi-method, longitudinal study. *Journal of Clinical Child and Adolescent Psychiatry, 46*(5), 721–731. https://doi.org/10.1080/15374416.2015.1063430

Porges, S. W. (2021). *Polyvagal safety: Attachment, communication and self-regulation*. W. W. Norton.

Schore, A. N. (2019). *Right brain psychotherapy*. W. W. Norton.

Silberg, J. L (2022). *The child survivor. Healing developmental trauma and dissociation* (2nd ed.). Routledge.

Skandrani, S., Harf, A., & El Husseini, M. (2019). The impact of children's pre-adoptive traumatic experiences on parents. *Frontiers in Psychiatry, 10*, Article 866. https://doi.org/10.3389/fpsyt.2019.00866

Steele, K., Boon, S., & van der Hart, O. (2017). *Treating trauma-related dissociation: A practical, integrative approach*. W. W. Norton.

Tangney, J. P., & Dearing, R. L. (2002). *Shame and guilt*. Guilford Press.

Thompson, R. A., Goodvin, R., & Meyer, S. (2006). Social development: Psychological understanding, self-understanding, and relationships. In J. L. Luby (Ed.), *Handbook of preschool mental health: Development, disorders, and treatment* (pp. 3–22). Guilford Press.

Tracy, J. L., & Robins, R. W. (2006). Appraisal antecedents of shame and guilt: Support for a theoretical model. *Personality and Social Psychology Bulletin, 32*(10), 1339–1351. https://doi.org/10.1177/0146167206290212

Young, P. (2015). *Understanding and treating chronic shame: A relational/neurobiological approach*. Routledge.

40
THE TRAUMA-FORMED DEFENSE AND SELF-PROTECTIVE SYSTEM

Ana M. Gómez

Introduction

Mary, a six-year-old, comes to therapy only because her parents are forcing her to do so. From the first session, she tells the therapists that she does not need to be there and that everything in her life is perfect. Mary's parents report extreme temper tantrums, nightmares, and frequent headaches without medical explanations. She also hates and refuses to use the word "feelings," insisting that she only feels happy. She completely denies any challenges, and reports that her life is wonderful.

Joe, an 11-year-old, cooperates and follows any invitations the therapist gives. He tells her exactly what she wants to hear. Joe reports quickly that he is feeling better and takes any opportunity to compliment his clinician, who believes Joe is doing very well during the sessions. However, every week, his parents report minimal shifts and progress in his anxiety and difficulty sleeping.

Skylar, a ten-year-old, comes to therapy because of severe trauma and spaciness. She was diagnosed with an attention deficit and put on medication that worsened the symptoms. Skylar disengages and detaches from any emotional content. However, at times, she engages in dangerous activities. She was caught stealing, and putting forks inside the power outlets at home, which seems exciting and thrilling to her.

Kelly, a 12-year-old, clings to her mother constantly. She refuses to have sleepovers or go to friends' birthday parties unless her mother is present. She feels jealous when her mother spends time with her siblings, and constantly fights with her family. When attending her therapy sessions, she demands that her mother sit with her throughout the session. She also refuses to engage in any playful activity unless her mother is involved.

George comes to therapy because of aggressiveness and extreme behavioral problems at school. George was born at an orphanage and adopted at the age of 5. When he comes to therapy, he wants to control everything and everybody, including the therapists. He becomes oppositional and belligerent if the clinician invites him to participate in playful activities. He wants to play video games and finds therapy utterly dull. George does not want the therapist to engage with or follow him in any way; if the therapist does, George becomes verbally, and sometimes physically, aggressive.

All the children described above hold multiple similarities: they all have been exposed to complex trauma and utilize strategies and defenses that represent their best attempt to attain homeostasis and survive. However, they can potentially stagnate the therapeutic process and prevent opportunities for connection, social engagement, and healing. The clinicians working with these children often report feeling defeated, frustrated, exhausted, and hopeless. Children like these also have the greatest potential of awakening the clinician's own unresolved trauma and defense system—that is, the clinician's forms of self-protection may become activated as they attempt to be the child's companion and bio-emotional regulator. Despite the clinician's best intentions, these children may push the therapist away; compulsively please them; become increasingly aggressive, dissociative, or sexual; control entire sessions; remain disengaged and avoidant; or utterly manipulate them.

These interactions often result in the clash between the child's protective system and the clinician's non-conscious defenses, ultimately leading to therapeutic failure.

When the autonomic nervous system (ANS) is in a constant state of defense and self-preservation, it becomes antagonistic, diminishing the effectiveness of treatment (Porges, 2021). As long as the child remains in defense mode, attempts of the clinician to support their healing can be blunted, and therapeutically addressing the defense mode thus becomes imperative.

Defining the Defense Mode: An Act of Recognition of the Self-Protective System

The human mind's attempt to escape suffering has been addressed by diverse approaches. However, there is no unifying theory encompassing the multiple biological systems involved, ranging from mechanisms of defense viewed through a psychoanalytic lens (e.g., denial, minimization), to the disorganization of inborn motivational systems, and to the cascade of rigid bio-behavioral states in the autonomic nervous system (ANS) resulting from chronic trauma exposure. Self-protective strategies are often given pejorative labels such as "resistance," "defensiveness," "opposition," and "maladaptive coping." Children with such defenses are sometimes called "impossible to work with" or "untreatable." Additionally, the child often carries the blame if they are not reaching the expected therapeutic goals. These definitions and divisions in responsibility share a blaming and pathologizing tone and approach.

This chapter offers a shame-free space to understand defenses while acknowledging their fundamental role in the survival of traumatized children, and humanity in general. Simultaneously, it recognizes the therapeutic challenges children's active defenders may create as well as their labor in preventing the healing of the wounds they protect, perseverating the suffering of these children. The reframing of trauma-forming defenses from "maladaptive" to "functional adaptations" (Wadsworth, 2015) made in the perpetual quest for safety and survival gives context and recognition to the suffering and struggles of these children.

Trauma results in synaptic architectures that hold the experiences of trauma and defenses against overwhelming affect that is stored in implicit-procedural memory (Schore, 2019). When the brain and associated biological systems cross sensitive developmental periods, children exposed to suboptimal and wounding environmental inputs are forced to grow and develop within these milieus. Children are pressed to rely on self-regulation even in the absence of well-developed psychobiological regulatory capacities. Thumb-sucking and gaze aversion, for example, are children's early emerging attempts to defend and protect against overwhelming stress in the absence of a caregiver's co-regulating forces. For children to develop a repertoire of coping, they need exposure to mild to moderate distress while experiencing the protective and regulating influences of their caregiver and age-appropriate scaffolding. The child who is without an emotional regulator and is exposed to severe, chronic stress is left to rely on developmentally primitive and rudimentary coping strategies that are limited and rigidly utilized (Wadsworth, 2015). As a result, the hypothalamic-pituitary-adrenal (HPA) axis may remain active across all situations, not just the ones associated with danger (Wadsworth, 2015), provoking the rigid self-regulatory and defensive strategies of either hypervigilance or avoidance. Even when the child has developed metacognitive, bio-affective, and behavioral capacities for regulation, the need to respond to threats rapidly activates their defenses, overriding conscious thinking capacities and wishes (Gilbert, 2001). In traumatized children, threats may come from both outside and within. The child's experience of abuse, neglect, or emotional unavailability becomes a biological imprint their mind defends against. The "threat" affect-regulating system governs what the traumatized child orients to in their inner and outer worlds (Gilbert, 2022). The neuroception of danger may be set off by the inner legacy left by trauma, which includes body-based inner cues. The child's inner world now has the power alone to activate the defense mode, as it carries the legacy of trauma.

When the child is in defense mode, the ventral vagus nerve is not optimally managing the ANS, rupturing the synergy and coordination between the sympathetic and dorsal vagus that is needed to support homeostasis (Porges, 2023). Safety has been compromised for children exposed to severe traumatization. As such, they find a false and distorted sense of security in the defense mode, which contains a cascade of offensive and protective forces—for example, "If I control everything and everyone, I will be safe," or "if I avoid feelings at all cost, I will not suffer." These defenses involve the activation of psychobiological systems and strategic active-energizing (fight and flight) or passive-inhibited (submission, immobilization, and passive avoidance) behaviors (Gilbert, 2001). In other words, hyper-reactive and hypo-reactive forces color defensive responses and adaptations to trauma. Gilbert (2001) identified common defensive behaviors resulting from trauma:

1. Defensive fights: children quickly become aggressive toward others as they perceive threats even in safe environments.
2. Escaping and avoiding: observed in children who use distance and disengagement in the presence of a threat.
3. Help-seeking: evident in children who constantly and frantically work on eliciting care and protection.
4. Submitting: seen in children who submit to deactivate threats and aggression from others.
5. Hiding and camouflaging: children avoid being seen and conceal self, feelings, and the inner world. They cut off interaction, such as by covering eyes and tuning away.
6. Demobilizing, long and short term: encompasses disengagement and freeze-faint responses. Long term, it results in a depressed mood and anhedonia.

These defensive behaviors are closely connected to the ANS defense cascade (fight, flight, freeze, flag, submit, and collapse) (Kozlowska et al., 2015), which can become obstructed or overactive in the presence of chronic occurrences of trauma. Trauma-formed defensive structures constitute a quiet complex phenomenon as multiple systems, such as the attachment system, the defense cascade of the ANS, and biological motivational systems, interact.

The Defense and Self-Protective System: Motivational Systems

Defensive goals and actions exist within an intricate matrix of motivational systems that are deeply affected by trauma and attachment disorganization. Some of the child's behaviors labeled as defensive are in fact driven by motivational systems in a state of dysregulation or inhibition. In order to protect and sustain life, the brain possesses motivational biological systems that move the individual into action to attain survival or prosocial needs. Multiple categories of motivational systems that generate distinct types of affective consciousness and behavioral goals have been proposed. For instance, Panksepp (1998) and Panksepp and Biven (2012) mapped seven inborn operational motivational systems that ensure survival and prosocial behaviors:

- Seeking (expectancy and curiosity, guides anticipatory learning, seeking things in the world, exploration)
- Care (nurturance, displays supportive behaviors)
- Fear/Anxiety (attachment separation and distress)

- Rage (anger)
- Panic/Grief (sadness)
- Play (social joy)
- Lust (sexual excitement)

Steele (2021) proposed nine multi-motivational systems:

- Attachment (security and safety)
- Caregiving (response to separation cry)
- Panic/loss (panic at loss of connection)
- Collaboration/cooperation
- Competition/ranking
- Sexuality (organized by lust, advanced goals of pleasure)
- Play (organized by joy, exploration and social connection)
- Defense (flight, fight, freeze and faint to defend)
- Predation (organized around killing or injuring another)

The child not only uses the typical defenses (fight and flight), but also engages the motivational systems in defensive ways (K. Steele, personal communication, December 20, 2023). Some of these systems are primitive and organized around survival, while others with later evolutionary developments are structured around prosocial behaviors supporting neocortical functions (van der Hart et al., 2006; Steele, 2021). These inborn systems are goal-oriented, and once the aim is attained and terminated, there is a signal that opens the opportunity for another system to initiate new goals and actions, which shows how closely they interact with one another (Steele, 2021). Once the action is fully completed, the joy of triumph and mastery emerges, which Pierre Janet referred to as "the act of triumph" (Ogden, 2019). For instance, during a moment of distress, a child will experience the activation of the attachment system, which motivates proximity seeking to the caregiver. Once the goal is reached (the child obtains the security, reassurance, protection, and regulation in the moment of distress), the attachment system is moved to the background in a "quiet" state (K. Steele, personal communication, December 20, 2023), and attachment behaviors are terminated. Once the child is regulated, having attained the act of triumph, the child resumes exploratory behavior (the exploratory system takes the foreground) until separation or another distressing event activates the attachment system to bring it into the foreground again (Beckes et al., 2015). Another example is a child who is able to engage their defense system when harassed at school and fight their attacker successfully, and thus experience a victorious completion of their fight response.

These motivational systems develop appropriately and congruently under the proper safety and security conditions. However, according to Liotti's (2017) multi-motivational theory, disorganized attachment and trauma during child development activate these systems in a disorderly fashion, resulting in tension and conflicts among them, which greatly impacts the defense system. In addition, children exposed to developmental trauma frequently do not reach the goal initiated by the activation of these motivational systems. As such, the act of triumph is frequently absent, which causes these systems to become overreactive and dysregulated, overinhibited, disorganized, and maladaptively combined with other systems and their associated goals (Steele, 2021). Let us take a look at this in real-life scenarios:

- The chronic activation of the fear and grief systems inhibits the play system, depriving the child of the integrative forces of joy and play (Panksepp, 1998). These children may be withdrawn during play or may frantically play, sometimes at the wrong times or in the wrong places. Panksepp

believed that these types of behaviors may be erroneously diagnosed as attention deficit and hyperactivity disorders, as the play system becomes overreactive in the presence of other children.
- A child exposed to abuse and violence without the completion of a fight response or regulating forces of the caregiver may be chronically fixated on defensive reactions of aggression or submission. In the presence of a minor stimulus, such as the request to clean up their room, the child may go into a complete activation of the defense system and a fight response, while another child may move into complete submission.
- In disorganized attachment and relational trauma, great tension arises between the attachment, caregiving, and competition/ranking systems, resulting in activation of the child's control strategies, either controlling-punitive or controlling-caregiving. This is often observed in children with disorganized attachment strategies. In the controlling-caregiving strategy, the care-seeking motivational system is inverted by the caregiving one. In the controlling-punitive strategy, the care-seeking is substituted by the competition/dominance system (Liotti & Liotti, 2019). The child seeking affiliation and attachment needs through the competition system never gets to experience the deep fulfillment that comes with collaboration, social engagement, and connection with others. As long as the goals are sought incongruently, the child is left with emptiness, loneliness, unfulfillment, dysregulation, and ineffective defensive strategies.
- The child who does not receive appropriate care and experiences chronic activation of their panic/loss system and separation anxiety without resolution may develop a frantic attachment-seeking defense to elicit caregiving behavior (Steele et al., 2017).
- The child who is sexually abused by an important attachment figure or experiencing emotional connection through sexual exploitation may have the attachment and sexuality systems maladaptively combined. The child may pursue attachment needs through the sexuality/lust system, never finding the fulfillment of attachment-related needs.
- In cases of sadistic and ritualistic abuse, the child will arrange their relational structures around dominance and submission while the ranking and attachment system are simultaneously activated (Gilbert, 1989).
- The child who seeks regulation and protection from an abusive and dysregulating caregiver would experience the simultaneous activation of two competing systems: the attachment system and the defense system of fight and flight (Main & Hesse, 1990). Both systems enter into tension and competition, and the child who is unable to fight or flee will enter into collapse, setting dissociative processes in motion (Liotti, 2017). Dissociation then becomes a survival and defense mechanism against powerful and consuming emotions, preventing them from penetrating consciousness.

In characterological dissociation, motivational structures serve as core organizers of the child's dissociative and defensive inner system of parts, which represent the compartmentalization and divisions of inhibited, over-activated, or dysfunctionally connected motivational systems (van der Hart et al., 2006). In characterological dissociation, altered states of consciousness emerge as a result of the disruption of neural processing and impairment of consciousness (Hill, 2021). The compartmentalization and sequestration of psychological structures such as trauma represent a defense against dysregulation (Hill, 2021). One part may hold the goal of desperately seeking connection while another holds the goal of pushing away and avoiding any possibilities for connection. Or a part may pursue attachment needs through sexual gratification while another may rigidly care for others. The lack of state integration (Siegel, 2020) and the dysregulation, rigidity, or absence of the connective tissue that links all of these systems and states cohesively and coherently will leave the child without the experience of a unified sense of self.

Defensive processes may also uncouple cognitive, emotional, and motivational systems that are typically linked together adaptively (Cortina, 2003), resulting in internal disorganization and distortions in mentalization, which is limited by the dominant motivational system. For example, in competition, the child focuses on power and control or submission, which colors the way they understand the motivation of others (K. Steele, personal communication, December 20, 2023). The child with an avoidant defensive strategy is another example of the delinking of cognitive, motivational, and emotional information processing usually integrated in children with secure attachment (Cortina, 2003). These children experience an assault to their attachment systems, and as a result, despite experiencing high autonomic activation when separated from their attachment figures, components of their attachment system become deactivated and delinked—that is, the action tendency that seeks the attachment figure and the emotional processing of information. The result is a child who does not seek comfort from the caregiver and focuses on toys rather than the attachment figure. Additionally, the recurrent activation of previously disrupted autonomic patterns that recruit defenses also blunts higher cognitive capacities and mentalization, preventing the child from witnessing their own stories and processing conscious experience. Instead, they are left with a wide range of trauma-based sensorimotor reactions (Ogden et al., 2006).

The distortions and tensions among the motivational systems, which are caused by experiences of disorganization and trauma, and the dysregulation or constriction of the ANS, lie at the core of the child's Internal Working Models (IWMs). These IWMs are not just cognitive representations; they also serve the homeostatic needs of the child and as such are radically embodied (Beckes et al., 2015). They serve as implicit and embodied anticipations of any future forming relationships, to which they will respond with the same defensive strategies. The relationship with a well-intended clinician may also set in motion these competing systems or parts coexisting in separateness, causing a constant "push and pull" in the therapeutic process, a competition for dominance and control, or a desperate attempt to please and elicit care from the therapist, potentially overriding the clinician's best attempt to engage the child.

Nevertheless, the defense system—with its typical fight-or-flight responses as well as the prosocial system that has become defensive—begins to reset when the child receives the corrective possibility of entering into a co-regulating, contingent, coherent, and safe relational environment. The safety and felt sense of belonging provided via the regulation of the attachment system dampens defenses, allowing these systems to reorganize coherently and congruently, which should be a fundamental goal of treatment.

Complex psychobiological processes exist underneath the defensive system with complex participation of biological circuitry in the brain and the nervous system. Understanding the complex psychobiological underpinnings of the human motivational matrix—the ANS, the attachment system, and trauma—can support clinicians' decision-making and selection of treatment methods for children exposed to chronic traumatization.

The Defense and the Attachment System

To add to the complexity of the defense system, we have to acknowledge the strong influence of the attachment system in the formation of defensive actions and strategies. The inborn attachment system has the hardwired goal of seeking connection to ensure safety, protection, and survival. The caregiver who promotes attachment security can attune to the infant's moment-to-moment demands for safety and contingently restore homeostasis and support internal organization. However, when the child's relational environment is demanding and wounding, strategies and adaptations have to be made by the child in the service of self-preservation. Insecure attachment and its accompanying working models represent chronic adaptations and a strategy to defend against shame, relational trauma, betrayal, and chronic misattunement (Hill, 2015). Whenever the insecure attachment system becomes activated, automatic defensive strategies are set in motion (Hill, 2015) as unclaimed and radically embodied fragments of implicit memories intrude into the child's mind in the present. Additionally, each insecure pattern has underlying over- and under-activated motivational systems.

Other intricate processes participate in defensive responses that emerge in the caregiver-child relationship and the child's attachment experiences. Bowlby (1969) proposed three sequential responses to separation from the primary attachment figure:

- Protest
- Despair (increased helplessness and mourning)
- Detachment (the child no longer seeks the caregiver for safety and protection; instead, they will become self-centered and preoccupied with material things such as toys, food, etc. The child will cease to show feelings and needs).

It is essential to note that these responses may become rigid, dysregulated, or constrained due to chronic disruptions in relational trauma that elicit defensive processes. The child's defensive developments can become entrenched and dysfunctional as they distort expressions of attachment needs, which no longer serve as signals that elicit comfort and care from caregivers (Schore, 2019). A child may be fixated on the *protest response*, while another may be stuck in the *detachment response*, even in the presence of a new caregiver who is responsive and attuned. The strategy that once aided the child in survival becomes the factor that sequesters new prospects of engagement, connection, and healing. Even though these are functional adaptations the child must make in the service of survival, later on, they may hinder the fulfillment of their deep-held longings for social engagement. Human connections become the source of danger—that is, these children implicitly anticipate in others the same rejection, enmeshment, abandonment, or abuse they initially experienced with wounding primary attachment figures. Just the prospect of connection and social engagement can set in motion a cascade of defensive states and actions.

Each category of insecure attachment provides a bio-emotional ecosystem to which the child must adapt. Each attachment pattern demands adaptations that allow the child's embodied mind to cohabit with and tolerate the caregivers' vulnerabilities (Hill, 2015) while maintaining self-organization (Sroufe et al., 2009). In order to elicit care and safety from a caregiver struggling with trauma responses, a strategy and form of self-protection must emerge in the child's system. These adaptations and defensive strategies for children affected by chronic traumatization become a lifelong struggle. Securely attached children balance the need to reduce threat and maximize environmental opportunities for affiliation, play, connection, and exploration. For these children, flexibility colors the use of defenses that are required to exist in a demanding world that holds numerous threats. The defense is used in the face of a threat and then concluded once the threat is terminated. Trauma-formed defenses, however, are rigid and relationally costly and may remain relentlessly activated even with the cessation of the threat. The neuroception of safety is never restored, thereby keeping the child in an eternal state of defense (Porges, 2011).

As the clinician addresses the child's trauma-formed defenses and attachment system, they must explore and acknowledge the central role that shame plays in complex trauma, dissociation, and defense formation. Shame is classified as an attachment emotion (Schore, 2019) and emerges early in the child's relational milieu as they place on themselves the responsibility for the parent's challenges and betrayal. This reversal in responsibility allows the child to remain in a relationship with the wounding caregiver. Shame and the defenses coexist within the child's dissociative matrix. The habituation of the defense cascade against threat increases in complexity when connected to an avoidance of pain and chronic shame and guilt (Steele et al., 2017). The activation of shame will result in the surge of defensive responses and strategies. Often, the dance between shame and defensive actions can inhibit therapeutic actions supporting healing.

Strategies Emerging from Preoccupied and Anxious Trauma

The child with anxious attachment develops adaptations so they can live and stay in a relationship with an unpredictable, undependable, and inconsistently available parent that promotes a symbiotic and enmeshed relationship (Cundy, 2017). The parent's intrusiveness and inconsistencies keep the child's attachment and defense system in a constant state of activation (Siegel, 2020). The anxious child uses the strategy of proximity seeking, clinginess, and role reversal to maintain engagement with an unreliable caregiver who moves in and out of connection in unpredictable ways. Nevertheless, the child remains committed to the caregiver, sacrificing their need for exploration and maintaining an under-activated seeking system. Insecure-anxious attachment patterns and presentations represent the birth of myriad strategies and forms of defense and self-protection that involve not only the attachment system but also other motivational systems that remain over- or under-activated. Approach and compulsive pleasing (high preoccupation and vigilance around acceptance and abandonment) may become primary ways of eliciting care and forming bonds with others.

At the center of the child's corresponding IWMs resides a pattern of autonomic activation put in motion often by the child's relational ecosystem. The anxious child carries the legacy of a highly mobilized and sensitized sympathetic system. The child may present with a strong, emotionally charged idealization of the caregiver that allows them to over-focus on the good about the parent while devaluating themselves. This will result in highly charged experiences of shame. While the infant struggles to adapt to a wounding relational environment, the older child must exist with its inner legacy, the resulting neuroception of danger, and the imprints left in their nervous system, motivational systems, and memory networks holding the wounding relational choreographies.

The inner structure of defense of the anxiety-driven child becomes active in the therapeutic process. The new relationship with a therapist intending to support the child's healing may be enough to activate the attachment system fully and, with it, the IWMs and their strategies, adaptations, and defenses. Hyperarousal, vigilance, the tendency toward enmeshment and symbiotic relationships, and the shame-rage cycle color the therapeutic encounters, posing a challenge to the therapist.

Strategies Emerging from Avoidant Trauma

The child relying on avoidance and self-sufficiency must live with a consistently dismissing, rejecting caregiver—non-reciprocal and emotionally unavailable. This child has to learn early in their lives that it is impossible to rely on their parent; thus, they must become self-sufficient and self-dependable, relinquishing the need for connection and relational modulation and instead relying on rudimentary forms of self-regulation. The child develops avoidance as a strategy to stay in relationship with a distant, cold, and often neglectful caregiver and to escape from shame (Cundy, 2019). Children avoidant in their attachment have to edit their feelings and deepest longings to maintain some level of connection with the caregiver. The result is a child who is cut off from their needs, emotions, and, ultimately, themselves. False positivity or severe emotional constriction/numbness becomes their refuge and defense as they attempt to fill in the gaps left by their impoverished and suboptimal relational environment. While the child may be emotionally and physiologically activated, their suffering will remain unrecognized, unacknowledged, unexpressed, and unseen even by themselves. The ANS will also be shaped by these early relational traumas, which may cause it to down-regulate and often move into the dorsal vagal state, becoming chronically withdrawn and hypo-aroused (Hill, 2015) without the modulating forces of the vagus nerve. The child's implicit expectations of any other human relationship will be influenced by these early experiences, with the same prospect of rejection and emotional unavailability, and the strategy of avoidance, disengagement, and detachment.

Because of the socio-emotional environment of the child exposed to trauma that causes avoidance, they may lack capacities to regulate sympathetic arousal (Hill, 2015). This results in strategies to defend against any type of arousal, including conflict, anger, or expanded experiences of joy. The child will use denial, minimization, and disengagement from any experiences or emotions perceived as vulnerable that exist outside their narrow window of affect tolerance. Even gaze aversion is associated not only with the avoidance of the dismissive caregiver's face, but also with the arousal generated by eye contact (Hill, 2015). Trauma-related phobias of affect and connection are present in children with an avoidant defensive mode, as they guard against intensity and the possibility of activating high arousal. They often refuse to connect to and share affective data, insisting that they do not need therapy or that their lives are just fine. They block any possibility for connection, remaining emotionally distant in any new forming relationship. At the same time, by engaging in thrilling, provoking activities, children with avoidant strategies who "feel too little" paradoxically attempt to have access to feelings they avoid at all costs. Ironically, they non-consciously attempt to up-regulate a system in shutdown by moving to exploration even in the presence of danger. These children had to exist within an emotionally constricted relational milieu with a narrow access to diverse affective and autonomic states.

In the service of self-sufficiency and avoidance, these children also tend to evade therapy at all costs—it activates IWMs and, with them, the strategy of avoidance. Avoidance wears several costumes, from "I do not know what I feel" and "I do not want to be here because I do not need therapy" to "My life is great" and "I've never had any challenges or difficulties."

The child relying on avoidance can thus miss out on potentially corrective experiences from an empathic companion. Clinicians may feel frustrated by these children's inner defenders, which will fight ferociously before sharing a feeling or acknowledging any vulnerability. Since these children often refuse the therapist's help, challenging their IWMs requires a gradual and consistent approach that titrates the access to affective data and promotes connection and regulation at a pace tolerable to the child.

Strategies Emerging from Disorganized Trauma

The child with disorganized attachment is caught in the dilemma of seeking protection and safety from the parent who is the source of both fear and dysregulation (Liotti, 2017). Due to fluctuating unpredictably between extreme hyper- and hypo-arousal and dissociation (Hill, 2015), this child is hard-pressed to develop a coherent template of their caregiver that activates both the attachment system and the defense system simultaneously (Liotti, 2017). The imbalance causes severe damage to the primary regulating system due to the neurochemical assault causing states to become uncoupled (Schore, 2003). Dissociation, in its multiple manifestations, becomes a defensive strategy and an organizing force of the child's embodied mind. Dissociation has been established primarily as an internal organization, and secondarily as a defense with the function of self-protection (van der Hart et al., 2006). Dissociation is defensively recruited to keep traumatic material and overwhelming affect away from consciousness, to avoid internally and externally generated shame, terror, and pain. As a defense, dissociation allows the child to compartmentalize affect and information, divide attention into multiple streams of consciousness, and create distance from the self (Fisher, 2017), all of which constitute important capacities of the mind to coexist with pain, terror, and shame. In characterological dissociation, motivational systems are primary organizers of dissociative self-states that remain over-activated or inhibited in ways that appear externally incoherent or disorganized yet have internal organization and consistency in how the child uses them (K. Steele, personal communication, December 20, 2023).

Treatment: Resetting the Biology of the Traumatized Mind and Reclaiming the Natural Rhythms of Being

This section aims to delineate the fundamental components of a multimodal approach in the therapeutic journey that draws from neuroscience, attachment theory, structural dissociation, and information processing to address the self-system of defense and protection. As our understanding of the psychological and neurophysiological processes at play that result from early and chronic traumatization increases, the field of psychotherapy is moving into an integrated, biopsychological science (Gilbert, 2009). This section will lay out the core therapeutic components that can be used to reset the defense mode.

Social engagement and inborn prosocial motivational systems are meant to move the human mind into growth and expansion, but disorganized attachment and trauma activate these systems in a disorderly manner. This causes them to become over-activated, inhibited, dysregulated, or maladaptively combined (Steele, 2021) across the dissociative continuum. The treatment clinicians deliver must have components that balance, reset, and repattern the growth-promoting vagus nerve and the inborn motivational systems. Clinicians especially work actively with the child's play, exploration/seeking, attachment and cooperation systems, and the parent's caregiving system. This vital work will move the child who is fixated on the defensive mode safely into self and co-regulation, connectedness, homeostasis, and social engagement. Safety is an essential treatment element that creates the foundation for regulating and balancing the defense and self-protective system, and as such it constitutes an essential therapeutic goal.

The Multiple Shades of Safety: The Mind of the Therapist and Their Relational, Mentalizing, and Engaging Capacities

We arrive at this section with a much deeper understanding of the sacrifices and adaptations that children exposed to polytraumatization and suboptimal environments have to make to ensure survival. The process of repatterning biological systems and rhythms, engaging the vagus nerve, and bringing homeostasis and coherence to the functioning of previously dysregulated or constricted motivational systems begins with restoring safety. This multifaceted and complex construct involves multiple layers: external, internal, and relational. In the therapeutic encounter, safety begins with the clinician's relational capacities for reciprocity, connectedness, coherence, and access to their engagement system.

Over the last 30 years of my clinical practice, I sometimes felt lost and hopeless as I worked to support the healing of children affected by severe traumatization. My therapeutic process has significantly added to my understanding of the intricacies of the human mind since I have become my own lab. In my travels through the endless layers of my human existence, I came face-to-face with my own defense and protective system. I began to observe my therapeutic tendencies when my young clients tapped into my own wounds and moved me non-consciously into survival and self-preservation mode. When this happened, strategies such as overdoing, trying harder, or working tirelessly to move these challenging children to the place I thought would be best for them overtook the therapeutic sessions; I didn't realize until then that this was my version of their journey and story—my own agenda, not theirs. I have come to understand that the clinician's unexplored mind may be a hindrance and do a disservice to the therapeutic journey of children affected by complex trauma. So, the first therapeutic suggestion is for the clinician to travel into their own mind. The acknowledgment of the clinician's own tendencies and vulnerabilities will break unhealthy socially held divisions between the clients (the wounded and traumatized) and the clinician (the "unwounded" and high-functioning). This is an invitation to clinicians to be open, to notice the children and the moments that stretch their regulatory capacities. These will be their least favorite clients, the ones who, when they look at their agenda for the day, make them feel a pit in their stomach, or fear, or a sense of mobilization, tension, and restlessness. They should also look at the clients who make them feel like a "superstar," those whom they look forward to seeing and cannot get enough of because they give them a sense of triumph and competency.

Then, clinicians are invited to notice their tendencies and responses when clients make them feel uncomfortable, activated, frustrated, tired, sleepy, hopeless, restless, and not good enough or in need of the reassurance of their clients. When these emotions and states arise, they can ask themselves: What do I do? Do I try harder? Do I overdo it and give the child a myriad of playful possibilities? Do I force the child into a technique I think will fix them? Do I disengage, detach, or even dissociate? Do I praise the child every time I am complemented, and non-consciously seek the child's acceptance? How does my ANS respond? Where am I in the defense cascade? How have my attachment experiences shaped my relational and regulatory tendencies in therapeutic relationships?

If the clinician follows the uncomfortable states and then lifts the veil, underneath they will find life affirming possibilities for development and expansion. Children affected by complex trauma have mastered the art of self-protection and, as such, are experts in detecting a clinician's defensive strategies and potential incongruencies. Once clinicians can see and sit with their inner happenings and compassionately befriend their own defenders and protectors, they can dance with various states of consciousness and their young clients' defense systems and reenactments.

Defenders are wise. When the clinician follows them, they find the child's deepest wounds underneath as they come in contact with the hardwired biological tendency of the human mind to adapt and survive. As the clinician brings gratitude and compassion to their own defense system and the various corners of the self that carry their wounds, they will also begin to see their young clients' protectors through the eyes of acceptance and compassion. This level of integration and awareness will support them as they walk into the unknowns occurring throughout the therapeutic encounters. They can more freely navigate the ups and downs of their nervous system and approach each client with curiosity and without judgment, which will give them an entrance into the child's embodied mind, their deepest wounds, and the most profound possibilities for healing and expansion. The clinician moves into an embodied practice of simultaneously holding space for different and incompatible realities. This becomes the essence and crux of an embodied state of connectedness and synchrony in psychotherapy.

Clinicians should also consider the parent's and child's intrapersonal and interpersonal organization within a cultural context. Oppressive and discriminatory practices may demand that the child and the parent maintain defensive postures and actions in the pursuit of survival. A nonjudgmental and culturally affirming approach that welcomes and accepts the child's cultural identities and multifaceted cultural dynamics will support fostering a safe relational environment.

Safety, Relational Regulation, and Challenging Insecure IWMs

So much has been said about being the bio-emotional regulator of the child suffering from complex trauma. On paper, it seems doable and easy to master, but in real life, sitting with moments of the unknown, uncertainty, and uncomfortableness that children with complex trauma bring is very challenging and yet at the heart of the therapeutic journey. Inevitably, trauma-based bottom-up or top-down processes will become activated as the clinician accompanies the child in their healing journey. However, to hold space for the client, the clinician—"the other mind"—must be at the receiving end. A playful activity, a processing session with EMDR therapy, or a somatic intervention may challenge the child's safety, and open up the defense system and the wounds it guards. In this vortex, the human mind (the client) needs "the other" (the clinician) to hold a safe relational space where integration, completions, and corrections of previously disrupted autonomic states become a possibility. In these vulnerable moments, the embodied mind longs for "the other" to hold the space and the intrinsic potentials for attachment repair and defensive completions. Human connections shape neural connections (Siegel, 2020); thus, secure relationships begin to reshape the inner world of the traumatized child living in the defense mode. Trauma leaves an imprint in the child's biology and so does relational safety, moments of shared coherence, homeostasis, belonging, and connection.

Many authors in this book have written about how the psychotherapeutic process is more about being than doing, and in being, we remain utterly in contact with ourselves and the moment. Techniques, psychoeducation, procedural steps, and protocols are welcome, but they need to be held and brought in coherently and cohesively by the clinician's embodied and intentional mind. The clinician's moment-to-moment decision-making while holding two different realities, the child's and their own, will give the therapeutic encounter greater congruency, reciprocity, and coherence. This invisible field of shared consciousness and possibilities holds the directive and non-directive therapeutic tools. The clinician's attuned mind will guide and support reflective communication and mirroring, the need for boundaries and structure or rest, and the joining in during a specific state to up- or down-regulate, to reset and repattern the nervous system and move it out of defensive mode, and to support the child and caregiver in creating new life-affirming meaning to their stories. However, the clinician's response and techniques are ultimately guided by awareness and consciousness.

The clinician must recognize the intricacies and complexities of creating safety and its multiple layers, from the removal of danger and threats from the child's environment to the establishment of relational safety with the child and caregivers. Safety is co-created each moment in the therapeutic relationship. Each moment demands an adaptation on the part of the clinician to meet the needs and requests for safety, reciprocity and synchrony (Hill, 2015). The clinician commits to moment-to-moment micro-adjustments to meet the child in the place where safety is a possibility. This ultimately begins to dim the defense system through the engagement of the vagus nerve and brain circuitry guiding prosocial behavior. When the clinician moves into connection, reciprocity, and regulation, they are moving away from survival, self-preservation, and the defense mode (Porges, 2011). Yet, they are not aiming to disarm and remove the defense and protective system, but rather to support its move into homeostasis and regulation, while still remaining active in the presence of danger.

Consistent relational regulation supports the child in eventually developing the capacity to modulate their own arousal and, with that, begin to repair and recalibrate physiological stress systems such as the HPA axis. Research shows that attachment-based and relational interventions intended to enhance children's capacities to regulate physiology and behavior produced changes in biological markers of the HPA in infants and toddlers in foster care (Dozier et al., 2008).

Resetting the Child's Relationship with Inborn Motivational Systems: Acts of Triumph and Completions

Children fixated on the threat cycle have typically experienced trauma early in their lives, during a time of significant brain growth and development, and as a result have dysregulated brain functions (Perry, 2013). The child's body may continue to signal danger even in the presence of safety, which shows the child's challenges in interoception and the capacity to assess safety and danger. Considering that the brain develops from the bottom up, interventions should follow these developmental lines (Perry, 2013). The clinician actively invites curiosity and with it the exploration and play systems. Sensorimodulating work that allows the child to discharge (Levine, 2015) and integrate defenses that are chronically activated across critical neurodevelopmental stages must also be part of the therapeutic repertoire. The higher brain cannot operate optimally if the lower brain is in a state of dysregulation (Perry, 2013).

When facing a threat, energy is mobilized to prepare the body to fight or flee. However, when these defensive responses are deprived of completeness, the old defensive and mobilized energy continues to exist in the individual's biology (Ogden et al., 2006; Levine, 2015). Clinicians can support the child with a sensitized fight-or-flight defense system to complete truncated and mobilized defenses existing in body-based holding patterns. Gradually inviting movement to highly mobilized or immobilized areas of the body and letting the body move in the way it longs, such as pushing, breaking free, opening and closing, or even fleeing and running, are all therapeutic embodiments that allow completions and the release of pent-up energy left by trauma (Levine, 2015). Caregivers can also participate to dyadically give the body the missing experiences of being physically held, rocked, and nurtured. This provides the opportunity not only for completion but also renegotiations that reset the structure of the biological actions in response to threat (Levine, 2015).

Within the clinician-child therapeutic encounters and the parent-child relationship, promoting and fully recognizing moments of repair will give the child the act of triumph they have been deprived of. Accompanying children through reflections and mirroring (verbal and nonverbal) to notice and fully embody these completions can begin to reorganize dysregulated, inhibited, or dysfunctionally combined motivational systems. Invite the child to slow down, perhaps using pretend slow-motion devices, to embrace the triumphant moment. Also, inquire about what it feels like, how the body wants to move, or what their voice wants to say to embrace the completions, repairs, and triumphs. Celebrations, "feeling" parties, and the use of figures physicalize the triumph. Overcoming adversity or a challenging project, or the body attaining greater strength, growth, and dexterity and arriving at the "I did it" moment (Steele, 2021) while in a relational environment that witnesses and accompanies these completions provide potent corrective experiences that begin to reorganize motivational systems structures around defense.

Children should also have access to attachment completions where the caregiver acknowledges and fulfills the child's unmet longings while honoring their intimacy threshold and window of affect tolerance. Trauma influences the relationship the child develops with their innermost needs, preventing them from attaining their deepest longings for belonging, affiliation, and social connection. Resetting and renegotiating the child's relationship with their needs, emotions, thoughts, behaviors, and, ultimately, themselves also moves the child out of defense mode and back into development and growth. When deprivation has colored the child's life, they may not tolerate the very thing they need and long for—defensive strategies may stand between the child and the fulfillment of unmet attachment needs. The clinician thus supports the child to connect to the need and the defender compassionately, to bring these inner polarities into consciousness. In the sand tray, the child can represent the longing on one side, and on the other side the part of them that wants to push away such offerings. In addition, clinicians may use attachment-based play strategies that direct the parent and the child to guess, explore, identify, and fulfill the child's needs (Gomez, in press). When the need is identified and met, clinicians should invite the child to savor the act of triumph somatically, affectively, behaviorally, and cognitively. The parent becomes the partner who supports the child's completions, repairs, and psychobiological renegotiations. As it develops, the child's interoceptive intelligence can direct behavior more efficiently to attain the act of triumph and experience the fullness and satisfaction that completions and repairs bring. It is relevant to highlight that these completions and acts of triumph have nothing to do with overdoing, overachieving, or grandiose accomplishments, which in some cases show only imbalances in these inborn motivational systems.

Mentalization and Higher Cognitive Capacities

Once regulation and the reestablishment of attachment bonds are in progress, the clinician invites the child's cognitive capacities to come online. Fonagy et al. (2002) distinguished between two affect-regulating systems: (1) the basic system, where the focus of regulation is a physiological and affective state, and (2) the complex system, where the aim is to regulate the self while actively utilizing mirroring and reflective function. The latter utilizes the parent's and child's mentalizing capacities; according to Fonagy and colleagues, the measure of one's mentalizing capacity is a crucial determinant of self-organization and affects regulation. The prefrontal cortex, which is also critical for self-regulation, has lengthy periods of maturation that extend into young adulthood (Dozier et al., 2008). Clinicians can capitalize on these biological systems to create neural pathways to reach the higher brain and higher cognitive faculties of mentalization and mindfulness. In this way, they can scaffold the child's self-regulatory capacities and downregulate the defense system when in the presence of safety. Inviting the child to embrace their emotions using analogies—suggesting it's like riding a wave (coming from the field of mindfulness) or a wild horse, petting a cat in distress, or engaging with an upset dog—while remaining present allows them to observe and "sit with" or "visit with" the dysregulated or constricted affect. Eckhart Tolle's (1999) well-known quote "You are the sky. The clouds are what happens, what comes and goes" can be playfully utilized with children to increase mindfulness to move out of defense and self-protection. The clinician can invite the child to observe and watch the clouds and thunderstorms without becoming them, by using movement and play. Mobilizing the play system, the child is invited to become the sky, dancing with the clouds while holding them, knowing their sun and moon are still behind them. The cloud dance turns into rambunctious thunder as the child is invited to let the pain, anger, or sadness go in and out as energy until it finds the portal and a channel to enter the world. It may be through their voice, painting, or creating a sandtray story, or just having a "tea party" or a gathering with their emotions.

The clinician's consistent presence, reciprocity, connectedness, and synchrony inevitably challenge the child and the parent's insecure and disorganized IWMs. At the same time, the clinician supports them in co-creating a new life-affirming meaning to their relational story. However, this process is not a quiet or smooth one. The mind seeks familiar over safe and synchronic relational offerings. New and different may be initially experienced as "weird" and unsafe. Part of the growth in therapeutic encounters is the repetitive challenging of IWMs that emerge from relational trauma, while simultaneously recognizing and working with the mind's threshold for intimacy. This must be a felt and ongoing experience clinicians enhance therapeutically through play, storytelling, and expressive arts therapies. The clinician supports the development of permanent safe relationships by playfully reminding the child that their safe relationships exist in them even when they cannot see them. To teach the child about connection, the caregiver can introduce the child to Karst's (2018) "Invisible String" that connects us all, and can be felt with their heart. The "heart jar" protocol (Gomez, 2013) also creates a safe space to experience connection: with permission from the child, the parent can fill their "heart jar" with verbal, nonverbal messages of appreciation, love, compassion, and gratitude. This therapeutic work of two minds and two bodies connecting in synergy can enhance new and lasting relational templates and inner representations of the self and others.

The integration of trauma memories with information processing approaches such as EMDR therapy (Shapiro, 2018) also supports the transformation and reorganization of the child's relationship to the implicit and explicit elements of their life stories and IWMs. Sandtray, expressive arts, and play therapy modalities provide space for children to represent "defenders" and initiate a dialogue with their inner world and themselves. The active work with defensive strategies is paramount within therapeutic approaches that aim to process and integrate traumagenic material. Defensive and protective self-states may prevent and block the access of trauma memories, and down-regulating these important defenders throughout treatment is pivotal.

Psychoeducation, Physicalizations, Therapeutic Embodiments, and the Defense System

Psychoeducation has been misunderstood and often used in a manner that causes children with short attention spans and dissociative symptoms to rapidly disengage. Nevertheless, children with long histories of neglect have a myriad of missing experiences and adaptive information, and benefit from developmentally appropriate psychoeducation. Even though developmental gaps are filled in primarily through corrective and reparative experiences of co-regulation and connection, psychoeducation can add to the richness of the therapeutic process. However, psychoeducation needs to be delivered using a titrated approach that provides repetitive, embodied, and patterned experiences and information. I call it "segmented embodied psychoeducation" (Gomez, 2021), which provides small kernels of information while inviting therapeutic embodiments, play, and social engagement. From this perspective, psychoeducation is more about providing the missing fabric from the quilt of the self than educating. Analogies, metaphors, movement, and play are interwoven and delivered in patterned routines. Psychoeducation also provides information that creates predictability and structure, thus contributing to building safety.

Animal Defenses and Play

A playful and metaphorical way of talking about defenses involves stories of animal protectors (Gomez, 2023b). The stories begin to open the door to the child's defenders while capitalizing on the containment and distance provided by play, movement, and metaphors. Animal cards, for example, may be used to demonstrate and normalize defenses, opening a pathway to explore what humans do to protect and defend. For instance, chameleons' colors change to help them blend in with their environment. The chameleon becomes an externalization and representation of the child's protector and defender; through it, the child can dialogue and develop a relationship with these inner defenders. The child and clinician can "play chameleon"—they can dress up, bring puppets, play in the sand tray, and use therapeutic embodiments of what it feels like to be compelled to change to the liking of others and not the self.

Another example of an animal defender is the ostrich, often a physicalization of avoidance, as this animal finds refuge in hiding, not knowing they are still uncovered and seen despite their efforts. It is similar to what the child utilizing avoidant strategies does, hiding from their feelings and themselves despite being visible through their reenactments. Through using ostrich movements, an ostrich hiding dance, or an ostrich hiding feelings, the child can realize their defenses and, hence, develop a relationship with them. Dissociative protective and defensive parts can unblend into puppets, sandtray figures, and costumes for their representation and movement into the outer world. The child, clinician, and sometimes the caregiver can dialogue, nurture, and promote greater connection between the child and their protective parts. As a result, the child expands their awareness and realization, ultimately developing a life-affirming and compassionate relationship with themselves.

Compassion, Rest, and Safety Checks

My book *The Visitor: A Book about Pain,* Defenses, and Love (Gomez, 2024) supports children in compassionately befriending defenses and looking beyond what they protect. Children are guided to befriend their inner world with all its shades and colors gradually and compassionately. Compassion is an essential component of any form of treatment (Gilbert, 2022). The child needs to experience and be the recipient of compassion in their relational milieu and playfully practice it during therapeutic sessions. For instance, I have trumpets that announce moments of self-compassion throughout the session, and pots in which we cook up self-compassion with ingredients such as kindness, love, and understanding. Metaphors also aid children in understanding the nature of their protective system. A story called "The North Pole" (Gomez, 2013) demonstrates that if we lived in the North Pole, we would have to protect ourselves from the cold, wearing heavy jackets and boots. These protectors are good and helpful. However, if we moved and ended up in a warm place during the summer, the jackets and boots would not serve us like when surrounded by snow. Instead, they would not let us enjoy the warm weather. We would need to get a much thinner jacket and keep the heavy one only for when the cold returns. Through this story, the clinician supports the child to befriend their defenders and relate to them flexibly. Children learn how to allow their protectors to work in different ways, and how to let them rest when they are safe. During sessions, the clinician and child can practice physicalizing the defense system and pendulating in and out of protection. The concept of "resting the protectors and defenders" is foreign for children who have lived in hypervigilance and defense mode most of their lives. However, over time, the clinician can invite the protectors to be present during therapeutic sessions, and also take short naps (which can be as short as a few seconds) or step aside so the child can "visit" a feeling that seems uncomfortable. A "resting space" may be created in the office so defenders and protectors have a place to rest while receiving reassurance of their importance.

When the child's sense of identity exists within a dissociative matrix, the self-system may be stuck in trauma time and defenses such as fight, flight, freeze, flag, and faint (Steele et al., 2017) as well as parts organized around over- or under-activated motivational systems. The clinician may use playful and embodied strategies that orient the child in time and space, move them out of trauma time, expand their field of present awareness, and allow them to experience groundedness in safety. "Embodied safety checks" to pacify the defense system may need to be done often, but as safety sets in the therapeutic relationship, they may happen less frequently. "The safety fairy," "the safety chair," or the "safety checker and thermometer" are playful ways of inviting interoception and befriending the vagus nerve and the neuroception of safety. The "safety chair" is a hanging chair where the child can rotate 360 degrees and have a total view and perspective of the space. Once the child has made their "safety checks," the clinician can invite them to savor the feeling of being safe and enhance their knowledge of safety with breathwork or, if doing EMDR therapy, by using a bilateral dual attention stimulus (BLS/DAS). Somatic interventions that increase interoceptive intelligence may be powerful, such as inviting the child to see how their body feels when safety is found versus when it is absent. Microphones can enhance the process by bringing in playfulness and interviewing the body about its narratives (Ogden & Gomez, 2013). The heart may be interviewed as well as the legs or stomach. The child can pendulate from the places where safety lives in the body to those places holding fear or shame (Ogden & Gomez, 2013). The clinician can actively use the motivational systems of play, attachment, and cooperation to repattern defenses.

Working Systemically

Even though state-change skills are necessary to support children's defense down-regulation, it is their increased tolerance of the affect they defend against and the modulation of its intensity that will most support the healing these children deserve (Hill, 2021). The therapeutic journey must honor the child's and the parent's window of affect tolerance and incorporate a gradual and titrated entrance into their emotional and somatic distress. All forms of relational trauma either constrict or dysregulate the child's affective system and their relationship with their emotions and body sensations, promoting the development and maintenance of defensive strategies. When the caregiver contains and tolerates the child's distressing experience and affect, the child will also begin to embrace these embodied affective states. In sum, the clinician and the caregiver work to increase regulatory capacities, containment, and emotional bandwidth so the child can experience a broader range of emotions and body sensations without having to defend against them.

Defenses are also passed from one generation to the other. To coexist with the vulnerabilities of their caregivers, infants and young children internalize their parents' defenses and strategies. These meta-defenses tend to be highly ingrained and have great rigidity. Involving a parent as an active therapeutic partner is paramount to changing these long-held patterns of self-protection and reestablishing safety. If the defenses strongly interfere with therapeutic healing, beginning to name the defenses and bring them into the field of consciousness and awareness of the parent when enough safety has been built will open the door for dyadic sessions. In these child–caregiver sessions, playful conversations about how multiple generations have coped and how hurts have been passed across generational lines will normalize and de-shame the wounds and strategy.

A helpful tool for this strategy is my story of "the traveling hurt," which contains "traveling companions" such as "the traveling feelings" and "traveling protectors and generational defenses" that guard and keep the pain and feelings away (Gomez, 2023a). Children learn that traveling hurts are guarded by traveling protectors that are shared by many generations. Active-energizing or passive-inhibited defensive strategies such as overdoing, perfectionism, control, manipulation, pleasing, frantic seeking of acceptance, and avoidance may be shared by multiple generations and not just the child. The act of naming the shared generational defense gives wounds and defenses collective recognition. Naming emotions has been found to decrease limbic activations, which led Dan Siegel (2020) to create the famous phrase "Name it to tame it." Naming the protectors and defenders while supported and surrounded by secured bonds provides the optimal milieu in which to gently soften the rigid walls created in the service of survival. The naming does not have to be verbal initially, but any form of externalization through sandtray figures, movement, and expressive arts therapy will begin the process of recognition. The traveling stories, wounds, and defenders can be witnessed, seen, acknowledged, and integrated as these rigid and defensive fences erode. The parent and the child are invited to dialogue with their shared defenders and to engage in therapeutic embodiments. If an ostrich represents avoidance, both the child and the parent can dance with the ostrich and create posters, sandtray worlds, or puppet shows depicting how the ostrich has lived with them and how they can renegotiate their relationship with it.

Parts Work and the Inner Dynamic

Clinicians should investigate whether defenses exist within a dissociative matrix or an ego state system. Whether the clinician uses standardized or non-standardized instruments, clinical interviews, or moment-to-moment observations, exploring what, when, and how the dissociative system becomes activated and how it moves into protection will give the clinician a view of the overall clinical landscape and the inner organization of the child and what they protect or defend from.

As unintegrated and unrealized aspects of the mind (Steele et al., 2017), dissociative parts represent inner storytellers that hold the traumatized child's non-realized life stories (Gomez, 2021). They contain cognitive, affective, and sensorimotor data that the mind defends against. If protections and defenses coexist within a compartmentalized inner milieu, the child's mind may endure endless inner battles that perpetuate the defense mode even when the child's environment is safe. Resolving inner conflict and increasing inner cooperation, communication, and awareness becomes a central therapeutic goal (Steele et al., 2017). The clinician works on promoting linkage among differentiated parts to create a functional whole at the nine domains of integration identified by Siegel (2020). Independently of the therapeutic approach the clinician utilizes, supporting the child in realizing, connecting, and dialoguing with their internal protectors will open greater access to their inner world and themselves.

The clinician honors the divided reality of the child without becoming lost in its subjectivity. Language such as "the different sides of you," "the parts of you," "the different ways in which you connect to yourself," and "the different colors of you" (Gomez & Paulsen, 2016) gives recognition to the inner system while supporting the realization that there is only "one child" holding these storytellers. Needless to say, sometimes the clinician and parent will communicate with parts to give reassurance, validation, and promote safety. As parts are externalized, the child can more easily dialogue with the inner storytellers that coexist in polarized states to support co-consciousness, interconnectedness, and collective synchrony amongst parts. A part may hold the desire to acknowledge a feeling, while another fights fiercely to cover it up and defend against it. A part may also idealize and maintain loyalty to the perpetrator while another feels rage against the offender. If the part holding the anger receives reassurance during a session, the one holding the loyalty toward the perpetrator may act out. The clinician reflects, both verbally and nonverbally, these polarities and inner conflicts to increase awareness, realization, and co-consciousness among parts as well as to repair the ruptures that resulted in such inner divisions and disputes. Increasing interoceptive awareness and supporting inner dialogues and negotiations among parts will quiet down the defense system, considering that conflicted inner relational dynamics and polarizations maintain dysregulation and prevent integration and realization.

Safety may also be challenging to attain, as each version of the child may hold a different idea of what is safe. In a state of psychobiological attunement, the clinician invites inner dialogues, compromises, and curiosity. Curiosity is an asset to integration and an antidote to dissociation. Curiosity creates the bridge to realization and the self. Remaining curious, present, reciprocal, and reflective will move the child gradually to greater levels of realization and safety.

Affect Tolerance

Even though state change skills are necessary to support children's regulatory capacities and defense downregulation, it is the increased tolerance for the affect they defend against and the modulation of its intensity that will most support the healing these children deserve (Hill, 2021, p. 171). The therapeutic journey must honor the child and the parent's window of affect tolerance and incorporate a gradual and titrated entrance into their emotional and somatic distress.

Time Orientation

According to Hill (2021) dysregulation engenders states of consciousness where there is loss of temporal perspective, over-immersion in experience, and loss of coherence which results in a sense of fragmentation. As long as the child's biology exists in trauma time (van der Hart et al., 2006), the defense system will remain active. Orienting the child frequently back into the present safety will dim the defensive repertoire. The clinician may invite parts to "time travel" through timelines or wearing the "time travel cape" to visit the present safety. "The hurt little self" or parts stuck in trauma time can tour the present to see what is different, what is safe, and in general how things have changed now that the trauma is over. Posters or a sandtray world depicting "this was me then and this is me now" (Gomez, 2013) can playfully orient the child to the present resources and safety. Needless to say, if the child is exposed to ongoing trauma, reestablishing safety should precede time orientation work.

Case Study

Lucy, a seven-year-old with a long history of domestic violence, abuse, and abandonment, always fought for control with her mother and therapists. Often, Lucy would wait for the clinician to deliver invitations that she would then reject while becoming agitated and angry. Lucy told the clinician loudly that she was the boss and that the clinician would have to obey any requests she made. The clinician's own father had been domineering and often pressured her to meet his needs. Lucy exhibited a control-punitive strategy where the care-seeking system became inverted with the competition-ranking system due to trauma.

The clinician began to experience a heavy sensation in her chest when Lucy commanded her obedience. The clinician playfully followed along, even though internally she felt a sense of resistance and anger. She noticed that she would disengage when Lucy became domineering and bossy, which would cause Lucy to escalate and become even more dominant. Lucy's ANS would move into mobilization and a fight response; at the same time, the clinician's social engagement system would disengage and move into defense. However, the clinician mindfully observed these bidirectional dynamics with Lucy and began to process this in her own therapy. She more actively began to witness her own forms of self-protection and defense, which consisted of disengaging, avoiding, and shutting down. She noticed her moments of activation and shutdown with Lucy, and as she did, she used breath, acceptance, and compassion to dive through the wave of these emotions to reconnect to herself and the present moment with Lucy. This allowed for a more open and genuine connection with Lucy, which began to touch Lucy's regulating systems—her ventral vagal, and her attachment system—co-creating greater levels of safety and providing the food needed for recalibrating Lucy's motivational systems and a space for repair. Lucy's disorganization in her attachment showed the simultaneous activation of her defense and attachment systems. The clinician made moment-to-moment adjustments to Lucy's requests for safety, connection, structure, and containment, which began to quiet down and dim the defense system, making connection possible.

The clinician also focused on safety and co-regulation with Lucy's mother, since she had extensive relational trauma. This started to engage the mother's vagus nerve to down-regulate her highly mobilized sympathetic system. Gradual changes were introduced to slowly increase structure at home to regulate sleep, rest, and eating. Dyadic sessions, where Lucy and her mother were invited to play and take turns being the leader, began to stimulate the cooperation system and reset the competition and ranking system. Lucy's strategy was represented by a captain hat. The clinician slowed down when Lucy was the boss and accomplished what she wanted so she could experience the act of triumph. Mirroring, celebrations, and the savoring of Lucy's completions colored the therapeutic sessions. Lucy felt empowered and began to enjoy sharing her "captain hat." The cooperation system was gradually stimulated and the parent and the child shared the joy of collaboration.

The clinician began to very gradually introduce small nuggets of "segmented psychoeducation," during which they played with animal cards depicting defenses. When Lucy played with the animal cards (Gomez, 2023b), she identified with the lion, who wanted everybody to do what he wanted. Lion dances, posters, and movements connected Lucy to her inner defender. One day, the clinician invited the voice of the left brain and wondered out loud if a side of Lucy did "lion's stuff," to which Lucy said, "Absolutely, yes." Lucy accepted invitations to connect, nurture, and give gratitude to her inner lion for its offerings. Curiosity was also invited, to stimulate the exploration system. When Lucy wore a lion costume, the clinician and Lucy invited the "wonder mind" to have a "moment of curiosity," which Lucy accepted. Both wondered what the lion wanted to do. As a storyteller, what stories did the lion carry? How was he helping Lucy to have a lion side in her? Lucy stated that the lion side of her kept her safe because she could not trust that others would be nice and safe with her. Lucy realized she longed to have friends, but her inner lion would push others away. Her competition, defense, and attachment systems had been affected by occurrences of trauma. Despite her longing to connect, when the connection was possible, even with a friend, Lucy's defense system was awakened along with old IWMs that pushed others away. Curiosity, compassion, and the co-regulating forces of the clinician and the mother softened the edges of Lucy's shame. Shame was named and invited so Lucy could get to know it. Lucy was encouraged and supported to visit and be with the shame, represented by a puppet. Lucy said shame could get cold and hot and poke and sink. Thermoregulation using stuffed animals that could be microwaved or frozen allowed Lucy to experience and play with the various temperatures of shame.

The clinician also engaged the lower brain through movement and sensory modulation activities, and, at the same time, supported the work with the left and higher brain through segmented playful psychoeducation, to increase mentalizing capacities so Lucy could hold her lion state in mind as well as her teddy bear side, which wanted to have friends. Both represented motivational systems in conflict. Both polarities with their competing forces were represented, witnessed, and dialogued with. Lucy was invited to communicate with the lion side of her to encourage cooperation one "little drop" at a time, and notice what it felt like to play and cooperate with others, starting with her mother and the clinician. The clinician, utilizing the forces of the play, collaboration, and attachment systems, began to regulate and integrate the competition and rage motivational systems, bringing greater balance and integration to Lucy's ANS and motivational systems.

As Lucy continued her therapeutic journey, she discovered that she also did "ostrich stuff" when hiding from her feelings, especially shame and the stories of trauma. The clinician and Lucy created forts to physicalize and represent her defensive strategy. Instead of trying to remove or strip Lucy of her defenses, she was supported in transforming her ongoing relationship with her protectors and inner world and increasing her emotional and somatic bandwidth. The clinician supported Lucy in making "negotiations" with the ostrich part of her. Lucy agreed to come out of the fort into a "feeling station," where the ostrich would step aside so Lucy could see and feel her emotions. Titration and pendulation served Lucy in gradually developing a relationship with her inner world and the stories of which she was phobic.

Lucy's life was also colored by role reversal and an overactive caregiving system stimulated very early in her life because she did not have access to adequate care. Her mother always felt incompetent and was unreliable and in and out of connection with Lucy. To coexist with her mother's vulnerabilities, Lucy's immature caregiving system became dysregulated and overactive as she cared for her mother. The attuned clinician worked therapeutically on rebuilding and scaffolding the mother's caregiving system so she could be the bigger, older, guiding, and wiser protector and co-regulator Lucy needed to reset her overactive caregiving system. Lucy's mother also agreed to do work with another clinician on her attachment traumas while continuing the dyadic work with Lucy. The mother's and Lucy's attachment systems became more regulated and integrated as they increasingly experienced relational safety, attachment completions, repair, and corrective experiences. Lucy's defensive and protective forces began to quiet down, creating an opening for her to access and develop a relationship with her inner world and herself. Time orientation work was routinely used to move Lucy out of trauma time and ground her in her present safety. She and her mother co-created a world in the sand tray depicting her life now with new helpers and friends, and a new emerging relationship with herself. Another tray depicted her past. Lucy and her mom playfully walked and danced back and forth, pendulating between the past and the present (Gomez, 2013). This work provided a portal into the acknowledgment and recognition of Lucy's traumatic memories.

Other therapeutic approaches such as EMDR therapy were also used to process trauma memories with Lucy and her mother. However, the foundational work with Lucy's defense system created the basis for further therapeutic work and opened portals into Lucy's inner world and, ultimately, herself. Lucy organically began to create stories in the sand tray and through puppet shows depicting her traumatic experiences. The gradual integration of the somatic, affective, and cognitive elements of her trauma, and the safety, co-regulation, connectedness and reciprocity of her relational milieu, began to reset her biology. This allowed her to dim her defense system, opening a psychobiological space through which she could connect and form safe and meaningful relationships with people at school and her siblings at home.

Conclusion

For the successful treatment of children affected by complex trauma and dissociation, it is paramount to acknowledge the children's underlying burdens that demand the formation of adaptations, defenses, and vital forces of self-protection. Understanding the complex psychobiological phenomena that underlie defense formation will support clinicians in their decision making, case conceptualization, and treatment delivery. Clinicians also need to recognize that trauma-forming defenses have the potential to block invitations for connection and co-regulation. The work with these defenders detailed in this chapter will enrich the therapeutic process and enhance its outcome.

References

Beckes, L., IJzerman, H., & Tops, M. (2015). Toward a radically embodied neuroscience of attachment and relationships. *Frontiers in Human Neuroscience, 9*, 266. https://doi.org/10.3389/fnhum.2015.00266

Bowlby, J. (1969). *Attachment and loss: Vol. 1*. Attachment. Basic Books.

Cortina, M. (2003). Defensive processes, emotions and internal working models: A perspective from attachment theory and contemporary models of the mind. In M. Cortina & M. Marrone (Eds.), *Attachment theory and the psychoanalytic process* (pp. 271–306). Whurr Publishers.

Cundy, L. (2017). *Anxiously attached: Understanding and working with preoccupied attachment*. Routledge.

Cundy, L. (2019). *Attachment and the defense against intimacy: Understanding and working with avoidant attachment, self-hatred, and shame*. Routledge.

Dozier, M., Peloso, E., Lewis, E., Laurenceau, J., & Levine, S. (2008). Effects of an attachment-based intervention on the cortisol production of infants and toddlers in foster care. *Development and Psychopathology, 20*, 845–859. https://doi.org/10.1017/S0954579408000400

Fisher, J. (2017). *Healing the fragmented selves of trauma survivors: Overcoming internal self-alienation*. Routledge.

Fonagy, P., Gergely, G., Jurist, E. L., & Target, M. (2002). *Affect regulation, mentalization, and the development of the self*. Other Press.

Gilbert, P. (1989). *Human nature and suffering*. Hove: Lawrence Erlbaum.

Gilbert, P. (2001). Evolutionary approaches to psychopathology: The role of natural defences. *Australian & New Zealand Journal of Psychiatry, 35*(1), 17–27. https://doi.org/10.1046/j.1440-1614.2001.00856

Gilbert, P. (2009). *The compassionate mind*. Little, Brown Book Group.

Gilbert, P. (2022). Introducing and developing CFT functions and competencies. In P. Gilbert & G. Simos (Eds.), *Compassion focused therapy* (pp. 243–272). Taylor & Francis Group. https://doi.org/10.4324/9781003035879-9

Gomez, A. M. (2013). *EMDR therapy and adjunct approaches with children: Complex trauma, attachment, and dissociation*. Springer.

Gomez, A. M. (2021). Dissociation in children: A multimodal approach to EMDR therapy. *Go With That magazine, 26*(4), 17–25.

Gomez, A. M. (2023a, January). *The EMDR parent-child & attachment specialist intensive program*. Agate Institute Programs, Phoenix, AZ.

Gomez, A. M. (2023b). *My helpers and protectors: Therapeutic cards that work with the self-protective system of children affected by trauma*. Agate Books.

Gomez, A. M. (2024). *The visitor: A book about pain, defenses and love*. Agate Books.

Gomez, A. M. (in press). *EMDR–sandtray-based therapy: Healing complex trauma and dissociation across the lifespan*. W. W. Norton.

Gomez, A. M., & Paulsen, S. (2016). *All the colors of me: My first book about dissociation*. Agate Books.

Hill, D. (2015). *Affect regulation theory: A clinical model*. W. W. Norton.

Hill, D. (2021). Dysregulation and its impact on states of consciousness. In D. Siegel, A. Schore & L. Cozolino (Eds.), *Interpersonal neurobiology and clinical practice* (pp. 169–194). W. W. Norton.

Karst, P. (2018). *The invisible string*. Scholastic.

Kozlowska, K., Walker, P., McLean, L., & Carrive, P. (2015). Fear and the defense cascade: clinical implications and management. *Harvard Review of Psychiatry, 23*(4), 263.

Levine, P. A. (2015). *Trauma and memory: Brain and body in a search for the living past*. North Atlantic Books.

Liotti, G. (2017). Conflicts between motivational systems related to attachment trauma: Key to understanding the intra-family relationship between abused children and their abusers. *Journal of Trauma and Dissociation, 18*(3), 304–318. https://doi.org/10.1080/15299732.2017.1295392

Liotti, G., & Gilbert, P. (2011). Mentalizing, motivation, and social mentalities: Theoretical considerations and implications for psychotherapy. *Psychology and Psychotherapy: Theory, Research and Practice, 84*(1), 9–25. https://doi.org/10.1348/147608310X520094

Liotti, G., & Liotti, M. (2019). Reflections on some contributions to contemporary psychotraumatology in the light of Janet's critique of Freud's theory. In G. Craparo, F. Ortu & O. van der Hart (Eds.), *Rediscovering Pierre Janet: Trauma, dissociation, and new context for psychoanalysis* (pp. 93–105). Routledge.

Main, M., & Hesse, E. (1990). Parents' unresolved traumatic experiences are related to infant disorganized attachment status: Is frightened and/or frightening parental behavior the linking mechanism? In M. T. Greenberg, D. Cicchetti & E. M. Cummings (Eds.), *Attachment in the preschool years: Theory, research, and intervention* (pp. 161–182). University of Chicago Press.

Ogden, P. (2019). Acts of triumph: An interpretation of Pierre Janet and the role of the body in trauma treatment. In G. Craparo, F. Ortu & O. van der Hart (Eds.), *Rediscovering Pierre Janet: Trauma, dissociation, and new context for psychoanalysis* (pp. 200–209). Routledge.

Ogden, P., & Gomez, A. M. (2013). Using EMDR therapy and sensorimotor psychotherapy with children. In A. Gomez (Ed.), *EMDR therapy and adjunct approaches with children: Complex trauma, attachment and dissociation.* (pp. 247–271). Springer.

Ogden, P., Minton, K., & Pain, C. (2006). *Trauma and the body: A sensorimotor approach to psychotherapy.* W. W. Norton.

Panksepp, J. (1998). *Affective neuroscience: The foundations of human and animal emotions.* Oxford University Press.

Panksepp, J., & Biven, L. (2012). *The archaeology of mind: Neuroevolutionary origins of human emotions.* W. W. Norton.

Perry, B. (2013). *Bonding and attachment in maltreated children: Consequences of emotional neglect.* fosteringandadoption.rip.org.uk/wp-content/uploads/2016/01/bonding-and-attachment-in-maltreated-children.pdf. Adapted in part from *Maltreated children: Experience, brain development and the next generation.* W. W. Norton.

Porges, S. W. (2011). *The polyvagal theory: Neurophysiological foundations of emotions, attachment, communication, and self-regulation.* W. W. Norton.

Porges, S. W. (2021). *Polyvagal safety: Attachment, communication, self-regulation.* W. W. Norton.

Porges, S. W. (2023). The vagal paradox: A polyvagal solution. *Comprehensive Psychoneuroendocrinology, 16*, Article 100200. https://doi.org/10.1016/j.cpnec.2023.100200

Schore, A. (2019). *The development of the unconscious mind.* W. W. Norton.

Schore, A. N. (2003). *Affect dysregulation & disorders of the self.* W.W. Norton.

Shapiro, F. (2018). *Eye movement desensitization and reprocessing: Basic principles, protocols, and procedures* (3rd ed.). Guilford Press.

Siegel, D. (2020). *The developing mind: How relationships and the brain interact to shape who we are* (3rd ed.). W. W. Norton.

Sroufe, L. A., Egeland, B. R., Carlson, E. A., & Collins, W. A. (2009). *The development of the person: The Minnesota Study of Risk and adaptation from birth to adulthood.* Guilford Press.

Steele, K. (2021). Beyond attachment: Understanding motivational systems in complex trauma and dissociation. In D. Siegel, A. Schore & L. Cozolino (Eds.), *Interpersonal neurobiology and clinical practice* (pp. 85–112). W. W. Norton.

Steele, K., Boon, S., & van der Hart, O. (2017). *Treating trauma-related dissociation: A practical integrative approach.* W. W. Norton.

Tolle, E. (1999). *The power of now: A guide to spiritual enlightenment.* New World Library.

van der Hart, O., Nijenhuis, E. R. S., & Steele, K. (2006). *The haunted self: Structural dissociation of the personality and treatment of chronic traumatization.* W. W. Norton.

Wadsworth, M. E. (2015). Development of maladaptive coping: A functional adaptation to chronic, uncontrollable stress. *Child Development Perspectives, 9*(2), 96–100. https://doi.org/10.1111/cdep.12112

41
SELF-HARM AND SUICIDALITY

Alexis E. Arbuthnott

Introduction

Self-harm and suicidality affect a large number of children. A meta-analysis (Liu et al., 2022) of the prevalence rates in community samples suggests that approximately 6% of children 12 years of age and younger have engaged in nonsuicidal self-harm, 15.1% have experienced suicidal ideation, 2.6% have made suicide attempts, and 0.79 per 1 million children have died by suicide. These rates reflect real suffering among children. Rates of self-harm among children with complex trauma are even higher (Beauchaine et al., 2019; Evans et al., 2017; Wamser-Nanney & Campbell, 2022).

This chapter provides an overview of the link between trauma and both self-harm and suicidality in children, frameworks for understanding self-harm and suicidality, and implications for clinicians working with children with complex trauma and self-harm or suicidality. Case examples are also provided at the end of the chapter to illustrate key concepts. Note that parts of this chapter, either as written here or updated with information specific to children, have been previously published (Arbuthnott, 2022) as part of a review of self-harm and suicidality among individuals with dissociative disorders.

Self-Harm and Suicidality among Traumatized Children

In this chapter, the term self-harm refers to nonsuicidal self-injury, which is behavior that intentionally harms one's own body for reasons that are not socially or culturally sanctioned, and that do not include suicidal intent (International Society for the Study of Self-Injury, 2018). Self-harm includes self-scratching, cutting, and burning, among many others methods. In children, self-harm may be of a more rudimentary form, such as biting the hands or lips to the point of pain or bleeding, self-pinching or slapping, or head banging. Suicidality broadly includes the full continuum of suicidal thoughts and behaviors, including passive thoughts of suicide (e.g., not wanting to be alive, wishing to go to sleep and never wake up), active thoughts of suicide (e.g., thinking of ways to die; suicide plans), suicide preparations (e.g., acquiring the means for suicide and writing suicide notes), suicide attempts (including aborted suicide attempts), and death by suicide. Self-harm and suicidal behavior overlap in that they both cause harm to the body, and unintended death can result from severe self-harm regardless of intent. In many cases, the degree to which intent is explicitly or implicitly suicidal may be unclear.

DOI: 10.4324/9781003350156-45

Even very young children may think about and engage in self-harm and suicidal behaviors. Children as young as preschool age may understand the finality and irreversibility of death, even if they do not fully grasp the body processes involved in dying (Wagner et al., 2022). However, the rates of self-harm and suicidality increase throughout the developmental period (Whalen et al., 2022). Although the average age of onset for self-harm is around 13 years, the onset of self-harm before age 12 is associated with more frequent self-harm, the use of a greater number of self-harm methods, and more severe self-harm in the future (Ammerman et al., 2018). Furthermore, self-harm and suicidality in childhood are associated with an elevated risk for self-harm, suicide, and substance-related deaths throughout adolescence and into adulthood (Hinshaw et al., 2012; Morgan et al., 2017; Whalen et al., 2022). Thus, prevention and intervention strategies are needed to mitigate this risk and turn self-harming and suicidal children toward a healthier developmental trajectory.

There is a paucity of empirical research on self-harm and suicidality among traumatized children, and no research to date on these topics includes children with dissociative disorders. Indeed, research on self-harm and suicidality in children younger than 12 years old is still in its infancy and has progressed little beyond identifying associated demographic characteristics. Nonetheless, the rates of self-harm and suicidality among traumatized children are consistently found to be elevated relative to the general population (see Beauchaine et al., 2019; Evans et al., 2017; Wamser-Nanney & Campbell, 2022). For example, the rates of suicide ideation and suicide attempts among children in the care of child protective services may be two and three times, respectively, those of children who are not in care (Evans et al., 2017). Post-traumatic stress symptoms have been associated with greater child- and caregiver-reported suicidality (Wamser-Nanney & Campbell, 2022), and may mediate the relation between child maltreatment and suicidal behaviors (McRae et al., 2022). Relative to children who experience suicidal ideation but have not made a suicide attempt, children who have attempted suicide report greater levels of dissociation, anger, and depression associated with traumatic experiences (Bodzy et al., 2016).

Child survivors of complex trauma may experience high levels of psychological pain resulting from the distressing life events they have endured. Furthermore, trauma during the developmental period disrupts development (see Herman, 1992; Silberg, 2021), which may interfere with the normative acquisition of healthy strategies for self-soothing, emotion regulation, problem-solving, and communication. Healthy strategies across these domains are initially learned through co-regulation and modeling with attuned caregivers, and later through explicit instruction and assistance. When caregivers are absent, abusive, or themselves lack healthy strategies across these domains, children do not have the opportunity to learn healthy strategies from their caregivers. Caregivers may actually model unhealthy emotion regulation strategies, which the child may then adopt for themselves. Trauma also dysregulates the nervous system, leading to increased emotion sensitivity, reactivity, and a slower return to baseline as a means of maintaining a readiness to respond to potential dangers. Taken together, trauma survivors experience higher levels of distress associated with a greater number and severity of current and lifetime cumulative stressors, while simultaneously having access to fewer healthy internal and external resources to manage these stressors.

Frameworks for Self-Harm

Frameworks linking self-harm to traumatic childhood experiences describe self-harm as a means to cope with the aftermath of trauma (Connors, 1996; Smith et al., 2014). It is the presence of trauma symptoms, rather than the exposure to trauma, that underlies later self-harm (Smith et al., 2014). Much of the information about self-harm in children is borrowed from the literature of self-harm in adolescents and adults, as similar psychological, social, and biological processes underlying self-harm are believed to be at work across the lifespan. However, developmental capacities (e.g., less developed cognitive abilities and executive functions) may also play a role, as discussed in more detail in Impact of Developmental Stage under Frameworks for Suicidality, below.

Research assessing the functions of self-harm generally group these functions into three broad categories (see Whitlock & Selekman, 2014): psychological functions, where self-harm is reinforced through intrapersonal or interpersonal consequences; social functions, where self-harm is used to meet a perceived interpersonal need; and biological functions, such as when self-harm is used to restore levels of endogenous opioids to homeostasis. Among trauma survivors, self-harm may also have the function of reenacting traumatic experiences (see Conners, 1996; Yakeley & Burbridge-James, 2018). There is a considerable amount of overlap between these functions, and self-harm often serves multiple functions simultaneously (Whitlock & Selekman, 2014). Furthermore, functions may change over time and the functions by which self-harm is maintained may differ from those for which it was originally used (Muehlenkamp et al., 2013; Nock, 2009; Whitlock & Selekman, 2014).

Psychological Functions

The psychological model (Nock, 2009) explains self-harm as being maintained through both intrapersonal and interpersonal functions, which are each composed of both positive (i.e., increasing something that is desired) and negative (i.e., removing something that is aversive or unwanted) reinforcers. Intrapersonal functions include using self-harm to generate sensations or feelings (e.g., anti-dissociation and generating a thrill or rush of energy), as well as the use of self-harm to escape from uncomfortable internal states (e.g., eliciting a dissociative state, shutting down unwanted emotions, and reducing internal tension). With respect to trauma symptoms specifically, self-harm may serve as a distraction from intrusive or disturbing thoughts or rumination, including self-critical, shaming, and suicidal thoughts (Ford & Gómez, 2015). Furthermore, self-harm may provide the child with an increased locus of control and a sense of self-efficacy. Interpersonal functions include the use of self-harm to influence others (e.g., to communicate distress in order to elicit care and obtaining resources or rewards) or to avoid punishment or expectations (e.g., preventing others from imposing demands, setting limits, or enforcing consequences). Interpersonal functions overlap with the social model of self-harm and are explored in more depth in the Social Functions section below.

Self-harm is also used to communicate distress both at an internal level (i.e., to themselves) and to other people (Muehlenkamp et al., 2013; Whitlock & Selekman, 2014). The central conflict of dissociation is the need to know and not know at the same time (Howell, 2011). Children with dissociative disorders are inherently disconnected from aspects of their internal experience, which often includes their own distress. When painful events and resulting emotions are ignored, denied, or invalidated by the people around them, children may dissociate their pain and internalize this invalidation. Self-harm may then be used to make invisible pain visible, or "real." Physical injury may be substituted for emotional injury, and distress related to internal conflicts may be acted out on the body (see Brand, 2001; Chefetz, 2017).

The Family Distress Cascade Theory (Waals et al., 2018) was originally developed for use with adolescents, but may also apply to preadolescent children. This theory highlights the bidirectional impact of child and caregiver behaviors in escalating distress within the family system in relation to the child's self-harm. In this model, the child's self-harm increases caregiver concern and distress, which causes the caregiver to react with controlling behaviors (e.g., increasing supervision and restricting privileges in an effort to maintain the child's safety). The preadolescent may experience these reactions as an intrusion of their privacy and a loss of autonomy, which then result in a corresponding increase in the child's self-harm frequency and severity. Caregivers may respond to this escalation of self-harm with further alarm and restrictions for the child, and thus this cascade is perpetuated.

In families with a history of abuse or neglect, self-harm may represent a means by which the child maintains autonomy over their body and choices.

Social Functions

The social model of self-harm describes self-harm as a tool to meet relational needs (see Whitlock & Selekman, 2014), including obtaining care (via expression of distress), influencing others, and social bonding. The use of self-harm to meet social needs can be understood within the context of disrupted attachment and learned behavior. The child either did not have the opportunity to learn healthy age-appropriate communication and problem-solving skills, or these skills were ineffective in getting their needs met within their environment. Thus, self-harm reflects the child's creativity in developing strategies to get their perceived needs met as effectively as they are able, with the resources they have available, within the context of their environment.

Self-harm may have a social bonding function (e.g., to fit in with others), particularly among older children. Social bonding may be more salient in the initiation of self-harm rather than its maintenance (Muehlenkamp et al., 2013). This highlights the potential social contagion effects associated with self-harm among children who are already at a higher risk (Jarvi et al., 2013), such as those with complex trauma. Thus, when a child is experiencing a high level of psychological pain and they are introduced to self-harm through interactions with their peers or through social media, they may perceive self-harm as a socially acceptable and effective way to manage their pain. Although a secondary gain may include a sense of connection with peers through shared experience, alternate functions (e.g., affect regulation and communication of distress) generally maintain self-harm in those who go on to engage in self-harm repetitively (Muehlenkamp et al., 2013).

Biological Functions

Biological models of self-harm highlight the neurobiological alterations that make people more vulnerable for using self-harm to down-regulate high arousal and tension (Groschwitz & Plener, 2012). Neuroimaging and neuroendocrine studies have shown that people who engage in self-harm may have neurobiological alterations affecting multiple biological systems, including those systems related to threat avoidance, learning and motivation, cognition (e.g., memory, perception, attention, and language), social processing, and arousal and biological regulation (see Schreiner et al., 2015). Many of these neurobiological alterations overlap with those altered through exposure to traumatic stress, particularly changes in the limbic system, hypothalamic-pituitary-adrenal axis, and key monoamine neurotransmitters. These biological changes map onto symptoms of hyperarousal, numbing, dissociation, and reexperiencing of trauma (Weiss, 2007).

On a biological level, self-harm can be surprisingly effective in reducing psychological pain, thus its appeal as a means of regulating painful affective states and reducing internal tension. Self-harm is often preceded by high emotional arousal and tension, and hyperarousal tends to be reduced following self-harm (Klonsky, 2007). The homeostasis model of self-harm suggests that people who engage in self-harm have lower baseline levels of endogenous opioids (perhaps due to chronic exposure to traumatic environments and adverse experiences), and the release of endogenous opioids via self-harm functions to regulate affect (see Bresin & Gordon, 2013).

Reenactment

Self-harm may serve as a means of attempting to differentiate between self and other, define and differentiate body boundaries, and master severe childhood trauma through psychophysiological reenactments (see Connors, 1996; Yakeley & Burbridge-James, 2018). A child who self-harms may use their own body to act out the violence they have witnessed or endured. For trauma survivors whose bodies have been violated, the act of self-harm may not only release negative affect and tension, but also symbolically relieve the child from the perceived badness inside themselves (e.g., cleansing or purification and atonement through self-punishment) or discharge rage onto a perpetrator. A child may feel it is safer to discharge their rage onto themselves rather than on a caregiver on whom they depend for survival. Furthermore, given the biological effects of self-harm in calming the nervous system, self-harm may come to be used as a substitute caregiver from which the child seeks soothing. Through this perspective, the child engaging in self-harm takes on the roles of the perpetrator, victim, and rescuer simultaneously as they act out traumatic events and inner conflict. These dissociative defenses are described in more detail elsewhere in this volume.

Frameworks for Suicidality

Suicidality has been studied predominantly in adults, a little bit in adolescents, and very little in children younger than 12 years old. Although the same mechanisms underlying self-harm are generally presumed to be at work throughout the lifespan, this is not necessarily the case for suicidality. Given the developmental differences between children, adolescents, and adults, the mechanisms underlying suicide in children are likely to have both similarities to those in adolescents and adults as well as differences unique to younger developmental stages. Theories developed to explain suicidality in adults may be a useful starting point in conceptualizing suicidality among children only when developmental capacities are also considered.

Theories of Suicide

There are a large number of theories explaining suicidality in adults (see Gunn & Lester, 2014, for a comprehensive overview of the various theories of suicide). It is important to note that these theories overlap. Rather than a single theory explaining all cases of suicidality, theories should be considered both complementary and supplementary to each other. Biological theories of suicide highlight the interaction between physiological vulnerabilities and psychosocial stressors. Cognitive-behavioral theories explain suicide as being driven by maladaptive cognitive styles (e.g., hopelessness, suicidal cognitive mode, state dependent memory, and perceptions of entrapment). Developmental and systems theories account for the role of social and family systems as causal factors in suicidality. Escape theories of suicide underscore the function of suicide as a means to escape from aversive states and situations (which trauma survivors may have in abundance).

Two theories of suicide have some research evidence suggesting that they may be applicable to adolescents (see Ayer et al., 2020, for a review): the interpersonal (or interpersonal-psychological) theory of suicide (Joiner, 2005; Van Orden et al., 2010), and the ideation-to-action framework (Klonsky & May, 2014, 2015). The interpersonal theory of suicide posits that suicidality arises when a person experiences unmanageable feelings of perceived burdensomeness and thwarted belongingness, and the person has the capability for suicide. Both perceived burdensomeness and thwarted belongingness reflect a sense of perceived social disconnection, with thwarted belongingness also including intense loneliness and a perceived lack of care. These are symptoms common among survivors of complex trauma.

The ideation-to-action framework (Klonsky & May, 2014, 2015) argues that suicide ideation and suicidal behavior are distinct processes with distinct explanations. Within this framework, pain and hopelessness contribute to suicide ideation. Connectedness serves as a protective factor against escalating suicide ideation. The shift from suicide ideation to suicide attempt is facilitated by an increase in the capacity for suicide, which results from changes in dispositional (e.g., pain sensitivity and blood phobia), acquired (e.g., habituation to experiences associated with pain and injury), and practical (e.g., concrete factors such as knowledge and access to lethal means) factors. The capability for the level of self-directed violence necessary for suicide may be acquired through exposure to other forms of violence against the body (e.g., abuse and assaults). Experiencing violence normalizes violence. Capacity for suicide may also be built up through increasingly severe self-harm. Indeed, self-harm is known to be a gateway to suicidal behavior, and it may confer a unique risk for future suicidal behavior independent of shared risk factors (Whitlock et al., 2013). The more severe the self-harm, where this self-harm is perceived as effective in meeting the person's needs, the less frightening suicide becomes.

Impact of Developmental Stage

Unfortunately, there are currently no solid frameworks explaining suicidality in children younger than 12 years old. Only demographic characteristics associated with suicidality have been detailed among children; empirical information about risk factors, prevention, and intervention for suicidality is lacking (see Ayer et al., 2020). Key variables associated with preadolescent onset suicidal behavior, when controlling for a variety of other psychosocial factors, include child maltreatment (Liu et al., 2022; Walsh et al., 2020), attention-deficit hyperactivity disorder (ADHD), and depressive disorders (Liu et al., 2022; Zelazny et al., 2021). Compared to adolescents who died by suicide in the United States, children who died by suicide were more commonly from marginalized populations, more often experienced relationship problems with family members and friends, were less likely to be depressed, and were more likely to have a diagnosis of ADHD (Sheftall et al., 2016). Among children with ADHD, those experiencing suicide ideation may have greater difficulties in both emotion regulation and executive functioning relative to children with ADHD who do not experience suicidal ideation (Uçur & Özcan, 2018).

The link between ADHD and suicidality in children is notable because of the overlapping symptoms between ADHD, post-traumatic stress disorder, and dissociative disorders (see Chapter 14 for more information about overlapping symptoms). In fact, one study assessing ADHD symptoms among abused children found that a large number of children fulfilled the criteria for ADHD after, but not before, trauma exposure (Endo et al., 2006). The authors postulated that this increase in ADHD symptoms following trauma exposure may reflect comorbid dissociative disorders. It is plausible that some of the research linking ADHD and suicidality, and particularly those studies examining traumatized children, may be better conceptualized through a dissociative lens. Regardless, the presence of emotion dysregulation, impulsivity, and lack of inhibition increases the likelihood that a child will act on urges for self-harmful behaviors when emotionally dysregulated (see Beauchaine et al., 2019).

Theories of suicide among children need to include the biological and social processes associated with this developmental stage that may make some children more vulnerable to suicidality. These processes are likely to include the child's pain, lack of connectedness, hopelessness, and neurobiological stage of development (e.g., developing cognitive abilities, impulse control, executive functions, and emotion regulation) (see Ayer et al., 2020). All of these factors are substantially impacted by trauma. Children with complex trauma may experience a greater amount of psychological pain and hopelessness owing to their painful life experiences and trauma symptoms, disruptions in their attachments and difficulties in relationships resulting from interpersonal trauma, and alterations in brain development due to neurobiological responses to traumatic experiences.

Clinical Implications

Given the strong associations between dissociation, self-harm, and suicidality, clinicians need to be mindful of the potential for severe self-harm and suicidality among children presenting with complex trauma or dissociation.

Risk Assessment

Clinicians should be familiar with procedures for thorough suicide risk assessments in children (American Academy of Pediatrics, 2023; Pettit et al., 2018). Reassessments over time are recommended as warranted. Several structured suicide screening measures exist (see Carter et al., 2018, for a review of assessment tools). Most suicide risk assessments ask about the presence and content of thoughts of self-harm and suicide, including whether the child has a history of self-harm and/or suicide attempts, a current suicide plan, access to the means to carry out their plan, and intent to follow through with their plan. Unfortunately, there is insufficient evidence to date that any structured suicide risk assessment measure is effective in identifying children who will attempt suicide or die by suicide (Carter et al., 2018; Viswanathan et al., 2022). However, the results of these measures may alert clinicians to an individual child's increased risk for self-harm and suicidality, and thus the need for more safety-focused interventions or closer follow-up. The combination of formal risk assessment and clinical judgment is necessary when responding to self-harm and suicidality.

The research is clear that asking about self-harm and suicide does not increase self-harm or risk of suicide in adults or youth (Gould et al., 2005; Viswanathan et al., 2022). Although this has not yet been examined specifically in children, developmentally sensitive and non-leading questions about the child's experience are necessary to assess risk. Open and nonjudgmental conversations about these topics reduce shame, open a pathway to understand the child's internal experience, and provide an opportunity to identify and teach alternate and healthier ways to help the child meet their needs.

How the clinician asks about self-harm and suicidality will impact the child's disclosure. Children who anticipate danger following a disclosure of self-harm or suicidality (e.g., being invalidated or misunderstood, eliciting uncomfortable emotions in caregivers, getting in trouble, other unwanted consequences such as hospitalization) are less likely to self-disclose. Equally problematic is when children anticipate assistance following their disclosure, but receive minimal concern or tangible help. For traumatized children, this may be a reenactment of a bystander effect in which people may have known about child abuse that was occurring but chose not to intervene. Thus, it is important that clinicians neither overreact nor underreact to disclosures of self-harm or suicidality. Instead, clinicians are encouraged to maintain a collaborative, compassionate, and curious stance that communicates to the child that their safety is important, that the child's behavior is understandable (though unhealthy) within the context in which it is being used, and that the clinician knows how to help and is willing to help.

Approximately 17% of preadolescents with suicidal ideation transition to attempting suicide (Liu et al., 2022). In addition to assessing for the presence and content of suicide ideation, clinicians need to be familiar with the child's baseline presentation and level of suicidality, and be vigilant for shifts away from this baseline. In general, three types of risk factors should be considered when assessing for suicide risk among children with complex trauma and dissociation: (1) risk derived from the child's demographics (e.g., trauma history, sex, gender, age, cultural marginalization, baseline level of dissociation and impulsivity, diagnoses, and family history of suicide); (2) risk relative to the child's baseline presentation (e.g., increases in depressive or trauma symptoms and acute increase in self-harm or suicide ideation); and (3) risk associated with current and foreseeable changes in social factors (e.g., life transition points, changes in the family system, relationships, and social supports), including increases in stressors and decreases in protective factors.

Chronic suicide ideation is not generally a mental health emergency unless accompanied by acute suicidal behaviors or an acute escalation in suicidal thoughts, plans, or intent. For many traumatized children, the thought that suicide is a potential option to escape their circumstances is protective; knowing there is a means of escape may provide the strength necessary to persevere. Similarly, self-harm may have an anti-suicide function whereby the release of tension and negative affect elicited through self-harm may decrease the intensity of suicidal thoughts and urges (see Kraus et al., 2020). However, self-harm may also act as a gateway to suicidality (Whitlock et al., 2013). Increasingly frequent or severe self-harm may signal that self-harm is no longer adequately fulfilling the function for which it was being used, or that self-harm is being generalized to serve additional functions beyond the initial purpose. This often reflects that the child's stressors or distress have increased beyond what they can manage through healthier means, and should alert caregivers to the child's need for additional supports. Escalating self-harm may also indicate rapidly increasing acquired capacity for greater self-harm and suicidal behavior.

Role of Caregivers and Family Systems

Parents and/or other primary caregivers are essential members of the treatment team. Parental support has been found to serve as a protective factor against suicide in children (Liu et al., 2022; Walsh et al., 2020). Many parents with children who self-harm report experiencing an increase in stigma and sense of isolation in relation to their child's self-harm, a loss of confidence in their parenting, and an increase in their own mental health concerns (see Arbuthnott & Lewis, 2015). Furthermore, mental health crises such as suicide attempts may be experienced by caregivers as traumatic. Given the bidirectional impact between the caregiver and child's distress (Waals et al., 2018), early intervention is essential in equipping caregivers to support their children in helpful ways and to minimize the cascade of distress between caregiver and child associated with the child's self-harm and suicidality. Key goals for working with caregivers include: the elimination of parenting behaviors that may be reinforcing the child's symptoms; reducing emotion invalidation, coercion, and maltreatment; increasing positive parent-child interactions; and increasing supervision (see Beauchaine et al., 2019).

Psychoeducation for caregivers can help destigmatize self-harm and reduce caregivers' alarm and distress. This may include information about distinguishing between the functions of nonsuicidal and suicidal behaviors, normative versus atypical behaviors across stages of development, developmental tasks across childhood, and the impact of trauma on both the child and their caregivers. Psychoeducation about acute trauma responses may also help normalize and mitigate caregivers' intense reactions to a child's mental health crisis.

Caregivers also have an important role in supporting the child's healthy development. Caregivers are central to helping the child generalize new skills to manage self-harm and suicidal urges beyond the clinician's office. As complex trauma is often intergenerational, parents may never have had the opportunity to develop these skills for themselves. Thus, it is imperative that parents and caregivers be included in the child's treatment plan and have the opportunity to learn alongside the child. Caregivers become responsible for modeling and reinforcing healthy emotion regulation skills (e.g., accurately identifying and responding to emotions in self and others, and tolerating distress), interpersonal skills (e.g., boundaries, communication, and collaboration), and developing sense of identity (e.g., increasing sense of competence and cohesion across self-states). Furthermore, the application of healthy strategies for managing emotions within the family's home may require the identification and cessation of unhealthy strategies and interactions that maintain the child's self-harm and suicidality. Finally, caregivers may benefit from referrals to mental health supports for themselves.

Maintaining Safety

A support plan (or safety plan) is a living document that outlines the child's and environment's resources for managing the child's intense distress and harmful urges, and is embedded in the child's larger treatment plan (see Pettit et al., 2018, for an overview of safety planning). In contrast to the traditional view of a safety plan as a piece of paper that lists coping skills and crisis phone numbers, support plans as described in this chapter are intended to help the child and caregivers understand the child's unique experience and respond in ways that effectively meet the child's specific needs.

Establishing and maintaining safety may be a complex process for traumatized children. Among children who experience divisions within their emerging sense of self, different aspects of the child's self may respond to the same safety-focused interventions in contradictory ways; what one aspect of the child's self finds soothing may be distressing for another. For example, some aspects of the child may feel soothed through connection with caregivers, whereas others feel threatened by this. Similarly, some aspects of the child may appreciate strategies to calm down the body (e.g., deep breathing and grounding through the five senses), whereas this level of somatic awareness may be overwhelming for others, and still others may increase their vigilance in response to suggestions that the child relax. Thus, creativity and moment-by-moment flexibility in co-creating safety is necessary when developing and implementing support plans with traumatized children.

Support plans should be created collaboratively with the child and their family and are updated when new information comes to light (e.g., insight into triggers and functions of unhealthy behaviors), or new resources are accessible (e.g., new skills acquired and additional family supports). Caregivers should always be involved in the development of a child's support plan. The younger the child, in general, the more important caregivers and other key adults in the child's life become in ensuring the child's safety. Many children and caregivers find it difficult to remember the components of their support plans, or even that they have a support plan, when children are in states of high distress. Thus, having the up-to-date plan written down and accessible (e.g., posted on the refrigerator and photo on a cell phone) is essential. Furthermore, some children benefit from multiple support plans tailored to different settings (e.g., home versus school).

Support plans should clearly outline the signs and symptoms indicating an increase in distress that may lead to a crisis. Identifying the child's triggers can help the child and caregiver anticipate difficult situations and validate the child's experience. Helping the child and caregivers identify the child's presentation (i.e., emotions, thoughts, sensations, urges, and behaviors) at baseline, when triggered and escalating, and when in crisis may be of value for matching the appropriate intervention to the child's level of escalation. In line with traditional safety plans, the support plan should also list strategies the child has learned for coping independently, effective methods of co-regulation, social contacts and social settings that can provide a distraction from suicidal and distressing thoughts, support people who can help resolve the crisis, and mental health professionals (e.g., clinicians) or agencies (e.g., crisis lines and hospital emergency departments) who can provide professional or crisis mental health supports. As an extension of the traditional safety plan, a support plan that acknowledges the complexity of the child's inner system can provide guidance for the child and caregivers around navigating the competing needs associated with different aspects of the child's self.

The child may have access to a wider variety of helpful de-escalation strategies when triggered and beginning to escalate versus when they are in crisis. In general, the younger the child, or the less developed their skills for independent self-regulation regardless of their age, the more co-regulation will be required by caregivers for de-escalation. Assisting caregivers to identify their child's emotional state and respond with appropriate methods for co-regulation is essential to an effective support plan. Note, however, that for traumatized children with attachment disruptions, the offer of co-regulation may initially be rejected by the child. Caregivers may need assistance to understand this rejection and continue to support the child despite this initial rejection. Over time, repeated experiences with co-regulation and progressive scaffolding of support toward self-regulation will help the child acquire the skills necessary to de-escalate themselves.

The role of the support plan in preventing crises, as well as in responding to crises, should be emphasized. There may be some merit to the child and caregiver's report that "nothing helps" when strategies are implemented only at very high levels of distress; at this point, the child may be too distressed to access or benefit from healthy coping strategies or co-regulation that may have been accessible and effective at lower levels of distress. During crises (i.e., the child is actively attempting to hurt themselves), the focus of the support plan shifts to managing the child's safety by managing the environment (e.g., removing unsafe items, reducing overstimulation, and decreasing demands on cognitive and executive functioning resources) until the child's distress begins to subside and they can reengage in co-regulation or self-regulation strategies. This is not the time for problem-solving or consequences, which should be delayed until the child's emotional state has returned to baseline and the child is able to engage in a debrief about the incident.

Caregivers are instrumental in reducing a child's access to lethal means for suicide, such as by removing or locking up medications, sharps, firearms, substances, or whatever means for suicide align with the child's specific suicide plan. The intention here is not to get rid of all potentially dangerous objects, but rather to remove access to those items that pose the greatest immediate risk of death, and to add an extra step between having thoughts of suicide and making a suicide attempt. Increasing the time it takes to obtain the means for suicide may reduce the impact of impulsivity on carrying out a suicide plan, and may provide enough time for the acute stressors to resolve, distress to reduce naturally, and support people to respond.

Stabilization Phase of Treatment

Serious self-harm and suicidal behaviors are unequivocally primary treatment targets during the treatment of traumatized children. Within the context of a phase approach to trauma treatment, self-harm and active suicidality reflect a need to stay in, or temporarily return to, the stabilization phase of treatment (see Chapter 15 for more information about the phase approach to treating complex trauma.) To date, there has been relatively little evidence that any particular intervention designed to target self-harm or suicidality is more effective than others for children (Busby et al., 2020; Hawton et al., 2015; Ougrin et al., 2015; Viswanathan et al., 2022; Witt et al., 2021). This does not mean that specialized interventions for self-harm and suicidality are not effective, but rather that they are not *more* effective than other interventions. This may reflect many different factors including improvements in treatment as usual over time, such as the incorporation of skills-based stabilization strategies into treatment as usual and the increased application of trauma-informed care in clinical settings. In general, interventions that target the child's emotion dysregulation are appropriate (see Beauchaine et al., 2019). Furthermore, among children who dissociate, identifying the self-states associated with self-harm and suicidality may provide opportunities for interventions involving these self-states. (Since a variety of appropriate interventions are outlined elsewhere in this book, they are not described again here.)

Given the complexity of symptoms and behaviors among traumatized children, it may be more helpful to conceptualize self-harm and suicidal behaviors as part of a complex trauma symptom constellation and to prioritize treating the underlying trauma. The logic behind this is that when the processes maintaining the symptom are addressed, the self-harm and suicidal behavior may naturally resolve. However, self-harm and suicidality are treatment targets in and of themselves; when these behaviors are reduced through the acquisition of healthier ways to cope with stressors, the child's quality of life and overall mental well-being naturally improve. When self-harm and suicidality are used to cope with trauma symptoms, the underlying trauma maintains the self-harm and suicidality. However, trauma processing—though essential for reducing the impact of the trauma on the child—is inherently destabilizing, which increases risk for self-harm and suicidality. Furthermore, self-harm and suicidality interfere with normative developmental opportunities (e.g., they may prevent the acquisition of healthy emotion regulation and interpersonal skills; hospitalization may interfere with school attendance and social activities; self-stigma may impact identity), and may themselves result in retraumatization (e.g., medical interventions to treat self-harm or suicide attempts, hospitalization and associated separations from caregivers). Thus, clinicians may need to hold both perspectives simultaneously: Self-harm and suicidality are used as a solution to trauma symptoms, but they also cause their own problems regardless of the underlying trauma; both the trauma and the self-harm and/or suicidality need to be directly addressed in tandem. This can be accomplished by moving back and forth between the three phases of trauma treatment, and returning to the stabilization phase whenever warranted.

Inpatient Care

Children may require admission to an acute inpatient mental health unit for a period of stabilization when safety concerns are unmanageable in the community. Although there is currently no data supporting the effectiveness of hospitalization in reducing suicide risk in children, an inpatient admission may ensure supervision and limit access to lethal means until the acute risk subsides (see Pettit et al., 2018). Other potential benefits of hospitalization include the opportunity for diagnostic clarification, more intensive opportunities for building or restoring skills, and rapid changes in medications to facilitate symptom reduction. The goal of inpatient care is generally rapid stabilization (Sharfstein, 2009), with the intention of returning the child to care in the community as quickly and as safely as possible.

While inpatient care can be potentially life-saving, it is not without risks. For children, hospitalization is often an acute separation from caregivers during a time of crisis. This separation may temporarily increase distress for both the child and caregivers. Clinicians should also be mindful of the risks of retraumatization associated with hospitalization, including perceived coercion, the use of seclusion and restraints, and the potential negative impacts of witnessing the behavior of other (often older) youth with severe mental health concerns. Children who dissociate may use dissociation as a means to cope with their distress associated with being hospitalized, which may reduce the effectiveness of inpatient interventions. Furthermore, the hospital environment may meet needs for the child or caregivers that are not being met in the community (e.g., safety, care or connection, supervision, reduction in demands and stressors, tangible needs such as access to food and shelter), which may lead to repeated admissions and difficulty generalizing stabilization from hospital to home. Indeed, the transition period immediately following discharge from inpatient care reflects a period of increased risk for suicide (Bojanić et al., 2020; Forte et al., 2019), and rapid follow-up with a community clinician is strongly recommended post-discharge (Bojanić et al., 2020).

Case Examples

These case examples were created through the amalgamation of features from many children and their families alongside details that have been changed or added to ensure anonymity. Note that the emphasis of these vignettes is on addressing the child's self-harm and suicidality. Aspects of treatment beyond those addressing self-harm and suicidality (e.g., trauma processing, medication managements, and addressing co-occurring mental health challenges) are not presented here, but can be assumed to occur both consecutively and in tandem with these interventions, as appropriate.

Self-Harm in a Young Child

Gus is a four-year-old boy who has witnessed physical and verbal aggression between his mother and father since birth. He was recently removed from the home due to neglect within the context of his parents' ongoing substance use, and he was placed in the care of kin. Gus has episodes where he screams and swears, slaps his face, and punches his thighs. These episodes tend to occur when Gus is scared or frustrated (e.g., when he does not get something that he wants, when caregivers attempt to set limits).

Treatment initially focused primarily on Gus's caregivers' parenting approaches. Caregivers were coached in increasing their caregiving consistency, emotion regulation, attunement, and opportunities for positive caregiver-child interactions. Caregiver behaviors that further escalated Gus's self-harm (e.g., yelling and making threats) and those that reinforced Gus's dysregulation (e.g., giving Gus what he was demanding to make him stop hurting himself) were targeted and decreased. With consistency in implementing new parenting strategies, Gus's verbal outbursts decreased in frequency and severity, and the self-harm ceased.

Suicidality in a School-Aged Child

Luz is an eight-year-old girl who was born with a life-threatening heart condition. She spent much of the first three years of her life in and out of the children's hospital. Luz required multiple surgeries to save her life, and she experienced several medical crises necessitating urgent and painful medical care. Luz's mother experienced post-partum depression that evolved into persistent depressive disorder, and her father received a diagnosis of post-traumatic stress disorder resulting from witnessing Luz's medical trauma. Luz is now a kind, empathic, and somewhat anxious child. For the past three months, Luz has been saying that she wishes she was not alive. Her primary trigger for the suicide ideation is feeling an acute disconnection from others, such as when disagreements occur in her relationships with friends, and while separating from her caregivers (e.g., transition into school each morning, when a parent leaves the home for an appointment). Luz was referred to the school counselor after writing a story about a group of friends who planned to die together by suicide.

The school counselor completed a suicide risk assessment and worked with Luz and her caregivers to establish a plan to support Luz's safety. Luz reported frequently thinking about death and dying. Although she had thought about a variety of ways that she might kill herself (e.g., overdosing on medications, stabbing herself or cutting her wrists, and drinking her caregivers' alcohol), she had never made a concrete suicide plan, and she denied having any intent to kill herself. She had also never engaged in any self-harm behaviors, though her caregivers noted that she had started taking more risks than usual (e.g., not wearing her helmet when she rides a bike and starting to cross the road without waiting for cars to stop). Luz was able to identify many reasons for living, and she displayed future-oriented thinking by excitedly describing her plans for the summer. Luz's suicide ideation reflected a high level of distress that warranted further intervention.

A plan to support Luz's safety was completed with Luz and her caregivers, and this plan was updated regularly throughout the intervention process. Luz's caregivers were encouraged to put away medications, sharps, and substances in the home. Due to her age, Luz spent little time unsupervised, and her parents increased the frequency with which they checked in with Luz. Luz, in turn, felt temporary relief when her parents provided reassurance, and she sought out her caregivers more frequently when distressed. Initially, the family noted that Luz's expressions of suicidal ideation increased dramatically as they attuned to Luz's emotional state, and her caregivers worried that the connection they gave Luz in response to these expressions was reinforcing them. Luz and her caregivers were encouraged to identify the information being communicated underneath the expressions of suicidal ideation and to respond to these needs rather than to the words themselves. For example, when Luz voiced the thought, "I wish I wasn't alive," her caregivers were able to re-label this for her: "You feel alone and very scared." At these times, Luz often then reflected on how alone and scared she must have been as a baby undergoing extensive medical treatment. Her caregivers provided compassionate attunement to her reflections. They took on the role of emotion coach, helping Luz find words to label what she was experiencing, using validation techniques to help her make sense of these feelings, orienting her to the safety and care within her current environment, and co-regulating her through activities to soothe and calm down her nervous system. The amount of support required from her caregivers progressively decreased as Luz became more adept at using strategies to help herself settle when distressed.

Self-Harm and Suicidality in a Preadolescent

Quinn is an 11-year-old youth who identifies their gender as nonbinary. They were apprehended by Child Protective Services and placed in foster care after being found during a raid on a drug house. Quinn appeared to be about three years old at the time they were found and had injuries consistent with physical and sexual abuse, as well as severe malnourishment. They were placed in a series of foster homes over the next three years, before finding a stable foster placement with dedicated caregivers. They were initially delayed in all developmental milestones, though had caught up to same-age peers in language and motor skills through the provision of supplemental speech-language therapy and occupational therapy supports. Quinn was reported to have difficulty with emotion regulation, attention, and impulsivity throughout elementary school. They often isolated themselves, were controlling of peers, tended to misperceive the behaviors of others as personal attacks, and had verbal outbursts when frustrated. They were diagnosed with ADHD at age 9, when they began to self-harm via superficially scratching themselves. Their self-harm progressively increased in frequency and severity over time. The more Quinn's caregivers attempted to increase their level of supervision and decrease Quinn's access to tools they could use to self-harm, the more resentful Quinn became toward their caregivers and the more they sought out opportunities to self-harm in secret. Quinn's caregivers felt burnt out and ineffective in managing Quinn's safety, and they requested an alternate placement for Quinn. Quinn was admitted to an acute inpatient mental health unit after a near-lethal suicide attempt one month after being moved to a group home.

While in hospital, Quinn's behavior alternated between calm withdrawal and periods of intense distress. Despite having access to little they could use to hurt themselves, when distressed they scratched their face with their fingernails, attempted to strangle themselves with their hospital attire, and ran head-first into the walls. Staff's attempts to verbally de-escalate Quinn were not effective. Once Quinn was in a dysregulated state, both connection with staff and the loss of this connection were noted to further escalate their distress, with Quinn simultaneously demanding to be left alone and demanding that staff not leave them. Furthermore, Quinn became physically aggressive toward staff who attempted to intervene to manage their safety. Chemical and mechanical restraints were initially required to prevent serious harm to both Quinn and staff. Quinn consistently reported that they intended to seriously harm and kill themselves, that they did not want to feel better, and that they did not want to learn any strategies or skills to help themselves. They rejected all mental health programming offered on the unit, disengaged from conversations about mental health topics, and refused to debrief about the self-harm incidents that occurred. In fact, they often denied that these incidents had occurred at all, and accused the staff of making up stories about Quinn's behavior. Staff quickly became disheartened with trying to help a youth who appeared to be unwilling to help themselves.

A behavior support plan was developed to assist staff to more effectively respond to Quinn's self-harm in hospital. Predictable triggers for the self-harm were identified, and included dysregulated co-patients and loud noises, staff shift changes, perceived invalidation, perceived failure, and perceived loss of agency. Care was taken to reduce the impact of triggers, such as by providing consistency in staffing, offering opportunities for agency and mastery, and increasing validation and appreciation of Quinn as a person. Staff intentionally shifted their focus from changing Quinn's behavior to building relationships with Quinn. When triggered, but not yet at a crisis level of escalation, Quinn was observed to de-escalate most effectively through nonverbal interactive physical activities, such as table tennis and basketball. Staff were assisted to understand Quinn's contradictory behavior and demands as a reflection of the inner conflicts among Quinn's different aspects of self. Parts language (e.g., "There is a part of you that really wants me to stay so that you are not alone with this, and there is a part of you that feels really threatened by my presence") and creativity in managing these dialectics (e.g., finding a balance in the physical distance between Quinn and staff that felt most comfortable to Quinn) increased Quinn's self-awareness of their inner conflicts.

Quinn eventually reported having a demon living inside them, to whom they ascribed responsibility for their self-harm. Staff modeled compassionate curiosity about Quinn's relationships with the demon, as well as the demon's own life experiences that had led it to hurt Quinn. Staff's validation, empathy, and respect for the dignity of all parts of Quinn provided the pathway for Quinn to begin to be able to tolerate their internal experiences and increased their ability to engage with strategies to self-soothe their distress and self-regulate their emotions. Quinn came to understand that the demon was actually a part of themselves, and they gained an appreciation for their mind's ability to create a means of surviving dehumanizing experiences. Quinn was then more prepared to engage in a collaborative plan to increase their safety.

Conclusion

Children with complex trauma are at a heightened risk for self-harm and suicidality. Unfortunately, there is a paucity of research outlining the mechanisms underlying self-harm and suicidality in children specifically. Some of the frameworks developed with adults and adolescents for understanding self-harm and suicidality can be applied to children, provided the neurodevelopmental and social processes unique to childhood are also incorporated into these models. Thorough risk assessments, strategies for maintaining safety, and interventions to increase stabilization are warranted to protect children's safety.

References

American Academy of Pediatrics. (2023). Screening for suicide risk in clinical practice. Retrieved May 30, 2023, from aap.org/en/patient-care/blueprint-for-youth-suicide-prevention/strategies-for-clinical-settings-for-youth-suicide-prevention/screening-for-suicide-risk-in-clinical-practice

Ammerman, B. A., Jacobucci, R., Kleiman, E. M., Uyeji, L., & McCloskey, M. S. (2018). The relationship between nonsuicidal self-injury age of onset and severity of self-harm. *Suicide and Life-Threatening Behavior, 48*, 31–37. https://doi.org/10.1111/sltb.12330

Arbuthnott, A. E. (2022). Non-suicidal self-injury and suicidality in dissociative disorders. In E. Christensen (Ed.), *Perspectives of dissociative identity response: Ethical, historical, and cultural issues* (pp. 89–118). HWC Press.

Arbuthnott, A. E., & Lewis, S. P. (2015). Parents of youth who self-injure: A review of the literature and implications for mental health professionals. *Child and Adolescent Psychiatry and Mental Health, 9*, Article 35. https://doi.org/10.1186/s13034-015-0066-3

Ayer, L., Colpe, L., Pearson, J., Rooney, M., & Murphy, E. (2020). Advancing research in child suicide: A call to action. *Journal of the American Academy of Child & Adolescent Psychiatry, 59*(9), 1028–1035. https://doi.org/10.1016/j.jaac.2020.02.010

Beauchaine, T. P., Hinshaw, S. P., & Bridge, J. A. (2019). Nonsuicidal self-injury and suicidal behaviors in girls: The case for targeted prevention in preadolescence. *Clinical Psychological Science, 7*(4), 643–667. https://doi.org/10.1177/2167702618818474

Bodzy, M. E., Barreto, S. J., Swenson, L. P., Liguori, G., & Costea, G. (2016). Self-reported psychopathology, trauma symptoms, and emotion coping among child suicide attempters and ideators: An exploratory study of young children. *Archives of Suicide Research, 20*(2), 160–175. https://doi.org/10.1080/13811118.2015.1004469

Bojanić, L., Hunt, I. M., Baird, A., Kapur, N., Appleby, L., & Turnbull, P. (2020). Early post-discharge suicide in mental health patients: Findings from a national clinical survey. *Frontiers in Psychiatry, 11*, 502. https://doi.org/10.3389/fpsyt.2020.00502

Brand, B. (2001). Establishing safety with patients with dissociative identity disorder. *Journal of Trauma & Dissociation, 2*(4), 133–155. https://doi.org/10.1300/J229v02n04_07

Bresin, K., & Gordon, K. H. (2013). Changes in negative affect following pain (vs. nonpainful) stimulation in individuals with and without a history of nonsuicidal self-injury. *Personality Disorders: Theory, Research, and Treatment, 4*(1), 62–66. https://doi.org/10.1037/a0025736

Busby, D. R., Hatkevich, C., McGuire, T. C., & King, C. A. (2020). Evidence-based interventions for youth suicide risk. *Current Psychiatry Reports, 22*, Article 5. https://doi.org/10.1007/s11920-020-1129-6

Carter, T., Walker, G. M., & Manning, J. C. (2018). Assessment tools of immediate risk of self-harm and suicide in children and young people: A scoping review. *Journal of Child Health Care, 23*(2), 178–199. https://doi.org/10.1177/1367493518787925

Chefetz, R. A. (2017). Issues in consultation for treatments with distress activated abuser/protector self-states in dissociative identity disorder. *Journal of Trauma & Dissociation, 18*(3), 465–475. https://doi.org/10.1080/15299732.2017.1295428

Connors, R. (1996). Self-injury in trauma survivors: Functions and meanings. *American Journal of Orthopsychiatry, 66*(2), 197–206. psycnet.apa.org/doi/10.1037/h0080171

Endo, T., Sugiyama, T., & Someya, T. (2006). Attention-deficit/hyperactivity disorder and dissociative disorder among abused children. *Psychiatry and Clinical Neurosciences, 60*(4), 434–438. https://doi.org/10.1111/j.1440-1819.2006.01528.x

Evans, R., White, J., Turley, R., Slater, T., Morgan, H., Strange, H., & Scourfield, J. (2017). Comparison of suicidal ideation, suicide attempts and suicide in children and young people in care and non-care populations: Systematic review and meta-analysis of prevalence. *Children and Youth Services Review, 82*, 122–129. psycnet.apa.org/doi/10.1016/j.childyouth.2017.09.020

Ford, J. D., & Gómez, J. M. (2015). The relationship of psychological trauma and dissociative and posttraumatic stress disorders to nonsuicidal self-injury and suicidality: A review. *Journal of Trauma & Dissociation, 16*, 232–271. https://doi.org/10.1080/15299732.2015.989563

Forte, A., Buscajoni, A., Fiorillo, A., Pompili, M., & Baldessarini, R. J. (2019). Suicidal risk following hospital discharge: A review. *Harvard Review of Psychiatry, 27*(4), 209–216. https://doi.org/10.1097/hrp.0000000000000222

Gould, M. S., Marrocco, F. A., Kleinman, M., Thomas, J. G., Mostkoff, K., Cote, J., & Davies, M. (2005). Evaluating iatrogenic risk of youth suicide screening programs: A randomized controlled trial. *JAMA, 293*(13), 1635–1643. https://doi.org/10.1001/jama.293.13.1635

Groschwitz, R. C., & Plener, P. L. (2012). The neurobiology of non-suicidal self-injury (NSSI): A review. *Suicidology Online, 3*, 24–32.

Gunn, J. F., III, & Lester, D. (2014). *Theories of suicide: Past, present and future*. Charles C Thomas Publisher.

Hawton, K., Witt, K. G., Salisbury, T. L. T., Arensman, E., Gunnell, D., Townsend, E., van Heeringen, K., & Hazell, P. (2015). Interventions for self-harm in children and adolescents. *Cochrane Database Systematic Review, 21*(12), CD012013. https://doi.org/10.1002/14651858.cd012013

Herman, J. L. (1992). *Trauma and recovery: The aftermath of violence—From domestic abuse to political terror.* Basic Books.

Hinshaw, S. P., Owens, E. B., Zalecki, C., Huggins, S. P., Montenegro-Nevado, A. J., Schrodek, E., & Swanson, E. N. (2012). Prospective follow-up of girls with ADHD into early adulthood: Continuing impairment includes elevated risk for suicide attempts and self-injury. *Journal of Consulting and Clinical Psychology, 80*, 1041–1051. https://doi.org/10.1037/a0029451

Howell, E. F. (2011). *Understanding and treating dissociative identity disorder: A relational approach*. Routledge.

International Society for the Study of Self-Injury. (May 2018). *What is self-injury?* Retrieved from https://www.itriples.org/aboutnssi

Jarvi, S., Jackson, B., Swenson, L., & Crawford, H. (2013). The impact of social contagion on non-suicidal self-injury: A review of the literature. *Archives of Suicide Research, 17*(1), 1–19. https://doi.org/10.1080/13811118.2013.748404

Joiner, T. E. (2005). *Why people die by suicide.* Harvard University Press.

Klonsky, E. D. (2007). The functions of deliberate self-injury: A review of the evidence. *Clinical Psychology Review, 27*(2), 226–239. https://doi.org/10.1016/j.cpr.2006.08.002

Klonsky, E. D., & May, A. M. (2014). Differentiating suicide attempters from suicide ideators: A critical frontier for suicidology research. *Suicide and Life-Threatening Behaviors, 44*(1), 1–5. https://doi.org/10.1111/sltb.12068

Klonsky, E. D., & May, A. M. (2015). The Three-Step Theory (3ST): A new theory of suicide rooted in the "Ideation-to-Action" framework. *International Journal of Cognitive Therapy, 8*(2), 114–129. https://doi.org/10.1521/ijct.2015.8.2.114

Kraus, L., Schmid, M., & In-Albon, T. (2020). Anti-suicide function of nonsuicidal self-injury in female inpatient adolescents. *Frontiers in Psychiatry, 11*, 490. https://doi.org/10.3389/fpsyt.2020.00490

Liu, R. T., Walsh, R. F. L., Sheehan, A. E., Cheek, S. M., & Sanzari, C. M. (2022). Prevalence and correlates of suicide and nonsuicidal self-injury in children: A systematic review and meta-analysis. *JAMA Psychiatry, 79*(7), 718–726. https://doi.org/10.1001/jamapsychiatry.2022.1256

McRae, E., Stoppelbeing, L., O'Kelley, S., Smith, S., & Fite, P. (2022). Pathways to suicidal behavior in children and adolescents: Examination of child maltreatment and post-traumatic symptoms. *Journal of Child & Adolescent Trauma, 15*, 715–725. https://doi.org/10.1007/s40653-022-00439-4

Morgan, C., Webb, R. T., Carr, M. J., Kontopantelis, E., Green, J., Chew-Graham, C. A., Kapur, N., & Ashcroft, D. M. (2017). Incidence, clinical management, and mortality risk following self-harm among children and adolescents: Cohort study in primary care. *BMJ 2017, 359*, j4351. https://doi.org/10.1136/bmj.j4351

Muehlenkamp, J., Brausch, A., Quigley, K., & Whitlock, J. (2013). Interpersonal features and functions of non-suicidal self-injury. *Suicide & Life-Threatening Behavior, 43*(1), 67–80. https://doi.org/10.1111/j.1943-278x.2012.00128.x

Nock, M. K. (2009). Why do people hurt themselves? New insights into the nature and functions of self-injury. *Current Directions in Psychological Science, 18*(2), 78–83. https://doi.org/10.1111/j.1467-8721.2009.01613.x

Ougrin, D., Tranah, T., Stahl, D., Moran, P., & Rosenbaum Asarnow, J. (2015). Therapeutic interventions for suicide attempts and self-harm in adolescents: Systematic review and meta-analysis. *Journal of the American Academy of Child & Adolescent Psychiatry, 54*(2), 97–107e.2. https://doi.org/10.1016/j.jaac.2014.10.009

Pettit, J. W., Buitron, V., & Green, K. L. (2018). Assessment and management of suicide risk in children and adolescents. *Cognitive and Behavioral Practice, 25*(4), 460–472. https://doi.org/10.1016/j.cbpra.2018.04.001

Schreiner, M. W., Klimes-Dougan, B., Begnel, E. D., & Cullen, K. R. (2015). Conceptualizing the neurobiology of non-suicidal self-injury from the perspective of the Research Domain Criteria Project. *Neuroscience and Biobehavioral Reviews, 57*, 381–391. https://doi.org/10.1016/j.neubiorev.2015.09.011

Sharfstein, S. S. (2009). Goals for inpatient treatment for psychiatric disorders. *Annual Review of Medicine, 60*, 393–403. https://doi.org/10.1146/annurev.med.60.042607.080257

Sheftall, A., Asti, L., Horowitz, L. M., Felts, A., Fontanella, C. A., Campo, J. V., & Bridge, J. A. (2016). Suicide in elementary school-aged children and early adolescents. *Pediatrics, 138*(4), Article e20160436. https://doi.org/10.1542%2Fpeds.2016-0436

Silberg, J. L. (2021). *The child survivor: Healing developmental trauma and dissociation* (2nd ed.). Routledge.

Smith, N. B., Kouros, C. D., & Meuret, A. E. (2014). The role of trauma symptoms in nonsuicidal self-injury. *Trauma, Violence, & Abuse, 15*(1), 41–56. https://doi.org/10.1177/1524838013496332

Uçur, Ö., & Özcan, Ö. (2018). The relationship of suicide ideation with emotional regulation and executive functions in children with attention-deficit/hyperactivity disorder. *Psychiatry and Clinical Psychopharmacology, 28*, 17.

Van Orden, K. A., Witte, T. K., Cukrowicz, K. C., Braithwaite, S. R., Selby, E. A., & Joiner, T. E. (2010). The interpersonal theory of suicide. *Psychological Review, 117*(2), 575–600. https://doi.org/10.1037/a0018697

Viswanathan, M., Wallace, I. F., Middleton, J. C., Kennedy, S. M., McKeeman, J., Hudson, K., Rains, C., Vander Schaaf, E. B., & Kahwati, L. (2022). Screening for depression and suicide risk in children and adolescents: Updated evidence report and systematic review for the US Preventive Services Task Force. *JAMA, 328*(15), 1543–1556. https://doi.org/10.1001/jama.2022.16310

Waals, L., Baetens, I., Rober, P., Lewis, S., Van Parys, H., Goethals, E. R., & Whitlock, J. (2018). The NSSI family distress cascade theory. *Child and Adolescent Psychiatry and Mental Health, 12*, 52. https://doi.org/10.1186/s13034-018-0259-7

Wagner, E., Gottipaty, A., Hunt, J. I., & Boekamp, J. R. (2022). Recognizing suicidal risk in very young children. *Rhode Island Medical Journal, 105*(4), 36–39. pubmed.ncbi.nlm.nih.gov/35476734

Walsh, R. F. L., Sheehan, A. E., & Liu, R. T. (2020). Suicidal thoughts and behaviors in preadolescents: Findings and replication in two population-based samples. *Depression and Anxiety, 38*(1), 48–56. https://doi.org/10.1002/da.23087

Wamser-Nanney, R., & Campbell, C. L. (2022). Suicidality among youth exposed to complex trauma. *Journal of Aggression, Maltreatment & Trauma, 31*(6), 715–733. https://doi.org/10.1080/10926771.2022.2068394

Weiss, S. J. (2007). Neurobiological alterations associated with traumatic stress. *Perspectives in Psychiatric Care, 43*(3), 114–122. https://doi.org/10.1111/j.1744-6163.2007.00120.x

Whalen, D. J., Hennefield, L., Elsayed, N. M., Tillman, R., Barch, D. M., & Luby, J. L. (2022). Trajectories of suicidal thoughts and behaviors from preschool through late adolescence. *Journal of the American Academy of Child & Adolescent Psychiatry, 61*(5), 676–685. https://doi.org/10.1016/j.jaac.2021.08.020

Whitlock, J., Muehlenkamp, J., Echenrode, J., Purington, A., Abrams, G. B., Barreira, P., & Kress, V. (2013). Nonsuicidal self-injury as a gateway to suicide in young adults. *Journal of Adolescent Health, 52*(4), 486–492. https://doi.org/10.1016/j.jadohealth.2012.09.010

Whitlock, J., & Selekman, M. D. (2014). Nonsuicidal self-injury across the life span. In M. K. Nock (Ed.), *The Oxford handbook of suicide and self-injury* (pp. 133–151). Oxford.

Witt, K. G., Hetrick, S. E., Rajaram, G., Hazell, P., Taylor Salisbury, T. L., Townsend, E., & Hawton, K. (2021). Interventions for self-harm in children and adolescents. *Cochrane Databased of Systematic Reviews, 3*(3), Article CD013667. https://doi.org//10.1002/14651858.CD013667.pub2

Yakeley, J., & Burbridge-James, W. (2018). Psychodynamic approaches to suicide and self-harm. *BJPsych Advances, 24*, 37–45. https://doi.org/10.1192/bja.2017.6

Zelazny, J., Stanley, B., Porta, G., Mann, J. J., Oquendo, M., Birmaher, B., Melhem, N., & Brent, D. A. (2021). Risk factors for pre-adolescent onset suicidal behavior in a high-risk sample of youth. *Journal of Affective Disorders, 290*, 292–299. https://doi.org/10.1016/j.jad.2021.04.059

42
COMPLEX TRAUMA AND DISSOCIATION IN THE FACE OF ONGOING STRESS AND TRAUMA
Child Refugees and Asylum Seekers

Safa Kemal Kaptan, Betül Yılmaz, Tania Bosqui and Trudy Mooren

Introduction

The literature pertaining to complex trauma and dissociation has expanded significantly in recent years, with a growing body of research shedding light on the risk and protective factors associated with diverse types of traumatic events (Lynn et al., 2022). Studies have also explored how children respond to complex traumatic experiences, with a focus on the effects of these experiences on well-being and their potential contribution to the development of further complexities and dissociation (DePierro et al., 2019; Choi et al., 2017; Haselgruber et al., 2021). Previous literature has also introduced new paradigms to advance clinical practices and developed new interventions that aim to address complex trauma and dissociation considering biological, psychological, and social dimensions (Arvidson et al., 2011).

This chapter focuses on forcibly displaced children, particularly refugees and asylum seekers, who endure stress and trauma, such as cumulative exposure to human rights violations, conflicts, loss, and the deprivation of necessities. The experiences of displaced groups are significantly meaningful, yet research on complex trauma and dissociation in displaced children is limited. Thus, the primary objective of this chapter is to address this research gap by discussing and describing the phenomena of complex trauma and dissociation among displaced children. By doing so, the chapter aims to enhance the reader's understanding of this specific population and the existing literature. This discussion also seeks to highlight the relevance of these issues within children and identify suitable models and interventions that can effectively meet the needs of clients, patients, or participants who have experienced displacement. The comprehensive summary in this chapter is also intended to assist professionals in optimizing their approach in healing displaced children who may face barriers to accessing care.

By synthesizing current knowledge, this chapter offers insights into the experiences of forcibly displaced children, emphasizing the importance of addressing complex trauma and dissociation within this context. We hope this chapter will raise awareness of the difficulties faced by displaced children who experience complex reactions to trauma and dissociation, thereby encouraging further attention and research in this field.

Understanding Forcibly Displaced Children

Various terms are employed to describe individuals who are forced to leave their homes or countries. As defined by the United Nations High Commissioner for Refugees (UNHCR), the term "refugee" describes a legal status granted to individuals who have been displaced from their country of origin and have sought refuge in another country. In contrast, the term "asylum seeker" refers to a person seeking refuge from another country, indicating that local authorities have not yet acknowledged their refugee status (UNHCR, 1951). These terms are often used interchangeably. Understanding the differences between refugees and asylum seekers is essential because different legal statutes entail varying rules and regulations that apply to different groups. Refugees, for example, are entitled to certain rights and benefits under international law, such as the right to work and access to education while asylum seekers are in the process of seeking such rights. This can have significant implications for mental health as uncertainty about future can lead to anxiety, stress, and emotional distress. Similarly, refugees, once recognized, typically have access to certain services, including mental health support while asylum seekers may have limited or no access to these services while their claims are pending, which can exacerbate mental health issues.

Although the recent increase in displacement is due to conflicts in countries like Syria and Afghanistan, as well as other factors such as human rights violations, hunger, and climate change, the global number of forcibly displaced individuals has been rising for decades (UNHCR, 2022). By July 2022, the global figure of forcibly displaced people had surpassed 100 million for the first time in history. According to the UNHCR, the current population includes approximately 35 million refugees, over 5 million asylum seekers, and around 63 million internally displaced people. Notably, children represent a considerable portion of the displaced population, with approximately 40% seeking refuge or asylum. Among them, more than 150,000 unaccompanied children have left their countries without an adult caregiver. Unfortunately, the numbers indicate no signs of improvement, as nearly 4.5 million children have been recently displaced internally or have crossed borders due to the conflict in Ukraine.

Displaced groups of all ages face a heightened risk of developing mental health difficulties. Displaced children are often regarded as the most psychologically vulnerable group, primarily due to limited access to resources and their developmental stage, which may impede their ability to cope with traumatic events. The current body of literature presents diverse findings regarding the prevalence and variety of common mental health difficulties in child refugees and asylum seekers. For instance, research indicates that the prevalence of post-traumatic stress disorder (PTSD) in displaced children in Europe varies between 19% and 53%, while the rates of depression range from 10% to 33%, and anxiety from 9% to 32%; and on a global scale, the prevalence of these mental health difficulties in displaced children averages at approximately 23%, 14%, and 16%, respectively (Blackmore et al., 2020; Kien et al., 2019). These variations in prevalence rates are usually explained by factors such as age, gender, country of origin, the methods used for mental health assessment, and the conditions present in host countries, including discrimination, limited resources, financial difficulties, language barriers, and other socioeconomic challenges (Andrade et al., 2023).

Exploring Complex Trauma and Dissociation in Child Refugees and Asylum Seekers

Complex trauma primarily encompasses interpersonal, repetitive, and prolonged events that cause direct harm, including various forms of abuse, usually occurring during sensitive developmental periods of an individual's life. However, there is currently no consensus within the field regarding the precise definition of psychological trauma, making it challenging to establish a clear distinction between psychological trauma and complex trauma. Compounding this challenge is the use of the term "complex" in studies, further contributing to ambiguity in understanding its meaning as uncertainty remains whether traumatic events or the resulting reactions or the therapy should be considered complex (Murray & El-Leithy, 2022).

Furthermore, forced displacement presents unique characteristics, as there are other complexities that demand careful consideration, such as intergenerational, collective, cultural, financial, and identity-related aspects of displacement. For example, existing literature often examines responses to trauma as "post-traumatic reactions," yet in many cases, forcibly displaced individuals do not have a distinct "post" period; instead, diverse types and degrees of traumatic events continue to replace one another over time. This implies a need for a new understanding of trauma in the context of forced displacement, as *what constitutes "post" in the life of refugees* is unclear, making comprehending the impact of such events more challenging when working with displaced children. Consequently, there are challenges in establishing a diagnostic criterion when the understanding of manifestations of distress remains limited. Therefore, any attempt in this field should delve into the multifaceted nature of "complex" at various levels to provide an overview of the challenges pertaining to displacement, the complexities associated with traumatic events, the reactions they elicit, and the complexity involved in treatment procedures.

Complex Trauma in the Context of Displacement

Within the context of forced displacement, child refugees and asylum seekers often encounter a series of complex traumatic events that occur in a cumulative and prolonged manner. Despite some variations, the journey of displacement typically follows three stages: (1) prior to their departure from their country of origin, (2) during their journey, and (3) during the process of integration into new societies and cultures in host countries. These stages are not always linear. Displaced individuals may go through several cycles and unique challenges, as the experiences and needs of displaced people at each stage vary depending on the reason for displacement, legal status, and the length of displacement (see Figure 42.1).

Before flight, displaced children may endure various terrifying experiences such as violence, torture, sexual abuse, war, conflict, forced labor, or being forcibly recruited as soldiers. They may also become victims of gender-based violence. The journey itself poses additional challenges. They may have to endure living in refugee camps, being separated from their family, losing their community, being detained, and experiencing further physical and sexual abuse by human traffickers. Moreover, despite families embarking on the journey with the hope of providing a better future for their children, caregivers themselves may have gone through traumatic experiences, which may trigger harsh practices and intergenerational trauma within their family (Sangalang et al., 2017). When they finally seek asylum in another country, refugee and asylum-seeking children may encounter ongoing stressors

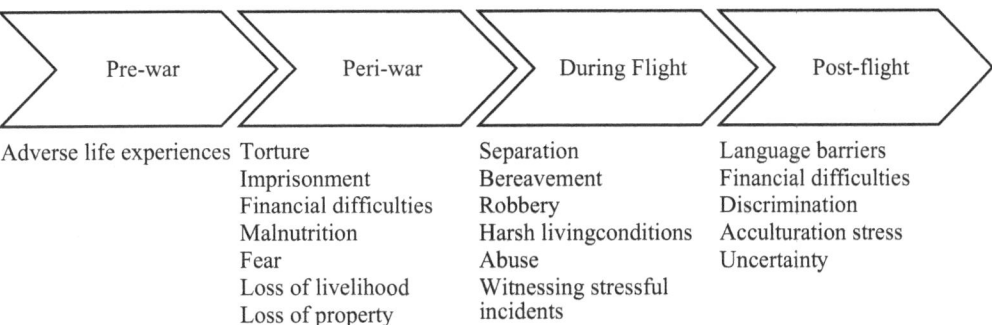

Figure 42.1 Stages of Displacement and Challenges. This Figure Illustrates the Stages of Displacement, and the Challenges Individuals May Encounter during Each Stage.

related to the asylum system and hostile policies against them, which result in further barriers to accessing support and integrating into society (Arakelyan & Ager, 2021).

Reactions to complex and cumulative traumatic events, however, can be influenced by several factors, including but not limited to the availability of resources and support systems, the presence of a caregiver, the resilience capacity of the child, and the child's developmental stage. The longevity of these experiences can also vary significantly, as some displaced children may endure them for a relatively brief period of time, perhaps a year or two. In contrast, others may endure prolonged suffering encompassing their entire childhood. These situations necessitate a lens through which to view lifelong trauma in the context of war and refugee status. As a result of such factors, the reactions of displaced children can manifest themselves in different forms, such as psychological, physical, neurological, and behavioral symptoms that may co-occur. Psychosomatic problems such as stomach aches, bodily pains, dizziness, and headaches are just some of the common ones. Displaced children may also struggle with post-traumatic stress symptoms such as reliving terrible events, avoiding distressing reminders, nightmares, and flashbacks. Difficulties controlling emotions and actions, sleep disruptions, and withdrawal from previously enjoyed activities can all occur. Fear, concern, anxiety, despair, and hopelessness may also be present, as well as difficulties with focus and memory.

The manifestation of these difficulties also varies across different age groups, as they experience and express these challenges in distinct ways. *Preschool children* may demonstrate their mental health distress through regressive behaviors (bed-wetting, thumb-sucking, and acting needy), temper tantrums, separation anxiety from parents, avoidance of their peers, trauma-related content in their play, and aggressive behaviors (hitting, kicking, biting). *Elementary school children* may face difficulties at school or with their peers. They may experience behavioral changes, characterized by hostility, impatience, and a pervading worry of something terrible happening. They may also show indicators of parental separation anxiety. *Middle and high–school–aged children* may feel shame, guilt, responsibility for past adverse life events, and helplessness. Previous experiences may alter their perspective on religion, culture, life, and self-identity. They can also demonstrate conduct problems and have trouble at school and with peers, family, and school staff.

Dissociation as a Reaction to Complex Trauma in the Context of Displacement

Wars, conflicts, and displacement are risk factors for developing complex trauma (Courtois, 2008). Displaced children face two types of complexities: displacement and the challenges of being a minority in host countries. The process of displacement can be traumatic in and of itself because it includes relocating to a different place and adjusting to a new culture, society, and way of life. Furthermore, being a minority in a new society might expose them to various issues, including discrimination, financial difficulties, and increased levels of anxiety and despair. Displaced children are usually piled up of negative life experiences, the absence of care (neglect) as well as the presence of threats that are detrimental to their development. As a result, these children also learn to be sensitive to cues predicting any threat of safety, which leaves them with a reduced capacity for abstract learning, reasoning, and reflecting.

The combination of a toxic environment and ongoing stress may lead to complex trauma, which may pave the way for dissociation. In displaced children, this means coping with PTSD-like symptoms as well as difficulties that hinder social, educational, and psychological development. Dissociative responses may, therefore, be regarded as part of the complexity of trauma, particularly when stressors have been numerous and the developmental environment has been challenging.

Dissociative experiences are also commonly acknowledged as coping mechanisms, and recent literature indicates a link between complex trauma and dissociation (Dorahy et al., 2022). In fact, dissociation has frequently been associated with PTSD despite it being essential to separate PTSD from dissociation as a coping mechanism (Schimmenti & Caretti, 2016). Separating PTSD from dissociation as a coping mechanism is crucial, as it enables a nuanced understanding of individual experiences, tailors appropriate interventions, and prevents the misinterpretation of symptoms that lead to inadequate support. Recent systematic reviews on mental health difficulties in displaced children, however, do not include dissociative experiences as a reaction to complex traumatic experiences (Blackmore et al., 2020; Frounfelker et al., 2019). Therefore, the studies below will only underline the limited understanding of dissociation in displaced children.

In one of the few studies examining trauma and dissociation among displaced children, Gušić et al. (2016) indicated an increased rate of dissociation among war-affected refugee children compared with non-war-affected children. The study also revealed that children whose parents had experienced war and poverty showed elevated levels of dissociation, suggesting that trauma's impact can extend beyond individual experiences and be transmitted generationally.

In their second study, Gušić et al. (2017) investigated dissociative experiences among 154 children in Sweden and reported that newly arrived children had symptoms of PTSD and dissociation nearly two times more than settled children. Furthermore, the study discovered a significant association between dissociative experiences and PTSD symptoms in all children.

A noteworthy investigation of 45 Syrian children living in refugee camps in Lebanon found significantly higher rates of dissociation compared with the local population with diagnosed clinical disorders (DeRaedt, 2018). In addition, the study indicated a positive correlation between age and dissociative tendencies among refugee children. This suggests that as refugee children grew older, their ability to disassociate increased, which can be attributed to several factors, including the ongoing nature of trauma, a lack of familial support, the inability to develop healthy coping mechanisms, and hindered neurological development (DeRaedt, 2018).

Additional studies have also pointed out that the likelihood of experiencing dissociation significantly increases during the process of migration, which was attributed to the lack of autonomy, security, and personal space in camp settings, leading to heightened stress levels (Harrell-Bond, 2000). It is suggested that complex trauma often disrupts a child's ability to self-regulate, primarily stemming from feelings of insecurity, which can significantly impact their developmental stage (Ford & Courtois, 2017). As a result, more than adults, children are more vulnerable to dissociation when they become victims of natural disasters or wars.

In their recent studies, Gušić et al. (2018) studied 40 war-traumatized refugee children with a shared number of traumatic experiences and other sociodemographic details, such as gender and residence status. Participants were grouped according to their levels of dissociative experiences: low level of dissociation, moderate level of dissociation, and high level of dissociation. Following semi-structured interviews, the study revealed that the children with higher levels of dissociation described a heightened emotional state characterized by extreme fear, grief, sadness and sudden crying, and a lack of coping skills. In the same line, those children in the high levels of dissociation group reported complete loss of control without any awareness. In contrast, children with low levels of dissociation were better at controlling their emotions. Compared with children with high levels of dissociation, children with low levels of dissociation were also better at using coping techniques more successfully, which included listening to music, praying, reading holy books, writing, visiting a real or imagined safe place, or seeking support from others. Moreover, the level of dissociation was also found to influence self-perception, as children with low levels of dissociation had a more positive self-image and more control over their lives. Children with high levels of dissociation regarded certain aspects of themselves and their experiences as "crazy" and "incomplete." The children with low levels of dissociation, however, were able to use their multiple selves as inner guidance and pleasant experiences. The study reported more differences between children with various levels of dissociation. Groups struggled with memory functioning, thoughts, cognitive abilities, concentration and attention, though child refugees with low levels of dissociation struggled less. All children reported having negative dreams and suffering psychosomatic pain. However, children with high levels of dissociation reported less control over the physical reactions of their emotions and pain, as this group reported not feeling physical pain when they were emotionally overwhelmed. Finally, regarding interpersonal experiences, children with high levels of dissociation reported having fewer close friends and disclosed physically and emotionally abusive controlling and neglectful interactions with their caregivers (Gušić et al., 2018).

The significance lies not only in evaluating the level of dissociation but also in assessing the type of dissociation, as it can have additional implications for a child's ability to cope with difficulties. Peritraumatic dissociation, for example, has been identified as a risk factor for developing PTSD-related symptoms (Lensvelt-Mulders et al., 2008). A recent study with nearly 200 children provided evidence of increased post-traumatic reaction in war-affected children who experienced greater peritraumatic dissociation. Dysfunctional trauma-related memory has also significantly mediated this association, indicating the role of memory fragmentation as a dissociative experience (Peltonen et al., 2017). This can be explained by an individual's awareness of the emotional aspects of the event without a full recall of the traumatic experience due to the fragmentation of the memory. This might also explain the moderating role of peritraumatic dissociation in poor treatment outcomes and indicates a greater risk for refugee children who exhibit peritraumatic dissociation than those who do not experience dissociation.

Another network analysis investigated the association between post-traumatic symptoms and other dissociative experiences—namely, depersonalization, derealization, amnesia, and compartmentalization—among mixed group samples, including refugees. They conducted both subgroup and pooled analyses, and the refugees reported similar results to the pooled outcome. However, the refugee group had significantly higher scores across dissociative experiences (Cardeña et al., 2022).

Studies have also uncovered new areas related to displacement, trauma, and dissociation. For example, a recent scoping review explored psychogenic non-epileptic seizures (also known as dissociative seizures) and reported a high incidence of epilepsy among war-affected children (Hallab & Sen, 2021).

These findings resonate with the concept of a further aspect of dissociation—namely, *resignation syndrome*. The syndrome was first identified in Sweden and has been described as a psychogenic stupor (ICD-9) and dissociative reaction (DSM-I) (Sallin et al., 2016). However, there is still no consensus on the diagnostic presentation, as suggestions range from conversion disorders (functional neurologic disorder), catatonia, epidemic hysteria, and dissociative states (von Knorring & Hultcrantz, 2020). The syndrome represents an extreme manifestation of dissociative responses to the possibility of re-exposure and despair in displaced children, often triggered when their parents' request for a residence permit was denied. A residency permit has been seen as the most effective treatment, yet due to its relation to legal procedures, authorities first investigated whether families were drugging their children. In many cases, the syndrome progresses from a general depressive state to lethargy, gradually and finally leaving displaced children in a long-standing tube-feeding state (Sallin et al., 2016). Despite its considerable impact, psycho-neuro-biological models have yet to comprehensively elucidate the underlying mechanisms of this condition (Kozlowska et al., 2021). However, the roots of resignation syndrome have been explored as a response to gain asylum in the host country, and as a sociocultural phenomenon. Remarkably, the syndrome represents the ultimate expression of despair in children, as a complex reaction to complex traumatic experiences.

Although there are noticeable attempts in the literature to understand the nature of dissociative experiences in displaced children, various other areas also require attention, such as attachment theory. Attachment difficulties are considered one of the ways to explain dissociation (Liotti, 2006). In one of the rare studies with displaced children, an association between parental post-traumatic distress and disorganized attachment style was found in refugee children (van Ee et al., 2016). Additionally, insecure attachment is associated with PTSD symptomology in refugee children; parental trauma has been indirectly associated with the overall well-being of refugee children through mechanisms such as insecure attachment, dysfunctional family communication, and maladaptive parenting styles (Flanagan et al., 2020). One study noted maternal attachment as a possible resilience factor in refugee children (Diab et al., 2015). However, evidence is absent for the role of attachment in dissociative experiences in displaced children, which is crucial, since displaced children may experience loss or separation from caregivers and family members or be detained in deportation centers (Sleijpen et al., 2022).

Dissociative experiences may also present through difficulties in the education setting. Due to an increased tendency to dissociate, displaced children may experience a lack of attention and present problems often translated as learning difficulties or attention-deficit disorders (Joshi & O'Donnell, 2003). Along with the language barrier, dissociative experiences may hardly be recognized in displaced students. Additionally, dissociation in displaced children plays a role in legal procedures; since their memories are fragmented and hold gaps, they may be unable to recall events to seek justice or acquire asylum status in the host country (Tufnell, 2003).

Case Examples: Different Responses to Trauma and Dissociation

Healthy dissociation can enable a refugee child to find a much-needed escape from surrounding complex traumatic stressors, some children may rely on dissociative coping styles for an extended period of time. Thus, understanding the various responses to trauma and dissociation is critical for services that suit individual needs. The following case studies offer the most salient presentations of displaced children and show numerous ways they respond to and negotiate their backgrounds. Sometimes their memory of the event is fragmented and confused by feelings of humiliation and confusion, making it difficult for them to explain and understand the experience adequately. Other times the complicated interaction of trauma and dissociation is evident, as well as their devastating influence on emotional well-being and daily functioning.

Dissociative Symptoms

A ten-year-old girl is still not sure what exactly happened. She frequently spaces out and feels disconnected from her surroundings. Not only does she find it difficult to talk about, but she also feels embarrassed and ashamed. Moreover, she does not know the words to use to talk about her experience. Also, she does not have a complete recollection of what has happened.

Emotional Dysregulation

A ten-year-old female asylum seeker usually experiences sudden aggression. She struggles to regulate her emotions and frequently lashes out at peers and caregivers. Her moods fluctuate rapidly, and she finds it challenging to calm down even after minor conflicts.

Avoidance

A 12-year-old refugee has become socially isolated since arriving in a new country. She avoids group activities, rarely interacts with her peers, and spends most of her time alone. She has lost interest in hobbies she once enjoyed and prefers to stay in her room, away from reminders of her traumatic past.

Re-Experiencing

A nine-year-old asylum seeker frequently has nightmares and flashbacks about the war he witnessed in his home country. He becomes highly anxious and frightened when hearing loud noises or seeing anything that reminds him of the conflict. These reminders trigger intense emotional distress, often leading to panic-like reactions.

Culture, Discourse and Displacement

Displaced children may be born into consecutive and potentially traumatic events, and their experiences may be interpreted through the lens of a culture they cannot relate to. However, existing models may not fully represent the experiences of displaced children as they are diverse, and not all groups are equally impacted by such challenges. Furthermore, not all refugees or asylum seekers experience mental health difficulties in response to the accumulation of adverse events. In fact, a significant percentage of displaced individuals overcome adversity without requiring professional assistance (Marley & Mauki, 2019), contrary to the prevailing narrative that portrays displaced individuals, including children, as *mentally broken*. For that reason, professionals must evaluate their cultural and professional priorities when working with displaced children and families and work collaboratively with clients by acknowledging and embracing cultural diversity.

Cultural factors can play an essential part in the expression of mental health difficulties; culture can improve the healing process and provide survivors with resources to cope with traumatic life experiences (Raghavan & Sandanapitchai, 2019) or prevent individuals or groups from addressing trauma in healthy ways (Dalgaard & Montgomery, 2015). Traumatic experiences might instill fear, leaving children on their own with the complex realities of life. In those cases, if a refugee child cannot find a source within the new culture to make sense of adverse life events, dissociative experiences may become their refuge.

An essential aspect of cultural sensitivity is being aware of perceiving refugees and asylum seekers as psychologically broken, as well as the power dynamics involved in attempting to "fix" them (Summerfield, 1999). It is vital to evaluate the underlying assumptions and narratives to prevent such damaging stereotypes and further marginalizing persons who have already undergone significant difficulties. Rather than approaching these groups from a deficit perspective, it is critical to use a culturally sensitive approach that acknowledges their innate strengths and resilience. This should include recognizing diverse backgrounds, experiences, and coping techniques, fostering a more balanced well-being assessment. Clinicians and researchers should advocate for including cultural and local knowledge and voices in theory, research, and practice (Benuto et al., 2021). Professionals should also highlight the need to collaborate meaningfully with displaced communities, honoring their experiences and encouraging them to be active participants in their healing by acknowledging that they are the experts of their lives (Lacroix & Sabbah, 2011). By embracing such concepts, professionals can change harmful discourses, challenge power inequities, and promote more culturally responsive and empowering methods.

Different Approaches and Therapeutic Strategies in Working with Child Refugees and Asylum Seekers

Trauma-focused mental health interventions for children affected by forced displacement have a growing and promising evidence base. Interventions vary widely in terms of aims, theoretical approaches, and implementation strategies. Aims include promotion, prevention, or treatment of mental health, and vary across social-ecological systems, targeting individuals or groups of children, their parents or caregivers, the family unit or groups of families, schools or communities, or broader socioeconomic structures around the child. In addition, interventions vary depending on the child's age, whether they are recently displaced, in transit, settled, or unaccompanied (Frounfelker et al., 2019). There is also variation in the theoretical underpinnings of interventions such as cognitive-behavioral, systemic, trauma-processing, play or expressive arts, and *how* they are delivered. Interventions may be implemented in homes, schools, community centers or outpatient clinics, and by specialist mental health professionals or non-specialist psychosocial workers trained and supervised through "task shifting." Therefore, intervention approaches also have an increasing focus on both the family and available caregiving systems surrounding children, to better address the wider attachment, interpersonal, and social determinants of child mental health given the particular links between parental complex trauma and "disconnected parenting" (van Ee et al., 2012). In addition, recent studies addressing community and structural and social disadvantages—such as food insecurity and cash transfer programs (Zimmerman et al., 2021)—also offer another novel approach to creating an environment where a refugee child can thrive.

Significant gaps in the evidence remain, however, for child refugees and asylum seekers with complex trauma and dissociative symptoms, and for those living in low- and middle-income countries and ongoing humanitarian emergencies (Barbui et al., 2020). Existing studies are also limited by small sample sizes and poor reporting of intervention aims and content (Cowling & Anderson, 2023).

Existing Therapies, Approaches, and Interventions in High-Income Countries

Evidence generated in high-income countries, predominantly in North America, Western Europe, and Australia, with refugees from numerous countries and contexts, demonstrates the effectiveness of various interventions for child trauma outcomes. Individual interventions that include *processing of trauma narratives*, like cognitive-behavioral therapy (CBT), trauma-focused cognitive-behavioral therapy (TF-CBT), narrative exposure therapy for children (KidNET), and eye-movement desensitization and reprocessing (EMDR) therapy, have strong evidence of effectiveness for PTSD and related symptoms, as well as for functional impairment, hopelessness, anger, behavioral problems, peer problems, and well-being, with evidence of maintaining gains at one-month follow-up (Tyrer & Fazel, 2014). Albeit with limitations to the quantity and methodological quality of the evidence, creative and expressive arts interventions, including play therapy, expressive writing, and sand play, have proved effective as a treatment for trauma symptoms, depression, anxiety, and peer problems (Tyrer & Fazel, 2014).

There is also a growing body of evidence supporting the effectiveness of parenting and family interventions. Parenting interventions that aim to support caregiver mental health and build parenting skills and capacity, and family interventions that aim to strengthen relationships and improve family functioning and cohesiveness, have shown effectiveness in child, caregiver, and family outcomes, such as child emotional and behavioral difficulties, parental PTSD, parenting, parenting stress, harsh discipline, parental empathy, and family communication—albeit with some mixed findings across studies (Bunn et al., 2022). For example, in the case of Somali Bantu and Bhutanese refugee families, a home-visiting intervention has shown effectiveness in reducing child trauma symptoms and diminishing family conflicts (Betancourt et al., 2020). Expressive arts interventions that include a dyadic parent-child component, such as Theraplay, have also proved helpful for parent-child relationship strengthening and reducing attachment disturbances (Cowling & Anderson, 2023).

However, it is essential to recognize that the concept of "family" may need to be redefined, as the caregiving system may shift in the context of displacement, requiring a newer understanding of who constitutes the family. Sometimes a community, another group of people, or a member of the extended family may assume responsibility for the child, which may influence the treatment. In such situations, establishing trust may take more time, as different networks may hold unique beliefs and expectations regarding child-rearing. Thus, non-traditional caregivers may require additional support and training to effectively fulfill their caregiving role, mainly if they have limited experience or knowledge in caring for children. Moreover, in situations where the child is receiving care from multiple caregivers or community members, it is crucial to facilitate coordination among all individuals involved to provide a sense of continuity and stability in the treatment journey. This may include considering strategies to maintain consistent relationships, minimizing transitions between caregivers, and addressing any emotional or psychological challenges associated with changes in caregiving arrangements.

More comprehensive and multi-component interventions also require further attention, as there is a clear need to address social determinants of mental health like acculturation stress, poor living conditions, and structural inequities. Such interventions may include holistic or joined interventions that address multiple layers affecting child mental health, or may directly advocate for families (Pacione et al., 2013). Some evidence does exist for these interventions. For example, trauma systems therapy, which aims to address children's emotional needs as well as their social environment, has proved effective for child depression and PTSD, as well as for reducing resource hardship. Families and Schools Together (FAST), a multi-system intervention that links parents with schools to promote child well-being, has shown evidence of effectiveness for child emotional and behavioral difficulties, parent-child relationships, and family cohesion, based on multiple randomized control trials in different countries (McDonald & Doostgharin, 2013). Another school-based, multi-tiered mental health program for refugees found improvements in PTSD and depression as well as a reduction in resource hardship, which was ongoing at the 12-month follow-up (Ellis et al., 2013). A more recent school-based intervention, somatic soothing and emotional regulation skill development, was designed to address various post-traumatic symptomatology and behavioral, somatic, and dissociative experiences, and showed improvements in children's confidence, communication, academic functioning, and social interactions (Mancini, 2020).

The following case highlights the importance of personalized treatments in meeting the varied needs of displaced children. The boy's traumatic experiences are processed through a combination of narrative approaches and EMDR therapy, allowing him to improve his emotional state. Furthermore, engagement of his caregivers promotes a sense of support and shared responsibility, which contributes to the healing process.

Case Example: An Example Treatment

A 12-year-old boy who has arrived in Europe as an unaccompanied minor is being referred for psychological assistance. His legal guardian worries about his concentration difficulties at school, his sleeping difficulties (awake during the night and walking through the house), and his depressed mood. He does not feel like doing anything or seeing other people and has no plans for the future. He constantly worries about his family, who is waiting in his home country. In addition, he is anxious about his younger brother—he is afraid that he will undertake the same dangerous journey and try to cross the Mediterranean Sea.

The boy agrees to psychological help. He is offered a combination of KidNET and EMDR therapies. Further, with the legal guardian, the therapist seeks contact with his parents to share his worries and sense of responsibility. He responds well to the trauma-focused therapy: together with the therapist, he draws a lifeline and organizes stones resembling memories of adverse events and flowers representing positive memories—for example, of people who have helped him during his travels—along the line. His narrated story is being written to create a book at the end. The stones representing memories of intrusive events are treated with EMDR therapy. The advantage of EMDR therapy is that he has the choice to talk or not; as long as he is focused on processing the memories, the procedure goes well. He finds it difficult, but definitely relieving. He is surprised by the result: the nightmares disappear, and he feels more at ease spending time with others. Due to the conversation with his parents in the legal guardian's presence, he feels entitled to spend leisure time with fun activities.

Existing Therapies, Approaches, and Interventions in Low and Middle-Income Countries

Despite the vast majority of refugees and asylum seekers living in low- and middle-income countries, and considerable additional challenges in levels of adversity and resource limitations, the evidence base for mental health interventions is far more limited than for refugees in high-income countries. Within the existing evidence base, similarly to high-income countries, individual interventions that include *processing trauma narratives* like KidNET, CBT, TF-CBT, and EMDR therapy are effective for treating symptoms of PTSD, including dissociative symptoms and functional impairment, with mixed evidence for depression and anxiety (Turrini et al., 2017). Some school-, community-, and camp-based interventions also have promising evidence, such as the Teaching Recovery Techniques (TRT) program delivered in schools in Gaza, Palestine, which was found to reduce PTSD-related symptoms. However, the treatment effect was moderated by peritraumatic dissociation (Qouta et al., 2012), indicating that children with elevated levels of dissociative symptoms during or immediately after traumatic exposure(s) benefited less from TRT intervention.

Parenting and family interventions also have a promising evidence base across low- and middle-income countries and contexts, with the number of studies growing exponentially over the last five years (Pedersen et al., 2019). This includes improvements in child trauma, depression, anxiety, behavioral problems, parent mental health and parenting, and family functioning and communication. Interventions with promising evidence include those that aim to improve parenting practices and capacity (Lee & Kim, 2022), as well as more comprehensive, multi-tiered interventions, such as the Happy Families intervention for refugee families in Thailand (Puffer et al., 2015) and the Strong Families Program in Afghanistan (Haar et al., 2020) that aim to address the social world of children.

However, interventions that address wider systemic influence on child mental health, particularly complex trauma and dissociation, lack research in low- and middle-income countries, despite strong evidence of the effect of daily stressors and poor living conditions on child mental health (Miller & Rasmussen, 2010).

Existing Therapies, Approaches, and Interventions in Ongoing Humanitarian Emergencies

Despite the desperately elevated levels of unmet need and significant differences in psychological processes during prolonged trauma exposure, there is a paucity of research on mental health interventions focused on treating complex trauma and dissociation for displaced children living through ongoing humanitarian emergencies. For example, the damaging effects of avoidant coping and mental inflexibility on psychological recovery are well established (Fledderus et al., 2010). Still, in Gaza, mental inflexibility in exposed children was associated with better psychological outcomes (Qouta et al., 2001). For children forced to serve in militias during the war in the Democratic Republic of Congo, appetitive aggression was associated with *fewer* trauma symptoms (Hecker et al., 2013). This perhaps reflects the need for children to concentrate on survival when amid life-threatening situations (Bosqui & Marshoud, 2018), and highlights the need for mental health interventions to be sensitive to context. In addition, the buffering effect of parent-child relationships and family functioning has also been found to be particularly important for children during armed conflicts (Harel-Fisch et al., 2010).

Evidence for a range of psychosocial interventions targeting children affected by armed conflict does indicate some effectiveness for trauma, internalizing and externalizing symptoms (Brown et al.,

2017), delivered predominantly by non-specialist trained and supervised community facilitators due to shortages of qualified mental health professionals. More specialist interventions, like KidNET and TF-CBT, have good evidence of effectiveness. For example, KidNET had positive effects on child PTSD and functioning for internally displaced people in camps in northern Uganda (Ertl et al., 2011), and TF-CBT had positive effects on PTSD for conflict-affected refugees in the Democratic Republic of Congo (McMullen et al., 2013). However, other interventions have mixed evidence. For example, the Early Adolescent Skills for Emotions (EASE) intervention, a transdiagnostic manualized program that incorporates evidence-based techniques, found no effect on child mental health in Lebanon (Brown et al., 2019), while the Common Elements Treatment Approach (CETA), another transdiagnostic intervention incorporating evidence-based techniques, found significant improvement in PTSD, internalizing and externalizing symptoms, in Somali refugee camps (Murray et al., 2018). A review of practice components of interventions with evidence of an effect on child mental health identified accessibility, psychoeducation, insight building, rapport building, cognitive and narrative processing, exposure, and relapse prevention as core components (Brown et al., 2017).

Beyond What Works: Accessibility and Acceptability

While the effectiveness of various studies can offer valuable insights into which approaches and techniques are most suitable for different groups, it is equally important to improve the accessibility and acceptability of these interventions.

In many countries, displaced children are significantly less likely to have access to mental health services, particularly for preventative or early interventions, but are inversely more likely to present to medical or emergency services with somatic symptoms (Fazel & Betancourt, 2018). These barriers to care encompass diverse factors, including disparities in help-seeking behaviors but also language proficiency, cultural competence of service providers, and attitudes toward and of providers (Jannesari et al., 2021). Conversely, facilitators to care, however, encompass community-level delivery (Kohrt et al., 2018), integration of services into primary care (Pacione et al., 2013), and the engagement of fathers as well as mothers (Cowling & Anderson, 2023). Enhancing accessibility also requires novel and innovative approaches, such as scaling up of interventions or, in other words, implementing low-intensity interventions. This approach can serve as a pathway for mental health professionals to increase the accessibility of their interventions as they transition from individual to group approaches.

Clinical Implications and Future Suggestions

The concerns raised earlier are substantial when it comes to the mental health and well-being of displaced children. To address these issues, clinicians should take a holistic approach that involves trust-building, cultural sensitivity, linguistic considerations, trauma-informed treatment, thorough assessment, and ongoing research. By applying these recommendations, clinicians can effectively support and intervene to improve the well-being of displaced children.

1 *Creating a safe environment and building trust:* Professionals should build trust with displaced children to create a safe environment. This can help relieve fear that may prevent children from sharing traumatic experiences.
2 *Culturally sensitive assessments*: Clinicians must be aware of displaced children's cultural and social backgrounds and adapt their evaluation procedures accordingly. It is critical to recognize that dissociative experiences present differently in diverse cultures. Clinicians should investigate markers of dissociative tendencies in children beyond Western understandings and conceptualizations of dissociation.

3. *Overcoming language difficulties*: Language barriers can prevent displaced children from expressing themselves effectively, making it challenging to identify aspects of dissociation. Professionals should be educated in working with interpreters and developing alternate communication methods, like play therapy or art therapy, to assist children in expressing their experiences.
4. *Clinician training*: Clinicians who work with displaced children should undergo training that addresses the cultural and political background of their experience. Understanding the unique issues refugees face and the practicalities of working with translators should all be part of this training. Moreover, clinicians should have developed sensitivity with regard to the variety of cultural backgrounds; they would do well to be acquainted with the Cultural Formulation Interview (Lewis-Fernández et al., 2016).
5. *Trauma- and dissociation-informed care*: Trauma-focused interventions should be made available to newly arriving refugees to prevent the development of further challenges. These therapies should address both their home and host country experiences. Thus, screening for trauma- and dissociation-related experiences in both host countries and throughout the asylum process is critical when planning services. Assessing post-settlement living conditions, familial ties, and environmental factors that may function as additional stressors should all be part of this process. A thorough assessment of the child's context can help guide treatment planning and ensure a comprehensive approach to their well-being.
6. *Research*: Additional studies on the prevalence, risk and protective factors, and interventions for dissociative tendencies in displaced children are required. To acquire a more profound knowledge of this population's experiences and needs, larger sample sizes, diverse sample groups, cultural-social backgrounds, and developmental stages should be included. This research can help shape evidence-based solutions tailored to the specific issues that displaced children confront.

Conclusion

While there is a dearth of research on this topic, the available studies suggest that cumulative and prolonged trauma during war, conflict, and displacement uniquely impacts children compared with other forms of complex trauma. Nonetheless, the findings must be interpreted and applied cautiously in clinical practice due to the scarcity and limitations of research in this area.

Despite the drastic consequences of war and violence, many children and families do their utmost to care for each other. However, for other refugee and asylum-seeking children, complex trauma and dissociation are a way of life, as they may be born into a world that lacks even the most basic human rights. Those children may exhibit a wide range of psychological, physical, and behavioral responses to complex trauma. While Herman (1992) explained dissociation as a "state-of-the-art" coping mechanism for individuals experiencing prolonged exposure to trauma, so far there has not been much attention given to dissociative experiences in refugee and asylum-seeking children.

Determining the best trauma- and dissociation-focused mental health intervention approaches for child refugees and asylum seekers depends on the child's context, culture, age, and presenting difficulties. In general, approaches that incorporate both individual and broader systemic interventions are likely to be most helpful, and interventions that include processing trauma narratives have the most robust evidence of effectiveness in reducing trauma-related symptoms. There are remaining gaps in the evidence, however, particularly related to dissociative symptoms, in low- and middle-income countries, and humanitarian emergencies, as our understanding of complex trauma and dissociation in displaced children is heavily based on studies involving children from non-refugee and non-asylum seeker populations. In addition, more work is needed to improve *access* to contextually and culturally relevant and evidence-informed interventions for displaced children.

References

Andrade, A. S., Roca, J. S., & Pérez, S. R. (2023). Children's emotional and behavioral response following a migration: A scoping review. *Journal of Migration and Health, 7,* Article 100176. https://doi.org/10.1016/j.jmh.2023.100176

Arakelyan, S., & Ager, A. (2021). Annual research review: A multilevel bioecological analysis of factors influencing the mental health and psychosocial well-being of refugee children. *Journal of Child Psychology and Psychiatry, 62*(5), 484–509. https://doi.org/10.1111/jcpp.13355

Arvidson, J., Kinniburgh, K., Howard, K., Spinazzola, J., Strothers, H., Evans, M., Andres, B., Cohen, C., & Blaustein, M. (2011). Treatment of complex trauma in young children: Developmental and cultural considerations in application of the ARC intervention model. *Journal of Child & Adolescent Trauma, 4*(1), 34–51. https://doi.org/10.1080/19361521.2011.545046

Barbui, C., Purgato, M., Abdulmalik, J., Acarturk, C., Eaton, J., Gastaldon, C., Gureje, O., Hanlon, C., Jordans, M., Lund, C., Nosè, M., Ostuzzi, G., Papola, D., Tedeschi, F., Tol, W., Turrini, G., Patel, V., & Thornicroft, G. (2020). Efficacy of psychosocial interventions for mental health outcomes in low-income and middle-income countries: An umbrella review. *Lancet Psychiatry, 7*(2), 162–172. doi.org/10.1016/S2215-0366(19)30511-5

Benuto, L. T., Newlands, R., Singer, J., Casas, J., & Cummings, C. (2021). Culturally sensitive clinical practices: A mixed methods study. *Psychological Services, 18*(4), 632–642. https://doi.org/10.1037/ser0000493

Betancourt, T. S., Berent, J. M., Freeman, J., Frounfelker, R. L., Brennan, R. T., Abdi, S., Maalim, A., Abdi, A., Mishra, T., Gautam, B., Creswell, J. W., & Beardslee, W. R. (2020). Family-based mental health promotion for Somali Bantu and Bhutanese refugees: Feasibility and acceptability trial. *Journal of Adolescent Health, 66*(3), 336–344. https://doi.org/10.1016/j.jadohealth.2019.08.023

Blackmore, R., Gray, K. M., Boyle, J. A., Fazel, M., Ranasinha, S., Fitzgerald, G., Misso, M., & Gibson-Helm, M. (2020). Systematic review and meta-analysis: The prevalence of mental illness in child and adolescent refugees and asylum seekers. *Journal of the American Academy of Child and Adolescent Psychiatry, 59*(6), 705–714. https://doi.org/10.1016/j.jaac.2019.11.011

Bosqui, T. J., & Marshoud, B. (2018). Mechanisms of change for interventions aimed at improving the wellbeing, mental health and resilience of children and adolescents affected by war and armed conflict: A systematic review of reviews. *Conflict and Health, 12*(1), 15. https://doi.org/10.1186/s13031-018-0153-1

Brown, F. L., de Graaff, A. M., Annan, J., & Betancourt, T. S. (2017). Annual research review: Breaking cycles of violence – A systematic review and common practice elements analysis of psychosocial interventions for children and youth affected by armed conflict. *Journal of Child Psychology and Psychiatry, 58*(4), 507–524. https://doi.org/10.1111/jcpp.12671

Brown, F. L., Steen, F., Taha, K., Aoun, M., Bryant, R. A., Jordans, M. J. D., Malik, A., van Ommeren, M., Abualhaija, A., Aqel, I. S., Ghatasheh, M., Habashneh, R., Sijbrandij, M., El Chammay, R., Watts, S., & Akhtar, A. (2019). Early Adolescent Skills for Emotions (EASE) intervention for the treatment of psychological distress in adolescents: Study protocol for randomised controlled trials in Lebanon and Jordan. *Trials, 20*(1), Article 545. https://doi.org/10.1186/s13063-019-3654-3

Bunn, M., Zolman, N., Smith, C. P., Khanna, D., Hanneke, R., Betancourt, T. S., & Weine, S. (2022). Family-based mental health interventions for refugees across the migration continuum: A systematic review. *SSM – Mental Health, 2,* Article 100153. https://doi.org/10.1016/j.ssmmh.2022.100153

Cardeña, E., Gušić, S., & Cervin, M. (2022). A network analysis to identify associations between PTSD and dissociation among teenagers. *Journal of Trauma & Dissociation, 23*(4), 432–450. https://doi.org/10.1080/15299732.2021.1989122

Choi, K. R., Seng, J. S., Briggs, E. C., Munro-Kramer, M. L., Graham-Bermann, S. A., Lee, R. C., & Ford, J. D. (2017). The dissociative subtype of posttraumatic stress disorder (PTSD) among adolescents: Co-occurring PTSD, depersonalization/derealization, and other dissociation symptoms. *Journal of the American Academy of Child & Adolescent Psychiatry, 56*(12), 1062–1072. https://doi.org/10.1016/j.jaac.2017.09.425

Courtois, C. A. (2008). Complex trauma, complex reactions: Assessment and treatment. *Psychological Trauma: Theory, Research, Practice, and Policy, S*(1), 86–100. https://doi.org/10.1037/1942-9681.S.1.86

Cowling, M. M., & Anderson, J. R. (2023). The effectiveness of therapeutic interventions on psychological distress in refugee children: A systematic review. *Journal of Clinical Psychology, 79*(8), 1857–1874. https://doi.org/10.1002/jclp.23479

Dalgaard, N. T., & Montgomery, E. (2015). Disclosure and silencing: A systematic review of the literature on patterns of trauma communication in refugee families. *Transcultural Psychiatry, 52*(5), 579–593. https://doi.org/10.1177/1363461514568442

DePierro, J., D'Andrea, W., Spinazzola, J., Stafford, E., van der Kolk, B., Saxe, G., Stolbach, B., McKernan, S., & Ford, J. D. (2019). Beyond PTSD: Client presentations of developmental trauma disorder from a national survey of clinicians. *Psychological Trauma: Theory, Research, Practice, and Policy, 14*(7), 1167–1174. https://doi.org/10.1037/tra0000532

DeRaedt, M. R. (2018). *Factors influencing pathological dissociative features in Syrian refugee children*. ProQuest. George Washington University ProQuest Dissertations Publishing. 10752363. proquest.com/openview/736b93360e1ecbd572c3c051efdf0eaa/1?pq-origsite=gscholar&cbl=18750

Diab, M., Peltonen, K., Qouta, S. R., Palosaari, E., & Punamäki, R. L. (2015). Effectiveness of psychosocial intervention enhancing resilience among war-affected children and the moderating role of family factors. *Child Abuse & Neglect, 40*, 24–35. https://doi.org/10.1016/j.chiabu.2014.12.002

Dorahy, M. J., Gold, S. N., & O'Neil, J. A. (Eds.). (2022). *Dissociation and the dissociative disorders: past, present, future*. Taylor & Francis.

Ellis, B. H., Miller, A. B., Abdi, S., Barrett, C., Blood, E. A., & Betancourt, T. S. (2013). Multi-tier mental health program for refugee youth. *Journal of Consulting and Clinical Psychology, 81*(1), 129–140. https://doi.org/10.1037/a0029844

Ertl, V., Pfeiffer, A., Schauer, E., Elbert, T., & Neuner, F. (2011). Community-implemented trauma therapy for former child soldiers in northern Uganda. *JAMA, 306*(5), Article 503. https://doi.org/10.1001/jama.2011.1060

Fazel, M., & Betancourt, T. S. (2018). Preventive mental health interventions for refugee children and adolescents in high-income settings. *Lancet Child & Adolescent Health, 2*(2), 121–132. https://doi.org/10.1016/S2352-4642(17)30147-5

Flanagan, N., Travers, A., Vallières, F., Hansen, M., Halpin, R., Sheaf, G., Rottmann, N., & Johnsen, A. T. (2020). Crossing borders: A systematic review identifying potential mechanisms of intergenerational trauma transmission in asylum-seeking and refugee families. *European Journal of Psychotraumatology, 11*(1), Article 1790283. https://doi.org/10.1080/20008198.2020.1790283

Fledderus, M., Bohlmeijer, E. T., & Pieterse, M. E. (2010). Does experiential avoidance mediate the effects of maladaptive coping styles on psychopathology and mental health? *Behavior Modification, 34*(6), 503–519. https://doi.org/10.1177/0145445510378379

Ford, J. D., & Courtois, C. A. (Eds.). (2017). *Treating complex traumatic stress disorders in children and adolescents scientific foundations and therapeutic models*. Guilford Press.

Frounfelker, R. L., Miconi, D., Farrar, J., Brooks, M. A., Rousseau, C., & Betancourt, T. S. (2019). Mental health of refugee children and youth: Epidemiology, interventions, and future directions. *Annual Review of Public Health, 41*, 159–176. https://doi.org/10.1146/annurev-publhealth-040119-094230

Gušić, S., Cardeña, E., Bengtsson, H., & Søndergaard, H. P. (2016). Types of trauma in adolescence and their relation to dissociation: A mixed-methods study. *Psychological Trauma: Theory, Research, Practice, and Policy, 8*(5), 568–576. https://doi.org/10.1037/tra0000099

Gušić, S., Cardeña, E., Bengtsson, H., & Søndergaard, H. P. (2017). Dissociative experiences and trauma exposure among newly arrived and settled young war refugees. *Journal of Aggression, Maltreatment & Trauma, 26*(10), 1132–1149. https://doi.org/10.1080/10926771.2017.1365792

Gušić, S., Malešević, A., Cardeña, E., Bengtsson, H., & Søndergaard, H. P. (2018). "I feel like I do not exist:" A study of dissociative experiences among war-traumatized refugee youth. *Psychological Trauma: Theory, Research, Practice, and Policy, 10*(5), 542–550. https://doi.org/10.1037/tra0000348

Haar, K., El-Khani, A., Molgaard, V., & Maalouf, W. (2020). Strong families: A new family skills training programme for challenged and humanitarian settings; a single-arm intervention tested in Afghanistan. *BMC Public Health, 20*(1), Article 634. https://doi.org/10.1186/s12889-020-08701-w

Hallab, A., & Sen, A. (2021). Epilepsy and psychogenic non-epileptic seizures in forcibly displaced people: A scoping review. *Seizure, 92*, 128–148. https://doi.org/10.1016/j.seizure.2021.08.004

Harel-Fisch, Y., Radwan, Q., Walsh, S. D., Laufer, A., Amitai, G., Fogel-Grinvald, H., & Abdeen, Z. (2010). Psychosocial outcomes related to subjective threat from armed conflict events (STACE): Findings from the Israeli-Palestinian cross-cultural HBSC study. *Child Abuse & Neglect, 34*(9), 623–638. https://doi.org/10.1016/j.chiabu.2009.12.007

Harrell-Bond, B. (2000). *Are refugee camps good for children?* Working Paper No. 29. UNHCR. unhcr.org/media/are-refugee-camps-good-children-barbara-harrell-bond.

Haselgruber, A., Knefel, M., Sölva, K., & Lueger-Schuster, B. (2021). Foster children's complex psychopathology in the context of cumulative childhood trauma: The interplay of ICD-11 complex PTSD, dissociation, depression, and emotion regulation. *Journal of Affective Disorders, 282*, 372–380. https://doi.org/10.1016/j.jad.2020.12.116

Hecker, T., Hermenau, K., Maedl, A., Schauer, M., & Elbert, T. (2013). Aggression inoculates against PTSD symptom severity—insights from armed groups in the eastern DR Congo. *European Journal of Psychotraumatology, 4*(1), Article 20070. https://doi.org/10.3402/ejpt.v4i0.20070

Herman, J. L. (1992). Complex PTSD: A syndrome in survivors of prolonged and repeated trauma. *Journal of Traumatic Stress, 5*(3), 377–391. https://doi.org/10.1007/BF00977235

Jannesari, S., Lotito, C., Turrini, G., Oram, S., & Barbui, C. (2021). How does context influence the delivery of mental health interventions for asylum seekers and refugees in low- and middle-income countries? A qualitative systematic review. *International Journal of Mental Health Systems, 15*, Article 80. https://doi.org/10.1186/s13033-021-00501-y

Joshi, P. T., & O'Donnell, D. A. (2003). Consequences of child exposure to war and terrorism. *Clinical Child and Family Psychology Review, 6*(4), 275–292. https://doi.org/10.1023/B:CCFP.0000006294.88201.68

Kien, C., Sommer, I., Faustmann, A., Gibson, L., Schneider, M., Krczal, E., Jank, R., Klerings, I., Szelag, M., Kerschner, B., Brattström, P., & Gartlehner, G. (2019). Prevalence of mental disorders in young refugees and asylum seekers in European countries: A systematic review. *European Child & Adolescent Psychiatry, 28*(10), 1295–1310. https://doi.org/10.1007/s00787-018-1215-z

Kohrt, B., Asher, L., Bhardwaj, A., Fazel, M., Jordans, M., Mutamba, B., Nadkarni, A., Pedersen, G., Singla, D., & Patel, V. (2018). The role of communities in mental health care in low- and middle-income countries: A meta-review of components and competencies. *International Journal of Environmental Research and Public Health, 15*(6), Article 1279. https://doi.org/10.3390/ijerph15061279

Kozlowska, K., Scher, S., Helgeland, H., & Carrive, P. (2021). Asylum-seeking children in shutdown: Neurobiological models. *Developmental Child Welfare, 3*(3), 282–309. https://doi.org/10.1177/25161032211036162

Lacroix, M., & Sabbah, C. (2011). Posttraumatic psychological distress and resettlement: The need for a different practice in assisting refugee families. *Journal of Family Social Work, 14*(1), 43–53. https://doi.org/10.1080/10522158.2011.523879

Lee, I.-S., & Kim, E. (2022). Effects of parenting education programs for refugee and migrant parents: a systematic review and meta-analysis. *Child Health Nursing Research, 28*(1), 23–40. https://doi.org/10.4094/chnr.2022.28.1.23

Lensvelt-Mulders, G., van der Hart, O., van Ochten, J. M., van Son, M. J. M., Steele, K., & Breeman, L. (2008). Relations among peritraumatic dissociation and posttraumatic stress: A meta-analysis. *Clinical Psychology Review, 28*(7), 1138–1151. https://doi.org/10.1016/j.cpr.2008.03.006

Lewis-Fernández, R., Aggarwal, N. K., Hinton, L., Hinton, D. E., & Kirmayer, L. J. (Eds.). (2016). *DSM-5 handbook on the cultural formulation interview*. American Psychiatric Association Publishing. https://doi.org/10.1176/appi.books.9781615373567

Liotti, G. (2006). A model of dissociation based on attachment theory and research. *Journal of Trauma & Dissociation, 7*(4), 55–73. https://doi.org/10.1300/J229v07n04_04

Lynn, S. J., Polizzi, C., Merckelbach, H., Chiu, C.-D., Maxwell, R., van Heugten, D., & Lilienfeld, S. O. (2022). Dissociation and dissociative disorders reconsidered: Beyond sociocognitive and trauma models toward a transtheoretical framework. *Annual Review of Clinical Psychology, 18*(1), 259–289. https://doi.org/10.1146/annurev-clinpsy-081219-102424

Mancini, M. A. (2020). A pilot study evaluating a school-based, trauma-focused intervention for immigrant and refugee youth. *Child and Adolescent Social Work Journal, 37*(3), 287–300. https://doi.org/10.1007/s10560-019-00641-8

Marley, C., & Mauki, B. (2019). Resilience and protective factors among refugee children post-migration to high-income countries: A systematic review. *European Journal of Public Health, 29*(4), 706–713. https://doi.org/10.1093/eurpub/cky232

McDonald, L., & Doostgharin, T. (2013). UNODC global family skills initiative. *Social Work and Social Sciences Review, 16*(2), 51–75. journals.whitingbirch.net/index.php/SWSSR/article/view/529

McMullen, J., O'Callaghan, P., Shannon, C., Black, A., & Eakin, J. (2013). Group trauma-focused cognitive-behavioural therapy with former child soldiers and other war-affected boys in the DR Congo: A randomised controlled trial. *Journal of Child Psychology and Psychiatry, 54*(11), 1231–1241. https://doi.org/10.1111/jcpp.12094

Miller, K. E., & Rasmussen, A. (2010). War exposure, daily stressors, and mental health in conflict and post-conflict settings: Bridging the divide between trauma-focused and psychosocial frameworks. *Social Science & Medicine, 70*(1), 7–16. https://doi.org/10.1016/j.socscimed.2009.09.029

Murray, H., & El-Leithy, S. (2022). *Working with complexity in PTSD*. Routledge.

Murray, L. K., Hall, B. J., Dorsey, S., Ugueto, A. M., Puffer, E. S., Sim, A., Ismael, A., Bass, J., Akiba, C., Lucid, L., Harrison, J., Erikson, A., & Bolton, P. A. (2018). An evaluation of a common elements treatment approach for youth in Somali refugee camps. *Global Mental Health, 5*, Article e16. https://doi.org/10.1017/gmh.2018.7

Pacione, L., Measham, T., & Rousseau, C. (2013). Refugee children: Mental health and effective interventions. *Current Psychiatry Reports, 15*(2), Article 341. https://doi.org/10.1007/s11920-012-0341-4

Pedersen, G. A., Smallegange, E., Coetzee, A., Hartog, K., Turner, J., Jordans, M. J. D., & Brown, F. L. (2019). A systematic review of the evidence for family and parenting interventions in low- and middle-income countries: Child and youth mental health outcomes. *Journal of Child and Family Studies, 28*(8), 2036–2055. https://doi.org/10.1007/s10826-019-01399-4

Peltonen, K., Kangaslampi, S., Saranpää, J., Qouta, S., & Punamäki, R.-L. (2017). Peritraumatic dissociation predicts posttraumatic stress disorder symptoms via dysfunctional trauma-related memory among war-affected children. *European Journal of Psychotraumatology, 8*(1), Article 1375828. https://doi.org/10.1080/20008198.2017.1375828

Puffer, E. S., Green, E. P., Chase, R. M., Sim, A. L., Zayzay, J., Friis, E., Garcia-Rolland, E., & Boone, L. (2015). Parents make the difference: A randomized-controlled trial of a parenting intervention in Liberia. *Global Mental Health, 2*, Article e15. https://doi.org/10.1017/gmh.2015.12

Qouta, S. R., El-Sarraj, E., & Punamäki, R.-L. (2001). Mental flexibility as resiliency factor among children exposed to political violence. *International Journal of Psychology, 36*(1), 1–7. https://doi.org/10.1080/00207590042000010

Qouta, S. R., Palosaari, E., Diab, M., & Punamäki, R.-L. (2012). Intervention effectiveness among war-affected children: A cluster randomized controlled trial on improving mental health. *Journal of Traumatic Stress, 25*(3), 288–298. https://doi.org/10.1002/jts.21707

Raghavan, S. S., & Sandanapitchai, P. (2019). Cultural predictors of resilience in a multinational sample of trauma survivors. *Frontiers in Psychology, 10*. https://doi.org/10.3389/fpsyg.2019.00131

Sallin, K., Lagercrantz, H., Evers, K., Engstrom, I., Hjern, A., & Petrovic, P. (2016). Resignation syndrome: Catatonia? Culture-bound? *Frontiers in Behavioral Neuroscience, 10*. https://doi.org/10.3389/fnbeh.2016.00007

Sangalang, C. C., Jager, J., & Harachi, T. W. (2017). Effects of maternal traumatic distress on family functioning and child mental health: An examination of Southeast Asian refugee families in the U.S. *Social Science and Medicine, 184*, 178–186. https://doi.org/10.1016/j.socscimed.2017.04.032

Schimmenti, A., & Caretti, V. (2016). Linking the overwhelming with the unbearable: Developmental trauma, dissociation, and the disconnected self. *Psychoanalytic Psychology, 33*(1), 106–128. https://doi.org/10.1037/a0038019

Sleijpen, M., Keles, S., Mooren, T., & Oppedal, B. (2022). Attachment insecurity in unaccompanied refugees: A longitudinal study. *International Journal of Migration, Health and Social Care, 18*(1), 66–82. https://doi.org/10.1108/IJMHSC-05-2021-0045

Summerfield, D. (1999). A critique of seven assumptions behind psychological trauma programmes in war-affected areas. *Social Science & Medicine, 48*(10), 1449–1462. https://doi.org/10.1016/S0277-9536(98)00450-X

Tufnell, G. (2003). Refugee children, trauma and the law. *Clinical Child Psychology and Psychiatry, 8*(4), 431–443. https://doi.org/10.1177/13591045030084002

Turrini, G., Purgato, M., Ballette, F., Nosè, M., Ostuzzi, G., & Barbui, C. (2017). Common mental disorders in asylum seekers and refugees: Umbrella review of prevalence and intervention studies. *International Journal of Mental Health Systems, 11*(1), 1–14. https://doi.org/10.1186/s13033-017-0156-0

Tyrer, R. A., & Fazel, M. (2014). School and community-based interventions for refugee and asylum seeking children: A systematic review. *PLoS One, 9*(5), Article e97977. https://doi.org/10.1371/journal.pone.0097977

UNHCR (UN Refugee Agency) (1951). *Convention relating to the status of refugees*. unhcr.org/about-unhcr/who-we-are/1951-refugee-convention

UNHCR (UN Refugee Agency) (2022). *Global trends forced displacement in 2022*. unhcr.org/global-trends-report-2022

van Ee, E., Kleber, R. J., Jongmans, M. J., Mooren, T. T. M., & Out, D. (2016). Parental PTSD, adverse parenting and child attachment in a refugee sample. *Attachment and Human Development, 18*(3), 273–291. https://doi.org/10.1080/14616734.2016.1148748

van Ee, E., Kleber, R. J., & Mooren, T. T. M. (2012). War trauma lingers on: Associations between maternal posttraumatic stress disorder, parent-child interaction, and child development. *Infant Mental Health Journal, 33*(5), 459–468. https://doi.org/10.1002/imhj.21324

von Knorring, A.-L., & Hultcrantz, E. (2020). Asylum-seeking children with resignation syndrome: Catatonia or traumatic withdrawal syndrome? *European Child & Adolescent Psychiatry, 29*(8), 1103–1109. https://doi.org/10.1007/s00787-019-01427-0

Zimmerman, A., Garman, E., Avendano-Pabon, M., Araya, R., Evans-Lacko, S., McDaid, D., Park, A.-L., Hessel, P., Diaz, Y., Matijasevich, A., Ziebold, C., Bauer, A., Paula, C. S., & Lund, C. (2021). The impact of cash transfers on mental health in children and young people in low-income and middle-income countries: A systematic review and meta-analysis. *BMJ Global Health, 6*(4), Article e004661. https://doi.org/10.1136/bmjgh-2020-004661

43
LISTENING TO THE BODY SPEAK
Conversion Issues and Functional Neurological Symptoms

Nicole Black

Introduction

For many years, the mental health field has struggled with its own dissociation of somatic symptoms and psychological symptoms. Historically, Pierre Janet included somatic dissociative symptoms in his theory of hysteria, a historical term now known as dissociation (Bowman, 2006; Janet, 1907; Nijenhuis, 1999). However, the realms of somatic dissociation and psychoform dissociation were categorically separated in the American Psychiatric Association's *Diagnostic and Statistical Manual of Mental Disorders* (*DSM*) with the release of the *DSM-III* and have remained that way with subsequent publications (American Psychiatric Association, 1980, 2013; Bowman, 2006; Cardeña & Nijenhuis, 2001; Steele et al., 2017).

Nijenhuis (1999) is credited with reconnecting the categories of psychoform dissociation and somatic dissociation. Over the years, many have called for the field of psychology to reunite these two realms formally within the *DSM* (Bowman, 2006; Cardeña & Nijenhuis, 2001; Nijenhuis, 1999; Ross, 2015), while others have highlighted issues with categorical differences between the *DSM* and the World Health Organization's International Classification of Diseases (ICD) (Steele et al., 2017). These categorical issues cause problems for clinicians who are struggling to conceptualize treatment for clients who are dealing with both somatic and psychological forms of dissociation. Researchers have attempted to reconnect the two constructs, but there continues to be a lack of practical applications for clinicians attempting to navigate presentations of both psychoform and somatic dissociation.

Psychoform and somatic (somatoform) dissociation are present in both dissociative disorders and functional neurologic disorders (FND). Often, clients with FND will experience psychoform dissociation such as derealization, depersonalization, and even dissociative amnesia, and these symptoms often occur around the time of the FND symptoms (American Psychological Association, 2013). For example, a client who has psychogenic nonepileptic seizures (PNES) often experiences derealization and depersonalization right before their psychogenic seizure occurs, and then will report amnesia for the episode after the episode has passed. Conversely, clients who have a dissociative disorder, especially dissociative identity disorder, will experience unexplained somatic symptoms such has headaches, transient loss of different bodily functions (i.e., blindness, inability to walk/move, or hearing loss) (International Society for the Study of Trauma and Dissociation, 2011).

Throughout this chapter, we will explore the intersectionality of psychoform and somatic dissociation and how the two are often present within the context of complex trauma disorders. This chapter will explore case conceptualization, treatment planning, and clinical applications for working with child clients with diagnostic presentations of both a dissociative disorder and FND. This chapter will keenly focus on conceptualizing and treating PNES in children using practical applications and will provide a case study to assimilate learning.

Functional Neurologic Symptom Disorder

Functional neurological symptom disorder is a *DSM-5* diagnosis that is also commonly called conversion disorder or FND for short. It is categorized in the *DSM-5* under "Somatic Symptom and Related Disorders." The first diagnostic symptom of FND is "one or more symptoms of altered voluntary motor or sensory functioning" (American Psychological Association, 2013, p. 318). There is evidence of an incompatibility between the symptoms of the patient and any recognized medical or neurological condition. The symptoms cannot be better explained by another mental health or medical condition and are not caused by the use of substances. Finally, the symptoms or deficits are causing clinically significant concerns for the client (American Psychological Association, 2013). Under this definition, clinicians may encounter clients with a variety of presentations, including PNES, choking, psychosomatic syncope, psychosomatic paralysis, speech issues like stuttering or slurred speech, and abnormal movements. Clients may also experience a mix of these presentations leading to a more complex presentation. As described above, FND is categorically separated from the dissociative disorders in the *DSM-5* even though many clients with dissociative disorders may also experience unexplained somatic symptoms or deficits, including PNES (American Psychological Association, 2013).

Psychogenic Nonepileptic Seizures

PNES have been documented in the literature for centuries (Bowman, 2006), and are defined as seizure-like activity that is without any organic neurological cause (Bowman & Markand, 2005). Again, PNES are a *symptom* that is categorized under FND within the *DSM-5* (American Psychiatric Association, 2013). PNES must be diagnosed by a medical doctor, typically a neurologist who completed video EEG monitoring, and are then subsequently treated by a mental health professional (Bowman, 2006).

Often, research on PNES is conducted by neurologists or psychologists/psychiatrists, which results in the research being categorically separated into medical journals, out of the reach of practicing mental health clinicals (Bowman & Markand; 2005; Lancman et al., 1994; Wyllie et al., 1999). Interestingly, many articles highlight dissociative phenomena present in clients with PNES (Bowman & Markand, 2005; Bowman & Coons, 2000; Bowman & Markand, 1996) and proper treatment for dissociative disorders is documented to lead to a notable reduction in PNES (Bowman & Coons, 2000). Unfortunately, based on this writer's experience, there seems to be a continued lack of attention to dissociative phenomenon when PNES are encountered in clinical practice.

Presentations of PNES

Quinn et al. (2008) reported that among a sample of therapists treating clients with PNES, the therapists conceptualized three categories into which PNES clients fell. Group one comprised clients with severe attachment trauma who had a variety of complex trauma symptoms, PNES being one of them. The clients in group one possibly also met criteria for a host of other mental health conditions, including PTSD and DID. The second group comprised clients who suffered from PNES but also experienced medical conditions such as traumatic brain injury or epilepsy. Lastly, the third group of clients was made up of those who experienced PNES but had no apparent history of trauma. This last group was understood to have poor emotional regulation skills. This chapter will focus on clients who fall under category one: those who experience PNES in the presence of a trauma-based mental health condition.

Psychogenic seizures can resemble a variety of different seizure types (Bowman & Markand, 2005). Behaviors during a PNES event may include (but are not limited to) pelvic thrusting, vocalizing, eye flutters, crying, shaking, flailing, and unresponsiveness to painful stimuli. PNES may occur during wakefulness or periods of sleep (Bowman & Markand, 2005). Although there are several symptoms that are common with PNES, there are no specific symptoms that are confirmatory for the diagnosis, and a diagnosis can be made only with EEG monitoring. Video-recorded EEG is considered the highest standard for diagnosing PNES (Bowman & Markand, 2005).

Some research and treatment models have resulted in harmful viewpoints on PNES presentations in children. Goodyer (1985) suggested that some children with PNES may be engaging in a sick role, thus resulting in their submission to ongoing medical exams and interventions. This view of children may easily result in providers taking a pejorative and dismissive stance with the child's symptoms. Additionally, this view of the child's condition would result in inappropriate behavioral modification interventions, missing a deeper underlying dissociative response that needs to be addressed clinically. Appropriate diagnosis, treatment planning, and case conceptualization remain vital in treating children with dissociative conditions, and will be discussed further below.

Diagnosis and Assessment

Unfortunately, there remains a lack of assessments appropriate for screening and assessing children for somatic dissociation. This undoubtably adds to the trouble in proper diagnosis and case conceptualization when both psychoform and somatoform manifestations of dissociative symptomatology are present. For example, clinicians will encounter troubles screening for somatoform dissociation present in child clients who are diagnosed with a dissociative disorder. Conversely, therapists of pediatric clients with FND may not be trained to screen for the presence of psychoform dissociative symptoms, including derealization, depersonalization, amnesia, or the presence of structural dissociation of the personality. For screening children, the Child Dissociative Checklist offers only one question about somatic symptoms (Putnam, 1990). Additionally, the Children's Dissociative Experiences Scale inquires about dizziness, stomach aches, and headaches, but does not ask about other known somatic dissociative symptoms (Stolbach, 1997; Stolbach et al., 2007).

With limitations in screening and assessment, child clinicians must become resourceful and creative in exploring and eliciting information that may lead to proper diagnosis of both psychoform and somatoform dissociation. Fortunately, child therapists tend to offer a great deal of creativity and ingenuity, especially play therapists. Play therapy encourages therapists to be creative, flexible, and adaptive as they explore ways to communicate through play. Child therapists should be sure to include questions for parents about somatic symptoms of children as part of any broader assessment, using the Adult Multidimensional Inventory of Dissociation (A-MID) Somatoform System Scale (Dell, 2006) or the Strengths and Difficulties Questionnaire (SDQ) (Nijenjuis et al., 1996) as a guide in symptom exploration. In addition, play therapists can utilize items like Gomez and Paulsen (2016) book *All the Colors of Me: My First Book about Dissociation* in order to explore symptoms. Therapists may also use the Dissociative Experiences Cards (Black, 2020), which depict images of somatic and psychoform dissociative phenomena that children may struggle to explain.

Treatment Planning

Multidisciplinary Approach

Working with FND, dissociative disorders, and PNES conditions requires a great deal of collaborative work with other professionals to support the client with the myriad of symptoms they experience. Somatic dissociation crosses the realms of mental health professions and medical professions, requiring support and collaborate efforts from many professionals who may lack education or clinical experience working with dissociative disorders or somatoform conditions. A dissociation-savvy therapist is the perfect candidate to help educate other professionals on somatic dissociation and will often assume the role of advocate for the client. Often, there is a need for advocacy or psychoeducation from professionals from occupational therapy, speech therapy, neurology, psychiatry, pediatric primary care, and within the educational system. Lastly, therapists may need to advocate for the child as part of psychiatric intervention in cases of excess medication (that may be contributing to psychopathology) or to provide psychoeducation about underlying dissociative organization of the internal system.

Family Environment, Dynamics, and Dysfunction

Research shows a strong relationship between family dysfunction and FND and PNES presentations (Lancman et al., 1994). Family dysfunction may present in the form of family conflict, abuse, neglect, or other familial issues. These issues may be representative of attachment trauma related to the family of origin, with trauma-related patterns of engagement repeating across generations. Likewise, dissociative disorders have a strong connection to childhood abuse, neglect, and attachment wounds, which have been found to originate within the family of origin (Steele et al., 2017).

Research into PNES suggests a strong connection between FND and familial issues (Bowman & Markand, 2005; Griffith et al., 1998; Lancman et al., 1994; Sawant & Umate, 2021). Lancman et al.'s (1994) study of 43 patients with a childhood onset of PNES concluded that "significant familial or personal distress was found in most of the cases," including conflict among the family and a history of sexual abuse (p. 406). The authors also found that stressful life events precipitated the onset of PNES (Lancman et al., 1994).

Including the child's family from the onset of diagnosis is of paramount importance and may give insight into dysfunctional family dynamics that have led to somatic manifestations of symptoms. Therapists working with these conditions should focus on developing an understanding of the child's strengths and weaknesses and how they relate to family dynamics. Support should be provided to bolster the young person's ability to communicate with supportive family members and identify family dysfunction that may need to be addressed further in family therapy.

Griffith et al. (1998) wrote about a variety of family dynamics that created "unspeakable dilemmas" for children who were experiencing PNES. The authors discussed how PNES was utilized as a "language of the body" to express double binds and suppressed emotions. These double binds often had to do with conflict within the family, abuse, domestic violence, or even custody issues. Therapists will need to carefully navigate these issues by starting out with a thorough assessment of family dynamics, parenting style, attachment style between family members, disciplinary methods, and history-gathering around familial events. Once these dynamics can be more readily understood, individual therapists can better support the child client with boundaries, affective expression, and other necessary tools to navigate home life. Individual therapists will also need to work closely with protective or supportive caretakers in order to mitigate stressful dynamics at home and provide supportive parenting and psychoeducation to caretakers. Individual therapists should also provide referrals for parental individual therapy and family therapy as appropriate so that families may better address intergenerational traumas or stressors and build communication skills within family therapy.

Other factors related to the family may be better addressed by social services and case management provided by other organizations, such as when there is a lack of resources, ongoing domestic violence or abuse, or other hardships that require systematic approaches to support the client. Some families may benefit from additional referrals to local organizations aimed at providing resources, case management, parenting support, or multidisciplinary approaches to complement the work of individual therapy. Other cases may necessitate referrals to child protective services in order to maintain the safety of the child in environments where there is found to be ongoing abuse or neglect.

Impact on Academic Functioning

Therapists who treat child clients with somatic dissociation, especially symptom presentations that include PNES, will need to provide recommendations for children in the classroom. Research indicates that children who experience PNES suffer academically and experience more academic stressors when they are symptomatic (Lancman et al., 1994). Often, these children will qualify for an individualized education plan, which will provide them with accommodations for testing and classroom participation. Beneficial accommodations might include copies of notes, extended or unlimited testing time, accommodations around testing format, and accommodations aimed at supporting emotional regulation in the classroom. Children struggling with somatic dissociation are also more likely to struggle with school attendance, school refusal due to stressors or avoidance issues, and absences due to an increase in medical and mental health appointments. Delayed diagnosis and treatment for clients who have complex presentations creates a further issue for these children. Lancman et al. (1994) reported that of their sample of children with PNES, there was a median delay in diagnosis of 3.5 years. During the long course of proper diagnosis, these children are also often subjected to multiple medical tests and extended hospitalizations (often at multiple hospitals), and provided with anticonvulsants while awaiting proper diagnosis and treatment, which may result in further traumatization. Children who have ongoing PNES activity may be subject to more hospitalizations or contact with emergency medical services when they experience seizure-like activity at school. This creates more obstacles for the child in an academic setting and will often lead to more stress and avoidance of academic environments. Ongoing collaboration and contact with school personnel will be of the highest importance when supporting children who have dissociative disorders with somatic symptoms.

Case Conceptualization and Practical Adaptations and Interventions with Children

Case conceptualization of clients with complex trauma and dissociation can often feel overwhelming, especially with the added layer of somatic or functional neurological symptoms. Working with children with these conditions can create an added layer of difficulty, as the clinician must explore symptoms and working through inner processes with a child who does not have the language or ability to fully express what they are experiencing internally. Furthermore, clinicians find an additional layer of difficulty when working with dysfunctional family systems, leaving them feeling overwhelmed and unskilled.

There are many theoretical lenses that may be utilized when working with children with symptom presentations that include somatic dissociation; however, it is of the utmost importance to develop a clear understanding of the child and the steps necessary to progress the child through their unique symptoms. It is recommended that the clinician layer pieces from different theoretical models in order to offer up a therapeutic approach that will be tailored to meet the needs of the client. Treatment for children with complex trauma and dissociative disorders should still follow the triphasic model of trauma treatment (Silberg, 2022).

During the initial phases of therapeutic work, it will also be important to assess and begin working with the child's family. It is crucial to explore the family unit and their strengths and weaknesses, and develop a list of therapeutic objectives to support the child in the broader context of the family unit.

Theoretical Modalities and Techniques for Therapeutic Work

An upcoming case study will give us insight into how therapists can incorporate elements of different therapeutic modalities to successfully treat clients with psychosomatic symptoms within a dissociative disorder. Once therapists have established comprehensive case conceptualization, they can begin to develop a dynamic and flexible treatment plan incorporating aspects of psychodynamic therapy, cognitive behavioral therapy, ego state therapy, EMDR therapy, somatic therapies, and hypnosis. These therapies can be easily adapted and implemented in playful ways to facilitate healing in children.

Play Therapy

For therapists who utilize play therapy, it is important to remain flexible and utilize both nondirective and directive play therapy interventions (Gil, 1991, 2017). Nondirective play therapy can be offered to build rapport with the child in the playroom and explore themes within the play. Children who have conversion or functional neurological symptoms may include play therapy themes or content around double binds, family conflict, reenactments or abuse scenes, helplessness, failed nurturing, need for control or lack of control, or even the inability to play freely due to being in a highly traumatized state. This can be explored with a variety of toys such as animals, dolls, a sand tray, or puppets. It is important that the clinician allow the child to speak through their play, so they may explore and begin to understand what cannot be spoken by the child.

TF-CBT Techniques

Trauma-focused cognitive behavioral therapy (TF-CBT) provides therapists with a useful framework from developing coping strategies that will be useful throughout the therapeutic process. Many researchers report that CBT is one the most effective forms of treatment for those who have PNES (LaFrance et al., 2014; Myers et al., 2021; Smith, 2014). TF-CBT offers stabilization techniques through the first four steps of the model—parenting skills/psychoeducation (for child and parent/family), relaxation skills, affective regulation skills, and cognitive coping skills—which fall into the stabilization and safety phase of the triphasic model. Following the preparatory phases of TF-CBT provides a solid structure for therapists to progress child clients through stabilization and safety, and helps ensure that each client is adequately prepared with the different tools that will be necessary before moving to trauma processing work.

PARENTING SKILLS/PSYCHOEDUCATION

Parenting skills and psychoeducation are a paramount first step when working with children who have been traumatized. This step is especially important when working with youth who have unexplained and sometimes frightening somatic complaints or a formal FND. Clinicians are encouraged to provide practical aspects of parenting children with trauma during this step, including appropriate ways to respond to trauma symptoms (or FND symptoms). Psychoeducation is also provided to both the child in an age-appropriate manner and the parents. Effective psychoeducation would include education on trauma symptoms, FND or somatic symptoms, dissociative symptoms, causes, methods of stabilization in the home, creating safety, and modifying any current parental behavior that may be inadvertently worsening symptoms.

RELAXATION SKILLS

Relaxation skills are a vital part of working with any child who has complex trauma or dissociative symptoms. These skills must be taught early in order to help the child regulate and gain a sense of mastery when faced with the activation of terrifying somatic symptoms. Often, children become increasingly afraid of somatic symptoms, especially PNES. During these episodes, children may be able to hear what is going on around them but be rendered completely unable to communicate with or control their bodies. This can result in a great deal of fear and panic, which leads to a high level of avoidance of anything that may be seen as a trigger for the somatic symptoms. These episodes may even lead children to fear that they are dying, due to the intensity of the somatic attacks and even repeated emergency medical treatment. Children will need to be provided with ample relaxation skills early in counseling. Utilizing these in session when the client observes a rise in bodily activation will help provide the child with a sense of mastery and reduce the phobia of bodily experiences.

Additionally, parents will need to be informed of these exercises, and therapists may model the use of relaxation techniques in order to help the child co-regulate through an attack of somatic symptoms. Some behavioral models of treatment for PNES encourage the parents to engage in positive and negative reinforcement of somatic symptoms such as PNES. In the book titled *Pediatric Psychogenic Non-Epileptic Seizures: A Treatment Guide*, the authors encourage therapists to coach the parents to leave the room when the child is having a PNES and return only when the PNES has subsided (Caplan et al., 2017). Other small studies of behavioral therapy interventions indicate a positive result from providing a reward- and consequences-based system to thwart PNES (Dworetzky & Baslet, 2017). Unfortunately, children with dissociative disorders or FND often have histories of attachment trauma, abuse, or neglect (Cook et al., 2005; Shanker & Sharma, 2023). For that reason, these methods of leaving a child alone when having a PNES or utilizing behavioral modification techniques involving the isolation of a child are not recommended and should be highly questioned. Children are not in conscious control of their body when these somatic episodes occur and are not utilizing these symptoms as a means of manipulation (Dworetzky & Baslet, 2017). Furthermore, there is great concern that this would further cause a sense of rejection, aloneness, or shame in children particularly with attachment traumas.

AFFECT REGULATION SKILLS

Often, children who have somatic dissociation, especially PNES, are diagnosed with alexithymia (Dworetzky & Baslet, 2017). This term may mislead newer clinicians into believing that the child is simply incapable of developing emotional connectedness or insight. However, alexithymia can be worked on therapeutically by paying close attention to the child's body and reflecting the child's current emotions and sensation back to them.

The focus in building affect regulation skills is on bolstering the child's ability to identify and manage different emotions. This portion of the treatment process works to broaden the child's emotional vocabulary and helps them learn various ways to express their emotions, especially verbally and in relation to trauma triggers or trauma material. Children are also taught self-soothing techniques and how to manage big feelings that arise. This is particularly useful for children who suffer from PNES.

Learning affect regulation skills allows children to help modulate and express their emotions instead of suppressing them, later leading to the PNES.

COGNITIVE COPING SKILLS

Cognitive coping skills help the child work through thinking errors that may be driving some behavior or worsening symptoms. These skills can include any of the variety of CBT skills, such as learning the Cognitive Triangle, working through thinking errors, or working on stopping negative thoughts. Clients can also be encouraged to keep track of the thoughts and triggers that kick off a flood of distressing thoughts. Unfortunately, younger children who lack metacognitive abilities will find developing cognitive coping skills more difficult. These skills or activities may be more useful for older children who have a better ability to track their own thoughts. Even still, children can be introduced to some basic cognitive coping skills to help aid in the development of metacognition.

Dissociative Symptom Interventions

CBT is cited by research as being a standard treatment for somatoform conditions, including PNES (Dworetzky & Baslet, 2017). However in this writer's experience, CBT, including TF-CBT, simply lacks the necessary tools and focus on treating the underlying dissociation that is present in many of these children. Furthermore, dissociative symptoms are frequently noted with functional conversion disorder symptoms such as PNES (Bowman, 2006; Bowman & Markand, 2005; Dworetzky & Baslet, 2017). For this reason, the clinician must assess thoroughly for derealization, depersonalization, and dissociation of the personality and provide appropriate interventions for treating these symptoms. When complex trauma and dissociative disorders are identified, CBT models of therapy will be inadequate for the treatment of the child and should not be used alone due to the fact that they do not address dissociative processes (Cohen et al., 2017). These dissociative symptom interventions need to include symptom identification, grounding, anchoring, and working with dissociative parts of the self through parts work, which will be described further in the next few sections.

Derealization and depersonalization can be identified in playful ways using resources like the Dissociative Experiences Cards or by using bibliotherapy, which will be discussed in more detail later in the chapter (Black, 2020; Gomez, 2013). Furthermore, grounding can be taught in playful ways using music, dance, scents like essential oils, slime, playdough, or the sand tray. Anchoring techniques can be taught in order to help anchor the child to the present. This can be facilitated in a variety of ways, including through sand trays, toys, or the use of transitional objects like marbles, personally made necklaces, worry stones, or trinkets that can be carried in the child's pocket. Utilization of these objects can be enhanced by incorporating hypnotic work while creating the transitional objects in the playroom.

Hypnotic Interventions

Throughout the course of therapy, there may be opportunities for therapists to incorporate clinical hypnosis. This would be useful when helping the child develop coping skills and explore symptoms, or when they need to prepare for upcoming stressful medical appointments or procedures. Hypnosis would also be useful throughout the course of treatment and can provide a foundational layer for working with dissociative parts of the self in therapy. Potential hypnotic techniques may include ideomotor signaling, hypnoprojectives, and hypnotic scripts that include guided imagery and hypnotic metaphors to deepen relaxation and a sense of mastery.

Ideomotor signaling can be used by the client to communicate subconscious "yes" or "no" responses with their fingers while in a hypnotic trance, and is useful in helping explore information that is stored within the subconscious mind (Hammond, 1992). Clinicians also may be faced with working with dissociative self-states that are nonverbal or unable to communicate for various reasons. These parts may present overtly with stuttering, selective mutism, bodily shutdown, or other somatic dissociative symptoms that result in an inability to communicate. Often, these symptoms are physiological representations of the child's internal conflict. Ideomotor signaling may be utilized to allow parts of the self that are triggering somatic symptoms, including PNES, to communicate without resorting to the use of triggering a dissociative shutdown.

Hypnoprojectives may be useful throughout therapy, but particularly in the process of identifying subconscious elements of PNES or another somatoform dissociative phenomenon. Furthermore, hypnotic guided imagery or hypnotic relaxation techniques are useful in speaking to the client's subconscious mind and aiding in the systematic relaxation of the client who is ailed by subconscious symptoms such as PNES. Children may be able to experience the benefits of hypnotic interventions in the form of bibliotherapy that utilizes hypnotic metaphors. This will be discussed more under the section on bibliotherapy.

Ego State Therapy Interventions

Ego state therapy work will be paramount when working with children who have dissociative disorders with somatic symptoms, including those with PNES (Bowman & Markand, 2006; Watkins & Watkins, 1997). Ego state work can be utilized to creatively explore functional neurological symptoms with the child, and parts of the self that are utilizing somatic experiences to communicate with the child.

Research conducted by Bowman and Markand (2006) revealed that after systematic questioning, almost half of the patients with PNES had a dissociated ego state that "[would] admit to causing the seizures" (p. 315). Anecdotally, somatic dissociation and PNES are utilized by various parts of the self to communicate internally. Also, somatic dissociation in children with dissociative disorders may be a form of somatic flashbacks from parts of the self that hold unintegrated trauma material. This can open up a window of exploration into parts of the self that may have conflicting feelings or hold unrealized trauma memories associated with the child's current life.

Furthermore, PNES may be utilized by various parts of the self as a means of managing affect and access to trauma material or intense, overwhelming emotions. Anecdotally, ego state exploration of clients with DID and FND with PNES presentation has revealed "gatekeeper" parts of the internal system utilizing PNES. Gatekeeper parts of the personality may utilize PNES as a means of shutting off, venting, or regulating the access of the "host" (adult part of the self) to emotions when the host becomes overwhelmed. This may happen when the client is fatigued, ignoring their body's need for rest, unable to manage stressors, unable to manage emotions, or coming too close to dissociated trauma material or emotions. When a gatekeeper part of the system is identified, it is important for clinicians to understand how this part of the self serves the overall functioning of the system. Clinicians will also need to explore triggers that activate this part's shutdown of the system and discover methods of internal communication between the gatekeeper and the host so that the client may begin to look inward for signs of fatigue, flooding, or need for regulation. Often, there is an internal struggle between dissociated parts of the self that are battling between doing too much or too little. Often, the host part wants to ignore their own fatigue, overwhelm, stress, or issues and continue to push forward in life, while other parts are forcing shutdown due to internal overwhelm. Maintaining a psychodynamic perspective while doing ego state work will be paramount (Watkins & Watkins, 1997). Facilitating this through ego state therapy will help the client self-regulate and begin to explore triggers to both dissociative responses and trauma material.

Somatic Interventions

Somatic interventions are a vital part of working with somatic dissociation (Levine, 2012). Incorporating body work will be necessary throughout the treatment process. Clients who experience somatic dissociation are often cut off from their bodies and trapped in a cycle of feeling too little (most of the time) and feeling too much (during somatic dissociation) (Nijenhuis, 1999; Steele et al., 2017). These cycles often exist because the client has learned to not feel as a means of coping, or as part of dissociating from traumatic material. Furthermore, clients who suffer from somatic dissociative symptoms, especially PNES symptoms, can develop a sort of phobia of the body. This often comes from the sense of being out of control of their body and unable to predict or control severe somatic symptoms that, for them, come on suddenly without any precursors or notice. The body thus becomes a source of distress to be ignored.

When working with child clients who have somatic symptoms, including PNES, it is important to help the client gently begin noticing what their body is telling them. Verbal labeling of emotions, particularly negative ones, can help children recover control over them. Torre and Lieberman (2018) refer to this idea as "affect labeling." In their research, an fMRI brain scan showed that this labeling of emotion decreased activity in the brain's emotional centers, including the amygdala. This dampening of the emotional brain allowed the frontal lobe (the reasoning and thinking center) to have greater sway over solving the problem (Torre & Lieberman, 2018). This practice should start early in the therapeutic process and with "gentle" curiosity, as children will often be detached and experience a high level of bodily phobia early in counseling. Therapists can begin by simply asking the child questions like, "What are you noticing in your body as you talk about that?" or "I wonder what your body feels right now?" Therapists should also help the child begin the process of identifying and naming different sensations in the body. This can be accomplished through the use of bibliotherapy, therapeutic games, or dolls or puppets in order to provide playful exploration of sensations while also offering the child the safety of distance.

Astute therapists will also pay close attention to the child's body as they talk about their life struggles or issues. As stated previously, these children often struggle with alexithymia. Therapists can help develop this ability by reflecting to the client what they are noticing in the child's body as the child speaks or plays. Furthermore, the therapist may ask the child to recount what happened earlier in the week when they had a somatic episode. Often, the child's body will begin to react to the verbalization of the event, but they will report having no emotions except possible fear of having another somatic event. Slow, gentle retelling of the event can help the therapist and child develop insight into possible triggers that led to the somatic episode and will also help the child reduce their anxiety and fear over the somatic symptoms themselves. Careful use of somatic pendulation and titration will also help children pace the work and reduce fear or apprehension as they become more in touch with their somatic experiences. Practicing this will help bolster the child's sense of mastery over their body and reduce phobia of bodily experiences. This practice should start early in the therapeutic process and increase gradually over time as the child develops a greater since of confidence. This will be paramount for helping the child integrate previously dissociated somatic material.

EMDR Interventions

EMDR therapy can be a useful tool to integrate when working with children who have complex trauma, dissociative disorders, or somatoform conditions. Like TF-CBT, EMDR therapy follows the triphasic model of trauma treatment and is an evidence-based therapy for the treatment of PTSD (Shapiro, 2001). EMDR's theoretical basis is called the adaptive information processing (AIP) model. This model states that memories are connected through memory networks and that current life triggers activate dysfunctionally stored material, thus causing unhelpful responses, or manifesting symptoms, in the moment (Shapiro, 2001). Case studies show that EMDR therapy has been efficacious in treating PNES in adolescents, as reported in research by Demirci and Sagaltici (2021), but this research has not yet been expanded to children. In their case studies, EMDR therapy was provided for five sessions with one client and four sessions with another, focusing on reprocessing targeted memories of PNES activity. Notably, both subjects in the case study were PNES-free when reevaluated six months after EMDR therapy was provided. Demirci and Sagaltici (2021) pointed out that both participants were able to connect their PNES events to earlier childhood memories associated with feeling excluded or being verbally and emotionally abused. While these case studies provide potential for future research and clinical application, their findings are limited. Unfortunately, there were only two samples provided in the case study, and it appears that EMDR therapy was applied rapidly in a hospital setting, which may not be generalizable to practitioners in outpatient care. Furthermore, the two case studies did not include participants who met criteria for complex trauma or exhibited criteria consistent with a dissociative disorder.

As illustrated in the proceeding case study, clinicians must take a slower and measured approach to applying EMDR therapy principles to those who have histories of complex trauma and meet the criteria for a dissociative disorder, which is supported and emphatically expressed in the EMDR manual by Francine Shapiro (2001, 2018), creator of EMDR therapy. In addition, Leeds et al. (2022) highlighted that EMDR therapy can disrupt dissociative barriers too quickly and cause flooding and destabilization. When working with children who have dissociative symptoms or disorders, or with histories of complex trauma, there is a need for extended preparatory work as well as stabilization and safety building techniques. EMDR therapy should be incorporated only with these clients as part of a more comprehensive treatment plan that includes other elements highlighted throughout this chapter. It should be emphasized that EMDR therapy should not be conducted with clients who have dissociative disorders and somatic dissociation (including PNES) without full understanding of the function of symptoms and how the dissociative system utilizes these symptoms to regulate or communicate needs within (Lemke, 2007). Furthermore, the client should be able to regulate themselves during the reprocessing phases of EMDR therapy without inducing a PNES event due to flooding of trauma material. There should also be adequate internal communication among dissociative parts of the self before starting EMDR therapy reprocessing (Lemke 2007; Shapiro, 2018). This is a vital aspect of remaining regulated. Triggering somatic dissociative symptoms during reprocessing, especially PNES, should be considered an indicator of intolerance for trauma material or possibly dissociative parts of the self using PNES in order to prevent dissociative barriers from being dismantled too quickly (Leeds et al., 2022; Shapiro, 2018). Child therapists utilizing EMDR are encouraged to explore adjunct approaches that may be integrated with standard protocol EMDR in order to facilitate healing. These approaches might include the use of sandtray therapy, puppets, and play therapy tools such as games, toys, or other tangible items that help facilitate titration and micro-processing of trauma materials (Gomez, 2013).

Bibliotherapy for Children with Complex Trauma, Dissociation, and Somatic Symptoms

There are numerous books that are useful when working with children who have trauma and dissociation. Bibliotherapy can provide a gateway to symptom exploration, discussion, and skills learning/building. Bibliotherapy also provides a window into difficult topics by allowing the child to explore an "other's" thoughts, feelings, dilemmas, and conflicts without having to discuss or disclose their own internal conflicts or struggles. This can create an opportunity for the therapist to help lower the child's internal defenses and introduce work that can be accomplished through hypnotic metaphors and ego state work. The following is a list of books that may be helpful for working with children who have complex trauma and somatic dissociation: *Healing Days: A Guide for Kids Who Have* Experienced Trauma

(Straus, 2013), *The Patchwork Quilt: A Book for Children about Dissociative* Identity Disorder (Clark, 2019), *Listening to* My Body (Garcia, 2017), Dissociative Experiences Cards (Black, 2020), *Harry the Hypno-potamus, Metaphorical Tales for the Treatment of* Children (Thomson, 2017), *All the Colors of Me: My First Book about Dissociation* (Gomez & Paulsen, 2016), *Brave Bart: A Story for Traumatized and* Grieving Children (Sheppard, 1998), *Dark, Bad Day...Go Away! A Book for Children about* Trauma & EMDR Therapy (Gomez, 2007), *Rob the Robin and the Bald Eagle* (Bray, 2015), and *A Terrible Thing Happened: A Story for Children Who Have Witnessed Violence or Trauma* (Holmes, 2000).

Case Study

The following case study is hypothetical to protect the confidentiality of clients.

Kassidy was a 12-year-old Hispanic girl who was referred to counseling after receiving a diagnosis of FND with PNES. She was a lively, high-achieving, compliant young lady who participated in sports and extracurriculars in her small town. Her mother described her as an obedient, focused, and helpful person who never got in trouble or had any issues at school or home. Kassidy lived at home with two older siblings and her mother. Her parents had divorced several years before, and her father was described as controlling with a short temper. She maintained contact with her father and described loving him but also feeling scared of his temper when she went to his house for visits.

One day, during sports practice, Kassidy was hit on the head by an object and was taken to the emergency department for evaluation. She received medical clearance at the hospital and was sent home. The next week during class, Kassidy fell out from her desk and began convulsing as if she were having a seizure. She was taken to the emergency room, where they determined that "nothing was wrong" and she did not have any physiological or organic cause for the seizure. Soon after this initial event, Kassidy began experiencing seizure-like activity multiple times daily, sometimes for an hour at a time, making it impossible for her to attend school. She began homeschooling due to the severity of her symptoms, and during the semester, she began experiencing paralysis, resulting in her need to use a wheelchair. The doctors could not find any medical reason to explain her paralysis, and she was told that the issue was "in her head." Her mother was told that Kassidy was "making up the symptoms" and that they should not feed into her behaviors.

Due to the complexity of her symptoms and her worsening condition, Kassidy's mother sought a second opinion at a major, nationally renowned diagnostic hospital, where they confirmed a diagnosis of FND and PTSD. During her time at the diagnostic hospital, Kassidy was noted to behave in a regressive manner, acting like a young child. Treating providers encouraged her mother to redirect or ignore this behavior and to take Kassidy's phone away as a negative consequence if she was experiencing PNES or other conversion symptoms. During her time at the clinic, Kassidy underwent a CBT-based treatment program aimed at redirecting these behaviors, providing psychoeducation of symptoms, and encouraging affective expression. She eventually completed the program and returned home to seek CBT in the community. Kassidy continued to have multiple PNES a week, but they lessened from 10 or 11 PNES events a day to five to six a week.

Once Kassidy returned home, she received general talk therapy from a couple of therapists without much success. She then transferred to a new therapist to receive EMDR treatment at the suggestion of her previous therapist. During her intake, Kassidy reported not knowing why she needed to be in counseling, and presented with alexithymia and severely blunted affect. Her mother reported that she is currently prescribed an antidepressant, a mood stabilizer, a sleep aid, and an antipsychotic to help with mood and sleeplessness. She reports that Kassidy's psychiatrist had tried various medications in the past several months. Due to the severe blunted affect, the therapist suggested that Kassidy and her mother speak to the psychiatrist about lowering or eliminating the antipsychotic so that therapy may be attempted with better access to Kassidy's emotions. Her reported only goal was to not have "seizures."

Mother and client provided historical information about the onset, duration, and frequency of symptoms as well as her bizarre behavior during her three-month hospital stay.

In addition to PNES, Kassidy experienced long periods of confusion after PNES events, such as tingling in her extremities, aches and pains, periods of involuntary jerking muscular movements, periods of transient paralysis, severe headaches, periods of being unable to speak, a choking sensation, racing heart, severe dizziness, and periods of severe stuttering or nonverbalization. She also reported transient, traveling tingling and pain throughout her body that crossed the midline of the body. All of these symptoms were thoroughly assessed by medical doctors and determined to be conversion-based symptoms. Kassidy reported feeling bad about her condition and that it was causing a lot of stress for her family. She reported that she would experience long periods of amnesia after her PNES and that she would be fatigued and confused afterward. Her PNES was debilitating to the point that she would be unable to complete schoolwork or other tasks after one occurred. She reported that she was not able to recall the three-month period of time when she was in a child-like state at the diagnostic hospital. She denied any history of verbal or physical abuse and reported having a happy childhood. She did admit that her dad would get angry at times, but that she loved him and enjoyed spending time with him on a regular basis. She admitted that her father used to yell, throw things, and hit the wall on a frequent basis.

During the intake, Kassidy was given the Child Dissociative Experiences Scale and Post-Traumatic Stress Inventory (Stolbach, 1997; Stolbach et al., 2007) and reported a score of 44. Further exploration of results indicated a high level of derealization, depersonalization, and amnesia symptoms. Kassidy's mother was provided with the Child Dissociative Checklist to fill out and asked about pertinent trauma history. Further diagnostic assessment and clinical interviewing resulted in a diagnosis of PTSD, DID, and FND.

Kassidy was seen for therapy on a weekly basis for two years. Her therapist conceptualized that Kassidy's psychogenic seizures were a way for her dissociative system to stop her from continuing (much of anything) when she was overwhelmed by external stressors. Since Kassidy was diagnosed with having DID as well as FND, her therapist focused treatment planning on treating the dissociative disorder with an understanding that the physiological symptoms were under the umbrella of the dissociative disorder.

With this understanding, the therapist conducted therapy following the triphasic model of trauma treatment using a psychodynamic framework, incorporating elements of ego state theory and hypnosis. Elements of EMDR were utilized in selective and strategic ways throughout the stabilization phase of treatment to help resource and stabilize dissociative parts of the self. Hypnotic interventions were utilized to create structure and promote internal communication and cooperation among dissociative self-states following Lemke's "Four C's model" (Lemke, 2007). Hypnotic and ego state work were utilized to help Kassidy explore the underlying causes of her symptoms. During treatment, Kassidy came to recognize that self-states were utilizing PNES and other somatic symptoms as a way to stop her from discussing emotions or topics or engaging in activities that would overwhelm her, cause anxiety, or potentially trigger PTSD symptoms in some way. She was also able to recognize that limb jerking, derealization, depersonalization, and tingling throughout the body were early warning signs of a possible PNES event and subsequently cues to begin grounding, deep breathing, or other regulating strategies to maintain her window of tolerance. In addition, eye rolling and periods of nonverbalization or stuttering were indicators of "switching" between dissociative self-states and self-state activity.

The first year and a half of therapy focused on stabilizing Kassidy's symptoms. Polyvagal and somatic experiencing principles of noticing the body, identifying sensations, and identifying nervous states were utilized in order to bolster Kassidy's ability to express her sensations, triggers, and physiological state throughout sessions (Levine, 2012; Porges, 2011), The therapist helped Kassidy develop a calm, safe place (Shapiro, 2018) for different parts of the self (Lemke, 2007) and helped her utilize the Container Exercise in order to manage trauma material without becoming flooded. The therapist focused on pacing therapy and allowing Kassidy to become in touch with her bodily sensations and emotions in a safe and manageable way using somatic and verbal titration and pendulation techniques to prevent her from becoming overwhelmed.

As Kassidy became more skillful in affective experiencing and expression, her PNES and other conversion symptoms quickly reduced over the course of a few months of treatment. Her therapist focused on reducing her phobias of inner experiences, physiological symptoms, and self-states (Steele et al., 2017). This was done through hypnotic interventions utilized to increase the cooperation of self-states during practical outside activities such as attending class, going to sports practices, and studying. Kassidy was then able to begin to explore self-states with increased comfort, resulting in a deeper understanding of dissociated thoughts, emotions, memories, and triggers. With increased awareness, Kassidy was able to gain further mastery over her symptoms, which resulted in less derealization, depersonalization, and amnesia. Over the course of therapy, Kassidy spontaneously reported recalling her previously amnesic time in the diagnostic hospital.

Kassidy's therapist focused on mapping out self-states of the system and how each part triggered or utilized somatic symptoms to communicate with Kassidy. Mapping also explored past traumas and fears held within the system that might continue to lead to conversion symptoms. After a year and a half of stabilization, Kassidy was able to begin working through identified targets associated with her father's anger outbursts that she witnessed and experienced during childhood. EMDR was utilized in this process with ego state theory–based modifications to help Kassidy communicate with parts of the self. Internal communication during EMDR processing was paramount to prevent flooding and maintain Kassidy's window of tolerance so that she would not experience a PNES during processing sessions. Nonverbal signals were utilized during the desensitization phase of EMDR to allow self-states to communicate a need to stop or pause processing without triggering a PNES.

As Kassidy progressed in therapy, her sessions were reduced to a biweekly basis while providing stress management and EMDR processing as needed. During this time, she suffered a brief setback when she tore a ligament in her ankle. When this happened, the doctors reported that she should be able to walk with only a brace and did not need to use crutches. However, Kassidy reported being unable to walk without crutches and that she would immediately fall if she tried to stand up unassisted. Hypnotic interventions focused on positive reinforcement of her ability to walk were utilized, and she was able to resume walking without intervention after a single therapy session. Therapy then focused on helping prepare her for her upcoming surgery to repair the ankle. Kassidy expressed worry about the surgery due to past surgeries resulting in months of unexplained pain, tingling, numbness, and other complications. Hypnosis was utilized again to prepare Kassidy for surgery with suggestions focused on her body healing fully and returning to complete ability. She was able to have surgery without a single complication afterward.

At the completion of her therapy, Kassidy had not had a PNES event in over six months, with the last PNES event lasting only a minute. She reported no amnesia symptoms, derealization, or depersonalization and said she felt integrated with her previously dissociated self-states.

Conclusion

Somatic dissociation, including PNES, can often overwhelm clinicians who are unfamiliar with the connection between somatoform and psychoform types of dissociation. However, with careful treatment planning and consideration, child therapists can provide a more comprehensive treatment approach. Clinicians can utilize a variety of treatment modalities and interventions in order to best support the healing of their clients. Careful interweaving of various therapeutic modalities can facilitate attention to what the body is saying to both child and clinician.

References

American Psychiatric Association. (1980). *Diagnostic and statistical manual of mental disorders* (3rd ed.). American Psychiatric Association.

American Psychiatric Association. (2013). *Diagnostic and statistical manual of mental disorders* (5th ed.). https://doi.org/10.1176/appi.books.9780890425596

Black, N. (2020). *Dissociative experiences cards* [Card game]. Self-Published.

Bowman, E. S. (2006). Why conversion seizures should be classified as a dissociative disorder. *Psychiatric Clinics of North America, 29*(1), 185–211. https://doi.org/10.1016/j.psc.2005.10.003

Bowman, E. S., & Coons, P. (2000). The differential diagnosis of epilepsy, pseudoseizures, dissociative identity disorder, and dissociative disorder not otherwise specified. *Bulletin of the Menninger Clinic, 64*, 164–180.

Bowman, E. S., & Markand, O. N. (2005). Diagnosis and treatment of pseudoseizures. *Psychiatric Annals, 35*(4), 306–316. https://doi.org/10.3928/00485713-20050401-05

Bowman, E., & Markand, O. (1996). Psychodynamics and psychiatric diagnoses of pseudoseizure subjects. *American Journal of Psychiatry, 153*(1), 57–63. https://doi.org/10.1176/ajp.153.1.57

Bray, M. (2015). *Rob the robin and the bald eagle* (J. Wheeler, Illus.). Artsake Publishing.

Caplan, R., Doss, J., & Plioplys, S. (2017). *Pediatric psychogenic non-epileptic seizures: A treatment guide*. Springer.

Cardeña, E., & Nijenhuis, E. R. (2001). Embodied sorrow. *Journal of Trauma & Dissociation, 1*(4), 1–5. https://doi.org/10.1300/j229v01n04_01

Clark, J. D. (2019). *The patchwork quilt* (M. Starling, Illus.). CreateSpace Independent Publishing Platform.

Cohen, J. A., Mannarino, A. P., & Deblinger, E. (2017). *Treating trauma and traumatic grief in children and adolescents*. Guilford Press.

Cook, A., Spinazzola, J., Ford, J., Lanktree, C., Blaustein, M., Cloitre, M., & van der Kolk, B. (2005). Complex trauma. *Psychiatric Annals, 35*(5), 390–398.

Dell, P. F. (2006). The Multidimensional Inventory of Dissociation (MID): A comprehensive measure of pathological dissociation. *Journal of Trauma & Dissociation, 7*(2), 77–106. https://doi.org/10.1300/j229v07n02_06

Demirci, O. O., & Sagaltici, E. (2021). Eye movement desensitization and reprocessing treatment in functional neurological symptom disorder with psychogenic nonepileptic seizures: A study of two cases. *Clinical Child Psychology and Psychiatry, 26*(4), 1196–1207. https://doi.org/10.1177/13591045211037276

Dworetzky, B. A., & Baslet, G. C. (Eds.). (2017). *Psychogenic nonepileptic seizures*. Oxford University Press.

Garcia, G. (2017). *Listening to my body* (Y. H. Tan, Illus.). Skinned Knee Pub.

Gil, E. (1991). *The healing power of play: Working with abused children*. Guilford Press.

Gil, E. (2017). *Posttraumatic play in children: What clinicians need to know*. Guilford Press.

Gomez, A. M. (2007). *Dark, bad day... go away! A book for children about trauma & EMDR* (C. S. Acosta, Illus.). A. M. Gomez. Self-published.

Gomez, A. M. (2013). *EMDR therapy and adjunct approaches with children: Complex trauma, attachment, and dissociation*. Springer.

Gomez, A. M., & Paulsen, S. (2016). *All the colors of me: My first book about dissociation* (S. Paulsen, Illus.). Agate Books.

Goodyer, I. M. (1985). Epileptic and pseudoepileptic seizures in childhood and adolescence. *Journal of the American Academy of Child Psychiatry, 24*(1), 3–9. https://doi.org/10.1016/s0002-7138(09)60403-9

Griffith, J. L., Polles, A., & Griffith, M. E. (1998). Pseudoseizures, families, and unspeakable dilemmas. *Psychosomatics, 39*(2), 144–153. https://doi.org/10.1016/s0033-3182(98)71361-1

Hammond, D. C. (1992a). *Handbook of hypnotic suggestions and metaphors*. Norton.

Holmes, M. M. (2000). *A terrible thing happened: A story for children who have witnessed violence or trauma* (C. Pillo, Illus.). Magination Press.

International Society for the Study of Trauma and Dissociation. (2011). Guidelines for treating dissociative identity disorder in adults (3rd rev.). *Journal of Trauma & Dissociation, 12*(2), 115–187. https://doi.org/10.1080/15299732.2011.537247

Janet, P. (1907). *L'automatisme psychologique: Essai de psychologie expérimentale sur les formes inférieures de l'activité humaine*. F. Alcan.

LaFrance, W. C., Baird, G. L., Barry, J. J., Blum, A. S., Frank Webb, A., Keitner, G. I., Machan, J. T., Miller, I., & Szaflarski, J. P. (2014). Multicenter pilot treatment trial for psychogenic nonepileptic seizures. *JAMA Psychiatry, 71*(9), 997–1005. https://doi.org/10.1001/jamapsychiatry.2014.817

Lancman, M. E., Asconapé, J. J., Graves, S., & Gibson, P. A. (1994). Psychogenic seizures in children: Long-term analysis of 43 cases. *Journal of Child Neurology, 9*(4), 404–407. https://doi.org/10.1177/088307389400900413

Lemke, W. (2007). Fostering internal cooperation through the use of imagery in the treatment of dissociative identity disorder. *Journal of Trauma & Dissociation, 8*(4), 53–68. https://doi.org/10.1300/j229v08n04_04

Levine, P. A. (2012). *Healing trauma: A pioneering program for restoring the wisdom of your body.* Sounds True.

Leeds, A. M., Madere, J. A., & Coy, D. M. (2022). Beyond the DES-II. *Journal of EMDR Practice and Research, 16*(1), 25–38.

Myers, L., Sarudiansky, M., Korman, G., & Baslet, G. (2021). Using evidence-based psychotherapy to tailor treatment for patients with functional neurological disorders. *Epilepsy & Behavior Reports, 16*, Article 100478. https://doi.org/10.1016/j.ebr.2021.100478

Nijenhuis, E. R. S. (1999). *Somatoform dissociation: Phenomena, measurement, and theoretical issues.* Van Gorcum.

Nijenhuis, E. R. S., Spinhoven, P., van Dyck, R., van der Hart, O., & Vanderlinden, J. (1996). The development and psychometric characteristics of the Somatoform Dissociation Questionnaire (SDQ-20). *Journal of Nervous and Mental Disease, 184*(11), 688–694. https://doi.org/10.1097/00005053-199611000-00006

Porges, S. W. (2011). *The polyvagal theory: Neurophysiological foundations of emotions, attachment, communication, and self-regulation.* W W Norton & Co.

Pullin, M. A., Webster, R. A., & Hanstock, T. L. (2014). Psychoform and somatoform dissociation in a clinical sample of Australian adolescents. *Journal of Trauma & Dissociation, 15*(1), 66–78. https://doi.org/10.1080/15299732.2013.828149

Putnam, F. W. (1990). Child dissociative checklist. *PsycTESTS Dataset.* https://doi.org/10.1037/t02069-000

Quinn, M., Schofield, M., & Middleton, W. (2008). Conceptualization and treatment of psychogenic non-epileptic seizures. *Journal of Trauma & Dissociation, 9*(1), 63–84. https://doi.org/10.1080/15299730802073676

Ross, C. A. (2015). Problems with DSM-5 somatic symptom disorder. *Journal of Trauma & Dissociation, 16*(4), 341–348. https://doi.org/10.1080/15299732.2014.989558

Sawant, N. S., & Umate, M. S. (2021). Dissociation, stressors, and coping in patients of psychogenic non-epileptic seizures. *Indian Journal of Psychological Medicine, 43*(6), 479–484. https://doi.org/10.1177/0253717620956460

Shanker, G., & Sharma, I. (2023). Study of determinants of somatoform disorders in children. *Cureus.* https://doi.org/10.7759/cureus.36447

Shapiro, F. (2001). *Eye movement desensitization and reprocessing: Basic principles, protocols, and procedures.* Guilford Press.

Shapiro, F. (2018). *Eye movement desensitization and reprocessing (EDMR) therapy: Basic principles, protocols, and procedures* (3rd ed.). Guilford Press.

Sheppard, C. H. (1998). *Brave Bart: A story for traumatized and grieving children.* Institute for Trauma and Loss in Children.

Silberg, J. L. (2022). *The child survivor: Healing developmental trauma and dissociation.* Routledge.

Smith, B. J. (2014). Closing the major gap in PNES research. *Epilepsy Currents, 14*(2), 63–67. https://doi.org/10.5698/1535-7597-14.2.63

Steele, K., Boon, S., & van der Hart, O. (2017). *Treating trauma-related dissociation: A practical, integrative approach.* W. W. Norton.

Stolbach, B. C. (1997). *The Children's Dissociative Experiences Scale and Posttraumatic Symptom Inventory: Rationale, development, and validation of a self-report measure.* [Doctoral dissertation, University of Colorado]. ProQuest Dissertations Publishing.

Stolbach, B. C., Dominguez, R. Z., Rompala, V., Fleisher, C., Gazibara, T., & Lawrence, G. (2007). Children's dissociative experiences scale and posttraumatic symptom inventory: A replication study. *PsycEXTRA Dataset.* https://doi.org/10.1037/e517322011-533

Straus, S. F. (2013). *Healing days: A guide for kids who have experienced trauma* (M. Bogade, Illus.). Magination Press.

Thomson, L. K. (2017). *Harry the hypno-potamus: More metaphorical tales for children.* Crown House Publishing.

Torre, J. B., & Lieberman, M. D. (2018). Putting feelings into words: Affect labeling as implicit emotion regulation. *Emotion Review, 10*(2), 116–124. https://doi.org/10.1177/1754073917742706

Watkins, J. G., & Watkins, H. H. (1997). *Ego states: Theory and therapy.* W. W. Norton.

Wyllie, E., Glazer, J. P., Benbadis, S., Kotagal, P., & Wolgamuth, B. (1999). Psychiatric features of children and adolescents with pseudoseizures. *Archives of Pediatrics & Adolescent Medicine, 153*(3), 244–248. https://doi.org/10.1001/archpedi.153.3.244

44
CHRONIC PAIN, MEDICAL ISSUES, AND COMPLICATED CLINICAL PRESENTATIONS

Christine C. Forner

Introduction

When asked to write a chapter on chronic pain, medical issues, and complicated clinical presentations in infants and children who are complexly traumatized, I was a bit overwhelmed. My mind went to those children I've worked with between the ages of 1 and 13 who were extremely reactive, who threw objects and themselves around. Or those children and infants who were extremely quiet and looked like ghosts, or those children who acted like perfect little adults. I think about the children who were forced to perform sex acts on adults, other children, or animals, and who were labeled as "difficult" kids. Or those who were made to eat and/or drink poisons and/or rotten food, who were later diagnosed with eating disorders. Or the children who spent much of their existence in hospitals undergoing massively painful procedures, while being told that what was happening was good for them and saving their lives, but with little to no consideration of how chronic pain affects every part of a tiny human and how this pain affects the development of their world.

When discussing how these children behave, the best descriptor is extreme. Extreme rage, extreme fear, extreme panic, extreme quiet, extreme good, extreme frozenness, extreme parentification, extreme sadness, extreme avoidance. These are hard cases to work with, and they require not only clinical expertise but also much internal self-awareness on the part of the clinician. Patience, tolerance, intuition, awareness, attunement, compassion, and excellent, healthy, age-appropriate boundaries are as necessary as any type of post-graduate continuing education course—perhaps more so. Basically, treatments that are unlike the original abuse all play a massive role in helping these small humans move through their trauma.

Sadly, these children are often accompanied by an adult who is a main contributor to the problem; or who has been given instructions by a medical professional who does not know about the extraordinary sensitivity infants and children have to being alone, to pain, and to human-to-human harm; or who is grossly under-resourced in being able to properly care for their child. This is a huge topic and one that could fill up an entire book all on its own. I could speak about what likely happens to infants and children who experience chronic pain and how this affects their development, or I could discuss what typically happens to infants and children when there are dangerous medical problems, and what complicated interventions, such as the impacts of being tied down or having to go through many surgeries, will have on their behavior. Or I could discuss what might be occurring inside a child when their parents are both active participants in the child's sexual abuse and producers of child sexual abuse material (CSAM). I could focus on one specific example and walk the reader through what might work to treat them, but unfortunately, it may not work for all children.

Sadly, there is no single intervention, except to meet the child where they are at, and then, in an ever-evolving, dynamic, moment-to-moment way, help them regulate what they are feeling. The difficulty is that there is no real step-by-step instructional manual for helping children with complicated medical issues, chronic pain, or these types of injuries. We are influenced by and live in a world that has billions of incidents of harm, abuse, cruel practices, harsh religious beliefs, impoverishment, ignorance in how to meet people's needs, and the objectification of infants, children, women, and large swaths of other people. The clinical worlds of psychology and psychiatry, and all the other healing professions that are heavily influenced by these areas, hold many beliefs about humans that are either misunderstood or false. It is hard for me to not write pages and pages of examples of how often this is evidenced in these fields and how these beliefs still dominate. The lobotomy, after all, did win a Nobel prize.

I often say that doing this type of clinical work is not all that complicated. I do not mean for this to sound glib. Humans grow best in safe and secure environments. The difficulty is knowing, exactly, what will make an infant or child experience safety and security and, conversely, what is happening that makes infants and children feel unsafe and insecure when they cannot verbalize. An added layer to this challenge is that much of the foundational information and ingrained biases about infant and child development has been and is still very incorrect. Psychology and medicine have yet to truly incorporate what we have learned about human trauma and attachment needs. Changing our perspectives is not easy. Uneducating ourselves, as most of us have been educated in the foundations of psychology, which heavily rely on the *mind* and the analysis of what someone is *thinking*, is hard. When working with infants and children, we cannot depend on words and thoughts as the primary source of information gathering.

So how do we gather the "data" we need from the infant or child that will inform us of what is creating the unsafe or insecure symptoms or experience, and then what do we need to do to help the child or infant get to a place of safe and secure? Our clinical task is interpreting their needs correctly and applying what will make the child experience and feel safety and security physiologically, not psychologically.

How Infants and Children Experience Pain

In an article in the *New England Journal of Medicine*, Anand and Hickey (1987) discussed pain and its effects on the human neonate and fetus. This medical influence that impacts how we comprehend, create treatment plans and goals, and orient our knowledge to the problems of the infant child are still pervasive in medicine, psychiatry, psychology, and social work. According to Anand and Hickey (1987),

> the evaluation of pain in the human fetus and neonate is difficult because pain is generally *defined as a subjective phenomenon* [emphasis added]. Early studies of neurologic development concluded that neonatal responses to painful stimuli were *decorticate in nature and that perception or localization of pain was not present* [emphasis added]. Furthermore, *because neonates may not have memories of painful experiences, they were not thought capable of interpreting pain in a manner similar to that of adults* [emphasis added]. On a theoretical basis, it was also argued that a *high threshold of painful stimuli may be adaptive in protecting infants from pain during birth* [emphasis added]. These traditional views have led to a widespread

belief in the medical community that the *human neonate or fetus may not be capable of perceiving pain* [emphasis added].

Strictly speaking, nociceptive activity, rather than pain, should be discussed with regard to the neonate, *because pain is a sensation with strong emotional associations* [emphasis added]. The focus on pain perception in neonates and confusion over its differentiation from nociceptive activity and the accompanying physiologic responses have obscured the mounting evidence that nociception is important in the biology of the neonate. This is true regardless of any *philosophical view on consciousness and "pain perception"* [emphasis added] in newborns ....

One result of the pervasive view of neonatal pain is that newborns are frequently not given analgesic or anesthetic agents during invasive procedures, including surgery [emphasis added]. Despite recommendations to the contrary in textbooks on pediatric anesthesiology, the clinical practice of inducing minimal or no anesthesia in newborns, particularly if they are premature, is widespread. Unfortunately, recommendations on neonatal anesthesia are made without reference to recent data about the development of perceptual mechanisms of pain and the physiologic responses to nociceptive activity in preterm and full-term neonates. Even Robinson and Gregory's landmark paper demonstrating the safety of narcotic anesthesia in preterm neonates cites *"philosophic objections"* [emphasis added] rather than any physiologic rationale as a basis for using this technique. Although methodologic and other issues related to the study of pain in neonates have been discussed, the body of scientific evidence regarding the mechanisms and effects of nociceptive activity in newborn infants has not been addressed directly.

(p. 1321)

It is notable that this paper is from 1987, and thankfully medical systems in the present tend to manage pain differently. But what is also notable is the subjective experience of children and the subjective interpretation of those experiences, which have not really changed. The notion that infants and young children do not "remember" as adults do somehow equates to the assumption that the person's years spent not remembering are filled with nothing or nothing notable. The still common notion that adult consciousness is the "gold standard" of perception and that all other types of consciousness are unimportant or invalid holds very true in our world. Yet this is just not the case: infants feel as adults do; they sense their inner sensations as adults do. However, adults can notice in ways that infants and children perhaps do not, and can also be disconnected from, dissociated from, and unempathetic toward an infant or child in pain.

The Central Nervous System

For the infant and child, the feeling of safety and security is directly related to the regulation or dysregulation of the central nervous system (CNS); organs don't speak in words, but in feelings. The difficult part is *how* to help an extremely injured child soothe and find safety when something extremely unsafe and mind-alteringly insecure happens. Our invaluable role, in many ways, is to "read" the body and the CNS. This means that our job is to be an interpreter of feelings, not words, or thoughts or memories. We must figure out what the crying, screaming, throwing, frozen, or reactive sensations and affect of the child are candidly communicating. It is our job as the regulated adult to then put these feelings and sensations into the accurate context, proper meaning, and appropriate language. It is only then that can we address the distress accordingly. To do this, we need to use our innate qualities of empathy, intuition, attunement, presence, and awareness. These needed skills are not taught in school, but they are the most needed tools for treatment. For many people, these characteristics have been dismissed and belittled. But because these skills are readily available, and if you know how to evoke them while in the same room as a terrified and pain-filled child, the solutions are usually simple. We need to get out of our head and dive deep into our intuition, which requires us to be extremely well regulated and open to being nurturing. This is in part achieved by the therapist using the innate capacities of secure attachment and mindfulness, a state that is being referred to as "securefulness," which is discussed later in this chapter (Danylchuk & Forner, 2022).

When the CNS is in a physiological state of regulation and the needs of the child have been met, the resulting safety and security can and do heal nearly every injury. This statement bears repeating. When the entire CNS, including the entire spinal column and facia and all the nerves that are connected to the CNS, is in a regulated state, which can only come from being properly nurtured, humans heal and grow. When the CNS is in a dysregulated state, humans cannot or will not have what is needed to grow. Dysregulation equates to a need, and if this need is not met, the infant's or child's body quickly goes into an emergency cascade response that always accompanies an inflamed CNS (Kozlowska et al., 2015). When a human is dysregulated, the whole body and mind orientate toward emergency survival and preventing death, which of course is not thriving and enhancing pro-social life. The neurobiological fact is that humans are hardwired to be regulated by regulated adults. But what if we were to exchange the word "regulation" with "nurtured"? That is what regulation is—to nurture that child, and nurturance in all of its layered nuances is the main tool of treatment. It is co-nurturing that leads to self-nurturing, and this is the task at hand. Nurturance is a powerful tool and, as stated, can and will heal most injuries; this is simply because infants and children are born to be nurtured.

To work with such hurt and sensitive, tiny humans, it is often easier to view the infant or child as a central nervous system (CNS) themselves. This electrical conduit, which is in every part of the human body, is where we start as a species. The feelings and sensations that are contained in the information highway are the foundation and core of who we are and what type of adult consciousness we have. The CNS is how electrical information is moved throughout the body to the mind and back again. The needs of the body travel both through electrical conduits and neurochemicals via sensorimotor and affective circuits (Barrett, 2020).

When an infant is born, the spinal cord and brain stem are two of the few structures that are well developed (Bellieni, 2019; Cerritelli et al., 2021; Lasselin, 2021; Perkeybile et al., 2019). At birth, an infant can feel and sense nearly the same or the exact same affective, feeling base information and sense perceptions as adults (Cerritelli et al., 2021). It is important to acknowledge that physical and affective emotional pain are perceived in the exact same areas of the brain (Vastag, 2003). This translates to children not really being able to differentiate between physical and psychological pain. The need for food, the pain of a broken bone, and the need for attention, connection, cuddles, and hugs are extremely similar feelings in the bodies of babies and small children. This can be deduced by both the anecdotal reports of adults who explore their early-life pain and suffering as well as the neurobiological response of dissociation. Affective, sensory pain and physical pain have the same or very similar pain perception. We know that actual fear and life threat is the same as perceived fear and life threat. A broken bone or a skin laceration in an infant or child, as far as pain perception is concerned, is no different from the pain of hunger, cold, and fear going uncared for.

Because infants run on 100% instinct mediated by lower regions of the brain (please see Chapter 11), there is no cognition, no abstract thinking, no external awareness. Infants and children cannot be mindful, self-soothe, or self-regulate/self-nurture—these are adult abilities. They cannot change how they feel on their own because their feelings originate as needs, which they cannot meet without an attachment system. Young children are unable to even know their own needs. An infant responds only to what the CNS, brain stem, and spinal cord instruct them to respond to. The CNS reacts only to need and survival. When infants are born, they have no control over their body and bodily functions. They cannot move, with intent, on their own for months. It takes at least a decade to control many fine motor functions. Survival is our primary basic need, and, thus, secure attachment (Bowlby, 1977;

Yilmaz et al., 2022). Expressing this need is our number one life-saving protection and defensive shield. And not receiving the care we require, or experiencing neglect and/or human-to-human harm, feeling equivalent to physical pain, is an unfathomable experience for an infant and child. It's like an animal's teeth, claws, speed, agility, or camouflage suddenly disappearing. It's an unbearable vulnerability that is communicated via pain.

As stated earlier, our needs are communicated through a sensorimotor reaction via a sensation (Ogden, 2021). The sensorimotor system is intimately connected to our affective circuitry—sensations are communicated via affect, or feelings (Hoemann et al., 2019; Quigley et al., 2021). Feelings are the mechanisms that publicize our internal needs. Sounds, cries, and, if all goes well, words and higher language follow (Gogtay et al., 2004; Lopez et al., 2008; Perrus et al., 2021; Wickrama et al., 2017). Born with the same feeling and sense perception of adults, infants are endlessly experiencing internal sensations and connected feelings. Yet they have no ability to modify, adjust, sidetrack, distract, or attend to their sensations and affective information. Again, infants and children cannot self-manage, understand, or regulate any of their internal biomechanics for many years after birth (Wesarg et al., 2020).

If the infant or child does not have their needs met, they will react quite quickly. They are designed to be instantly soothed and regulated. If there is no answer to their call for help, they will rapidly become scared and go into an emergency survival state. If soothed, the child will return to homeostasis. If the needs are not met, the infant almost immediately has an emergency response that consists of a full neuronal attachment cry. When this happens, the autonomic nervous system (ANS) and CNS instantly become electrically charged and inflamed (Kendall-Tackett, 2009; Kendall-Tackett et al., 2003; Porges, 1998, 2003, 2011), which is experienced as pain (Diseth, 2006). If you have ever had inflammation or a pinched nerve, this is likely a similar feeling to that of the attachment cry response. This may explain why a child who was left alone but is later picked up after an attachment cry/attack pulls away from their caregiver. The touch and holding stops a dissociative reaction to the pain of attachment/detachment inflammation. It could also explain why some people feel pain when touched.

The infant or child who is left alone in chronic pain, with unmet needs, or who is being harmed by others, will quickly make the neurobiological assumption that their needs will not or cannot be met. If this happens often, the infant or child will experience terrifying feelings of abandonment and vulnerable aloneness. Because they are too little to run or too ineffectual or incapable of fight, often dissociation is the only way to manage this legitimate, scientifically proven, unbearable pain (Schore, 2022). Dissociation is the only way for an infant to survive abandonment; it is a last-ditch effort of coping. They are quiet and still until hopefully another human comes along to rescue them or to numb out the pain of prolonged suffering.

Our goal is to help the child who is in pain to be relieved of that pain, no matter what the source of it is. We do this usually through comfort, soothing, settling, safe and secure touches, rocking, and holding. We must be aware, however, that soothing, nurturing, and care can overwhelm the infant or child and eliminate the emergency cascade response and dissociation, leaving the infant or child to feel, with full clarity, the neuronal activation and inflammation of dysregulation. If we go through the healing process too fast, the infant or child will have no option but to return to an emergency response. We need to provide care in doses the infant or child can tolerate. This is the art of the work we are trying to achieve.

How do we move the body to a place of healing, where the pain is felt and soothed, without reinforcing the emergency response that is always accompanied with pain? Our intuition as clinicians can and will guide us. If you are stuck or afraid in a session or getting overwhelmed by the child's stuck behavior, take a moment to bring your attention inside your own body. Take a deep breath, nurture yourself by saying something like, "I'm okay, and I have the ability to settle this child. I can do this," or other supportive language. Calm yourself down and then ask, "What does this child in front of me need?" When you are calm, regulated, and self-nurtured, the answer will be there, inside your own intuitive knowing. The process of you calming down in and of itself will help. Your centering, safety, compassion, and willingness to be with this child will do many things to help. This process then becomes a "rinse and repeat" type of intervention. We keep doing this until the soothing is more dominant, or just as consistent as the chronic pain.

Dissociation in Infants and Children with Complex, Chronic Pain

Dissociation is a massive biomechanical event inside the human body and mind. We are often taught that the child somehow chooses this response or has some semblance of agency over this process. Simply put, dissociation happens or it doesn't, and occurs before fear can be registered (Lanius et al., 2018). It is neurochemically and neuroelectrically driven (Guérin-Marion et al., 2020; Lanius et al., 2018; Lebois et al., 2022), and seems to have a few main "jobs." It is a physical, mental, and awareness anesthetic, and it freezes movement and action. Dissociation, the emergency cascade defense of inaction, put the brakes on the sympathetic, emergency cascade defenses for action, which is the bullet train of fight and flight. It is one of the most powerful reaction systems in a human body, and utilized only when the possibility of death is imminent. This notion needs to be highlighted. Dissociation occurs only when the CNS deems that the next thing to happen following danger is death. This is not the land of the dying, where there is still some possibility of survival if action is taken. No, that is based in adult thought. What I am speaking of is the land of the dead, where no action is best. This is the place where helplessness, hopelessness, and inability are the only options. An infant's or child's body will typically do two things in this state—the first is to be despondent or quiet, a very common reaction in adopted infants. The other response is clinging and a hyper-focus on attachment.

Dissociation, and the multitude of inactive defenses that humans experience, is fueled by natural opioids and cannabinoids, in conjunction with instantly scattering information systems so that the integration of "data" like sensing and thinking cannot occur. Certain structures cut off sensorimotor and affective information, sort of like an internal brain shutoff valve, as our only way to escape (Kozlowska et al., 2015; Lanius et al., 2018; Mobbs et al., 2009). Dissociation prevents the realities that are causing the pain, terror, and abandonment from being known. The mechanisms for dissociation start in the periaqueductal gray (PAG) under the insula, amygdala, and other traditionally known fear response centers (Lanius et al., 2018). On the outside, dissociation may be undetectable in infants and children, but inside the body are the simultaneous needs to be very close and to pull away. Disorganized play, relating skills, affect, and attachment are common responses. As dissociation is the most common response to the lack of attachment, it can play a large part in disorganized attachment styles (Lyons-Ruth, 2015).

A way of translating this into a clinical example is to consider the child who is internally terrified and in pain, whose body is experiencing a near-death feeling but is not actually in the mouth of the tiger. Because attachment is our primary defense strategy as a species, the child will continually adapt their outward behaviors and actions in an attempt to remain attached when attachment is difficult or impossible because the parent/s attachment abilities are not engaged or the parents are dissociated themselves. As the child moves from one survival tactic to another, they develop various relating maneuvers, such as soothing the parent, cleaning things, being overly concerned with the adults around them, or they may move from one action defense to another, all under a dissociative umbrella.

What seems to be a unique human trait is that infants and children can survive harsh conditions even if they are prolonged, but surviving is very different from thriving. The main reason humans can both appear engaged but still be dissociated is that the only other system more powerful than dissociation is the attachment system. Attachment and bonding are inflexible for our species (Bowlby, 1977). The child who is in a chronically unnurtured state will be in pain, as their CNS is always inflamed.

This child will not be able to express their internal affect/feelings because of dissociation and the pain that occurs when they are no longer dissociating. A pained child can be one who has not been able to express their most basic need of safety and security. This holds especially true if the child has been victimized by organized abuse.

The Complex Problem of Working with Children with Chronic Pain and Complex Medical Presentations

As stated above, the focus of our work with complexly traumatized children in pain is learning the narrative of sensations and affect inside each child we are working with, as this is where change begins for the child. Clinicians must be comfortable with how affect drives everything, which includes being comfortable with intensely uncomfortable feelings or sensations inside of themselves. This is an oxymoronic task at best, and a vicariously traumatizing undertaking at worst, in a patriarchal, misogynistic world. Our job is to help infants and children with terror and pain by caring for them, not getting rid of their feelings. nurture them and meet the need they are requesting. Care is a strange declaration in misogynistic, patriarchal systems. Hugs and cuddles from a therapist have been frowned upon or totally removed from the clinical setting. Touch is almost universally sexualized. The loving hug between people is not typically viewed as a necessary regulation instrument. Yet it is known, through Havening especially (Ruden, 2011), that touch can produce healing, reparative, and restorative delta waves, as well as other benefits (Harper et al., 2009; Ruden, 2011).

As mentioned earlier, our task in clinically assisting young people is to regulate (self-nurture) ourselves first, then help the person in front of us, so that they learn how to eventually regulate (self-nurture) themselves. The clinician's own self-regulation and self-nurturing are key in working with infants and children who experience chronic pain and complex medical issues. Because the concepts and language of dysregulation are quite abstract, speculative, and heavily influenced by our own experiences, we can hear the words the child might be speaking and not really know from a felt sense both on the part of the child and on the part of the clinician what that word could mean. For example, one aspect of regulation requires being safe. "Safe" is an extremely subjective word and experience. What one might deem safe and okay, another could experience as unsafe and not okay. Being safe also requires being secure. My meanings of these words include the known science of the physiological and neurobiological aspects of mindfulness (Danylchuk & Forner, 2022). They also include the biomechanics of dissociation—not the commonly understood mental version of dissociation, but the full-body driven dissociation. Our current definitions of dissociation are very adult, and cognitively oriented. As has been explored in other chapters in this volume, children experience dissociation much differently than adults do. The DSM-5 does not cover the symptoms of pain, chronic pain, unrelenting terror, overworking emergent attachment systems, and the impact of being constantly afraid on our bodies and developing mind. If it did, most of what we call mental illness would likely not exist.

When working with these complex cases, it is important to hold in the back of your mind that violence is not intrinsic. A simple yet massive piece of evidence to counter the notion that humans were and are inherently violent is that dissociation, complex trauma, and post-traumatic stress disorders are rampant (Kate et al., 2020). If violence was innate in us, then we would have inborn ways that could or would deal with it. It would not be so brutally deleterious to every part of our bodies and mind. We know that humans cannot tolerate violence (Schore, 1994, 2019), but somehow we have been able to manage in very unnatural, dangerous conditions. In many ways, shame and the physical and psychological pain that go along with violence and neglect are the same language as self-hated or self-distain. We are not supposed to dislike ourselves or others. We are not supposed to fear other humans. Our task with our clients is to learn how the harm was felt and experienced in each child so that we can then figure out what needs are being evoked, and then try to meet these needs. Our response is to communicate to the child through our sensations, feelings, actions, and words that we really do have their back and are on their side. To feel another on the inside of us, as we do when neurobiologically empathic who is feeling us on their insides, and then returns these feelings with positive feelings is how kids work. Feeling is how children "talk" and communicate and is designed to be a two way shared "highway",

Changing How We Work with Complicated Medical Presentations and Chronic Pain in Children

Our clinical mission is to learn, interpret, and understand the clues and data that are communicated, via movement and affect (rather than words), by the infant and/or child about what is wrong with them. Our main undertaking is to then either help the adults around that child meet the needs of the child, or for us to meet the child's needs directly. When a child's needs are met, the body goes into an entirely different state of being from when their needs are not being met. This includes chronic pain. I realize we cannot get rid of some types of chronic pain, but a child who is treated in a medical system that teaches its practitioners to be intellectual, logical, and emotionally stoic so they do not get attached is going to feel a lot different with this type of from the child treated by a professional who is capable of healing touch, like Havening or therapeutic swaddling, swaying, and holding within an attitude of compassion, tenderness, respect, and dignity, all while being also shame-sensitive and dissociation-aware (Salter & Hall, 2022). A child who feels loved and connected while in a state of pain responds to the world and those around them vastly different from a child who feels alone, removed, and in pain. A child who is in chronic physical pain and is responded to with tenderness and compassion from a responsible other who is concerned with their co-regulation/co-nurturance does not have to attend to the emergency and terrifying experience of perceived aloneness and abandonment. This child will have an entirely different experience than a child who is left alone. These two children, even if they had the exact same experiences, are going act, speak, and be very different based on their treatment.

I do acknowledge that using the language "its not terribly complicated" might sound trivial. In no uncertain terms is the harm and neglect of a young human being okay, in any way. As uncomplicated as our main goal is, achieving this goal is extremely, and often, unimaginably hard. Working with harmed humans is hard, because the injuries we are talking about are not from tiger attacks or the occasional natural disaster. Animal predation is fairly simple to heal as humans have a lot of innate body and affect physiological, unconscious functions such as shaking, sweating, crying, yawing, sneezing, sleeping, moving, taking actions and many other biological responses to deal and manage these types of emergency events. But many of these healing/processing responses are different for humans than other animals.

Our need for others is not just about safety in numbers. Others are needed to shape our sense of self, they are needed to regulate/nurture/soothe/process all our bodily functions, including the emergency cascade responses. Others are needed to assist with managing co-consciousness and the side-effects of having long-term memory (perceived threat). Our attachment is not just about being physically safe, it is really about the need for others input into our existence, for us to fully exist. It is all the nuances of attachment as a defense. Attachment, for human, not only helps us avoid predation and threat, but it is also the "other" who nurtures and help us move from cascade emergency responses, that are affectively and sensorily painful and frightening, to a neuronally different state of safe and secure again. It is others who help us process the information that occurs while we are coming out of a cascade defense. It is the other who is needed that assist with the experience of post-emergency association, through safe grief and secure loss. It is others who help prevent PTSD, DD's and many other mental health problems from occurring in the first place.

Emergency responses in our clients will continue if they do not get help. Without help, dissociation or other cascade defenses that are used to continually survive will be activated when safety, security, nurturance, and regulation are not present. Once a person is in a perpetual state of survival, healing will always feel threatening because the pain is real, the threat is current, stuck, and frozen inside the body. This also means that the trust and the utilitarian need for others will be broken. The only reason someone is in a dissociated state is that no one helped that person out of it. This is experienced as a fundamental species betrayal. The innate "social contract" of our species, to nurture each other and help soothe, has been broken, and this is hard to repair—especially if you as a clinician have not healed your own trauma, or if the you are in an emergency response yourself.

It is unending pain and terror that drives all dissociation. Our task is to help heal the pain by nurturing, soothing, and attaching to the pained, silenced, or ignored aspects of that child. We do this by providing mindful care, which instantly drops dissociation barriers, as all the feelings and need for regulated help come flooding out. When working with children with complex medical presentations and chronic pain, we must consider that soothing, comfort, and attention all bring forth the pain of the emergency response. Care can feel like it hurts in the case of human harm. For example, perhaps the child you're working with was hugged by their father after he raped them. In this situation, a hug that should be for healing and a part of secure attachment is now a booby-trapped and associated as a part of the abuse.

One of my clients was a six-year-old boy who presented as quiet and reserved. He tightly held on to a Spider-Man figure. I noticed that when I moved my body, his body stiffened, and I also felt scared and on guard. I knew these were not my feelings but his (from my human attribute of empathy). Listening to my intuition and being attuned, I could tell that this child needed the feeling of protection and to contain it. My problem was to figure out how I could get under the fear and reach his physiological need for human connection. Empathy and interoception, attunement, intuition, and differentiating my feelings from his all informed my clinical decisions.

In this case, I used transitional objects—stuffed animals. When I asked him if one of the animals could hang out with him and help him feel like there was something warm and soft between him and the world, his choice was a large, fluffy lion. I said to him, "Your body seems scared" (I was trying to help him put words and meaning to his inner physiology of fear). His body changed when the stuffy was introduced. I then highlighted what a difference the stuffed animal made by stating out loud, "Ah, that seemed to do something. Does it feel different inside of you?" Again, I was helping him put words and meaning to his inner physiology of the sensorimotor and affective "data" influencing his behavior. I labeled the difference I saw and drew his attention to the change (the start of self-nurturing). He relaxed. This, for him, was the beginning of learning that after feelings of fear, relaxing feelings can and do follow, just as he can learn the difference between comforting hugs and hurtful hugs.

To get the best view of what is happening in a child's inner world, the typical adult-like projection that is so often placed onto children's behaviors and internal experiences must be deconstructed and replaced with a better comprehension of what is really happening inside infants and children. Infants and children communicate via movement, impulses, and sounds for at least the first three years of life. The processes of thinking and the words that go with those thoughts are often decades away from an infant's or child's repertoire of self-expression and awareness. For example, how does a child describe the pain of juvenile rheumatoid arthritis? How can a child articulate, in any real, meaningful way, the pain of sexual abuse? How does a child coherently describe the inner experience of both physical pain or chronic illness and sadistic sexual abuse—which, by the way, is often a common cluster of experiences? How can a child accurately describe the land mines of odd attachment and pain that come with a parent who has Munchausen syndrome by proxy or practices fanatical religious behavior? It is impossible for them to do so, for so many reasons.

These convoluted concepts are experienced as feelings and sensations to a child. They end up get labeled as they are experienced: "Something is wrong (with me), I am/feel bad, I am unlovable, I'm disgusting." They get experienced through the process of dissociation ("This is not happening to me"). They are labeled by the ones doing the harm: "This pain is necessary to help you heal," "This is good for you," "This is what love is," "This is what you deserve," "You are disgusting, bad, horrible, my play thing," "I own you," "I brought you into this world, and I can take you out."

As clinicians, we must, in many ways, view language and words as a leaf on a tsunami. They are not as important as what our young clients are feeling. We must learn to give credence and credibility to the way each child moves, the pitches of their screams, the frequency of their silence, the direction of their eyes. We must learn the specific language of sensory information, movements, and feelings of each individual child.

This is the challenge of working with this clinical population. How does a therapist, healer, or helper gain enough insight and information from the sensorimotor and affective data the child or infant is expressing and then accurately and cohesively interpret these inner experiences so as to find a real neurobiological, needs-meeting solution?

Feeling and sensing are humans' first language. The feelings infants and children have are very real, very important, and vital in communicating their needs. Feelings, sensations, and the felt sense inside of their bodies, like chronic pain, terror, or frozen dissociation, are part of the affective narrative of the infant or child. This narrative will look like frustration, rejection of a parent's hugs and cuddles, repetitive behavior, tummy aches, headaches, screaming, kicking, extreme quietness, gazing off into the distance, being inconsolable, thrashing, fawning over or hyper-focus on the adults around them, difficulty engaging with other children, hitting, choking, and slapping other people, hyper-independence, and so much more. These actions and reactions all tell a story. A kicking child might mean a terror response, or it could mean a need to run or push. All these movements and affect have information within them that help us get a better understanding of what is happening inside the child. The most amazing part of this form of communication is that as adults we have the proverbial "Rosetta Stone" inside of us, but it will only work if we are in a place of regulation/self-nurturance. This is another piece that makes this work hard. Staying regulated while a child is literally melting down, when words don't work, is hard.

Again, to do this best, we as clinicians and researchers must learn about ourselves first. We must learn about our internal worlds of sensorimotor and affective information. We must discover if we are dissociated, triggered, or full of biases when we are around infants and children, and work on these issues. We must find absolute comfort, internal safety, and security as a baseline for ourselves and these children. The hardest part in working with infants and children in pain is learning how to find absolute or nearly absolute CNS regulation within us. This is a very hard part of this work.

Necessary Paradigm Shifts in Working with Infants and Children Who Have Chronic Pain, Medical Issues, and Complicated Clinical Presentations

Humans are a curious neurobiological species. There are what one might call "rules" or biological imperatives that are dictated by our genetic and epigenetic information. Evolution made us the unique species we are. These biomechanical, neuroelectrical, and neurochemical musts are absolutes for our species. The one basic rule that every living creature must follow is to be, and to stay, alive. In strange ways, for humans, everything revolves around this basic principle. The strangeness resides in the uniquely evolved homo sapiens defense of being tame or domesticated (Belyaev, 1979; Hare, 2017). We use safety from others, instead of safety in ourselves. We evolved to be cared for, throughout our whole lives, by other people. It is this need for care from others, more than we can create on our own, that is one of the main differences in our species. We are the only animals, that we are aware of, that use *being cared for* as our one and only protection from predation and as an encourager of life.

As adults, we are equipped to consciously regulate our inner bodies and minds as well as regulate our young. This is our primary protection as a species: being regulated in a large group of other people who help regulate other people. The need for others to help us reach our adult developmental milestones is our one and only defense mechanism (Kenkel et al., 2019). Instead of claws, sharp teeth, camouflage, speed, or thick skin, we evolved with empathy, attunement, self- and co-regulation, and awareness of self and others, and this is fostered through safe and secure relationships with others (Emmott & Page, 2021).

This basic rule plays a huge part in therapy with infants and children. They need to experience an other who is regulated, empathic, attuned, and aware, and who can be present with the infant's or child's intense affect and be able to fully regulate themselves as well as the child. Your regulation is the foundation to their regulation. These are dexterities that are not typically discussed in postsecondary institutions. Learn to understand your own regulated/self-nurtured baseline and then trust that this is what is needed to help these children.

What Care Is Like in a Mindful/Secure Attached Environment: Treatment

The evidence of how astounding the state of mindfulness is and of how this state is the same as that of someone who is securely attached is overwhelming (Snyder et al., 2012). The impressive functions of the ventral medial prefrontal cortex, the default mode network, and the salient stress network when in a mindful state support the conclusion that they could only have developed in a safe and secure environment (Forner, 2019a; Hölzel, Carmody, et al., 2011; Hölzel, Lazar, et al., 2011; Kang et al., 2013; Lazar et al., 2000, 2005; Luders et al., 2009; Siegel, 2017). Full mindfulness and secure attachment come from structures that are developed in only two ways: by growing and developing around mindful people, or by practicing some type of mindful or meditative method many times a day. Fear, lack, suffering, pain, and terror prevent these brain structures from growing, developing, or working as they are designed to. When we are in a mindful, safe, secure, regulated state, it will impact others who are not, in tangible, triggering, potent ways. Mindfulness, or secure care, eliminates dissociative barriers.

As stated above, but worth repeating, dissociation is in many ways the body's natural anesthetic, whereby powerful natural opioids and cannabinoids are secreted to manage physical and psychological chronic pain (Lanius, 2015; Lanius et al., 2006, 2014, 2018). When this pain happens and no help occurs, an infant's or child's body will "read" this as aloneness on some level. And for infants and children, being alone equates to a real, actual vulnerability of death.

Evolutionarily, abandonment equals the huge risk of being eaten. The fear is felt as that of imminent death because that is what is happening. That infant is literally and neurobiologically moving into emergency responses of dying and death. The child, in looking for help, feels pain. To assist in healing these wounds, we have to understand that the offering and presenting of innate, empathic care is what the feelings and needs, which are alive and well underneath the dissociative barrier/s, are seeking. Like all feelings, emergency responses are part of communicating our needs. The big feelings that are scary and painful are seeking care.

When children first come to be helped, their suffering and pain will be expressed first, which may not look to us as though they are accepting of the help and support we offer. Despite this, they need to be met with gentleness while the pain works its way out of their bodies. In other words, we have to help children and infants feel their painful feelings, and not reject the feelings or pull away. We do this with safe touches, holding, protecting, shhh-ing, and rocking, all of which we teach to the caregiving system, and offer transitional objects that are comforting and soothing, befriending, and that teach them about psychological and physical pain. Our adult fear and discomfort, if we do not self-regulate, will teach the child to be fearful and uncomfortable, as well as add to their dysregulation. Our soothing, comfort, gentleness, and regulation will teach the child what this feels like, what it is experienced as, what needs to be done to handle (regulate) the feelings.

Humans are born with these innate ways of helping injured infants and children heal. As mentioned above, a better word for mindfulness in this work with children is *securefulness*. Danylchuk & Forner (2022), describe securefulness as follows.

> Securefulness is a combination of the theory and research surrounding secure attachment and the theory, research, and best practices of trauma-informed mindfulness. Securefulness is a new concept which recognizes the connections between the biopsychosocial process of attachment and the neurological, psychological, and social impacts of mindfulness practices.
>
> *(p. 387)*

Securefulness hypothesizes that the state of mindfulness, different from ordinary consciousness, is the groundwork of what is required for meaningful change (Cahn & Polich, 2006; Goleman & Davidson, 2018; Shapiro, 1980; Siegel, 2017). Mindfulness is an embodied state, where the mind is not focused on just thoughts but also on sensations, affective information, and intuition. In a therapeutic context, the same brain structures that are responsible for mindful states are engaged during interactions with the infant or child. The state of mindfulness is incredibly powerful and one of the few, if not the only, therapeutic interventions that change not only the function of the brain but also its structures (Forner, 2019b; Hölzel, Carmody, et al., 2011; Kang et al., 2013; Lazar et al., 2000, 2005; Luders et al., 2009). There are very few interventions that alter the structure of the brain (Manthey et al., 2021). This speaks to the power of mindfulness for both the clinician and child, and, if possible, the parent/s as well. The states of mindfulness and secure attachment, which are basically the same thing, play a huge part in the development of a mature, fully developed adult. Infants and children expect every adult to be like this.

In my practice with infants and children, I have found it helpful to use the Five S's found in the book *The Happiest Baby on the Block* (Karp, 2015), which are swaddling, swaying, shushing, sucking, on the side. For infants, this is rather easy; for children, I have to follow the child's comfort and tolerance level, or encourage the parent to use these skills, but the goal is to eventually get to a place where you can safely and securely wrap a child in a blanket or weighted blanket, on their side, with rhythmic sounds of waves or heart beats playing, or by patting them on their back with your hand in gentle, soothing ways, and letting them lie down on their side while sucking a candy or soother. I try to help them feel safe by asking them to feel, not think about, what their bodies are doing. I try to help them by lying on the floor with them and, with permission, writing letters, numbers, or shapes on their back to help them feel their bodies settling. I try to soothe the feelings of terror or dissociation and help them feel settled, comforted, and regulated. And, if possible, I always invite the caregivers in the room to teach them how to settle and soothe themselves first, then soothe their children.

Conclusion

We live in a world that is dominated by top-down practices, where intellect and cognition have the top billing in human understanding, and feelings are usually met with repugnance. This is a direct consequence of misogynist, patriarchal societies, a consequence of cultures that are extremely dysregulated, and in which the collective memory of how to regulate our infants has been lost. If we view infants and children as instinctual beings who feel and sense just as adults do, then perhaps everything could or would change. If we viewed our infants as beings who feel as adults do but who can do absolutely nothing about their feelings except rely on those around them for help, perhaps this too might change things. If there was more acknowledgment that the infant's or child's expressed feelings are a guide to how to help them, then perhaps we would view things from the bottom up, where the body and feelings are more important or equally as important as the mind.

Our young communicate using the narrative of the body, its feelings and sensations. Our job as clinicians is to learn the language of each child's affective information as it manifests somatically, because that affective information is letting us know what is needed. Hunger needs food, thirst needs water, fear needs soothing, attention needs attention, shame or "I am not a good enough human" needs connection, terror needs safety, and insecurity needs security. Our children make sense. It is our task to follow their logic and help them learn to regulate themselves and what is happening in their bodies. Our task is to meet their needs, and to recognize that, for humans, the needs to be assured and reassured, comforted, soothed, safely and securely touched, and neuronally settled are as vital as food and air. This is what heals traumatized infants and children, and this is what we all thrive on.

References

Anand, K. J., & Hickey, P. R. (1987). Pain and its effects in the human neonate and fetus. *New England of Medicine, 317*(21), 1321–1329. https://doi.org.10.1056/NEJM198711193172105

Barrett, L. F. (2020). *Seven and a half lessons about the brain.* Houghton Mifflin.

Bellieni, C. V. (2019). New insights into fetal pain. *Seminars in Fetal and Neonatal Medicine, 24*(4), Article 101001. https://doi.org/10.1016/j.siny.2019.04.001

Belyaev, D. K. (1979). Destabilizing selection as a factor in domestication. *Journal of Heredity, 70*(5), 301–308.

Bowlby, J. (1977). The making and breaking of affectional bonds: I. Aetiology and psychopathology in the light of attachment theory. *British Journal of Psychiatry, 130*(3), 201–210. https://doi.org/10.1192/bjp.130.3.201

Cahn, B. R., & Polich, J. (2006). Meditation states and traits: EEG, ERP, and neuroimaging studies. *Psychological Bulletin, 132*(2), 180–211. https://doi.org/10.1037/0033-2909.132.2.180

Cerritelli, F., Frasch, M. G., Antonelli, M. C., Viglione, C., Vecchi, S., Chiera, M., & Manzotti, A. (2021). A review on the vagus nerve and autonomic nervous system during fetal development: Searching for critical windows. *Frontiers in Neuroscience, 15*, Article 721605. https://doi.org/10.3389/fnins.2021.721605

Danylchuk, L., & Forner, C. (2022). Securefulness: A care-centered approach to therapy. In E. Christensen (Ed.), *Perspectives of dissociative identity response: Ethics, historical and cultural issues.* (pp. 387–416). HWC Press.

Diseth, T. H. (2006). Dissociation following traumatic medical treatment procedures in childhood: A longitudinal follow-up. *Development and Psychopathology, 18*(1), 233–251. https://www.cambridge.org/core/journals/development-and-psychopathology/article/abs/dissociation-following-traumatic-medical-treatment-procedures-in-childhood-a-longitudinal-followup/ECAA20FCEA4F9B00C58AF28543CAD9AF

Emmott, E. H., & Page, A. E. (2021). Alloparenting. In T. Shackelford & V. A. Weekes-Shackelford (Eds.), *Encyclopedia of evolutionary psychological science* (pp. 210–223). Springer.

Forner, C. (2019a). Mindful attachment: An organic way to work with children who have been through complex trauma and neglect. *Frontiers in the Psychotherapy of Trauma and Dissociation, 3*(1), 91–106. https://doi.org/10.46716/ftpd.2019.0027

Forner, C. (2019b). What mindfulness can learn about dissociation and what dissociation can learn from mindfulness. *Journal of Trauma & Dissociation, 20*(1), 1–15. https://doi.org/10.1080/15299732.2018.1502568

Gogtay, N., Giedd, J. N., Lusk, L., Hayashi, K. M., Greenstein, D., Vaituzis, A. C., Nugent, T., Herman, D. H., Clasen, L., Toga, A., Rapoport, J. L., & Thompson, P. (2004). Dynamic mapping of human cortical development during childhood through early adulthood. *Proceedings of the National Academy of Sciences of the United States of America, 101*(21), 8174–8179. https://doi.org/10.1073/pnas.0402680101

Goleman, D., & Davidson, R., (2018). *Altered traits: Science reveals how meditation changes your mind, brain and body.* Avery.

Guérin-Marion, C., Sezlik, S., & Bureau, J. F. (2020). Developmental and attachment-based perspectives on dissociation: Beyond the effects of maltreatment. *European Journal of Psychotraumatology, 11*(1), Article 1802908. https://doi.org/10.1080/20008198.2020.1802908

Hare, B. (2017). Survival of the friendliest: Homo sapiens evolved via selection for prosociality. *Annual Review of Psychology, 68*, 155–186. https://doi.org/10.1146/annurev-psych-010416-044201

Harper, L., Rasolkhani-Kalhorn, T., & Drozd, F. (2009). On the neural basis of EMDR therapy: Insights from qEEG studies. *Traumatology, 15*(2), 81–95. https://doi.org/10.1177/1534765609338498

Hoemann, K., Xu, F., & Barrett, L. F. (2019). Emotion words, emotion concepts, and emotional development in children: A constructionist hypothesis. *Developmental Psychology, 55*(9), 1830–1849. https://doi.org/10.1037/dev0000686

Hölzel, B. K., Carmody, J., Vangel, M., Yerramsetti, S. M., Gard, T., & Lazar, S. W. (2011). Mindfulness practice leads to increases in regional brain gray matter density. *Psychiatry Research Neuroimaging, 191*(1), 36–43. https://doi.org/10.1016/j.pscychresns.2010.08.006

Hölzel, B. K., Lazar, S., Gard, T., Schuman-Oliver, Z., Vago, D., & Ott, U. (2011). How does mindfulness meditation work? Proposing mechanisms of action from a conceptual and neural perspective. *Perspectives on Psychological Science, 6*(6), 537–559. https://doi.org/10.1177/1745691611419671

Kang, D. H., Jo, H. J., Kim, S. H., Jung, Y. H., Choi, C. H., Lee., U. S., An, S. C., Jang, J. H., & Kwon, J. S. (2013). The effect of meditation on brain structure: Cortical thickness mapping and diffusion tensor imaging. *SCAN, 8*, 27–33. https://doi.org/10.1093/scan/nss056

Karp, H. (2015). *The happiest baby on the block: The new way to calm crying and help your newborn baby sleep longer* (Revised and updated 2nd ed.). Bantam.

Kate, M.A., Hopwood, T., & Jamieson, G. (2020). The prevalence of dissociative disorders and dissociative experiences in college populations: A meta-analysis of 98 studies. *Journal of Trauma & Dissociation, 21*(1), 16–61. https://doi.org/10.1080/15299732.2019.1647915

Kendall-Tackett, K. (2009). Psychological trauma and physical health: A psychoneuroimmunology approach to etiology of negative health effects and possible interventions. *Psychological Trauma: Theory, Research, Practice, and Policy, 1*(1), 35–48. https://doi.org/10.1037/a0015128

Kendall-Tackett, K. A., Marshall, R., & Ness, K. E. (2003). Chronic pain syndromes and violence against women. *Women and Therapy, 26*, 45–56. https://doi.org/10.1300/J015v26n01_03

Kenkel, W. M., Perkeybile, A. M., & Carter, C. S. (2019). The neurobiological causes and effects of alloparenting. *Developmental Neurobiology, 77*(2), 214–232.

Kozlowska, K., Walker, P., McLean, L., & Carrive, P. (2015). Fear and the defense cascade: Clinical implications and management. *Harvard Review of Psychiatry, 23*(4), 263–287. https://doi.org/10.1097/HRP.0000000000000065

Lanius, R. A. (2015). Trauma-related dissociation and altered states of consciousness: A call for clinical, treatment, and neuroscience research. *European Journal of Psychotraumatology, 6*, Article 27905.

Lanius, R. A., Boyd, J. E., McKinnon, M. C., Nicholson, A. A., Frewen, P., Vermetten, E., & Spiegel, D. (2018). A review of the neurobiological basis of trauma-related dissociation and its relation to cannabinoid- and opioid-mediated stress response: A transdiagnostic, translational approach. *Current Psychiatry Reports, 20*(12), Article 118. https://doi.org/10.1007/s11920-018-0983-y

Lanius, R., Lanius, U., Fisher, J., & Ogden, P. (2006). Psychological trauma and the brain: Toward a neurological treatment model. In P. Ogden, K. Minton & C. Pain (Eds.), *Trauma and the body: A sensorimotor approach to psychotherapy* (pp. 139–161). W. W. Norton.

Lanius, U. F., Paulsen, S. L., & Corrigan, F. M. (2014). *Neurobiology and treatment of traumatic dissociation: Towards an embodied self.* Springer.

Lasselin, J. (2021). Back to the future of psychoneuroimmunology: Studying inflammation-induced sickness behavior. *Brain, Behavior, & Immunity – Health, 18*, Article 100379. https://doi.org/10.1016/j.bbih.2021.100379

Lazar, S., Bush, G., Gollub, R., Fricchione, G., Gurucharan, K., & Benson, H. (2000). Functional brain mapping of the relaxation response and meditation. *NeuroReport, 11*(7), 1581–1585. https://doi.org/10.1097/00001756-200005150-00042

Lazar, S., Kerr, C., Wasserman, R., Gray, J., Greve, D., Treadway, M., & Fischl, B. (2005). Meditation experience is associated with increased cortical thickness. *NeuroReport, 16*(17), 1893–1897. https://doi.org/10.1097/01.wnr.0000186598.66243.19

Lebois, L. A., Kumar, P., Palermo, C. A., Lambros, A. M., O'Connor, L., Wolff, J. D., Baker, J., Gruber, S., Lewis-Schroeder, N., Ressler, K. J., Robinson, M. A., Winternitz, S., Nickerson, L. D., & Kaufman, M. L. (2022). Deconstructing dissociation: A triple network model of trauma-related dissociation and its subtypes. *Neuropsychopharmacology, 47*, 2261–2270.

Lopez, B., Schwartz, S. J., Prado, G., Campo, A. E., & Pantin, H. (2008). Adolescent neurological development and its implications for adolescent substance use prevention. *Journal of Primary Prevention, 29*(1), 5–35. https://doi.org/10.1007/s10935-007-0119-3

Luders, E., Toga, A. W., Lepore, N., & Gaser, C. (2009). The underlying anatomical correlates of long-term meditation: Larger hippocampal and frontal volumes of gray matter. *Journal of Neuroimaging, 45*(3), 672–678. https://doi.org/10.1016/j.neuroimage.2008.12.061

Lyons-Ruth, K. (2015). Dissociation and the parent–infant dialogue: A longitudinal perspective from attachment research. *Attachment, 9*(3), 253–276.

Manthey, A., Sierk, A., Brakemeier, E. L., Walter, H., & Daniels, J. K. (2021). Does trauma-focused psychotherapy change the brain? A systematic review of neural correlates of therapeutic gains in PTSD. *European Journal of Psychotraumatology, 12*(1), Article 1929025. https://doi.org/10.1080/20008198.2021.1929025

Mobbs, D., Marchant, J. L., Hassabis, D., Seymour, B., Tan, G., Gray, M., Petrovic, P., Dolan, R. J., & Frith, C. D. (2009). From threat to fear: The neural organization of defensive fear systems in humans. *Journal of Neuroscience, 29*(39), 12236–12243. https://doi.org/10.1523/JNEUROSCI.2378-09.2009

Ogden, P. (2021). The different impact of trauma and relational stress on physiology, posture, and movement: Implications for treatment. *European Journal of Trauma & Dissociation, 5*(4), Article 100172. https://doi.org/10.1016/j.ejtd.2020.100172

Perkeybile, A. M., Carter, C. S., Wroblewski, K. L., Puglia, M. H., Kenkel, W. M., Lillard, T. S., Karaoli, T., Gregory, S. G., Mohammadi, N., Epstein, L., Bales, K., L., & Connelly, J. J. (2019). Early nurture epigenetically tunes the oxytocin receptor. *Psychoneuroendocrinology, 99*, 128–136. https://doi.org/10.1016/j.psyneuen.2018.08.037

Perrus, K., Sisk, C. L., & Romeo, R., D. (2021). Review: Coming of age: The neurobiology and psychobiology of puberty and adolescence. *Journal of Youth Adolescence, 50*, 1738–1740. https://doi.org/10.1007/s10964-021-01439-7

Porges, S. W. (1998). Love: An emergent property of the mammalian autonomic nervous system. *Journal of Psychoneuroendocrinology, 23*(8), 837–861. https://doi.org/10.1016/S0306-4530(98)00057-2

Porges, S. W. (2003). The polyvagal theory: Phylogenetic contributions to social behavior. *Journal of Physiology & Behavior, 79*(3), 503–513. https://doi.org/10.1016/S0031-9384(03)00156-2

Porges, S. W. (2011). *The polyvagal theory: Neurophysiological foundations of emotions, attachment, communication and self-regulation*. W. W. Norton.

Quigley, K. S., Kanoski, S., Grill, W. M., Barrett, L. F., & Tsakiris, M. (2021). Functions of interoception: From energy regulation to experience of the self. *Trends in Neurosciences, 44*(1), 29–38.

Ruden, R. (2011). *When the past is always present: Emotional traumatization, causes, and cures*. Routledge.

Salter, M., & Hall, H. (2022). Reducing shame, promoting dignity: A model for the primary prevention of complex post-traumatic stress disorder. *Trauma, Violence, & Abuse, 23*(3), 906–919. https://doi.org/10.1177/1524838020979667

Schore, A. (1994). *Affect regulation and the origin of the self*. Lawrence Erlbaum Associates.

Schore, A. N. (2019). *The development of the unconscious mind*. W. W. Norton.

Schore, A. N. (2022). Attachment trauma and the developing right brain: Origins of pathological dissociation and some implications for psychotherapy. In M. J. Dorahy, S. N. Gold & J. A. O'Neil (Eds.), *Dissociation and the dissociative disorders* (2nd ed., pp. 177–208). Routledge.

Shapiro, D. H. (Ed.). (1980). *Meditation: Self-regulation strategy and altered state of consciousness* (1st ed.). Routledge. https://doi.org/10.4324/9780203785881

Siegel, D. (2017). *Mind: A journey to the heart of being human*. W. W. Norton.

Snyder, R., Shapiro, S., & Treleaven, D. (2012). Attachment theory and mindfulness. *Journal of Child and Family Studies, 21*, 709–717.

Vastag, B. (2003). Scientists find connections in the brain between physical and emotional pain. *JAMA, 290*(18), 2389–2390. https://doi.org/10.1001/jama.290.18.2389

Wesarg, C., Van Den Akker, A. L., Oei, N. Y., Hoeve, M., & Wiers, R. W. (2020). Identifying pathways from early adversity to psychopathology: A review on dysregulated HPA axis functioning and impaired self-regulation in early childhood. *European Journal of Developmental Psychology, 17*(6), 808–827. https://doi.org/10.1080/17405629.2020.1748594

Wickrama, K. A. S., O'Neal, C. W., & Holmes, C. (2017). Towards a heuristic research model linking early socioeconomic adversity and youth cumulative disease risk: An integrative review. *Adolescent Research Review, 2*, 161–179.https://doi.org/10.1007/s40894-017-0054-3

Yilmaz, H., Arslan, C., & Arslan, E. (2022). The effect of traumatic experiences on attachment styles. *Anales de Psicología/Annals of Psychology, 38*(3), 489–498. https://doi.org/10.6018/analesps.489601

45
"MIND CONTROL" IN RITUALISTIC AND OTHER EXTREME AND DISSOCIATION-SAVVY ABUSE

Ellen Lacter

Introduction

This chapter describes the nature of "abusive mind control," the psychological manipulations that abusers systematically inflict on victims, usually beginning in early childhood, to control their minds and behavior, and a discussion of psychotherapeutic approaches to help victimized children and adolescents to work to overcome these controls.

The content of this chapter is a synthesis of information obtained from the following sources: (1) my work with child, adolescent, and adult clients, (2) qualitative research with psychotherapists reporting personal histories of ritualistic abuse and mind control (Lacter et al., 2012), (3) accounts and memoirs of other therapist-survivors and victim-activists, (4) colleagues whose work I know through consultation, and (5) research and professional writings on ritualistic abuse and abusive mind control (Becker et al., 2007; Lacter, 2011; Miller, 2012; Noblitt & Noblitt, 2014; Salter, 2017; Schröder et al., 2020; Sinason, 2018).

Note: The material in this chapter has the potential to cause the reader significant psychological distress as it describes abuse that is highly systematic, sadistic, and extreme.

The Nature of Abusive Mind Control

Definition

Abusive mind control, aka *programming*, can be defined as psychological manipulations systematically inflicted on victims, usually beginning in early childhood, intended to control victims' behavior long-term or life-long. Mind control aims to produce thoughts, beliefs, perceptions, memories, pain, terror, and other emotional, somatosensory, and physiological states, to compel behaviors that serve abuser objectives, including execution of acts that violate victims' volition, principles, and instinct for self-preservation.

Application of Mind Control to Victims' Dissociated Self-States

Abusers systematically apply mind control strategies to dissociated "self-states," aka "identities," within their victims. This includes self-states that they systematically induce to form, as well as self-states previously established in victims' minds through either mind control or organic defensive dissociative processes. Abusers confine mind control to dissociated self-states to prevent "normative-life" self-states – that is, those who typically control conscious executive mental functions – from encoding their abuse and from discovering their programmed self-states, the internal effects of the mind control, and the behaviors executed under mind control.

In recovery, usually years later, when normative-life self-states may recall the mind control inflicted upon their dissociated self-states, they can apply executive mental functions, including critical thinking and purposive action, to overcoming mind control's effects and control.

Proposed Classification of Subtypes of Abusive Mind Control

In this section, I propose a classification of subtypes of mind control strategies. I describe the strategies that abusers apply in each subtype to psychologically manipulate their victims, including examples from child, adolescent, and adult survivors. The purpose of distinguishing amongst these subtypes is to make each form understandable within well-established psychological mechanisms, and thereby, less ominous and more manageable in recovery.

Conditioning

Conditioning victims' thoughts and behavior may be the most common method of "installing" mind control. It generally includes abuse or torture, and is applied in three forms:

OPERANT CONDITIONING

In abusive mind control, operant conditioning, that is, punishment and reward, is used to shape the thoughts and behavior of designated self-states. A particular focus is to condition victims to squelch any attempt at disclosure and to prevent victims from receiving help and protection. One common set-up is to manipulate a child to develop trust in a particular individual in order to encourage the child to risk disclosing the abuse to this person. Unbeknownst to the child, this person is connected to the abuser network. When the child makes the disclosure, the abusers severely punish the child and make such statements as: "We know everything you think and we see and hear everything you do. There is no escape."

Hans Ulrich Gresch, a German psychologist, Cold War mind control survivor, and author of a book on abusive mind control (Gresch, 2010), provided me with the following complex example of operant conditioning (personal communication, 2008). In a training session, his abusers were programming his "mediator" self-state, whom his abusers named "Peter Munk," to internally maintain the obedience of all of his other programmed self-states. This strategy used operant conditioning by proxy to train Peter Munk to allocate memories as follows:

> The flower game: Forget me and forget-me-not – A perpetrator confronts the child with a list of common words like cow, flower, chair, or so. Every word is connected with "forget me" or "forget-me-not". The list becomes longer and longer. The child is punished if he/she remembers or forgets the wrong words. Then the day of the big test comes. Target child [Peter Munk] is not tested, but another, expendable child. The test is staged as a ritual, maybe a Satanic ritual. When the tested child makes a mistake, the master of ceremonies kills this expendable child with a knife in front of the eyes of the target child.

CLASSICAL CONDITIONING

In classical conditioning within mind control, abusers expose the victim to an unconditioned stimulus paired with the stimulus they seek to condition, in order to evoke a conditioned response to the conditioned stimulus alone. For example, abusers classically condition designated self-states in victims to associate sexual or physical abuse/torture with positive emotions. To accomplish this, they may administer a psychoactive drug (e.g., cocaine), to induce the unconditioned response of euphoria. While drugged, the child is sexually or physically abused. The designated self-state now associates the conditioned stimulus of abuse with positive affect, the desired conditioned response.

FEAR CONDITIONING

Fear conditioning is a form of classical conditioning and a mainstay of mind control. Abusers apply abuse, often torture-level (unconditioned stimuli), to a designated dissociated self-state to induce fear, terror, pain, or other noxious psychophysiological responses, such as, nausea, dizziness, or spinning sensations (unconditioned responses). The abusers then apply the stimulus they seek to condition, for example, a hand signal, touch, code, image, color, sound, words, or speaking the name they have assigned to the dissociated self-state (the conditioned stimulus), to produce such feelings as fear, terror, and pain (a conditioned response).

The abusers will later use conditioned stimuli alone, such as the hand signal or calling out the self-state's name, to activate or "trigger" the noxious response in the self-state who was subjected to this fear conditioning. Once activated, the self-state re-experiences the torture inflicted on it (the unconditioned stimuli) and the associated feelings, such as pain and/or fear (unconditioned responses). The pain and fear prime the self-state to comply with all directives in an effort to appease the abusers. The fear and pain tend to "spill over" into normative-life self-states, who may feel compelled to perform particular behaviors with no idea of the source or reason. Since the advent of the Internet, abusers commonly deliver "trigger" stimuli via email, texts, pop-ups, and the like, containing coded messages, disappearing messages, and images on electronic devices.

Neuroscientist Joseph Le Doux's work on fear-conditioning helps us understand the power of abusive mind control. In his book, *The Emotional Brain*, LeDoux (1996) explains that, "stimuli associated with the danger or trauma become *learned triggers* that unleash emotional reactions in us" (p. 150). Fear-conditioned responses operate "independently of consciousness" in the implicit memory system rather than in the more conscious explicit memory system. They occur quickly, instinctually, and with relative automaticity, in response to perceived threat to physical or psychic survival. Accordingly, victims of mind control experience rapid fear-conditioned noxious responses and behavioral compulsions with little or no ability to understand their source or to suppress them.

COMBINED OPERANT AND FEAR CONDITIONING

Mind control abusers often combine fear conditioning with operant conditioning to compel victims to execute involuntary behaviors. For example, the abusers combine fear and operant conditioning to compel a designated self-state in a victim to perform a specific sexual act on cue. The abusers first pair electroshock torture with the display of a picture of an apple. They then quickly command the victim to perform the sex act. Upon compliance, they reward the victim with praise. When the abusers later seek to compel the victim to perform this act, they display the picture of an apple.

The programmed self-state becomes activated and feels compelled to perform the sexual act to avoid electroshock and to win favor.

Similar combinations of fear and operant conditioning are used to compel many forms of compliance, acts of violence, self-harm, suicidality, and more. For example, a fear-conditioned self-state may have also been operant-conditioned to report the victim's activities to the abusers and to self-injure upon any failure to report in on schedule. In response to any effort to defy this programming, this self-state may self-injure, or normative-life self-states may experience a perplexing ego-dystonic compulsion to self-injure.

Deception

Deception may be the second most commonly applied strategy in the installation of mind control. Deception includes use of lies, trickery, film, virtual reality, holograms, staged scenarios, and impersonation to cause dissociated self-states to perceive feigned events to be real. Abusive mind control usually begins in early childhood, in turn exploiting the magical thinking and high hypnotizability of young children. Programmers know that perceptions and beliefs "installed" in the first four years of life will "stick," especially if stored in self-states dissociated from normative-life self-states.

When installing deceptions, abusers often simultaneously induce confused, suggestible, dream-like, mental states to impede the normal cognitive processes that might otherwise allow victims to discern the deceptions. Methods that increase suggestibility include hallucinogens, electrical stimulation of particular brain regions, and torture itself. Torture primes victims into states of intense, narrow attention to environmental cues, especially to the abusers on whom they depend for their survival. A psychologist-survivor explained to me: "Fear focuses attention intensely and survival information is encoded deeply."

Deceptions commonly reported by survivors include the following:

a Abusers place a child in front of a mirror, project an image of an eye onto the child's forehead, and tell the child that this is their all-seeing eye, the eye of a demon, or something similar, that it transmits everything the child says, does, and thinks back to the abusers, and that any disobedience will be punished.
b Abusers use similar illusions to deceive victims into believing that they have placed bombs in their bodies that will detonate if they disobey any directives. In one scenario, the abusers place the child in a cage and tell the child that they have placed a bomb inside of the child's body and the same kind of bomb in a bunny that is in another cage. The abusers instruct both the child and bunny to stay in their cages until they tell them to exit. Then, the abusers open both cages. When the bunny exits the cage, the abusers shoot it and tell the child that the bunny exploded because it disobeyed them. The abusers may also tell the child that their all-seeing eye controls the bomb. This technique combines use of illusion and operant conditioning by proxy– punishment of the bunny.
c Abusers stage pseudo-surgeries to deceive victims into believing that they have placed microchips in their brains that transmit all of their thoughts back to the abusers. This strategy often includes a staged operating room, abusers dressed in surgical scrubs, a tray of surgical tools, a small cut made with a scalpel that the child can see in a mirror, etc.
d Similar strategies are used to deceive victims into perceiving a variety of other monitoring and harmful objects within their bodies, including demons, replicas of the abusers, snakes, spiders, devices that contain toxins, etc.
e Abusers use film, virtual reality, and the like, to deceive designated self-states into believing that they are victims in Nazi death camps to be punished for any disobedience. The abusers may

deceive other self-states into believing that they are death-camp executioners, to cause them to believe themselves evil, murderers, and/or Nazis. Many survivors who initially believed they were tortured in Nazi concentration camps later realized that these memories were in black and white with flashing numbers that counted down at the beginning of the memory. They then realized that they had been forced to watch a WWII Nazi film.

f   Abusers deceive victims into believing that they are watching live-stream video of victims being punished with torture or death for their own failure to obey abuser directives. Abusers may use the same illusion to make victims believe that their thoughts killed the victims on screen.

g   Abusers impersonate non-abusive relatives, teachers, therapists, etc., to deceive victims into believing that these potential protectors have abused them, belong to the abuser network, and/or sanctioned their abuse. Additionally, abusers may use such platforms as video, holograms, and virtual reality to create the illusion that protective adults are present at abusive events and sites.

Hypnosis

Hypnosis is another mainstay of abusive mind control. Abusers use hypnotic suggestions and commands to install thoughts, perceptions, and beliefs in dissociated self-states. Like deception, hypnosis relies on the exploitation of victims' suggestibility. Young children are naturally highly suggestible, easily hypnotized, and compliant with adults. Abusers can also induce high suggestibility in older children, adolescents, and adults through the use of drugs, brain stimulation, and torture. Receptiveness to hypnosis "involves the intentional evocation of a special state characterized by focused attention" (Putnam & Carlson, 2002). Torture sharply focuses victims' attention on the demands of the abusers.

An anonymous survivor provided the following example of the successful use of abusive hypnotic suggestions with a young victim. These events were registered in dissociated self-states. Until the normative-life self-state consciously remembered these events, this child was paralyzed by the sight of maggots.

> [T]here was beating and rape at the [abusers' house] that generally ended with the body having to clean up the rotten fruit [filled with maggots]. There was the same basic message… every time. They told her the maggots were the first sign they knew the body was talking. They [the abusers] would send that [the maggots] to the body. [They said] It was the first warning… "The truth of speaking out carries on the wings of the flies." Then, the flies would bring back the warning [the maggots]… They said, "Flies are not of nature; they are witnesses to death, that's what creates the maggots, to eat the dead body."

Hypnotic commands are often used to induce the formation of new dissociated self-states. An adolescent whom I will call "Tammy" provided me with the following example of a simple and effective mind control strategy. Tammy was enrolled in a preschool controlled by abusers, unbeknownst to her family. One day, during reading circle, the abusers transported Tammy off-site, where they tortured her for the first time. When they finished, they commanded: "When you are here, you are Janie. When you go back to school and at home, you are Tammy. Tammy will only remember that you were in reading circle." The abusers' directive to form a new identity capitalized on Tammy's need to banish from consciousness the horrors that had just been inflicted, to dissociate from her pain, terror, and helplessness. This strategy immediately induced "Janie" to form, and caused Tammy to be amnesiac for Janie and the abuse, a division that became more deeply entrenched with each subsequent abuse episode.

Survivor Lynn Schirmer (2008) described her abusers use of the *Tin Man* in the *Wizard of Oz* film to cause her dissociated self-states to develop dissociative amnesia and confusion about her abuse memories:

Elements of the *Wizard of Oz* movie were used in programming, especially the bit (in my case) about having no brain. Generally this was used to remind major alters inside of their limitations, that they can't access certain parts or memories, and calls up programming that induces a hazy air-headed feeling. They actually played the little *Tin Man* song in the lab room.

Carol Rutz, victim of the CIA's MK-ULTRA mind control program and author of, *A Nation Betrayed* (Rutz, 2001), explained that her mind control was initially applied with torture, but later accomplished with hypnosis alone, exploiting formerly installed "triggers" (Rutz, 2003):

All the programming that was done to me by the CIA and Illuminati was trauma-based using things like electroshock, sensory deprivation, and drugs. Later the trauma wasn't necessary, only hypnosis accomplished with implanted triggers and occasional tune-ups....

(approx. para. 57)

Manipulation of Attachment Needs

Mind control abusers take ready advantage of children's basic needs for attachment, nutritional sustenance, touch, and so on, in order to develop bonds between the abusers and victims' dissociated self-states.

Commonly, much of a child's foundational programming is applied by mothers, fathers, and other close familial abusers.

Svali, mind control survivor, former "programmer," and author of, *How the Cult Programs People* (1996, 2024a, 2024b), explained that her abusers conditioned babies to associate nurturing and attention with nighttime and rituals, and abandonment with daytime and a time of no rituals, so that the infant "eventually will associate cult gatherings with feelings of security" (Chap. 4).

Many survivors describe that familial abusers and non-familial abusers systematically develop sexual attachment bonds with particular self-states to further exploit them. They systematically eroticize victims, starting in infancy, with sexual stimulation, often combined with pharmaceutical aphrodisiacs. Some survivors report that their abusers indoctrinated particular self-states to believe that sex is love, and that any adult, such as a protective parent, who is not sexual with them does not love them.

Non-familial abusers may designate themselves as "Daddy" or "Mommy" as they induce new self-states to form, and systematically dole out basic needs of food, comfort, affection, and rescue from abuse to these self-states to reward compliance and build emotional bonds and loyalty to the abusers.

Rutz (2001) recalled MK-ULTRA director, Sidney Gottlieb, using drugs and hypnosis to induce a new self-state to form, naming her, "Baby," and instructing her:

"I am your mammer and your papper. You love only me, and I am the only one who loves you. I feed you and hold you, and you are mine alone"... Our baby part grew to love and depend on "Daddy Sid" as her only source of love and nourishment. From that day forward, a deep bonding took place... No matter what experiment he was to make me a part of, I would love and remain loyal to the man who my baby alter considered the sole supplier of the basics of life, food, and love.

(p. 19)

Consistent with attachment theory, Gresch (personal communication, 2010) believes that identity develops within significant relationships. For self-states induced to form within torture, the programmer is the significant other to whom the child attaches. This relationship is all they know; it is their "normal." Accordingly, these self-states define themselves by the interactions within that molding process, including internalizing the abuser's messages, beliefs, and conditioning. By design, these self-states have no motives of their own, except to avoid torture through complete submission, identification with, and loyalty to, their abuser, consistent with the psychodynamics of Stockholm Syndrome (Goddard & Stanley, 1994). These very young self-states will do anything for any crumbs of affection or attention, including following abuser directives when not in the abuser's presence, a primary goal in mind control. Mind control abusers also develop bonds between victims and co-victims, spouses, the victim's own children, etc., across the life-span in order to weaponize these bonds. In her book, Never Give Up Part Two: The Struggle, Svali (2024b) describes how her abusers powerfully thwarted her efforts to escape their network for decades by threatening to punish particular abusers for her defiance and by killing victims in a "sibling group" that they had formed in her early childhood.

Coerced Perpetration

Coercion of victims to harm and kill other victims is another mainstay of abusive mind control. It is a highly effective means of manipulating victims' minds to form additional dissociated self-states: 1) who will define themselves as evil, irredeemable, unworthy of being with people other than the abusers; 2) whom the abusers claim to be initiates into the abuser group; 3) whom the abusers claim to be accomplices and murderers (the abusers may threaten to release video of their "crimes" to the authorities); 4) who are forced to harm or kill others in abusive rituals; 5) whom the abusers define as assassins used to kill people who threaten to expose or interfere with abuser network operations, and; 6) who may be exploited in the production of sadistic child abuse and torture materials.

A primary goal of coerced perpetration is to cause victims to believe that they harmed and killed others of their own free will. This is easily accomplished through torture and Machiavellian set-ups comprised of false choices between two reprehensible options. The abusers completely control the setting. Suicide is never an option.

Many forms of torture cannot be endured for even a moment. Electroshock is particularly effective because abusers can inflict shock remotely with hand-held devices as they direct victims to harm or kill other victims. When victims hesitate or resist directives, the abusers typically prolong the torture of the second victim, blame the first victim for this suffering, then coerce the first victim to complete the act.

In her book, *Quest for Love: Memoir of a Child Sex Slave* (2022), Anneke Lucas described how her abusers applied this strategy the first time they coerced her to kill. First, they told her that as a reward, she could choose a puppy from a litter to keep. After allowing her to bond with the puppy for two days. they ordered her to stab it to death. When she refused, her abusers tortured the puppy in front of her as punishment. She stabbed it to stop their torture. She then felt responsible for its death, as her abusers had intended. Thereafter, whenever they directed her to kill, she describes that it felt like a *mercy killing* (personal communication, April 20, 2023).

Another often-reported tactic is to direct a victim to harm or kill another victim under the threat of killing the victim's loved one or pet or killing multiple victims.

Another tactic is to force a young child to kill a baby or animal, then to immediately, as a group, feign horror, shock, and moral outrage that the child did such a thing, and to label the child a murderer. At that moment, a new self-state is likely to form who has no memory of the coercion applied moments before, but who knows only that they did something unforgivable.

Many survivors report that their abusers subjected them to days-long torture to induce rage-filled dissociated identities to form, whom they could then exploit to kill others. Svali (1996) explained:

> The child is severely beaten, for a long period of time, by the trainer, then told to hit the other child in the room, or they will be beaten further. If the child refuses, it is punished severely, the other child is punished as well, then the child is told to punish the other child. If the child continues to refuse, or cries, or tries to hit the trainer instead, they will continue to be beaten severely, and told to hit the other child, to direct its anger at the other child. This step is repeated until the child finally complies…The child will be taught that this is the acceptable outlet for the aggressive impulses and rage that are created by the brutality the child is constantly being exposed to.
>
> *(Chap. 4, para. 26)*

I have identified four types of dissociated self-states that mind control abusers induce to form through torture-coerced harm, each representing a deeper break in self-agency and loss of self:

1. Self-states consumed with soul-crushing guilt, shame, and self-hatred,
2. Emotionally numb robotic self-states who obey directives like a hammer in the abusers' hands,
3. Self-states who experience harm to others as the entirety of who they are, and whom may feel pride in fulfilling the tasks demanded and praised by the abusers,
4. Self-states who release rage when they are forced to commit violence, who achieve a "high" from feeling powerful, but who are unconsciously driven by pent-up terror, pain, helplessness, tension, and rage toward their abusers. This also relates to the kill-or-be-killed survival response that soldiers experience in combat and that often results in devastating moral injury (Shay, 1994).

Manipulation of Identification with the Aggressor

Identification with the aggressor is a well-established defense against unbearable feelings of helplessness and fear of annihilation.

As children are horribly abused, their minds often spontaneously form dissociated self-states who endure the abuse and retain the memory of the unbearable pain, terror, helplessness, shame, heartbreak, shock of exposure to unmitigated human cruelty, and rage toward their abusers.

Other self-states often form who align with the motives of the abusers on whom their survival depends. They adopt the position of top dog, seek to feel powerful by harming others, and scorn the weak, helpless underdog. They displace unconscious rage toward their abusers onto other victims and the self. This often extends to terrorizing victimized self-states within.

Programmers systematically build upon these responses to develop abuser-aligned self-states. Svali (1996) described one of these strategies:

> Many trainers will put themselves in the person, over the internal programmers or trainers… The survivor may be horrified to find a representative of one of their worst perpetrators inside, but this was a survival mechanism…The survivor may mimic accents, mannerisms, even claim the perpetrator's life history as their own.
>
> *(Chap. 13)*

Many abusers falsely promise designated self-states that they will earn positions of power and reduced abuse in exchange for loyalty. For example, ritualistic abusers commonly tell designated self-states that they have been "chosen" for priest or priestess positions. These self-states are often amnesiac for their abuse, but eventually recall that they had to prove that they could "take more pain" than other victims to earn this status.

Programmers often work to develop victims who ultimately choose to be abusers. Svali (1996, Chap. 10) related that her abusers subjected children to "betrayal programming" to destroy all loving bonds and create a world limited to "hated, hateful, sadistic persecutors." Her abusers gave young children adult "saviors" only to have these "saviors" later betray them, and also gave them so-called "twins" with whom to bond, but then later forced the children to hurt or kill them, all to build a "willing" persecutor.

Otto Kernberg (1994) stated that the antisocial personality develops in a world of sadistic persecutors. This accurately depicts the world of mind control victims:

> The antisocial personality proper may be conceived of as a personality so dominated by hatred that primitive, split-off idealizations are no longer possible; the world is populated exclusively by hated, hateful, sadistic persecutors. One can triumph in such a terrifying world only by becoming a persecutor, the sole alternative to destruction and suicide.
>
> *(p. 38)*

Deprivation of Basic Needs

Deprivation of basic needs includes extended periods of sensory deprivation, social isolation, physical restraint, starvation, thirst, exposure to hot or cold elements, and the like. Radical sensory deprivation often begins in earliest infancy and is often done at the hands of the infant's mother, who may or may not also be programmed. This deprivation may include the absence of human contact, starvation, confining the baby to a dark space, slapping the baby's hands for reaching for touch, and binding their limbs. The objective is to extinguish all attachment-seeking and any subjectively experienced sense of having psychological or physical needs. This strategy appears to be aimed at making the mind of the child like a blank canvas on which to apply mind control. It primes the victim to bond to abusers as the only source of sustenance, stimulation, and relatedness and to deeply orient to abusers' demands, including sexual and physical abuse and hypnotic commands.

Sensory deprivation is also often used prior to programming sessions to cause victims' minds to crave stimulation and human contact, apparently to induce greater receptivity to programming.

Direct Terrorization

Direct terrorization is an age-old, effective means of controlling victims in most organized crime. It includes torture-level abuse, threats of harm to others, particularly loved ones, and abductions. One threat to kill a protective and loving adult can effectively secure silence and compliance from a child for decades. The effectiveness of the threat is compounded by the child having repeatedly witnessed the abusers' capacity for violence, often including murder.

Although direct terrorization does not rely on manipulation of dissociated self-states, terrorized children tend to defensively relegate these experiences to dissociated self-states. In abusive mind control, terrorization is systematically applied to designated self-states to secure compliance apart from the awareness of normative-life self-states.

Indoctrination/Enculturation

Many abuser networks claim to embrace religious, political, and scientific, ideologies, including:

- Ritualistic abuse networks that incorporate spiritual beliefs and practices into their abuse. They may perform human or animal sacrifices and sexually abuse children to propitiate their deities or spiritually empower themselves. They may incorporate Judeo-Christian practices, invert them, or hold other beliefs. These networks are often familial and transgenerational.

- Politically motivated networks, such as established nation-states (e.g., Project MKULTRA; see United States Senate, 1977) and ethnic- and religious-superiority/hate groups, that work to develop intelligence operatives and military forces.
- Child sexual abuse and torture networks that seek to legitimatize pedophilia.
- Networks that seek to control the human mind in the name of science.

Such abusers indoctrinate and enculturate victims into their ideologies. Some abusers are true believers in their ideologies and employ mind control techniques to prevent normative-life self-states from ever discovering or disclosing them. In some cases, abusers only feign ideological beliefs to control their victims.

Spiritual Abuse

Ritualistic abuser networks use abusive rituals to cause victims to feel spiritually controlled by themselves or by the deities they worship or claim to worship. Practices commonly reported by survivors include the following.

a Abusers place semen, blood, saliva, breath, or other bodily substances inside of a child's body or on the surface, and claim that this has accomplished a spiritual "attachment," that part of the abuser's spirit now resides within. Victimized children believe this unequivocally because they are young, terrorized and indoctrinated into their abusers' beliefs. The child now perceives the abuser to control them internally, including repeating claims spoken within the abuse, e.g. "You are mine," "You will obey," "You are evil," etc. Abusers further claim that the sites of abuse on the child's body have become portals attached to astral pathways through which the abusers send their spirits, their deities, curses, and so on.

Victims describe abusers performing spiritual "transfers" primarily with their own children within life-long abuse, then finally on their death beds when they seek to "transfer" the remainder of their spirit into their progeny. Victims report that their abusers believe that their descendants serve as living vessels for their spirits until their prophesied apocalypse, when the deities that they have worshiped will give them human bodies again and they will live in Paradise on Earth for all eternity.

b Abusers worship Judeo-Christian or pre-Christian deities, for example, Celtic, Nordic, Germanic, Greek, Roman, Egyptian, and others. They believe that they appease, gain favor with, and empower their deities through inflicting great pain on others, human sacrifice, and child sexual abuse.

c Abusers manipulate victims to surrender to their deities. One strategy is to confine a child to a coffin with limited air supply for an extended period. When the child is near death, a new self-state forms. The abusers tell this new self-state that it has died, but can be born again to the deity the abusers worship. When the child agrees, an abuser dressed as a frightful demon, or some such figure, removes the child from the coffin, breathes air into their mouth, claims to be their savior, to forever control their life force, and assigns the self-state a new name to "baptize" it into the group's religion.

d Much effort is placed on sabotaging victims' faith in a loving God and preventing victims from finding support and community in mainstream religions. For example, a child is bound to a cross for hours, as the abusers taunt, "Where is your God now?"

e Rituals are held in mainstream houses of worship to defile them and/or to empower the abusers' own deities in the spiritual realm.

f The abusers "marry" designated self-states to frightening deities in rituals to terrorize these self-states or make them feel bound together in evil. Children are married to adult abusers to form long-term sexual and emotional bonds to each other and to the abuser network. Young child victims are also married to each other to bond them to each other and the abuser group. When a victim's abuse continues into adulthood, such illegitimate marriages may continue within abuse events, while they may have another, or the same, spouse in their normative lives.

Formal Programming

Formal programming is the application of mind control strategies to construct inner landscapes that sequester victims dissociated self-states internally, thereby controlling the relationships between self-states so as to set victims up against themselves.

Formal programming is largely accomplished by the "installation" of the perception of physical "structures" in victims' inner landscapes or in their bodies, beginning in early childhood, to organize, sequester, and conceal dissociated self-states from each other. Structures may include (a) locations that confine self-states, such as castles, torture facilities, concentration camps, pyramids, cemeteries, forests, trees, and two- and three-dimensional grids, (b) barriers to separate groups of self-states, such as walls, floors, lids or "caps," chasms, mountains, and bodies of water, and (c) devices that store large bodies of information, such as computers and files.

Many programmed self-states perceive themselves as trapped within such structures, reliving the torture used in their abusive mind control.

Survivors explain that torture, illusions, and hypnosis are used to install structures. For example, a programmer projects a grid on a child's chest and commands, "This grid is in your chest," "Amy, go to cell C-5."

An anonymous survivor-colleague provided the following explanation of complex programming strategies to develop an "overseer" of multiple other self-states.

> First, her programmers tortured her to induce multiple new self-states to form, assigned each a name, and conditioned each to perform a particular function, e.g., to be sexually violated in multiple ways and to appear to enjoy it. Then, they developed an "overseer." They used virtual reality technology to cause another self-state to believe that she was happily tending a garden of flowers. They assigned each flower a name that corresponded with the names of the sexually-violated self-states. Then, they instructed her: "You have the important job of making sure the flowers behave and of punishing them if they have bad thoughts." Then, they played recordings of actual abused children voicing pain, begging the abusers to stop, etc. They increased the pitch and speed to create an illusion of little flowers protesting. Then, they instructed the "overseer" that the flowers were misbehaving, and she must hurt them. When the "overseer" resisted, they tortured her until she complied. The abusers then sexually violated the "overseer," which activated the sexually-violated self-states. Their common pain made them highly accessible to each other. The programmers then commanded the sexually violated self-states to announce their names as they commanded the overseer to take the garden to them and to place each named flower over each child of the same name. The programmers then commanded the "overseer" to continue to tend the garden. Now, the "overseer" believed she was overseeing and punishing flowers when they misbehaved. In fact, she was punishing human self-states whenever they failed to comply.

Survivor Patricia Baird Clark (2001) described the use of models and hypnosis to install her inner world:

> A child may be... shown a castle... She spends several days in the castle going through painful, terrifying rituals in many of the rooms. She is forced to memorize the castle's entire layout. There will be a small replica of the castle much like an architectural model... Once this has

been memorized, she is subjected to magic surgery. A tiny replica of the castle is shown to the child and she is told that it is being placed inside. The castle is now "within"... In this person's inner world she can now walk through the rooms and this castle has become as real to her in the spiritual dimension as it had been in the physical world.

In subsequent rituals... the alters formed will be assigned to live in various rooms. These rooms are guarded by demons and booby traps are placed in strategic places so there is no escape... These castles have cold, dark dungeons filled with rats and snakes along with torture rooms....

(pp. 126–127)

Such illusions and commands become classically conditioned with the torture of the painful rituals. The induced survival-driven psychological state causes such structures to be perceived as very real. In his book, *Dialogues with Forgotten Voices* (2000), Harvey L. Schwartz stated:

The power of all statements made during and immediately after abusive episodes while the victim is in an altered state will be enhanced by the absence of an operative critical consciousness (Conway, 1994) and by the indelible connection with intense fear, intolerable anxiety, or mind-shattering dread.

(p. 318)

Skills Training

Large abuser networks train dissociated self-states within their victims, beginning in early childhood, in skills and knowledge bases needed to further and conceal their operations. These skills include medicine; technology; military and intelligence; law; multiple language proficiency; human, weapons and drug trafficking; and abusive mind control.

Training in each skill is confined to separate dissociated self-states whose sole function is to apply their training. Torture is often applied to compel fast and accurate learning. One survivor-colleague described how her programmers "placed" skills-trained self-states in separate holding cells in her inner world. When the abusers wanted to exploit a self-state's training, another self-state programmed to temporarily pair self-states together linked it with a third self-state who applied the skill. This strategy is intended to prevent victims from accessing their skills for their own use.

Abusers induce normative-life self-states to work in professions where they can apply their skills legitimately, while other self-states use these positions to further the gains of the abuser group. Still other self-states apply their skills solely within the criminal operations of the network.

Therapy Approaches with Children and Adolescents

The Sociological Backdrop to Treatment

Child abuse has always been under-reported. In *Recognising and Responding to Child Maltreatment*, Gilbert et al. (2009), reviewed the data on the prevalence of child abuse and concluded:

Few maltreated children come to the attention of child-protection agencies, indicating failure of professionals to recognize maltreatment, failure to report, and failure of agencies to investigate or substantiate maltreatment.

(p. 167)

A review of ten retrospective studies indicated that only one-third of adults revealed their child sexual abuse to anyone during childhood and only 10%–18% recalled that their cases had been reported to the authorities (London et al., 2005). Most studies demonstrate that when the perpetrator is a family member, the rate of disclosure of abuse is even lower and delays in disclosure are even longer (Lemaigre et al., 2017; Olafson & Lederman, 2006). Research suggests that ritualistic abuse networks tend to include family members (Schröder et al., 2020).

Dissociative amnesia is a powerful factor in low rates of abuse disclosure. The incidence of dissociative amnesia for childhood sexual abuse ranges from 19% to 38% (van der Kolk, 2014, Chap. 12, note 18). There is substantial evidence that abuse is commonly dissociated into adulthood (Barlow et al., 2017; McElvaney, 2013). In mind control abuse, programmers systematically further sequester abuse memories to dissociated self-states.

Beginning in 1992 and continuing to the present day, widespread disinformation campaigns have: (1) misrepresented reports of child abuse as "false allegations" and "false memories" (Nelson, 2016; Salter, 2022), (2) discounted the validity of dissociative amnesia as a response to child abuse, (3) misrepresented the diagnosis of dissociative identity disorder as the product of bad therapy, (4) attributed recovered memories of child abuse to therapist influence, and (5) branded reports of ritualistic abuse as born of a "witch-hunt" or "moral panic" (Cheit, 2014).

Many researchers and psychotherapists in the field of child abuse make a credible case that these campaigns, often referred to as "the child abuse backlash" and "memory wars," have had profoundly harmful social effects, including: (1) public skepticism about the prevalence of child abuse, (2) reduced protection of abused children by government agencies, (3) reticence among psychotherapists to use established psychotherapeutic approaches to recall and resolve trauma, (4) reduced capacity within victim-survivors to trust their own memories, and (5) wide-scale skepticism about the existence of ritualistic abuse (Conway, 2022; Nelson, 2016; Richardson, 2015; Salter, 2022).

Due to the above-described psychological and sociological factors, most children who have been subjected to abusive mind control never come to the attention of the authorities; nor do they ever receive psychotherapy. However, in recent years, victims appear to be recalling their abuse at younger ages due to the availability of information on extreme abuse and dissociation on the Internet.

In cases in which extreme and systematic abuse is identified in childhood and a protective parent (or caregiver) is bringing the minor to therapy, there is still substantial risk that abuse is ongoing. Unbeknownst to protective parents, other perpetrators may still be abusing the child, such as extended family members, nannies, teachers, or clergy. In some cases, perpetrators access children through cell phones and computers, without the knowledge of protective parents.

In cases of separation or divorce, a protective parent may share physical custody of their children with an ex-partner who is still abusing the children. Yet, they may be powerless to protect their children from this abuse. Most family courts have a strong bias toward shared custody and tend to view child abuse allegations in custody disputes as fabricated. Furthermore, research indicates that family courts often retaliate against parents who seek to protect their children from ex-partners by reducing their physical custody (Meier et al., 2019). Some protective parents are aware of this family court bias and thus do not report the abuse to the court.

Clearly, it is tragic that many children suffer ongoing abuse while they are in therapy, and that this is even more likely when the abuse is extreme. It is also tragic that a therapist's report of suspected child abuse to the appropriate child protection authorities may endanger the child further due to failures to substantiate the abuse or provide protection, and retaliation by perpetrators who still have access to the child. However, it also true that children are usually brought to therapy by protective parents who can actively participate in the therapy process and support their children's needs at home.

Due to this sociological backdrop and the associated risk factors, psychotherapists who work with children and adolescents who have been subjected to abusive mind control and ritualistic abuse must carefully weigh the following considerations when selecting treatment approaches and interventions: (1) the child may be suffering ongoing abuse or be at significant risk, (2) facilitation of disclosure of the abuse may be contraindicated, (3) the therapist and protective parent may have no means to protect the child.

Therapists must also consider whether "normative life" self-states would be harmed by recalling their abuse. Clients can become extremely destabilized. Programmed self-states can be activated to punish other self-states, to self-injure, or to report memories and disclosures to their abusers. Therefore, much of the work of therapy with victims of abusive mind control must be disguised in symbolic play and metaphor. Only when children are safe and have adequate support can this abuse be addressed directly.

Non-Directive Play Therapy

Non-directive play therapy is a powerful treatment approach with children who have suffered mind control abuse. It is a platform within which all of a child's dissociated self-states can find self-expression without being directly identified or exposed. Symbolic expression in pretend play additionally side-steps programming to not remember, not tell, and not defy the abusers.

Children's imaginative play is fueled by the drive for mastery. Children unconsciously create dramas that exist on the cusp of the knowable and unknowable, the tolerable and intolerable. In the world of pretend, children can represent their fears and needs with enough psychological distance to be able to work to triumph over their trauma. It is a miniature and magical world that they fully control. They are no longer small, afraid, defeated, and alone. They are empowered. They can have allies and protectors. They can achieve a corrective denouement. For all of these reasons, abused children tend to use imaginative play at older ages than non-abused children.

My approach to play therapy is much like Landreth's *Child-Centered Play Therapy* (2012): I unconditionally accept all of the child's play, I verbally track the actions and overtly expressed emotions of all play characters, and I do not directly relate the play content to the child's feelings or the events in the child's life. However, I modify some of the methods of *Child-Centered Play Therapy*. For many abused children, shame and fear of harm have a looming, constant presence, especially when their abuse was extreme. I have found that abused children feel safer and less guarded when I focus more on their play dramas than on directly relating with them, especially early in treatment.

In doing so, I place myself eye-level with the toys and become completely absorbed and captivated in the child's pretend drama as if I am watching a play. I take my attention off the child and largely avoid eye contact. I suspend disbelief. My goal is for the child to become fully immersed in the creative process, for all self-consciousness to melt away, and for the child's inner world to spontaneously unfold before both the child and me, with unexpected twists and turns, much like in a dream. While I verbally track the actions of all figures in a child's play to demonstrate deep interest and attentiveness, my reflections primarily support the characters that I judge to represent the child. I verbalize their feelings, needs, and wishes, and I do not reflect the needs or wishes of figures whom I judge to represent the child's abusers. Children who have been invaded physically and mentally through abuse, especially extreme abuse, have little sense of self and little capacity to identify and express their feelings and needs. I have found that support for self-representational figures helps abused children build self-awareness and a belief that their needs and wishes matter, and helps them direct this awareness into self-advocacy and empowered action.

I also work to facilitate resolutions at critical junctures when I judge that a child's drama may be re-traumatizing (see Lenore Terr on posttraumatic play, 1990). If a child figure freezes in fear in face of an assailant in a drama, I may say, "I wonder what the tiger cub wishes," or "Pause! I wonder what could help!" I may quietly place a toy jail or protective figure, like an elephant, on the periphery of the drama to suggest possible forms of help. In cases in which a child appears deeply panicked, I may actually place the elephant between the tiger cub and assailant. If a child plays with human figure dolls, but this "hits too close to home" to contain the anxiety in the metaphor of the drama and work it thorough to a resolution, I may suggest that we play with animal figures. Synergetic Play Therapy, covered in this volume by Lisa Dion, LPC, RPT-S, is a relatively new approach to play therapy that builds upon *Child-Centered Play Therapy and* works to facilitate trauma resolution in many of the ways I describe.

Case Example

The following case illustrates the power of pretend play with a three-year-old girl who had suffered ritualistic abuse. A highly sensitive and protective mother brought this child to therapy. The child was terrified to take a bath no matter how shallow the water level. She could tolerate only sponge baths. She feared bathrooms, pools, running water, and feces. She would eat no brown food.

In therapy, this child liked to play in a water basin with Play-Doh™. She dropped the Play-Doh™ in the basin and squished it. She mixed it with water in a cup to make "mud." She shook this mixture together in baby bottles. She used only green and blue Play-Doh™. She described the wet Play-Doh™ as "gross," but continued this play for many sessions.

She then began to wash the hair of two little girl dolls in the basin, enjoying this for some time. Then she suddenly began lifting the dolls by their feet and dropping them in the water, head first. The happy affect disappeared. She appeared to be in a dissociative trance, perhaps in an alternate self-state. Concerned that she might be reliving terrible abuse without any support, I watched for only a few moments and then asked, "Do they like that or are they scared?" She replied, "Scared." I responded with compassion for the dolls.

At home, she challenged herself to overcome her fear of water. She watched her mother bathe her little brother. She finally decided she was ready to take a bath. Then she spontaneously and directly told her mother that "the bad people" put feces on her.

In therapy, she continued to put Play-Doh™ in the water basin, plopping it like feces dropping into a toilet and squashing it with her hands. She put Play-Doh™ on the outside of a small bottle and rinsed it off with cups of water, stating, "I'm rinsing her off." I provided quiet support, reflecting her actions and her enjoyment in washing the Play-Doh™ off of the bottle. Then, one day, she said, "The bad people put poop on my face." She then told her mother the bad people put her in water filled very high, upside-down. Many survivors of extreme abuse report similar punishment with feces and drowning in water to condition them not to disclose their abuse.

This highly symbolic play allowed this child to work at her own pace to overcome the horror of her cruel abuse. First, she unconsciously worked to master her fear of water and feces by playing in a water basin with green and blue Play-Doh™, colors very different from that of feces. Then, she worked to master her fear of baths by repeatedly washing the hair of two little girl dolls. Next, in a trance or alternate self-state, she unconsciously reenacted a memory of torture as she dunked the dolls head-first into the water. I intervened with a question to interrupt the reliving of this abuse and vicariously communicate compassion to her through the dolls. Then she told her mother that her abusers had put feces on her. Her play then changed to washing Play-Doh™ off bottles, symbolically washing feces off of herself as many times as she needed. Then, she could finally tell her mother more about this abuse and be comforted directly.

If this child had not been protected, but instead was suffering ongoing abuse, her play may not have led to a disclosure. However, in the sanctity of the playroom, her needs and wishes could be respected and find full expression. She and her alternate self-states could experience complete self-agency. She could symbolically: (1) work to master her fear of feces, (2) vicariously give herself safe baths, (3) experience the therapist's compassion for her, via the dolls, in regard to having been submerged in water, (4) internalize the implied message that she deserved not to be abused, and (5) wash the feces off herself (the bottle) as many times as she needed.

The play therapy process is sacred and delicate. Children must feel deeply accepted and valued to be able to express themselves freely, without internal censorship. The therapy process can be easily undermined if a parent and therapist discuss the child's behavioral problems and behavioral strategies in the child's presence. I conduct these conversations alone with the parent.

This is a critical issue in extreme abuse. Abusers blame victims for the horrible things they do to them, coerce them to harm others, and make them believe themselves to be evil. Furthermore, these children are unable to control much of their behavior. They erupt in explosive rage before they can inhibit it. Dissociated self-states execute programmed or abuse-reactive behaviors outside of the awareness of normative self-states. All of these issues result in stores of self-condemnation, self-hatred, and suicidality. Any attribution of willful wrongdoing, or even a focus on behavioral problems, can cause these children to feel more intrinsically bad, blameworthy, and morally irredeemable. When children feel hopeless of ever being seen as innocent and good by the therapist and parent, these relationships suffer devastating damage.

Full-Body Role Play

Mind control abuse seeks to completely rob victims of their own volition, to reduce them to puppets. Many adult survivors of extreme abuse freeze in response to any perceived threat, and experience severe depersonalization and disconnection from their bodies. In full-body role play, children can express their needs and wishes both emotionally and physically. They can experience themselves in their bodies and be mobilized and empowered.

Shoot-and-die role play is a common choice of many abused children. It creates a great sense of safety, especially in early sessions. The child shoots the therapist and the therapist falls to the ground, reliably, over and over. The child quickly understands that the therapist poses no threat.

Police play is also a common choice. A life-size jail is my most popular therapy supply. I spend a lot of time locked up in there, as do my life-size dummies! Children usually designate the "bad guys" as robbers rather than violent criminals to achieve enough psychological distance. When protective parents can participate in sessions, children often make them their second-in-command.

As children feel increasingly comfortable, they usually move into full-body revenge play. They assault the dummies. They release rage. They often exact retributive justice, inflicting on the dummies forms of abuse that may be only thinly disguised from the abuse done to them.

I sometimes suggest forms of physical play that encourage embodied self-agency. I give children a water gun, and as they squirt me, I run away in feigned fear as I try to shield myself with a towel. I suggested to a very young child who was ritually abused that he push me down as I stood in front of my couch. Years after therapy concluded, I talked to him on the phone. He said to me with a tone of nostalgia, "Remember when I pushed you?" "Yes," I said, "I do."

All of these methods can be used with children who are not currently safe to help them preserve or develop a sense of self-worth and to internalize the belief that they deserve to be safe.

Art Therapy

Art therapy, like play therapy, is a means by which children can symbolically represent traumatic material and bypass much "forget/don't tell" programming. Play and art often act in concert to allow children to work through extreme abuse. A small boy who had been ritualistically abused would first empower himself against particular abusive events in highly disguised pretend play. After some time, he would instruct his protective mother to draw a picture of that event. Then, he would ask his mother to show the drawing to me. We could then talk about what happened, sharing our sadness, compassion, and outrage with the boy.

Collage is a particularly powerful therapeutic tool for victims of all ages of mind control and other extreme abuse. Collage does not require conscious selection of images. Clients need only select the images that "call to them." Multiple self-states tend to spontaneously contribute images. A non-interpretive stance facilitates uncensored expression by all parts of the self. Early in therapy, a ritualistically abused young teen pasted only five images on a piece of paper. As she told me about them, she realized that five dissociated identities had each selected a self-image.

Sand tray therapy is much like a three-dimensional collage. Deeply dissociated material tends to find uncensored expression. A pre-teen who was still being abused created a tray of particular ancient structures that later, when he was a young adult, were revealed to be central programmed structures in his internal world. Many older adolescents and adults explicitly depict abusive events in the sand. This permits non-verbal expression by dissociated and programmed self-states.

Stories and Metaphor

Like play and art, metaphor and stories can be used to send therapeutic messages to dissociated, programmed self-states without normative self-states needing to consciously understand the intervention. This is of particular value with children and adolescents who are not safe and with clients who cannot yet tolerate directly addressing their memories and fears.

One of my most rapid successful interventions occurred in a case in which I had never met the children or parents. The parents contacted me seeking resources to help their children who had been ritualistically abused in a preschool. For two years, we corresponded via sporadic emails. When the children were school-aged, the parents wrote again, explaining that one of the children had been badly triggered by a movie and was now suffering increased separation anxiety, insomnia, and anger. The other child was suffering increased symptoms as well. I emailed back to suggest that it might help to write metaphorical stories that represent children seeing through the tricks used in their abuse, disguising all the players and the abuse. I wrote:

> So, say you wrote (or found something similar) a story about a bad dragon who stole all the acorns from all the forest animals, and three little squirrels saw him doing it, and he told them that they better not tell anyone and that he was magic and could always see everyone and hear everyone, and he would know if they ever told on him and he'd blow fire on them. Then the little squirrels were so scared and hid underground and would not even talk to each other about it and pretended it never happened so they would not have to feel afraid. And now they felt scared all the time and didn't know why and there were hardly any acorns left, etc. And the Momma and Papa squirrels were so worried because their children looked so sad and scared. Then one day, the little squirrels were up in a tree, and they saw the dragon stealing acorns, and they saw an owl throw one down on the dragon's head. And then the dragon was mad, "Who did that?" and the dragon looked around and could not see the owl and the dragon could not see the squirrels. So, then the squirrels smiled at each other because they saw with their very own eyes that the dragon was not magic after all and that he told lies to scare everyone. And they ran home and told the whole story to the Momma and Papa squirrels. And they all moved to a forest where there were only nice animals, etc.

> This kind of thing can get them [the children] questioning, not consciously, but internally. I know this seems small, and it is in some ways, but it can plant a seed inside that can grow.

The father quickly wrote back:

> This worked! [Child] is back in [child's] own bed... The story provides... great comfort... [Child] is now asking for us to tell the story before bed... Thank you very much....

I believe that presenting these concepts in story form gave the children enough psychological distance from this threatening material to allow them to evaluate and understand their current safety without activating their fear. In addition, stories and metaphors are processed largely in the right brain, where so much trauma memory is stored (Schore, 2019).

Films, literary works, and historical events can also be used to communicate helpful messages to programmed self-states. For example, if a therapist suspects that a child was coerced to abuse other victims, the child can be engaged in a philosophical discussion about the Holocaust. In the Nazi death camps and Eastern European ghettos, victims were forced into moral dilemmas very similar to those of mind control victims, involving starvation, torture, and being forced to harm others.

The central event in the film, *Sophie's Choice*, involves a Nazi officer who demands that Sophie give up one of her children to be sent to the death camps, or he will take them both. Horrified, she hands him one child and is then plagued by her "choice" for a lifetime, blaming herself for the outcome. A therapist can engage victims of suspected coerced perpetration in a friendly debate about this scene, posing Socratic questions, etc. In so doing, the therapist is hoping to reach, to "talk through to," as many dissociated self-states as possible, even if normative self-states are unaware they exist. Victims may argue that Sophie could have done something different. However, this dialogue is likely to reach the programmed self-states who most need to hear it, planting seeds of self-compassion and self-forgiveness without normative-life self-state(s) ever having to remember this trauma. In one case, I used a similar historical reference with a young adolescent. When this individual came back into therapy in adulthood, this reference had become the person's internal "safe place."

The experience of child soldiers also directly compares to victimization within extreme abuse, especially with regard to coerced perpetration and the development of violent self-states (see Harvey Schwartz's treatise, *The Alchemy of* Wolves and Sheep, 2013). The therapist could recommend to adolescent victims that they read Ishmael Beah's memoir, *A Long Way Gone: Memoirs of a Boy Soldier* (2006). Even without normative self-states accessing their memories, programmed self-states could be helped to understand their violent responses and to work toward self-forgiveness.

Direct Abuse-Focused Work

When children are safe and have developed some capacity to consciously recall their abuse and dialogue about it, therapy can begin to include direct abused-focused work. The younger the child, the lower the capacity for such work. Young children need to spend most of their therapy time in self-expressive play and art so they can regulate the distance from traumatic material. Even when incorporating abuse-focused work into therapy with young children, it is usually necessary to do this with play, art, and stories to reduce anxiety, sustain the child's interest, and help the child register the concepts in long-term memory.

A common strategy in abusive mind control is to attempt to destroy relationships with loving and protective adults, including deceiving victims into believing that these adults sanctioned or participated in the abuse. For example, a young preschool child was taken to an abusive ritual by a teen-age baby-sitter. Prior to ever leaving the teenager alone with her child, the mother had her visit a few times so she could watch their interaction. She noticed no concerns. However, the abusers made the child believe that her protective mother had allowed the abuse. The child was frightened and confused. With the mother participating in the therapy session, I asked the child to pick dolls to be herself, her mother, and the sitter. I asked her to show me how the baby-sitter acted when Mommy was home, and we all talked about how nice she acted. I took a photograph of that scene and of each successive event: the mother leaving, the sitter taking the child to a ritual, the sitter bringing her home, and the sitter acting nice again. Then I called the sitter a "mean tricker." The use of dolls and the provision of an illustrated storybook helped this child see through the trick.

Even with adolescents, direct processing of material as frightening and cruel as ritualistic abuse and mind control is made more tolerable if it incorporates fiction and even humor. A teen-age client wrote the following story about his abusers' use of impersonation and torture-conditioning to train his abused self-states to lie to his protective parents when they asked him if anyone had hurt him. This, and many other forms of abusive mind control, succeeded in terrorizing and silencing this young man, and preventing his parents from detecting his abuse, for most of his childhood.

Once upon a time there was a little boy, and his name was Pancakes. And when he had just come off the griddle, Pancakes had some very bad people in his life who did very bad things to him. And their names were Shitake and Portobello. Sometimes the very bad people would take him to very bad places. In these very bad places, they would do very bad things to him. They would hurt him and teach him how to lie. After they hurt him very badly, they would have someone who looked like his Mama, named Waffles, ask him if he got hurt. If he could not convince the person who looked like Waffles that he did not get hurt, they would hurt Pancakes again. After they hurt Pancakes again, they would have the person who looked like Waffles ask him again if he got hurt. After doing this several times, they brought in someone who looked like French Toast, his Dad. And they would continue the same pattern with the person who looked like French Toast. After many times of going to the very bad place and getting very good at lying, the real Waffles and the real French Toast finally got Pancakes away from the very bad people. Many, many, breakfasts later, Pancakes realized that he did not have to lie, and that if he told the truth, he would not get hurt. Even though he knows this, he still has a hard time not lying, but he is doing his very best to learn to tell the truth.

In later adolescence and young adulthood, victims become more able to do direct work to make conscious and overcome the psychological manipulations within their mind control abuse. It is grueling work. The victim's heart rate is usually accelerated. Victims may chew on ice, squeeze a ball, or hug a plush bear the whole time. Some adolescent and young adult victims feel more contained by having a third-party present for support, ideally a protective parent. Many hundreds of dissociated self-states (polyfragmented self-state systems) may participate over time. The therapist is alert to when a new self-state comes forward and must usually initiate the dialogue, e.g.: "Hello. Were you watching me from the inside? Have I met you before? If you would like to talk to me about something, I'd like to help you."

The beginning dialogue can take the form of playing Twenty Questions. Simple yes-no questions are generally easier to tolerate as self-states come forward for the first time. Questions informed by knowledge of mind control abuse help build a framework for self-states to disclose more about their abuse: "How many adults were there?", "Were you forced to do anything against your will?", "Did any new parts form in this event?", "What words did the abusers speak?", "Were they trying to make you believe something about yourself, about someone else?"

Once the manipulations of programmed self-states have been made conscious, these self-states can be relocated from their sites of torture in the inner landscape to an internal place of healing.

In the limited space of a chapter in a book, I am able to provide only representative examples of therapeutic interventions with victims of abusive mind control. Psychologist Joyanna Silberg presents many more interventions, both symbolic and abuse-focused, in her book *The Child Survivor* (2022). Chapter 15 specifically addresses victims of systematic and highly sadistic abuse.

It is also not within the scope of this chapter to elaborate further on therapy approaches with adults to overcome the effects of abusive mind control. This is discussed in significant depth elsewhere (see Lacter, 2011).

Ongoing Consultation with Child's Caregivers/Protective Parents

Children and adolescents who have been subjected to abusive mind control generally experience severe psychological and behavioral symptoms, especially once normative self-states have recalled and disclosed their abuse, and programming to not remember or tell about the abuse has become activated. They are typically plagued by multiple phobias, including things as ordinary as food, water, and colors, making daily functioning a great challenge. Their dissociated self-states suddenly "come forward" into executive control and relive torture-level abuse in flashbacks in which they are completely disoriented, may not recognize the parent, and are inconsolable. They often feel physically threatened, and react with violence against caregivers, teachers, or other children. They may be too fearful and behaviorally dysregulated to attend school outside of the home. They may resist sleep because of terrifying posttraumatic nightmares. They commonly have self-states who have been programmed to sabotage relationships with protective parents, to harm their siblings, to maintain contact with their abusers, and to comply with their abusers' directives. Many of these children require 24-hour close supervision to protect them and other family members. All of this causes extreme psychological distress and exhaustion for caregivers/protective parents.

The child's therapist must provide regular support and a great deal of psycho-education to these caregivers/protective parents as they deal with these intense symptoms that the child has no capacity to regulate independently. The therapist must help them understand the origin of these symptoms, to not react with anger to challenging behaviors, to not morally condemn children for destructive behaviors that they cannot inhibit, and to learn how to dialogue with the many dissociated self-states that are routinely activated into executive control.

When a child has a meltdown or violent tantrum, sometimes the best a caregiver can do is to not react with panic or anger, but to simply wait it out while holding in mind that the child may be in another self-state, a flashback, or the like. The child may need to become physically exhausted before they can orient to the present surroundings and perceive the caregiver's benevolence. These challenges generally last for many years with many set-backs along the way. Caregivers usually need a therapist for themselves, in addition to ongoing contact with the child's therapist, to support them and to problem-solve as they navigate this arduous process.

Conclusion

Overcoming mind control abuse is life-long work. Therapists are transformed by this work, having learned of incomprehensible and systematic sadism. This fills us with sorrow, righteous rage, and deep respect for the victims. We draw from this well as we sit with victims and survivors to help them know that they have always been worthy of love, kindness, and protection.

References

Barlow, M. R., Pezdek, K., & Blandón-Gitlin, I. (2017). Trauma and memory. In S. N. Gold (Ed.), *APA handbook of trauma psychology: Foundations in knowledge* (pp. 307–331). American Psychological Association. https://doi.org/10.1037/0000019-016

Beah, I. (2006). *A long way gone: Memoirs of a boy soldier*. Sarah Crichton Books.
Becker, T., Karriker, W., Overkamp, B., & Rutz, C. (2007). Extreme abuse survey project. Retrieved June 12, 2010, from extreme-abuse-survey.net
Cheit, R. E. (2014). *The witch-hunt narrative: Politics, psychology, and the sexual abuse of children*. Oxford University Press. https://doi.org/10.1093/acprof:oso/9780199931224.001.0001
Clark, P. B. (2001). *Restoring survivors of satanic ritual abuse: Equipping and releasing God's people for spirit-empowered ministry*. Bairdspong Publications.
Conway, A. (1994). Trance formations of abuse. In V. Sinason (Ed.), *Treating survivors of Satanist abuse* (pp. 254–264). Routledge.
Conway, A. (2022). The abuse of science to silence the abused. In V. Sinason & A. Conway (Eds.), *Trauma and memory: The science and the silenced* (pp. 54–67). Routledge.
Gilbert, R., Kemp, A., Thoburn, J., Sidebotham, P., Radford, L., Glaser, D., & Macmillan, H. L. (2009). Recognising and responding to child maltreatment. *Lancet, 373*(9658), 167–180. https://doi.org/10.1016/S0140-6736(08)61707-9
Goddard, C. R., & Stanley, J. R. (1994). Viewing the abusive parent and the abused child as captor and hostage: The application of hostage theory to the effects of child abuse. *Journal of Interpersonal Violence, 9*(2), 258–269. https://doi.org/10.1177/088626094009002008
Gresch, H. U. (2010). *Hypnose bewusstseinskontrolle manipulation: Bewusstseinskontrolle durch persönlichkeitsspaltung*. Elitär Verlag.
Kernberg, O. F. (1994). Aggression, trauma, and hatred in the treatment of borderline patients. *Psychiatric Clinics of North America, 17*(4), 701–714.
Lacter, E. (2011). Torture-based mind control: Psychological mechanisms and psychotherapeutic approaches to overcoming mind control. In O. B. Epstein, J. Schwartz & R. Wingfield (Eds.), *Ritual abuse and mind control: The manipulation of attachment needs* (pp. 57–142). Karnac.
Lacter, E., Karriker, W., Sinason, V., & Ball, T. (October 22, 2012). Therapists reporting histories of ritual abuse trauma: Preliminary results on beneficial and detrimental treatment approaches. International Society for the Study of Trauma and Dissociation 29th Annual Conference, Long Beach, CA.
Landreth, G. L. (2012). *Play therapy: The art of relationship* (3rd ed.). Routledge/Taylor & Francis Group.
LeDoux, J. (1996). *The emotional brain: The mysterious underpinnings of emotional life*. Simon & Schuster.
Lemaigre, C., Taylor, E. P., & Gittoes, C. (2017). Barriers and facilitators to disclosing sexual abuse in childhood and adolescence: A systematic review. *Child Abuse & Neglect, 70*, 39–52. https://doi.org/10.1016/j.chiabu.2017.05.009
London, K., Bruck, M., Ceci, S. J., & Shuman, D. W. (2005). Disclosure of child sexual abuse: What does the research tell us about the ways that children tell? *Psychology, Public Policy, and Law, 11*(1), 194–226. https://doi.org/10.1037/1076-8971.11.1.194
Lucas, A. (2022). *Quest for love: Memoir of a child sex slave*. Unconditional Books.
McElvaney, R. (2013). Disclosure of child sexual abuse: Delays, non-disclosure and partial disclosure. What the research tells us and implications for practice. *Child Abuse Review, 24*(3). https://doi.org/10.1002/car.2280
Meier, J. S., Dickson, S., O'Sullivan, C., Rosen, L., & Hayes, J. (2019). Child custody outcomes in cases involving parental alienation and abuse allegations. *GWU Law School Public Law Research Paper No. 2019-56; GWU Legal Studies Research Paper No*, 2019-2056. https://doi.org/10.2139/ssrn.3448062
Miller, A. (2012). *Healing the unimaginable: Treating ritual abuse and mind control*. Karnac.
Nelson, S. (2016). *Tackling child sexual abuse: Radical approaches to prevention, protection and support*. Policy Press.
Noblitt, J. R., & Noblitt, P. P. (2014). Empirical and forensic evidence of ritual abuse. In *Cult and ritual abuse: Narratives, evidence, and healing approaches* (3rd ed., pp. 52–78). Praeger. Available in full on the internet. endritualabuse.org/empirical-and-forensic-evidence-of-ritual-abuse/
Olafson, E., & Lederman J. C. (2006). The state of debate about children's disclosure patterns in child sexual abuse cases. *Juvenile and Family Court Journal, 57*(1), 27–40. https://doi.org/10.1111/j.1755-6988.2006.tb00112.x
Putnam, F. W., & Carlson, E. B. (2002). Hypnosis, dissociation, and trauma: Myths, metaphors, and mechanisms. In D. Bremner & C. Marmar (Eds.), *Trauma, memory, and dissociation* (pp. 27–55). American Psychiatric Press.
Richardson, K. (2015). Dissecting disbelief: Possible reasons for the denial of the existence of ritual abuse in the United Kingdom. *International Journal for Crime, Justice and Social Democracy, 4*(2), 77–93. https://doi.org/10.5204/ijcjsd.v4i2.228

Rutz, C. (2001). *A nation betrayed: Secret Cold War experiments performed on our children and other innocent people*. Fidelity Publishing.

Rutz, C. (2003). Healing from ritual abuse and mind control, a presentation at the Sixth Annual Ritual Abuse, Secretive Organizations and Mind Control Conference, August 8–10, 2003. Retrieved December 3, 2023, from ritualabuse.us/smart.conference/conf03/healing.from.ritual.abuse.and.mind.control/

Salter, M. (2017). Organized abuse in adulthood: Survivor and professional perspectives. *Journal of Trauma & Dissociation, 18*(3), 441–453. https://doi.org/10.1080/15299732.2017.1295426

Salter, M. (2022). Finding a new narrative: Meaningful responses to "false memory" disinformation. In V. Sinason & A. Conway (Eds.), *Trauma and memory: The science and the silenced* (pp. 130–141). Routledge.

Schirmer, L. (2008). Personal communication.

Schore, A. N. (2019). *Right brain psychotherapy*. Norton.

Schröder, J., Nick, S., Richter-Appelt, H., & Briken, P. (2020). Demystifying ritual abuse - insights by self-identified victims and health care professionals. *Journal of Trauma & Dissociation, 21*(3), 349–364. https://doi.org/10.1080/15299732.2020.1719260

Schwartz, H. (2000). *Dialogues with forgotten voices: Relational perspectives on child abuse trauma and the treatment of severe dissociative disorders*. Basic Books.

Schwartz, H. (2013). *The alchemy of wolves and sheep: A relational approach to internalized perpetration for complex trauma survivors*. Routledge.

Shay, J. (1994). *Achilles in Vietnam: Combat trauma and the undoing of character*. Atheneum Publishers/Macmillan Publishing Co.

Silberg, J. (2022). *The child survivor: Healing developmental trauma and dissociation*. Routledge.

Sinason, V. (2018). Sexual sadism in ritual abuse: The dilemma of the perpetrator. In A. Sehgal (Ed.), *Sadism: Psychoanalytic developmental perspectives*. Routledge. https://doi.org/10.4324/9780429445408-4

Svali. (1996). The Illuminati: How the cult programs people. Svali 1st Series. Retrieved April 4, 2023, from bibliotecapleyades.net/sociopolitica/esp_sociopol_illuminati_svali01a.html

Svali (2024a). *Never Give Up: The Autobiography of a Survivor of Ritual Abuse and Mind Control*, Independently published.

Svali (2024b). *Never Give Up Part Two: The Struggle*. Independently published.

Terr, L. (1990). *Too scared to cry: Psychic trauma in childhood*. Basic Books.

United States Senate. (August 3, 1977). Project MKULTRA, the Central Intelligence Agency's program of research into behavioral modification. Joint hearing before the Select Committee on Intelligence and the Subcommittee on Health and Scientific Research of the Committee on Human Resources, United States Senate, ninety-fifth Congress, first session. Published by the *New York Times*. nytimes.com/packages/pdf/national/13inmate_ProjectMKULTRA.pdf

van der Kolk, B. A. (2014). *The body keeps the score: Brain, mind, and body in the healing of trauma*. Viking.

46
PSYCHIATRY AND PHARMACOLOGY

Darren Bingham, Helen Milroy, Guilia Pace, Pradeep Rao and Alix Woolard

Introduction

Dissociation refers to the mental process where an individual disconnects from their thoughts, feelings, memories, and in some cases, their identity. Dissociation can be a useful and often essential coping mechanism during ongoing traumatic events or times in a person's life. Though it is a useful short-term strategy, if used as a coping mechanism in the long term, it can interfere with daily functioning and many studies have shown trauma-related persistence dissociation to be a risk factor for later psychopathology (Cudzik et al., 2019; Dorahy et al., 2014; Loewenstein, 2018; Şar et al., 2017; Silberg, 2000). Dissociation following complex trauma is related to the presentation of symptoms that are often diagnosed as post-traumatic stress disorder (PTSD), depression, schizophrenia, substance abuse, attention-deficit hyperactivity disorder (ADHD), and eating disorders, to name only a few (Ford & Connor, 2009; Hall, 2022; Kulacaoglu et al., 2017). The overlapping nature of these dissociative symptoms with other psychopathology has led to treatment methods that may further impede healing from the trauma. Furthermore, dissociative disorders related to complex trauma are associated with a high burden of illness and a poor quality of life, with symptoms being linked to self-injurious and suicidal behaviors, and interpersonal and relational difficulties (Cudzik et al., 2019; Dorahy et al., 2014; Loewenstein, 2018).

In order to live a healthy and fulfilling life, it is important for individuals of all ages who experience chronic dissociation to receive treatment to help them process and heal from past trauma, learn new coping skills, regain a sense of control over their thoughts and emotions, integrate identities if they experience this phenomenon, and support development to get back on track. This chapter will address the principles and modalities of psychiatric treatment used with children who experience dissociation as a result of histories of complex trauma. Descriptions of dissociation are covered in other chapters in this volume.

The goal of therapy with children who struggle with dissociation is to help them understand the underlying causes of their dissociation in a developmentally appropriate way and develop healthy coping skills, and to support the integration of dissociated parts of self into a more cohesive, functional whole. Medications may also be prescribed to manage co-occurring symptoms or conditions such as anxiety or depression. With appropriate assessment and treatment, children who experience dissociation can learn to manage their symptoms and live a more fulfilling life.

There are, however, several issues with the treatment of dissociation in children. Although it is generally agreed that dissociative disorders predominantly arise due to complex and pervasive trauma that occurs during childhood, there are still issues with assessment and diagnosis, and there is no single treatment that is currently viewed as the gold standard for the treatment of dissociation in childhood and adolescence (Dorahy et al., 2014; Loewenstein, 2018; Silberg, 2000). Another issue is that for many individuals, the identification and treatment of dissociation occurs later in life despite the origin of dissociative symptoms occurring during childhood (Gillig, 2009). In fact, children have a greater capacity to dissociate compared to adults, with symptoms reaching a peak between 9 and 12 years of age (Diseth & Christie, 2005). Non-pathological dissociative symptoms (such as daydreaming) are common in most children, meaning that pathological dissociation can be difficult to differentiate in children with unknown histories of complex trauma, and may therefore go undiagnosed. Adding to the issue of misdiagnosis and underdiagnosis of dissociation in children is that some mental health professionals are not familiar with symptoms related to dissociative disorders in children (Diseth & Christie, 2005). Many studies report on treatment methods for dissociative disorders that are diagnosed in adulthood; however, an individual may have been living with the traumatic experiences and dissociative symptoms since childhood (for a review, see Woolard et al., 2024). This is particularly concerning given that early detection, diagnosis, and treatment for dissociative disorders demonstrates better outcomes for children and adolescents when compared to adults treated for dissociative disorders stemming from childhood maltreatment (Dorahy et al., 2014; Loewenstein, 2018; Myrick et al., 2012; Spitzer et al., 2006). Nevertheless, professionals and researchers in this field do agree on two principles of the treatment of dissociation in children following histories of complex trauma.

1 Treatments need to be developmentally appropriate and specific, and each child needs to have a complex assessment prior to treatment to determine individual needs.
2 Treatments will typically involve a phase-oriented approach, building on the child's skills as they become more integrated.

Two sources have described use of the SARI model (Frederick & McNeal, 1993; Phillips & Frederick, 1995), which outlines a useful method for phasic therapy and has been suggested as a valuable base for treating populations of children experiencing dissociation. The four phases are: (1) ensuring *safety* and *stabilization*, (2) *accessing* the trauma, (3) *resolving* the trauma, and (4) *integration* of the child's identity.

Guidelines have also been suggested for clinicians and therapists to use when working with children who experience dissociation as a result of complex trauma (for a review, see Diseth & Christie, 2005; Kluft, 1999; Putnam & Loewenstein, 1993; Steiner et al., 2003; Woolard et al., 2024), which include:

- Helping the child integrate their emotions, cognitions, and behaviors, especially in instances where they may be triggered.
- Encouraging the child to build skills and focus on strengths.
- Promoting self-acceptance and self-knowledge.
- Helping the child resolve or accept conflicting feelings, identifications, expectations, and behaviors that may be facilitated by play, imagery, or narrative.
- Working toward desensitizing the child to traumatic memories.
- Promoting and encouraging the child to regulate and express their emotions.
- Promoting healthy attachments and relationships.

Building on these guidelines and the SARI model are a range of psychotherapeutic treatments, as well as adjunctive treatments and pharmacotherapy, that can be used with this population. Below, we outline the most common treatment methods used with children who experience dissociation, as well as the somewhat scarce literature that supports the use of each treatment. As dissociation becomes more widely accepted in the medical and allied health fields, more research is becoming available on the use of these treatments. Hopefully, in the coming years, more rigorous clinical trials will be reported, and our evidence base will lead us to stronger, gold-standard treatments for these child populations.

Current Treatments Used with Children with Complex Trauma and Dissociation

As outlined in the SARI model, the first goal in the treatment of dissociation in children is to provide a safe environment for the child, which supersedes any other therapeutic treatment. Literature reports that the more successful approaches are facilitated by open-minded therapists with flexibility and creativity, and who do not rely on a sole therapeutic model (Herman, 2015; Putnam, 1997; Steiner et al., 2003). A gentle, non-judgmental, and open therapeutic stance is needed when working with children, and a connection must be made with the whole child across all internal states.

The typical treatment protocol for dissociation in children with complex trauma involves a combination psychotherapy, pharmacotherapy, and family therapy (which may include caregivers and foster families, depending on circumstances). If the child is engaging in dangerous, self-injurious, or harmful behavior, or is at risk and needs a safe environment, then inpatient or residential treatment may be necessary.

It is also important to note that often the management and treatment of dissociative disorders requires a multidisciplinary team that needs to function in a well-coordinated manner. Psychiatrists, psychologists, social workers, occupational therapists, and speech pathologists need to work together to improve the child's outcomes. The child will do better in the long run if the multidisciplinary team works with the child's family and school to provide a holistic approach to treatment.

Commonly Used Psychotherapeutic Techniques in the Treatment of Dissociation

Psychoeducation: generally speaking, psychoeducation is a cornerstone of most therapeutic treatments, and an important part of trauma treatment. Psychoeducation is important in the treatment of children who experience dissociation for the following reasons:

1. *Understanding the impact of their trauma*: Children who have experienced trauma often do not understand the impact it has had on their mental and physical health. Educating children in a developmentally appropriate way can help them understand how trauma has affected their emotions, thoughts, and behaviors.
2. *Normalizing reactions*: Psychoeducation can help children understand that their reactions to trauma are normal responses to an abnormal situation. This can help them feel less isolated and reduce shame and self-blame.
3. *Reducing stigma*: Many children feel stigmatized or ashamed of their experiences, and psychoeducation can help them understand that trauma is a common experience, and that seeking treatment is a sign of strength, not weakness.

4 *Building coping skills*: Psychoeducation can help children learn coping skills to manage their symptoms and improve their functioning. By understanding the nature of their condition, children can develop realistic expectations about treatment and the time it may take to see improvement.
5 Finally, psychoeducation can empower children to take an active role in their treatment and recovery.

Trauma-focused cognitive behavioral therapy (TF-CBT): TF-CBT is a type of psychotherapy that helps individuals overcome the effects of trauma by addressing unhelpful thoughts, feelings, and behaviors related to the traumatic event(s) (see Chapter 25 for more information).

Schema-focused cognitive behavioral therapy: Schema-focused cognitive behavioral therapy is a type of psychotherapy that focuses on identifying and addressing long-standing, negative patterns of thoughts, feelings, and behaviors (known as schemas) that develop early in life and impact one's daily functioning and relationships (Kennerley, 1996; Khosravi, 2020). If a child has experienced maltreatment early in life, then their schemas are known as "maladaptive"—that is, from their interpersonal trauma, the child has learned patterns of thoughts, feelings, and behaviors that are unhelpful (and often self-critical). Schema-focused cognitive behavioral therapy integrates elements of cognitive behavioral therapy, attachment theory, and psychodynamic principles to help individuals understand and change their maladaptive schemas and coping styles (Bricker et al., 1993).

Dialectical behavior therapy (DBT): DBT was originally developed to treat individuals with borderline personality disorder (BPD), but it has since been used to treat a range of mental health disorders including PTSD and dissociation (Groves et al., 2012). DBT is based on the theory that people who struggle with emotional dysregulation have difficulty managing their emotions and are often in intense emotional states that are difficult to control; as such, DBT can be helpful for young people who have experienced trauma and are triggered by external events.

Eye movement desensitization and reprocessing (EMDR): EMDR, developed by Shapiro (2001), is a treatment method that posits that the two hemispheres of the brain function autonomously and that bilateral stimulation (through eye movements, audio signals, or tapping on parts of the body) facilitates rapid left-right integrated processing (see Chapter 20 for more information).

Trauma-focused acceptance and commitment therapy (TF-ACT): TF-ACT is a type of psychotherapy used to help those who have experienced trauma with psychological flexibility and aims to allow individuals to develop psychological flexibility in order to accept unpleasant thoughts and emotions without them affecting their behavior (Harris, 2021). TF-ACT encompasses six principles that contribute to psychological flexibility: contact with the present moment, acceptance, diffusion (i.e., separating from our cognition), self-as-context (i.e., perspective taking or the "noticing" self), values, and committed action (Harris, 2021).

Family Systems therapy (FS): FS therapy is a type of psychotherapy that focuses on treating issues within the context of a family unit. Provided the child has a family unit that is safe to engage with in therapy, this type of therapeutic technique can help examine the family's structure, communication patterns, and relationships, and work to change negative patterns and develop healthier ways of interacting with one another. Within the context of a child who experiences dissociation, FS therapy involves encouraging family members to accept all aspects of the child and improve the communication that occurs between family members that may trigger dissociative states in the child (Silberg, 2000; Waters, 1996). FS therapy also helps caregivers process guilt or denial around traumatic events.

Mentalization-based therapy: Mentalization is the ability to imagine the mental states, intentions, and reasons for behaviors of others and ourselves (Bateman & Fonagy, 2013). Mentalizing is essential for the development of attachment and emotional regulation in children (Ensink et al., 2016). There has been recent evidence to suggest that mentalization is related to the experience of dissociation, and lower ability to mentalize may even be a risk factor leading to dissociation (Ensink et al.,

2017). Mentalization is thought to be developed through early interactions with primary caregivers, and thus adverse experiences that take place within contexts where caregivers are able to help the child mentalize are less likely to result in trauma-induced symptoms. Furthermore, when a primary caregiver generates adverse experiences for the child (i.e., maltreatment), they are likely to do so as a result of a limited capacity to mentalize the child's experience, or to avoid engaging with the suffering they are inflicting. Therefore, opportunities for talking about mental states are minimal, frequently resulting in the caregiver inhibiting the development of mentalizing in the child (Allen et al., 2008). Mentalization-based treatment (MBT) focuses on stabilizing the sense of self, sustaining mentalizing within the therapeutic relationship context, and helping the patient maintain optimum arousal during intense emotional states around other people (Allen et al., 2008). Similar to other therapeutic treatments, MBT involves a detailed assessment and an individual, group, and/or family therapy component. The therapist stance is integral to the efficacy of treatment outcomes. For children and adolescents, focusing MBT on the child as well as on the parents is essential in order to foster the development of a virtuous mentalizing cycle, allowing for mental states to be made sense of in a relational context.

Psychodynamic psychotherapy: The origins of psychodynamic psychotherapy are rooted in Freud's psychanalytic theory (for the history, please refer to the chapter on a trauma-informed psychoanalytic approach), which emphasized unconscious conflict and the release of repressed emotion. However, in recent decades, it has evolved into an approach that emphasizes intrapersonal and relational therapeutic processes (Spermon et al., 2010). Psychodynamic psychotherapy is based in models of attachment, which are often interrupted in children who experience dissociation and may be used as the overarching frame for psychotherapy. The psychodynamic treatment model encourages emotion regulation and tolerance and relies on the relationship between the therapist and the child (American Psychiatric Association, 2010). The therapist will typically build on established attachment models with the child and increase the child's tolerance to emotions, as well as build insight. The therapist will promote acceptance and a cohesive sense of self by inquiring about alter identities or states and will then move on to object- and self-representation by non-judgmentally acknowledging coherence in the child's shifts in identity and the use of these shifts as a defence mechanism. Common across psychodynamic models of therapy is the concept of the therapist's awareness of their own emotional regulation and reactions to the patient, or countertransference (Spermon et al., 2010). In psychodynamic psychotherapy, the therapist is an important source of recovery, unlike in other therapeutic methods where they are instead a pathway to recovery. The therapist must be aware of the transference and countertransference dynamics that are playing out in the therapeutic space, and these dynamics can inform the therapist about reenactments of roles from the original trauma that the patient replays within the therapeutic relationship (e.g., perpetrator, victim, rescuer, etc.).

Adjunctive Therapeutic Techniques

Mindfulness-based techniques: Mindfulness is typically used as a practice to encourage being present and in the moment, which children who experience dissociation often struggle with. Mindfulness can be used to help children regulate distressing emotions and their responses to triggering situations that remind them of their trauma (Zerubavel & Messman-Moore, 2015). Some examples of mindfulness-based activities include mindful breathing (focusing on the breath, helpful for panic and anxiety), the body scan (particularly useful for children who tend to experience depersonalization and derealization), mindful movement (see yoga, below), meditation (e.g., loving-kindness and compassion meditations). Mindfulness has been suggested as particularly useful when children experience detachment (in the form of depersonalization and derealization), absorption (daydreaming, spacing out, having a distorted perception of time), or self-fragmentation (amnesic barriers, separate personality states) (Zerubavel & Messman-Moore, 2015). Mindfulness is suggested to be about knowing and awareness, whereas dissociation is about the opposite (Forner, 2019). Mindfulness with children who have experienced trauma should be a slow approach, as intense emotions may be triggered in the process of association. Clinicians working with children experiencing dissociation need to be aware that the dissociation came about as a survival instinct, and that moving too quickly into mindfulness will trigger dissociation (Forner, 2019). Mindfulness is suggested to be used within a developmental framework, whereby the child needs to learn to reach mindfulness milestones before progressing.

Yoga: Yoga has been found to be an effective practice for individuals who have histories of trauma, as it provides a holistic approach to healing the mind and body (Macy et al., 2018). As trauma can have a significant impact on the nervous system, yoga is reported to help regulate the nervous system, reducing the impact of trauma on the body and mind. Additionally, the physical postures and breathing techniques used in yoga can help release tension and promote relaxation. Yoga also emphasizes mindfulness, which can help children who are struggling to stay grounded (a particular issue with dissociation) to become more aware of their thoughts and emotions and develop greater self-awareness and self-compassion. Obviously, this treatment method needs to be developmentally appropriate, but it can also be used as a fun and useful skill for children. Overall, yoga can be a valuable tool for children and young people to help them manage symptoms and promote healing. Practitioners should be aware of poses, or potential triggers, that may arise for individuals with experiences of trauma (e.g., avoiding the use of certain terms like "corpse pose," avoiding props like straps that might remind the individual of experiences etc.) (for more guidelines, see Davis et al., 2022).

Clinical hypnosis: Clinical hypnosis is one of the techniques often reported in small studies or case studies with children who dissociate following complex trauma (Coons & Bowman, 2001; Fink, 1992). It should be noted that clinical hypnosis is a topic debated by clinicians, and some do not support the use of this treatment with dissociative populations. Use of clinical hypnosis requires in-depth training, and advanced training to work with children and dissociation. Clinical hypnosis reportedly accesses the ego state and promotes integration (Diseth & Christie, 2005), and it can also reportedly contain intense emotions, strengthen the ego state, and educate and support the child (Kluft, 1985). Phase-oriented clinical hypnosis claims to help individuals manage their trauma and overcome feelings of helplessness. The specifics of the phases are a topic of debate; however, all models of clinical hypnosis for dissociative patients recognize that recovery via this treatment should occur in progressive stages, and the establishment of a sense of internal and external safety is essential before exploration of the trauma can happen (Sau Kuen Kwan, 2009). Some models posit that phases should consist of (1) forming a therapeutic alliance, (2) exploring traumatic memories, and (3) personality reintegration or rehabilitation (Herman, 2015), whereas others follow the SARI principles, with the four phases of (1) ensuring *safety* and *stabilization*, (2) *accessing* the trauma, (3) *resolving* the trauma, and (4) *integration* of the child's identity (Phillips & Frederick, 1995).

Art therapy: Art therapy can be a useful adjunct to psychotherapy, and some experts have even suggested that art therapy for children experiencing dissociation can be especially helpful, as the child enters a "flow" or altered state that allows them to tap into unconscious material that may be expressed in their artwork (Shirar, 1996) (see Chapter 32 on Expressive Arts Therapies for more information).

Externalization or storytelling: The therapist may use externalization as a tool to allow the child to access traumatic memories with a level of detachment, or by suggesting the child try to tell their story without expecting emotional and cognitive reintegration (i.e., allowing space for other identities to help in storytelling) or as if the story is happening to a third person. This may allow the child to increase their distress tolerance. Often, children have different parts of themselves that play different roles, which can be helpful in therapy, and the therapist should try to identify the different parts. Some common parts include feeling parts, playmates, helpers, denial parts, attachment needing parts, parts that carry sexual trauma, parts of different genders, spiritual parts, and core parts (Shirar, 1996). It should be noted, though, that while this technique can be useful early on in therapy, the primary goal should be to help the child integrate dissociative behavior that is impacting functioning.

Pharmacotherapy in Dissociation and Trauma in Children and Adolescents

It's important to note that treatment approaches should be tailored to each individual's unique needs and preferences and may involve a combination of different techniques. Typically, these psychiatric techniques are used in conjunction with pharmacology and the treatment approaches listed above and in other chapters of this book. Clinicians working in this area often state that medication alone is not sufficient for the treatment of dissociation and trauma in children. A comprehensive approach that includes psychotherapy, family therapy, or other adjunctive treatments, is necessary for the best outcomes.

The literature in the field of pharmacotherapy for trauma and dissociative symptoms is generally sparse. Additionally, there is even less of an evidence base for the use of psychotropic medications for these conditions in children. There are no specific medications approved for the treatment of complex trauma and dissociation. However, medications may be used under strict supervision to address specific symptoms associated with these conditions, such as depression, anxiety, and sleep disturbances.

Pharmacotherapy in PTSD Treatment

Evidence-based pharmacotherapy for PTSD in adults includes SSRIs (selective serotonin reuptake inhibitors) as first-line treatment. Indeed, paroxetine and sertraline are the only two medications approved by the FDA for the treatment of PTSD in adults. A Cochrane review in 2006 (Stein et al., 2006) concluded that medications were effective for core symptoms of PTSD in adults and recommended considering them as part of the treatment armamentarium. While SSRIs were not shown to be more efficacious or better tolerated than other classes of medications, they had the greatest number of effective trials. Negative studies also exist and Friedman and colleagues (2007) found that there were no significant differences between sertraline and a placebo in the treatment of PTSD in US veterans, although they did note that sertraline was well tolerated by the cohort. While the study did attempt to examine moderating variables that could have affected the results, it was not powered to do so, so no definitive conclusions could be drawn.

In the child and adolescent population, the evidence is even less robust. Despite the poor evidence base, a survey in 2001 found that about 95% of practitioners used medications for treating childhood PTSD, usually in combination with psychological therapies (Cohen et al., 2001). Most studies conducted in this population have not found any benefits of SSRIs (Cohen et al., 2007; Robb et al., 2008; Robert et al., 2008) in the treatment of PTSD in this cohort. The studies, however, have been characterized either by short duration or SSRIs being used as adjunctive treatments. A small 12-week open-label trial in eight children found that citalopram was effective in reducing some symptoms of moderate to severe PTSD (Seedat et al., 2001). SSRIs are likely to find broader acceptability in children due to their broad-spectrum activity on associated symptoms such as anxiety, depression, and obsessive compulsive disorder as well their reasonable safety profile. The evidence is even weaker for other serotonergic agents such as nefazodone and buspirone. In modern pharmacopoeia, tricyclic antidepressants have largely been replaced by SSRIs in children due to their better safety profile and may be considered as second- or third-line agents. Imipramine has been shown to have some beneficial effect on sleep-related flashbacks and insomnia in a small study treating acute stress disorder in children with burns (Robert et al., 1999). Of note, there are no medications approved by the FDA for the treatment of PTSD in children and adolescents.

A few other psychotropic medications have been investigated in the treatment of PTSD including adrenergic agents such as clonidine, antipsychotics, and anxiolytics. Two open-label trials have investigated the role of clonidine in children with PTSD and found some benefit, especially in reducing arousal symptoms of PTSD (Harmon & Riggs, 1996; Perry, 1994). A more recent open-label study of extended-release guanfacine prescribed for traumatic stress symptoms in children with ADHD concluded that it was beneficial for trauma-related symptoms in children with ADHD; however, this study included only 19 participants over eight weeks (Connor et al., 2013).

Risperidone was investigated as an adjunctive treatment in chronic military-related PTSD in adults but it was not found to be efficacious after a six-month treatment block (Krystal et al., 2011). However, a 2013 meta-analysis of an adult population (Watts et al., 2013) that reviewed eight studies of risperidone in PTSD concluded that the drug was effective as a monotherapy in contrast to use as an augmentation when participants had an inadequate response to another agent. This meta-analysis also found that topiramate and venlafaxine were effective in the treatment of PTSD. The α1-adrenoreceptor antagonist prazosin has also been investigated primarily for disordered sleep in PTSD with inconsistent efficacy demonstrated (Khachatryan et al., 2016; Raskind et al., 2018) in two studies. Benzodiazepines such as alprazolam have not been demonstrated to have any efficacy in PTSD and, indeed, may result in harm, including worsening of symptoms of PTSD, worsening of psychotherapy outcomes, aggression, depression, and substance use (Guina et al., 2015). Therefore, the use of benzodiazepines is relatively contraindicated for this condition and is not recommended. One retrospective study (Hartberg et al., 2018) found that oral ketamine was a "promising pharmacologic adjunct" for treatment-resistant depression and PTSD in adults, but more research is needed before it can be recommended as a suitable therapeutic option.

A newly emerging field is that of psychotherapy assisted by psychoactive agents such as methylenedioxymethamphetamine (MDMA) in the treatment of PTSD. The rationale is that traditional psychotherapy may result in increased anxiety during the process of flooding, when the client relives the trauma in psychotherapy. MDMA is postulated to reduce anxiety and increase euphoria, which allows for an increased sense of trust and a better working alliance between the therapist and the client (Mithoefer et al., 2011). A recently conducted randomized double-blind, placebo-controlled phase 3 trial (Mitchell et al., 2021) investigated MDMA-assisted therapy for severe PTSD and found that three doses of MDMA given in conjunction with manualized therapy over a course of 18 weeks resulted in improvement in symptoms of PTSD. A previously conducted meta-analysis compared the cumulative effect size of MDMA-assisted psychotherapy studies with those of prolonged exposure therapy and found that MDMA-assisted psychotherapy had both higher effect sizes and lower dropout rates compared to prolonged exposure therapy for PTSD. To our knowledge, no trials of psychedelic-assisted psychotherapy have yet been conducted with children and adolescents.

A recently concluded systematic review (Astill Wright et al., 2019) of the role of pharmacotherapy in the prevention and early treatment of PTSD included two studies of propranolol in the treatment of PTSD, focused on the child and adolescent population. No beneficial effects were seen in either study. Hydrocortisone as a preventative treatment was found to be a viable consideration for adults, but there were no corresponding studies with children.

Pharmacotherapy in the Treatment of Dissociative Disorders

The role of pharmacotherapy in the treatment of dissociative disorders is even less clear than in the treatment of PTSD, even in the adult population. A review (Somer et al., 2013) investigating evidence-based treatments in adults for depersonalization-derealization disorder found some inconsistent evidence for the efficacy of lamotrigine and no efficacy for fluoxetine. A more updated systematic review conducted in 2019 investigating the role of pharmacotherapy for dissociative disorders found some evidence for the efficacy of paroxetine and naloxone in controlling depersonalization symptoms and dissociative symptoms comorbid with PTSD. The authors noted the high level of heterogeneity of the five randomized control trials (RCTs) included in the review. Dissociative symptoms are also found in a diverse range of psychiatric disorders and a diagnosis of dissociative disorder is in itself heterogenous, which makes it difficult to conduct studies. Over 20 years ago, the International Society for the Study of Trauma and Dissociation Taskforce (ISSTD, 2011) noted that there were no controlled studies on the use of medications with dissociative disorders in children, adolescents, or adults. They noted that pharmacotherapy was noted to have some benefit as an adjunct to psychotherapy for targeted symptoms such as incapacitating anxiety, insomnia, and depression, among others. Medications were recommended for treatment of comorbid conditions including ADHD, PTSD, obsessive compulsive disorder, and major depression.

The evidence base for pharmacotherapy for the treatment of dissociative disorders is still limited and the use of psychotropic medications in this children and adolescents requires careful consideration of risks and benefits. It is important to note that medication should always be prescribed and monitored by a qualified health care professional and used in conjunction with other therapeutic approaches for the treatment of complex trauma and dissociation.

Overall, while there may be a role for medications in children with symptoms of trauma and dissociation, any decision regarding prescribing medications must be made after careful consideration of the phenomenology as well as other differential diagnoses and psychosocial factors. The current evidence suggests that medications may be useful for the treatment of comorbid conditions and, in some circumstances, suitable for symptomatic relief following a thorough assessment of all factors. In these circumstances, medications must be initiated and monitored only under specialist oversight with frequent reviews to evaluate efficacy and emergence of adverse effects.

The following are several practitioner tips for prescribing medications for children and adolescents with symptoms of dissociation and trauma:

1 Prescribing medication for children with symptoms of trauma and dissociation must always follow a detailed assessment and evaluation of the child, usually in a specialist setting or, at a minimum, under specialist oversight.
2 Medications are not considered to be first-line agents for treatment of dissociation and trauma symptoms in children.
3 There is reasonable evidence of the benefit of medications for the treatment of comorbid conditions such as depression.
4 Some evidence exists for the use of medications to provide symptomatic relief for trauma and dissociative symptoms, but this must be initiated and monitored only under specialist oversight.

Case Study: Marcus[1]

Background

At the time of referral, Marcus was a ten-year-old boy presenting with externalizing behavior, school refusal, problems in class at school like "zoning out," and behavioral issues at home.

Marcus had a long history of primarily externalizing behavior both in the home and school environments. He had been suspended from school multiple times due to his behavior, which included aggression toward both peers and teaching staff. Staff were unable to easily identify triggers to his dysregulated behavior; however, he was described at these times to appear different physically, with some staff saying that it appeared that even his eye color changed when he was distressed (pupillary dilation). He was described as being unreachable and would not respond to any verbal commands or gestures. He often missed instructions in class and found it very difficult to complete any work. He often referred to himself as "dumb" and "stupid" in this context.

At home, Marcus presented with similar difficulties, often having physical altercations with his siblings, which had been increasing in frequency and intensity. His mother was having difficulty getting him to school with his increasing school refusal. Marcus had witnessed severe domestic violence perpetrated by his biological father toward his mother, which, along with multiple Violence Restraining Order infringements, had resulted in his father's incarceration. At the time of Marcus's referral, his father had recently been released from prison. Marcus's mother had also experienced family domestic violence (FDV) growing up in her family of origin. She had experienced FDV during her pregnancy with Marcus and reported having significant post-natal depression, which had not been formally treated. Marcus's sister (eight years old) is known to the local child and adolescent mental health services and is currently being treated for anxiety and obsessive compulsive disorder.

Initial Assessment

Following triage and a review of the referral information, the possibility of Marcus having a developmental trauma presentation was considered, and it was noted that in relation to this diagnosis, the team would have to be mindful that there may be dissociation present as part of his presentation.

Initial assessments are an important time to get an understanding of a young person and their family's struggles and strengths. It is imperative that the family be engaged in such a way that they experience a sense of safety and control when retelling their narratives of their experiences. In an attempt to give young people a sense of control in the meeting, a full explanation of who we are and what we do with young people at our service is given. We recognize out loud how difficult it can be to tell their story, and give them strategies for what to do and say if they feel the topic of conversation is becoming overwhelming for them (e.g., "put up your hand and tell us to stop"). This has been successful in keeping young people in the room (physically and mentally), giving them an experience of agency and a sense of containment, and trust that the adults are listening and responding to their needs in the moment. The intent is to reduce anxiety from the outset and prevent any dysregulation or dissociation that would result.

Treatment Plan

The psychiatric recommendations for Marcus were assessment and identification of any comorbid mental health difficulties, specifically depression and anxiety, and monitoring these during his attendance. After completing the initial assessment, Marcus engaged with the day program and attended three days a week while still being engaged with his mainstream school on the other days of the week.

Children attending this program have significant mental health difficulties as well as education struggles and/or school refusal. The vast majority of children have experienced significant trauma. Children are fully assessed by the multidisciplinary team (MDT), from the departments of psychiatry, psychology, occupational therapy, social work, and speech pathology. The MDT recommended ongoing monitoring of symptoms. Typically, patient engagement and response to the non-pharmacological interventions would then be the major determinant of whether pharmacological intervention would be considered as an adjunct to reduce anxiety or depressive symptoms enough to allow for better engagement in the non-pharmacological interventions. In this case, medication was not needed, as Marcus was able to engage and improve without it.

The day program included individualized and group support in the following areas:

- Social communication
- Emotion and behavior regulation

- Creative expression
- Healthy coping and stress management
- Movement and physical activity

Marcus and his family were engaged in the therapeutic program, which includes a fully systemic intervention for young people and their families. This includes attendance by parents at therapeutic crisis intervention for families, which helps parents manage and deal with crises through a trauma-focused lens and provides ongoing one-to-one parenting support, case management, and family work, if indicated. The young person will attend the group program, family therapy if indicated, as well as one-to-one work with a clinician. Regular MDT review and formulation is informed by observations in one-to-one and group work in the program. During the program, Marcus was able to attend but showed high levels of separation anxiety from his mother, especially in the mornings. Additional staff support was required to give reassurance and co-regulation to allow him to proceed during the program. Marcus was noted to act "silly and impulsively" in the program's class on a frequent basis, with non-specific triggers in the class contributing to his behaviors. He would often appear to be resistant and speak to staff in accents and mimicking the languages of French, Russian, and Italian, though he did not know how to actually speak these languages. He was also noted to be "zoning out," staring into the distance at times in the classroom and finding it difficult to maintain his concentration and attention in the group and education sessions. Marcus usually responded that he had been daydreaming when interrupted but could not describe any specific place or thing that he had been daydreaming about. It was recognized that dissociation was a highly likely diagnosis due to his presentation.

Once dissociation was recognized by the team, strategies were to give psychoeducation to Marcus and his mother about dissociation and the impact that it was having on him. Analogies of how dissociation can be like "a pressure valve going off when we are overwhelmed" and finding it "all too much" are useful and easily understood by young people. It is also important to discuss dissociation as part of a normal spectrum—for instance, it can happen to anyone, but when someone has had the intense experiences related to trauma that Marcus has had, it can be unhelpful and impact how people function in a negative way. For young people like Marcus who are not conscious of their "zoning out," adults around them (such as his mother) need to be able to recognize and respond to the young person when they start zoning out. Coming up with a plan for how to do this alongside the young person is very important. The strategies may include lightly touching the young person on the shoulder or calling out their name. When they appear to be present once again, employing some grounding techniques to help reorient them is important; they can be simple things (e.g., list five things you can see, feel, and touch), but you may need to reduce the number of things the child must manage, depending on their development and the severity of the dissociation, so they do not feel overwhelmed and turn to dissociation once again. When settled, exploring with the young person how they felt prior to their dissociative experience can help them recognize the early signs of dissociation and ultimately use grounding exercises themselves.

Upon transitioning out of treatment, Marcus displayed a vast improvement in emotional and behavior regulation, as well as a decrease in dissociative symptoms. Further exploration of his difficulties through therapy revealed the meaning behind some of his fixed behavioral patterns, especially his use of accents. He was able to reveal that each accent related to a specific overwhelming emotion that he was experiencing. He explained that a French accent meant he was sad, a Russian accent meant that he was angry, and an Italian accent meant that he was anxious. At the start of his time in the program, he was adamant that he could speak these languages fluently, despite it being clear he was unable to speak them and had no knowledge of them. With increased emotional literacy and skills built in seeking help and support for his feelings, as well as explicit supportive discussions about no longer needing his French, Russian and Italian parts to communicate his distress, Marcus gradually worked toward ceasing the use of these dissociative behavior strategies. Concurrent to Marcus's attendance in the day program, his parents were seen by case coordinators to do individual and family work. This was an opportunity to understand the unique needs of the family. Through the relationship that was built with the case coordinator, the mother's mental health could be explored, and following encouragement she was able to engage with treatment for her own mental health, which had a significant impact on her ability to be present for Marcus. Psychoeducation was also provided to Marcus's mother, so that she could also identify dissociation in the home environment and employ the strategies that had worked with Marcus in the day program. His mother's improved mental health provided a much stronger sense of safety for Marcus and his sister, with a related improvement in his mental health and dissociation.

Case Study: Vivienne

Background

At the time of referral, Vivienne was a 12-year-old girl with a two-year history of fluctuating mood, difficulties sleeping due to frequent nightmares, poor appetite, lack of interest in previously enjoyed activities, social withdrawal, anxiousness, suspiciousness, and feeling like she was "going crazy." She had stopped attending school regularly and after about six months of school refusal, she had started attending a care school that was better able to accommodate her needs. She had only a few friends, whom she described as "acquaintances," and one close friend with whom she had frequent relational ruptures. She complained she was unable to feel any feelings, and that often the world around her felt distant and she couldn't tell whether or not what she was experiencing was real (hence thinking of herself as crazy). She often forgot things that had happened and struggled to memorize information, which had been quite problematic at school. She engaged in chronic self-harm (i.e., cutting, burning, head banging) and reported that the reasons for this included her desire to have a break from feeling so deeply hopeless, to punish herself, and to feel something when she felt empty and numb. Vivienne had attempted suicide by overdosing and jumping into traffic, which required emergency department presentations and an inpatient admission. Over the last two years, Vivienne had received treatment in community outpatient services, engaging inconsistently and superficially. In the last six months, she had begun attending therapy more regularly and had expressed a stronger wish to get more intense help.

Historically, Vivienne had experienced a period of marked generalized anxiety, with constant preoccupations about her physical health and that of her loved ones, somatic symptoms, and school refusal, around the age of 7. This had coincided with Vivienne needing medical treatment for an episode of juvenile rheumatoid arthritis that resolved within a year but required high doses of steroids and several hospital admissions.

Two years prior to her physical illness, Vivienne's family had mourned the sudden loss of her father due to a heart attack. Following his death, Vivienne and her mother relocated multiple times, and her mother had several short-lived relationships, until she stabilized with the man who was her current partner, when Vivienne was 8, and with whom she had a son when Vivienne was 10.

Vivienne, her brother, her mother, and her stepfather had been living together in a stable accommodation for two years. Both parents were employed. When Vivienne was 11 years old, in the context of one of her inpatient admissions, she disclosed that at age 7, one of her mother's previous partners had sexually interfered with her. The incident had been reported to the police and was undergoing court proceedings by the time Vivienne began attending therapy.

Vivienne's mother described them as doing well prior to the death of Vivienne's father, but admitted to having suffered with anxiety as a teenager herself and with post-natal depression following Vivienne's birth. She had no awareness of her biological parents' (Vivienne's maternal grandparents) physical or mental health, as she had been adopted in early childhood. Vivienne's biological father had no known mental health conditions, but his mother (Vivienne's paternal grandmother) had received treatment for what appeared to be a psychotic episode and had had a very traumatic life, escaping the Holocaust.

Initial Assessment

On admission to an MBT and therapeutic community-based day program (Gilbey et al., 2023), Vivienne was medicated with a combination of a low-dose antipsychotic to aid her sleep and an SRRI antidepressant. She found that the antidepressant possibly reduced her degree of overthinking about situations, but did not alleviate many other symptoms. The antipsychotic had improved her initial insomnia but had not resolved her nightmares. In the past, she had trialed two other antidepressants with very limited benefit, and melatonin for sleep, which had caused her nightmares to feel more vivid.

In her one-on-one meeting, Vivienne shared that she had an extremely negative view of herself, with ongoing self-doubt, confusion about what she liked/disliked and her wants, and a tendency to act how she imagined others would want her to. "I am like a chameleon," she reported.

She invested a lot in one person, her best friend, for whom she thought she also had romantic feelings, pleasing them so they would stay close. However, in most cases the relationship would break down, leaving Vivienne feeling abandoned and experiencing periods of isolation, poor functioning, and increased self-harm urges.

In spite of her desire for closeness, Vivienne noticed being highly anxious about the way other people behaved with her, feeling they were untrustworthy and unpredictable, if not harmful in the way they could use their knowledge of her against her. In this context, she worked hard to read other people, predict their intentions, and act in ways that wouldn't impact her negatively. For this reason, she had not experienced sharing her mind and opening up about her difficulties as easy, except in instances when she became extremely close to someone, but then she would be overly trusting and get exploited. When she was alone, everything felt too intense and unbearable to Vivienne, and this triggered wishes of death.

Relationships in the family were explored on meeting Vivienne's parents, which revealed an enmeshment between mother and daughter. Vivienne's mother had difficulty reading Vivienne's mental states and precursors to self-harm episodes, which led to her disengaging and isolating, dismissing Vivienne's needs. Vivienne's parents had problems reflecting on difficult events in Vivienne's life, ignoring them as if they had not taken place.

Vivienne had an ambivalent view of her stepfather: on the one hand, she perceived him as having brought back stability to the family, but on the other, she saw him as getting in the way of the relationship between her and her mother, and as favoring his biological child. The stepfather revealed difficulty in knowing how to position himself in relation to Vivienne and her mother, and perceived that since Vivienne's symptoms had been exacerbated, he had been pushed to the side even further.

Vivienne's current presentation was understood as being the result of a number of bio-psychosocial factors, including genetic loading for emotional difficulties, intergenerational trauma, disrupted attachment, repeated losses (both physical and emotional) that severely compromised Vivienne's as well as the broader system's functioning, and childhood sexual abuse with ongoing repercussions.

Treatment Plan

The treatment plan included attendance at the intensive day program with therapeutic community and mentalization-based treatment models, offering:

- Twice weekly individual therapy
- Weekly group therapy
- Parenting support for crises management
- Family therapy
- Education support
- Creative therapies
- Psychiatric management and medication review

The therapeutic approach focused on the following steps:

- Psychoeducation on the nature of developmental trauma and how this was manifesting for Vivienne, holding a specific focus on her dissociative symptoms
- Managing dissociative symptoms through grounding techniques
- Focusing on sleep with sleep hygiene and medication review
- In individual therapy:
  - Shifting focus from other to self: Vivienne was excessively preoccupied with aspects concerning others, with likely underdeveloped awareness of self-experiences; intense emotions were not tolerated and resulted in immediate search for action (i.e., self-harm) or disconnection (i.e., dissociation)
  - Exploring current mental states in relation to past traumas to learn what those events were leaving in the here and now
  - Giving Vivienne an experience of being understood, in the "making sense" process, for her to rebuild trust in relationships and tolerate easier access to emotions without the need for defensive mechanisms such as dissociation to emerge as strongly
- In group therapy:
  - Fostering capacity to notice dissociation and its triggers and use the support of group members to regain awareness; practicing flexible movement between focus on other people's experiences and self
- With mother:
  - Supporting mother to gain awareness of her own trauma responses and attachment style and model for Vivienne increasing dialogue around personal experiences, practicing personal sharing and increased explicit communication with partner/family
- In family therapy:
  - Strengthening Vivienne's alliance with her brother
  - Balancing closeness/distance between Vivienne and her mother

Vivienne and her family engaged well within a six-month intervention time. Some aspects continued to be problematic (i.e., sleep), and Vivienne continued to feel intense emotions and not trust others fully as well as being unclear about herself; however, the intensity of her feelings and the degree of rigidity in her personality style had reduced, and overwhelmingly she made several improvements, including:

- Reduced dissociative symptoms
- Greater awareness of function of symptoms as protective mechanisms and strategies to manage them
- Reduction in self-harm urges, mediated by increased tolerance for emotional intensity and greater dialogue within trusted relationships
- Increased opportunities for managing emotional overwhelm with other people rather than in isolation
- Increased social openness
- Reduced hypervigilance and social isolation
- Improved view of self with engagement in creative arts and pursuit of related educational courses

Although medication had assisted initially in response to anxiety and insomnia, it was not thought to be necessary in the long term. Medication was slowly withdrawn without ill effects. Vivienne and her mother had a good understanding of the role of medication if anxiety and/or depression recurred in the future.

Vivienne's family also reported increased dialogue in the family, improved family function with the strengthening of Vivienne's alliance with her brother, and increased dialogue between Vivienne and her stepfather. Vivienne's mother accessed her own therapy, which enabled a more balanced separation between Vivienne and her mother, and her mother reported finding it a beneficial way to support the processing of her own traumas.

Conclusion

Because many children and young people who present with dissociation following complex trauma may have experienced improper diagnosis and treatment in their time, it is important to start with a thorough assessment, and appropriate treatment will depend on the individual child's needs and developmental level. We have outlined many treatment options that medication may be used to adjunctively support, with varying amounts of empirical support, that can be used depending on the child's symptoms, needs, and environment. Most experts agree that for children experiencing dissociation, the most important factor to establish early on is safety in the therapeutic relationship, and this must be the starting point for any treatment plan. As the child has likely experienced stress and uncertainly in their life, a therapeutic alliance built on trust and hope is essential for the child's healing.

A combination of psychotherapy, adjunctive therapy, and pharmacotherapy can be used depending on the child's age, symptoms, and needs, and can be adjusted throughout the course of therapy. The ultimate goal when working with children who experience dissociation has historically been integration and supporting getting development back on track, which includes other goals related to emotion regulation, processing trauma, building strong, trusting interpersonal relationships, and being able to better function in everyday life, including learning at school. The treatment of children who experience dissociation is rarely short, often involving years of treatment at different developmental ages and stages, use of a multidisciplinary team approach, and patience and dedication on the part of the therapist or treating team.

Note

1 The case studies in this chapter are hypothetical.

References

Allen, J. G., Fonagy, P., & Bateman, A. W. (2008). Treating attachment trauma. In *Mentalizing in clinical practice* (pp. 211–239). American Psychiatric Association Publication.

American Psychiatric Association. (2010). Psychodynamic psychotherapy brings lasting benefits through self-knowledge. apa.org/news/press/releases/2010/01/psychodynamic-therapy

Astill Wright, L., Sijbrandij, M., Sinnerton, R., Lewis, C., Roberts, N. P., & Bisson, J. I. (2019). Pharmacological prevention and early treatment of post-traumatic stress disorder and acute stress disorder: A systematic review and meta-analysis. *Translational Psychiatry, 9*, Article 334. https://doi.org/10.1038/s41398-019-0673-5

Bateman, A., & Fonagy, P. (2013). Mentalization-based treatment. *Psychoanalytic Inquiry, 33*(6), 595–613. https://doi.org/10.1080/07351690.2013.835170

Bricker, D., Young, J. E., & Flanagan, C. M. (1993). Schema-focused cognitive therapy: A comprehensive framework for characterological problems. In K. T. Kuehlwein & H. Rosen (Eds.), *Cognitive therapies in action: Evolving innovative practice* (pp. 88–125). Jossey-Bass/Wiley.

Cohen, J. A., Mannarino, A. P., Perel, J. M., & Staron, V. (2007). A pilot randomized controlled trial of combined trauma-focused CBT and sertraline for childhood PTSD symptoms. *Journal of the American Academy of Child & Adolescent Psychiatry, 46*(7), 811–819. https://doi.org/10.1097/chi.0b013e3180547105

Cohen, J. A., Mannarino, A. P., & Rogal, S. (2001). Treatment practices for childhood posttraumatic stress disorder. *Child Abuse & Neglect, 25*(1), 123–135. https://doi.org/10.1016/s0145-2134(00)00226-x

Connor, D. F., Grasso, D. J., Slivinsky, M. D., Pearson, G. S., & Banga, A. (2013). An open-label study of guanfacine extended release for traumatic stress related symptoms in children and adolescents. *Journal of Child and Adolescent Psychopharmacology, 23*(4), 244–251. https://doi.org/10.1089/cap.2012.0119

Coons, P. M., & Bowman, E. S. (2001). Ten-year follow-up study of patients with dissociative identity disorder. *Journal of Trauma & Dissociation, 2*(1), 73–89. https://doi.org/10.1300/J229v02n01_09

Cudzik, M., Soroka, E., & Olajossy, M. (2019). Dissociative identity disorder as a wide range of defense mechanisms in children with a history of early childhood trauma. *Current Problems of Psychiatry, 20*(2), 117–129. https://doi.org/10.2478/cpp-2019-0006

Davis, L., Aylward, A., & Buchanan, R. (2022). Trauma-informed yoga: Investigating an intervention for mitigating adverse childhood experiences in rural contexts. *Educational Studies, 58*(4), 530–559. https://doi.org/10.1080/00131946.2022.2102495

Diseth, T. H., & Christie, H. J. (2005). Trauma-related dissociative (conversion) disorders in children and adolescents: An overview of assessment tools and treatment principles. *Nordic Journal of Psychiatry, 59*(4), 278–292. https://doi.org/10.1080/08039480500213683

Dorahy, M. J., Brand, B. L., Şar, V., Krüger, C., Stavropoulos, P., Martínez-Taboas, A., Lewis-Fernández, R., & Middleton, W. (2014). Dissociative identity disorder: An empirical overview. *Australian & New Zealand Journal of Psychiatry, 48*(5), 402–417. https://doi.org/10.1177/0004867414527523

Ensink, K., Bégin, M., Normandin, L., Godbout, N., & Fonagy, P. (2017). Mentalization and dissociation in the context of trauma: Implications for child psychopathology. *Journal of Trauma & Dissociation, 18*(1), 11–30. https://doi.org/10.1080/15299732.2016.1172536

Ensink, K., Normandin, L., Plamondon, A., Berthelot, N., & Fonagy, P. (2016). Intergenerational pathways from reflective functioning to infant attachment through parenting. *Canadian Journal of Behavioural Science/Revue canadienne des sciences du comportement, 48*, 9–18. https://doi.org/10.1037/cbs0000030

Fink, D. (1992). The psychotherapy of multiple personality disorder: A case study. *Psychoanalytic Inquiry, 12*(1), 49–70. https://doi.org/10.1080/07351699209533882

Ford, J. D., & Connor, D. F. (2009). ADHD and posttraumatic stress disorder. *Current Attention Disorders Reports, 1*(2), 60–66. https://doi.org/10.1007/s12618-009-0009-0

Forner, C. (2019). What mindfulness can learn about dissociation and what dissociation can learn from mindfulness. *Journal of Trauma & Dissociation, 20*(1), 1–15. https://doi.org/10.1080/15299732.2018.1502568

Frederick, C., & McNeal, S. (1993). From strength to strength: "Inner strength" with immature ego states. *American Journal of Clinical Hypnosis, 35*(4), 250–256. https://doi.org/10.1080/00029157.1993.10403016

Friedman, M. J., Marmar, C. R., Baker, D. G., Sikes, C. R., & Farfel, G. M. (2007). Randomized, double-blind comparison of sertraline and placebo for posttraumatic stress disorder in a Department of Veterans Affairs setting. *Journal of Clinical Psychiatry, 68*(5), 711–720. https://doi.org/10.4088/jcp.v68n0508

Gilbey, D., Brealey, G., Mateo-Arriero, I., Waters, Z., Ansell, M., Janse Van Rensburg, E., De Gouveia Belinelo, P., Milroy, H., Pace, G., Runions, K., Salmin, I., & Woolard, A. (2023). The effectiveness of a day hospital mentalization-based therapy programme for adolescents with borderline personality traits: Findings from

Touchstone—Child and Adolescent Mental Health Service. *Clinical Psychology & Psychotherapy, 30*(6), 1303–1312. https://doi.org/10.1002/cpp.2854

Gillig, P. M. (2009). Dissociative identity disorder: A controversial diagnosis. *Psychiatry, 6*(3), 24–29.

Groves, S., Backer, H. S., van den Bosch, W., & Miller, A. (2012). Dialectical behaviour therapy with adolescents. *Child and Adolescent Mental Health, 17*(2), 65–75. https://doi.org/10.1111/j.1475-3588.2011.00611.x

Guina, J., Rossetter, S. R., DeRhodes, B. J., Nahhas, R. W., & Welton, R. S. (2015). Benzodiazepines for PTSD: A systematic review and meta-analysis. *Journal of Psychiatric Practice, 21*(4), 281–303. https://doi.org/10.1097/PRA.0000000000000091

Hall, H. (2022). Dissociation and misdiagnosis of schizophrenia in populations experiencing chronic discrimination and social defeat. *Journal of Trauma & Dissociation*, 1–15. https://doi.org/10.1080/15299732.2022.2120154

Harmon, R. J., & Riggs, P. D. (1996). Clonidine for posttraumatic stress disorder in preschool children. *Journal of the American Academy of Child & Adolescent Psychiatry, 35*, 1247–1249. https://doi.org/10.1097/00004583-199609000-00022

Harris, R. (2021). *Trauma-focused ACT: A practitioner's guide to working with mind, body, and emotion using acceptance and commitment therapy.* New Harbinger Publications.

Hartberg, J., Garrett-Walcott, S., & De Gioannis, A. (2018). Impact of oral ketamine augmentation on hospital admissions in treatment-resistant depression and PTSD: A retrospective study. *Psychopharmacology, 235*(2), 393–398. https://doi.org/10.1007/s00213-017-4786-3

Herman, J. L. (2015). *Trauma and recovery: The aftermath of violence—From domestic abuse to political terror.* Hachette.

ISSTD. (2011). Guidelines for treating dissociative identity disorder in adults (3rd revised). *Journal of Trauma & Dissociation, 12*(2), 115–187. https://doi.org/10.1080/15299732.2011.537247

Kennerley, H. (1996). Cognitive therapy of dissociative symptoms associated with trauma. *British Journal of Clinical Psychology, 35*(3), 325–340. https://doi.org/10.1111/j.2044-8260.1996.tb01188.x

Khachatryan, D., Groll, D., Booij, L., Sepehry, A. A., & Schütz, C. G. (2016). Prazosin for treating sleep disturbances in adults with posttraumatic stress disorder: A systematic review and meta-analysis of randomized controlled trials. *General Hospital Psychiatry, 39*, 46–52. https://doi.org/10.1016/j.genhosppsych.2015.10.007

Khosravi, M. (2020). Child maltreatment-related dissociation and its core mediation schemas in patients with borderline personality disorder. *BMC Psychiatry, 20*(1), 405. https://doi.org/10.1186/s12888-020-02797-5

Kluft, R. P. (1985). Hypnotherapy of childhood multiple personality disorder. *American Journal of Clinical Hypnosis, 27*(4), 201–210. https://doi.org/10.1080/00029157.1985.10402608

Kluft, R. P. (1999). An overview of the psychotherapy of dissociative identity disorder. *American Journal of Psychotherapy, 53*(3), 289–319. https://doi.org/10.1176/appi.psychotherapy.1999.53.3.289

Krystal, J. H., Rosenheck, R. A., Cramer, J. A., Vessicchio, J. C., Jones, K. M., Vertrees, J. E., Horney, R. A., Huang, G. D., Stock, C., & Veterans Affairs Cooperative Study No. 504 Group. (2011). Adjunctive risperidone treatment for antidepressant-resistant symptoms of chronic military service-related PTSD: A randomized trial. *JAMA, 306*(5), 493–502. https://doi.org/10.1001/jama.2011.1080

Kulacaoglu, F., Solmaz, M., Ardic, F. C., Akin, E., & Kose, S. (2017). The relationship between childhood traumas, dissociation, and impulsivity in patients with borderline personality disorder comorbid with ADHD. *Psychiatry and Clinical Psychopharmacology, 27*(4), 393–402. https://doi.org/10.1080/24750573.2017.1380347

Loewenstein, R. J. (2018). Dissociation debates: Everything you know is wrong. *Dialogues in Clinical Neuroscience, 20*(3), 229–242.

Macy, R. J., Jones, E., Graham, L. M., & Roach, L. (2018). Yoga for trauma and related mental health problems: A meta-review with clinical and service recommendations. *Trauma, Violence, & Abuse, 19*(1), 35–57. https://doi.org/10.1177/1524838015620834

Mitchell, J. M., Bogenschutz, M., Lilienstein, A., Harrison, C., Kleiman, S., Parker-Guilbert, K., Ot'alora G., M., Garas, W., Paleos, C., Gorman, I., Nicholas, C., Mithoefer, M., Carlin, S., Poulter, B., Mithoefer, A., Quevedo, S., Wells, G., Klaire, S. S.,…, & Doblin, R. (2021). MDMA-assisted therapy for severe PTSD: A randomized, double-blind, placebo-controlled phase 3 study. *Nature Medicine, 27*(6), Article 6. https://doi.org/10.1038/s41591-021-01336-3

Mithoefer, M. C., Wagner, M. T., Mithoefer, A. T., Jerome, L., & Doblin, R. (2011). The safety and efficacy of {+/-}3,4-methylenedioxymethamphetamine-assisted psychotherapy in subjects with chronic, treatment-resistant posttraumatic stress disorder: The first randomized controlled pilot study. *Journal of Psychopharmacology, 25*(4), 439–452. https://doi.org/10.1177/0269881110378371

Myrick, A. C., Brand, B. L., McNary, S. W., Classen, C. C., Lanius, R., Loewenstein, R. J., Pain, C., & Putnam, F. W. (2012). An exploration of young adults' progress in treatment for dissociative disorder. *Journal of Trauma & Dissociation, 13*(5), 582–595. https://doi.org/10.1080/15299732.2012.694841

Perry, B. D. (1994). Neurobiological sequelae of childhood trauma: Posttraumatic stress disorders in children. In M. M. Murburg (Ed.), *Catecholamine function in posttraumatic stress disorder: Emerging concepts* (pp. 253–276). American Psychiatric Press.

Phillips, M., & Frederick, C. (1995). *Healing the divided self: Clinical and Ericksonian hypnotherapy for post-traumatic and dissociative conditi*ons (pp. xix, 371). W. W. Norton.

Putnam, F. W. (1997). *Dissociation in children and adolescents: A developmental perspective.* Guilford Press.

Putnam, F. W., & Loewenstein, R. J. (1993). Treatment of multiple personality disorder: A survey of current practices. *American Journal of Psychiatry, 150*(7), 1048–1052. https://doi.org/10.1176/ajp.150.7.1048

Raskind, M. A., Peskind, E. R., Chow, B., Harris, C., Davis-Karim, A., Holmes, H. A., Hart, K. L., McFall, M., Mellman, T. A., Reist, C., Romesser, J., Rosenheck, R., Shih, M.-C., Stein, M. B., Swift, R., Gleason, T., Lu, Y., & Huang, G. D. (2018). Trial of prazosin for post-traumatic stress disorder in military veterans. *New England Journal of Medicine, 378*(6), 507–517. https://doi.org/10.1056/NEJMoa1507598

Robb, A. S., Cueva, J. E., Sporn, J., Yang, R., & Vanderburg, D. (2008). Efficacy of sertraline in childhood PTSD. 55th Annual Meeting of the American Academy of Child and Adolescent Psychiatry Meeting, October 28–November 2, Chicago, IL.

Robert, R., Blakeney, P. E., Villarreal, C., Rosenberg, L., & Meyer, W. J. (1999). Imipramine treatment in pediatric burn patients with symptoms of acute stress disorder: A pilot study. *Journal of the American Academy of Child and Adolescent Psychiatry, 38*(7), 873–882. https://doi.org/10.1097/00004583-199907000-00018

Robert, R., Tcheung, W. J., Rosenberg, L., Rosenberg, M., Mitchell, C., Villarreal, C., Thomas, C., Holzer, C., & Meyer, W. J. (2008). Treating thermally injured children suffering symptoms of acute stress with imipramine and fluoxetine: A randomized, double-blind study. *Burns: Journal of the International Society for Burn Injuries, 34*(7), 919–928. https://doi.org/10.1016/j.burns.2008.04.009

Şar, V., Dorahy, M., & Krüger, C. (2017). Revisiting the etiological aspects of dissociative identity disorder: A biopsychosocial perspective. *Psychology Research and Behavior Management, 10*, 137–146. https://doi.org/10.2147/PRBM.S113743

Sau Kuen Kwan, P. (2009). Phase-orientated hypnotherapy for complex PTSD in battered women: An overview and case studies from Hong Kong. *Australian Journal of Clinical and Experimental Hypnosis, 37*(1), 49–59. hypnosisaustralia.org.au/wp-content/uploads/journal/AJCEH_Vol37_No1_MAY09.pdf

Seedat, S., Lockhat, R., Kaminer, D., Zungu-Dirwayi, N., & Stein, D. J. (2001). An open trial of citalopram in adolescents with post-traumatic stress disorder. *International Clinical Psychopharmacology, 16*, 21–25. https://doi.org/10.1097/00004850-200101000-00002

Shapiro, F. (2001). *Eye movement desensitization and reprocessing: Basic principles, protocols, and procedures* (2nd ed., pp. xxiv, 472). Guilford Press.

Shirar, L. (1996). *Dissociative children: Bridging the inner and outer worlds*. W. W. Norton. onlinelibrary.wiley.com/doi/abs/10.1002/jts.2490100417

Silberg, J. L. (2000). Fifteen years of dissociation in maltreated children: Where do we go from here? *Child Maltreatment, 5*(2), 119–136. https://doi.org/10.1177/1077559500005002004

Somer, E., Amos-Williams, T., & Stein, D. J. (2013). Evidence-based treatment for depersonalisation-derealisation disorder (DPRD). *BMC Psychology, 1*(1), 20. https://doi.org/10.1186/2050-7283-1-20

Spermon, D., Darlington, Y., & Gibney, P. (2010). Psychodynamic psychotherapy for complex trauma: Targets, focus, applications, and outcomes. *Psychology Research and Behavior Management, 2010*(3), 119–127. https://doi.org/10.2147/PRBM.S10215

Spitzer, C., Barnow, S., Freyberger, H. J., & Grabe, H. J. (2006). Recent developments in the theory of dissociation. World Psychiatry.

Stein, D. J., Ipser, J. C., Seedat, S., Sager, C., & Amos, T. (2006). Pharmacotherapy for post traumatic stress disorder (PTSD). *Cochrane Database of Systematic Reviews, 2006*(1), CD002795. https://doi.org/10.1002/14651858.CD002795.pub2

Steiner, H., Carrion, V., Plattner, B., & Koopman, C. (2003). Dissociative symptoms in posttraumatic stress disorder: Diagnosis and treatment. *Child and Adolescent Psychiatric Clinics of North America, 12*(2), 231–249. https://doi.org/10.1016/S1056-4993(02)00103-7

Waters, F. S. (1996). Parents as partners in the treatment of dissociative children. In J. Silberg (Ed.), *The dissociative child: Diagnosis, treatment, and management* (2nd ed., pp. 273–295). Sidran Press.

Watts, B. V., Schnurr, P. P., Mayo, L., Young-Xu, Y., Weeks, W. B., & Friedman, M. J. (2013). Meta-analysis of the efficacy of treatments for posttraumatic stress disorder. *Journal of Clinical Psychiatry, 74*(6), e541–e550. https://doi.org/10.4088/JCP.12r08225

Woolard, A., Boutrus, M., Bullman, I., Wicken, N., De Gouveia Belinelo, P., Solomon, T., & Milroy, H. (2024). Treatment for childhood and adolescent dissociation: A systematic review. *Psychological Trauma: Theory, Research, Practice, and Policy*. https://doi.org/10.1037/tra0001615. https://psycnet.apa.org/search/display?id=a56c9e94-e33a-3393-00c2-cf3666fae038&recordId=1&tab=PA&page=1&display=25&sort=PublicationYearMSSort%20desc,AuthorSort%20asc&sr=1

Zerubavel, N., & Messman-Moore, T. L. (2015). Staying present: Incorporating mindfulness into therapy for dissociation. *Mindfulness, 6*(2), 303–314. https://doi.org/10.1007/s12671-013-0261-3

47
CONCLUSION

Jillian Hosey and Ana M. Gómez

How the Past and Present Inform the Future

After over 40 years of combined experience in the treatment of severely traumatized and dissociative children, this book represents an effort to address the collective challenges child therapists face when it comes to the multifaceted phenomena of childhood complex trauma and dissociation. Through the collective knowledge, experience, and wisdom of various experts and pioneers in the field, this volume covers important considerations across theory, assessment, research, and clinical practice to educate clinical professionals, students, and researchers alike, regardless of their level of experience and expertise. Organized to provide both an informative and a practical approach, therapeutic strategies and resources grounded in relevant theory are offered throughout the book, giving treating professionals a greater sense of agency and direction as they face their most challenging cases. In offering a rich compendium of the ways in which manifestations of complex trauma and dissociation in children are and can be understood and treated, we endeavor to reawaken, challenge, and reinvigorate the field, to inspire new explorations into the magnitude and impact of complex trauma on the developing mind. In reaching beyond this volume and the additional references provided throughout, we also encourage readers to review new and emerging research on the neurological effects of trauma and maltreatment (Ireton et al., 2024; Teicher et al., 2016), dissociation and dissociative disorders (Dimitrova et al., 2021; Lebois et al., 2021; Reinders et al., 2014), fetal and infant consciousness (Bayne et al., 2023), and epigenetics (Yehuda & Lehrner, 2018).

We do recognize, however, the confinements of any single source to fully depict the profundity of this subject matter. Even the most exhaustive volumes cannot encapsulate the complexity inherent in this field. The intricate interplay of neurobiological, psychological, cultural intersectionality, and environmental/relational dynamics encompassing childhood trauma and dissociation transcends the frontiers of any singular discourse. We hope this book inspires interest in the exploration and development of multiple areas that are beyond the scope of this volume. The following are some of the recommended advancements needed in the area of childhood complex trauma and dissociation.

Advancing Assessment and Diagnosis

The field grapples with critical challenges, compounded by the lack of comprehensive assessment measures to assess polysymptomatic dissociation and other comorbidities in children that

Conclusion

are often misunderstood and under-reported. Dissociative symptomatology, whether chronic or acute, needs clear differentiation from acute stress disorder, PTSD, adjustment disorders, mood disorders, and other chronic dissociative clinical presentations (Şar, 2022). The current diagnostic framework offered by the DSM-5 falls short in addressing child-specific dissociation and complex trauma-related diagnostic categories, contributing to the ongoing challenges regarding the refinement and study of treatment outcomes (Silberg & Dallam, 2023). In addition to the research recommendations proposed in Chapter 2, Şar et al. (2012) add the importance of including "an age-sensitive clinical evaluation stage to screening studies on children and adolescents in the community" (p. 183). To complicate issues of assessment and diagnosis further, complex trauma and dissociation are transdiagnostic phenomena, with multiple symptoms, displays, and variations presenting across various conditions and diagnoses. Critical questions that ask what makes a child develop dissociation versus an anxiety disorder, how we can understand the differentiating factors, and whether existing self-report instruments can provide information on the nuances of dissociative processes and experiences across diagnostic categories require deeper exploration. Further, how does this relate to issues of misdiagnosis, comorbidity, and the role of dissociative phenomena across the spectrum of child mental health challenges? Transdiagnostic inquiry and study would support a greater understanding of the relationships between dissociation, child maltreatment, and different types of childhood mental health challenges and diagnoses.

Despite the established connections woven through this volume that propose a link between trauma and dissociation, with trauma serving as either a root cause or a driving force, epidemiological studies of dissociation and dissociative disorders in children continue to be minimal compared to the adult literature (please see Chapter 2 in this volume). Increased attention to the multidimensional impacts of child maltreatment in undergraduate studies across helping professions and related disciplines is needed. By increasing the dissemination of knowledge, we hope that interest in the study of dissociation in childhood is stirred, creating space for much-needed qualitative and quantitative research in the areas covered in this volume. In alignment with recommendations for further research into the study of adult dissociation (Şar & Ross, 2023), our child population would also benefit from similar studies that look at, but are not limited to, (a) the more silent forms of traumatization and their relationship to the development of dissociative symptomology in childhood; (b) neurobiological studies into developmental trauma and dissociative symptomology in childhood; (c) the relationship between individual and interactional psychopathology within family systems; (d) treatment outcomes; and (e) the relationship between community violence, trauma, and dissociation in childhood. Studies that pay attention to the role of hypnotizability as a mediating factor in the development of childhood dissociation (see Chapter 7), despite the controversy it has brought, are also needed to better understand the neurobiological and phenomenological underpinnings of childhood dissociation.

Further, considering the interconnectedness of assessment/diagnosis as a pathway to effective treatment delivery, changes and advancements in these areas will significantly influence clinical practice. Without the full recognition of complex trauma/DTD and CPTSD in children as diagnostic categories in childhood, funding may not be allocated to the research and treatment of complex trauma and dissociation across institutions. Additionally, children's developmental divergences, the spectrum of trauma exposure that exhibits a nuanced array of presentations, and the range of dissociative presentations and severity will yield treatment and assessment variations. We need research to critically explore and examine individual differences (Woolard et al., 2024), to in turn support effective treatment. Some authors propose a multimodal approach to address the various areas and domains of a child's functioning (Gomez, 2012; Woolard et al., 2024).

Advancing Treatment

We assert that the field also needs much greater delineations of the nuances of delivering treatment across multiple settings, which includes consistent early identification practices. Boyer et al. (2022) assert that, typically, "People living with DDs spend an average of 5 to 12.4 years actively engaged in treatment before receiving an accurate diagnosis" (p. 78). These authors further remind us that "untreated dissociation puts the aging child at risk for the development of more severe impairments in functioning over time due to worsening symptoms" (p. 81), which is a high cost for individuals, communities, systems, and societies as a whole. In outpatient or private practice settings, clinicians need substantial training to engage in the assessment of trauma and dissociation with children who present with severe and perplexing symptoms; however, these settings are often unequipped for the child whose needs require a higher level of care than outpatient treatment can provide. For many children presenting with severe symptomatology, inpatient treatment may not be optimal due to: financial constraints, lack of accessible insurance and financial resources, and concerns related to re-traumatization within systems that are not attuned to trauma-specific needs and presentations. While inpatient treatment facilities offer the greatest containment, the forced separation of the child from their relational environment can reactivate and set in motion internal working models and memory systems holding traumatogenic data and trauma-formed patterns of nervous system activation, in turn exacerbating the child's symptomatology. However, for the child that our system completely misses or provides ineffective treatments, inpatient facilities often become the last resource and a source of hope. There is a lack of sufficient studies that show the effectiveness of residential treatment for dissociative children exposed to complex traumatization and the maintenance of therapeutic changes after discharge. We need to conduct further studies to develop consistent continuums of care and treatment. For many children on the severe side of the dissociative spectrum, residential treatments are the only option to avoid hospitalizations, stop abusive and chaotic family systems, prevent suicide attempts, closely monitor self-harm, and improve medication management (Butler & McPherson, 2007).

An understanding of what facilitates or hinders outpatient treatment retention in dissociative children is another area of treatment research that is needed. For example, with increased social isolation, parental stress, losses, and family illnesses brought up by the COVID-19 pandemic, a deterioration in mental health in individuals across the lifespan, including children, has occurred (Loades et al., 2020; Rauschenberg et al., 2021). The scarcity of statistics on the effectiveness and retention of inpatient and outpatient treatment that takes into consideration the residual impact of the COVID-19 pandemic and its influence on child dissociation speaks to a need to identify dynamic, more effective treatment components that lead to increased access, engagement, and retention.

Addressing the gaps requires a multifaceted approach that elucidates the developmental trajectories and impact of early exposure to ongoing trauma and the emergence of dissociation in children. Early identification can potentially mitigate the long-term consequences of the untreated legacy of trauma in the pediatric population. Schools are a venue to consider regarding accessibility, familiarity, and as a relational milieu that can support children who would otherwise not receive adequate treatment. Schools have traditionally been underutilized as a first line of detection and treatment for complex traumatization even though studies are reporting significant success in trauma-specific interventions in school settings (Dorado et al., 2016). However, the specific elements contributing to change and positive outcomes remain unclear (Overstreet & Chafouleas, 2016). Attention to processes that support early recognition is a critical factor in preventing escalations in symptomatology and a lifelong trajectory into more severe forms of dissociation (Woolard et al., 2024; Silberg & Dallam, 2023).

Conclusion

Another area needing attention is the cultural context within which dissociation is defined, assessed, and treated across treatment settings. Some authors call for a perspective that considers the intergenerational effects of colonization, oppression and power imbalances, displacement, forced immigration, and enslavement (Mullan, 2023) as part of the multiple manifestations of complex trauma and dissociation in our children. Critical inquiry into how children's unique cultural backgrounds and interrelated experiences impact responses to trauma, as well as how they manifest and report dissociative experiences, is needed.

We encourage a stance of cultural humility in how we explore systems of power and dominance and how they have influenced our mental health definitions, models, and treatment guidelines. According to Somer (2006), "Ideas about self, the soul, and the nature of reality influence the way societies view the etiology of dissociative experience" (p. 214). Somer further states that a culture may consider the self to be continuous, which is different from a society that considers this construct illusory. The study of the cultural variants of dissociation requires a cross-cultural perspective that spans interdisciplinary collaborations beyond just mental health scholars into anthropology and beyond (Mullan, 2023; Somer, 2006). Research that investigates the relationship between culture, trauma, and the full spectrum of dissociation in children is paramount (Krüger, 2020). Furthermore, research and inquiry that delves deeper into the intersections of social identity, childhood trauma, and dissociation is lacking, including, but not limited to considerations across gender identity, religion, and (dis)abilities. The psychobiological underpinnings of children with identities that deviate from binary social conceptions and expressions (Diamond, 2020), especially the ones with dissociative identities have not been adequately studied.

We also call on scholars, practitioners, researchers, and stakeholders to approach the examination of child complex trauma and dissociation with intentionality, humility, and openness. There are areas of treatment that would benefit from further exploration and expansion in the field of integrative mind-body methodologies that include, but are not limited to, tai chi, qigong, yoga, Reiki, meditation, dance/rhythm movement, breathwork, music, and sound therapy, to determine their effectiveness and feasibility with this population. A literature review of 199 controlled trials (RCTs) of integrative body-mind-spirit interventions from 2004 to 2014 showed promising results with a variety of mental health conditions in adults (Yee et al., 2018). A study conducted on traumatized youth ages 12–21 in residential treatment demonstrates the effectiveness of yoga in building self-regulatory capacities (Spinazzola et al., 2011). Trauma-sensitive yoga has also been developed as an adjunct treatment for individuals affected by trauma (Emerson, 2015). However, control studies with children affected by trauma and experiencing dissociation are absent in this field. How and what integrative and holistic approaches may benefit children affected by complex trauma and dissociation is an area of growth in clinical practice that requires support from empirical study and advancement.

Energy-based interventions and the connection between quantum theory and human psychology are unexplored and even stigmatized despite scientific discoveries in physics within the realm of quantum theory. This area remains controversial, as it challenges conventional theories of the human mind and a medical model highly reliant on chemicals to promote healing. However, these interdisciplinary and ancient perspectives are beginning to receive attention from great minds in our field. For example, Siegel (2023) stated that the mind is the flow of energy and information and "as an emergent property of energy flow, mind emerges not just from within our bodies, but between the body and the world" (p. 89). Siegel further states that electromagnetic energy flows in every neural representation and each bottom-up and top-down transaction of the nervous system. According to Siegel, this energy flow of the mind is *shared* within individuals, nature, and everything in existence. This dynamic dance of energy among all that exists intertwines a dynamic tapestry of interconnectedness. We wonder about the role of consciousness and how the clinician's mind fundamentally influences the psychological states of the client's experience and the co-creation of their reality. It is worth igniting critical thinking in this area to expand our understanding of human consciousness and venture into new healing possibilities for children that extend beyond conventional paradigms and approaches.

Other Important Considerations

Several unaddressed issues demand additional attention, which include, but are not limited to, the use of telehealth, issues regarding aggression, and legal issues and implications. As therapy shifted outside of in-person spaces during the COVID-19 pandemic out of necessity, the use of telehealth with children became a popular alternative that allowed the continuity of treatment. Telehealth provides greater accessibility; eliminates barriers related to transportation, mobility, and financial resources; and supports continuity of care. It also makes it easier to involve the caregivers and enhance the child's relational milieu. However, the use of screens can inhibit the ability to attune to the whole child and hold the therapeutic space, and assumes that families have consistent access to technological resources. Studies on the use of telehealth with children with histories of complex trauma and dissociation are scarce, calling for a need to further explore its effectiveness, efficiency, and the specific therapeutic adaptations that support it.

Aggression directed at others is an additional symptom that often manifests in varying degrees in children chronically exposed to interpersonal trauma (Guo et al., 2024). Aggression is a multi-layer phenomenon that is interconnected with psychological, biological, and social systems, making it a highly nuanced behavior in children with histories of complex trauma and symptoms of dissociation. To better support treatment delivery, we recommend expanding the literature and research on aggression and its relationship to complex trauma and dissociation, including issues related to attachment to the perpetrator and perpetrator introjection.

Finally, many children affected by complex trauma are found in the foster care and judicial systems (Greeson et al., 2011; Kisiel et al., 2014, 2020). The lives of these children are nuanced by frequent ruptures, inconsistent caregiving, and disruptions in attachment as they face multiple placements. Children of incarcerated parents, in foster care, or adopted from orphanages face shame and embarrassment, financial hardship, marginalization, and, at times, parentification as they are forced to assume the caregiver's role in addition to other forms of trauma. The legal system plays a crucial role in overseeing children's welfare, making placement decisions, terminating parental rights, guardianship, case oversight, and more. Our personal experience with hundreds of children and our journeys in family court lead us to wonder how much the legal system is adequately trained to understand the nuances of complex trauma and dissociation (see Paulson et al., 2023). We have witnessed innumerable instances in which reunification or unsupervised visits with perpetrators were granted prior to the appropriate therapeutic work to ensure the safety and stability of the child, or times when the welfare system frequently moved children from foster home to foster home, despite clinical recommendations against such changes. We have also encountered incredible child advocates, judges, and guardians who have assumed heroic roles as stakeholders and protectors of these children. However, these social structures are often inconsistent, lose funding, or are characterized by the absence of complex trauma and dissociation-informed practices. Considering that judges, guardians ad litem, court-appointed advocates, case managers, and decision-makers are entrusted with the responsibility of safeguarding the well-being of our most vulnerable children impacted by trauma, further explorations into the functioning of these structures are paramount. Ensuring that children's voices are heard is a responsibility we have as a field, and as such, we hope this topic is further addressed in future editions, literature, and research to ensure change.

In the ever-evolving landscape of child complex trauma and dissociation, our exploration in this volume has endeavored to be comprehensive and extensive. However, the depth and breadth of the field comprise a multitude of factors across numerous domains that need further exploration.

Conclusion

We consider it imperative to mentor newer clinicians, academics, and researchers entering the field to support the growth and development of the treatment of childhood complex trauma and dissociation for future generations. We hope to be able to pass on the torch and share it with our readers to continue expanding and refining what is known while delving deeper into unexplored areas. Together, we can grow and create better outcomes for our most vulnerable children while supporting their growth and development and influencing their health and well-being. We remain committed to amplifying children's voices and advocating for systemic change so children can heal and thrive. We hope to empower future generations of clinicians to be guided by sound research and theoretical constructs while cultivating cultural humility, social justice, self-reflection, and compassion in their therapeutic endeavors.

References

Bayne, T., Frohlich, J., Cusack, R., Moser, J., & Naci, L. (2023). Consciousness in the cradle: On the emergence of infant experience. *Trends in Cognitive Sciences, 27*(12), 1135–1149. https://doi.org/10.1016/j.tics.2023.08.018

Boyer, S. M., Caplan, J. E., & Edwards, L. K. (2022). Trauma-related dissociation and the dissociative disorders: Neglected symptoms with severe public health consequences. *Delaware Journal of Public Health, 8*(2), 78–84. https://doi.org/10.32481/djph.2022.05.010

Butler, L. S., & McPherson, P. M. (2007). Is residential treatment misunderstood? *Journal of Child and Family Studies, 16*(4), 465–472. https://doi.org/10.1007/s10826-006-9101-6

Diamond, L. (2020). Gender fluidity and nonbinary gender identities among children and adolescents. *Child Development Perspectives, 14*(2), 110–115. https://doi.org/10.1111/cdep.12366

Dimitrova, L. I., Dean, S. L., Schlumpf, Y. R., Vissia, E. M., Nijenhuis, E. R. S., Chatzi, V., Jäncke, L., Veltman, D. J., Chalavi, S., & Reinders, A. A. T. S. (2021). A neurostructural biomarker of dissociative amnesia: A hippocampal study in dissociative identity disorder. *Psychological Medicine, 53*(3), 805–813. https://doi.org/10.1017/S0033291721002154

Dorado, J. S., Martinez, M., McArthur, L. E., & Leibovitz, T. (2016). Healthy environments and response to trauma in schools (HEARTS): A whole-school, multi-level, prevention and intervention program for creating trauma-informed, safe and supportive schools. *School Mental Health, 8*(1), 163–176. https://doi.org/10.1007/s12310-016-9177-0

Emerson, D. (2015). *Trauma-sensitive yoga in therapy: Bringing the body into treatment.* Norton Professional Books.

Gomez, A. M. (2012). *EMDR therapy and adjunct approaches with children: Complex trauma, attachment, and dissociation.* Springer Publishing.

Greeson, J. K. P., Briggs, E. C., Kisiel, C. L., Layne, C. M., Ake, G. S., III., Ko, S. J., Gerrity, E. T., Steinberg, A. M., Howard, M. L., Pynoos, R. S., & Fairbank, J. A. (2011). Complex trauma and mental health in children and adolescents placed in foster care: Findings from the National Child Traumatic Stress Network. *Child Welfare, 90*(6), 91–108.

Guo, Z., Hu, Q., Chen, J., Hong, D., Huang, Y., Lv, J., Xu, Y., Zhang, R., & Jiang, S. (2024). The developmental characteristics of proactive and reactive aggression in late childhood: The effect of parental control. *Aggressive Behavior, 50*(1), e22112. https://doi.org/10.1002/ab.22112

Ireton, R., Hughes, A., & Klabunde, M. (2024). A functional magnetic resonance imaging meta-analysis of childhood trauma. *Biological Psychiatry: Cognitive Neuroscience and Neuroimaging, 9*(6), 561–570. https://doi.org/10.1016/j.bpsc.2024.01.009

Kisiel, C. L., Fehrenbach, T., Torgersen, E., Stolbach, B., McClelland, G., Griffin, G., & Burkman, K. (2014). Constellations of interpersonal trauma and symptoms in child welfare: Implications for a developmental trauma framework. *Journal of Family Violence, 29*(1), 1–14. https://doi.org/10.1007/s10896-013-9559-0

Kisiel, C. L., Torgersen, E., & McClelland, G. (2020). Understanding dissociation in relation to child trauma, mental health needs, and intensity of services in child welfare: A possible missing link. *Journal of Family Trauma, Child Custody & Child Development, 17*(3), 189–218. https://doi.org/10.1080/26904586.2020.1816867

Krüger, C. (2020). Culture, trauma and dissociation: A broadening perspective for our field. *Journal of Trauma & Dissociation, 21*(1), 1–13. https://doi.org/10.1080/15299732.2020.1675134

Lebois, L. A. M., Li, M., Baker, J. T., Wolff, J. D., Wang, D., Lambros, A. M., Grinspoon, E., Winternitz, S., Ren, J., Gönenç, A., Gruber, S. A., Ressler, K. J., Liu, H., & Kaufman, M. L. (2021). Large-scale functional brain network architecture changes associated with trauma-related dissociation. *The American Journal of Psychiatry, 178*(2), 165–173. https://doi.org/10.1176/appi.ajp.2020.19060647

Loades, M. E., Chatburn, E., Higson-Sweeney, N., Reynolds, S., Shafran, R., Brigden, A., Linney, C., McManus, M. N., Borwick, C., & Crawley, E. (2020). Rapid systematic review: The impact of social isolation and loneliness on the mental health of children and adolescents in the context of COVID-19. *Journal of the American Academy of Child & Adolescent Psychiatry, 59*(11), 1218–1239. https://doi.org/10.1016/j.jaac.2020.05.009

Mullan, J. (2023). *Decolonizing therapy: Oppression, historical trauma, and politicizing your practice*. Norton Professional Books.

Overstreet, S., & Chafouleas, S. M. (2016). Trauma-informed schools: Introduction to the special issue. *School Mental Health, 8*(1), 1–6. https://doi.org/10.1007/s12310-016-9184-1

Paulson, T., Perrin, B., Maunder, R. G., & Muller, R. T. (2023). Toward a trauma-informed approach to evidence law: Witness credibility and reliability. *The Canadian Bar Review, 101*(3), 496–545.

Rauschenberg, C., Schick, A., Goetzl, C., Roehr, S., Riedel-Heller, S. G., Koppe, G., Durstewitz, D., Krumm, S., & Reininghaus, U. (2021). Social isolation, mental health, and use of digital interventions in youth during the COVID-19 pandemic: A nationally representative survey. *European Psychiatry, 64*(1), e20. https://doi.org/10.1192/j.eurpsy.2021.17

Reinders, A. A. T. S., Willemsen, A. T. M., den Boer, J. A., Vos, H. P. J., Veltman, D. J., & Loewenstein, R. J. (2014). Opposite brain emotion-regulation patterns in identity states of dissociative identity disorder: A PET study and neurobiological model. *Psychiatry Research: Neuroimaging, 223*(3), 236–243. https://doi.org/10.1016/j.pscychresns.2014.05.005

Şar, V. (2022). Dissociation across cultures: A transdiagnostic guide for clinical assessment and management. *Alpha Psychiatry, 23*(3), 95–103. https://doi.org/10.5152/alphapsychiatry.2021.21556

Şar, V., Middleton, W., & Dorahy, M. J. (2012). The scientific status of childhood dissociative identity disorder: A review of published research. *Psychotherapy and Psychosomatics, 81*(3), 183–184. https://doi.org/10.1159/000333361

Şar, V., & Ross, C. A. (2023). A research agenda for the dissociative disorders field. In M. J. Dorahy, S. N. Gold & J. A. O'Neil (Eds.), *Dissociation and the dissociative disorders: Past, present, future* (2nd ed., pp. 793–810). Routledge. https://doi.org/10.4324/9781003057314

Siegel, D. J. (2023). *Intraconnected: Mwe (me + we) as integration of self, identity, and belonging*. Norton Professional Books.

Silberg, J., & Dallam, S. (2023). Dissociative disorders in children and adolescents. In M. J. Dorahy, S. N. Gold & J. A. O'Neil (Eds.), *Dissociation and the dissociative disorders: Past, present, future* (2nd ed., pp. 433–447). Routledge. https://doi.org/10.4324/9781003057314

Somer, E. (2006). Culture-bound dissociation: A comparative analysis. *Psychiatric Clinics of North America, 29*(1), 213–226. https://doi.org/10.1016/j.psc.2005.10.009

Spinazzola, J., Rhodes, A. M., Emerson, D., Earle, E., & Monroe, K. (2011). Application of yoga in residential treatment of traumatized youth. *Journal of the American Psychiatric Nurses Association, 17*(6), 431–444. https://doi.org/10.1177/1078390311418359

Teicher, M. H., Samson, J. A., Anderson, C. M., & Ohashi, K. (2016). The effects of childhood maltreatment on brain structure, function and connectivity. *Nature Reviews Neuroscience, 17*(10), 652–666. https://doi.org/10.1038/nrn.2016.111

Woolard, A., Boutrus, M., Bullman, I., Wickens, N., Gouveia Belinelo, P. d., Solomon, T., & Milroy, H. (2024). Treatment for childhood and adolescent dissociation: A systematic review. *Psychological Trauma: Theory, Research, Practice, and Policy*. https://doi.org/10.1037/tra0001615

Yee, L. M., Xiafei, W., Chang, L., Salome, R., & Susan, T. (2018). Outcome literature review of integrative body–mind–spirit practices for mental health conditions. *Social Work Research, 42*(3), 251–266. https://doi.org/10.1093/swr/svy018

Yehuda, R., & Lehrner, A. (2018). Intergenerational transmission of trauma effects: Putative role of epigenetic mechanisms. *World Psychiatry, 17*(3), 243–257. https://doi.org/10.1002/wps.20568

INDEX

Note: **Bold** page numbers refer to tables and *italic* page numbers refer to figures.

abandonment 40, 45, 48, 107, 157, 209, 221, 292, 293, 295, 296
Abrams, M. P. 96
abuse 31, 34, 259, 628; betrayal 61; childhood 108, 110, 114–116, 188, 364, 452, 696, 811; domestic violence 189; emotional 32, 39, 79, 108, 189, 197, 200; intrafamilial/extrafamilial 113; neglect 39, 41, 42, 62, 108, 110, 189, 302, 628; physical 32, 39, 59, 62, 79, 108, 189, 793; psychological 255, 354; sexual 31, 32, 39, 59, 65, 67, 79, 108, 189, 302, 311, 318, 793; *see also* child sexual abuse (CSA)
Acute Stress Checklist for Children (ASC-K) 216
adaptive information processing (AIP) model 365, 702, 817
adjunctive therapeutic techniques for dissociation treatment 865–867; art therapy 866; clinical hypnosis 866; externalization/storytelling 866–867; mindfulness 865–866; yoga 866
Adlerian play therapy 316
Adler-Tapia, R. L. 316
Adolescent Dissociative Experiences Scale (A-DES) 214
Adult Attachment Interview (AAI) 40, 42, 66, 604, 710, 715
adverse childhood experiences (ACEs) 2, 31, 58, 59, 522, 533, 673, 675, 676, 679, 686
affective neuroscience 170, 739
affect regulation 63–64, 174, 366; adaptive 65; assessment 68; attachment, adversity, and 65; attachment, dissociation and 66–68; importance of 64–65; maladaptive 65; skills 814–815
affect regulation assessment: Difficulties in Emotion Regulation Scale (DERS) 68; Emotion Regulation Checklist (ERC) 68

aggressive states 295, 296
Ainsworth, Mary 61, 66, 108, 130, 346; attachment theory 108, 130; Strange Situation Procedure (SSP) 66
Aitken, K. J. 647, 650
Akay-Sullivan, S. 116
Allen, J. G. 40
All the Beauty and the Bloodshed (Goldin) 632
All the Colors of Me: My First Book about Dissociation (Gomez and Paulsen) 810
Alpha-Down training 463
altered states of consciousness 23, 45, 62, 96
Amédée, L. M. 498
American Academy of Child and Adolescent Psychiatry (AACAP) clinical guidelines 462
American Psychological Association (APA) 90, 503, 660
American Veterinary Medical Association (AVMA) 503
amnesia 4, 76, 77, 91–93, 112, 197–199, 208, 240
amygdala 125, 158
Anand, K. J. 825
Andor, Karen 561, 569, 570, 573
Andreas-Salomé, Lou 312
animal and brain network activity 26–27
animal-assisted education (AAE) 503
Animal-Assisted Interventions (AAI) 502, 503
animal-assisted therapy (ATT) 501–518; animal partner selection to address dissociation and hyperarousal 517–518; definition 503; Neurosequential Model© *see* Neurosequential Model© (NM); relational patterns *see* relational patterns in ATT sessions; theory and tenets of 502–504
Anna Freud Centre 315

Index

Anna Freud Centre for Children and Families 315, 613
anterior cingulate cortex (ACC) 30
apparently normal personality (ANP) 157
Aquerone, Stella 317
arousal model training approach 467–469
arousal regulation/dysregulation 42, 398, 399
Arthur, Andrew 309
art therapy 69, 612–633, 854–855, 866; advocacy and meaning making 632; art expression, implicit and explicit mentalization 629–632, *630*; case example 618–621, 624, 626–627, 630–632; cautions and considerations working with children 614; complications in treating developmental trauma 612–613; exploring attachment and developmental needs timeline 625–627, *627*; history-gathering and container timelines 617–618, *619*; integrated into phase-oriented treatment-phase 616–617, *617*, 627, 632; precautions using art media and 614–615; psychic split and finding meaning 628–629; psychoeducation 622–625, *623*, *625*; recommendations 613–614; strengths and resources development 620–621; therapeutic relationship, art making in 615–616
assessment phase in EMDR therapy 375–381, 384–385; desensitization, installation and body scan 377; EMDR interweave 380–381; exploration and processing of trauma 375–376; platform for processing 376–377; reevaluation and closure 381; titration continuum 377–379
The Association for Play Therapy (APT) 520, 521, 526
Association of Child Psychotherapists, UK 316
attachment: behaviors 131; and caregiving systems 710–711; disruption 2, 62, 79, 178, 257, 473, 539, 638, 782; fear and 60–61; motivational system 42; phobia 47; prenatal 62; secure 346, 347; seeking 82; styles *see* attachment styles; trauma and dissociation 711–713; wounding 469, 471, 474
attachment-based assessment 66–67; Adult Attachment Interview 66, 604; Attachment Q-Set 67; Maternal–Fetal Attachment Scale 66; Postpartum Bonding Questionnaire 66; in practice 67–68; standardized 66; Strange Situation Procedure 66
Attachment Q-Set 67
attachment styles 61–62; defensive-avoidance 67; disorganized/disoriented 30, 32, 34, 61–62, 67, 79, 82, 96, 131–132, 177, 193, 209, 328, 345–348, 646; insecure 63, 67, 328; insecure-anxious/ ambivalent 61, 130, 346, 347; insecure-avoidant 61, 66, 130, 346, 347; insecure-disorganized/ disoriented 96, 130; insecure-resistant 66; secure 60–63, 65–67, 130, 298; unresolved 62
attachment system and defense 757–760; anxious attachment, child with 759; avoidant trauma, child with 759–760; disorganized trauma, child with 760
attachment theory 2, 57–59, 108, 130–131, 345, 346, 710; adversity and affect regulation 65; affect regulation and dissociation 66–68; and neuroscience 316
attachment theory of STM 292–298; Bowlby's five stages of psychological responses 293–298; Bowlby's internal working models (IWMs) and dissociated self-states development 292; traumatic grief and mourning 292–293
attachment trauma 2, 38–49; alterations in biological regulatory systems 42–43; child maltreatment and 38–39, 347; definition 39–41; dysregulation of mental functions and self-states 43–45; as hidden epidemic 41; mentalization failures 47; pathogenic beliefs 47–48; and psychopathology 38–41, 43, 44, 48; relational dysregulation 46–47; states of detachment and dissociation 45–46
attachment video-feedback intervention (AVI) 345–359; Attachment Biobehavioral Catch-up intervention 352; disorganization and dissociation 346–351, *351*; dysregulated parental behavior and its reduction 348–351, **350**, 354–355, *355*; Infant/Child-Parent Psychotherapy 351; parent-child-oriented approach 352; with parents and young children 351–354; phases and parents' progression 353–354, *354*; post-AVI observations of behavior 359; pre-AVI observation of behaviors 355–358; support-oriented approach 351; trauma-focused cognitive behavioral therapy 352; Video-Feedback Intervention to Promote Positive Parenting and Sensitive Discipline 352
attention-deficit hyperactivity disorder (ADHD)/ ADD 209, 242, 243, 256, 257, 462, 468, 779
Atypical Maternal Behavior Instrument for Assessment and Classification system (AMBIANCE) 349, 354
autism spectrum disorder (ASD) 237, 256–259; *vs.* developmental trauma disorder (DTD) **258**
autobiographical memory 5, 26, 32, 38, 41, 44, 77, 607
autohypnotic model 93–101; attachment, tonic immobility, and shock 96–98; contemporary phenomenological data 98–99; context 93–95; genetic, epigenetic, and neurobiological correlates 98; links from functional neuroimaging 99–100; overview 93–95; pathological/normative dissociation 95–96
automatisms 93
autonomic navigation 162
autonomic nervous system (ANS) 56, 64, 65, 150, 175, 177, 441–443, 602, 695, 753; child's symptoms and 576; and Polyvagal Theory 143–144; tracking of activation/deactivation cycles using physical games 456–457
autonomic patterns in trauma 159; high levels of sympathetic and dorsal vagal 159; prolonged

Index

sympathetic irritability 159; stuck in dorsal vagal, afraid of sympathetic 159; stuck in sympathetic, afraid of dorsal vagal 159
Axline, Virginia 525, 526, 529
Ayres, Anna Jean 397; Ayres Sensory Integration (ASI) 397; Ayres Sensory Integration Fidelity measure 397; sensory integration therapy 397
Ayres Sensory Integration (ASI) 397

Baby Book, The (Sears and Sears) 125
background feeling 169–171, 179
background orientation 169–171, 179
Badenoch, Bonnie 125, 129, 134, 140, 162, 582; "Becoming a Therapeutic Presence in the Counseling Room and the World in IPNB and Clinical Practice" 129; *Being a Brain Wise Therapist* 125
Baita, S. 744
Barabasz, A. 95
Barach, P. M. 96
Barlow, M. R. 99
Barlow, Wilfred 404
Barnier, A. J. 98
baroreflex 144, 145, 149; characteristics of 144
Barthel, K. 404
Bateman, Anthony 613, 628
Bateson, G. 34
The Battered Child Syndrome 324
battle neurosis 94
Baylin, Jon 153, 156, 159, 328; *Brain-Based Parenting* 156
"Becoming a Therapeutic Presence in the Counseling Room and the World in IPNB and Clinical Practice" (Badenoch) 129
behavioral state modulation 30
behavioral therapy 539
Behrens, T. E. J. 27
Being a Brain Wise Therapist (Badenoch) 125
Bellevue Diagnostic Interview for Dissociation in Children and Adolescents (BDID-C) 220
Bentovim, Arnon 318
Bentzen, Marianne 443
benzodiazepines 868
Berger, Hans 462, 464
Berman, P. S. 266, 273; organizational features to treatment plan 273
Bernard, Claude 583
Betrayal Blindness Questionnaires 118
Betrayal Trauma: The Logic of Forgetting Childhood Abuse (Freyd) 108
betrayal trauma theory (BTT) 107–119; betrayal blindness 108, 118; conceptualizing as separable dimension 109–110; context 108–109; knowledge isolation 108, 110, 112, 113, 118; overview 108–109; trauma of interpersonal betrayal 110; *see also* high betrayal trauma in childhood
Bevin, L. 524

bibliotherapy for somatic symptoms 818–819
bilateral dual attention stimulus (BLS/DAS) 365, 369, 371, 379–381, 383, 384, 767
biofeedback 461
Biofeedback Certification International Alliance (BCIA) 462
biological imperative 149, 452, 592, 833
biological paradox 131–132, 209
biological regulatory systems, alterations in 42–43
Bion, Wilfred 62
biopsychosocial formulation 267, 276
bipolar disorder 24, 209, 237
Biven, L. 398, 754
Bliss, E. L. 90
Bliss, Eugene 94
blocked trust and blocked care 328
Bluhm, R. L. 463
body map research of emotion-related sensations 456–457
Bodynamic Somatic Psychotherapy 403–404
Booth, Phyllis 560
borderline personality disorder (BPD) 39, 864
bottom-up therapeutic approaches 7, 271, 274
Bowen, Murray 426, 699; Bowen theory 699
Bowers, K. S. 96
Bowlby, John 58, 108, 130, 292, 293, 303, 315, 317, 324, 345, 346, 701, 710, 758; attachment-seeking behaviors 131; attachment theory 58, 108, 130, 292, 345, 710; incompatible internal working models 293; internal working models (IWMs) and dissociated self-states development 292; sequential responses to separation 758
Bowlby's five stages of psychological responses 293–298; appeals for help 295–296; case study 297–298; despair, withdrawal, regression, and disorganization 296–297; hostility 294–295; reorganization of behavior toward new object 297; thought and behavior directed with parent 293–294; *vs.* Waters' STM five stages **294**
Bowman, E. S. 816
bradycardia 145, 147
Braffman, W. 90
Brain-Based Parenting (Hughes and Baylin) 156
brain connectivity 43, 44
Brand, Bethany 618; *Finding Solid Ground* 618
Brand, B. L. 276
Braun, B. G. 4, 267
Breuer, Josef 93, 309, 310
Bridges, S. K. 598
Brief Betrayal Trauma Survey 111
Brief Dissociative Experiences Scale (DES-B) 215
Briere, J. N. 32, 651
British Psycho-Analytical Society 314
Bromberg, P. 649
Brown, Daniel 615, 625, 682
Bryan, J. 678
Bryson, Payne 129; *Power of Showing Up, The* 129

Buckner, R. L. 100
Burlingham, Dorothy 57
Burn, Robert 56; "Man Was Made to Mourn: A Dirge" 56
Burt, C. 434
Butler, L. D. 98

California Evidence-Based Clearinghouse for Child Welfare (CEBC) 532
The California Evidenced-Based Clearinghouse (CEBC) 521
Calming Womb Family Therapy Model (CWFTM) 62, 690–705; attachment, definition 690; bonding 690, 691, 701; challenges 692–693; client and womb baby dyad wellness see client and womb baby dyad wellness; collaborative pre-perinatal trauma-informed team approach see collaborative pre-perinatal trauma-informed team approach; conception 691; hidden trauma, dissociative phenomena, and pregnancy 695–697; high-risk conditions see high-risk conditions in pregnancy; integration of EMDR therapy and see prenatal EMDR-CWFTM framework; multigenerational family therapy see multigenerational family therapy; post-birthing 705; preconception 690–691; pregnancy 692; prenatal treatment myths and clarifications see prenatal treatment myths and clarifications; reversing prenatal inertia 705; in utero developmental guidance see in utero developmental guidance; womb baby, definition 690
Campagner, D. 98
Cannon, Walter 583; *Wisdom of the Body, The* 583
Caplan, R.: *Pediatric Psychogenic Non-Epileptic Seizures: A Treatment Guide* 814
Cardeña, E. 4
caregivers' responses for healthy psychological development 58, 60, 64–65
caregiving motivational system 81
caregiving system 2, 69, 81, 82, 647–650, 710–711
Caretti, V. 40, 47
Carr, N. 34
Cascade of Care in TraumaPlay model 547–549; nurturer 547; safe boss 547; story keeper 548
case conceptualization 264–270, **277–281**; considerations in 265–266; models of 266–268; through trauma and dissociation 268–270
Center for Play Therapy 526
Center for Youth Wellness Adverse Childhood Experiences Questionnaire (CYW-ACE-Q) 216
Centers for Disease Control and Prevention (CDC) 59
Champagne, Tina 393
Charcot, Jean-Martin 23, 89, 93, 95, 96, 309, 311, 318
Charles, Liz 146
Checklist of Indicators of Trauma & Dissociation in Youth (CIT-DY) 214–215
Chen, C. 26

Child/Adolescent Dissociative Checklist (CADC) 215
Child And Adolescent Needs And Strengths (CANS) 217–218
Child and Adolescent Trauma Screen (CATS) 216
Child Behavior Checklist (CBCL) 217; CBCL-3 214, 225, 354
child-centered play therapy (CCPT) 520–535; case example 533–534; children's traumatic experience 522–524; conceptualization 533–534; definition 520; evidenced-based approaches 521, 524, 532, 534; needs of children experiencing complex trauma and dissociation 524–525; research 532–533; theories 521; toys *see* therapeutic toys
child development 59, 64, 66, 107, 111, 116, 149, 199, 268, 312, 400, 443, 486, 492, 524, 825
Child Dissociative Checklist (CDC) 17, 19, 206, 810
Child Dissociative Experiences Scale 820
Child Guidance Clinic 312
Childhood Antecedents of Multiple Personality Disorder (Richard) 4
childhood non-betrayal trauma 113
Childhood Trauma Questionnaire 354
child maltreatment 38–39, 108, 347; dimensional impact of 39; nature of 38; representing attachment trauma 39; *see also* state-related effects of child maltreatment
child refugees and asylum seekers 791–803; accessibility and acceptability 802; case examples 797–798, 800–801; complex trauma and dissociation in 792–794; context of displacement, complex trauma and dissociation in *793*, 793–798; culture, discourse and displacement 798; definition 791–792; forcibly displaced children 791–803; high-income countries, therapies and interventions in 799–801; humanitarian emergencies, therapies and interventions in 801–802; improving mental health and well-being 802–803; low and middle-income countries, therapies and interventions in 801
children's developmental stages, DDP interventions at *333*, 333–343; with parent and child at early school age 336–340; as parent-child psychotherapy with preadolescent 340–343; with parents of preschool child 333–336
Children's Dissociative Experiences Scale And Post-Traumatic Symptom Inventory (CDES/PTSI) 215–216, 226, 810
Children's Perceptual Alteration Scale (CPAS) 215
child sexual abuse (CSA) 108, 110, 222, 311, 736, 825, 848, 851
Child Stress Disorders Checklist 216
Chiu, S. 462
Choi, K. R. 192
Christie-Sands, J. 97
chronic pain 824–836; dissociation in infants and children with 829–830; infants and children

Index

experiencing 825–826; related to central nervous system (CNS) 826–829; state of mindfulness and securely attached environment 834–835; working with children have medical issues and complicated medical presentations 830–834
chronic trauma/traumatization 1–3, 6, 9, 189, 690
CIA's MK-ULTRA mind control program 844
Ciaunica, A. 169
Cintron, G. 193, 211
Circle of Security paradigm 131
Clark, Patricia Baird 849
Cleveland, J. M. 98, 99
client and womb baby dyad wellness 701–702; prenatal bonding 701; pre-perinatal self-regulation 701–702
clinical hypnosis 89, 96, 101, 311, 815, 866
Clinic for Nervous and Difficult Children 591
clonidine 868
co-creation 127, 329, 883
cognitive-behavioral approaches 34
cognitive-behavioral therapy (CBT) 75, 799
cognitive interventions 160
cognitive skills 64, 346, 486, 493, 494, 815
collaborative motivational system 81
collaborative pre-perinatal trauma-informed team approach 700
collage therapy 855
collapsed immobility 98, 176, 177, 442, 461, 468, 476
Color-Your-Heart 221
Comas-Díaz, L. 676
Common Elements Treatment Approach (CETA) 802
comorbidities 6, 74, 228, 269, 275, 368, 779, 869, 880
compartmentalization 45, 46, 76, 114, 190, 191, 199
compassionate self 747–750
compassion-focused therapy (CFT) 739–744; emotional regulation systems 742–743, 746–747; exploration and coping with shame 743–744; self-regulation skills 743, 747–750; therapeutic relationship/psychoeducation 741–742, 746
competition/ranking motivational system 82–84; dominance 83; submission 82–83
competitive aggression 83
complex post-traumatic stress disorder (CPTSD) 39, 216, 218, 318, 325, 498; diagnosis 239, 240; systems and ethical issues in assessment 222–223
complex trauma 40; definition 2–3, 189, 202; symptoms 187, 189, 191; treatment for 68–69; Type I 2, 189; Type II 2, 189; Type III 2, 189; *see also individual entries*
complex trauma-informed assessment using HOT model 223–228; challenges and limitations 227–228; clinical case example 223; cognitive functioning 225; depressive symptoms 225; dissociative symptoms 225–226; formulation and diagnoses 227; history (H) 224; imaginary friends 226–227; measures 224; observations (O) 224–225; outcomes 227; projective testing 226;

sexualized behaviors 225; testing (T) 225–227; trauma exposure 225; trauma symptoms 225
Complex Trauma Task Force 613
compromised mentalization 47
conditioning victims' thoughts 840–842; classical conditioning 841; combined operant and fear conditioning 841–842; fear conditioning 841; operant conditioning 840
"Confusion of Tongues between adults and the child-The Language of Tenderness and of Passion" (Ferenczi) 311
Conroy, J. 533
consent 20, 210, 376, 463, 470, 652, 659, 703
controlling caregiving strategies 81–83
controlling punitive strategies 82, 83
Cook, A. 49, 155, 191, 271
Cooper, L. M. 92
co-regulation 191, 329, 371, 577–578
Corrigan, F. M. 97, 98
Crenshaw, Kimberle 677
Crittenden, Patricia 400; Dynamic Maturational Model of Attachment and Adaptation (DMM) 400
Cruz, D. 268
Cultural Betrayal of Black Women and Girls, The (Gómez) 110
culturally responsive framework and orientation 679–681; cultural attunement to physiological impact of trauma 680–681; cultural comfort 680; cultural opportunities 679–680; of intersectionality 681
culturally responsive treatment planning 681–684; expressive-based techniques 683–684; multicultural toys and materials 682–683; working with caregivers 682
culture(al): attunement to physiological impact of trauma 680–681; betrayal 110; comfort 679, 680; humility 679; opportunities 679–680

Daglar, G. 691
Dales, S. 578
Dallam, S. 93, 201
Damasio, A. R. 170, 317, 453
Dana, Deb 150, 159, 162
Daniels, A. D. 678
Danylchuk, L. 835
DARVO (deny, attack, and reverse victim and offender) 116
Daws, Dilys 317
Dearing, R. L. 735
deception 842–843
Deco, G. 27
deep brain reorienting (DBR) 167–179; background feeling 169–170; background orientation 169–170; early-life shock and pre-attachment wounding 174–179; innate connection system (ICS) 167–174; sensory-affective orienting 170–174

deep breathing 69, 782, 820
default mode network (DMN) 100, 463, 474
defense mode and self-protective system 752–772; affect tolerance 769; animal defenses and play 766; attachment system *see* attachment system and defense; case study 769–771; child's relationship with inborn motivational systems 763–764; compassion, rest, and safety checks 766–767; defensive behaviors resulting from trauma 754; definition 753; mentalization and higher cognitive capacities 764–765; motivational systems 754–757; parts work and inner dynamic 768–769; psychoeducation, physicalizations and therapeutic embodiments 766–767; recognition 753–754; safety, relational regulation, and IWMs 762–763; therapist and caregiver work systemically 767–768; time orientation 769; treatment 761
defensive aggression 83
defensive-avoidance attachment styles 67
Delacroix, Eugene 632
Delafield-Butt, J. T. 171
D'Elia, D. 522
Dell, Paul F. 4, 31, 89, 90, 94–99; "the essence of hypnosis" 31
Demirci, O. O. 818
Dennis, C. 691
Department of Child and Family Welfare (DOCFW) 658, 659, 667–668
depersonalization 45, 62, 74–75, 98, 132, 175, 190, 194–197, 199, 240; disorder 197; and eating behaviors 196; feeling numb, encopresis, and enuresis 195–196; and self-harm 195; shock-induced 174, 175
depersonalization/derealization disorder (DPDR) 197
derealization 45, 62, 74–75, 98, 175, 190, 196–197, 199, 240; in self-perception 197; shock-induced 174, 175
despair 82, 134, 293, 294, 296–297, 344, 745, 794
Despine, Antoine 206, 318
detachment states 45–46
Developing Mind: Toward a Neurobiology of Interpersonal Experience, The (Siegel) 130, 392
developmental psychopathology 46, 64
developmental theory of STM 298–301, *300*; case study 300–301; Erickson's model *vs.* 299–300
developmental trauma 2, 40, 153, 179, 189, 328; standardized clinical interviews for 219; *see also* art therapy
developmental trauma disorder (DTD) 2, 187, 208; *vs.* autism spectrum disorders (ASD) **258**; diagnosis 238–240
Developmental Trauma Disorder Structured Interview for Child (DTD SI-C) 219
Developmental Trauma Disorder Structured Interview for Parent/Caregiver (DTD SI-P/Care) 219

Diagnostic and Statistical Manual of Mental Disorders (DSM) 238, 240, 260; DSM-5 2, 92, 187, 189, 199, 208, 216, 220, 227, 238, 239, 242; DSM III 310, 808; DSM-IV 19, 238
Diagnostic Classification of Mental Health and Developmental Disorders of Infancy and Early Childhood 238
dialectical behavior therapy (DBT) 494, 864
Dialogues with Forgotten Voices (Schwartz) 850
diathesis-stress model 79, 98
differential and co-occurring diagnoses 242–243, **244–252**, 255; case example 243, **253–254**, 253–255; emerging personality 254; developmental considerations in 243; of neurodevelopmental disorders 256–257
differentiation of the self, concept of 699
Difficulties in Emotion Regulation Scale (DERS) 68
direct terrorization 847
Disconnected and Extremely Insensitive Parenting (DIP) behavior coding system 349
discrete behavioral states/states of being model 23–35, 288–289, 293, 299, 642; in animals 26–27; concepts of 24–27; metacognitive and executive functions 28; modulation 27–28; origin and evolution 23–24; parental state-altering behaviors and parent-child state interactions 28; sense of self and personal identity 29; state-related effects of child maltreatment *see* state-related effects of child maltreatment; states at birth, new states, and new pathways 27; for treatment 33–35; value of 35
Diseth, T. H. 97
disinhibited social engagement disorder (DSED) 240
disorders of extreme stress not otherwise specified (DESNOS) 238
disorganized/disoriented attachment 30, 32, 34, 42, 61–62, 67, 79, 82, 96, 131–132, 177, 193, 209, 328, 345–348, 645–646; behaviors of children with 67
disorganized play 646–647
dissociated self-states 207, 292, 821, 839–845; types of 846
dissociation 3–5, 45–46, 73–85; as alterations in attention and awareness 73–74, **78**; as alterations in perception 73–75, **78**; bidirectional model of 4; Branch A 99, 100; Branch B 99, 100; clinical diagnosis of 18–19; continuum 189–191, *190*, 199; definition 3–5, 92–93; *vs.* dissociative symptoms 73–75; as dorsal vagal activation 74, 75, **78**; epidemiology 18–19; etiology of 191, 883; future research on 19–20; standardized clinical interviews for 219; structural *see* structural dissociation; treatment 68–69; *see also individual entries*
dissociation assessment: dissociative symptoms and disorders 207; indicators for 208–209; rationale and process 206–207; standardized tools

212–213; using history, observation, and testing (HOT) framework 209–211; *see also* complex trauma-informed assessment using HOT model
Dissociation in Children and Adolescents: A Developmental Perspective (Putnam) 23
dissociation screening: Adolescent Dissociative Experiences Scale 214; Brief Dissociative Experiences Scale 215; Checklist of Indicators of Trauma & Dissociation in Youth 214–215; Child/Adolescent Dissociative Checklist 215; Child Dissociative Checklist 206, 214, 810; Children's Dissociative Experiences Scale And Post-Traumatic Symptom Inventory 215–216, 226, 810; Children's Perceptual Alteration Scale 215; indicators for 208–209; measures 213–214
dissociation theories 93; descriptive models 93; explanatory/descriptive models 93; explanatory models 93
dissociative amnesia (DA) 26, 112, 113, 189, 197–198, 242
dissociative disorders 31–32, 39, 99, 113; advancing assessment and diagnosis 880–881; advancing treatment 882–884; dissociative symptoms and 207–208; maltreatment types and 32
dissociative disorders in adults: epidemiology of 17–18
Dissociative Disorders Interview Schedule (DDIS) 17, 18
Dissociative Experiences Cards 810
Dissociative Experiences Scale (DES) 18, 19
dissociative identity disorder (DID) 3, 17–18, 20, 26, 79, 94, 132, 140, 190, 198–199, 208, 241, 242, 268, 325; hypnotizability of 99, 100; as multiple reality disorder 24; origins 31–32; switch process in 23
dissociative multiplicity 99, 240, 243
dissociative symptomatology 4, 6, 174, 272, 384, 810, 881
dissociative symptoms 187–189; amnesia/memory confusion 197–198; categories 191–192; depersonalization 194–197; derealization 196–197; dissociative disorders and 207–208; dissociative identity disorder 198–199; domains 191; emotion regulation 202; hyperactivity 200–201; imaginary playmates 201; perpetrator introjects 200; psychoform and somatoform symptoms 202; regressed states and hearing voices 201–202; in school-aged children 193–194; self-diagnosis among youth 256; sexually inappropriate behavior 200; shame and trauma 202–203; sleep difficulties 200; in young and preschool-aged children 192–193
dissociative table technique 602
Dodson, John Dillingham 167, 465
Dorahy, M. J. 32
dorsal PAG (DPAG) 176, 177
dorsal raphe nucleus (DRN) 168, 178
dorsal vagal collapse 147–149, 154, 155, 158, 159, 407
dorsolateral prefrontal cortex (DLPFC) 30
Dosenbach, N. U. F. 100
double-bind communication 34
Downey, L. 276
Draw-A-Person (DAP) 221
DTD Field Trial Study Group 219
Dual Attention Stimulus (DAS) 371–372
Dubossarsky, H. 27
dyadic developmental psychotherapy (DDP) 160, 163, 328–344; evidence base for 343; interventions with parent and child at early school age 336–340; intervention with parents of preschool child 333–336; as parent-child psychotherapy with preadolescent 340–343; principles, attitude, and practice *329*, 329–331, *331*; working with culture, experience, and identity 331–333
Dynamic Core for Kids 402–403
Dynamic Interpersonal Therapy (DIT) 315
Dynamic Maturational Model of Attachment and Adaptation (DMM) 400–401
dysfunctional interpersonal circularities 48
dysphoric affects 30, 32
dysregulated parental behavior 348–351, **350**, 354–355, **355**; Atypical Maternal Behavior Instrument for Assessment and Classification system (AMBIANCE) 349; Disconnected and Extremely Insensitive Parenting (DIP) behavior coding system 349; disconnected behaviors category 349; extremely insensitive behaviors category 349; Frightening/Frightened parental behavior system (FR) 349

Early Adolescent Skills for Emotions (EASE) intervention 802
early-life sensory experiences 169, 170
early-life shock 168, 169, 171, 174–179
early-life shock and pre-attachment wounding 174–179; induced derealization and depersonalization 175; neurochemical dissociation 175; structural dissociation 175
early relational traumas 40, 47, 65, 112–114
Ecker, B. 592, 598
EDUCATE Model 271, 273–274
ego identity 298, 299
ego states 74–76, **76**, 84
Ego State Therapy 94, 816
"Eight Essentials of Healthy Attachment" 448–449
electroencephalogram (EEG) 461, 462, 465
Ellenberger, Henri 94
Elliott, David 615, 625
EMDR therapy for FND 817–818
Emotional Brain, The (Le Doux) 841
emotion/emotional: dysregulation 61, 65, 194, 290, 486, 493, 694, 698, 705, 797, 864; regulation 65, 68, 69, 75, 77, 84, 187, 202; skills 64, 118, 493

emotional personality (EP) 157
emotional systems in brain 64
Emotion Regulation Checklist (ERC) 68
emotion tolerance 75, 96, 457, 616, 640, 743, 764
Endo, T. 19
epistemic distrust 613
epistemic freezing 47
epistemic trust 641
Erickson, Milton 23
Erickson's model *vs.* STM 299–300
Erikson, Erik 298, 299, 556; developmental therapy and psychosocial stages 299; ego identity 298, 299
European Society for Trauma and Dissociation (ESTD) 207, 272
explicit memories 445–446
expressive and creative therapies 393
expressive-based techniques 683–684
exteroception 540, 543, 594
Eye Movement Desensitization and Reprocessing International Association (EMDRIA) Conference 125
eye movement desensitization and reprocessing (EMDR) therapy 291, 364–386, 631, 799, 864; adaptive information processing model 365; assessment *see* assessment phase in EMDR therapy; case study 382; circular phase approach to 366; client history and treatment planning 366–368; Constant Installation of Present Orientation and Safety 378; EMDR Group Parent Empowerment Protocol 370–371; Group-Traumatic Episode Protocol 370; history and research 364–365; multimodal-integrative approach to 366; phases 366–386; preparation *see* preparation phase in EMDR therapy; processing 385–386; Recent Traumatic Episode Protocol 378; Resource Development and Installation Protocol 370
Eys, P. van 209

factitious disorders and malingering 255; case example 255
Fagan, J. 206
The Family Distress Cascade Theory 776
family projection process 699
family systems theory of STM 301–304; case study 302–304
family systems (FS) therapy 864
Farina, B. 42
fearful (appeasing) strategies 83
Feedback-Informed Treatment (FIT) 669
Feiler, T. 157
Feldman, R. 174
Felitti, Vincent 59
Ferenczi, Sándor 311, 312; "Confusion of Tongues between adults and the child-The Language of Tenderness and of Passion" 311

fight-or-flight response *see* sympathetic state
Finding Solid Ground (Brand) 618
Fisher, J. 398, 430, 433, 437, 563, 569, 570; *Sensorimotor Psychotherapy: Interventions for Trauma and Attachment* 430
Fisher, S. F. 179, 194
Fisler, R. E. 522
Fitzpatrick, M. 661–664
flashbacks 24, 29, 32, 46, 75, 82, 158, 193, 222, 240
Flavell, S. W. 26
Fonagy, Peter 315, 319, 613, 628, 641, 764
Foo Fighters 125
Ford, J. D. 202
formal programming 849–850
Forner, C. 835
Four Factor theory of dissociative disorders 94
Four Ps 267, 276–277
Fraiberg, Selma 317; "transformation of affect" 317
Franz, Shepherd Ivory 94
Franzen, Jonathan 38; *Purity* 38
Fraser, G. A. 602
Frazier, J. A. 462
Freud, Anna 57, 312, 314–319, 324, 520
Freud, Sigmund 93, 309–313, 324, 520
Freyd, J. J. 99, 108, 109, 111, 112, 115, 116; *Betrayal Trauma: The Logic of Forgetting Childhood Abuse* 108; two-dimensional model for traumatic events 109, *109*, 115
Frightening/Frightened parental behavior system (FR) 349
frontoparietal/central executive network (CEN) 99, 100
frontoparietal network (FPN) 99, 100
full-body role play 854
Fuller, Buckminster 575
functional magnetic resonance imaging (fMRI) 27, 452, 463, 466
functional neurologic disorder (FND) 809–821; case conceptualization and practical adaptations and interventions 812–819 *see also* therapies and interventions for FND; case study 819–821; diagnosis and assessment 810; multidisciplinary approach in treatment planning 811–812 *see also* multidisciplinary approach in FND treatment; psychogenic nonepileptic seizures (PNES) symptom *see* psychogenic nonepileptic seizures (PNES)
Fung, H. W. 113

Gangopadhyay, N. 171
Gardner, G. G. 91
Gaskill, R. L. 524
Gazzillo, F. 273
Gendlin, Eugene 446
Generation Alpha: complex trauma and dissociation in 730–731
George, C. 82

"ghosts in the nursery" 62, 317
Gilbert, Paul 739, 753; compassion-focused therapy (CFT) 739–744
Gilbert, R.: *Recognising and Responding to Child Maltreatment* 850
"Gingerbread Girl Body Map" 454–455
Giolas, M. H. 19
Gobin, R. L. 111
Goldin, Nan 632; *All the Beauty and the Bloodshed* 632
Golding, K. S. 163, 329, 331
Goldsmith, R. E. 117
Gómez, A. M. 640; *All the Colors of Me: My First Book about Dissociation* 810; *Visitor: A Book about Pain, Defenses, and Love, The* 766
Gómez, J. M. 110; *Cultural Betrayal of Black Women and Girls, The* 110
"good enough mother," concept of 59, 60
Goodhart, S. P. 94, 95
Goodyer, I. M. 810
Gottlieb, Sidney 844
Grant, E. M. 163
Grasso, D. J. 273
Green, J. G. 38
Greenwald, Ricky 625
Gresch, H. U. 840, 845
grief 34, 82, 293, 296, 434, 438, 508, 516, 594, 642, 695, 702, 710, 715, 755
Griffith, J. L. 811
Gross, J. J. 202
Guerney, L. F. 526
Guidelines for the Assessment and Treatment of Children and Adolescents with Dissociative Symptoms and Dissociative Disorders 272
Guidelines for the Evaluation and Treatment of Dissociative Symptoms in Children and Adolescents 222, 271
Guidelines for Treating Dissociative Identity Disorder in Adults 271
Gušić, S. 795
Gutierrez, B. 680

Hahamy, A. 27
Hampstead Clinic 312, 315
Happiest Baby on the Block, The (Karp) 835
Hardy, K. V. 424
Harris, Martha 315
Hart, O. van der 46, 175, 324, 569
Hartzell, M. 125; *Parenting From the Inside Out* 125
Havighurst, S. S. 276
Healing the Fractured Child: Diagnosis and Treatment of Youth with Dissociation (Waters) 269
heart rate variability (HRV) 144–145, 149
Hebb, Donald 466
Hébert, M. 202, 498
Heide, K. M. 2, 189
Heinicke, C. M. 296

helpless caregiving 82
Henderson, S. W. 267, 275
Henrich, J. 332
Herbert, J. 464
Herman, J. L. 803; *Truth and Repair: How Trauma Survivors Envision Justice* 117
Herman, Judith 324
Hesse, E. 96, 347–349
Hickey, P. R. 825
hierarchy of response (second polyvagal principle) 147, 147–149; danger and fight-or-flight response 148–149; life threat and collapse 147–148; safety and social engagement system 149
high betrayal trauma in childhood: adaptive knowledge isolation as means of preserving attachment relationships 111–113, 115–116; adult survivors, dissociation research in 113–114; child survivors, dissociation research in 114–115; impact 111–112; linear recovery and knowledge isolation fluctuations 116–117; monitoring knowledge isolation and maintaining connections to healthy supports 117; prevalence and risk 110–111; research on 118–119
high-risk conditions in pregnancy 694–695; anxiety 695; disempowerment 694; hormonal-physiological shifts 694; prenatal humiliation 694; stress 694–695
Hilgard, Ernest 23, 92, 95; neodissociation theory of hypnosis 95
Hilgard, Josephine 98
Hill, D. 769
Hillman, S. 67
hippocampus 27, 30, 38, 125, 126, 442, 445, 463
Hippocrates 243
Hirshberg, L. M. 462
Hoeft, F. 99
Holmes, E. A. 4
homeostasis 6, 8, 9, 291, 364, 368, 369, 380, 381, 383, 398, 442, 511, 576, 582–585
homeostatic mechanism, dissociation as 583–585
Hopenwasser, K. 408, 647, 651
Hopkins, Juliet 317
horizontal integration 127, 592
Hostinar, C. E. 434
House-Tree-Person (HTP) 221
Howe, N. 725
Howell, Elizabeth 3, 324, 648, 651
How the Cult Programs People (Svali) 844
Huet, V. 615
Hug-Hellmuth, Hermine von 312; "Play Therapy" 312
Hughes, Daniel 152, 153, 156, 328, 329, 331, 569; *Brain-Based Parenting* 156
Hulette, A. C. 19, 114, 115
human beings as social beings 57
Huolman, M. 201
hyper-arousal behaviors 200–201, 517–518

hypnosis 90, 95, 310, 311, 843–844; abilities 91, 92, 98; autohypnosis 90; capacities 89, 94, 95, 98, 101; definition 90; and dissociation 92–93, 99; formal 95; heterohypnosis 90–92; highly hypnotizable individuals 94, 95; neodissociation theory of 95; self-hypnosis 90
hypnotically induced paralysis 96
hypnotizability 90–92, 95; children's response to 91–92; and dissociation 89; sex-based differences in 91; and traumagenic experience 98
hypothalamic-pituitary-adrenal (HPA) axis 148, 753
hysteria 94, 309, 310; aetiology of 318
hysterical neurosis 94

Iacoboni, M. 577
ideation-to-action framework of suicide 778–779
identity: alterations 99, 190, 199, 202, 206, 214, 217, 220, 222, 243; confusion 190, 199, 202, 217, 220, 444; development 187, 268, 524, 599; disruption 31; states 24, 26, 268
Imaginary Companion [IC] toys 201
Imaginary Friends Questionnaire 226
imaginary playmates 201, 226–227
imaginative play and identities 31
implicit association task (IAT) 118
implicit memories 41, 43–45, 47, 48, 445–446
Incomplete Sentences 221
independence and autonomy 662, 665
informed consent 223, 659, 660, 704
innate alarm system (IAS) 167, 174, 176
innate connection system (ICS) 167–174, 179; sensory-affective orienting and 170–174
innate defense system (IDS) 167, 168, 174
insecure-anxious/ambivalent attachment 61, 130, 346, 347
insecure attachment 63, 67, 328
insecure-avoidant attachment 61, 130, 346, 347
insecure-disorganized/disoriented attachment 96, 130
insecure-resistant attachment 66
Inside-Outside Technique 221
integrated developmental treatment model 268
integration 126–127, 140–142; characteristics of 128; of consciousness 127, 132, 135–136; development of 129; horizontal 127; interpersonal 127, 134–135; memory 128; narrative 128; state 128, 140, 141; temporal 128; transpirational 128; vertical 127, 137–138, 141
integration phase in PRACTICE components 497–498; conjoint child-parent sessions 497; enhancing safety and future development 497–498
integrative treatment approach 73, 274–275
intergenerational trauma 675, 725–732; baby boomers 726; Generation Alpha 729–731; Generation X 726–727; Generation Y 727–728; Generation Z 728–729; limitations and future research 731–732; turnings 725
internal states 26, 47, 128, 200, 294, 299, 579, 776, 863

Internal Working Models (IWMs). 59, 65, 710, 715, 757, 759, 760, 762–763; of self and others 79
International Classification of Diseases (ICD) 238, 240, 260, 808; 11th revision (ICD-11) 189, 216, 238, 239, 242, 345; ICD-10 318
International Psychoanalytic Association 310, 312
The International Society for Neuroregulation and Research (ISNR) 461
International Society for Sandplay therapy 316
The International Society for the Study of Trauma and Dissociation (ISSTD) 198, 206, 222, 271, 272, 366, 591, 869
The International Society for the Study of Trauma and Dissociation (ISSTD) Child Trauma Task Force 613
International Society for Traumatic Stress Studies (ISTSS) 434, 613
International Trauma Questionnaires: Child and Adolescent Version (ITQ-CA) 216
interoception 132, 151, 594, 607
interoceptive awareness and empowerment 452–456; case study 454–456; drawing and coloring sensation/emotion body maps to track body reactions 453–454; grounding 453; inviting exploration through mutual tracking in SE sessions with art and/or movement 454–456; teaching ANS tracking of activation/deactivation cycles using physical games 456–457
interpersonal betrayal 110
interpersonal integration 127, 134–135
interpersonal/interpersonal-psychological theory of suicide 778
interpersonal neurobiology (IPNB) 124–142, 366, 391; attachment 130–132; chaos and rigidity 127; complex systems 126; connecting mind and body 136–137; dissociation through 132–133; integration *see* integration; paradox of impossible 133–134
interpersonal relationship 47, 68, 83, 116, 203, 269, 304, 474, 498, 639, 713, 737, 750, 875
interpersonal trauma 2, 40, 48, 108, 109, 115, 197
interpersonal violence 117, 229, 293
intersectionality 677; ADDRESSING framework 681; culturally informed and responsive exploration of 681
in utero developmental guidance 697–698; definition and practice 697–698; prenatal therapeutic alliance 698
Isobel, S. 40, 675
Itzkowitz, Sheldon 324

Jackson, Hughlings 44
Jacobs, J. 92
Jacobs, L. 92
James, William 23
Janet, Pierre 3, 44, 89, 91, 95, 114, 311, 318, 366, 591, 755, 808

Jenkins, M. A. 502; *Transforming Trauma: Resilience and Healing Through Our Connections With Animals* 502
Jernberg, Ann 560
Jerry, P. 578
Jiang, H. 99
Jones, Caroline Okell 317
Jones, Ernest 312
Journal of Abnormal Psychology 93
Journal of Child and Adolescent Psychiatric Clinics of North America 462
Jung, Carl 23, 310, 312, 318

Kabat-Zinn, Jon 424
Kahlo, Frida 632
Kalff, Dora 316, 591; *Sandplay, A Psychotherapeutic Approach to the Psyche* 316
Kamiya, Joe 462, 467
Karadag, M. 365
Karaosmanoğlu, H. A. 158
Karp, H.: *Happiest Baby on the Block, The* 835
Kate, M. A. 17, 18
Keith-Spiegel, P. 664
Kelly, C. T. 425
Kempe, Henry 324
Kennell, J. H 62
Kernberg, Otto 847
Kestly, Teresa 582
Kiddie Schedule for Affective Disorders and Schizophrenia-Present and Lifetime Version (K-SADS-PL) 219
Kihlstrom, J. F. 95
Kim, P. Y. 675
Kinetic Family Drawing (KFD) 221
Kirsch, I. 90
Klaus, M. H. 62
Klein, Melanie 58, 312, 314–317, 324, 520
Kluft, Richard 4, 24, 93, 94, 206, 311, 325, 641; *Childhood Antecedents of Multiple Personality Disorder* 4; Four Factor theory of dissociative disorders 94
knowledge isolation 108, 110, 112, 113, 118; linear recovery and fluctuations 116–117; as means of preserving attachment relationships 111–113, 115–116; monitoring and maintaining connections to healthy supports 117
Kolk, B. A. van der 2, 152, 433, 522, 524, 540, 696
Kringelach, M. L. 27
Kulkosky, P. J. 463

Landin-Romero, R. 365
Landreth, G. 520, 525, 526, 529, 530, 534; ACT model 530
Lanius, Ruth 29, 149, 158, 452, 463
Lanktree, C. B. 651
Laszloffy, T. A. 424
Lawson, D. M. 116

Lebois, L. A. M. 98, 99, 158
Le Doux, Joseph 317, 841; *Emotional Brain, The* 841
Leeds, A. M. 818
Leslie, C. E. 675
Levine, Peter A. 152, 155, 159, 441, 442, 445, 457
limbic system 60, 64
Liotti, G. 96
Liotti, M. 46, 347, 348, 645
Liu, S. 197
locus coeruleus (LC) 168, 174–178
Loewenstein, R. J. 23, 24, 26, 93
logical binds 33–34; double-bind 34
London, P. 92
Lorenz, Konrad 59
Lowenfeld, Margaret 316, 590, 591
Lucas, Anneke 845; *Quest for Love: Memoir of a Child Sex Slave* (Lucas) 845
Lyons-Ruth, Karlen 32, 349, 562, 569

MacLean, Paul 443
Madlon-Kay, S. 26
Main, Mary 30, 34, 59, 130, 317, 345–349, 711
Malchiodi, C. A. 393
Manassis, K. 638
Manfield, Philip 625
"Man Was Made to Mourn: A Dirge" (Burn) 56
Marcher, Lisbeth 403; Bodynamic Somatic Psychotherapy 403
Marci, Carl 581
Marek, S. 100
Markand, O. N. 816
Marques, J. C. 26
Martin, A. 267, 275
Masson, J. 324
Maternal–Fetal Attachment Scale (MFAS) 66
Mause, Lloyd de 325
McAlister, S. 34
McCormick, D. A. 27
McGilchrist, I. 592
McMahon, P. P. 206
memory confusion 197–199
memory reconsolidation (MR) 590, 598
Menon, V. 99, 100
mental absorption 73, 373
mental disorders diagnosis: case example 240, **241**; classifications 238, **239**; complex/developmental trauma disorders 238–240; differential and co-occurring 242–243, **244**–**254**, 255; dissociative disorders 240–242; factitious disorders and malingering 255
mental functions, dysregulation of 43–45
mentalization 8, 43–47, 75, 315, 592, 628, 631–632
mentalization-based therapy 864–865
mentalizing skills 84, 392, 628
Mesmer, Franz Anton 23
metacognition 29
methylenedioxy methamphetamine (MDMA) 868

Midolo, L. R. 46
Mikulincer, M. 58
Miller, Alice 324
Miller, J. E. 434
Miller, William 23
mind control abuse 839–850; application to victims' dissociated self-states 839–840; coerced perpetration 845–846; conditioning victims' thoughts 840–842; deception 842–843; definition 839; deprivation of basic needs 847; direct terrorization 847; formal programming 849–850; hypnosis 843–844; identification with aggressor 846–847; indoctrination/enculturation 847–848; manipulation of attachment needs 844–845; skills training 850; spiritual abuse 848–849; therapy approaches to *see* therapy approaches to mind control abuse
mindfulness 69, 740, 835, 865–866
Minnesota Multiphasic Personality Inventory 463
Minuchin, Salvador 426
Mitchell, T. W. 93
momentary and transient failures of integrative/inhibitory functioning 44
Monastra, V. J. 462
moral defence 324
Moreno, P. 741, 743
Morgan, A. H. 92, 98
Moro reflex 404–405, *405–406*
Motivational Interviewing 668–669
motivational systems in structural dissociation 79–84; caregiving 81; collaborative 81; competition/ranking 82–84; dissociative parts and 83–84; play 83; separation cry, panic and loss 81–82; sexual 83
multicultural orientation (MCO) 679
multicultural toys and materials 682–683
Multidimensional Inventory of Dissociation-Adolescent Version (A-MID) 220, 810
multidisciplinary approach in FND treatment 811–812; family environment, dynamics, and dysfunction 811–812; impact on academic functioning 812
multigenerational family therapy 699–700; Bowen theory and application 699; gender preference and expectations 700; traumatic transference 699–700
multiple personality disorder 4, 93, 190; *see also* dissociative identity disorder (DID)
multisensorial experiences 174–176, 178, 179
Myers, L. 157

nameless dread 62
narrative exposure therapy for children (KidNET) 799, 802
narrative integration 128
Nathanson, Daniel 622; "compass of shame" 622–625; *Shame and Pride: Affect, Sex, and the Birth of the Self* 622

National Association of Social Workers 660
The National Center for Child Trauma Stress Network 192
National Center for Health Statistics 452
The National Child Traumatic Stress Network 270, 488
National Health Service, UK 311, 312, 315
Nation Betrayed, A (Rutz) 844
Neff, K. 740
neurobiology 3, 9, 99, 398, 399; mechanisms 68; structures 59; *see also* interpersonal neurobiology (IPNB)
neurobiology in STM model 290–292; applying neuroception with dissociative children 290–291; case study 291–292
neuroception (first polyvagal principle) 81, 145–146, 151, 160; characteristics of 146; concept 290–291; with dissociative children 290–291
neurochemical dissociation 97, 175
neurodevelopmental disorders 209, 237, 242; differential and co-occurring diagnoses of 256–257; and trauma 256–257
neuro-developmental treatment (NDT) 402, *403*
neurodivergence 256–260; case examples 257–259; differential diagnoses 256–257; neurodevelopmental disorders and trauma 256–257; trauma and dissociation among children with developmental disabilities 259
neurofeedback training (NFT) 179, 460–479; age ranges 471–472; approaches and theories 465–467; arousal model 467–469; brain regions for 472–474; case study 469–479; considerations 470–471; disordered arousal 468; frequency and amplitude 464–465; functional magnetic resonance imaging 452, 463, 466; history and research of 462–464; infra-low frequency approach 466; Low Energy Neurofeedback System 466; low-resolution electromagnetic tomographic analysis 467; QEEG (quantitative) guided neurofeedback 467; slow cortical potential neurofeedback 467; Z-Score training 467
neuroplasticity 426, 461, 525
Neurosequential Model© (NM) 366, 511–517; brainstem and rhythmic, patterned, repetitive sensory input 513–514; clinical applications of 512; diencephalon 514–515; limbic system 515–516; neocortex 516–517; practical strategies and interventions 512–513; state-dependent functioning 511–512
New England Journal of Medicine 825
New York Philharmonic 125–127
Nijenhuis, E. 157, 202, 561, 808
Nilsson, D. 196
non-directive play therapy 852–853
non-linear dynamical systems theory 26
Norcross, J. C. 274
normative dissociation 188, 207, 268

numbing 29, 45, 62, 195–197, 240
Nur, N. 691
Nurcombe, B. 272, 273; treatment planning styles 272–273

observing ego 29
obstetric and gynecological (OB-GYN) procedures 695
occupational therapy (OT) 389, 395; case study 389–390; practice in mental health and childhood trauma 389; *see also* Psycho-Sensory Intervention® (PSI)
Occupational Therapy Act 395
Ochoa, L. G. 675
Ochs, Len 466
Oedipus Complex 311
Ogawa, J. R. 217
Ogden, P. 398, 430, 437; *Sensorimotor Psychotherapy: Interventions for Trauma and Attachment* 430
Oosterman, M. 42
oppositional defiant disorder (ODD) 237, 240, 257
orbitofrontal cortex (OFC) 30
Orne, M. 95
Orvaschel, H. 265
other specified dissociative disorder (OSDD) 19, 242, 253, 254
Othmer, Siegfried 466
Othmer, Sue 466
Out, D. 349, 350
Oxford College of Arts and Therapies 615

Paikin, D. 96
Pain, C. 398
panic and loss motivational system 81–82
Panksepp, Jaak 64, 398, 524, 754
Pappenheim, Bertha 310
parent-child relationship 28, 30; parental trauma impact on 58; in ventral vagal state 150
Parent-Infant private clinic 317
Parenting From the Inside Out (Siegel and Hartzell) 125
Parisette-Sparks, A. 736
paroxetine 867
pathogenic beliefs 47–48; in attachment trauma 47–48
pathological dissociation 65, 79, 89, 93–95, 192, 207, 215, 228, 268
pathological mourning 292, 310
Paulsen, S.: *All the Colors of Me: My First Book about Dissociation* 810
Pediatric Psychogenic Non-Epileptic Seizures: A Treatment Guide (Caplan et al.) 814
Peltonen, K. 201
Peniston, E. G. 463
periaqueductal gray (PAG) 168, 174–178
peritraumatic dissociation 97, 98, 154, 796, 801

perpetrator introjects 200
Perry, B. D. 393, 511, 512, 524, 641; *see also* Neurosequential Model© (NM)
Perryman, K. 532, 533
Peterson, C. 712
Peterson, G. 4
pharmacotherapy for complex trauma and dissociation 867–869; for dissociative disorders 868–869; for post-traumatic stress disorder (PTSD) 867–868
physiological arousal 42, 488, 491, 681
Piaget, J. 520, 556
Picasso, Pablo 632
Piontelli, Alessandra 172
Pittman, J. F. 298
Play-Doh™ 853
playfulness, acceptance, curiosity and empathy (PACE) 163, 330, 337–339
play motivational system 83
play therapy 34, 69, 138, 150, 813; *see also* child-centered play therapy (CCPT)
"Play Therapy" (Hug-Hellmuth) 312
Pocket Guide to Interpersonal Neurobiology (Siegel) 125, 128
Poels, M. 691
polysymptomatic dissociation 880
polytraumatization 2, 761
Polyvagal Theory and complex trauma 152–160; autonomic patterns 159; disrupts child's integration 154–156, *156*; fragmentation and structural dissociation 156–159; resets nervous system 152–154, *153*; treatment fails without addressing social engagement 159–160; *see also* social engagement system
Polyvagal Theory/Principle 65, 144–147, 391, 404, 443, 591–592; autonomic nervous system and 143–144; autonomic state as intervening variable 151–152; dissolution 150–151; heart rate variability (HRV) and 144–145; hierarchy of autonomic response *147*, 147–149; neuroception 145–146; ventral vagal complex as communication and co-regulation circuit 149–150, *151*
Pope, K. S. 664, 666
Porges, Stephen 144–145, 147, 149–151, 159–161, 290, 391, 404, 443, 457; *see also* Polyvagal Theory
posterior cingulate cortex (PCC) 463
Postpartum Bonding Questionnaire (PBQ) 66
post-traumatic stress disorder (PTSD) 2, 24, 79, 157, 211, 216, 219, 237, 238, 240, 257, 259, 463, 498; pharmacotherapy for 867–868; in pregnancy 695; in Preschool Aged Children 216
Post-Traumatic Stress Inventory 820
Potter, A. E. 711
Power of Showing Up, The (Siegel and Bryson) 129
PRACTICE components **484**, 485–498; integration phase *see* integration phase in PRACTICE

components; overview 488–489; stabilization phase *see* stabilization phase in PRACTICE components; trauma narration phase *see* trauma narration phase in PRACTICE components
pre-affective shock 97, 175, 176, 178, 179
pre-attachment wounding 168, 169; early-life shock and 174–179
prefrontal cortex 28, 30, 57, 64, 126
prenatal attachment 62–65; affect regulation 63–65; case example 63, 64
prenatal EMDR-CWFTM framework 702–703; trauma and dissociative phenomena methodology 702–703
prenatal treatment myths and clarifications 703–705; cautions 704; complex presentations 705; recommendations 704
preparation phase in EMDR therapy 368–375, 383–384; affect tolerance 372–373; client's dual attention 374–375; creating safety 368–370; defenses 375; Dual Attention Stimulus 371; psychoeducation 370–371; skill building 372; state-change and self-regulatory capacities 372; therapeutic relationship 370; working with dissociation 373–374
Prescott, D. 660, 664
primary intersubjectivity 57
Prince, Morton 93
procedural memory 442, 445, 446, 560, 563
processing trauma narratives 799, 801
professional boundaries and professional ethics 658–671; abstain from personal gain 661; boundary crossings and violations 664–665; decision-making 666–668; definitions 660–661; elements of ethical codes 660–661; empathy, validation, and shame 663; exploring upstream 670; illustration 658–660; independence and autonomy 662–663; meditation on 670–671; neutrality 662; preventing problems 668–670; principles 665–666
progressive muscle relaxation 69, 486, 492
Projective Storytelling (PST) 221
projective testing 220–221; drawings 221 *see also* Color-Your-Heart; Draw-A-Person (DAP); House-Tree-Person (HTP); Inside-Outside Technique; Kinetic Family Drawing (KFD); Incomplete Sentences 221; Rorschach Inkblot Method (RIM) 220–221; storytelling 221 *see also* Projective Storytelling (PST); Roberts Apperception Test (RAT-C); Sexual Projective Card Set (SPCS); Tell-Me-A-Story test (TEMAS)
proximity seeking and survival system 59–61, 346; case example 61; clinical example 60; fear and danger 60–61
Psychical Mechanism of Hysterical Phenomena 310
Psychoanalytic Disagreements in Child and Adult Work 314–317

psychoanalytic psychotherapy 309–325; child analysis and 311–313; composite clinical examples 317–324; definition of trauma and its relationship to 309–311; dissociation, complex PTSD and DID 318–324; infant and family 317–318; transference and countertransference components of 313–317; trauma-informed analytical work 318
psychodynamic psychotherapy 865
psychoeducation 370–371, 491, 741–742, 746, 766–767, 813–814, 863–864; shame 622–625, *623*, *625*
psychoform/somatoform dissociation 46, 98, 196, 202–203, 808, 810; *see also* functional neurologic disorder (FND); psychogenic nonepileptic seizures (PNES)
psychogenic nonepileptic seizures (PNES) 808–810
Psychological Automatism theory 3
psychological mechanism 29, 840
Psycho-Sensory Intervention® (PSI) 390–397, *392*; assessment and treatment in practice 407–409, 414–415, 417; case study 417, 420; clinician's self-awareness 392; complex childhood trauma in posture and movement systems 404–407, *405–406*; contributing frames of reference to 396, **396**; definition 390–391; Dynamic Maturational Model of Attachment and Adaptation 400–401; neurobiologically informed 391; OT Sensory Integration frame of reference 397; play-based activities 393; postural and movement frames of references 401–404; postural and movement interventions 395; psychotherapy 395–396; regulation through relationship 392–393; sensory-based interventions 393; sensory integration 397; trauma-sensitive 391
Psycho-Sensory Intervention® (PSI) assessment and treatment 407–409, 414–415, 417; boundaries 414, 417; creating safety in first session 408–409; sensory-based options and clinical reasoning for usage 409, **410–413**, 414; theory into practice 407–408; using posture and movement system as intervention 414, *414*, *415*, **415–417**
psychotherapeutic techniques for dissociation treatment 863–865; dialectical behavior therapy 864; eye movement desensitization and reprocessing 864; family systems therapy 864; mentalization-based therapy 864–865; psychodynamic psychotherapy 865; psychoeducation 863–864; schema-focused cognitive behavioral therapy 864; trauma-focused acceptance and commitment therapy 864; trauma-focused cognitive behavioral therapy 864
psychotropic medications 160, 253, 867–869
Purity (Franzen) 38
Purvis, Karen 502
Putnam, Frank W. 4, 23–29, 33, 34, 89; *Dissociation in Children and Adolescents: A Developmental*

Perspective 23; *Way We Are: How States of Mind Influence Our Identities, Personality and Potential for Change, The* 23; *see also* discrete behavioral states/states of being model

Quest for Love: Memoir of a Child Sex Slave (Lucas) 845
Quinn, M. 809

racial trauma 674, 676
Ratcliffe, M. 169
Ray, D. C. 524, 532; *Therapist's Guide to Child Development: The Extraordinary Years, A* 524
reactive attachment disorder (RAD) 240
Reck, C. 691
Recognising and Responding to Child Maltreatment (Gilbert) 850
reflective functioning 62, 77, 81, 82, 352, 596, 643, 715
Reinders, A. S. 158
Reiss, Helen 581
relational dysregulation 46–47, 191
relational environment 7, 47, 59, 373, 606, 638, 646, 757, 759, 762, 882
relational patterns in ATT sessions 504–511; avoid labeling behaviors 507–508; balancing needs of animal partner and child 510–511; exit and wait to connect plan 505–506; maintaining focus on present relationship 506; navigating relationships 508; navigating sickness and death of animal partners 508–509
relational safety 9, 153, 187, 210, 368–370, 441, 542, 592, 593, 598, 763, 771
relational trauma 2, 298, 501, 518, 647, 712, 756; caregiver-induced 2; childhood 111–114; chronic 79; complex 152, 160; early 40, 47, 65
relaxation skills 483, 492, 813, 814
repetitive night terrors 450–451
resignation syndrome 796
respiratory sinus arrhythmia (RSA) 144
reticular activating system (RAS) 398
revictimization 111, 115, 191, 489
Riordan, J. P. 452; "Toddler Trauma: Somatic Experiencing, Attachment and the Neurophysiology of Dyadic Completion" 452
risperidone 868
ritualistic abuse *see* mind control abuse
Roberts Appercetion Test (RAT-C) 221
Robertson, J. 293
Rogel, A. 464
Rogers, Carl 504, 525, 579; *Way of Being, A* 579
Rorschach Inkblot Method (RIM) 220–221
Ross, M. 26
Rothschild, B. 563
Russell, Jo 319
Rutz, Carol 844; *Nation Betrayed, A* 844

Sachs, R. 267
Sagaltici, E. 818
salience network (SN) 99, 100
Sanders, B. 19
Sandplay, A Psychotherapeutic Approach to the Psyche (Kalff) 316
sandtray therapy 316, 590–609, 855; attachment patterns and tendencies 605–608; creating safe space 592–594, *593*; developmental perspective on 608; dissociative parts and inner relational dynamics 602–603; history of 590–591; identity integration 599–600; integrative and phase-oriented approach to 591–592; nervous system states in 603–605; research 591; stabilization, resourcing, capacity building, and repatterning of ANS 594–596, *595–596*; systemic and dyadic 596–597; trauma memories integration 597–598; for treating dissociative children 600–602; working with caregivers during processing and identity integration 598–600
Santoro, G. 46
Şar, V. 3, 32, 188
SARI model for trauma and dissociation treatment 861–875; adjunctive therapeutic techniques *see* adjunctive therapeutic techniques for dissociation treatment; case studies 869–875; pharmacotherapy *see* pharmacotherapy for complex trauma and dissociation; psychotherapeutic techniques *see* psychotherapeutic techniques for dissociation treatment
Satir, Virginia 301–303, 426
Sawyer, S. 660, 664
Scaer, Robert 444
schema-focused cognitive behavioral therapy 864
Schimmenti, A. 40, 47
Schirme, Lynn 844
Schoonover, T. J. 532
Schore, Allan 65, 68, 96, 292, 316, 391, 463, 578, 592, 639, 641, 651
Schottelkorb, A. A. 532
Schowalter, J. 648
Schutz, C. A. 464
Schwartz, Harvey L.: *Dialogues with Forgotten Voices* 850
Scott, C. 32
scripts 624–625, 627, 642, 646, 739, 815
Sears, M. 125; *Baby Book, The* 125
Sears, W. 125; *Baby Book, The* 125
secure attachment 60–63, 65–67, 130, 298, 346, 347
securefulness 827, 835
selective serotonin reuptake inhibitors (SSRIs) 867
self and personality integration 77, 79
self-compassion 336, 738–740, 744, 766, 767, 866
self-harm and suicidality 62, 63, 774–787; among traumatized children 774–775; biological model 777; case examples 784–787; depersonalization and 195; impact of developmental stage 779;

inpatient care 784; maintaining safety 782–783; psychological model 776–777; reenactments 777–778; risk assessment 780–781; role of caregivers and family systems 781; social model 777; stabilization phase of treatment 783–784; theories 778–779
self-modulation of states: maladaptive attempts of alcohol and drugs 30–31
self-referential memory 109, 111, 113, 114
self-regulation 150, 191, 270–272, 398, 402, 425, 433, 444, 489, 492
self-soothing 27, 35, 68, 69, 187, 200
self-states 43–46, 291, 293, 296, 299, 300, 602, 840, 841
Seligman, M. E. P. 712
Semi-structured Clinical Interview for Dissociative Symptoms and Disorders (SCID-D) 220
semi-structured clinical interviews 66, 212, 218–220, 715, 716, 795
Seng, J. 695
Sensations, Images, Body Behaviors, Affects, and Meanings (SIBAM) model 441, 443, 446, 447, 450
sensation-tracking activities: drawing and coloring sensation/emotion body maps to track body reactions 453–454; inviting exploration through mutual tracking in SE sessions with art and/or movement 454–456; teaching ANS tracking of activation/deactivation cycles using physical games 456–457
sense of self 24, 29, 32, 62, 76, 77, 79, 84, 170, 171, 174, 187, 298
sensorimotor directionality 172, 173, 177
sensorimotor intentionality 171–173, 177
Sensorimotor Psychotherapy and family interventions 424–439; difficulties with communication 427–429; fostering resilience 434–436; overview 425–426; responses to boundaries 436–438; self-regulation 431–434; setting and/or respecting boundaries 430–431
Sensorimotor Psychotherapy: Interventions for Trauma and Attachment (Ogden and Fisher) 430
sensory-affective orienting 170–174
sensory integration therapy 390, 397
sensory-motor issues 257
sensory systems: processing related to complex childhood trauma and dissociation 398–399, **399–400**; and their functions 393, **394–395**
separation cry 81–82
sertraline 867
sexual motivational system 83
Sexual Projective Card Set (SPCS) 221
shame and guilt 34, 48, 82, 83, 202–203, 735–750; case example 746–750; in child complex trauma and dissociation 736–738; compassion-focused therapy (CFT) for children *see* compassion-focused therapy (CFT); EMDR therapy with parents 744–745

Shame and Pride: Affect, Sex, and the Birth of the Self (Nathanson) 622
shame psychoeducation 622–625, *623*, *625*; case example 624; Nathanson's compass of shame in sand 623–625
Shapiro, Francine 364, 374, 376, 378, 592, 818
Shaver, P. R. 58
Sherman, Cindy 632
Shewfelt, M. 650
shutdown response *see* dorsal vagal collapse
Sidis, B. 94, 95
Siegel, D. 125, 128–130, 135, 140, 154, 155, 159, 591, 883; *Developing Mind, The* 130; metaphor of Wheel of Awareness 135; *Parenting From the Inside Out* 125; *Pocket Guide to Interpersonal Neurobiology* 125, 128; *Power of Showing Up, The* 129
Siegel, Daniel 391, 392, 453; *Developing Mind: Toward a Neurobiology of Interpersonal Experience, The* 392
Sierra, M. 197
Silberg, J. L. 5, 93, 95, 192, 198, 201, 202, 208, 209, 222, 238, 268, 271, 273, 274, 276, 325, 642, 643, 651, 736
Sim, L. 217
Simonov, P. V. 96
Slade, A. 60, 644
sleep difficulties 200, 470, 678
Smith, D. 661–664
social brain of child 57
social engagement face-heart circuitry 149, 150
social engagement system (SES) 151, 153, 443, 602; and dissolution 145, 147; neurocepting safety and 149; passive and active pathways regulation 160–162, *161*; polyvagal-informed treatment of complex trauma and dissociation 162–163; trauma treatment failure without 159–160; ventral vagal 154, 155
Society for Psychophysiological Research 145
sociocultural determinants of complex trauma and dissociation 673–686; anti-oppressive lens 677, 684–686; case study 684–686; children from Black, Indigenous, and people of color (BIPOC) backgrounds 673–676, 678, 686; of complex trauma & dissociation 674; culturally responsive framework, orientation and treatment planning *see* culturally responsive framework and orientation; culturally responsive treatment planning; cultural views and mental health 674–675; family lens 678; intergenerational trauma 675; intersectionality lens 677–678; proposed approaches and therapeutic strategies 678–679; puppet play 683; racial trauma 676
Soffer-Dudek, N. 99
Solms, Mark 317, 319
Solomon, E. P. 2
Solomon, J. 30, 34, 82, 189, 347

somatic experiencing (SE) 160, 163, 441–457; body map research of emotion-related sensations 456–457; case study 446–448, 450–451; complex trauma and dissociation through 443–444; definition 442–443; dissociation and freeze/immobility 444–446; "Eight Essentials of Healthy Attachment" for co-regulation 448–449; emBODY tool 441, 456; Gestalt techniques with 450; Gingerbread Body Map 441, 453, 454, 456, 457; global/partial dissociation/freeze 451; with play therapy to prevent post-surgical toddler trauma 451–452; repetitive night terrors 450–451; Resilience Roadmap 441, 442, 452–457; self-regulation through interoceptive awareness 452–456; SIBAM model to access dissociated implicit memory 446

Somer, E. 99, 883

Spiegel, D. 4

spiritual abuse 848–849

Spitz, Rene 57, 58

Springham, N. 615

Squeglia, L. M. 30

stabilization phase in PRACTICE components 489–494; enhancing safety 489–491; psychoeducation 491; relaxation, affect modulation and cognitive coping skills 492–494

standardized clinical interviews 218–220; for developmental trauma 219 see also Developmental Trauma Disorder Structured Interview for Child (DTD SI-C); Developmental Trauma Disorder Structured Interview for Parent/Caregiver (DTD SI-P/Care); for dissociation 219–220 see also Bellevue Diagnostic Interview for Dissociation in Children and Adolescents (BDID-C); Multidimensional Inventory of Dissociation-Adolescent Version (A-MID); Semi-structured Clinical Interview for Dissociative Symptoms and Disorders (SCID-D); for trauma 218–219; see also Kiddie Schedule for Affective Disorders and Schizophrenia-Present and Lifetime Version (K-SADS-PL)

star theoretical model (STM) 287–304, *288*, 325; attachment theory of *see* attachment theory of STM; case study 289–290; developmental theory of *see* developmental theory of STM; family systems theory of *see* family systems theory of STM; neurobiology in *see* neurobiology in STM model; Putnam's theoretical model of discrete behavioral states 288–289

state change disorders 23, 24

state-dependent functioning 511–512

state-dependent learning and memory (SDLM) 25–26, 28

state integration 128, 140, 141

state-related effects of child maltreatment 29–33; traumatic alterations of state pathways 29–33; traumatic states creation 29

states: at birth, new states and pathways 27; definition 24; state-dependent learning and memory (SDLM) 25–26; state-space 24–25, *25*; switches 26, 35; types of 24

states of being (SoB), definition 24; *see also* self-modulation of states

states of consciousness 23, 24, 28, 29, 44, 45, 62, 220, 464, 631, 769

Steele, Howard 319

Steele, Kathy 156, 158, 755

Sterman, M. B. 167, 462

Story Stem Assessment Profile (SSAP) 67

storytelling 333, 866–867

Strange Situation Procedure (SSP) 30, 34, 42, 66, 96, 347

Strauss, W. 725

Strengths and Difficulties Questionnaire (SDQ) 810

stress-induced analgesia 175–177

structural dissociation 45, 75–85, **78**, 114, 175; as deficit and defense 77; developmental pathways to 77, 79; *vs.* dissociative symptoms 73–77; *vs.* ego states 75–76, **76**; fragmentation and 156–159; motivational systems in *see* motivational systems in structural dissociation; primary 157, 569; secondary 569; symptoms 77; tertiary 569; treatment implications 84–85

Structured Clinical Interview for DSM-IV Dissociative Disorders (SCID-D) 17

structured clinical interviews 17, 212

Substance Abuse and Mental Health Services Administration (SAMHSA) 521, 522

substance-use disorders 24, 30–31

superior colliculus (SC) 168, 175–178

supracortical dissociation 168, 174–176, 179

Svali 844–846; *How the Cult Programs People* 844

Swales, D. 696

sympathetic adrenal medullary (SAM) axis 148

sympathetic nervous system 75, 143, 147, 148, 176, 177, 187, 404

sympathetic state 147–149, 152, 154, 155, 158, 159, 404

symptomatology 187–203; complex trauma 187; depersonalization 194–196; derealization 196–197; dissociation 187–189; dissociation continuum 189–191, *190*; dissociative amnesia/memory confusion 197–198; dissociative identity disorder (DID) 198–199; dissociative symptom categories 191–192; domains of symptoms 191; eating behaviors 196; emotion regulation 202; encopresis and enuresis 195–196; feeling numb 195–196; hyperactivity 200–201; imaginary playmates 201; perpetrator introjects 200; psychoform/somatoform symptoms 202; regressed states and hearing voices 201–202; in school-aged children 193–194; self-harm 195; self-perception, depersonalization and derealization in 197; sexually inappropriate behavior 200; shame and trauma 202–203; sleep difficulties 200; trauma types 189; in young and preschool-aged children 192–193

synergetic play therapy (SPT) approach 575–588; case study 586–588; child's symptoms and ANS activation 576; concept of attachment to self 582–583; dissociation as homeostatic mechanism 583–585; and dissociative states 576, 585; goals of 576; mindfulness and co-regulation 577–578; therapist as external regulator modeling and co-regulating child's integration and re-patterning of ANS 578–579; therapist as toy in playroom 581; therapist's opportunity to experience child's experience 577; therapist supporting child in getting in touch with their authentic self 580–581; therapist supporting child in integrating their perceptions of perceived challenging events and thoughts in their lives 580; therapist's verbal and nonverbal signals allowing child to feel safe in relationship and engage in reflective awareness 579–580

synergetics 575

Systematic Touch Inventory 224

Tangney, J. P. 735
Target, Mary 319
Tart, Charles 23
Tavistock Clinic 315–318, 324
Tavistock Clinic Baby Observation course 315
Tavistock model 313
Teaching Recovery Techniques (TRT) program 801
Tedeschi, P. 502; *Transforming Trauma: Resilience and Healing Through Our Connections With Animals* 502
Teicher, M. H. 30
telehealth 884
Tell-Me-A-Story test (TEMAS) 221
temporal integration 128
Tereno, S. 352
Terr, L. C. 2
terror 132, 136, 155, 157, 159, 188, 190, 193, 195, 198, 200, 328, 417, 450, 451, 511, 642, 711, 760
Tesla, Nikola 464
therapeutic relationship 395, 637–653; affect scripts 624–625, 627, 642, 646, 739, 815; all behavior as communication 639–640; disorganization in developing 647; disorganized attachment 645–646; disorganized play 646–647; enactments and reenactments 649–650; language 652–653; operationalizing right-brain to right-brain communication 651–652; play, relational self and healing 642–645; sense of safety and trust 640–642; therapists' use of self 650–651; transference and countertransference 648–649; working with nuanced relational challenges 647–653
therapeutic toys 526–532; limits 530–531; objectives and skills 529; principles 528–529; themes 531

therapies and interventions for FND 813–819; play therapy 813; trauma-focused cognitive behavioral therapy (TF-CBT) 813–815

Therapist's Guide to Child Development: The Extraordinary Years, A (Ray) 524

Theraplay process 560–573; Behavior Assessment System for Children, Third Edition 561; case conceptualization 561–563; child in 565–566; core elements 563–565; levels of integrative work 569–573; Marschak Interaction Method 561, 562, 564, 570; Parenting Relationship Questionnaire 561; Structural Dissociation model 569; therapist in 568–569; Trauma-Informed Stabilization Treatment 569, 570, 572, 573; working with parents 566–568

therapy approaches to mind control abuse: art therapy 854–855; case example 853–854; consultation with child's caregivers/protective parents 858; direct abuse-focused work 856–858; full-body role play 854; non-directive play therapy 852–853; sociological backdrop 850–852; stories and metaphor 855–856

Thomas, Dylan 164
Thompson, G. S. 163
Thompson, R. A. 202
3P Factor Theory of Multiple Personality Disorder 267
Tinbergen, Nikolaas 59
titration continuum: distance 379; frequent time orientation 378; gradual entrance into memory 379; manipulation of speed and length of BLS/DAS 379; memory segmentation 378–379; micro-processing 379; pendulation/oscillation strategy 378; time titration 379
Tokophobia 705
Tolle, Eckhart 765
tonic immobility (TI) 96–98, 148, 177
top-down therapeutic approaches 7, 271, 274
touch/touching 172–174
toxic shame 622
trait dissociation 154
trait vulnerability 44, 45
trance elicitation technique 92
trance logic 95
transcranial magnetic stimulation (TMS) 75
transdiagnostic approaches 267; biopsychosocial formulation 267, 276; Four Ps 267, 276
Transforming Trauma: Resilience and Healing Through Our Connections With Animals (Tedeschi and Jenkins) 502
transgenerational transmission of trauma: attachment, traumatic experiences, and dissociation 711–713; attachment and caregiving systems 710–711; caregiver attachment and parenting styles 715–717; EMDR and working with parts 718–720; resources identification 718; traumatization and vicarious dissociation in context of parental

relationship 713–714; treatment considerations 714–715; treatment planning with parents 717–718
transitional identities 193, 201
transpirational integration 128
trauma: cumulative 2, 40; definition 309; intergenerational 675; as intrapsychic phenomenon 109–110; and memory systems 445–446; psychic 310, 311; psychoanalysis and its relationship to 309–311; racial 676; shame and 202–203; standardized clinical interviews for 218–219 *see also* Kiddie Schedule for Affective Disorders and Schizophrenia-Present and Lifetime Version (K-SADS-PL); unresolved 209, 292, 304, 348, 675, 694, 709, 710
trauma-focused acceptance and commitment therapy (TF-ACT) 864
trauma-focused cognitive behavioral therapy (TF-CBT) 483–498, 539, 799, 802, 813–815, 864; affect regulation skills 814–815; applications for complex trauma and dissociation 487–488; bibliotherapy 818–819; caregiver involvement 485; cognitive coping skills 815; effectiveness research 487, 498; ego state therapy interventions 816; EMDR interventions 817–818; gradual exposure to traumatic content 484–485; hypnotic interventions 815–816; parenting skills/psychoeducation 813–814; PRACTICE components *see* PRACTICE components; principles of 483–485; relaxation skills 814; somatic interventions 817
trauma narration phase in PRACTICE components 494–496
TraumaPlay as integrative play therapy model 539–557; addressing thought life 546, 556; assessment and augmentation of coping 543, 553–554; assessment phase 551–552; Cascade of Care and therapist roles *see* Cascade of Care in TraumaPlay model; case example 549, 551–556; Circle of Security Protocol 540, 547; continuum of disclosure 545; dissociation 547; emotional literacy 544–545, 555; enhancing safety and security 543, 552–553; enhancing self-regulation 543–544; experiential mastery play 545–546; framework *541–542*, 541–543; mapping tool *550*; Nurture House Dyadic Assessment 544, 548, 549; origins and development 539–540; parents as partners 544; play-based gradual exposure/trauma narrative work 545–546, 555–556; positive meaning of post-trauma self 546, 556; soothing physiology 543, 554; therapeutic influences and practices 540–541; trauma narrative 546; trust-based relational intervention 540, 547
trauma-related altered states of consciousness (TRASC) 29
trauma-related phobias 77, 85, 372
Trauma-Sensitive Practice® (TSP) 391

trauma-specific screening measures 216–218; Acute Stress Checklist for Children 216; Center for Youth Wellness Adverse Childhood Experiences Questionnaire 216; Child And Adolescent Needs And Strengths 217–218; Child and Adolescent Trauma Screen 216; Child Behavior Checklist 217; Child Stress Disorders Checklist 216; International Trauma Questionnaires: Child and Adolescent Version 216; PTSD in Preschool Aged Children 216; Trauma Symptom Checklist for Children 216–217, 354; Trauma Symptom Checklist for Young Children 216–217; UCLS Brief Screen for Child/Adolescent PTSD 216
Trauma Symptom Checklist for Children (TSCC) 216–217, 354
Trauma Symptom Checklist for Young Children (TSCYC) 216–217
traumatic attachment *see* attachment trauma
traumatic disintegration 43–45
traumatic events, Freyd's two-dimensional model for 109, *109*, 115
traumatic memory 44, 82, 84, 85, 109, 157–158, 198, 318, 375, 384, 404, 445, 484, 496, 564, 613, 652, 694, 717
traumatic states: alterations of state pathways 29–32; creation 29; identity 31
treatment approach and planning 270–283, **277–281**; guidelines 271–272; phased-oriented approach to 270–271, 366; principles 271; styles and goals 272–273
treatment planning for child dissociation 273–276, 281, 282; clinical example 276–277, 281, **282–283**; integrative treatment 274–275; pacing and length 276; setting 275–276; systemic approach 276
Trevarthen, Colwyn 57, 173, 174, 647, 650, 652; primary intersubjectivity 57
Trickett, P. K. 19
triphase model of trauma treatment 613, 614
triple network model of psychopathology 99–100
Tronick, E. 651
Truskauskaite-Kuneviciene, I. 31
Truss, A. 209
Trust-Based Relational Intervention (TBRI) 502
Truth and Repair: How Trauma Survivors Envision Justice (Herman) 117
Tuber, S. 643
Type I complex trauma 2, 189
Type II complex trauma 2, 189
Type III complex trauma 2, 189

UCLS Brief Screen for Child/Adolescent PTSD 216
umbrella breathing *415*
UN convention on the Rights of the Child 318
United Nations High Commissioner for Refugees (UNHCR) 791

unperceived pregnancy, definition 705
unresolved attachment 62, 348, 349
unstructured clinical interviewing 221–222
U.S. Department of Health and Human Services (USDHHS) 110

vagal paradox 145
Vandenberg, B. 92
ventral vagal state 147, 149, 150, 157, 162, 163
ventral vagal system 75, 83, 152, 380, 604, 694
ventral vagus nerve 65, 754
ventrolateral PAG (VLPAG) 176, 177
Verhage, M. L. 348
vertical integration 127, 137–138
virtuosos 91
Vischer, A. F. W. 352
Visitor: A Book about Pain, Defenses, and Love, The (Gómez) 766
Vogt, R. 295
Vonderlin, R. 113

Wade, M. 434
Waiess, E. A. 525
Waller, G. 196
Wampold, B. E. 274
Waterbury, M. 19, 20
Waters, F. S. 5, 193, 196, 200, 209, 222, 269–271, 274, 276, 325; *Healing the Fractured Child: Diagnosis and Treatment of Youth with Dissociation* 269
Watkins, John G. 92, 94, 95
Watts, L. L. 660

Way of Being, A (Rogers) 579
Way We Are: How States of Mind Influence Our Identities, Personality and Potential for Change, The (Putnam) 23
Wesselmann, D. 711
Wieland, S. 5
Wills, C. 113
Wilson, A. E. 26
window of diagnosability 208, 243
window of tolerance 75, 85, 134, 140, 195, 200, 271, 303, 330, 376, 379, 385, 392, 432, 435, 544, 578, 580, 585, 629, 737
Winnicott, Donald 59, 62, 316, 324, 616, 638, 640, 641
Wisdom of the Body, The (Cannon) 583
Wizard of Oz (film) 844
Wolff, P. H. 27
Woodbourne Children's Diagnostic Treatment Center 19
Woody, E. Z. 96
Woolard, A. 270, 274
Wyrwicka, W. 462

Xu, Y. 27

Yarger, H. A. 352
Yerkes, Robert M. 465, 467
Yerkes-Dodson law 466, 467
yoga 145, 449, 554, 866, 883
Young, E. 325, 738

Zeeman, L. 434

Printed in the United States
by Baker & Taylor Publisher Services